Handbook
of Nutrition
and Diet

FOOD SCIENCE AND TECHNOLOGY

A Series of Monographs, Textbooks, and Reference Books

Handbook of Nutrition and Diet

Babasaheb B. Desai

Mahatma Phule Agricultural University
Rahuri, India

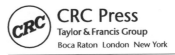

CRC Press
Taylor & Francis Group
Boca Raton London New York

CRC Press is an imprint of the
Taylor & Francis Group, an **informa** business

CRC Press
Taylor & Francis Group
6000 Broken Sound Parkway NW, Suite 300
Boca Raton, FL 33487-2742

First issued in paperback 2019

© 2010 by Taylor & Francis Group, LLC
CRC Press is an imprint of Taylor & Francis Group, an Informa business

No claim to original U.S. Government works

ISBN-13: 978-0-8247-0375-2 (hbk)
ISBN-13: 978-0-367-39827-9 (pbk)

Visit the Taylor & Francis Web site at
http://www.taylorandfrancis.com

and the CRC Press Web site at
http://www.crcpress.com

To the memories of
Vikas and Varsha

Preface

The science of nutrition interprets the relationship of food to the functioning of living organisms. Nutrition and diet are concerned with the intake of food, digestive processes, the liberation of energy and the elimination of wastes, as well as all the syntheses that are essential for maintenance, growth, and reproduction. Nutrients, whether naturally occurring or synthesized, are necessary for the normal functioning of organisms, and include carbohydrates, lipids, proteins, vitamins and minerals, water, and some unknown substances.

Whereas the nutritionist translates the science of nutrition into optimal nourishment for people, the dietitian is concerned with both the science and art of human nutritional care, an essential component of the health science. The treatment of disease by diet modification lies within the province of both the physician and the dietitian.

Food is a source of energy and of about 45 to 50 essential nutrients, including vitamins and minerals, required for the development and maintenance of human life. It has been established that the lack of adequate quantities of essential nutrients results in clinical manifestation of several physical and mental disorders in humans. Clinical malnutrition can result from a variety of factors, such as an imbalance of nutrients, inability to eat, malabsorption, loss of endogenous nutrients, or multisystem dysfunction producing clinical complications that may lead to morbidity and mortality. During the last couple of decades, nutrition and diet-related health disorders and diseases have increased significantly.

The aim of the *Handbook of Nutrition and Diet* is to present comprehensive principles of nutrition, food science and technology, and diet and human health in a lucid and simple manner to point out how this knowledge can be utilized to maintain normal, healthy bodies with a high degree of vigor. Part I emphasizes various food nutrients and their functions in the human body, body composition, energy needs, and recommended daily allowances (RDAs). Part II describes various food sources and their acceptability; foods of plant, animal, and microbial origin; potential protein sources; food processing and preservation methods; food additives and nutrification; food labeling, quality assurance, and food safety; and food transportation, distribution, and marketing. Part III of the book deals with food consumption and utilization, describing adequacy of diet, food digestion, absorption, metabolism, and excretion of wastes; endocrine systems and regulation of food intake; evaluation of food and nutritional status; and dietary allowances and goals. The last part, Part IV, discusses nutritional management of various human disorders and diseases—including heart and circulation disorders, cancer, diabetes, and diseases of the bones, teeth, skin, hair, kidneys, and liver. The relationship of diet to nervous system disorders and mental health is covered, in addition to the nutritional management of underweight babies and the treatment of alcoholism, the management of inherited metabolic disorders and gastrointestinal diseases, as well as minor disorders such as sepsis, hemopoiesis, anemias, asthma, and food allergy. The handbook concludes with an integrated approach to food, nutrition, diet, and health.

The *Handbook of Nutrition and Diet* is devoted to the needs of students, teachers and professionals in the areas of food science and technology, nutrition, and health, and it has been designed to become a standard reference book for the food scientists, nutritionists, dietitians, and various others involved in food industry, agriculture, and medicine.

I would like to express my deep sense of gratitude to my teacher and guide, Professor D. K. Salunkhe, for encouraging me to write this volume; Dr. U. D. Chavan and Mr. Ashok Karande, Librarian, Mahatma Phule Agricultural University, Rahuri, for their help making the extensive literature and new information readily available; and Ms. Ranjana Rasal for her help in typing. I would like to thank my wife, Vilasini, and daughter, Savita, for their patience and understanding during the writing of this book.

Babasaheb B. Desai

Contents

1
Introduction

I. NUTRIENTS FOR HUMAN HEALTH

Food is the most basic prerequisite of living organisms. Food builds the body, provides energy for living and working, and regulates the mechanisms essential for health and survival of life. Food thus constitutes the foundation of health of humans and animals. According to a report on *Health for All*: *An Alternative Strategy* (1), human health is a function not only of medical care but of the overall integrated development of society—cultural, economic, educational, social, and political. It also depends on a number of supportive services, nutrition, improvement in environment, and health education.

Food being the basic vehicle of satisfying man's hunger, it is intimately woven into the physical, economic, psychological, intellectual, and social life of human beings. Our food has several dimensions, the most obvious being the quantitative one. Insufficiency of food leads progressively from mild discomfort to severe hunger and ultimately to death. Its qualitative dimension is equally important, because low-quality or improper diets lead to malnutrition and diseases. Food affects health, life span, physical fitness, body size, and mental development. Food also has a cultural dimension. The food habits of people are part of their cultural and emotional life, and preferences for foods are ingrained. People may cling for generations to their food habits, which may become rituals and patterns of daily routine life. A satisfying meal soothes both the body and mind and determines quality of human life.

From the dietitian point of view, good nutrition involves an accounting of calories and other essential nutrients, such as amino acids, vitamins, and minerals. Approximately 45 essential nutrients are needed by the human body, though it is likely that a few more may be added to the list. These essential nutrients can be supplied in many ways, although it is not clear what combination of foods is optimal. It is known, however, that no universal food will satisfy all nutrient requirements. Relatively few species of plants and animals are edible and have been found by experience to be tolerable. Humans consume a variety of these species, for no single species provides the full spectrum of our complex needs. Agricultural produce, such as cereals, pulses, oilseeds, fruits, and vegetables, as well as animal products (meat, eggs, and milk primarily) constitute the food or its raw materials. When consumed, foods undergo physicochemical changes during digestion to supply energy and various other nutrients required by the body. However, foods are also subject to numerous adverse physiochemical and microbiological conditions; spoilage and production of toxic factors cause several diseases and disorders of health when such foods are consumed. Advances made in the areas of processing, preservation, and storage of foods have minimized such maladies.

A. Nutrients in Foods

According to the laws of thermodynamics, the human body exchanges both mass and energy from the environment: mass for growth and replacement of wornout parts and for reproduction, and energy to fuel the biochemical processes taking place in the body and for various types of works. Food provides both the mass and energy. The system operates under the steady-state conditions—i.e., without a net gain or loss of mass or energy—so that the expenditure is balanced by the intake, meeting the demand by the supply. Too little intake leads to hunger and starvation, too much of it will result into obesity and other related disorders. Food and feeding, seemingly very simple and straightforward phenomena, are indeed very complex and as subjects of scientific studies involve disciplines such as biology, biochemistry, medicine, nutrition, and psychology (2).

Food nutrients (when consumed in adequate amounts) fulfill various functions of the body. The nutrients present in the foods may be classified into the following six broad categories:

1. Carbohydrates
2. Proteins
3. Lipids (fats and oils)
4. Vitamins
5. Minerals
6. Water

The human body requires 17 vitamins and 24 mineral elements; it contains about 54% to 62% water, 15% to 17% proteins, 14% to 25% fat, 5% to 6% mineral matter, and about 1% carbohydrates. Though carbohydrates, broad groups of food nutrients, represent the smallest proportion in the human body (about 1%), they make up the bulk of our diet and constitute the chief source of energy (about 70%). Carbohydrates are burned in animal cells (biological respiration) using oxygen to produce energy. They help in the utilization of proteins and fats for more complex functions than production of energy. The carbohydrates consumed in excess of the body's needs are converted into fats (and glycogen) to be used when needed. Starches and sugars are the main sources of carbohydrates in our diet and are obtained from cereal grains such as wheat, rice, corn, sorghum, and millet as well as from tubers such as potato, sweet potato, and cassava. Sugarcane, beets and fruits provide sugars and sweetness to the diet.

Proteins are the major source of building material for the body and play an important role as structural constituents of the cellular membranes. Proteins function in the maintenance and repair of worn tissues. Enzymes, which are primarily proteins, are biological catalysts necessary for various biochemical reactions. The food value and quality of proteins is determined by the nature and amount of amino acids (essential amino acids). Proteins, if necessary, may be used to produce energy.

Both animal and plant tissues contain proteins, e.g. meat, fish, poultry, eggs, milk, cheese, pulses and food grains such as oilseeds and cereals. Soybeans contain about 40% protein on dry weight basis. Certain nuts and seeds are a rich source of storage proteins, whereas most fruits and vegetables are poor sources of proteins.

Lipids (oils and fats) are the most concentrated source of food energy, furnishing more than two times the energy of either carbohydrates or proteins. They contain lower proportion of oxygen and higher content of hydrogen than carbohydrates. About 30% of the body's energy is met by the food lipids. Excessive calories supplied to the body are stored as fats. In plants, fats are mainly confined to cytoplasmic membrane or may be present as reserve material. Fats are concentrated in oilseeds such as peanut, sunflower, safflower; in fruits such as avocado and olive; and the germ of cereals. Milk, butter, and adipose tissue of animals are also rich source of fats.

Vitamins can be considered as accessary nutrients, required for the proper utilization of bulk nutrients—carbohydrates, fat, and proteins—and are responsible for the maintenance of good health. Vitamins and minerals are the constituents of enzymes functioning as catalysts in the regulation of most biochemical processes.

Vitamins are not uniformly distributed in plants and animal tissues, their content depending on the condition of growth, stage of maturity, handling, processing and storage of plant and animal products. Fruits and vegetables are rich sources of most vitamins, minerals, and dietary fiber.

Minerals act as catalysts in many biochemical reactions of the body. They also function in the growth and development of bones (calcium [Ca] and phosphorus [P]) and other structural parts, muscular contraction, transmission of messages through nerves, as well as in the digestion and utilization of other food nutrients. Certain minerals (Ca, P, iron [Fe], manganese [Mg], and sulfur [S]) are required in relatively larger quantities; others, such as zinc (Zn), copper (Cu), iodine (I), cobalt (Co) and fluoride (F) are required in smaller amounts. Minerals are widely distributed in both plant and animal foods, their content varying greatly according to the medium of growth. Like vitamins, minerals also can be added to foods.

Water is second only to oxygen in importance to the body. It is an ideal medium for transportation of the dissolved nutrients and elimination of waste products from the body. In addition to water consumed as such, body needs of water can be met through foods and metabolic water. Some foods such as fruits, vegetables, milk, and soft drinks contain a high percentage of water. Also, biological oxidation of carbohydrates, fats, and proteins yields metabolic water in the body.

According to Manay and Shadaksharaswamy (3), food is more than the content of its nutrients. Besides nutrition, food has played important roles throughout the history of the human race. People have stolen for it, even killed other people over it. Explorers have searched the world for new foods and scientists have been rewarded for their research. Food also has been responsible for the gain and loss of fortunes. Food is a source of power. Wars have been won by blocking food supplies to the enemy. In the home, families use food as a reward or punishment.

Food is a source of security: by storing enough food tides people over the periods of scarcity. It is a symbol of hospitality and friendship throughout the world. Food is an outlet for emotion. One may eat or overeat as a relief from tension, whereas anger and frustration may turn one against food. Thus, food is much more than a substance supplying nutrients for health. It is the sum of human culture and traditions, emotional outlets, gratification of pleasure, and a relief from stress, a means of communication, security, and status, all interwoven into the fabric of life, and unconsciously expressed in our likes and dislikes for foods. The psychological and emotional reactions to food cannot be easily justified through scientific facts about nutrition (3).

Various food nutrients and their functions are described in Part I, Chapters 2 through 8.

II. BODY COMPOSITION

The weight of the human body increases about 20-fold during its growth and development from baby to adult. Barring the oxygen coming from the respired air, all the remaining mass enters the body through food and water, in addition to the material gained during intrauterine growth from the mother's diet. Thus, the human or animal body is literally what is consumed in the form of food or drinks, i.e., one is what one eats.

The typical chemical composition of the bodies of both the sexes of human beings is shown in Table 1. Water is the major constituent of the human body, followed by fat or protein, mineral matter, and carbohydrates. Garrow et al. (4) noted that some of the most severely malnourished children contained the highest amount of protein in proportion to the body weight. The effects of

Table 1 Composition of Human Body (%)

Nutrients	Man	Woman
Water	60–62	54
Protein	17	15
Fat	14	25
Minerals	6	5
Carbohydrates	1	1
Vitamins	Trace	Trace

Source: Ref. 32.

Table 2 Composition of Human Body and Fat-Free Tissue as Influenced by Growth, Malnutrition and Obesity

Components	Fetus (20–25 wk)	Premature baby	Full-term baby	Infant (1 year)	Adult man	Malnutritioned infant	Obese
Body weight (kg)	0.3	1.5	3.5	20	70	5	100
Water %	88	83	69	62	60	74	47
Protein %	9.5	11.5	12	14	17	14	13
Fat %	0.5	3.5	16	20	17	10	35
Remainder %	2.0	2.0	3	4	6	2	5
Fat-free weight (kg)	0.30	1.45	2.94	8	58	4.5	65
Water %	88	85	82	76	72	82	73
Protein %	9.4	11.9	14.4	18	21	15	21
Na (mmol/kg)	100	100	82	81	80	88	82
K (mmol/kg)	43	50	53	60	66	48	82
Ca (g/kg)	4.2	7.0	9.6	14.5	22.4	9.0	64
Mg (g/kg)	0.18	0.24	0.26	3.5	0.5	0.25	0.5
P (g/kg)	3.0	3.8	5.6	9.0	12.0	5.0	12.0

Source: Ref. 5.

growth, malnutrition, and obesity on the composition of body and of fat-free tissue are shown in Table 2. The embryo has a very high percentage of water, which decreases with maturation, with a significant shift in the distribution of water from extracellular (with Na^+ as a chief cation) to intracellular (with K^+ as the chief cation) states. The concentration of protein and electrolytes increase with decreasing proportion of water during the aging process. Fat is deposited mostly during the last trimester of pregnancy and during the first year of extrauterine life.

Severe malnutrition hinders normal gains in body weight, slowing down the chemical maturation of the body (5). A severely undernutritioned child or the one who has starved to death will have less protein and more water than normal in the lean tissues, but because they have little fat, the percentage of protein relative to body weight may actually be higher than normal. Garrow (5) therefore stressed the importance of considering separately changes in the fat content of the body, and the changes in the composition of fat-free component. According the Pace and Ruthbun (6), the water and protein content of the fat-free body of a series of guinea pigs ranging from lean to obese animals was little influenced by the amount of its fat content.

During the 1950s and 1960s, several studies on the analysis of the chemical composition of the human body were reported (7–13). The water, protein, and potassium contents of fat-free bodies as influenced by the age and those of the selected organs like skin, heart, liver, kidneys, brain and muscle are given in Table 3. The fat-free tissue has about 725 g of water, 205 g of protein, and 69 mmol of potassium per kilogram, but there is a considerable variation between individual bodies. The fat-free skin has a very different water and potassium content from other body organs such as brain or muscle (Table 3).

A. Body Fat

Based on the assumption that the fat and the fat-free tissues of the body have a fairly constant composition, efforts have been made to measure the energy stores of the individual indirectly, through in vivo methods of determining fat and fat-free mass. Behnke et al. (14) employed body specific gravity (density) as an index of obesity. Allen et al. (15) also measured the density of human tissues.

The excess weight of sportspersons (e.g., football players) may be due to their extra muscle and not fat; the latter tends to lower the body density. Human fat at body temperature has a density of 0.900 g/cm and that of a-fat-free tissue is around 1.100 g/cm (16). Thus, a person having body weight as fat will have an average body density of 1.00. Any mixture of fat and lean tissue will result in body density varying from 0.90 to 1.10. Using these assumptions, it is possible to calculate the fat percentage of a body with an average density. Streat et al. (17) pointed out that in very fatty or severely malnourished persons, the hydration of the fat-free body is altered, which may cause a small error in the estimation of body fat from density (5).

It is rather difficult to estimate accurately the volume of the tissues of a living person. This is often done by submerging the subject in water and measuring the volume of water displaced or the apparent weight loss. Garrow et al. (18) used a tank with a plastic cover in which the subject stands up to the neck in water, and the volume of air remaining under the cover is measured. By knowing the volume of water and of the whole tank, the volume of the subject can be calculated.

Table 3 Water and Protein Content, Potassium and K:N Ratios of the Fat-Free Bodies of Different Age and Some Organs

Age (years)	Water (g/kg)	Protein (g/kg)	Remainder (g/kg)	Potassium (mmol/kg)	K:N Ratio (mmol/kg)
Fat-free whole bodies					
25	728	195	77	71.5	2.29
35	775	165	60	—	—
42	733	192	75	73.0	2.38
46	674	234	92	66.5	1.78
48	730	206	64	—	—
60	704	238	58	66.0	1.75
Mean	725	205	71	69.0	2.05
Selected organs					
Skin	694	300	6	23.7	0.45
Heart	827	143	30	66.5	2.90
Liver	711	176	113	75.0	2.66
Kidneys	810	153	37	57.0	2.33
Brain	774	107	119	84.6	4.96
Muscle	792	192	16	91.2	2.99

Source: Ref. 5.

B. Body Water

Body water of a living human subject can be measured by giving a dose of water labeled either with tritium (^{3}H) or deuterium (^{2}H) or ^{18}O. The concentration of the radioactive isotope of hydrogen or oxygen after the equilibrium is measured in a scintillation counter or by using an isotope ratio mass spectrometer to measure the enrichment of stable isotope (^{2}H, ^{18}O) in the equilibrated sample [19]. The dose of labeled isotope can be given orally diluted in 100 ml of tap water. The isotopic equilibration takes about 3 hours; during this period no food or drink is given to the subject. A small error of about 1% to 2% may occur through loss of isotope in urine during equilibration period and due to exchanges of labeled hydrogen with labile organic hydrogen atoms and water hydrogen, which can be ignored. By obtaining an estimate of total body water (TBW, kg), fat-free mass (FFM, kg) can be calculated by the following formula [6]:

$$FFM = TBW/0.73,$$

on the assumption that FFM is 73% water. The fat content of a person can then be obtained by deducting fat-free mass from the body weight.

C. Body Potassium, Calcium, and Nitrogen

Potassium is labeled with the natural radioactive isotope ^{40}K, each gram of potassium emitting about three gamma rays of high energy (1.46 MeV) each second. Total body potassium can be estimted by detecting the gamma rays by suitable equipment. Having estimated total body potassium (TBK, mmol), the FFM (kg) can be calculated for women and men from formulas, FFM = TBK/60 and FFM = TBK/66, respectively, assuming that fat-free tissue of women and men contains 60 and 66 mmol K/kg, respectively (1g K = 25.6 mmol).

Garrow [5] described a technique of neutron activation to estimate body Ca or N along with K. The subject is irradiated with a beam of fast neutrons whose energy is captured by atoms in the body, some of which become short-lived radioactive isotopes, notably ^{43}Ca and ^{15}N, emitting radiation at characteristic energy bands.

Efforts have been made to derive equations to estimate the fat and fat-free mass of the body from the measurements of selected lengths and circumferences. Thus, skinfold thickness and indexes relating weight to height can be measured by using these equations (anthropometry).

Most of the body's fat lies immediately under the skin, and thickness of a skin fold at the strategic sites indicates the amount of subcutaneous fat [20]. Biceps, triceps, subcapular, and suprailiac are the best sites used under the established system for measuring body fat by skinfold thickness [21,22]. The Harpenden Caliper (Holtain Ltd., Bryberian Crymmych, Pembrokeshire) has been designed to keep the surface of the jaws applied to the skin surface parallel and exert a constant pressure.

D. Frame Size

Skeletal size is not essentially related to the body weight in some people. Attempts to use measurements of frame size to estimate body fat based on weight and height measurements have not succeeded [23,24].

Methods of estimating frame size depend on the difference in electrical conductivity of lean tissue (which, being an electrolyte solution, is a good conductor) and fat (non-conductor). Conway et al. [25] employed a newer technique of infrared interactance to estimate body composition. Light from a sophisticated monochromator in the range of 700–1000 nm is shone onto the skin surface at selected sites, and the spectrum of wavelengths reflected is analyzed by computer.

Fat and lean tissue have different interactive spectra, from which lean to fat ratio at the test sites can be calculated.

Scanning techniques such as computer-assisted tomography can be used to obtain valuable information about the relative proportion of fat, subcutaneous or intra-abdominal (26). In this technique, x-rays are emitted in a narrow beam from a source that travels in a semicircle around the subject and the energy passing through the body is recorded by a detector which is mounted diametrically opposite the x-ray source to gather a large amount of information. A suitably programmed computer can reconstruct the pattern of absorbing material within the slice. Since fat, water, lean tissue, and bone have different absorption characteristics, the computer-assisted tomograph displays on video screen the distribution of these tissues within the slice. By performing serial scans at different levels of the body from head to feet, it is possible to build data on the volume of the different types of tissue and their distribution in the body. This equipment is quite expensive to buy and maintain. Two other techniques—nuclear magnetic resonance and photon absorptiometry—are also used to get lean to fat ratio in the soft tissue and bone mineral in limb section. Unlike in tomography, the radiation dose used in these techniques is low and non-damaging to the tissues (5).

Creatine is hydrolyzed nonenzymatically to creatinine. About 98% of all the creatine in the body is found in muscle, as creatine phosphate. According to Talbot (27), 17.9 kg of skeletal muscle contributes to 1 g/day of urinary creatinine. Thus, by analyzing the creatinine content of the urine of the subject, collected for 24 hours, it is possible to estimate the muscle mass, provided the subject is kept on a meat-free diet for several days.

An amino acid, histidine, is methylated during the synthesis of actin in the body muscle, but when the latter is broken down, the methyl-histidine cannot be recycled and is excreted quantitatively in the urine. In subjects with normal rates of turnover of muscle protein, the excretion of 3-methylhistidine in urine provides a index of muscle mass. Rennie and Millward (28) demonstrated, however, that in abnormal physiological states such as myopathies, non-muscle sources of 3-methylhistidine (e.g., platelets, the intestine) can invalidate the accuracy of this method of estimating muscle mass.

The ratio of circumference of waist to that of the buttocks or thigh can be used to measure the fat distribution (see Chapter 26).

Measurement of fat loss by balance techniques such as energy balance or nitrogen balance done carefully in a metabolic ward over several weeks produce more reliable results. These investigations are rather tedious and expensive and were seldom carried out. (18). However, for a group of people ranging in body fat from 10 to 50 kg, many of the methods described above can serve to rank them reliably in order of their body fat.

III. SOURCE OF FOODS

In prehistoric times, humans lived as hunters and gatherers, obtaining their food from wild animals and plants. They depended on fruits, nuts, roots, and other plant foods as well as meat from animals and fish from seas and rivers. Gradually, humans learned to domesticate plants and animals to provide food. Plant domestication began in China around 10,000 B.C., followed by India, the eastern Mediterranean region, and Africa. Wheat and barley were among the first crops grown from the wild grasses. Simultaneously, livestock such as cows, sheep, and goats were domesticated, milk probably being the first animal product used as food. Small farming communities developed around the river basins, followed by the development of agricultural skills and resulting supply of sufficient food, its preservation, storage, and processing, leading to the emergence of urban civilization and bigger cities.

Today, several categories of foods are available including, fruits, vegetables, cereals, pulses, oilseeds, nuts and their range of products, beverages, spices, milk and milk products, eggs, meat, poultry, sea foods, sugar, and confectionery products. These foods are described in Part II of this volume under *Foods from Producers to Consumers* (Chapters 9 through 12), and their processing, preservation, quality, safety, transportation, distribution, and marketing are dealt with in Chapters 13 through 17. Food consumption and utilization in terms of adequacy of diet, digestion, absorption, metabolism, and excretion of waste products; endocrine systems and regulation of food intake, evaluation of food and nutritional status, and dietary allowances and goals are described in Part III of this volume (Chapters 18 through 22).

IV. FOOD, DIET, HEALTH, AND AGING

Food, diet and nutritional factors have been known to influence host susceptibility, immune functions, and other defensive measures against several infectious diseases. A complex reciprocal interrelationship has been envisioned between infection and immune functions (29). Nutritional depletion and weakened host defences are being recognized as expected sequelae of acute infectious disorders, and conversely the presence or development of an infectious process is anticipated in patients with malnutrition, both before and during nutritional rehabilitation.

Throughout human history, the search for the means to prevent or slow down the aging process has followed three main lines (30): (a) removing waste products and cleansing impurities, (b) using plant and animal products as medicine, and (c) compensating for decrease in various hormones, vitamins, and other chemicals in the body. The popularity of various spas and water therapies, even in modern times, is an example of the first type of anti-aging aproach for which there is no real scientific basis (31). Some experimental support from laboratory and/or clinical trials is available for various herbal and other medicinal plant and animal products, as nutritional supplements. Replacement therapy, especially hormonal replacement therapy as an anti-aging treatment, has been used and misused for quite some time (32).

In the inaugural address of the Fourth International Congress on *Essential Fatty Acids and Eicosanoids*, held July 20–24 1997, in Edinburgh , Scotland, Ian A. D. Bouchier, Chief Scientist of the Scottish Office of Department of Health, said that essential fatty acid (EFA) and eicosanoids play important roles in health and disease. Bouchier cited pregnancy, inflammation, coronary heart disease, cancer, and animal husbandry as areas in which EFA and eicosanoids can play a role. This congress discussed a vast range of topics, including vascular disease, brain function, gene expression of eicosanoids, models in cell culture, development in utero and early life, infant nutrition, eicosanoid receptors, alcohol abuse, inflammation and the immune function response, diabetes, cancer, and schizophrenia (33).

According to Krishnaswamy (34), disease and dietary habits are closely linked and several functional foods can either prevent or cure disease. Currently such foods are of great public health significance because they also promote positive health and nutrition. Reviewing Indian functional foods and their role in prevention of cancer, Krishnaswamy (34) concluded that yellow and green vegetables, *Allium* vegetables (garlic), fruits and spices such as turmeric have several nutrient and non-nutrient components (antioxidants, antimutagens, and anticarcinogens) that can prevent cancer in humans. Expected benefits of incomporating such functional foods liberally into diets may not only lower the risk of cancer but also reduce the risk of other chronic diseases, such as cardiovascular disease and cataract, and perhaps delay the aging process (34) Ramarathnam et al. (35) isolated and characterized endogenous plant antioxidants that are thought to inhibit lipid peroxidation and offer protection against damage to membrane functions. Antioxidants have been isolated from conventional food sources, such as tea (green and black), sesame, and wild rice and from other plant sources, such as rice hull, and crude plant drugs. Ramarathnam et al. (35) have provided data on new types of water-soluble and lipid-soluble plant antioxidants and have discussed the biological activity and functionality of these antioxidants.

According to Akoh (36), health-conscious individuals are modifying their dietary habits and eating less fat. Consumer acceptance of any food product depends upon taste—the most important sensory attribute. Although consumers want foods with minimal-to-no fat or calories (37), they also want the foods to taste good. Because several foods formulated with fat replacers do not compare favorably with flavor of full-fat counterparts, it is difficult for most people to maintain a reduced fat dietary regimen. Food manufactures thus continue to search for the elusive ideal fat replacer that tastes and functions like conventional fat without the potential adverse health impact. Akoh (36) has reviewed the key characteristics and functions of fat replacers that are commercially available today and a few that are under development.

The fourth edition of *Nutrition and Your Health: Dietary Guidelines for Americans* recommends that consumers should choose a diet with most of the calories from grain products, vegetables, fruits, low-fat milk products, lean meats, fish, poultry, and dry beans, and with fewer calories from fats and sweets. This latest *Dietary Guidelines* from the USDA and U.S. Department of Health and Human Services stresses the importance of exercise. In response to these guidelines and health goals, the food industry has introduced a variety of innovative food products designed to help the American public lower its fat intake. Gershoff (38) has recently reviewed the physical characteristics and safety considerations of these products, as well as their association with chronic disease prevention. According to Gershoff (38), the availability of a wide array of low-fat foods, some using fat substitutes, has the potential for expanding the ways in which people, with the assistance of health care providers, can control their weight. Although these foods may be misused by some, their potential value to those with weight, lipid, and associated chromic disease problems should not be discounted.

Although the normal liver has considerable ability to regenerate, advanced liver disease can significantly reduce this ability. According to Corish (39), in compensated liver disease, all efforts should be made to maintain nutrition status. In decompensated liver disease, symptoms of decompensation may require therapeutic dietetic interevention. Early nutrition assessment and dietetic intervention in the management of malnutrition, ascites, encephalopathy, and esophageal varices are mandatory and have shown reduced morbidity and mortality in these patients.

A meta-analysis of 13 case-control studies has shown that intakes of dietary fiber and risk of colon cancer are inversely associated. Weaker associations were observed between the risk of colon cancer and dietary intake of ascorbic acid and beta-carotene (40). Dietary fibers are consumed from cereals, fruits, and vegetables, but are also added in the purified form to food preparations. They have different structures and chemical compositions and are of varying nutritional and technological interest. Although many studies have confirmed the nutritional benefits of dietary fibers, the results depend on the types of dietary fibers studied or on the experimental conditions used. Thebaudin et al. (41) have described the technological properties of dietary fibers according to their botanical origin and physical characteristics, discussing the main application of insoluble dietary fibers in the food industry.

Despite a general lack of evidence for the carcinogenic effects of *trans* fatty acids, some recent research and popular media have suggested a possible association. Reviewing the literature, Ip and Marshall (42) concluded that the available scientific data do not support the relationship between the intake of *trans* fatty acids and risk for cancer. There is, however, good and increasing evidence that diet is related to the risk of cancers of colon and rectum. This evidence centers around the intake of saturated fat or animal fat as increasing risk and the intake of fiber and vegetable products as decreasing risk. The clinical trials that are currently under way are evaluating dietary restriction of fat intake and supplementation of fiber and fruit and vegetable intake. There is also a good evidence that fat intake might be related to the risk of prostate cancer; most of this evidence is focused on the consumption of saturated fat and on fats of animal origin (42).

Several nutrient deficiency diseases exist that could be effectively prevented by proper attention to the diet, e.g., anemias (iron, folate, vitamin B$_{12}$), goiter (iodine) and rickets/osteomalacia (vitamin D). Table 4 shows some of the proposed linkages between certain chronic diseases and dietary factors.

New evidence concerning the benefits and risks associated with particular aspects of dietary fat is constantly emerging in both scientific literature and the popular media, leading to growth of controversies about these findings. At the invitation of the FAO and WHO, an international group of experts in nutrition, public health, and food science and technology gathered in Rome from October 9 to 25, 1993, to consider the latest scientific evidence on dietary fats and oils. A series of recommendations about dietary fats and oils was made to assist policy makers, health care specialists, the food industry, and consumers (43).

Animals that are well fed and cared for are usually healthier than those that are not; nutritionists have long been concerned with minimum nutrient requirements for maximal growth rate and maintenance. Investigations have now begun to search for the nutritional requirements that are necessary to provide optimal health. Sophisticated immunological methods have allowed researchers to define indicators of resistance to diseases, such as cell-mediated immunity, lymphocyte functions, and macrophage functions. The combination of such immunological tools with the classic methods of nutrition research may enable us to know how food and dietary constituents influence each of these cellular immune systems to gain an overall understanding of the relationship between food, diet, and health. Part IV of this volume is devoted to the clinical nutrition and relationship between diet, nutrition, and various diseases and disorders of human beings, such as high cholesterol and heart diseases; cancers; obesity and diabetes; diseases of bones, teeth, skin, and hair; and diseases of kidney and liver (Chapters 23 through 28). The nutritional management of gastrointestinal diseases, inherited metabolic disorders, underweight babies, alcoholic disorders, and disorders such as trauma, sepsis, hematopoiesis and anemias, are dealt with (Chapters 29 through 33). Chapters 34 and 35 describe the relationship of diet and nutrition with nervous system disorders and human behavior, respectively. The book concludes with an elaborate final chapter on an integrated approach to human dietetics and health.

Table 4 Summary of Certain Chronic Diseases and Other Health Problems with Possible Dietary Links

Disease	Dietary excess	Dietary deficiency
Heart disease	Saturated fats	Antioxidant nutrients n-3 fatty acids
	Total fats	Dietary fiber
Hypertension	Salt	Calcium
	Total fat (?)	Potassium
Diabetes (non-insulin-dependent)	Energy intake (link via obesity)	Antioxidant nutrients
	Total fat	Dietary fiber
	Meat (?)	
	Salt (?)	
Gallstones	Energy intake (link via obesity)	Dietary fiber
	Salt (?)	Vitamin D/calcium
	Animal protein (?)	
Dental disease	Sugar	Fluoride
		Dietary fiber (?)
Arthritis	Total energy (linked to obesity)	General dietary deficiencies (?)
	Alcohol	

Source: Ref. 44.

REFERENCES

1.   ICSSR, A Report of a Study Group on Health for All: An Alternative Strategy, set up jointly by the Indian Council of Social Science Research and Indian Council of Medical Research, Indian Institute of Education, Pune, 1981.

2.   Hoff, J.E., and J. Janick, Introduction, *Food Readings from Scientific American*, W.H. Freeman and Co., San Francisco, 1973, p. 1.

3.   Manay, N.S., and M. Shadaksharaswamy, Foods: Facts and Principles, Wiley Eastern Ltd., New Delhi, 1987.

4.   Garrow, J.S., R. Smith, and E.E. Ward, *Electrolyte Metabolism in Severe Infantile Malnutrition*, Pergamon Press, Oxford, 1968, p. 1.

5.   Garrow, J.S., Composition of the body, *Human Nutrition and Dietetics*, 9th ed. (J.S. Garrow and W.P.T. James, eds.), Churchill Livingstone, London, 1993, p. 12.

6.   Pace, N., and E.N. Rathbun, Studies of body composition: Water and chemically combined nitrogen content in relation to fat content, *J. Biol. Chem. 158*: 685 (1945).

7.   Mitchell, H.H., T.S. Hamilton, F.R. Steggerda, and H.W. Bean, The chemical composition of the human body and its bearing on the biochemistry of growth, *J. Biol. Chem. 158*: 625 (1945).

8.   Widdowson, E.M., R.A. McCance, and C.M. Spray, The chemical composition of the human body, *Clin. Sci. 10*: 113 (1951).

9.   Forbes, R.M., A.R. Cooper, and H.H. Mitchell, The composition of the adult human body as determined by chemical analysis, *J. Biol. Chem. 203*: 359 (1953).

10. Forbes, G.B., and A.M. Lewis, Total sodium, potassium and chloride in adult man, *J. Clin. Investigation. 35*: 596 (1956).

11. Forbes, R.M., H.H. Mitchell, and A.R. Cooper, Further studies on the gross composition and mineral elements of the adult human body, *J. Biol. Chem. 223*: 969 (1956).

12. Dickerson, J.W.T., and E.M. Widdowson, Chemical changes in skeletal muscle during development, *Biochem. J. 74*: 247 (1960).

13. Widdowson, E.M., and J.W.T. Dickerson, The effect of growth and function on the chemical composition of soft tissues, *Biochem. J. 77*: 30 (1960).

14. Behnke, A.R., B.G. Feen, and W.C. Welham, The specific gravity of healthy men; body weight and volume as an index of obesity, *J. Am. Med. Assoc. 118*: 495 (1942).

15. Allen, T.H., H.J. Krzywicki, and J.E. Roberts, Density, fat, water and solids in freshly isolated tissues, *J. Appl. Physiol. 14*: 1005 (1959).

16. Keys, A., and J. Brozek, Body fat in adult man, *Physiol. Rev. 33*: 245 (1953).

17. Streat, S.J., A.H. Beddoe, and G.L. Hill, Measurement of body fat and hydration of the fat-free body in health and disease, *Metabolism. 34*: 509 (1985).

18. Garrow, J.S., S. Stalley, R. Diethelm, Ph. Pittet, R. Hesp, and D. Halliday, A new method of measuring the body density of obese adults, *British J. Nutr. 42*: 173 (1979).

19. Halliday, D., and A.G. Miller, Precise measurement of total body water using trace quantities of deuterium oxide, *Biomedical Mass Spectrometry. 4*: 82 (1977).

20. Edwards, D.A.W., Observations of the distribution of subcutaneous fat, *Clin. Sci. 9*: 259 (1950).

21. Durmin, J.V., G.A. Womerslay, and J. Womerslay, Body fat assessed from body density and its estimation from skinfold thickness: measurement on 481 men and women from 16 to 72 years, *British J. Nutr. 32*: 77 (1974).

22. Womerslay, J., and J.V.G.A. Durmin, A comparison of the skinfold method with extent of overweight and various weight-height relationships in the assessment of obesity, *British J. Nutr. 38*: 271 (1977).

23. Himes, J.H., and C. Bouchard, Do the new Metropolitan Life Insurance weight-height tables correctly assess body frame and body fat relationships? *Am. J. Public Health, 75*: 1076 (1985).

24. Rookus, M.A., J. Burema, P. Deurenberg, and W.A.M. Wiel-wetzels, Van der, The impact of adjustment of a weight-height index (W/H^2) for frame size on the prediction of body frames, *British J. Nutr. 54*: 335 (1985).

25. Conway, J.M., H. Norris, and C.E. Bodwell, A new approach for the estimation of body composition: Infrared interactance, *Am. J. Clin. Nutr. 40*: 1123 (1984).

26. Kvist, H., B. Choudhury, U. Tylen, and L. Sjostrom, Total and visceral adipose-tissue volume derived from measurements with computed tomography in adult men and women: predictive equations, *Am. J. Clin. Nutr. 48*: 1351 (1988).

27. Talbot, N.B., Measurement of obesity by the creatinine coefficient, *Am. J. Dis. Children. 55*: 42 (1938).

28. Rennie, M.J., and D.J. Millward, 3-Methylhistidine excretion and the urinary 3-methylhistidine/creatinine ratio are poor indicators of skeletal muscle protein breakdown, *Clin. Sci. 65*: 217 (1983).

29. Beisel, W., Nutrition, infection, specific immune responses, and nonspecific host defenses: A complex interaction, *Nutrition, Disease Resistance and Immune Function* (R.S. Watson, ed.), Marcel Dekker, New York, 1984, p. 3.

30. Rattan, S.I.S., Is gene therapy for aging possible? *Indian J. Exp. Biol. 38*: 233 (1998).

31. Austad, S.N. *Why we age?* John Wiley and Sons Inc., New York, 1997.

32. Raheena Begum, M., *A Textbook of Foods, Nutrition and Dietetics,* 2nd revised ed., Sterling Publishers, Pvt. Ltd., New Delhi, 1991.

33. Anonymous, Essential fatty acids, ecosanoids have a vital role in health, summary of the proceedings of the Fourth International Congress on *Essential Fatty Acids and Eicosanoids*, July 20–24, 1997, Edinburgh, Scotland, *INFORM 8*: 1016 (1997).

34. Krishnaswamy, K., Indian functional foods: Role in prevention of cancer, *Nutr. Rev., 54*: 5127 (1996).

35. Ramarathnam, N., T. Osawa, H. Ochi, and S. Kawakishi, The contribution of plant food antioxidants to human health, *Trends Food Sci. Technol. 6.*: 75 (1995).

36. Akoh, C.C., Fat replacers, *Food Technol. 52*: 47 (1998).

37. Miller, G.D., and S.M. Groziak, Impact of fat substitutes on fat intake, *Lipids. 31*: 293 (1996).

38. Gershoff, S.N., Nutrition evaluation of dietary fat substitutes, *Nutr. Rev. 53*: 305 (1995).

39. Corish, C., Nutrition and liver disease, *Nutr. Rev. 55*: 17 (1997).

40. Dwyer, J., Dietary fiber and colorectal cancer risk, *Nutr. Rev. 51*: 147 (1993).

41. Thebaudin, J.Y., A.C. Lefebvre, M. Harrington, and C.M. Bourgeois, Dietary fibres: Nutritional and technological interest, *Trends Food Sci. Technol. 8*: 41 (1997).

42. Ip, C., and J.R. Marshall, *Trans* fatty acids and cancer, *Nutr. Rev. 54*: 138 (1996).

43. FAO, Fats and oils in human nutrition: Report of a Joint Expert consultation (WHO/FAO), Paper 57, 1994. *Nutr. Rev. 53*: 202 (1995).

44. Barasi, M.E., Health and promotion policy, *Human Nutrition: A Health Perspective*, Oxford University Press, New York, 1977, p. 305.

2
Water

I. WATER IS LIFE

Water is the predominant constituent of all living organisms. The physical and chemical properties of water are central to biological structure and function. The solvent and reactant properties of water thus undoubtedly appear to have influenced the evolution of life on earth (1). In Sanskrit literature, water has rightly been called as *jeevan*, meaning life.

Water makes up more than about 70% of the weight of most organisms. It pervades all living cells and is an excellent medium for the transport of nutrients from one part to another as well as for the enzyme-catalyzed reactions of the metabolism. Water is not only the solvent in which metabolic reactions occur, it directly participates in many chemical reactions such as hydrolysis and condensation reactions. The first living organisms most probably arose in the primeval oceans and their further evolution was shaped by the most unusual and unique properties of water. All aspects of cell structure and function appear to have adapted to the physicochemical properties of the universal solvent, water.

Thus, second only to oxygen, water is crucial to the existence of all living organisms; they can live without food for a few weeks but for only a few days without water. Being an integral part of animal and vegetable tissues, water serves as an excellent medium for the cellular reactions. It functions in the digestion, absorption, transport of nutrients, and excretion of waste products. Water helps to maintain the electrolyte balance and temperature of the body. It is either a reactant or a product in many of the reactions.

Water is the basic molecule of life, forming the natural environment of the cells. It constitutes an interface for exchanges that occur between living and nonliving regions, thus connecting the physical world with the biological one. Water is widely distributed in its solid, liquid, or gaseous state and is a predominant constituent of foods and drinks, such as fruits and vegetables (around 90%), milk (87%), meat (60–75%) and dried fruits (20–30%). Even dried foods such as cereals, pulses, and other grains also contain appreciable amounts of water. Water influences the appearance, texture, and flavor of foods. It is involved in most of the changes taking place during cooking and processing. It is also related to the spoilage and deterioration of food by favoring the growth of undesirable microorganisms. Shelf life of many foods can be enhanced by keeping the water activity of foods to its minimum.

II. UNIQUE PROPERTIES OF WATER

Water is a liquid at room temperature because hydrogen bonds between water molecules provide enough cohesive force to hold them together. Polar substances dissolve readily in water because they can replace energetically favorable water-water interactions with even more favorable water-solute interactions (hydrogen bonds and electrostatic forces). Conversely, nonpolar compounds are poorly soluble in water because they interfere with favorable water-water interactions and thus tend to cluster together in aqueous solutions.

The melting point, boiling point, and heat of vaporization of water are higher than those of most other common solvents (Table 1). These unique properties of water are due to the strong attractive forces between the adjacent water molecules, giving the liquid water great internal cohesion. Water would be gaseous at normal temperatures if it had no high boiling point, making the life processes difficult. The high specific heat (heat required to raise temperature by one degree celsius) of water ensures that it heats up very slowly, which is of considerable biological significance. Owing to its high specific heat, water helps to keep the temperature of living organisms fairly constant. Barring liquid ammonia, the specific heat of most other substances is less than that of the water (Table 2).

Water also has a very high latent heat of fusion or melting (number of calories required to convert one gram of solid at freezing point into liquid at the same temperature) (Table 2). This

Table 1 Melting Point, Boiling Point, and Heat of Vaporization of Water and Some Other Common Solvents

Solvents	Melting point (°C)	Boiling point (°C)	Heat of Vaporization (J/g)[a]
Water [H_2O]	0	100	2260
Methanol [CH_3OH]	−98	65	1100
Ethanol [CH_3CH_2OH]	−117	78	854
Propanol [$CH_3(CH_2)OH$]	−127	97	687
Butanol [$CH_3(CH_2)_3OH$]	−90	117	590
Acetone [$CH_3CO\ CH_3$]	−95	56	523
Hexane [$CH_3(CH_2)_4CH_3$]	−98	69	423
Benzene [C_6H_6]	6	80	394
Butane [$CH_3(CH_2)_2CH_3$]	−135	−0.5	381
Chloroform [$CHCl_3$]	−63	61	247

[a] The heat of energy required to convert 1.0 g of a liquid at its boiling point, at atmospheric pressure, into its gaseous state at the same temperature. It is a direct measure of the energy required to overcome attractive forces between molecules in the liquid phase.
Source: Ref. 1.

Table 2 Specific Heat and Latent Heat of Fusion of Selected Substances

Substance	Specific heat (Calories)	Latent heat of fusion (Calories)
Water	1.00	80
Methanol		16
Ethanol	0.60	—
Benzene	—	30
Acetic acid	—	45
Chloroform	0.24	—
Liquid ammonia	1.23	—

Source: Ref. 2.

has great significance in the biological world. A large amount of heat is abstracted from water before it freezes, the excess heat released being responsible for preventing water from freezing in the living cell.

Water has a very high surface tension (force acting on the water surface), so it has a high capillary action for its movement in the soil and plant cells. Water movement through plants is also aided by its viscosity and tensile strength, higher than many other solvents. Water has a very high dielectric constant (ability of a substance to oppose attraction of unlike charges), which enables it to be an universal solvent, dissolving salts and many nonionizable organic molecules. Finally, water has a high transmission of visible light, which enables plants to carry out photosynthesis under submerged conditions. Water allows light to penetrate and reach deeply seated plant tissues. Various other physical properties of water, such as density (g/cm^3), 0.9987 (°C), 1.0000 (4°C), 0.9910 (15°C); dielectric constant, 80.0; saturation vapor pressure (mm Hg), 12.78 (15°C); surface tension ($ergs/cm^2$), 72 (20°C); viscosity (g/cm/sec) 1.1404×10^{-3} (15°C); thermal conductivity, (cal/cm/sec) 1.42×10^{-3} and tensile strength, (mm Hg/cm^3) 10.64×10^{ms3}, make it an ideal medium for conducting various life processes (2).

The water molecule has a special geometrical structure. Each hydrogen atom of a water molecule shares an electron pair with the oxygen atom. The shapes of the outer electron orbitals of the oxygen atom dictate the geometry of the water molecule, forming a rough tetrahedron, with a hydrogen atom at each of two corners and unshared electrons at the other two. The H-O-H bond angle being 104.5° (slightly less than 109.5° required to form a perfect tetrahydron), the nonbonding orbitals of the oxygen atom compress the orbitals shared by hydrogen.

The oxygen nucleus is more electronegative than that of the hydrogen, resulting in unequal sharing of electrons between H and O and consequently two electric dipoles in the water molecule. This gives rise to a hydrogen bond because of electrostatic attraction between the oxygen atom of one water molecule and the hydrogen of another. These hydrogen bonds are weaker (20 kJ/mol bond energy) than the covalent bonds (460 kJ/mol), and the lifetime of each hydrogen bond is less than 1×10^{-9}s, although most of the molecules in the liquid water are hydrogen bonded at any given time. The very large number of hydrogen bonds between molecules, however, confers great internal cohesive force to the liquid water.

Because of the tetrahedral geometry of water, each molecule forms hydrogen bonds with as many as four neighboring water molecules (on an average 3.4 molecules). To break the large number of hydrogen bonds in the lattice structure of ice requires much thermal energy, which accounts for the relatively high melting point of water. When ice melts or water evaporates, heat is taken up by the system (1)

H_2O (S)	H_2O (L)	H = +5.9 kJ/mol
H_2O (L)	H_2O (g)	H = +44.0 kJ/mol

Thus, during melting or evaporation, the entropy of the aqueous system increases, with an increase in the disorderliness of molecules moving from solid to liquid or from liquid to gaseous state.

Hydrogen bonds can also form between an electronegative atom (oxygen or nitrogen) and a hydrogen atom covalently bonded to another electronegative atom in the same or another molecule. However, hydrogen atoms covalently bonded to carbon atoms (not electronegative) do not form hydrogen bonding. This accounts for the high boiling point of butanol (117°C) compared to that of butane (–0.5°C). The polar hydroxyl groups of butanol can form hydrogen bonds with other butanol molecule. Similarly uncharged polar biomolecules such as sugars can readily dissolve in water because of the formation of many hydrogen bonds between the hydroxyl groups or the carbonyl oxygen of the sugar and water molecules. Thus, alcohols, aldehydes, and ketones as well as compounds containing N-H (proteins and nucleic acids) can form hydrogen bonds with water. Also, because water is a polar solvent, it dissolves most of the charged or polar biomolecules like amino acids and salts.

Having effectively adapted to their aqueous environment, living organisms have evolved means of exploiting the unusual properties of water. The high specific heat of water, for example, permits organisms to maintain a relatively constant temperature, despite the fluctuation of the air temperature and generation of heat as a by-product of catabolic reactions in the body. Certain vertebrates use the high heat vaporization of water to lose excessive body heat through evaporation of water in the form of sweat. Plants can transport dissolved nutrients from roots to the leaves in the process of transpiration because of the high degree of internal cohesion of liquid water contributed by hydrogen bonding. Aquatic organisms have survived because of a unique property of water: ice has lower density than liquid water at 4°C. Thus ponds and oceans freeze from the top down, and the layer of ice at the top can insulate the water below from frigid air, preventing the ponds and oceans (and the organisms) from freezing solid. Many of the physical and biological properties of the cellular macromolecules such as proteins and nucleic acids have been derived from their interactions with the water molecules.

The availability of water to living organisms and their habitat appears to have modified the molecular pathway for nitrogen excretion. Differences in the molecular form in which nitrogenous products are excreted depend on the variation in the anatomy and physiology of different organisms in relation to their habitat, based on availability of water. Thus, bacteria and free-living protozoa excrete their nitrogen in the form of toxic ammonia into their aqueous environment, in which it will be diluted and made harmless. In the ammonotelic bony fishes also, ammonia is rapidly cleared from the blood at the gills by the large volume of water passing through these respiratory structures. These organisms therefore do not require complex urinary cycles to excrete ammonia. The terrestrial species, which have comparatively lesser amounts of water available, have evolved the ability to convert toxic ammonia to less toxic urea through the urea cycle. The birds and reptiles that have the least amount of water available and that live in the arid environments convert amino nitrogen into uric acid, the relatively insoluble and least toxic semisolid substance, as their nitrogenous excretary product. The biosynthesis of uric acid (purine) is a complex energy-requiring process developed in these terrestrial organisms for the purpose of conserving the limited amount of water available to them.

III. WATER BALANCE AND ELECTROLYTE BALANCE

Water makes up approximately 72% of the human body i.e. about 45 liters in an average 70 kg man, of which about 30 liters is an intracellular fluid (ICF) and the remaining occurs as an extracellular fluid (ECF). Of the latter, around 3 liters constitutes plasma water within the intravascular space. Smaller portions of the ECF also occurs as cerebrospinal fluid, fluids in the eye and ear, and intestinal secretions, having slightly different ionic structures owing to their selective properties (3).

Almost the entire osmolality of body fluids is contributed by three monovalent electrolytes—sodium (Na^+), potassium (K^+), and chloride (Cl^-)—and their deposition within the body determines the volume of ICF and ECF; K^+ is predominantly found intracellularly, along with magnesium and phosphate, and Na^+ and Cl^- are found mainly in ECF. The average concentrations of Na^+, K^+, and Cl^- in men and women, as analyzed by the neutron activation method, were 47 and 43 (Na^+), 26 and 25 (K^+), and 28 and 28 (Cl^-), respectively (4,5).

Unlike other nutrients, water and monovalent ions are not stored in the body: they are kept at a very constant level by a precise balance between intake and output, mainly through urinary losses.

A. Water Balance

Water intake comprises water drunk and that present in foods consumed, and metabolic water formed in the body; water output consists of water lost as urine, as sweat from the skin, in feces, and, to a lesser extent, from the lungs. The typical water balance of a healthy young man leading a sedentary life in a temperate climate is shown in Table 3 (6). The volume of water drunk as fluid is roughly equal to the volume of the urine output, and these figures represent only about one-half of the total water taken in or lost.

According to Wrong (3), the serial measurement of body weight is a easier way of determining changes in body water with a reasonable degree of accuracy than a clinical water balance. Daily weight measurements are especially useful in following the response to treatment of fluid-overloaded or depleted subjects.

Of the six components of water balance (Table 3), only two—fluid intake and urine volume—are controlled by homeostatic mechanisms responsive to the state of body water. A water deficit results in increased osmolality of all body fluids, including that of the plasma circulating in the brain, which in turn stimulates the thirst center and the osmoreceptor, the centers intimately connected, functionally and structurally, to cause thirst by releasing the antidiuretic hormone vasopressin. This hormone also acts on receptors in the renal collecting tubule to cause increased water absorption and reduced urinary volume. The reverse process occurs when the body has an excessive amount of water. This mechanism is quite sensitive and precise and comes into action with deficits and excesses of only about 200–300 ml water, so that the total body water in a normal healthy person (70 kg), drinking fluids as dictated by thirst alone, varies by not more than 500 ml. Also the changes in the plasma osmolality that produce these effects are negligibly small.

Because the water balance is regulated by both the thirst and the release of hormone vasopressin, both of these mechanisms respond to ECF osmolality, the latter being in osmotic equilibrium with ICF osmolality. Thus, the total amount of body water is ultimately determined by the amount of osmotically active solute present, i.e. by the quantities of Na^+ and K^+ and their accompanying anions in the body. Wrong (3) has described various mechanisms by which the body controls these amounts.

Table 3   The Daily Water Balance of a Young Man Leading a Sedentary Life on a Diet Providing 8.8 MJ (2110 kcal) Daily (Mean of 5 Daily Measurements)

		Water (ml/day)
Intake		
Water content of solid food		1115
Liquid drunk		1180
Metabolic water		279
	Total	2574
Output		
Urine		1294
Fecal water		56
Evaporative water loss		1214
	Total	2565
	Water balance	+ 9

Source: Ref. 6.

B. Electrolyte Balance

The balance of Na^+, K^+ and Cl^- can be measured with greater ease than for water, because these ions do not volatilize appreciably and are neither created nor destroyed in the body. Thus, it is only necessary to determine dietary intake of these electrolytes through use of food tables or by analysis of a diet, and that lost in urine, feces, or any other body secretions.

Correction of abnormal balances of Na^+, K^+, and Cl^- by the body takes longer to complete than the corrections in the water balance (2–4 hours). The regulation of Na^+, K^+ and Cl^- balance is precise, but takes 2 to 5 days to complete or even longer if the initial disturbance is marked. Changes in the volume of body water may also occur as secondary responses to changes in its osmolality. It is a common experience of many people to become conscious of increased thirst after the consumption of salted fish or other salty products. This is due to the response of the thirst center to increased ECF osmolality caused by the extra load of sodium chloride. As a result more water is drunk, and simultaneously increased vasopressin release causes a reduction in the urine flow initially. ECF osmolality is thus returned to normal by the newly conserved water, but at the expense of an increase in ECF volume. During the next 2 to 3 days, the extra water, Na^+, and Cl^- are all slowly excreted through urine, bringing the ECF volume to its normal level (3).

1.   Electrolyte Intake

The amounts of dietary intake of Na^+ and Cl^- vary to a greater extent than those of K^+ because of the significant but large amount of common salt consumed as well as other compounds containing Na^+, and Cl^- (e.g. baking powder, citrate and tartrate in soft drinks, sulfites used as preservatives, and flavoring agents, such as monosodium glutamate) consumed in small quantities. Sanchez-Castillo et al. (7) showed that the ratio of urinary Na^+ and Cl^- in human subjects consuming their usual intake was 1.03, indicating identical excretion of the two ions. This meant that the intake of the two ions was also nearly identical. Sanchez-Castillo et al. (7) also demonstrated that nearly 85% of the dietary salt intake (on an average about 9 g or 155 mmol/day) was from foodstuffs purchased from the market and the remaining 15% was added during domestic cooking or at the table.

Foods such as cereals, vegetables, and fruits contain little Na^+, and Cl^-, but meats and fish contain larger amounts of these minerals. Cow's milk has about 22 mmol of Na^+ and Cl^-, most of which is lost in the whey when cheese is prepared from it. Most commercial cheeses contain large amounts of added salt, as do most other processed foods, such as meat, fish, pickles, spices, soups, sauces, and bread. K^+, an essential elements for all organisms, is present in all foods in their unprocessed forms. Also, K^+ is an intracellular ion, so it is present in large amounts in highly cellular tissues like animal meat and certain fruits like banana, tomato, citrus, and potato (see Table 3 in Chapter 7) (8).

Na^+ and Cl^- are essential constituents of all forms of animal life. Both ions are found only in soluble compounds and have been leached out of the earth's surface by rain water into the oceans. Animals have developed efficient mechanisms to conserve their body Na^+ and Cl^-, including a salt appetite, which is most marked in herbivorous animals consuming plants that often contain insignificant amounts of Na^+ and Cl^-. According to Denton (9), the salt appetite is primarily for Na^+ rather than for Cl^-. Salt appetite means both a craving to consume salt, and an enhanced ability to detect traces of salt by taste. Both of these aspects are increased by the physiological stimulus of Na^+ deficiency.

The normal physiological requirement for salt has not been accurately established, but is probably less than 10 mmol/day and may increase as a result of physiological losses during lactation, menstruation, parturition, and heavy sweating. The average salt intake, however, is about 20 times higher than 10 mmol/day, so the retention of an efficient salt appetite becomes biologically irrelevant, though occasionally seen in certain diseased conditions leading to severe Na^+ depletion.

2. *Electrolyte Output*

Electrolytes are lost from the body through urine, sweat, and the alimentary tract. The kidney excretes excesses of Na^+, Cl^-, and K^+ taken in the diet to regulate the volumes of ECF and ICF. The renal capacity to excrete Na^+ and Cl^- ranges from 0.5 to as high as 1000 mmol/day (2000-fold), depending on the needs of the body. Na^+ appears to be the prime mover, accompanied by Cl^-, to preserve the acid-base (pH) equilibrium.

The control of Na^+ excretion is probably achieved by mechanisms that are responsive to changes in ECF volume or one of its critical components, rather than to changes in ECF Na^+ concentration. Renal control of K^+ excretion has a lower range than that of Na^+, and Cl^-. Definite symptoms of K^+ deficiency may be developed with total K^+ deficits of 700–1200 mmol, at which urinary excretion falls to 7–12 mmol/day and the plasma K^+ to less than 3.5 mmol/l. The upper limits of urinary K^+ excretion values have not been determined.

Sweat contains low concentrations of electrolytes (Na^+, 45; K^+, 10; and Cl^-, 30 mmol/l, on average). Na^+ and Cl^- concentrations fall at high sweating rates or when heavy sweating continues for several days. Increased aldosterone possibly reduces Na^+ concentration in the sweat. Fecal losses of electrolytes through the alimentary tract are very negligible compared to urinary losses (3).

C. Body Deficits and Excesses

Dehydration usually means deficiency of water, combined with that of Na^+, as indicated by decreased ECF volume. Wrong (3) preferred to use terms "water depletion" and "saline or ECF depletion" to mean losses of pure water and isotonic salt and water, respectively.

Water deficit often implies a defect in either thirst/drinking mechanism or in the osmoreceptor/antidiuretic mechanism or both. The water deficiency may become more severe when insensible water loss is increased by a high ambient temperature, fever, or respiratory exertion.

Water-deficit symptoms include severe thirst (providing the hypothalamic thirst center is functioning), scanty and highly concentrated urine (as long as vasopressin production is not impaired and renal tubules are responsive), dizziness, and muscle twiching, followed by coma when the condition is severe. Some other recognized complications are cerebral venous thrombosis and persistence of neurological deficits leading to irreversible brain damage, even after the relief of water deficit.

Increased plasma concentration of Na^+, Cl^- and osmolality (more than 148 mmol/l of Na^+ and over 315 mmol/kg, osmolality) aid in the diagnosis. Despite high plasma Na^+, urinary Na^+ is often low, due to decreased ECF volume. The ECF Na^+ concentration controls renal Na^+ excretion. Severe water deficit can destroy the thirst center and result in the release of vasopressin caused by hypothalamic disease.

While milder water deficits can be treated by oral water, desmopressin (DDAVP) is used when the osmoreceptor/vasopressin mechanism is disturbed. Intravenous fluid containing 2.5 to 5.0% dextrose may be used when appropriate, because pure water will cause hemolysis. Total body water deficit can be calculated from the degree of elevation of plasma Na^+, assuming that the defect is distributed over total body water. In some cases it is advisable to lower the plasma Na^+ concentration slowly to the normal range over the first 48 hours of treatment or longer (3).

Overhydration or body water excess refers to an edamatous state in which Na^+ and water are retained by the body in isotonic proportions (saline excess or ECF excess), water retention in most cases being only secondary to Na^+ retention. An excess of body water alone is less common and is described as "water intoxication" when it develops rapidly. It may be caused by excessive intake of water or the failure of water diuresis, or both.

Clinical features are most marked when the water excess develops rapidly and include symptoms such as nausea and vomiting followed by confusion, muscle cramps, convulsions, and coma. Depression of plasma Na^+, Cl^-, and osmolality are very useful signs of water excess.

Treatment of severe cases of water excess is aimed at increasing plasma Na^+ and osmolality to normal levels, both by withholding dilute fluids and providing hypertonic saline (2–5%) intravenously, coupled with a high-ceiling diuretic like furosemide to increase sodium excretion in a dilute urine. The plasma Na^+ must not be raised too rapidly (at a rate faster than 0.7 mmol/l/hr) or elevated completely to normal values, to avoid complications (3).

IV. WATER, PH, AND BUFFERS

Water ionizes very slightly to form H^+ and OH^- ions, and in dilute aqueous solutions, the concentrations of H^+ and OH^- ions are inversely related by the formula $Kw = (H^+ (OH^-) = 1 \times 10^-14$ M^2 (at 25°C). The hydrogen ion concentration of biological systems is often expressed in terms of pH, which is the negative logarithmic value (p) of the hydrogen ion activity, that can be measured by H^+-sensitive glass electrode in a pH meter. Thus, pH helps to know the acidity or basicity of the aqueous solutions. Acids are recognized as proton donors and bases as proton acceptors; and a conjugate acid-base pair consists of a proton donor (Ha) and its corresponding proton acceptor (A^-). The tendency of an acid (HA) to donate protons is expressed by its dissociation constant Ka ($Ka = (H^+) (A^-)/(HA)$, or by the function pKa, defined as $-\log Ka$. Thus, the pH of a solution of a weak acid is quantitatively related to its pKa, and to the ratio of the concentrations of its acid and base species by the Henderson-Hasselbalch equation (1).

A conjugate acid-base pair can act as a buffer and resist changes in pH; its capacity to do so is greatest at a pH equal to its pKa. Many biomolecules have characteristic functional groups that contribute to buffering capacity. Carbonate and phosphate type buffering systems are important to living organisms. The catalytic activity of biological catalysts (enzymes) is strongly influenced by pH and it is essential that the environments in which they function are buffered against large changes in pH. Cellular organisms maintain a specific and constant cytosolic pH to keep biomolecules in their optimal ionic state—usually near pH 7.0. In multicellular species, the pH of the extracellular fluids such as blood must also be tightly regulated. For example, the human blood plasma has a pH close to 7.40, and is maintained around this value by the buffering system of the blood, containing proteins made of amino acids with their functional groups that are either weak acids or weak bases. In disease conditions such as diabetes, the pH of blood may fall to 6.8 or below due to acidosis, leading to irreparable cell damage and death. In other diseases, blood pH may rise to lethal levels. Several aspects of cell structure and function are thus influenced by pH, the activity of enzymes being the most sensitive to pH. The enzymes show the maximal catalytic activity at a specific pH value, called the optimum pH; on either side of this value their catalytic activity usually declines sharply.

V. NUTRITIONAL ASPECTS OF WATER

The significance of water in the digestion of food, absorption and transportation of food nutrients, and excretion of waste products from the body has been well recognized.

A. Bound Water

In addition to its free state, water is also present in foods (and living systems) in the bound form, owing to the presence of solutes and biological structures that determine the intensity of binding. The water activity, however, depends on the more mobile water molecules that are present in the least bound states. The bound water, which behaves differently from free water, is often grouped into four major types (I to IV), though there are intermediate types of boundness.

Type IV has full water activity and exists only in its free (boundless) state. Type III bound water is found physically entrapped in the tissue matrix and in solutions. It represents the majority of water present in plant cell sap and animal tissues and foods. The activity of type III bound water is only slightly less than that of free water. This type of bound water is available for the growth of microorganisms in foods, enzymatic activity (hydrolytic reactions), and nonenzymatic browning. This water can be easily removed by reducing moisture content to about 12% to 15%.

Type II water is more firmly bound, with substantially reduced water activity. Although it permits hydrolytic type of enzymatic reactions and nonenzymatic browning, elimination of this water (3 to 7% moisture content) arrests microbial growth and most other types of biochemical reactions.

Type I water is very firmly bound, with the least water activity. This type of water can be removed partially by dehydrations but not by freezing. The degree of binding being very high, reactions that depend on Type I water cannot be measured. At this stage, however, reactions such as oxidative rancidity are enhanced (10).

1. The Changing Role of Water Binding in Nutrition

Twenty years ago, water binding was defined as the result of a protein-fat-water gel state and was improved by using ingredients or manufacturing processes that affected the emulsion made between the components. Terms like water binding and moisture retaining were used to describe the ability of an emulsion to keep the water in place in a variety of uses. Today, water binding is considered an alternate term for other properties that describe the use of water as a plasticizer, the crystalline state of water in mixed food systems, and the ability of water to interact with the mixed food systems. In this context, water binding refers to the ability of a food system to retain water in a stable state throughout the shelf life of a food (11). According to Katz (11), water binding has achieved nutritional significance in reduced-fat systems because of changes in balance between food components occurring during removal of fat from a conventional food. Bacterial growth characteristics change in high-water-phase systems, thus limiting the kinds of food systems that can use water as a plasticizer.

The water-holding capacity of gels is influenced by a variety of compounds such as minerals (calcium, sodium, potassium, and phosphate) in protein-containing gels made from materials like whey-protein. With a decrease in the amount of lipid in these protein gels, the cohesiveness of the gel is increased, decreasing the moisture-retention capacity of the product at normal processing and holding temperatures; this is attributed to the fact that lipids act as an emulsifier, forming a tighter emulsion when fat level is higher.

Stabilizing the water phase in combination foods has a great nutritional significance. In low-fat, filled baked foods, for example, it has a different role than in conventional baked foods, where the fat phase surrounding baked food changes the possibility that the filling will alter the whole water balance. A thermostable filling system with less than 15% fat has been reported (U.S. Patent No. 5, 529, 801, Crompton and Knowles Corpn., Stamford, Conn). Primarily a water-based system, it uses an ultrahigh surface-area cellulose that is activated by shearing. The cellulose presumably binds water, because the cellulose defibrillates itself, forming distended and dislocated microfibrils, exposing a large number of hydroxyl groups which in turn provide interparticle association and hydrogen binding between fibrils and microfibrils in the hydrophilic continuous phase of the filling. The special treatment of cellulose (Avicel PH 101 from FMC Corp., Philadelphia) provides extra water binding capacity. By shearing the mixture, the viscosity can be decreased for the proper filling during production. Fats and emulsifiers can be added at low levels, to provide good mouthfeel and texture. The reduced fat content of the filling thus makes possible the low-fat cookies and snacks that are so high in demand.

Starch-based and shear-processed products, such as Stellar^R, potato-based maltodextrin, and C* delight, with a high concentration of large-molecular-weight amylose, used in low-fat cheese for water binding and strength, have been introduced.

One difficulty often encountered in the preparation of low-fat cookies is crisp texture. The additional moisture used to provide a dough that will machine well interacts with the gluten in the wheat flour, causing rubberiness. This can be avoided by coating the flour with a fat in the new formula, thus preventing absorption of water by the gluten (U.S. Patent No.5, 492, 710, Nabisco Inc.). Use of "weak" flours like white rye flour, rice flour, and corn flour to replace part of the wheat flour has been suggested. These flours are provided in a very small particle size to prevent grittiness.

The reduction of fat in the cookies makes them taste sweeter than the amount of sweetener would normally produce. The patent suggests addition of sorbitol to mask the sweetness, add bulk, reduce cookie spread, and coat the flour particles to decrease starch gelatinization, improving the crumb texture. Sorbitol also acts as a water binder, providing additional functionality.

Carbohydrates in their conventional forms (starches, fibers in whole fruits, grains, and vegetables) are used to adjust water-binding activity in food products. The physicochemical forms of these products can be modified by physical shearing, chemical addition of active groups, or enzymatic reduction in chain lengths.

Products used for binding water or influencing humectancy of foods include raisin paste, oat bran, corn germ, and apple and citrus concentrates. The water-binding compounds present in these products are glucose, fructose, starches, pectin, fiber, betaglucans, and other components.

Other researchers have suggested use of Actinidia (kiwifruit) as a source of a fiber-rich fruit concentrate to shear-thicken and provide the viscosity of a fat-containing ingredient in low-fat foods (M.J. Rossiter, U.S. Patent 5,665,413, New Zealand). The kiwifruits are heated whole, then communuted and deodorized to remove the bitter taste, followed by homogenization and shearing. The kiwifruit concentrate can also be used in low-fat dairy products. According to Katz (11), it is difficult to determine whether it is the interactions between some of the components or a single component that is responsible for improved water binding in these combination system products. The research being done in this vital area of nutrition will help us understand the role of interactivity and structure with water holding.

REFERENCES

1. Lehninger, A.L., D.L. Nelson, and M.M. Cox, *Principles of Biochemistry*, 2nd ed., CBS Publishers and Distributors, Delhi, 1993.
2. Trehan, K., *Biochemistry*, Wiley Eastern Ltd., New Delhi, 47, 1987, p. 47.
3. Wrong, O., Water and monovalent electrolytes, *Human Nutrition and Dietetics* (J.S. Garrow and W.P.T. James, eds.), 9th ed., Churchill Livingstone, 1993, p. 146.
4. Cohn, S.H., A. Vaswani, I. Zanzi, J.F. Aloia, M.S. Roginsky, and K.J. Ellis, Changes in body chemical composition with age measured by total-body neutron-activation, *Metabolism 25*: 85 (1976).
5. Ellis, K.J., A. Vaswani, I. Zanzi, and S.H. Cohn, Total body sodium and chlorine in normal adults, *Metabolism 25*: 645, (1976).

6. Passmore, R., A.P. Meiklejohn, A.D. Dewar, and R.K. Thow, Energy utilization in overfed thin young men, *British J. Nutr. 9*: 20 (1955).
7. Sanchez-Castillo, C.P., S. Warrender, T.P. Whitehead, and W.P.T. James, An assessment of the sources of dietary salt in a British population, *Clin. Sci. 72*: 95 (1987).
8. Paul, A.A., and D.A.T. Southgate, *McCance and Widdowson's The Composition of Foods*, 4th ed., HMSO, London, Elsevier, Amsterdam, 1978.
9. Denton, D., *The Hunger for Salt*, Springer Verlag, Berlin, 1982.
10. Manay, N.S., and M. Shadaksharaswamy, *Foods: Facts and Principles*, Wiley Eastern Ltd., New Delhi, 1987.
11. Katz, F. (ed.) The changing role of water binding, A Special Report, *Food Technol.* 51(10): 64, (1997).

3

Carbohydrates

I. INTRODUCTION

Carbohydrates are the most abundant biomolecules produced on the earth; photosynthetic plants and algae convert over 100 billion metric tons of CO_2 and H_2O into sugars, starches, and cellulose-like substances. These are polyhydroxy aldehydes or ketones and their derivatives or substances that yield such compounds on hydrolysis. Most carbohydrates have the empirical formula $(CH_2O)_n$; some do not conform to it, while others contain in addition to C, H, and O, elements such as nitrogen, phosphorus, or sulfur. Three major size classes of carbohydrates are monosaccharides, oligosaccharides, and polysaccharides, the word *saccharide* meaning sugar. Monosaccharides are simple sugars consisting of a single polyhydroxy aldehyde or ketone unit; oligosaccharides consist of short chains of few (two to eight) monosaccharide units joined together by characteristic glycosidic linkages. The most abundant monosaccharide and disaccharide found in nature are glucose (fruit sugar) and sucrose (cane sugar). The latter consists of two 6-carbon sugars, D-glucose and D-fructose joined covalently. All common mono-and disaccharides have names ending with the suffix "-ose". Most oligosaccharides do not occur as free entities but are joined to nonsugar molecules such as lipids or proteins (glucoconjugates). The polysaccharides are the high-molecular-weight, long-chain compounds containing hundreds or thousands of monosaccharide units, either in linear or branched chain fashions. The most abundant polysaccharides found in nature are starch and cellulose, which consist of recurring units of D-glucose but differ in the type of glucosidic linkage (1).

II. BIOLOGICALLY IMPORTANT CARBOHYDRATES

In addition to simple carbohydrates, such as glucose, galactose, fructose, and mannose, and a range of oligosaccharides and polysaccharides, such as starches and celluloses, living organisms contain a variety of derived carbohydrates in which a hydroxyl group in the parent compound is replaced with another substituent, or a carbon atom is oxidized to a carboxylic acid (e.g., glycolipids and glycoproteins). In sugar amines (glucosamine, galactosamine, and mannosamine), the hydroxyl group at C-2 of the parent compound is replaced with an amino group. The amino group may be condensed with acetic acid, as in *N*-acetylglucosamine, which forms part of many structural polymers of bacterial cell walls. The substitution of a hydrogen for the hydroxyl group at C-6 of galactose or mannose produces fucose or rhamnose, respectively, forming deoxy sugars found in the complex oligosaccharides of glycoproteins and glycolipids.

Aldonic acids are produced when the carbonyl (aldehyde) carbon of a monosaccharide is oxidized to a carboxylic acid (e.g., gluconic acid from glucose) and oxidation of carbon at the other end of carbon chain forms the corresponding uronic acids (e.g., glucuronic acid from glucose). Both aldonic and uronic acids form stable intramolecular esters, known as lactones. *N*-acetylneuraminic acid (sialic acid), a nine-carbon derivative of *N*-acetyl mannosamine, is a component of many glucoproteins and glycolipids found in higher animals.

Sugar phosphates are relatively stable at neutral pH and bear a negative charge. These highly charged molecules are not diffused out of the cell without the help of specific transport systems. Phosphorylation of sugars activates them for subsequent chemical transformation in the metabolism.

Chitin is a linear homopolysaccharide containing repeated units of *N*-acetyl-D-glucosamine in beta-glycosidic linkage. Chitin forms extended fibers similar to those of cellulose, and like cellulose is not digested by vertebrates. It is the principal component of the hard exoskeletans of insects, lobsters, and crabs and probably the second most abundant polysaccharide, next to cellulose, in nature. The more rigid component of bacterial cell walls is a heteropolymer of alternating beta-(1–4) linked *N*-acetylglucosamine and *N*-acetylmuramic acid units. The cross-linked peptidoglycan is degraded by the enzyme lysozyme, which hydrolyzes the glycosidic bond between the two types of polymers, killing the bacterial cells.

The extracellular matrix of the animal tissues that holds the cells of a tissue together and provides a porous pathway for the diffusion of nutrients and oxygen to individual cells, contains an interlocking meshwork of heteropolysaccharides and fibrous proteins. The former are a family of linear polymers composed of repeating disaccharide unit of a uronic acid with either *N*-acetylglucosamine or *N*-acetylgalactosamine (glycosaminoglycans). In some glycosaminoglycans, one or more of the hydroxyls of the amino sugar are esterified with sulfate. The latter combine with carboxylate groups of the uronic acids to give glycosaminoglycans a very high density of negative charge. These molecules assume an extended conformation in solution to minimize the repulsive forces among neighboring charged groups, consequently resulting in a viscous solution of long, thin molecules of glycosaminoglycans. The latter get themselves attached to extracellular proteins to form proteoglycans, containing about 55% of the polysaccharide (2).

Another glycosaminoglycan, hyaluronic acid (hyaluronate) of the extracellular matrix of animal tissues, has alternating units of D-glucuronic acid and *N*-acetylglucosamine. These are high-molecular-weight (more than one million) compounds, forming clear, highly viscous lubricants of the synovial fluid of joints and giving the vitreous character of the vertebrate eye its jellylike consistency. Hyaluronate also constitutes a central component of the extracellular matrix of cartilages and tendons, contributing to their tensile strength and elasticity.

Proteoglycans are composed of a very long strand of hyaluronate, attached to numerous protein molecules at about 40 nm intervals. Each core protein is bound covalently to many short-chain glycosaminoglycan molecules, such as chondroitin sulfate, keratan sulfate, heparan sulfate, and dermatan sulfate. Interwoven with these proteoglycans are the fibrous proteins, collagens and elastin, forming a cross-linked meshwork that gives the extracellular matrix strength and resiliency.

Proteins and certain lipids may be covalently attached to oligosaccharides to form glycoproteins and glycolipids, most proteins secreted by eukaryotic cells being glycoproteins. The biological significance of these compounds has not been fully elucidated. The hydrophilic clusters of carbohydrate alter the polarity and solubility of the proteins or lipids. The physical effects of carbohydrates on protein structure have been implicated, apart from more specific biological functions. Many of the proteins of plasma membranes are glycoproteins, with their oligosaccharide moieties (1% to 70%) located on the external surface of the membrane; e.g., glycophorin of the erythrocyte membrane contains about 60% carbohydrate by weight in the form of 16 oligosaccharide chains (60 to 70 monosaccharides) covalently attached to residues near the amino terminus polypeptide chain. Many of the glycoproteins are soluble; some are carrier proteins and immunoglobulins (antibodies) in the blood of vertebrates, and others are found within the lysosomes, playing vital roles in disease resistance.

Like glycoproteins and proteoglycans, other conjugated carbohydrates such as glycolipids and lipopolysaccharides are also constituents of the cellular membranes; e.g., in gangliosides, the polar head group is a complex oligosaccharide containing sialic acid (N-acetylneuraminic acid) and other monosaccharide units. Lipopolysaccharides are major components of bacterial outer membranes. They are the dominant surface features of gram-negative bacteria (*E. coli* and *Salmonella typhimurium*), which are the prime targets of the antibodies produced by the immune system in response to bacterial infection (antigen). The lipopolysaccharide of certain bacteria is toxic to humans and other animals, dangerously lowering blood pressure; in humans, a shock syndrome can occur with *Staphylococcus aureus* poisoning (1).

III. NUTRITIONAL ASPECTS OF CARBOHYDRATES

A. Dietary Sources of Carbohydrates

The three major constituents of foods are carbohydrates, proteins, and lipids, with small amounts of vitamins, minerals, pigments, flavoring substances, and enzymes. Water is also present in foods in varying quantities. These constituents give foods their structure, texture, color, flavor, and nutritive value.

Carbohydrates are widely distributed in nature in the form of sugars, starches, celluloses, and other complex substances. They provide a major part of the energy in human diets: about 80% to 85% of the energy for the people of developing countries and about 40% to 45% of the energy of the more affluent Western world, though neither of these extremes is desirable nutritionally. Englyst and Kingman (3) distinguished two types of polysaccharides from plant foods: the storage polysaccharide, starch, and the cell wall or chemically related structural polysaccharides that do not contain alpha-glycosidic linkages, called non-starch polysaccharides (NSP). Cereal grains, pulses and other seeds, root vegetables and stem vegetables such as potato, sweet potato, cassava, and plantains contain large amounts of starch, constituting the world's most important starchy foods; NSP is the principal and readily measurable food component termed as dietary fiber.

Animal tissues also contain a starch-like substance—glycogen, a storage polysaccharide. The amount of carbohydrate in animal tissues is comparatively small in relation to their fat and protein content and is not important in dietary terms. The main types of food carbohydrates in the human diet are shown in Fig. 1. The proportions of starch, sugar, and NSP (dietary fiber) in the diet are highly variable (Fig. 2) for the people of different communities in the world.

1. Monosaccharides and Disaccharides

Fruits and vegetables contain variable amounts of glucose and fructose, the latter being the major constituent of honey. Natural foods do not contain abundant glucose and fructose, but they can be made as invert sugars from sucrose by hydrolysis and used in a number of food preparations and pharmaceuticals. Fructose is sweeter than sucrose, whereas glucose is only half as sweet as sucrose. Mannose is uncommon in foods but is present in manna or lichens, which in drought curl up into light balls from which a bread can be made (3).

Pentoses are present in small amounts as constituents of the macromolecules in the cells of both plant and animal foods, and thus are not important as a source of dietary energy. Ribose and deoxyribose are constituents of ribonucleic acid (RNA) and deoxyribonucleic acid (DNA) and are synthesized naturally by plants and animals.

Sucrose is the most abundant disaccharide found in nature and is extracted commercially from cane and sugar beet and from certain other minor sugar crops (4). Table sugar (99% pure

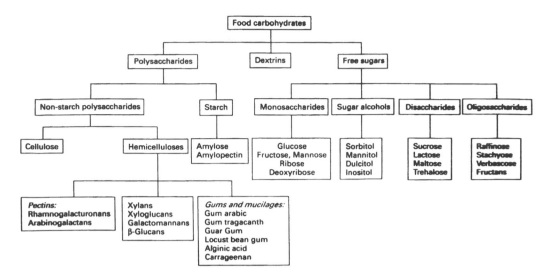

Figure 1   The principal carbohydrates in the human diet (from Ref. 3).

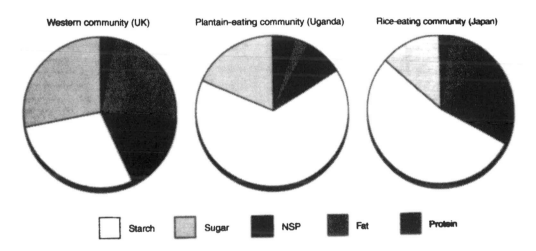

Figure 2   Percentage nutrient intake in three communities with different dietary intakes (from Ref. 3).

sucrose) is the major dietary source of this disaccharide and is also present to a lesser extent in most fruits and vegetables. It is readily hydrolyzed by mineral acids and an enzyme, sucrase (invertase), present in the brush border of the small intestine, into glucose and fructose.

Lactose is a milk sugar made up of glucose and galactose. During childhood, lactose is readily hydrolyzed by the enzyme lactase, but in adulthood certain ethnic groups lose the ability to produce lactase, causing a disorder, lactose intolerance (see Chapters 16 and 19).

Maltose is a hydrolysis product of starch and comprises two glucose molecules. It is present in malted (sprouted) wheat and barley, from which malt is extracted commercially for use in brewing and in the manufacture of malted foods.

Trehalose, like sucrose, is a non-reducing disaccharide, made of two glucose units bound in alpha-(1-1) glycosidic linkage; it is found in mushrooms to the extent of about 15% on a dry-weight basis. It is a major constituent of the circulating fluid (hemolymph) of insects. Humans still possess the specific enzyme, trehalase, for its hydrolysis, suggesting that fungi and insects were more important foods for primitive peoples than for today's modern societies.

Contrary to previous claims that simple sugars may have adverse effects on several metabolic conditions involved in the etiology of obesity, cardiovascular disease, and diabetes mellitus, Black and Saris (5), on the basis of available literature, concluded that there was no consistent evidence to implicate differences in simple and complex dietary carbohydrates in the etiology of these human diseases. Moreover, there are indications that simple carbohydrates may have beneficial effects on glucose tolerance and blood lipid spectrum. These findings require further research work.

2. Oligosaccharides and Sugar Alcohols

The important oligosaccharides found naturally occurring in pulses (beans and peas) are raffinose, stachyose, and verbascose, containing glucose, fructose, and galactose. These oligosaccharides are not hydrolyzed by human endogenous enzymes, and, like NSP, they are fermented in the large intestine, producing gases such as carbon dioxide, hydrogen, and methane and volatile fatty acids such as acetic, propionic, and butyric acids.

Fructans are a group of oligo- and polysaccharides containing fructose residues attached to a single glucose molecule; the chain length varies from 3 to 50 units, depending on the food source. Shorter-chain fructans predominate in cereals and a longer-chain fructan, known as inulin, is found in Jerusalem artichokes. Other food sources of fructans include onions, garlic, and asparagus. The trisaccharides, for the most part, are not hydrolyzed in the stomach and intestine and may be excreted in the urine if absorbed directly. Most of the fructans are fermented in the large intestine.

Sugar alcohols occur naturally and can also be manufactured industrially. Sorbitol, for example, found naturally in fruits such as cherries, is made commercially from glucose by aldose reductase, which reduces the aldehyde group (CHO) to the alcohol (CH_2OH) in the glucose molecule. Sorbitol, being less sweet (60% as sweet as sucrose), is used in dietetic foods such as soft drinks and confectioneries for diabetics. It is absorbed from the gut more slowly and converted to fructose in the liver, and thus, has less effect on blood glucose levels. However, daily intakes of more than 50 g/day of sorbitol may lead to diarrhea in diabetic patients.

On reduction, mannose and galactose yield mannitol and dulcitol, respectively, which have a range of uses in the food industry. Mannitol is commercially extracted from a seaweed growing on the British coasts (3). Inositol, a cyclic alcohol with six hydroxyl groups, is present in the bran of cereals and many other foods. Hexaphosphate ester of inositol is a phytic acid present in some pulses and other foods. Phytic acid decreases the absorption and utilization of certain micronutrients such as calcium, iron, and zinc in the small intestine (see Chapter 7).

3. Polysaccharides

Starch is the principal storage polysaccharide of staple foods such as cereals, potatoes, cassava, and plantains. It is present in granular form in characteristic shapes specific to each species. Amylose is a linear polysaccharide containing alpha-(1–4) type of glycosidic linkage; amylopectin is a brached-chain polysaccharide with 15–30 alpha-(1–4) linked glucose units in each branch, the branches being joined by alpha-(1–6) type of glycosidic linkage. The relative amounts of amylose and amylopectin vary among different plant sources, from about 2% amylose in waxy cornstarch to around 80% in high-amylose cornstarch. Most other starches contain 15% to 35% amylose.

The semi-crystalline structures of amylose and amylopectin in the starch granules make them relatively insoluble in water and retards their digestion by pancreatic amylase. However, when starch is heated in aqueous solution and the crystalline structure is disrupted, the polysaccharide chain takes up a random conformation that causes swelling and thickening of starch matrix (gelatinization). Such starch is readily hydrolyzed by the digestive amylases. On cooling, the gelatinized starch begins to recrystallize itself, a process known a retrogradation, which is very rapid for amylose but takes a longer time (several days) for amylopectin. The latter is known to be responsible for the staling of bread.

Englyst and Kingman (6) classified starch for human nutritional purposes (Table 1).Three fractions of starch, defined in physicochemical terms and determined in vitro, demonstrate the probable behavior of starchy foods within the digestive tract. Rapidly digestible starch (RDS) is primarily amorphous and more dispersed and is found in starchy foods cooked by moist heat (bread, potato). Slowly digestible starch (SDS) is thought to be completely digested in the small intestine. This type is poorly accessible to enzymes e.g., partly milled grain or seeds, highly dense foods like pasta, and granula starch in raw foods. Resistant starch (RS) is the starch that is potentially resistant to digestion in the small intestine and therefore undergoes fermentation in the large intestine. The amounts of RDS SDS, and RS in foods vary greatly and depend partly on the source of starch, but largely on the type and extent of processing the food has undergone (3) (Table 2).

Dextrins are the degradation products of starch, wherein the glucose chains are partially hydrolyzed. These constitute the main source of carbohydrate in the proprietary preparations (liquid glucose) used as oral supplements for tube feeding. Liquid glucose contains a mixture of dextrins, maltose, glucose, and water. Having less osmotic effects than glucose or sucrose, the dextrins are less likely to cause osmolar diarrhea.

Glycogen is an animal starch present in the liver and muscle tissues where it is stored as readily available energy reserve. It is hydrolysed by pancreatic amylase to glucose. In most animal foods, it is a negligible source of dietary carbohydrate.

B. Role of Carbohydrates as Dietary Fibers

Dietary fiber has not been defined correctly in chemical terms, which has led to delay in developing accurate methods of its measurement and misinterpretation of the studies on dietary fiber in human nutrition. Hipsley (7) estimated dietary fiber as the material derived from the plant cell wall in foods. Trowell (8) defined dietary fiber as the skeletal remains of plant cells that are resist-

Table 1   Classification of Starch for Nutritional Purposes

Type of starch	Example of occurrence	Probable digestion in small intestine
Rapidly digestible starch (RDS)	Freshly cooked starchy food	Rapid
Slowly digestible starch (SDS)	Most raw cereals	Slow but complete
Resistant starch (RS), physically inaccessible starch	Partly milled grains and seeds	Resistant
Resistant starch granules	Raw potato and banana	Resistant
Retrograded amylose	Cooked potato after cooling, bread, cornflakes, etc.	Resistant

Source: Ref. 6.

Table 2 In Vitro Digestibility of Starch in Some Foods (% of Total Starch Present in Food)

Food	RDS (%)	SDS (%)	RS_1 (%)	RS_2 (%)	RS_3 (%)
White flour	49	48	—	3	t
Shortbread	56	43	—	—	1
White bread	94	4	—	—	2
White spaghetti	52	43	3	—	3
Banana biscuits	39	23	—	38	t
Potato biscuits	47	27	—	25	1
Haricot beans	18	42	18	9	12
Pearl barley	41	41	9	—	2

RSD = rapidly digestible starch
SDS = slowly digestible starch
RS = resistant starch
t = trace
Source: Ref. 3.

ant to digestion by man's enzymes. However, Cummings and Englyst in 1978 proposed that dietary fiber should be measured as the non-starch polysaccharides (NSPs) in plant foods (9). Englyst et al. (10) defined dietary fiber as non-starch polysaccharide (NSP) for the purpose of food labeling, because this gave the best index of plant cell-wall polysaccharide and was in keeping with the original concept of dietary fiber.

The dietary fiber that resists digestion in the small intestine would logically include NSP, lactose (in many ethnic groups), oligosaccharides such as raffinose, stachyose, and others, a small amount of lignin, organic acids such as oxalate and tartate, Maillard reaction products, some fat, hairs, bone, grit and such other insoluble materials, and a highly variable amount of starch and protein, depending on the processing. In addition to these, certain synthetic products such as lactulose, polydextrose, neosugar, and others resistant to pancreatic amylase may also be included as dietary fiber. Such a broad definition of dietary fiber is clearly very different from the original concept (3).

The factors that influence resistance of foodstuffs to digestion include—apart from the chemical structure and food processing—a number of other factors not related to the food per se: e.g., extent of chewing, transit time through the stomach and small intestine, and the amount and type of other food components in the meal. The extent of digestion in the small intestine and digestibility vary greatly among individual population groups and subjects. Thus, defining dietary fiber as the material resisting digestion in the small intestine is not analytically as accurate as NSP, which appears to be a more reliable index of plant cell-wall polysaccharides, in keeping with the original concept of dietary fiber.

Southgate (11) put forth the concept of unavailable carbohydrates, which was further modified by Englyst and his associates by evolving a procedure for the measurement of NSP as an index of dietary fiber. In this method, starch is completely removed enzymatically, and NSP is measured as the sum of its constituent sugars released by acid hydrolysis. The sugars may be determined by using gas-liquid chromatography (12) or high-performance liquid chromatography (13) to obtain values for individual monosaccharides, or even by rapid colorimetric technique (14). Values for total dietary fiber as well as for soluble and insoluble dietary fiber may be obtained. Cellulose content also can be measured separately by using a small modification.

The values of dietary fiber of a foodstuff may vary considerably according to the method of analysis (Table 3). The estimation of crude fiber in animal feed trial studies measures only a small

Table 3 Comparison of Dietary Fiber Values Obtained by Different Methods

Sample	Crude fiber	NDF[a] method	Southgate (Ref. 11)	Prosky et al. (Ref. 15)	Mongeau and Brassard (Ref. 17)	Englyst et al. (Ref. 10)
White bread	1.7	2.4	4.4	3.5	3.0	3.0
Wholemeal bread	5.1	10.6	14.2	8.8	9.2	6.6
Porridge oats, raw	2.0	6.9	7.7	10.5	11.0	8.2
Shredded wheat cereal	3.6	13.4	13.3	10.4	11.1	9.0
Sweetcorn kernels	2.2	7.9	13.5	7.7	7.8	5.9
Onion	6.1	7.6	18.0	16.9	17.3	16.7
Carrots, raw	5.7	9.2	28.7	25.4	23.4	23.4
Cabbage, raw	8.4	14.2	28.4	23.3	20.7	21.0
Apples	3.7	7.6	12.7	14.6	14.2	13.4
Oranges	2.7	3.7	12.6	12.8	13.7	13.5

[a]NDF = Neutral detergent fiber.
Source: Refs. 17, 41, 42.

proportion of dietary fiber (mainly cellulose) that resists hydrolysis with acid and alkali. Thus, it severely underestimates dietary fiber in foods. The NDF (neutral detergent fiber) method, measuring selectively insoluble fraction of dietary fiber, also tends to underestimate the total fiber present in the foods, especially in fruits and vegetables that are sources of soluble non-starch polysaccharides. Higher values of dietary fiber are obtained by the Southgate (11) method and the enzmatic-gravimetric methods of Prosky et al. (15,16) as well as by the Mongeau and Brassard (17) method, because these methods include substances other than the non-starch polysaccharides measured directly by the Englyst et al. (10) procedure.

According to Thebaudin et al. (18), the fiber content of different foods varies greatly, e.g., cereal products, 2.0% (white rice) to 42.0% (wheat bran); dried vegetables, 2.0% (chickpeas) to 25.5% (beans); dried fruits and nuts, 5.0% (walnuts) to 18.3% (figs); fresh fruits, 0.5% (most fruit) to 3.0% (pears); and green vegetables, 1.4% (most vegetables) to 5.3% (garden peas).

Fiber-rich ingredients can be used in foods only if the product has good sensory characteristics, regardless of the nutritional benefits of the fibers. The hydration properties of dietary fibers determine their optimal usage levels in foods because a desirable texture must be retained. The hydration properties are often described by parameters such as water holding capacity (WHC), water-binding capacity (WBC), swelling, and solubility. Values for swelling, WHC, and WBC are not relevant for soluble polysaccharides, instead they are attributes of insoluble polysaccharides (19). The electric charge influences the solubility of polysaccharides significantly. The presence of charged, dissociated uronic acid, sulfate or pyruvate groups, for example, tends to favor solubilization of the polymers. This effect depends on the pH, temperature and concentration of other components in water, such as salts or sugars. The influences of the origin and particle size of dietary fibers on their swelling properties and WBC are shown in Table 4. Sugar-beet and apple fibers exhibit high WBC values. Increasing the particle size of the fibers increases the WBC. The WBC of fibers can have technological interest (e.g., increased yield of food) as well as nutritional interest, because increased water retention increases the orocecal transit time.

Estimation of different components of the diet as a measure of dietary fiber has led to considerable confusion and misinterpretation in research and food labeling of dietary fiber, resulting in different RDAs. The Prosky method includes the part of the starch retrograded during food processing and also 'lignin'-type substances as dietary fiber, thus giving higher values than the

Table 4 Functional Evaluation of Vegetable Materials That are Rich in Fiber According to Their Particle Size

Properties	Apple		Pea		Wheat		Sugarbeet		Carrot
Particle size (mean, μM)	80	600	80	600	600	80	600	80	80
TDF content (w/w, dry mass)	70	90	90	90	60	60	75	75	50
WBD (g water/g fiber)	4.5 ± 0.2	3.5 ± 0.2	2.7 ± 0.2	3.5 ± 0.2	3.1 ± 0.2	2.5 ± 0.2	10 ± 0.2	5 ± 0.2	3.8 ± 0.2
FAC (g fat/g fiber)	1.3 ± 0.1	1 ± 0.1	0.9 ± 0.1	1 ± 0.1	2.3 ± 0.1	1.3 ± 0.1	5 ± 0.1	1.5 ± 0.1	1.2 ± 0.1
Swelling (cm^3)[a]	9 ± 0.5	5.5 ± 0.5	5 ± 0.5	5.5 ± 0.5	7.5 ± 0.5	4 ± 0.5	10 ± 0.5	10 ± 0.5	7.5 ± 0.5
Texture[b] after heat treatment (Newtons)	30 ± 2	5.5 ± 0.5	5 ± 0.5	5.5 ± 0.5	0.5 ± 0.1	0.2 ± 0.01	25 ± 0.5	25 ± 0.5	6 ± 0.1

[a]Volume of dispersion (water + fiber) when equilibrium is obtained
[b]Measured by a penetrometric method in a medium of 90% water, 15% fiber
TDF = Total dietary fiber,
WBD = Water-binding capacity
FAC = Fat-absorption capacity.
Source: Ref. 18.

Englyst method (Table 3). The physiological effects of the material measured by this technique have not been understood and are likely to be different from that of the dietary fiber measured solely as NSP.

Prosky's AOAC method (15) consists largely of retrograded amylose and represents the portion of the starch measured as resistant starch (RS). This type of starch is thought to escape digestion in the human small intestine, as does dietary fiber. Testing of the digestibility of different types of starch in humans has now revealed that retrograded amylose (RS_3) represents only a small proportion of the total amount of starch escaping digestion in the small intestine.

Substances other than NSP and different types of starch escaping digestion in the human small intestine are certain proteins, lactose, free sugars and oligosaccharides, raffinose, and stachyose. Thus, inclusion of any type of starch with dietary fiber does not appear to be warranted on the basis of escaping digestion (3).

A suggestion that retrograded amylose (RS_3) may have a fecal bulking effect has been argued on the basis that several other food components (protein, free sugars, and oligosaccharides) also have bulking effects, either directly or through bacterial fermentation (20). Also, the amount of RS_3 in starchy foods varies greatly according to processing factors, such as source of starch, water content, pH, heating temperature and time, number of heating and cooling cycles, freezing, and drying (21). These authors further argued that the amount of RS_3 found in normal cooking is nutritionally insignificant for most foods. If RS_3 is included as dietary fiber, food manufacturers may raise the RS_3 content of some foods substantially to boost sales through a claim of high dietary fiber content, apart from causing food labeling problems. Thus, different apparent "dietary fiber" values will be obtained for the same food if it is hot, cold, frozen, or dried before analysis. The Prosky method employs one or more of these treatments prior to analysis. The dietary fiber values obtained by the Prosky method thus do not reflect the RS content of the food as eaten but instead that produced by storage and pretreatment of the sample; e.g., the RS measured in a cooled or dried potato sample will be different from the value obtained for the potatoes eaten hot. Thus, food processing primarily influences RS_3, and not NSP.

The material measured as lignin also may result in large overestimations of dietary fiber, especially in processed foods, though when measured accurately, lignin would be quantitatively insignificant in the human diet. Lignin is not a carbohydrate and its physiological significance (in animal studies) is very different from that of NSP. Englyst et al. (10) therefore suggested that, unlike in the Prosky method, lignin should not be measured with NSP and not be included in the analytical definition of dietary fiber. According to Cummings et al. (22), lignin is quantitatively a minor component of the human diet.

According to Asp et al. (23), dietary fibers do not constitute a well-defined chemical group, but are a combination of chemically heterogenous substances such as celluloses, hemicelluloses, pectins, lignins, gums, and polysaccharides from seaweeds or bacteria. The most widely accepted definition is a physiological one, in which dietary fibers correspond to the vegetable cell-wall residues that are resistant to enzymatic hydrolysis in the small intestine. A chemical definition describes dietary fibers as non-starch polysaccharides. Most commonly, however, dietary fibers are regarded as oligosaccharides, polysaccharides, and the (hydrophilic) derivatives that cannot be digested by the human digestive enzymes to absorbable components in the upper alimentary tract, including lignins (24).

The single most important factor that dictates fecal weight in the West is dietary fibers, where constipation is a common problem and it can be treated with dietary fibers. The physiological effects depend on the type of dietary fibers, either insoluble or soluble. Insoluble fibers, such as wheat bran and cellulose, increase stool weight and frequency, soften feces, increase fecal bulk, and reduce intestinal transit time (25). Cereal fibers more effectively increase stool weight than fruit fibers. Soluble fibers such as pectins do not markedly change colonic function or decrease intestinal transit time, and they are completely digested by the gut microflora (26).

Increasing evidence since 1980 indicates that there are distinct benefits to human health from increasing the intake of complex carbohydrates, which can be grouped into two main areas (27):

1. In the small intestine, where consumption of starchy foods has an effect to reduce and delay the magnitude of the glycemic response after a meal (28).
2. In the large intestine, where starch resistant to degradation by human digestive enzymes (resistant starch) is fermented, producing short-chain fatty acids and other products that may have a role in maintaining the health of the colonic mucosa (29).

Englyst et al. (30) have developed a procedure to analyze the different components in their nutritional classification, which will prove very useful in determining the likely physiological effects of eating certain types of starchy foods. For the past three or four decades, starch has had a very negative image, being perceived as fattening or merely as a filler. The information on the health benefits of starch as a nutrient will help to promote its increased consumption. Already some segments of the food industry have recognized the growing interest in starchy foods and are trying to address the lack of interest in this food component, and to encourage a renewed enthusiasm for foods containing starch. Advertisements with phrases such as "Rediscover Baked Beans" (31), "Potatoes contain large amounts of an ingredient essential for a healthy balanced diet—starch" (32), and "Dismissed in the past as 'storage,' starch is now recognized by nutritionists as the healthiest form of energy" (33) are good examples of renewed interest in the starch in the United Kingdom and North America. Potatoes are being referred as "Britain's Buried Treasure." The term complex carbohydrate, rather than starch, defies definition and is not analyzable. Thus, it is far more meaningful to refer to starch itself, to educate consumes about the problems with its image in the past, and with increasing knowledge of its health benefits, to promote its consumption in the future. According to Stephen (27), it may be a much more difficult goal to achieve than the reduction in fat intake, but as the accumulating evidence suggests, there may be many health benefits from taking on this challenge.

1. Food Sources of Dietary Fibers

Englyst et al. (34) reported the total, soluble, and insoluble dietary fiber contents of 178 fruits and vegetables and 114 cereal products. The total and soluble NSP and the composition of total NSP of some foods are shown in Tables 5 and 6, respectively. By employing gaschromatographic techniques, dietary fiber can be separated into cellulose and noncellulosic polysaccharides (NCP) with values for the individual constituent sugars (Table 6), which have different physiological roles in human nutrition. Wheat bran has a higher content of total NSP, with a majority of insoluble part (Table 5). Cereals generally have greater portion of NCP xylose than arabinose, but contain only traces of uronic acids. This is in contrast to fruits and vegetables, where arabinose, especially soluble NCP arabinose, predominates. Also, fruits and vegetables have generally higher content of uronic acids (from pectin).

2. Major NSP Polysaccharides

Cellulose, hemicelluloses, pectins, beta-glucans, and gums and mucilages are the main polysaccharides constituting NSP. Cellulose, the major component of cell walls of plants, is the high-molecular-weight polymer containing up to 10,000 glucose units, linked by beta -(1–4) glycosidic bonds. Strong inter- and intramolecular hydrogen-bonding between cellulose chains are responsible for the formation of microfibrils and fibers and development of highly stable crystalline structures. The low chemical reactivity of cellulose thus explains its characteristic physical properties. Hemicelluloses are heterogenous, branched polymers of hexoses, pentoses, and uronic acids found in all plant cell walls. These are short-chain polymers, containing about 50 to

Table 5 Total and Soluble Non-Starch Polysaccharide (NSP) Contents of Some Foods (g/100 g)

	Total NSP		Soluble NSP
Food	Fresh weight	Dry weight	Dry weight
Wheat bran	36.0	41.1	4.2
White bread	1.6	2.7	1.6
Rye bread	7.3	13.3	6.7
Oatmeal	6.6	7.4	4.1
Cornflakes	0.9	0.9	0.4
Potato	1.2	6.4	3.8
Beans, French	3.1	30.4	12.7
Carrots	2.4	19.5	11.4
Cabbage	2.9	24.4	11.8
Tomato	1.1	18.8	7.4
Apples	1.7	12.5	5.4
Oranges	2.1	15.0	9.8

Source: Ref. 3.

Table 6 Composition of Non-Starch Polysaccharide[a] of Some Foods (g/100 g dry weight)

		Non-Cellulosic polysaccharides							
Food	Cellulose	Rha	Fuc	Ara	Xyl	Man	Gal	Glc	UAC
White bran	8.2	—	—	9.9	17.7	0.3	0.8	3.0	1.2
White bread	0.2	—	—	0.8	1.2	0.1	0.1	0.3	—
Rye bread	1.2	—	—	3.5	5.8	0.1	0.3	2.3	0.1
Oatmeal	0.4	—	—	0.9	1.3	0.1	0.2	4.2	0.3
Cornflakes	0.3	—	—	0.1	0.3	—	—	0.1	0.1
Potato	2.0	0.1	—	0.4	0.1	—	2.2	0.6	1.0
Beans, French	11.1	0.3	—	2.3	1.7	1.4	4.1	0.6	8.9
Carrots	6.4	0.7	—	2.0	0.3	0.4	3.4	0.1	6.2
Cabbage	8.0	0.7	—	4.6	1.0	0.5	2.7	0.1	6.8
Tomato	7.5	0.3	—	0.9	1.0	1.3	1.7	0.4	5.7
Apples	4.2	0.3	0.2	1.7	0.8	0.3	1.0	0.3	3.7
Oranges	3.4	0.3	—	2.2	0.6	0.4	1.8	0.1	6.2

Rha = Rhamnose, Fuc = Fucose   Ara = Arabinose   Glc = Glucose
Xyl = Xylose   Man = Mannose   Gal = Galactose   UAC = Uronic acid

[a] Cellulose is present in the insoluble NSP fraction, but non-cellulosic polysaccharides are present in both the fractions. Foods with substantial uronic acid content have these predominantly in the soluble fraction of NSP.

The monosaccharides are found in either the soluble or insoluble polysaccharides.

A dash (—) indicates only trace quantities of the monosaccharide.

Source: Ref. 3.

2000 units of sugars, varying according to plant source. Xylans are polymers of xylose with the side chains of arabinose and glucuronic acid, often found in cereals such as wheat, rye, and barley. In contrast, legumes are characterized by galactomannans, consisting of a mannose backbone with glucose and galactose side chains. The xyloglucans with a glucose backbone and xylose branches are associated with cellulose found in the plant tissues.

Pectins are branched polymers found in fruit and vegetables. Two predominant types are rhamnogalacturonans, the polymers of rhamnose and galacturonic acid with branches of galactose and arabinose; and arabinogalactans, which are the galactose chains with the short arabinose side chains. The uronic acid groups of pectins are often partly esterified with methoxyl groups. The beta-glucans are the water-soluble polymers of glucose linked with beta-(1–3) and beta-(1–4) bonds. The glucose chains are branched, with a low degree of polymerization. Oats and barley are rich sources of beta-glucans, which are implicated to have an important property of cholesterol reduction.

Gums are water-soluble viscous polysaccharides, containing 10 to 30 thousand units of glucose, galactose, mannose, arabinose, rhamnose, and their uronic acids, which may be methoxylated or even acetylated. Gums are commercially extracted and used in the food industry as emulsifiers, stabilizers, and thickeners, e.g., gum arabic from acacia tree (*Robinia pseudacacia*) and gum tragacanth from *Sterculia* and *Khaya* species. Examples of galactomannans are guar gum and locust bean gums, the storage polysaccharides of the Indian cluster bean and the locust or carob bean, respectively.

Mucilages are D-galacturonic acid–containing polymers found in seeds and roots and are thought to prevent desiccation. Algae and seaweeds are sources of mucilages used as food additives. Alginic acid, extracted from brown seaweeds, is a polymer of mannuronic and guluronic acids and is used as thickening and stabilizing agent in ice creams and confectioneries (3).

Rickard and Thompson (35) reported that flaxseed is the richest known plant source of the n-3 fatty acid, alpha-linolenic acid (more than 50% of the fatty acids present in the oil fraction), as well as of lignan precursors, and contains high amounts of soluble fiber. These components appear to contribue to the benefical health effects observed for flaxseed in chronic diseases.

3. Synthetic Carbohydrates

Polydextrose is a synthetic carbohydrate consisting of randomly cross-linked glucose polymers of different types. It is manufactured by thermal polymerization of glucose in the presence of citric acid and sorbitol. Polydextrose is available in two forms: an off-white amorphous powder and a light yellow aqueous solution; both are non-sweet and tasteless, having functional properties similar to sucrose. Polydextrose is not digested in the small intestine and enters the colon, where approximately 30% is fermented by the intestinal bacteria to volatile fatty acids and CO_2; the remainder is excreted in the feces (36).

A mixture of short-chain fructose-base oligosaccharides (3–5 residues) synthesized from sucrose by the fungal enzyme beta-fructofuranosidase is called *neosugar*. It is used in cooking like sucrose but is only half as sweet, and like polydextrose is not digested by endogenous human digestive enzymes. It can get fermented by certain bacterial strains such as *Bifidobacterium* spp. Neosugar gives about 1.5 kcal of energy per gram, compared with 4 kcal/g from sucrose (3).

4. Intake of Dietary Fiber

According to Bingham et al. (37), the average daily intake of dietary fiber in the United Kingdom is around 12 g, both for men and for women, though there is considerable individual variation in the consumption of NSP. The omnivorous diet of some people may contain as much as 30 g of dietary fiber per day. Fruits, vegetables, and cereals constitute approximately 10%, 48%, and 38%, respectively, of source of dietary fiber in the diet of British people (38).

According to Englyst and Kingman (3), intakes of dietary fiber in the affluent countries have decreased in the recent times with an increase in the use of the processed foods. The average intake of NSP by the American people is slightly higher than that of the British, and it is considerably higher in men than in women. The sex difference could be attributed to higher caloric intake by the men. The people of Denmark, Finland, and Japan have NSP intakes similar to those of the British people, although rural communities in these countries tend to consume more fiber in their diets than the urban population. In the developing tropical countries, the dietary fiber intake of people eating rice as a staple food (China, India, South America) are similar to Western intakes. However, the amount of starch escaping digestion in these areas may be substantial and of great importance for large-bowel physiology (see Chapter 19).

A meta-analysis of 13 case-control studies suggested that intake of dietary fiber and risk of colon cancer were inversely associated (39). Weaker associations were observed between risk of colon cancer and dietary intake of ascorbic acid and beta-carotene (40). There is a need to focus research on explaining the mechanism of action of dietary fiber. Do high intakes of fiber alter the adenoma polyposis sequence? Do they alter microbial metabolism or the colonic milieu? Does fiber exert physical effects related to altered transit time or absorption of carcinogens or other harmful substances? Does fiber alter mucosal cytokinetics or influence gut enzymes or hormone production? These questions are not likely to yield to epidemiological approaches and will require direct observation and experimentation.

In countries whose populations ingest low-calorie, high-fiber diets, there is evidence of growth retardation primarily due to negative zinc balance. Virtually all fibers bind cations such as Zn, Ca, and Mg. A diet too high in fiber may lead to a mineral imbalance. It is easy to overshoot fiber in the diets of elderly people whose energy intake is normally low. Expert panels convened in Canada and the United States have arrived independently at similar suggestions for fiber intake, i.e. 10 to 13 g of fiber per 1000 kcal. These amounts provide about 20 to 35 g of dietary fiber for the average healthy adult. The ratio of insoluble to soluble fiber should be about 3 to 1.

C. NUTRITIVE AND NONNUTRITIVE SWEETENERS

Sugars are a fairly good source of calories. Apart from their nutritive value, sugars have several other functions, such as humectants (absorption of moisture from air), plasticizers, texturizing agents, flavoring agents, and sweeteners. The flavor-producing function of sugars depends on the reactions sugars undergo when they are subjected to heat during sterilization, cooking, and dehydration. The sweetness of sugars depends on their ability to form hydrogen bonds with water, other polar compounds, and among themselves (2).

All sweet-tasting compounds are thought to have a unit consisting of two electronegative atoms A and B, with a hydrogen atom covalently bonded to A. Thus, AH is a proton donor group, and B is a proton acceptor group. The distance between AH and B is about 3A°. The sweetness of a compound is the result of the concentrated intermolecular H-bonding phenomenon, which uses the adjacent OH-groups of a sugar molecule as a AH-B unit to interact with a geometrically commensurate AH-B unit on the receptor site. On the receptor site, an amino acid residue (probably lysine) of a sweet-sensitive protein provides the AH-B unit. Sugars differ in their sweetness because of the variation in the stereochemical position between the two hydroxyl groups in a sugar molecule. When the effective distance constituting an AH-B unit is too great, the hydroxyl groups are not able to bond effectively to the taste bud; and if too close, they form intramolecular bonds, diminishing the sweetness in both cases.

The chemical interaction with the receptor site described above is a "bipartite AH-B interaction," which is associated with the sweetness of the compound. High intensity of sweetness is associated with a tripartite AH-B interaction, the third component, ψ (psi) is involved in such tripartite interaction. The ψ-group in glucose is the methylene C-6 carbon atom. The tripartite interaction results in hydrophobic and lipophilic characters that determines the relative sweetness of compounds. A tripartite fit results in a stronger interaction with the receptor site or may activate an otherwise inert or relatively inert AH-B unit on the compound.

Like sweetness, bitterness also results from the stereochemistry of stimulus molecules. When the sugar molecules are chemically modified, the resulting derivatives are almost bitter, sweet, or bittersweet, e.g. sucrose octacetate is very bitter. When the sugars are chemically modified, one "end" of the molecule (third and fourth hydroxyl groups of the glucopyranoside) elicits sweetness and the other end (first and second hydroxyl groups, ring oxygen atom and primary alcoholic group of glycopyranoside) elicits bitterness. In the bittersweet compounds, the sweet-eliciting ΛH-B systems are not involved in modification. Such substances may be polarized on taste receptors in such a way that one end elicits sweetness and the other bitterness. The evidence for the proximity of sweet and bitter sites in the compounds has been obtained. The relative sweetness of some sweeteners compared with that of sucrose (taken as 100) is as follows:

Sweetener	Relative sweetness (sucrose = 100)
Sucrose	100
Lactose	40
Maltose	50
D-Galactose	60
D-Glucose	70
D-Fructose	110
Invert sugar	70–90
D-Xylose	70
Sorbitol	50
Mannitol	70
Dulcitol	40
Glycerol	80
Glycine	70
Sodium-3-methyl-cyclopentyl sulfamate	1500
Sodium cyclohexyl-sulfamate (Cyclamate)	3000–8000
Sodium saccharin	20000–70000
5-Nitro-propoxy-aniline (P-4000)	400000

Sucrose is thus an ideal sweetener in many ways: it is colorless and water soluble and has a pure taste—not mixed with overtones of bitterness or saltiness—and it is rich in calories.

Synthetic, nonnutritive sweeteners with less than 2% of the caloric value of sucrose have been developed as an alternative to sucrose for diabetics and overweight persons who must restrict their intake of sugar. Saccharin (sodium ortho-benzenesulfonamide) was the first synthetic sweetener used; it is about 300 times sweeter than sucrose, in concentrations up to 10% of sucrose solution. Saccharin often leaves a bitter and unpleasant aftertaste and eventually was banned in most countries for it was shown to be carcinogenic.

Cyclamates (sodium and calcium salts of cyclamic acid cyclohexane sulfamate), which are about 30 times sweeter than sucrose, have been found to be better nonnutritive sweeteners. Unlike saccharin, they leave no unpleasant after taste. Cyclamates were extensively used in the manufacture of soft drinks and other low-calorie liquid foods and dietetics, but their use also has been banned—high doses of these compounds were found to produce bladder cancer in rats, probably by forming cyclohexylamine, a known carcinogen.

Newer, more effective nonnutritive sweeteners ranging from 10 to 3000 times the sweetness of sucrose have been discovered, e.g. glycyrrhizic acid obtained from the roots of the leguminous plant *Glycyrrhiza glabra* (licorice). The sweet taste of glycyrrhizic acid can be detected at one-fiftieth the threshold taste level of sucrose. It is used extensively in confectioneries, beverages, and tobacco products. Neohespiridine dihydrochalcone isolated from citrus peels is about 2000 times sweeter than sucrose.

Low-calorie sweeteners have also been isolated from two tropical African fruits, kutemfe and serendipity berry. Kutemfe contains two proteins, thaumatin I and II, and is about 100,000 times sweeter than sucrose. The proteinous substance obtained from serendipity berries, known as monellin, is as sweet as the sweeteners obtained from kutemfe. These sweeteners, however, are unstable to heat and lose their sweetness at pH 2, at ambient temperatures. Another potentially useful low-calorie sweetener is aspartame (methyl diester of l-aspartic acid and l-phenylalamine), about 180 to 200 times sweeter than sucrose, with similar taste characteristics. Aspartame is available under its trade names: "Nutrasweet" when added to foods and "Equal" when sold as powder. Aspartame has never been linked with cancer, although some complaints have been filed with the FDA by individuals claiming adverse reactions to aspartame, such as headaches, dizziness, seizures, nausea, and allergy. A disease called phenylketonuria (PKU) limits a person's ability to metabolize phenylalanine. Therefore, labels on products containing aspartame warn people with PKU not to use the product.

The newest alternate sweetner in the United States is acesulfame (Sunette), approved by the FDA in July 1988. Acesulfame is 200 times sweeter than sucrose. It is used in chewing gums, powdered drink mixes, gelatins, puddings, and non-dairy creamers. It does not contribute any calories to the diet because it is not digested by the body.

REFERENCES

1. Lehninger, A.L., D.L. Nelson, and M.M. Cox, Carbohydrates, *Principles of Biochemistry*, 2nd ed., CBS Publishers and Distributors, New Delhi, 1993, p. 298.
2. Manay, N.S., and M. Shadaksharaswamy, *Foods: Facts and Principles*. Wiley Eastern Ltd., New Delhi, 1987, p. 15.
3. Englyst, H.N., and S.M. Kingman, Carbohydrates, *Human Nutrition and Dietetics* (J.S. Garrow and W.P.T. James, eds.), Churchill Livingstone, London, 1993, p. 38.
4. Salunkhe, D.K., and B.B. Desai, *Postharvest Biotechnology of Sugar Crops*, CRC Press, Boca Raton, FL, 1986.
5. Black, E.E., and W.H.M. Saris, Health aspects of various digestible carbohydrates, *Nutr. Res. 15*: 1547 (1995).
6. Englyst, H.N., and S.M. Kingman, Dietary fiber and resistant starch: A nutritional classification of plant polysaccharides, *Dietary Fiber* (D. Kritchevsky, C. Bonfield, and J.W. Anderson, eds.), Plenum Publishing Co., New York, 1990.
7. Hipsley, E.H., Dietary fibre and pregnancy toxaema, *British Med. J. 2*: 420 (1953).
8. Trowell, H., Ischaemic heart disease and dietary fiber, *Am. J. Clin. Nutr. 25*: 926 (1972).
9. James, W.P.T., and O. Theander, *The Analysis of Dietary Fiber in Food*, Marcel Dekker, New York, 1981, p. 258.
10. Englyst, H.N., H.W. Trowell, D.A.T. Southgate, and J.H. Cummings, Dietary fiber and resistant starch, *Am. J. Clin. Nutr. 46*: 873 (1987).
11. Southgate, D.A.T., Determination of carbohydrates in foods. II. Unavailable carbohydrates, *J. Sci. Food Agri. 20*: 331 (1969).
12. Englyst, H.N., M.E. Quigley, G.J. Hudson, and J.H. Cummings, Determination of dietary fibre as non-starch polysaccharides by gas-chromatography, *Analyst 117*: 1707 (1992).

13. Quigley, M.E., and H.N. Englyst, Determination of neutral sugars and hexosamines by high-performance liquid chromatography with pulsed amperometric detection, *Analyst 117*: 1715 (1992).

14. Englyst, H.N., and G.J. Hudson, Dietary fiber and starch: Classification and measurement, *Dietary Fiber in Human Nutrition* (G.A. Spiller, ed.), CRC Press, Boca Raton, FL, 1992.

15. Prosky, L., N.G. Asp, I. Furda, J.W. De Vries, T.F. Schweizer, and B.F. Harland, Determination of total dietary fibre in foods and food products: interlaboratory study, *J.A.O.A.C. 68*: 677 (1985).

16. Prosky, L., N.G. Asp, T.F. Schweizer, J.W. De Vries, and I. Furda, Determination of insoluble, soluble, and total dietary fibre in foods and food products: interlaboratory study, *J.A.O.A.C. 71*: 1071 (1988).

17. Mongeau, R., and R. Brassard, A comparison of three methods for analysing dietary fibre in 38 foods, *J. Food Comp. Anal. 2*: 189 (1990).

18. Thebaudin, J.Y., A.C. Lefebvre, S. Cagnet, and C.M. Bourgeois, Les Fibres Alimentaires. Interet Nutritionnel et Interet Technologique, *La Bretagne Agroaliment 5*: 4 (1995).

19. Thibault, J.F., M. Lahaye, and F. Guillon, Physico-chemical properties of food plant cell walls, *Dietary Fibre: A Component of Food* (T.F. Schweizer and C.A. Edwards, eds.) Springer-Verlag, 1992, p. 21.

20. Cummings, J.H., and H.N. Englyst, Fermentation in the human large intestine and the available substrates, *Am. J. Clin. Nutr. 45*: 1243 (1987).

21. Englyst, H.N., and J.H. Cummings, Improved method for measurement of dietary fiber as non-starch polysaccharides in plant foods, *J.A.O.A.C. 71*: 808 (1988).

22. Cummings, J.H., H.N. Englyst, and R. Wood, Determination of dietary fibre in cereals and cereal products collaborative trials. Part 1: Initial trial, *J.A.O.A.C. 23*: 1 (1985).

23. Asp, N.G., T.F. Schweizer, D.A.T. Southgate, and O. Theander, Dietary fibre analysis, *Dietary Fibres—A Component of Food* (T.F. Schweizer and C.A. Edwards, eds.), Springer-Verlag, 1992, p. 57.

24. Thebaudin, J.Y., A.C. Lefebvre, M. Harrington, and C.M. Bourgeois, Dietary fibres: Nutritional and technological interest, *Trends Food Sci. Technol. 8*: 41 (1997).

25. Staniforth, D.H., I.M. Baird, J. Fowler, and R.E. Lister, The effects of dietary fibre on upper and lower gastrointestinal transit times and fecal bulking, *J. Int. Med. Res. 19*: 228 (1991).

26. Van Dokkum, W., A. Wesstra, R. Luyken, and R.J.S. Hermus, The effect of high animal protein diet on mineral balance and bowel function of young men, *British J. Nutr. 56*: 341 (1988).

27. Stephen, A.M., Increasing complex carbohydrate in the diet: Are the benefits due to starch, fiber or decreased fat intake? *Food Res. Intl. 27*: 69 (1994).

28. British Nutrition Foundations, Complex carbohydrates in foods, The Report of the British Nutrition Foundations Task Force, Chapman and Hall, London (1989).

29. Englyst, H.N., and J.H. Cummings, Resistant starch, a 'new' food component: A classification of starch for nutritional purposes, *Cereals in a European Context* (I.D. Morton, ed.). First European Conf. On Food Science and Technology, Ellis Horwood, Chichester, 1987, p. 221.

30. Englyst, H.N., S.M. Kingman and J.H. Cummings, Classification and measurement of nutritionally important starch fractions, *European J. Clin. Nutr. 46* (Suppl. 2): 533 (1993).

31. Canadian Bean Council, Rediscover baked beans (advertisement), Canadian Bean Council, *Homemaker's Mag.* Jan/Feb, 1991, p. 74.

32. Potato Marketing Board, Potatoes, Britain's buried treasure (advertisement) Potato Marketing Board, *Good Housekeeping* (UK), April, 1992a, p. 193.

33. Potato Marketing Board, Potatoes, Britains buried treasure (advertisement), Potato Marketing Board, *Good Housekeeping* (UK), May, 1992b, p. 175.

34. Englyst, H.N., S.A. Bingham, S.A. Runswick, E. Collinson, and J.H. Cummings, Dietary fiber (non-starch polysaccharides) in fruit, vegetables and nuts, *J. Hum. Nutr. Diet. 1*: 247 (1988).

35. Rickard, S.E., and L.U. Thompson, Health effects of flaxseed mucilage, lignans, *INFORM. 8* (8): 860 (1997).

36. Torres, A., and R.D. Thomas, Polydextrose and its application in foods, *Food Technol.*: July, 1981, p. 44.

37. Bingham, S.A., D.R.R. Williams, and J.H. Cummings, Dietary fibre consumption in Britain: new estimates and their relation to large bowel cancer mortality, *British. J. Cancer. 52* L: 399 (1985).

38. Bingham, S.A., J.H. Cummings, and N.T. McNeil, Intakes and sources of dietary fiber in British population, *Am. J. Clin. Nutr. 32*: 1313 (1979).

39. Dwyer, J.T., Dietary fiber and colorectal cancer risk, *Nutr. Rev. 51*: 147 (1993).

40. Howe, G.R., E. Benito, R. Castelleto, et al., Dietary intake of fibre and decreased risk of cancers of colon and rectum: evidence from the combined analysis of 13 case control studies. *J. Natl. Cancer Inst. 24*: 1887 (1992).

41. Van Soest, P., Fiber analysis tables, *Am. J. Clin. Nutr. 31*: 5281 (1978).

42. Paul, A.A., and D.A.T. Southgate, *The Composition of Foods*, 4th ed., HMSO, London, 1978.

4
Lipids

I. INTRODUCTION

Lipids, including oils and fats, are a chemically diverse group of compounds that are insoluble in water and have a variety of functions. Oils and fats are the principal stored forms of energy in many organisms, with phospholipids and sterols making up approximately half the mass of biological membranes. Other crucial lipids are enzyme cofactors, electron carriers, light-absorbing pigments, hydrophobic anchors, emulsifying agents, hormones, and intracellular messengers (1).

The fatty acids found in fats and oils are highly reduced hydrocarbon derivatives whose cellular oxidation is highly exergonic. They are carboxylic acids with hydrocarbon chains of 4 to 36 carbons, which may be either fully saturated and unbranched or unsaturated with the presence of one or more double bonds. A few fatty acids contain three-carbon rings or hydroxyl groups. Some of the naturally occurring fatty acids along with their common names derived from Latin or Greek and systematic names specifying chain length and number of double bonds, melting point, and solubility at 30°C are shown in Table 1. A saturated lauric acid (Latin *laurus*, laurel plant) with 12 carbons is named 12:0 (n-dodecanoic acid), and a saturated 16-carbon palmitic acid (Greek *palma*, palm tree) is named 16:0 (n-hexadecanoic acid). The 18-carbon oleic acid with one double bond is 18:1. The positions of double bonds are indicated with superscript numbers, e.g., a 20-carbon fatty acid with one double bond between C-9 and C-10, (C-1 being the carboxyl carbon) and another between C-12 and C-13, is designated as 20:2 ($\Delta^{9,12}$). Most commonly occurring fatty acids have even numbers of carbon atoms in a linear chain of 12 to 24 carbons (Table 1). The even number of carbon atoms in these compounds reflects the mode of their synthesis, which involves condensation of 2-C acetate units. Most monounstured fatty acids have their double bond between C-9 and C-10, the other double bonds being usually after C-12 and C-15 positions and are in the *cis* configuration.

The physical properties of the fatty acids and their derivatives are influenced by the length and degree of unsaturation of the hydrocarbon chain, the nonpolar hydrocarbon chain primarily acccounting for their poor solubility in water. The water solubility decreases with an increase in the length of the fatty acyl chain and a decrease in the number of double bonds. The polar carboxylic acid group accounts for the slight solubility of short-chain fatty acids in water.

The length and degree of unsaturation of the hydrocarbon chain of fatty acids and lipids also influence their melting points (Table 1). At the ambient temperature (25°C), the saturated fatty acids from C-12 to C-24 have a waxy consistency, whereas the unsaturated fatty acids of the same lengths are oily liquids. Free rotation around each C-C bond in the fully saturated fatty acids enables great flexibility and more stable conformation of the fully extended hydrocarbon chain with minimum stearic hindrance from the neighboring atoms. Such molecules can pack together tightly as the result of van der Waals forces with the atoms of neighboring molecules. The pres-

Table 1 Some Naturally Occurring Fatty Acids

Carbon skeleton	Structure	Systematic name	Common name (derivation)	Melting point (°C)	Solubility at 30°C (mg/g solvent)	
					Water	Benzene
12:0	$CH_3(CH_2)_{10}COOH$	n-Dodecanoic acid	Lauric acid (Latin *laurus*)	44.2	0.063	2600
14:0	$CH_3(CH_2)_{12}COOH$	n-Tetradecanoic acid	Myristic acid (Latin *Myristica* genus nutmeg)	53.9	0.024	874
16:0	$CH_3(CH_2)_{14}COOH$	n-Hexadecanoic acid	Palmitic acid (Greek *Palma*)	63.1	0.0083	348
18:0	$CH_3(CH_2)_{16}COOH$	n-Octadecanoic acid	Stearic acid (Greek, *Stear*, hard fat)	69.6	0.0034	124
20:0	$CH_3(CH_2)_{18}COOH$	n-Eicosanoic acid	Arachidonic acid (Latin *Arachis*, genus legume)	76.5		
24:0	$CH_3(CH_2)_{22}COOH$	n-Tetracosanoic acid	Lignoseric acid (Latin *lignum* wood, cera, wax)	86.0		
16:1 (Δ^9)	$CH_3(CH_2)_5\ CH{=}CH\ (CH_2)_7COOH$		Palmitoleic acid	-0.5		
18:1 (Δ^9)	$CH_3(CH_2)_7\text{-}CH{=}CH\ (CH_2)_7COOH$		Oleic acid (Greek *oleum* oil)	13.4		
18:2 ($\Delta^{9,12}$)	$CH_3(CH_2)_4\ CH{=}CHCH_2\ CH{=}CH\ (CH_2)_7\ COOH$		alpha-Linoleic acid (Greek *linion*, flax)	-5		
18:3 ($\Delta^{9,12,15}$)	$CH_3(CH_2)\ CH{=}CHCH_2\ CH{=}CHCH_2\ CH{=}CH\ (CH_2)_7COOH$		Linolenic acid	-11		
20:4 ($\Delta^{5,8,11,14}$)	$CH_3\ (CH_2)_4\ CH{=}CHCH_2\ CH{=}CHCH_2\ CH{=}CHCH_2\ CH{=}CH(CH_2)_3\ COOH$		Arachidonic acid	-49.5		

Source: Ref. 1.

ence of one or more *cis* double bonds interferes with this tight packing and results in less stable aggregates. The lower melting points of the unsaturated fatty acids can be attributed to the lower energy required to disorder the poorly ordered arrays of fatty acids due to the presence of double bonds.

II. BIOLOGICALLY IMPORTANT LIPIDS

A. Storage and Structural Lipids

In vertebrate animals, free fatty acids circulate in the blood bound to a protein carrier, cerum albumin. However, fatty acids are mostly present as derivatives of carboxylic acid in the form of esters and amides, thus rendering them more nonpolar and less soluble in water.

Common oils and fats are the simplest lipids occurring as triacylglycerols or triglycerides, composed of three same or different fatty acids, each ester-linked with a glycerol molecule. Simple triglycerides (containing the same fatty acid in all three positions) are named after the component fatty acid, e.g., triglycerides of 16:0, 18:0 and 18:1 are called tristearin, tripalmitin, and triolein, respectively. The names of mixed triglycerides are given by specifying the name and position of each fatty acid.

The triglycerides are nonpolar (polar hydroxyls of glycerol and polar carboxylates of fatty acids being bound in ester linkages), hydrophobic molecules with poor solubility in water. Triglycerides constitute depots of metabolic fuel for most eukaryotic cells. Specialized cells of the vertebrates (adipocytes or fat cells) can store large amount of triglycerides as fat droplets, nearly filling the entire cell. Seeds of many plants also contain triglycerides to provide energy and biosynthetic precursors during seed germination.

The carbon atoms of fatty acids are more reduced and in a more concentrated form than those of sugars, so the oxidation of triglycerides yields more than twice as much energy per gram than carbohydrates. Also, because triglycerides are hydrophobic and unhydrated, an organism carrying fat as fuel does not have to bear the extra weight of water of hydration associated with stored polysaccharides. In humans, fat tissue (adipocytes) occurs under the skin, in the abdominal cavity, and in the mammary glands. Obese people may have 15 to 20 kg of triglycerides deposited in their adipocytes, sufficient to provide energy for several months. The human body, however, can supply less than a day's energy in the form of glycogen, though the latter serves as a quick source of metabolic energy because of its ready solubility in water.

In addition to serving as stored energy, the fat deposited under the skin of animals forms an insulation layer protecting them against very low temperatures—e.g., seals, walruses, penguins, and polar bears are amply padded with triglycerides. The low density of triglycerides stored in the body of sperm whales helps to match the buoyancy of their bodies to that of their surroundings during deep dives in the cold water.

Vegetable oils, dairy products, and animal fats are mixtures of simple and mixed triglycerides occurring in nature. Most vegetable oils are composed of triglycerides with unsaturated fatty acids and therefore are liquids at room temperature; animal fats containing only saturated fatty acids such as tristearin are white greasy solids at room temperature (Table 2). Lipid-rich foods exposed to oxygen in air for long periods may spoil and become rancid. The oxidative cleavage of the double bonds in unsaturated fatty acids gives rise to aldehydes and volatile short-chain carboxylic acids, resulting in off-flavor and unpleasant taste (oxidative rancidity).

Triglycerides can be easily hydrolyzed with acids or alkalis. Heating of oil or fat with NaOH or KOH produces glycerol and Na^+ or K^+ salts of fatty acids, known as soaps, which are able to solubilize or disperse water-insoluble materials by forming microscopic aggregates

Table 2 Fatty acid Composition of Three Natural Food Fats[a]

Oil or fat	Physical state at room temperature (25°C)	Fatty acids (%)[b]				Unsaturated
		Saturated				
		C_4–C_{12}	C_{14}	C_{16}	C_{18}	C_{16} + C_{18}
Olive oil	Liquid	< 2	< 2	13	3	80
Butter	Solid (soft)	11	10	26	11	40
Beef fat	Solid (hard)	< 2	< 2	29	21	46

[a] These fats consist of mixtures of triacylglycerols; they differ in their fatty acid composition and thus in their melting points.
[b] Values are given as percentage of total fatty acids.
Source: Ref. 1.

(micelles). Lipids can also be hydrolyzed by a range of lipases at neutral pH. Lipases in the intestine aid in the digestion and absorption of dietary fats (see Chapter 19).

Waxes are esters of long-chain fatty acids (14 to 36 carbons) with long-chain alcohols (16 to 30 carbons), having higher melting points (60 to 100°C) than those of the triglycerides. Waxes are the chief storage form of metabolic fuel in marine animals. Their water-repellent properties and firm consistency are important in the natural world. Skin glands of marine vertebrates secrete waxes to protect the hair and skin and to maintain them pliable, lubricated, and waterproof. Birds such as waterfowl secrete waxes from their preen glands to make their feathers water-repellent. The leaves of many tropical plants are coated with a wax layer to protect them against parasites and excessive transpiration. Biological waxes have several important aplications in the pharmaceuticals, cosmetics, and other industries. Beeswax, lanolin (from lamb's wool), carnauba wax (from a Brazilian palm tree) and spermaceti wax (from whales) are widely used in lotions, ointments, and polishes.

The biological cellular membranes are a double layer of lipids (constituting a barrier for polar molecules and ions) and proteins, the composition depending upon the species, cell type, and organelle. Membrane lipids are amphipathic, the orientation of hydrophobic and hydrophilic regions directing their packing into membrane bilayers. Three general types of membrane lipids are (a) glycerophospholipids, with hydrophobic regions composed of two fatty acids linked to a glycerol, (b) sphingolipids, with a single fatty acid attached to a fatty amine, sphingosine, and (c) sterols, characterized by a rigid system of four fused hydrocarbon rings. The hydrophilic moieties in these compounds may be a single OH-group at one end of the sterol or more complex groups, such as charged alcohols and phosphates. A range of membrane lipids with diverse functions results from various combinations of fatty acid "tails" and polar "heads." Lehninger et al. (1) have described various types of membrane lipids found in living organisms, the arrangement of lipids in membranes and their structural and functional roles. Certain inherited human diseases can arise from abnormal accumulations of membrane lipids, e.g. Tay-Sachs disease, which affects brain cells: a specific ganglioside accumulates in the brain and spleen due to the lack of the lysosomal enzyme hexosaminidase A that hydrolyzes a specific bond between an N-acetyl D-galactosamine and a D-galactose residue in the polar head of the ganglioside. The partially degraded ganglioside thus accumulates in the brain, causing nervous system degeneration.

B. Steroids, Isoprenoids, and Other Active Lipids

The storage lipids (more than 50% mass of an adipocyte) and structural lipids (5 to 10% of the dry mass of most cells) are the major cellular constituents. However, both classes of these lipids have a *passive* role in the cell. Whereas the storage lipids are oxidized for energy, membrane lipids form impermeable barriers that separate cellular compartments. Apart from these, another group of lipids have specific and essential biological functions. Although relatively minor cellular components on a mass basis, the third group of lipids includes hundreds of steroids, with the four-ring steroid nucleus (more polar than cholesterol), and a large number of isoprenoids, synthesized from a 5-carbon 'isoprene' unit. The latter group includes fat-soluble vitamins A, D, E, and K, used in making the fatty material essential for the normal growth of animals, as well as numerous biological pigments. Other more active lipids are those serving as essential cofactors for enzymes, as electron carriers, or as intracellular signals.

Steroid hormones constitute a major group of the male and female sex hormones, and the hormones of the adrenal cortex, cortisol and aldosterone, all having an intact steroid nucleus. They are synthesized in one tissue and carried in the bloodstream to the target tissues, where they bind to highly specific receptor proteins and trigger changes in gene expression and metabolism. Very low concentrations of these steroid hormones (10^{-9} M or less) are needed to produce effects on target tissues (see Chapter 20).

Phosphatidylinositol and its phosphorylated derivatives, which are components of the plasma membranes of all eukaryotic cells, serve as a reservoir of messenger molecules, released inside the cell when certain extracellular signals interact with specific receptors in the plasma membrane—e.g., activation of a specific phospholipase in the membrane, when the hormone vasopressin binds to receptor molecules in the plasma membranes of cells in the kidney and the blood vessels. The phospholipase breaks the bond between glycerol and phosphate in phosphatidylinositol-4, 5-biphosphate, releasing inositol-1, 4,5-triphosphate and diacylglycerol. The former causes the release of Ca^{2+} from the cell membranes and activation of a variety of Ca^{2+}-dependent enzymes and hormonal responses. Diacylglycerol binds to and activates protein kinase C, which transfers phosphate groups from ATP to several cytosolic proteins, thereby altering their enzymatic activities (1).

Eicosanoids are fatty acid derivatives with a range of hormone-like actions on various animal tissues where they are produced. They have various reproductive functions and are involved in the inflammation, fever, and pain associated with injury or disease; in the formation of blood clots; in the regulation of blood pressure; in gastric acid secretion; and in many other processes important to human health and diseases. Eicosanoids are derived from a 20-carbon polyunsaturated fatty acid, arachidonic acid. Three classes of eicosanoids are: (a) prostaglandins, (b) thromboxanes, and (c) leukotrienes.

The Fourth International Congress on Essential Fatty Acids and Eicosanoids (2) has discussed advances made in the areas of eicosanoid regulation and function. The molecular structure of prostaglandin syntheses and the interactions and structural requirements for different fatty acid substrates were described. The relationship between eicosanoids and the immune response has been explored at a molecular level, and the role of eicosapentenoic acid (EPA) in angiogenesis has been described. The latest pharmacological information about the basic classes of eicosanoid receptors and their subdivision was reviewed and the splice variants that give rise to different activities in signal transduction pathways were described. A further study of the role of long-chain PUFA retroversion in regulating eicosanoid production in humans and animals was urged. A better understanding of this process could aid our understanding of how the body partitions the bioactive fatty acids for structural use and eicosanoid production, and, on the applied side, will facilitate the optimization of long-chain, n-3 fatty acid enrichment of food products and formation of long-chain fatty acid supplement (2).

According to Newton (3), marine plants are the primary source of n-3 PUFA in the food chain. Fish and other marine animals who feed on these plants are able to elongate and desaturate the parent essential fatty acid into longer-chain PUFA. Therefore, most fish have quite high levels of both EPA and docosahexenoic acid (DHA) (Table 3) (28).

The prostaglandins (recognized first in the prostate gland) contain a five-membered carbon-ring, originally part of the chain of arachidonic acid. Prostaglandins have been known to influence a wide range of cellular and tissue functions by regulating the synthesis of the intracellular messenger molecule 3'-5'-cyclic AMP (cAMP), which mediates the action of many hormones. Some prostaglandins stimulate contraction of the smooth muscle of the uterus during labor or menstruation, and others affect blood flow to specific organs, the wake-sleep cycle, and the response of some tissues to hormones, such as epinephrine and glucagon. A third group of prostaglandins elevate body temperature (produce fever) and cause inflammation, resulting in pain.

The thromboxanes (thrombocytes), isolated first from blood platelets, have a six-membered ring containing an ether. They act in the formation of blood clots and in the reduction of blood flow to the site of a clot. Leukotrienes (noticed first in leukocytes), containing three conjugated double bonds, are powerful biological signals—e.g., they induce contraction of the muscle lining the airways to the lung and their overproduction causes asthmatic attacks. The strong contraction of the smooth muscles of the lungs occurring during anaphylactic shock may be part of the potentially fatal allergic reaction in persons hypersensitive to bee stings, penicillin, or other agents (1).

The fat-soluble vitamins A, D, E and K are dealt with elsewhere (see Chapter 6). Other isoprenoid derivatives, ubiquinone and plastoquinone, function as electron carriers in the phosphorylation reactions of mitochondria and chloroplasts. In most mammalian tissues, ubiquinone, also known as co-enzyme Q, has 10 isoprene units. Plastoquinones, plant equivalents of ubiquinone, serve as electron carriers, accepting either one or two electrons and reducing either one or two protons.

Dolichols are isoprenoids found in animals (17 to 21 isoprene units), bacteria (11 units) and fungi and plants (14 to 24 units). They have strong hydrophobic interactions with membrane

Table 3   Total EPA and DHA Content of Selected Fish

Fish	g/100 g sample[a]
Atlantic mackerel	2.5
Atlantic salmon, farmed	1.8
Pacific herring	1.7
Atlantic herring	1.6
Lake trout	1.6
Bluefin tuna	1.6
Sturgeon	1.5
Anchovy	1.4
Sprat	1.3
Sardines, canned, drained	1.1

EPA = Eicosapentenoic acid.

DHA = Docosahexenoic acid.

[a] Amounts specified may vary slightly according to season and food availability.

Source: Ref. 28.

lipids, anchoring the attached sugars to the membranes, where they take part in sugar-transfer reactions (1).

III. NUTRITIONAL ASPECTS OF LIPIDS

Gurr (4) has reviewed the nutritional aspects of food lipids, including triacylglycerols, phospholipids, glycolipids, sterols (cholesterol), and fat-soluble vitamins. In assessing the roles of dietary lipids in health and disease, it is important to put fat in perspective with other dietary components and diet as well as with the environmental factors. Western diets have changed drastically during the past century, compared with diets to which the body had become accustomed during the evolution of human race. This is probably a major cause of many ills affecting the developed world (5). According to Gurr (4), the human body is very adaptable and homeostatic mechanisms ensure that its cells, tissues, and organs adapt to changes in nutrient intakes by subtle changes in the amounts and activities of enzymes in the metabolic pathways and by changes in membrane composition as well as in the numbers and activities of membrane receptors and other regulatory proteins. The notion that a single "primitive" diet is appropriate for all human beings does not fit easily with the knowledge that diets apparently consistent with good health and well-being vary enormously throughout the world, with several-fold differences in the fat intakes and types of fats consumed. Also, life expectancy and general health have steadily improved in the industrialized countries and this fact is often forgotten in the enthusiasm for branding dietary fat as a major killer. Although a reduction in fat intake may be a distinct advantage for many people, especially for those finding difficulty in maintaining energy balance, there is a danger that in this obsession with dietary fat, other more important lifestyle factors are forgotten, e.g. smoking, too little exercise, and raised blood pressure. Thus, the role of fat must be seen in perspective, and it should not be concluded that widespread changes in dietary fat consumption will lead inevitably to freedom from the so-called diseases of affluence. The key to a good diet is variety (4).

Fat calories appear to be more fattening than carbohydrate calories and the reasons for this are complex. The main cause is the body's inability to increase fat oxidation rapidly in response to increases in fat consumption. Instead, fat is put into limitless stores. By contrast, when carbohydrate intake exceeds its limited storage capacity, the excess is readily oxidized. In the longer term, fat oxidation adjusts to the higher body fat stores, bringing intake and oxidation into equilibrium and resulting in a new stable weight.

The influence of dietary cholesterol on plasma cholesterol is still a subject of debate. The U.S. dietary guidelines clearly emphasize the importance of dietary cholesterol as determinant of plasma cholesterol, whereas in Europe the scientific evidence has generally been interpreted to indicate that it plays a minor role, if any (6). An analysis and review of 68 human intervention studies that examined the effect of dietary cholesterol on plasma cholesterol showed that there is an effect, but it is small compared with the influence of saturated fatty acids (SFA). A mean change of 100 mg/day dietary cholesterol causes a change of only 2.3 mg/100 ml plasma cholesterol, and somewhat larger reductions could be achieved by relatively modest reductions in body fat (4).

A. Dietary Sources of Fats

Animal adipose tissue fat, milk fat, eggs, fish oils, muscle meats, vegetable oils, and some green vegetables are the important dietary sources of oils and fats in the human diet. Ruminant adipose tissue fat (beef and mutton fat) is less variable than that of pigs and poultry, because 90% of the unsaturated fatty acids in the animal diets are hydrogenated to saturated fatty acids by the rumen microorganisms. The animal fat contains a higher proportion of saturated and monounsaturated fatty acids, and a lower proportion of *trans* unsaturated and branched fatty acids. *Trans* double bonds are formed by isomerization of the *cis* double bonds during the enzyme-catalyzed hydrogenation process brought about by rumen microorganisms (7,8).

Variation in the adipose tissue fatty acid composition can occur, depending on the animal species and feed-type—e.g., feeding sheep a diet rich in barley leads to much higher proportions of branched chain fatty acids, and results in a softer carcass fat. Ruminant dairy cows may be fed with fat supplements or crushed oil seeds to improve their production efficiency (9).

The adipose tissue fat composition can be altered more effectively by feeding animals with "protected" fat in which the treated fat particles resist hydrogenation in the rumen (10). These products are also thought to be useful for people on lipid-lowering diets. However, these products are costly and susceptible to oxidative deterioration. Watts et al. (11) suggested that the problem of lipid lowering in the diets may be approached more effectively by using lean meat, which provides primarily structural fat with a high P/S ratio.

Cow's milk and dairy products contribute nearly 24% of the fat in the diet of the population of the United Kingdom, although there is a decreasing trend in the use of full-fat milk, low-fat milk being preferred. Milk fat is composed of triglycerols in an emulsion of fat globules, stabilized by a surrounding membrane composed of proteins, phospholipids, and cholesterol. Fat globules are also associated with small amounts of cholesterol esters and fat-soluble vitamins A, D, and beta-carotene. Milk fat has a higher proportion of short- and medium-chain saturated fatty acids, long-chain saturated and monounsaturated fatty acids, and very small proportions of polyunsaturated fatty acids (PUFA) (Table 4).

Butter, a commonly used food fat, contains about 15% water as an emulsion in oil. The composition of milk fat does not normally vary greatly as compared with that of the margarines. Feeding cattle with high-fat oat supplements or crushed oilseeds has been shown to increase the proportion of oleic acid in the milk fat and provide a product with a higher unsaturated to saturated (u/s) fatty acid ratio (8). Cream is an emulsion of milk fat in water, whose textural properties and amount of fat in the diet depend on the total concentration of fat in the emulsion. Fat emulsions markedly enhance the palatability of food.

Eggs provide an average of 6 to 7 g of triacylglycerols and phospholipids and 250 to 300 mg of cholesterol in the human diets. The egg-fat has a high nutritive value and egg-yolk lipoproteins can improve textural properties of bakery products.

Lean fish store their reserve fat as triacylglycerols in the liver (e.g., cod), whereas fatty fish like mackerel and herring store fat in their flesh. Both fish oils are rich in fatty acids with 20 or

Table 4 Fatty Acid Composition of Some Animal Storage Fats Used as Foods (g/100 g of Total Fatty Acids)

Food fat	4:0–12:0	14:0	16:0	16:1	18:0	18:1	18:2	20:1 22:1	LC PUFA	Others
Lard (I)	0	1	29	3	15	43	9	0	0	0
Lard (II)	0	1	21	3	12	46	16	0	0	1
Poultry	0	1	27	9	7	45	11	0	0	1
Beef suet	0	3	26	9	8	45	2	0	0	7
Lamb	0	3	21	4	20	41	5	0	0	6
Milk (cow)	13	12	26	3	11	29	2	0	0	4
Milk (goat)	21	11	27	3	10	26	2	0	0	0
Egg york	0	0	29	4	9	43	11	0	0	4
Cod-liver oil	0	0	13	13	3	20	2	18	20	5

LC PUFA = Long chain polyunsaturated fatty acids.
Source: Ref. 8.

more carbon atoms, some of which contain five or six double bonds. However, wide variation in fatty acid composition can occur depending on the species, the diet, and season of the year (also see Chapter 11).

Muscle meats mainly contain fats in the form of phospholipids and free cholesterol. However, muscles may be infiltrated with storage triglycerides (marbling) in many meat animals. More than 85% of the total fatty acids of muscle fat consist of palmitic, stearic, oleic, linoleic, and arachidonic acids (Table 5). The composition of marble fat resembles that of adipose tissue (12).

Most oilseeds store their fat as triacylglycerols in the endosperm (e.g., soybean, rape, sunflower), as do fleshy fruits in the exocarp (e.g., avocado), and palm fruits, both in the exocarp (palm oil) and in the endosperm (palm kernel oil). Seed oils vary widely in their fatty acid composition and predominate in palmitic, stearic, oleic, and linoleic acids (Table 6) (29). The coconut and palm kernel oils, like milk fat, contain an unusual proportion of saturated fatty acids of medium chain length (C-8 to C-14). Seed oils also provide phospholipids, chlorophylls, carotenoids, tocopherols, and plant sterols, such as beta-sitosterol, which remains unabsorbed by the human gut. Certain vegetable oils contain unusual fatty acids that when ingested in large amounts have toxic or undesirable metabolic effects, e.g., 22-carbon monoenoic erucic acid present in rapeseed (Table 6). Zero-erucic-type varieties of rapeseed are now available.

Leaves of foods like lettuce, cabbage, and other green vegetables provide most of the alpha-linolenic acid in the human diet. Five fatty acids accounting for more than 90% of total fatty acids are palmitic, hexadecanoic, oleic, linoleic, and alpha-linolenic acids (Table 5).

B. Source of Energy, Palatability, and Essential Nutrients

Triacylglycerols represent a very concentrated form of fuel with a gross energy value of 38 kJ/g. For most people, foods are more palatable if they have substantial fat content. In the affluent countries where food is abundant, palatability is a major factor in choosing food. Indeed, most food is selected on the basis of its price, appearance, and taste rather than its nutritive value or health-giving properties. According to Gurr (8), the latter aspect of food is now beginning to assume greater importance for consumers than before.

Fats contribute palatability to foods by improving response of the mouth to their texture (mouthfeel), and by the olfactory responses of taste in the mouth and aroma in the nose (flavor). Mouthfeel is determined by the way in which fat is associated with other food components in the form of emulsions (e.g. butter, cream, and milk are all different types of emulsions of milk fat, but each causes a different sensation in the mouth) which is more pleasant than that obtained by

Table 5 Fatty Acid Composition of Some Animal Storage Fats Used as Foods (g/100 g of Total Fatty Acids)

Food	16:0	16:1	18:0	18:1	18:2	18:3	20:4	LC PUFA	Others
Beef (muscle)	16	2	11	20	26	1	13	0	11
Lamb (muscle)	22	2	13	30	18	4	7	0	4
Lamb (brain)	22	1	18	28	1	0	4	14	12
Chicken (muscle)	23	6	12	33	18	1	6	0	1
Chicken (liver)	25	3	17	26	15	1	6	6	1
Pork (muscles)	19	2	12	19	26	0	8	0	14
Cod (flesh)	22	2	4	11	1	Trace	4	52	4
Green leaves	13	3	Trace	7	16	56	0	0	5

LC PUFA = Long-chain polyunsaturated fatty acids.
Source: Ref. 12.

Table 6 Fatty Acid Composition of Selected Vegetable Oils Used in Foods

Oil	8:0	10:0	12:0	14:1	16:0	18:0	18:1	18:2	18:3	20:1 + 22:1	Others
Avocado	0	0	0	0	20	1	60	18	0	0	1
Coconut	8	7	48	16	9	2	7	2	0	0	1
Corn	0	0	0	1	14	2	30	50	2	0	1
Olive	0	0	Trace	Trace	12	2	72	11	1	0	2
Palm	0	0	Trace	1	42	4	43	8	Trace	0	2
Palm kernel	4	4	45	18	9	3	15	2	0	0	0
Peanut	0	0	Trace	1	11	3	49	29	1	0	6
Rape (high erucic)	0	0	0	Trace	4	1	24	16	11	4.3	1
Rape (low erucic)	0	0	0	Trace	4	1	54	23	10	Trace	8
Safflower (high oleic)	0	0	0	0	5	2	73	17	1	0	2
Safflower (high linoleic)	0	0	0	0	6	3	15	73	1	0	2
Soybean	0	0	Trace	Trace	10	4	25	52	7	0	2
Sunflower	0	0	Trace	Trace	6	6	33	52	Trace	0	3

Source: Refs. 12, 29.

eating a pure fat. Flavor or aroma is due to low-molecular-weight volatile compounds derived from lipids, which after their lipolysis, oxidation, and microbial or thermal decomposition generate short-chain fatty acids, aldehydes, ketones, lactones, and other volatile compounds.

Dietary lipids also provide certain essential fatty acids and the fat-soluble vitamins, which must be taken in the diet, since these essential nutrients cannot be made by the human body. Burr and Burr (13) demonstrated that acute deficiency states could be produced in rats by feeding them fat-free diets, which could be eliminated or prevented by adding only certain specific fatty acids to the diet. It was also shown that fatty acids related to linoleic acid were the most effective in preventing the disease that is characterized by skin symptoms such as dermatosis, the skin becoming leaky to water. Growth is retarded, reproduction impaired, followed by degeneration or impairment of functions in other body organs. The essential fatty acid (EFA) deficiency is characterized by changes in the fatty acid composition of many tissues, especially the biological membranes, impairing their functions. Mitochondria lose their efficiency at producing metabolic energy by oxidizing fatty acids. Soderhjelm et al. (14) described EFA deficiency in man. When 400 human infants were fed milk formulas containing different amounts of linoleic acid, clinical and chemical signs of EFA deficiency could be noticed in the subjects fed with diets containing less than 0.1% of the dietary energy as linoleic acid. The skin abnormalities were very similar to those seen in rats, and the signs of deficiency disappeared by providing linoleic acid in the diet (15).

Gurr (8) pointed out that until recently attention has been devoted almost entirely to linoleic acid (18:2), the significance of alpha-linolenic (18:3) just being recognized. Thus, some infant formulas are being supplemented with alpha-linolenic acid to give a ratio of 18:2 (n-6) to 18:3 (n-3) of about 5:1. Also, human milk (but not infant formulas) contains small amounts of long-chain polyunsaturated fatty acids, principally arachidonic (20:4) and docosahexenoic (22:6, n-3) acids (DHA). These are derived from linoleic and alpha-linolenic acids, respectively, by further chain elongation and desaturation. These are required for the very active brain development occurring at the infant stage. About 50% of the dry weight of brain is composed of lipids, of which upto 50% are the long-chain polyunsaturated fatty acids. It is likely that premature babies need to be supplied with dietary long-chain polyunsaturated fatty acids, and it is not known whether full-term babies given formula also need these fatty acids in their diet (8).

Collins et al. (16) established an unequivocal case of EFA deficiency in an adult man. The patient (adult of 44) who had all but 60 cm of his bowel removed surgically, was fed intravenously with a liquid diet containing no fat. After 100 days he developed a scaly dermatitis. Biochemically EFA deficiency can be diagnosed before the appearance of skin lesions by noticing tissues fail to produce arachidonic acid (20:4) and produce an excessive amount of all-*cis*-20:3 fatty acid. The ratio of triene to tetraene (20:3 to 20:4) measured in plasma phospholipids is a biochemical index of EFA status. In healthy persons, this ratio is around 0.1 or less, and may rise to 1.0 in severe EFA deficiency. Press et al. (17) used this ratio to diagnose EFA deficiency in three patients with chronic disease of the small bowel who had been treated with low-fat diets but not given intravenous feeding. They responded positively to the application of lipids containing a high proportion of linoleic acid to the skin. Holman and Johnson (18) used a more sophisticated method of serum fatty acid profiling to pinpoint subtle defects in polyunsaturated fatty acid metabolism, wherein a whole spectrum of unsaturated fatty acids, including positional and geometric isomers, is analyzed.

Overt EFA deficiency in man is noticed only when less than 1% to 2% of dietary energy, or 2-5 g of linoleic acid is given to an adult. More may be needed during pregnancy and lactation, although the body contains considerable stores in the adipose tissue. Even a higher intake (10% of energy) is desirable in view of its effects in lowering the concentration of cholesterol in the blood.

The essentiality of linolenic acid for man remains to be established fully. Holman et al. (19) described a case of a young girl displaying neurological symptoms 4 to 5 months after being on total parenteral nutrition, having as the fat component only linoleic acid and a minute quantity of alpha-linolenic acid. The neurological symptoms disappeared when safflower oil was replaced by soybean oil, containing a higher proportion of alpha-linolenic acid. Bierve et al. (20) also provided evidence for alpha-linolenic acid deficiency in elderly patients fed by gastric tube.

The human body cannot make either linoleic or linolenic acid and these must come from the diet. A large proportion of the lipids of the brain, and of specialized tissues such as the retina, are composed of polyunsaturated fatty acids of the n-3 family derived from dietary alpha-linolenic acid. Thus, it is reasonable to assume the essentiality of linolenic acid for man. However, only small amounts of this fatty acid are required in human diets (21,22). The essential roles of linoleic and linolenic acids as the components of biological membranes and as precursors of physiological active metabolites (eicosanoids) have been discussed (22).

According to Bouchier (23), essential fatty acids and eicosanoids play important roles in human health and disease. Bouchier cited pregnancy, inflammation, coronary heart disease, cancer, and animal husbandary as areas in which EFA and eicosanoids can play a role. The Fourth International Congress on Essential Fatty Acids and Eicosanoids held from July 20 to 24, 1997, in Edinburgh, Scotland, covered a vast range of topics, including vascular disease, brain function, gene expression of eicosanoids, models in cell culture, development *in utero* and early life, infant nutrition, eicosanoid receptors, alcohol abuse, inflammation and the immune response, diabetes, cancer, and schizophrenia. It was noted that until recently Scottish residents had the highest rate of premature deaths from ischemic heart disease in the world, and although there has been improvement in the mortality and morbidity data, Scotland continues to have the second-highest mortality rate for coronary heart disease (CHD) in Western Europe. Researchers are now assessing local risk factors and exploring dietary fat issues and the complex roles lipids play in the body.

Numerous presentations in the Congress addressed recent advances concerning the role of polyunsaturated fatty acids in the regulation of tumor cell growth. It was pointed out that novel diol formulations of gamma-linolenic acid (GLA) and eicosapentanoic acid (EPA) were selectively incorporated into tumors without the complication of patient hemolysis (a loss of RBCs) normally associated with intravascular fatty acid administration. The increase in UVB-induced immunosuppression and carcinogenesis could be related to increased levels of linoleic acid in the diet (UVB refers to a specific ultraviolet bandwidth). It was indicated that PUFAs inhibit pancreatic cancer cell growth and this process appeared to be clearly oxidative, although the exact mechanism, or whether PUFAs can discriminate against cancer cells versus healthy cells, remains to be elucidated, and if they can, PUFAs would be the perfect cancer treatment (2). This work also showed that monounsaturated fatty acids promoted cancer cell growth, while the addition of antioxidants protected pancreatic cancer cells from cell death. Antioxidants may prevent tumor induction but may not be helpful after a tumor has formed.

Rat studies showed that docosahexenoic acid (DHA) prevents chemotherapy-induced hair loss without protecting leukemic cells. The explanation for such selective protection needs further research (2).

Although there is interest in incorporating long-chain PUFAs in infant formulas, it is vital first to determine if their addition is necessary or safe. The most common DHA dose in infant studies is 0.3% of total fatty acids, the amount typically found in human breast milk in countries eating a Western diet. It was further pointed out that in full-term infants, effects are not found at one year of age by feeding DHA with or without arachidonic acid (AA), and data from premature infant trials are equivocal. It is possible that requirements change with gestational development. Thus, the premature infant may need more DHA than term infants, infants of less than 32 weeks' gestation being most at risk (2).

It was observed that premature infants supplemented with DHA, but not AA, had poor growth, which did not occur with full-term infants. Thus, some nutritionists favor combination of AA and DHA in supplementation. DHA certainly appears to be associated with physiological benefits to infants born at less than 32 weeks' gestation. However, as these infants are most at risk of adverse effects from feeding n-3 long chain PUFA, all long-chain PUFA requirements need to be reestablished in a broader nutritional framework.

A WHO Lactation Study investigating lactating women in Thailand and Hungary reported that mothers eating a high-fat diet had lower DHA levels in their breast milk than those of mothers on a low-fat diet. Perhaps the wrong models are being used for infant formula. Currently, the recommended level of DHA is based on levels found in breast milk from mothers eating a Western, high-fat diet (2).

According to Gerald Hornstra of Maastricht University, the Netherlands, neonatal head circumference is negatively related to maternal consumption of linoleic acid. In fact, research indicates, the higher the linoleate in the mother's diet, the lower the levels of long-chain PUFA in the infant. The current EFA and long-chain PUFA intakes may need a better balance to optimize brain development. It has been cautioned, however, that this conclusion is based on epidemiological data and needs further follow-up (2).

A 16-site study was conducted throughout the United States and Canada to see if DHA plus AA affected growth and visual acuity in premature infants. The premature infants were given formula supplemented with either algaderived DHA or algal DHA plus fungal-derived AA, followed by conventional infant formula not containing long-chain PUFA. The study divided the infants into four groups: a control, DHA-supplemented, DHA plus AA–supplemented, and human milk, with the different formulas fed during gestational weeks 32 to 36. Infants were monitered for 57 weeks. Those fed the DHA-AA combination gained as much weight as those on human milk. Although the human milk–fed infants had the best visual acuity, all infants studied had acceptable visual acuity. Algal DHA and fungal AA given at human milk levels are safe for the intended use, and there was no evidence of any adverse effects (2).

In another study with PUFA supplementation and its effects on growth and neurodevelopment in premature infants, it was indicated that premature infants were able to desaturate and elongate n-3 and n-6 PUFA at a rate similar to or higher than those of full-term infants. A dose-response study with full-term infants in which AA was added to formula containing DHA showed that the balance of DHA and AA in infant tissue reflected the balance of these in the diet, regardless of whether provided from human milk or infant formula. However, because human milk composition varies according to geographic area due to local diets, infant formula manufacturers must decide which breast milk to mimic. Results from a series of studies have shown evidence that infants' EFA levels will improve if their mothers increase their EFA intake during pregnancy; the best outcome was when mothers received both DHA and AA supplements (2).

The Shunt Occlusion Trial (SHOT) was conducted to see if EPA and DHA might prevent graft occlusion that commonly occurs after coronary artery bypass surgery. SHOT participants— 610 patients undergoing coronary artery bypass—were randomized into four groups and were given antithrombic agents: warfarin, warfarin plus 4 g/day of n-3 fatty acids, aspirin or aspirin plus 4 g/day of n-3 fatty acids. The patients were monitered for a year. The n-3 fatty acids were given in a 2:1 ratio of EPA to DHA, with the addition of vitamin E. The findings indicated that n-3 fatty acids helped to prevent occlusion in patients who had undergone vein grafts. This study has now recommended increasing n-3 fatty acid intake in these patients. The n-3 fatty acids, however, do not prevent restenosis after coronary angioplasty. Although a 1995 meta-analysis from relevant clinical trials showed significant reduction of restenosis after n-3 fatty acid supplementation, a double-blind placebo-controlled trial of 388 patients showed more occurrence of restenosis in the n-3–treated group than in the placebo group. Supplementation with 5.1 g of highly concentrated n-3 PUFA a day for 6 months, initiated at least 2 weeks prior to coronory angioplasty, did not reduce restenosis incidence. Some other studies also have shown that n-3 fatty acids failed to prevent restenosis (2).

A study conducted in Norway has reported that n-3 fatty acids plus simvastatin were beneficial in patients with combined lipidemia. This combination, which is already being used in therapy for patients in Norway, has been recommended.

Gary Nelson of the USDA's Western Human Nutrition Center in San Francisco reported that a metabolic ward trial with 10 men showed that dietary DHA lowered triglycerides in the absence of dietary EPA. The trial was undertaken to help address the controversy concerning the effects of DHA versus EPA. The assumption that EPA is the active agent and DHA is innocuous has been disproved. However, the dietary DHA is rapidly retroconverted to EPA in humans, so EPA may be the active substance that lowers plasma triglycerides in vivo (2).

A Japanese study has shown that the n-6/n-3 ratio and minor components of fats and oils affect the survival time of stroke-prone spontaneously hypertensive rats. A low n-6 to n-3 ratio was beneficial, perhaps indicating a hypotensive effect. Minor components in some vegetable oils and hydrogenated oils, however, appeared to shorten survival time. Researchers are still investigating the possible mechanism for the observed antiarrhythmic effects provided by n-3 PUFA. It has been hypothesized that possible alterations in electrophysiology are linked to changes in membrane fluidity (2).

A multicenter study of dietary *trans* alpha-linolenic acid (ALA), serum lipids, and platelet aggregation in healthy European men was conducted. A total of 88 men took part in the studies at three medical centers in France, Holland, and Scotland. All participants were fed a trans-free oil (neutralized, degummed, bleached rapeseed/canola oil) during the first 6-week period. During the second 6-week period, one group received low *trans* oil (0.1 g, created by mixing the *trans*-free oil with highly isomerized sunflower oil), and another was fed high *trans* oil (1.7 g, made from a highly isomerized rapeseed/canola oil plus vitamin E). These different oils were given in such products as margarines, cookies, and cheeses. Results showed no significant differences in platelet response, triglycerides, or total cholesterol between men on either diet. Although there were no major differences in the fatty acid composition of plasma triglycerides, there were higher *trans* 18:3 and *trans* 20:5 levels in those on the higher trans diet. An increase in high density lipoprotein cholesterol in those fed the low-trans diet may have been confounded as it might be a further washout effect, or the amount of dietary fat rather than the composition of the fat, may be a factor. Thus, *trans* fatty acids administered for a short period cannot be expected to have major effects (2).

According to Norman Salem Jr. of the National Institute on Alcohol Abuse and Alcoholism, Rockville, Maryland, alcohol alters PUFA composition and metabolism. Studies have indicated a marked increase in alcohol-induced EFA degradation. It has been hypothesized that the prooxidant challenges posed by alcohol intake as well as diets low in EFA and antioxidant nutrients lead to lower levels of tissue long-chain PUFA. This contributes to multiple organ system pathologies observed in alcoholics. Another study conducted in the United Kingdom suggested that impaired DHA assimilation may contribute to pathogenesis of fetal alcohol syndrome, and that maternal dietary DHA supplementation might be useful in reducing the severity of ethanol-induced brain damage.

Research work concerning schizophrenia has revealed decreased levels of AA and DHA in RBC membranes of schizophrenic patients. Phospholipid breakdown in the cerebral cortex of these patients was evident. A double-blind placebo-controlled trial comparing oils enriched with EPA, DHA, or a placebo in treating symptomatic schizophrenic patients on neuroleptic medication in the United Kingdom indicated that patients treated with EPA, but not DHA or the placebo, showed significant improvement in their symptoms.

Researchers have been cautioned not to overlook docosapentenoic acid (DPA) when considering positive health effects linked to n-3 fatty acids. Seal oil, which was a major component of the Eskimo diet, contains 10 times as much DPA as fish oil does, and DPA also is found in human breast milk. Enriching infant formulas only with DHA may be a mistake. The retroconversion of DHA may go to EPA, and not to DPA. The role of DPA in infant nutrition has created immense fascination. DPA accumulates from the pathway from ALA, and it is incorporated in brain tissues (2).

It has been suggested that EFA metabolism impairment, particularly in the conversion of linoleic acid to GLA, leads to a loss of dihomogamma-linolenic acid and then AA, resulting in diabetic complications. The efficacy and safety of GLA in managing patients with diabetic sensorimotor neuropathy has been tested. Those receiving GLA improved compared with those in the placebo group. Evidence indicates that the deficit in GLA formation is important in the development of diabetic complications.

According to Newton (3), the typical Western diet, which is low in long-chain n-3 fatty acids and high in long-chain n-6 fatty acids, may not supply the appropriate balance for optimal metabolism. This imbalance is thought to cause a variety of disease symptoms, ranging from cardiovascular disease, hypertension, inflammatory and autoimmune disorders to depression and disrupted neurological functions. In the area of cardiovascular disease, new research on arrhythmias is exciting and shows that application of n-3 fatty acids can produce rapid results. In addition, n-3 fatty acids are showing benefits in preventing restenosis following angioplasty in about one-half of the reported studies. Significant research in infant nutrition indicates that long-chain PUFAs are "conditionally essential" for growth and development. Adequate intake of DHA and AA is critical during pregnancy, lactation, and infancy for proper development of the fetus and infant. Premature babies are particularly at risk for inadequacies. Thus, many specialist groups are recommending that infant formulas include long chain fatty acids at levels matching breast milk. Recommendations by many academic and government bodies propose that daily intakes of long-chain n-3 fatty acids be increased as a step in reducing certain chronic diseases (3).

C. Cholesterol and Lipoproteins

Cholesterol is the main sterol of animal tissues, present as the free alcohol or as cholesteryl esters with fatty acids. Cholesterol plays a vital role in stabilizing the hydrophobic interactions within animal membranes by inserting itself between the fatty chains in the bilayer. Animals consuming diets relatively rich in polyunsaturated fatty acids tend to accumulate a higher proportion of these acids in the membrane bilayer. The fluidity of the membranes can be maintained constant when the proportion of cholesterol to phospholipids is higher (24). The fluidity of the membranes must be maintained within certain limits for their metabolic functions. Cholesterol seems to be the only sterol that allows proper functioning of animal membranes. Because plant membranes have little or no cholesterol, dietary cholesterol comes almost entirely from animal foods.

In addition to its role as a membrane constituent, cholesterol serves as a precursor for bile acids (with hydrophilic side chain at C-17) that act as detergents in the intestine, emulsifying dietary fats to make them more readily accessible to digestive lipases. Sterols are also necessary to make a range of steroid hormones, produced from cholesterol by oxidation of its side chain at C-17 (1). Cholesterol was isolated from gallstones in 1784; since then, 13 Nobel prizes have been awarded to scientists who devoted their careers to research involving the role of cholesterol in biological membranes, its remarkable biosynthetic pathway, and its role as a precursor to various steroid hormones.

Most of the cholesterol in vertebrates is synthesized in the liver. A small fraction of cholesterol is incorporated there into the hepatocyte membranes, and most of it exported in the form of either bile acids or cholesterol esters. Bile acids and their salts are the hydrophilic cholesterol derivatives synthesized in the liver and aid in lipid digestion. Cholesterol esters are formed and stored in the liver or transported to other tissues that use cholesterol. All growing animal tissues require cholesterol for membrane synthesis, and some organs, such as gonads and adrenal glands, use cholesterol for the production of steroid hormones. Cholesterol is also a precursor of vitamin D.

Cholesterol and its esters, such as triacylglycerols and phospholipids, are essentially insoluble in water. These lipids must be transported from the liver (place of synthesis) and intestine (place of absorption) to various other tissues where they may be stored or consumed. They are carried in the blood plasma from one tissue to another as plasma lipoproteins, the molecular aggregates of specific carrier proteins (apolipoproteins) with various combinations of phospholipids, cholesterol, cholesteryl esters, and triacylglycerols. Different combinations of lipid and protein produce particles of different densities, ranging from very low-density lipoproteins (VLDL) to very high-density lipoproteins (VHDL), which can be separated by ultracentrifugation (Table 7) (1,30).

The chylomicrons are the largest lipoproteins and the least dense, containing a high proportion of triacylglycerols. They are synthesized in the smooth endoplasmic reticulum of epithelial cells that line the small intestine, and move through the lymphatic system, entering the bloodstream. Chylomicrons thus carry fatty acids obtained from the diet to the tissue where they are stored or consumed as fuel. When the diet contains more fatty acids than are needed immediately as fuel, they are converted into triacylglycerols in the liver and, by combining with specific apolipoproteins, are converted into VLDL. The excess carbohydrate in the diet can also be converted into triacylglycerols in the liver, and exported as VLDLs. In addition to triacylglycerols, the VLDLs also contain some cholesterol and cholesteryl esters (Table 7). These lipoproteins are transported in the blood from the liver to adipose tissue, where triacylglycerols are hydrolyzed to free fatty acids. The latter are taken up by adipocytes to resynthesize triacylglycerols from them and store the products in intracellular lipid droplets.

The loss of triacylglycerols converts VLDL to low-density lipoproteins (LDL), which are very rich in cholesterol and its esters. The LDLs carry cholesterol to peripheral tissues having specific surface receptors that mediate the uptake of cholesterol and its esters. The high-density lipoproteins (HDL) are synthesized in the liver as small, protein-rich particles containing relatively low cholesterol and its esters. After release into bloodstream, the HDLs collect cholesteryl esters from other circulating lipoproteins. A mature, cholesterol-rich HDL returns to the liver to unload the cholesterol, some of which is converted into bile salts (1).

Table 7   Some Properties of the Major Classes of Human Plasma Lipoproteins

Lipoprotein	Density (g/ml)	Composition (wt. %)				
		Protein	Free cholesterol	Cholesteryl esters	Phospholipids	Triacylglycerols
Chylomicrons	<1.006	2	1	3	9	85
VLDL	0.95–1.006	10	7	12	18	50
LDL	1.006–1.063	23	8	37	20	10
HDL	1.063–1.210	55	2	15	24	4

Source: Ref. 1, as modified by Kritchevsky (Ref. 30).

Cholesterol synthesis is a complex, energy-expensive process, regulated by several factors. In mammals, it is regulated by intracellular cholesterol concentration and by hormones, glucagon and insulin, the rate-limiting step in the pathway being conversion of beta-hydroxy-beta-methylglutaryl-CoA (HMG-CoA) into mevalonate, catalyzed by HMG-CoA reductase. The latter enzyme is hormonally regulated through phosphorylation. This enzyme exists in phosphorylated (inactive) and dephosphorylated (active) forms. Whereas glucagon stimulates phosphorylation (inactivation), insulin promotes dephosphorylation, activating the enzyme to favor cholesterol synthesis.

Unregulated cholesterol production can lead to serious disease. When the sum of cholesterol synthesized in the body and that obtained in the diet exceeds the body's needs (membranes, bile salts, steroids), pathological accumulation of cholesterol in blood vessels (atherosclerotic plaques) develops in humans, resulting in obstruction of blood vessels (atherosclerosis), leading to heart failure from occluded coronary arteries. Atherosclerosis has been linked to high levels of cholesterol in the blood, especially to high levels of LDL-bound cholesterol. A negative correlation exists between HDL levels and arterial disease.

Familial hypercholesterolemia is a human genetic disease in which blood levels of cholesterol are very high. The individuals afflicted by this disease may develop severe atherosclerosis during childhood. The LDL receptor in these cases being defective, the receptor-mediated uptake of cholesterol does not take place. Thus, cholesterol obtained in the diet is not cleared from the blood and its accumulation leads to the formation of atherosclerotic plaques. Endogenous synthesis of cholesterol continues even in the presence of excessive cholesterol in the blood because the extracellular cholesterol cannot enter the cytosol to regulate intracellular synthesis. According to Lehninger et al. (1), two natural products derived from fungi, *lovastatin* and *compactin* are being used successfully to treat patients with familial hypercholesterolemia. Both of these products are competitive inhibitors of HMG-CoA reductase and can therefore inhibit synthesis of cholesterol.

D. Lipid Peroxidation, Plant Food Antioxidants, and Human Health

As humans grow older, they became less active, have an increased probability of illness, and experience a loss of optimum function of all physiological systems. At sexual maturity, an age-dependent process sets in, progressing gradually, leading to the eventual death of the individual. Lipid peroxidation and formation of free radicals such as superoxide (O_2^-), a hydroxyl (OH), hydrogen peroxide (H_2O_2), and singlet oxygen ($^1O_2$) are thought to be involved in the aging process (25).

Ramarathnam et al. (25) have isolated and characterized endogenous plant antioxidants that are believed to inhibit lipid peroxidation and offer protection against oxidative damage to membrane functions. Antioxidants have been isolated from conventional food sources, such as tea (green and black), sesame, and wild rice, and also from other plant sources, such as rice hulls and crude plant drugs. These authors provided data on new types of water-soluble and lipid-soluble plant antioxidants and have discussed their biological activity and functionality. Ramarathnam et al. (25) concluded that lipid peroxidation in vivo has been indicated to be the primary cause of many of the cardiovascular diseases such as atherosclerosis and also the culprit in cancer and aging. Consumers, especially in the Western world, were advised in the 1980s to reduce their fat intake and to increase consumption of food sources that would provide more dietary fiber. The current emphasis is on drastically reducing the intake of red meat and increasing the intake of fresh fruits and vegetables. Consumers all over the world are becoming increasingly health conscious and are prepared to educate themselves about nutrition. The concern about the safety of synthetic antioxidants such as butylated hydroxy toluene (BHT) and butylated hydroxyanisole (BHA) that have been used widely for many years to retard lipid oxidation has resulted in increased search for natural antioxidants. Many spices have been shown to have an antioxidative effect in foods. Madsen and Bertelsen (26) have reviewed literature on the antioxidative effects of spices. Spice is a dried plant material that is added to impart flavor to the food. Rosemary and sage were the most effective antioxidants in lard. Both of these spices were also found to have a low redox potential in an oil-in-water emulsion. Clove was the most effective spice with antioxidant properties (26).

Food tannins have been associated with human health as a double-edged sword because of their cancer-preventing as well as antinutritional properties. Vegetable tannins are water-soluble phenolic compounds that precipitate alkaloids, gelatin, and other proteins in addition to phenolic reactions. They are present in plants, fruits, wines, and teas and are consumed in appreciable amounts every day.

Tannins bind epithelial cells and cause precipitation, and can induce liver damage. They also damage the mucosal lining of the gastrointestinal tract, alter excretion of certain cations, and increase loss of proteins and essential amino acids. They inhibit virtually every digestive enzyme and reduce bioavailability of iron and cobalamin (B_{12}).

Some tannins, however, are antimutagenic against a number of mutagens such as benzapyrene, benzoanthracene, and nitroso compounds. Tannins have antimicrobial activity and inhibit many fungi, bacteria, and viruses. Medical herbs containing tannins as active compounds have shown inhibition of carcinogenesis, host-mediated anti-tumor activity, anti-viral activity, and inhibition of lipid peroxidation and lipoxygenase, xanthine oxidase, and monoamine oxidase. Induction of endogenous lipid peroxidation by xenobiotics through generation of free-radical species results in alterations of cellular functions, genotoxic damage, and tumor initiation. Tannins may act as antioxidants to scavenge the free radicals and stop damaging reactions. Tannins and their related compounds may also inhibit the metabolic activation enzymes for xenobiotics. Thus, while tannins are beneficial to health as a result of their antimutagenic activity, they may also have carcinogenic, hepatoxic, and antinutritional activity. Therefore it is not advisable to ingest a large quantity of tannins because of their potential adverse health effects. However, consumption of a small quantity of the right kind of tannin may be beneficial (27). Fish oil supplementation, particularly if used in conjunction with tocopherol, does not compromise an individual's plasma antioxidant status. These findings allay safety concerns that have deterred the use of oil in such products as infant formula (2).

A new GC, NICI (methane) MNS assay has been developed to measure the excretion of a malondialdehyde (MDA)-lysine adduct to determine the interaction of PUFA peroxidation with proteins in vivo. It has been shown that severe atherosclerosis is not associated with increased whole body lipid peroxidation yielding MDA-lysine adducts, although cigarette smoking is (2). According to Howard R. Knapp of the Department of Internal Medicine and Pharmacology, University of Iowa, further research using pharmacologic manipulation of MDA-lysine adduct formation will expand our understanding of the relationship between lipid oxidation and disease processes in humans.

REFERENCES

1. Lehninger, A.L., D.L. Nelson, and M.M. Cox, Lipids, *Principles of Biochemistry*, 2nd ed., CBS Publishers and Distributors, New Delhi, 1993, p. 240.
2. Anonymous, EFA, Eicosanoids have vital role in health, a short summary of the Proceedings of the Fourth International Congress on Essential Fatty Acids and Eicosanoids, July 20–24, 1997, Edinburgh, Scotland, *INFORM. 8* (10): 1016 (1997).

3. Newton, I.S., Long chain fatty acids in health and nutrition, *J. Food Lipids. 3*: 233 (1996).
4. Gurr, M.I., Lipids and nutrition, *Lipid Technologies and Applications* (F.D. Gunstone and F.B. Padley, eds.), Marcel Dekker, New York, 1997, p. 79.
5. WHO, Nutrition and Prevention of Chronic Diseases, World Health Organization Study Group, *Tech. Rep. Ser. 797*, World Health Organization, Geneva, 1990.
6. McNamara, D.J., Relationship between blood and dietary cholesterol, *Meat and Health: Advances in Meat Research*. Vol. 6 (A.M. Pearson and T.R. Dutson, eds.), Elsevier, London, 1990, p. 63.
7. Gurr, M.I., and J.L. Harwood, *Lipid Biochemistry: An Introduction*, Chapman and Hall, London, 1991.
8. Gurr, M.I., Fats, *Human Nutrition and Dietetics* (J.S. Garrow and W.P.T. James, eds.), Churchill Livingstone, London, 1993, p. 77.
9. Wiseman, J. (ed.), *Fats in Animal Nutrition*, Butterworths, London, 1984.
10. McDonald, I.W., and T.W. Scott, Foods of ruminant origin with elevated content of polyunsaturated fatty acids, *World Rev. Nutr. And Diet. 26*: 144 (1977).
11. Watts, G.F., W. Ahmed, and J. Quiney, et al., Effective lipid-lowering diets including lean meat, *British Med. J. 296*: 235 (1988).
12. Gurr, M.I., *Role of Fats in Food and Nutrition*, Elsevier Applied Science Publishers, London, 1992.
13. Burr, G.O., and M.M. Burr, A new deficiency disease produced by rigid exclusion of fat from the diet, *J. Biol. Chem. 82*: 345 (1929).
14. Soderhjelm, L., H.F. Wiese, and R.T. Holman, The role of polyunsaturated fatty acids in human nutrition and metabolism, *Progress in Chemistry of Fats and Other Lipids, 9:* 555 (1970).
15. Hensen, A.E., M.E. Haggard, A.N. Boelsche, D.J.D. Adam, and H.F. Wiese, Essential fatty acids in infant nutrition: clinical manifestation of human linoleic acid deficiency, *J. Nutr. 66*: 565 (1958).
16. Collins, F.D., A.J. Sinclair, J.P. Royle, D.A. Coats, A.T. Maynard, and R.F. Leonard, Plasma lipids in human linoleic acid deficiency, *Nutrition and Metabolism 13*: 150 (1971).
17. Press, M., H. Kikuchi, T. Shimoyama, and G.R. Thompson, Diagnosis and treatment of essential fatty acid deficiency in man, *British Med. J. 2*: 247 (1974).
18. Holman, R.T., and S.B. Johnson, Essential fatty acid deficiencies in man, *Dietary Fats and Health* (E.G. Perkins and W.J. Visek, eds.), Am. Oil Chemists' Society, Champaign, Illinois, 1983.
19. Holman, R.T., S.B. Johnson, and T.F. Hatch, A case of human linolenic acid deficiency involving neurological abnormalities, *Am. J. Clin. Nutr. 35*: 617 (1982).
20. Bierve, K.S., I.L. Mostad, and L. Thoresen, Alpha-linolenic acid deficiency in patients on long-term gastric tube feeding: estimation of linolenic acid and long-chain unsaturated n-3 fatty acid requirements in man, *Am. J. Clin. Nutr. 45*: 66 (1987).
21. Zollner, N., Dietary linolenic acid in man: an overview, *Progress in Lipid Res. 25*: 177 (1986).
22. British Nutrition Foundation, Unsaturated fatty acids: Nutritional and physiological significance, Report of the British Nutrition Foundation's Task Force, Chapman and Hall, London, 1992.
23. Bouchier, A.D., Inaugural address at the Fourth International Congress on Essential Fatty Acids and Eicosanoids, July 20–24, 1997, Edinburgh, Scotland, *INFORM 8* (10): 1016 (1997).
24. Edwards-Webb, J.D., and M.I. Gurr, The influence of dietary fats on the chemical composition and physical properties of biological membranes, *Nutrition Res. 8*: 1297 (1988).
25. Ramarathnam, N., T. Osawa, H. Ochi, and S. Kawakishi, The contribution of plant food antioxidants to human health, *Trends Food Sci. Technol. 6*: 75 (1995).
26. Madsen, H.L., and G. Bertelsen, Spices as antioxidants, *Trends Food Sci. Technol. 6*: 271 (1995).
27. Chung, K.T., and Wei, C.I., Food tannins and human health: A double-edged sword, *Food Technol. 51* (9): 124 (1997).
28. Nettleton, J.A., n-3 fatty acids: composition of plant and sea food sources in human nutrition, *J. Am. Diet. Assoc. 91*: 331 (1991).
29. Mattson, F.H., and S.M. Grundy, Comparison of dietary saturated, monounsaturated and polyunsaturated fatty acids on plasma lipids and lipoproteins in man, *J. Lipid Res. 26*: 194 (1985).
30. Kritchevsky, D., Atherosclerosis and nutrition, *Nutr. Int. 2*: 290 (1986).

5
Proteins

I. INTRODUCTION

Like water, proteins have a central place in the cell. Proteins constitute the structure of living organisms and catalyze cellular reactions. The genetic information present in the DNA segment (gene) is expressed in the form of a protein. Proteins are thus among the most fundamental biological macromolecules and have versatile functions. Cells contain thousands of different proteins, each with a specific function or biological activity, including enzymatic catalysis (biological catalysts), molecular transport, nutrition, cell or organismal defense and motility, structural roles, regulation of metabolism, and many others.

Proteins are composed of very long polypeptide chains having 100 to 2000 amino acid residues joined together by peptide linkage. Some proteins have more than one polypeptide chains (subunits). Whereas simple proteins yield only amino acids on their hydrolysis, conjugated proteins in addition have some other non-protein component such as a metal ion or organic prosthetic group like a carbohydrate or lipid.

Proteins differ in their size, shape, binding affinities, charge, etc.; these properties are used in their analysis and purification. Proteins can be separated and visualized by electrophoretic methods. All proteins found in the natural world are made by the same set of about 20 amino acids. Their differences in the functions result from the variations in the composition and sequence of the amino acids in the polypeptide chain.

The structures of 20 amino acids differ as the result of their different side chain, as well as variation in their size and charge. Whereas some groups in the branched chain and aromatic amino acids are hydrophobic, in most other amino acids they are hydrophilic. These side chains have an important bearing on the stabilization of protein structure, and are closely involved in many other aspects of protein function. Attractions between positive and negative charges pull different parts of the molecule together. Hydrophobic groups tend to cluster together in the center of globular proteins, while hydrophilic groups remain in contact with water on the periphery. The thiol groups in cysteine form sulfur-sulfur bonds, which are crucial in the formation of primary structure. The hydroxyl and amino groups of amino acids can get attached to oligosaccharide side chains which are a feature of many mammalian proteins. Histidine and the dicarboxylic amino acids (glutamate and aspartate) are critical ion-binding proteins, such as the calcium-binding proteins and iron-binding proteins.

Certain amino acids achieve their final structure only after their precursors are incorporated into the polypeptide, e.g. hydroxyproline and hydroxylysine residues of the collagens, and methylated histidines and lysines of actin and myosin proteins. Hydroxyproline and hydroxylysine are critical components of the cross-linking of collagen chains, leading to their rigid and stable structures. The role of the methylated amino acids in contractile protein function remains to be elucidated. Eight of the 20 amino acids found in proteins are nutritionally essential because the structures of these amino acids cannot be made in the body of animals, and therefore must be provided in the diet.

The amino acid sequences of proteins can be determined by fragmenting them into smaller pieces using specific reagents, and then establishing the amino acid sequence of each fragment by the Edman degradation method. By placing the peptide fragments in the correct order by finding sequence overlaps between fragments generated by different methods, the amino acid sequence of the original polypeptide chain can be established.

Homologous proteins from different species of organisms show sequence homology, i.e. certain positions in the polypeptide chains contain the same amino acids, regardless of the species, though in other positions the amino acids may differ. The invariant residues of amino acids are evidently essential to the function of the protein. The degree of similarity between amino acid sequences of homologous proteins from different organisms correlates with the evolutionary relationship of the species (1).

Each protein has a unique three-dimentional structure, reflecting its function. The protein structure is stabilized by multiple weak interactions. Primary protein structure is established by amino acid sequence and location of disulfide bonds, secondary structure refers to the spatial relationship of adjacent amino acids, and tertiary structure is the three-dimentional conformation of an entire polypeptide chain. The quaternary structure of protein involves the special relationship of multiple polypeptide chains.

Proteins are classified as fibrous and globular proteins. Fibrous proteins primarily have structural roles. The stability of structural proteins, forming alpha-helix or beta-conformation, is established by their amino acid content and by their relative placement in the sequence. In structural proteins such as keratin and collagen, a single type of secondary structure (alpha-helix, beta-conformation, or beta bend) predominates. The polypeptide chains are supertwisted into ropes and combined in larger bundles to provide the needed strength. The structure of elastin also permits stretching.

Globular proteins have more complicated tertiary structures and may contain several types of secondary structure in the same polypeptide chain. Globular proteins are compact, with their hydrophobic amino acids located in the protein interior. Different proteins often differ in their tertiary structure. Three-dimensional protein structure can be destroyed by treatments (e.g., heat) that disrupt weak interactions, a process called denaturation, which also destroys protein function. Thus, protein structure and function have a very close relationship. Certain denatured proteins can renature spontaneously to produce functional protein (e.g., ribonuclease), which shows that the tertiary structure of a protein is determined by its amino acid sequence.

The quaternary structure refers to the interaction between the oligomeric subunits of proteins or large protein assemblies, e.g. four subunits of hemoglobin exhibit cooperative interactions on oxygen binding, these effects being mediated by subunit interactions and conformational changes.

II. NUTRITIONAL ASPECTS OF PROTEINS

A. Protein Turnover

Garlick and Reeds have demonstrated, in a highly simplified way, the exchange between the body protein and free amino acid pool (2). In this scheme, all the proteins in the body tissues and circulation are lumped together into a single pool "body proteins," and the free amino acids dissolved in the body fluids are put together in a second pool "free amino acids." There is a continual degradation and resynthesis of proteins, known as "protein turnover." Free amino acids are also supplied to the pool by the gut from the absorbed dietary proteins and the de novo synthesis of non-essential amino acids. Similarly, some of the amino acids may be lost from the pool by oxidation, excretion, or conversion to other metabolites (2).

The net loss or gain of body protein mass depends on the balance between the degradation and resynthesis of proteins in the body. The protein mass of the body remains in balance when both of these processes are equal. The loss of protein mass results from the excess of degradation over synthesis, which may occur due to stimulation of protein degradation, inhibition of protein synthesis, or a combination of both processes. The amount of a single protein or that of the whole body is regulated by altering the rates of their synthesis and degradation.

The control of protein metabolism by nutrients and hormones and its alteration in pathological states have been areas of intensive research work during the past few decades. A variety of techniques have been developed to assess the control and integration of protein metabolism in the whole organism, which range from methods of evaluating the net gains and losses of protein from body tissues to techniques for assessing amino acid fluxes and protein turnover rates.

The protein status of an individual can be assessed by sequentially measuring certains aspects of body composition (see Chapter 1) and comparing the values with population estimates. Often the body mass is measured as lipid and nonlipid components. Four characteristics of lean tissue (fat-free mass) that are used to estimate cellular or protein mass include the following:

1. The densities of lean tissues and fat stores are different, which can be known by measuring specific gravity of the body, and that of lean and fat tissues, separately.
2. The concentration of water in the lipid stores is much less than that in lean tissue. Measurement of body water gives valuable information on lean-fat relationships.
3. Cells have high K concentration, and measurement of body K content is an indication of cellular (and hence protein) mass.
4. The electrical properties of lean and fat tissues being different, measurement of the conductivity or impedance are used to derive conductive volume of the body, which is also a measure of the fat-free body mass.

All these techniques are used to provide valuable information to support classic studies based on balance methods (2).

1. Nitrogen Balance

Nitrogen is the predominant constituent of proteins and can be estimated accurately by classic methods such as the Kjeldahl procdure. The "nitrogen balance" technique has been extensively employed to study individual protein turnover. Nitrogen balance is the algebraic sum of N intake and N loss via the urine, feces, and skin; the sum is zero at N equilibrium. Positive N balance indicates that body protein is being deposited, and negative N balance shows loss of protein from body. However, the nitrogen balance does not reveal anything about body's protein mass, concentration, distribution, or function (2).

The nitrogen excretion in the urine and feces is not constant throughout the day, or even between days, because one does not eat continuously. Also, the urea pool in the body is large and turns over with a half-life of around 12 hours. Thus, it may take two days for a change in urea synthesis (i.e., nitrogen balance) to be fully reflected in the urine. The delay in the urea pool and the day-to-day variation in nitrogen excretion suggest that protein turnover by this method can be properly assessed only after prolonged collection of urine, at least over 72 hours. The start and end of the balance measurements are therefore defined by the appearance of some external marker dye in the feces. Other errors in this method include difficulty in accurately measuring the quantities of nitrogen lost in sweat. Reports based on a limited number of studies indicate values as high as 1g N and as low as 90 mg N for adults, accounting for 8% and 1%, respectively, of the current estimates for the amount of protein-nitrogen needed by adults to achieve nitrogen balance. Thus, measured nitrogen balance tends to overestimate protein deposition and underestimate protein loss.

Infant diets, such as human milk, contain significant quantities of non-protein nitrogen, therefore dietary protein has more nitrogen than accounted for in nitrogen balance. Also, the utilization of nitrogen in the non-protein pathways can lead to nitrogen retention, but not protein retention. For these reasons nitrogen balance appears to be only a crude method of studying the body's protein balance or its turnover (2).

2. Measurement of Protein/Amino Acid Turnover in Whole Body

Animal experiments using radioactive isotopes (^{14}C, ^{3}H, and ^{35}S) or human experiments using stable isotopes (^{13}C, ^{2}H, and ^{15}N) have been employed to study protein turnover in the whole body. These techniques are based on the concept that body protein metabolism can be represented by a simplified model. One such technique involves continuous infusion of a carbon-labeled amino acid (^{13}C-1-leucine) given intravenously over a period of few hours for the isotope enrichment, wherein the ratio of labeled to total molecules, expressed on atom percent basis, exceeds the natural abundance, rising to a plateau value (A max). The latter is used to compute the rate of turnover (Q) of the free leucine in the body as:

$$Q = i/A \ max$$

where the term 'i' is the rate of infusion of the isotope. This equation assumes that at plateau the rates of entry and exit from free leucine pool are equal for both labeled and unlabeled molecules, and they are in steady state. The 'Q' is also known as flux rate, apperance rate, or irreversible loss rate. The appearance of leucine can be partitioned into intake from the diet (I) and entry from the degradation of body protein (D), de novo synthesis being zero (leucine is an essential amino acid). Similarly, loss of leucine from free leucine pool also can be partitioned into protein synthesis (S) and other pathways of metabolism (O), of which only oxidation to CO_2 and urinary N are taken to be significant. Since the entry and exit are equal in the steady state:

$$Q = I + D = S + O$$

By knowing the flux rate (Q), it is possible to calculate the rate of whole body protein degradation (D), because the dietary intake (I) of leucine is known. By assessing the production of labeled CO_2 in the breath, the rate of leucine oxidation (O) also can be measured, to calculate the rate of whole-body protein synthesis. Thus, by this method, rates of metabolism of an individual amino acid by oxidation and by the synthesis and degradation of body protein can be determined more accurately; a similar approach is used with ^{15}N, usually given in the form of ^{15}N-glycine. Because of transamination, this label serves as a tracer for total free amino acid nitrogen, instead of for an individual amino acid (2).

3. Tissue and Organ Balance Techniques

Techniques based on measurements using samples of tissue or organ are more invasive than those for the whole body. Protein synthesis in a tissue can be measured isotopically by assessing incorporation of a labeled amino acid into protein of the tissue under study. This method requires that the isotope enrichment of the free amino acid at the site of protein synthesis be monitored throughout the incorporation period, which is difficult because of the compartmentation of free amino acid pools within cells. Thus, such measurements cannot reliably be made on plasma or tissue free amino acids. Garlick et al. (3) minimized this problem by giving the label as a large, non-tracer dose or by measuring amino acid bound to transfer RNA. In vivo protein synthesis in tissues can also be studied by measuring the amount of ribosomes in the tissue. Ribosomes are extracted from a tissue biopsy and centrifuged to separate them into aggregates of polysomes, sites of protein synthesis. Wernerman (4) employed decreases in the ratio of polysomal to non-polysomal RNA as well as the total amount of ribosomes in the tissue as indicators of a decrease in the rate of protein synthesis in traumatized patients.

It is difficult to assess protein degradation in individual tissues in humans, but in animals it can be estimated by knowing the rates of synthesis and growth of tissue protein. The rates of degradation in certain human tissues can be estimated through balance techniques across limbs or organs and in muscle by measuring the urinary excretion of 3-methylhistidine, which is found only in the actin and myosin of muscle, where it is synthesized by methylation of specific histidine residues of the proteins. The 3-methylhistidine released after degradation of proteins is not incorporated into protein and is excreted quantitatively in the urine, serving a direct measure of the rate of actin plus myosin degradation. According to Sjolin et al. (5), this method was found to be totally noninvasive and very useful in protein turnover studies of patients, although the results cannot be solely equated with the degradation of skeletal muscle, because smooth muscle (e.g., the gut) contains 3-methylhistidine.

Amino acids exchange between tissues, especially when a tissue has a discrete blood supply, which allows all the blood entering and leaving to be sampled. It is thus possible to measure the total uptake or output of amino acids and other nutrients by limbs or organs. The forearm or leg may be used to represent the metabolism of skeletal muscle, and arterial and hepatic vein catheters can be used to study the liver and intestine. Abumrad et al. (6) employed this method to demonstrate the role of the liver in the metabolism of amino acids from the diet.

The organ balance technique measures only the net balance of amino acid in a tissue, however by adding isotopically labeled amino acid it is possible to estimate simultaneously the synthesis and degradation of tissue protein (3,7).

Rates of catabolism of amino acids cannot be determined by measuring nitrogen excretion. Breath measurements of $^{13}CO_2$ production serves as an index of total amino acid catabolism, when the labeled amino acid is not limiting in the diet. Unlike nitrogen balance, this method is rapid because there is little delay between a change in amino acid catabolism and a change in labeling of breath CO_2. This approach can be used to study more dynamic aspects of the regulation of amino acid catabolism (2).

4. *Factors Influencing Protein Turnover*

a. Growth and Maturity. The rate of protein turnover of the adult whole body, of around 200–300 g/day, corresponds to approximately 3–4 g/day/kg of body weight. In young babies and children, the rates expressed on the basis of g/day/kg are very high, viz., 17.4 (newborn/premature), 6.9 (infants of about 1 year), 3.0 (young adults), and 1.9 (elderly) (9). Age thus gradually decreases the protein turnover during growth. Similar changes with age take place for both dietary protein requirements and metabolic rate. The relationship between protein turnover rate and mature body weight has been well established in mammals ranging widely in body size. However, changes in protein synthesis, expressed in terms of protein requirement and basal metabolic rate from birth to senescence, result more from differences in the stage of maturity. Immature animals in general show higher rates of both synthesis and degradation of protein than more mature (adult) ones.

Animal immaturity is characterized by the higher capacity for growth, which is strongly related to the synthesis and degradation of cellular and structural proteins (turnover). Animal studies have shown that protein turnover in individual tissues is also higher in the newborn than in adults, with pronounced changes in muscle tissue. An approximately 10-fold decline in the protein synthesis rate is observed during the first few weeks of life in rats. A slower fall in protein degradation is noticed as the rate of growth declines, the synthesis and degradation rates becoming equal at maturity (zero growth). Because of the prolonged period of development and very slow growth of humans compared with most other animal species, such changes are likely to be much less pronounced in humans.

    b. Diet and Starvation. Garlic and Reeds (2) separated dietary factors influencing protein turnover into (a) acute responses, such as those occurring after individual meals, and (b) chronic effects that may accompany a prolonged change in the diet. Dietary intake mostly being taken as discrete meals, with intervals of fasting, the normal state of the body is divided into two phases: (a) absorptive period, during which the dietary nutrients are actively absorbed from the gut, and (b) post-absorptive period, occurring after the completion of absorption and before the next meal. In the latter state, body uses its stores of nutrients and is in the catabolism state, with continuation of oxidation of amino acids, despite the absence of their intake. This results in the loss of tissue protein, notably of skeletal muscle and the splanchnic area. The drain of amino acids may continue, despite the body's ability to recycle most of the amino acids from protein degradation back into the synthesis of new proteins. The loss occurs because of a need for the precursors of gluconeogenesis, and the continued synthesis of many compounds requiring amino acids as precursors. The proteins lost during fasting and starvation are replenished after feeding.

    The anabolism accompaning feeding in the adult is brought about mostly by decline in the rate of whole-body protein degradation, rather than by an increased protein synthesis. This is in contrast with the pronounced increase in protein synthesis when food is given to infants or animals during their rapid growth stage. There is also an increase in the rate of amino acid oxidation if the meal supplies plentiful protein. After the dietary amino acids are absorbed by the intestine, some are diverted for protein synthesis, while others such as glutamine are selectively oxidized. Most of the amino acids are passed and extracted in the liver, which is reflected in the much higher peak in amino acid concentrations of the portal blood after protein ingestion than those measured routinely in venous blood samples. The extracted hepatic amino acids serve to enhance the protein content of the liver by inhibiting protein degradation, while the protein synthesis is continued. The production of secretory proteins such as serum albumin also increases. Amino acids escaping extraction by the liver are mostly utilized for the synthesis of muscle proteins, which are the largest protein reserve of the body. The three branched-chain amino acids, viz., leucine, isoleucine, and valine, are not extracted by the liver to the same extent as the others, and are extensively oxidized in the muscle peripheral tissues.

    With a decline in the rate of amino acid absorption from the diet, protein turnover shifts, and a net flow of amino acids from body proteins begins. Many of the amino acids coming from net protein degradation in the muscle pass directly to the liver for gluconeogenensis. The glycogen reserve of liver being limited (one day's supply), post-absorptive supply of glucose from amino acids is vital. The branched-chain amino acids, found abundantly in dietary proteins, are trans-aminated in muscle to form alanine and glutamine, which in turn are passed on to the liver to serve as precursors for glucose and urea.

    The post-absorptive state may progress into starvation if another meal is not forthcoming. The loss of protein then is restricted by minimizing the need for glucose. The ketone bodies are used as main oxidative substrate in place of glucose for a period of about one week or so, with a concomitant reduction in the oxidation of amino acids and urinary nitrogen excretion, which may fall from 12 g/day in well-nourished subjects to about 3 g/day in the fully adapted starved state. Starvation is also accompanied by a substantial fall in the protein synthesis of most tissues, especially the skeletal muscle, where its degradation also is depressed. Thus, the fall in both synthesis and degradation of body proteins limits both the protein loss and energy expenditure needed to maintain these processes. During the terminal phase of starvation, when the energy supplies have been substantially exhausted, proteins are diverted to be used as fuels, resulting in their rapid degradation.

c. Pathological Disorders. Injury, infection, burns, and cancer-like diseases invariably result in a loss of body protein, the ensuing negative nitrogen balance being proportional to the degree of trauma undergone during such pathological disorders. The nitrogen excretion may range from a few grams of nitrogen per day after minor or moderate surgery to more than 30 g N/day with severe burns, the value corresponding to a loss of about 1 kg of lean tissue per day. The persistance of such condition for more than a few days may lead to impaired recovery and threaten survival. This metabolic response is aggravated by starvation, which often accompanies trauma. The effects of trauma and starvation on protein metabolism are different, however; starvation brings about the loss of protein from most tissues to a similar extent, whereas trauma results in pronounced loss of skeletal muscle, with preservation of the visceral protein mass. Also, the adaptation that limits glucose utilization and protein loss during starvation does not occur in severe trauma (see Chapter 34).

The rates of both protein synthesis and degradation increase under the disease condition with the increase in degradation predominating, resulting in net loss of total body protein. The increase in protein synthesis occurs in the liver and in the cells of the immune system, whereas it is depressed in the skeletal muscle. The loss of protein from the relatively non-essential organs such as muscle provides substrates (amino acids) required for the repair of the injured or affected tissue (wound healing) and for activating the host defense mechanism, including enhancement in the synthesis of a series of plasma proteins by the liver, e.g., fibrinogen, C-reactive protein, and alpha-1-acid glycoprotein.

Attempts have been made to clinically reverse the loss of body protein by nutritional means, either through oral or intravenous infusion of nutrient mixtures in very sick patients. This substantially reduces the nitrogen losses, but muscle mass is often not regained until the underlying pathology is treated successfully. Because of their chemical instability and insolubility in water, certain amino acids (e.g., glutamine, tyrosine, cysteine) cannot be given in the free form; alternative forms such as dipeptides and mixtures enriched with certain amino acids are being tested— e.g., branched amino acids are used to reverse the amino acid imbalance experienced during liver failure and to enhance muscle anabolism. Mixtures of amino acids have also been designed to minimize nitrogen excretion for use in kidney failure, by replacing some of the essential amino acids with their keto acid analogues (2).

d. Metabolic Hormones. Anabolic hormonal factors are responsible for modulating deposition of nutrients after feeding and for growth, and catabolic hormones mediate tissue loss during starvation and trauma. Insulin, the most notable anabolic hormone, secreted by beta-cells of the pancreas in response to the increased plasma glucose concentration after meals, is a major factor in controlling the retention of absorbed protein. In vitro studies with animal tissues have shown that insulin stimulates protein synthesis in skeletal muscle and inhibits its degradation in both muscle and liver tissues. Infusion of insulin into growing rats stimulates muscle protein synthesis within a few minutes. Even an increase in the concentrations of amino acids, especially the branched-chain amino acids (leucine, isoleucine, and valine) induce effects similar to those of the insulin in vitro. These two factors appear to act synergistically in the intact animal to initiate the response to feeding. The levels of insulin are much reduced during starvation and malnutrition, thus partially mediating the loss of body protein.

Glucagon, a hormone secreted by alpha-cells of the pancreas, increases in quantity during fasting. This catabolic hormone promotes gluconeogenesis in the liver from free amino acids and lactate, and the effect is very rapid. Thus, glucagon balances insulin in the precise control of the body's responses to feeding and fasting. According to Garlick and Reeds (2) the ratio of insulin to glucagon concentration appears to be more important than the absolute level of either of these hormones.

Cortisol, a steroid hormone produced by the adrenal cortex, has effects similar to but slower (2 to 4 hours) than those of glucagon. It directly decreases muscle protein synthesis and increases protein degradation. Trauma and injury increase secretion of cortisol, as do glucagon and adrenaline. These three together are known as "stress hormones," and they are thought to be responsible for mediating many, though not all, metabolic responses to trauma, such as the high rate of gluconeogenesis and the mobilization of muscle protein (see Chapter 34).

A new group of hormones, known as the cytokines, have been found to be produced by activated macrophases, particularly in response to local injury. These are involved in organizing the metabolic and immunological events following trauma. For example, a tumor necrosis factor, cachectin, when injected brings about fever and negative nitrogen balance. This factor stimulates liver protein synthesis and inhibits muscle protein synthesis in rats. Whether these effects are direct or mediated through cytokine-like hormones remain to be elucidated.

B. Requirements of Amino Acids and Proteins

The subject of requirements of protein and essential amino acids by humans has been debated, and current RDAs are being reexamined (10–12). The term 'human protein requirement' has often been used in an ill-defined way, and protein nutritionists have generally followed two different approaches to assess the body's requirements:

1. The first method depends on using the relationship between protein intake and body protein status, i.e., nitrogen retention, weight gain, and linear growth. This approach tries to assess the body's requirements in terms of dietary protein supply.
2. The second, more direct, biological approach defines requirements in terms of the rates of metabolic pathways, i.e., tissue growth, amino acid catabolism, and protein turnover.

Whereas the first approach defines requirements in practical terms, as dietary allowances, the second approach defines them in biological terms, as amino acid needs. Both approaches, however, recognize explicitly that amino acid needs are primarily a function of physiological and reproductive status. The first approach tends to give higher requirements than the second one. Dietary protein not being absorbed with 100% efficiency, there is always some extra amino acid catabolism associated with the surge in plasma and tissue amino acid concentrations after a protein meal; thus the two approaches used to assess protein and amino acid requirements are bound to produce different results (2).

Earlier, amino acids were grouped into two nutritional classes, essential (indispensable) and non-essential (dispensable) amino acids, essential being those whose structures cannot be synthesized by the animal body and therefore must be provided in the diet. With more recent information available on the intermediary metabolism of non-essential amino acids, they are being defined more accurately as truly non-essential and conditionally essential (13). Non-essential amino acids are now more rigidly defined as those synthesized either by reductive amination of a keto acid by NH^+_4, or by transamination of a carbon chain synthesized in the central pathways of carbon metabolism, i.e., EMP and TCA cycle. Thus, only glutamate, aspartate, and alanine are regarded as truly non-essential amino acids. The second class, conditionally essential amino acids (Table 1), are now defined as those derived from the metabolism either of other amino acids or of other complex nitrogenous metabolites. The synthesis of these amino acids does not involve transamination. Amino acids such as methionine and cysteine as well as phenylalanine and tyrosine are closely interrelated with each other both metabolically and nutritionally, so that these amino acids are often considered in pairs in many formulations of RDAs. However, it is known that only the thiol group of cysteine is derived from methionine, whereas its carbon and nitrogen atoms come from serine. Similarly, both arginine and proline require the supply of excess amounts of glutamate and aspartate, and histidine depends on adenine and glutamate as its precursors (Table 1). It has also been established that amino nitrogen is not freely interchanged between all amino acids. The nitrogen from serine, lysine, and threonine, for example, is not readily transferred to glutamate, aspartate, or alanine. Thus, conditionally essential amino acids in principle may be required to be provided in the diet of the animals, unless abundant amounts of their precursors are available for their synthesis in the body at the rates needed to confer nutrition and health. Also, in certain physiological circumstances, such as in newborn babies, the enzymes involved in the complex synthetic pathways of the amino acid may be present in inadequate amounts. In such situations, too, the amino acid in question will have to be considered a dietary essential one.

In addition to its requirement for the maintenance of protein turnover, and a variety of products of amino acid metabolism, dietary protein is also needed to build new tissue during the growth phase; the extra amino acids needed appear to approximate the amino acid composition of the newly synthesized protein during growth (Table 2).

The details of the amino acid and protein requirements during growth and maintenance for different categories of population are dealt with in Chapters 19 and 22.

Table 1 Precursors of Conditionally Essential Amino Acids

Amino acid	Precursors
Cysteine	Methionine, serine
Tyrosine	Phenylalanine
Arginine	Glutamine/glutamate, aspartate
Proline	Glutamate
Histidine	Adenine, glutamine
Glycine	Serine, choline

Source: Ref. 2.

Table 2 Body Protein Composition of Amino Acids as Compared with Growth Pattern in Pigs (g Amino Acid/16 g N)

Amino acid	Body protein	Growth pattern
Leucine	6.9	7.8
Threonine	4.2	4.7
Lysine	7.8	6.8
Methionine	2.1	1.9
Cysteine	1.9	1.7
NEAA/EAA	52/48	54/46

Source: Refs. 15, 16.

C. Traditional and Nontraditional Food Proteins

Plants, animals, and microorganisms all serve as sources of food proteins. Most proteins are required to be processed or modified before they can be consumed by humans.

Animal proteins, including those coming from meat, milk, eggs, and fish have been regarded as high-quality proteins in the human diet. Meat, the edible muscle of cattle, sheep, and swine, is usually designated as red meat (beef) or light (lamb and pork), or dark red when it contains red-colored myoglobin. Adult mammalian muscle, stripped of all external fat, contains about 18% to 20% protein on a weight basis. On the basis of origin and solubility, proteins may be categorized as myofibrillar (49% to 55%), sarcoplasmic (30% to 34%) and stroma (connective tissue) (10% to 17%) of the total protein content.

The protein content of mammal milks ranges from 2.0% to 5.4% depending on the species, and cow's milk is about 3.5% protein. Milk proteins are often designated as (a) casein, a heterogenous group of phosphoproteins that are insoluble in water and account for 80% of total milk proteins, and (b) whey proteins, which make up about 20% of the total proteins and are soluble in water.

Poultry egg contains about 13% to 14% protein, two-thirds of which is present in the egg-white; proteins are readily denatured and become coagulated with agents such as heat. Yolk is a mixture of different lipoproteins and phosphoproteins.

The protein content of fish may vary from 10% to 21%. Fish muscle is similar to the skeletal muscle of mammals, both structurally and functionally, but the former has a shorter shelf life. Much of the instability of fish proteins is due to the presence of enzymes in the reddish brown muscle of fish, which continue to remain active after harvest.

Cereal food grains contain about 6% to 20% protein, e.g. rice (7%–9%) and wheat (12%–15%). These proteins are present in the embryo, germ, bran or seed coat, and the endosperm. The germ proteins are predominantly either albumins or globulins, with several associated enzymes. The endosperm proteins of wheat are mostly prolamines, gliadins, and glutelins. Rice contains high levels of glutelins and low prolamine. Cereal proteins have generally been regarded to have low nutritional quality, because they lack certain essential amino acids, such as lysine.

Pulses (legumes) contain about 20% to 25% proteins, and soybeans contain about 40% to 42% protein. These proteins are mostly concentrated in aleurone layers, the subcellular granules of the cotyledon cells. Most seed proteins are globular. Seed proteins are often low in lysine content, most pulses being deficient in methionine, tryptophan, and threonine. They also contain certain antinutritional factors, such as protease inhibitors, which must be subjected to appropriate heat treatments to destroy or inactivate them.

Fresh vegetables and fruits are not rich sources of proteins and often contain less than 1% protein. Potatoes contain about 2% proteins, which are considered of high quality, because of their relatively higher levels of lysine and tryptophan.

Apart from the traditional food proteins described above, nontraditional sources such as microorganisms have been exploited for the production of proteins, known as single cell proteins (SCPs) (see Chapter 12). Two yeast species viz., torula yeast (*Candida utilis*) and brewer's yeast (*Saccharomyces carlsbergensis*) have been utilized to produce human food proteins. Brewer's yeast is collected after beer fermentation; torula yeast grows well on sulfite waste liquor (waste product from paper industry) and wood hydrolysates by utilizing pentoses as a carbon source. These yeasts contain around 50% proteins on a dry-weight basis. They are deficient, however, in their methionine content, and by adding 0.3% methionine, their biological value can be increased to over 90%. The nucleic acid content of yeast foods, being relatively insoluble, may lead to formation of kidney stones or aggravate arthritic or gouty conditions (14).

Certain yeast strains (*Candida lipolytica*) can grow on petroleum products as a carbon source. A commercial product (Toprina) made by this procedure has been found to be safe toxicologically. Similarly, a product named Pruteen has been manufactured by using the bacterium *Methylophilus methylotrophus*, which can oxidize methane or methanol and use them as a source of carbon and energy.

Two algal genera, *Chlorella* (green algae) and *Spirulina* (blue-green algae) can be grown under controlled conditions to produce 50% to 60% protein on a dry weight basis. Barring low methionine content, algal proteins contain all other amino acids. Higher proportions of algal protein in the human diet however have been reported to cause nausea, vomiting, and abdominal pain, though its poor digestibility can be eliminated through processing.

Food fungi (mushrooms) contain about 27% protein on a dry-weight basis and are commercially grown and used as nutritious vegetable foods. Proteins can also be extracted from green plant leaves and used as food; the dried product is around 50% to 70% protein. The nutritional value of leaf proteins is much higher than the other plant proteins and they are rich in lysine content. The cost, yield, and palatability of most of these non-traditional proteins obtained either from microbial or plant sources have not yet made them commercially successful products (see Chapter 12).

D. Protein Quality

The nutritional quality of proteins depends on their amino acid composition, digestibility, and absorptive ability. A high-quality protein should supply all essential amino acids in proper proportions and help growth, repair of damaged tissues, reproduction, and health of the organism. Protein quality is often determined by biological methods, such as conducting nitrogen balance experiments on animals. Biological value (BV) of a protein is one such useful measure of protein quality. It is based on the nitrogen retained in the body in relation to nitrogen absorbed by the body. Another measure of protein quality, protein efficiency ratio (PER), relates weight gain in animals to protein consumed with a reference protein. The net protein ratio (NPR) is defined as the weight gained by the test group of animals plus the weight lost by the non-protein group (given a diet with no protein), divided by the protein consumed. The net protein utilization (NPU) is similar to NPR except that body nitrogen, rather than body weight is used, i.e., NPU = (N retained/Food N) × 100. NPU thus incorporates both BV and digestibility of food because it relates food nitrogen rather than absorbed nitrogen to nitrogen retained. The biological value of an ideal protein taken as 100, the values for common foods used in the human diet have following biological values; egg (95), cow milk (84), fish (76), meat (74), rice (78), wheat (66), maize (60), peanut (55), and pulses (49–63).

REFERENCES

1. Lehninger, A.L., D.L. Nelson, and M.M. Cox, Proteins, *Principles of Biochemistry*, 2nd ed. CBS Publishers and Distributors, New Delhi, 1993, p. 134.
2. Garlick, P.J., and P.J. Reeds, Proteins, *Human Nutrition and Dietetics* (J.S. Garrow and W.P.T. James, eds.), Churchill Livingstone, London, 1993, p. 56.
3. Garlick, P.J., J. Wernerman, M.A. McNurlan, and S.D. Heys, Organ-specific measurements of protein turnover in man, *Proc. Nutr. Soc. 50*: 217 (1991).
4. Wernerman, J., Ribosome profiles from human skeletal muscle as a measure of protein synthesis, *Clin. Nutr. 10*: (Suppl-6) (1991).
5. Sjolin, J., H. Stjernstrom, S. Henneberg, et al., Splanchnic and peripheral release of 3-methylhistidine in relation to its urinary excretion in human infection, *Metabolism 38*: 23 (1989).
6. Abumrad, N.N., P. Williams, M. Frexes-Steed, et al., Inter-organ metabolism of amino acids in vivo, *Diabetes/Metabolism Rev. 5*: 213 (1989).

7. Wernerman, J., and E. Vinnars, The effect of trauma and surgery on interorgan fluxes of amino acids in man, *Clin. Sci. 73*: 129 (1987).

8. Young, V.R., Kinetics of human amino acid metabolism, nutritional implications and some lessons, *Am. J. Clin. Nutr. 46*: 709 (1987).

9. Young, V.R., W.P. Steffee, P.B. Pencharz, J.C. Winterer, and N.S. Scrimshaw, Total human body protein synthesis in relation to protein requirements at various ages, *Nature 253*: 192 (1975).

10. Beaton, G.H., and A. Chery, Protein requirements of infants: a reexamination of concepts and approaches, *Am. J. Clin. Nutr. 48*: 1403 (1988).

11. Millward, D.J., and J. Rivers, The nutritional role of indispensable amino acids and the metabolic basis for their requirements, *European J. Clin. Nutr. 42*: 367 (1988).

12. Young, V.R., D.M. Bier, and P.L. Peller, A theoretical basis for increasing current estimates of the amino acid requirements in adult man with experimental support, *Am. J. Clin. Nutr. 50*: 80 (1989).

13. Laidlaw, S.A., and J.D. Kopple, Newer concepts of the indispensable amino acids, *Am. J. Clin. Nutr. 46*: 593 (1987).

14. Manay, N.S., and M. Shadaksharaswamy, *Foods: Facts and Principles*, Wiley Eastern Ltd. New Delhi, 1987, p. 42.

15. Reeds, P.J., Amino acid needs and protein scoring patterns, *Proc. Nutr. Soc. 49*; 489 (1990).

16. Fuller, M.F., R. McWilliam, T.C. Wang, and L.R. Giles, The optimum dietary amino acid pattern for growing pigs. 2. Requirements for maintenance and for tissue protein accretion, *British J. Nutr. 62*: 255 (1989).

6
Vitamins

I. INTRODUCTION

Vitamins are low-molecular-weight organic substances required in small amounts in the diets of higher animals for normal growth, maintenance of health, and reproduction. All animals need vitamins, but not every vitamin is required by all animals; e.g., vitamin C is needed only by humans, guinea pigs, monkeys, some birds, and some fish that lack the enzyme gulonolactone oxidase, which is required to make 1-ascorbic acid from glucose via D-glucuronic acid. Plants and microorganisms can synthesize all vitamins.

Vitamins are a group of heterogeneous substances that differ widely in their chemical nature and function. They are usually classified on the basis of their solubility in water and fats as water-soluble and fat-soluble vitamins. The latter group includes vitamins A, D, E, and K, found in foods associated with lipids. The water-soluble vitamins are ascorbic acid (vitamin C) and the vitamins of the B complex group—nitrogenous organic substances of varied chemical structures.

Vitamins have a range of functions in different animals. They regulate metabolism, help to convert carbohydrates and fats into energy, and assist in the build of body structure, such as formation of bones and teeth. Most vitamins of the B complex group have coenzyme functions. Vitamins taken in excess of the body's needs are useless; excess water-soluble vitamins are excreted mainly in the urine. However, the excess fat-soluble vitamins are stored in the body and could become toxic in very large excess.

Requirements for vitamins differ during growth and maturity, additional quantities being needed under special circumstances such as pregnancy and lactation. The actual daily requirements may also vary depending on inheritance, microbial flora of the intestine, and eating habits. Thus, the recommended daily allowances (RDAs) of vitamins may also differ from one country to other. The standards have been set by organizations such as FAO/WHO, MRC (Medical Research Council, UK), and NRC/NAS (Nutritional Research Council, National Academy of Sciences, USA).

Vitamins are distributed widely in natural foods; some foods are richer in certain vitamins and poor in others. Vitamin deficiency rarely occurs in persons eating a wide variety of natural foods. Green leafy vegetables, fruits, whole grain cereals, pulses, and nuts are fairly rich sources of different vitamins. Milk, eggs, and meat are good sources of the vitamin B complex group, but the organ meats, such as liver and kidney, are richer.

Vitamins are lost in various ways. Food processing involving blanching, cooking, heating, irradiation, and removal of water (drying), as well as trimming and peeling, can cause significant losses of vitamins and minerals. Most water-soluble vitamins may be lost during cooking through leaching. Vitamins lost during food processing may be added by fortification; the added vitamins may be either synthetic or natural. Vitamins may also be lost during storage of food.

II. FAT–SOLUBLE VITAMINS

A. Vitamin A (Retinol)

Vitamin A exists in three forms in animals: retinol, retinal, and retinoic acid, and as carotenoids in its provitamin form in many fruits and vegetables, in the form of orange-yellow pigments. Among a number of nutritionally useful carotenoids, beta-carotene is most effective as a source of vitamin A. Because only a part of the carotene in plants is converted to vitamin A in the animal body (about 25%), the concentration of vitamin A is often expressed in international units (IU) or retinol equivalents, which takes into account the actual amount of vitamin A available. Being heat-stable, vitamin A is not lost during cooking and processing, but it may be destroyed by exposure to oxygen or to sources of ultraviolet light, including sunlight. Fats are equally likely to turn rancid under the same conditions, so when fatty substances go rancid, most of their vitamin A value is likely to be lost.

McCollum and Davis (1) first isolated fat-soluble vitamin A from fish liver oils, and its structure was fully elucidated in 1930. The biological conversion of beta-carotene to vitamin A was demonstrated only recently (2).

Vitamin A (all *trans*-retinol, vitamin A1 alcohol) is the parent of a group of chemical compounds known as retinoids, both natural and synthetic, having structural features similar to vitamin A, including an extensive system of conjugated double bonds (Fig. 1). Beta-carotene is the principal compound among carotenoids having vitamin A value. The majority of these naturally occurring compounds are not converted to vitamin A: those most commonly found in human diets, such as lycopene and lutein, are absorbed from the intestine unchanged and are found in the circulation. Most carotenoids are thought to serve as singlet oxygen quenches, and as antioxidants, unlike retinol (3).

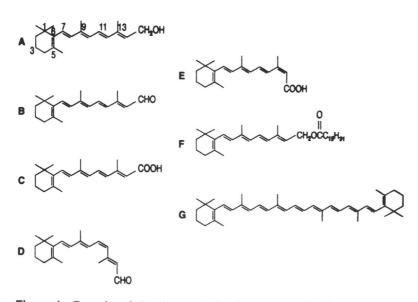

Figure 1 Formulas of vitamin A and related compounds. A. All-*trans*-retinol, approved numbering system. B. All-*trans*-retinal. C. All-*trans*-retinoic acid. D. 11-*cis*-retinal; E. 13-*cis*-retinoic acid, F. Retinyl palmitate, G. All-*trans*-beta-carotene. (From Ref. 3.)

1. Sources and Requirements

Dairy products such as milk, butter, cheese; egg yolk; some fatty fish; and the liver of farm animals and fish, especially the liver oils of cod, halibut, and shark, are the richest sources of vitamin A, used as dietary supplements. Certain fruits and vegetables with dark green leaves contain carotenes. Barring carrots and sweet potatoes, starchy roots contain little carotene. Yellow fruits such as papayas, mangos, apricots, and peaches are good sources of beta-carotene. The oils of certain palm trees are the richest source of provitamin A; in tomatoes, most of the carotenoid is present in the form of non-provitamin lycopene (Table 1).

As is true of other nutrients, the requirements for vitamin A in animals vary according to age, sex, and some other factors. Vitamin A requirements, or RDAs, are often expressed in units that allow for the differing potency of retinol and the provitamin carotenoids. This unit is the retinol equivalent (RE) with the following relationships:

1.0 microgram RE = 1.0 microgram retinol

= 6.0 micrograms beta-carotene

= 12.0 micrograms other provitamin carotenoids

= 3.3 international units (IU) retinol

= 9.9 international units (IU) beta-carotene

Thus, one IU of retinol is equivalent to 0.3 microgram of retinol, and one IU of beta-carotene equals 0.6 microgram of beta-carotene. The variations in the recommended dietary intakes (RDIs) published by national and international organizations can be attributed to differences in the body weights used for reference adults (4) (see Chapter 8).

The mean intake of vitamin A in the form of beta-carotene and retinol differs considerably in different parts of the world (5). The daily intakes of vitamin A recommended in Europe are 666 RE beta-carotene and 531 RE retinol, as compared to 725 and 170 in Africa, 564 and 103 in Asia, and 437 and 483 in the United States, respectively. Care must therefore be excercised in the use of food composition tables when estimating vitamin A values of foodstuffs. The method of analysis used also contributes to variations in the reported values of vitamin A content of foods. Whereas the earlier methods employed have often over-estimated the beta-carotene content of foods because of the inclusion of inactive carotenoids, more recent techniques employing high-performance liquid chromatography (HPLC) can estimate individual carotenoids and retinoids separately to give accurate results and are increasingly used in dietary analysis.

Table 1 Plasma Vitamin A Levels and Vitamin A Status

Status	Plasma vitamin A	
	(Micromol/liter)	(Microgram/dl)
Deficient	Less than 0.35	Less than 10
Marginal	0.35–0.70	10–20
Satisfactory	0.70–1.75	20–50
Excessive	1.75–3.5	50–100
Toxic	More than 3.5	More than 100

Source: Ref. 3.

2. *Physiological and Biochemical Functions*

Preformed vitamin A in foods is present predominantly as retinyl ester, which together with carotenoids aggregates with other lipids during digestion in the stomach. In the duodenum, lipids are hydrolyzed by pancreatic lipases, and bile salts facilitate micelle formation and their transfer across the intestinal villi. In the presence of adequate fat intake, about 80% of vitamin A is absorbed by the body. Absorption of carotenoids primarily depends on the presence of bile salts which is around 50% of the absorption of vitamin A. Conversion of beta-carotene and other carotenoids into vitamin A occurs mainly at the intestinal mucosal cells, the major pathway being the oxidative cleavage of the central 15, 15' double bond (6). Retinol is then transported to the liver and target cells through various pathways, as described by Blomhoff et al. (7). According to these authors, holo-retinol-binding protein (holo RBP), consisting of 1:1 complex of all *trans*-retinol and RBP (mol. wt.21,000), is the major form of circulating vitamin A released from the liver and taken up by the target cells. In contrast, circulating carotenoids, about 15% to 30% of which are beta-carotenes and the remainder mainly non-provitamin carotenoids, are transported by various classes of lipoproteins (LDLs and HDLs).

According to Sauberlich et al. (8), vitamin A is depleted from the liver at a relatively low rate of around 0.5% per day, though within the body it is in a high dynamic state; the half-life of holo-RBP bound to transthyretin is about 11 hours (9).

Vitamin A is metabolized in various ways in the body. Retinal is reversibly reduced to retinol and irreversibly oxidized to retinoic acid in many tissues (10). Retinol is conjugated, forming Schiff bases with e-amino groups of proteins, such as in the important interaction between 11-*cis*-retinal and opsin and the opsin proteins (rhodospin in the rods for night vision and porphyropsins in the cones for day and color vision) in the eye. The carotenoids and vitamin A may also become isomerized as in the conversion of all-*trans* to 11-*cis*-retinol in the eye (11). Specific retinoid-binding proteins are involved in the transport and metabolism of retinol, retinal, and retinoic acid. These specialized proteins also help to protect the vitamin A forms from oxidation and the lipid structures of membranes from surface action of vitamin (3).

Retinoic acid has been found to be powerful morphogen in embryonic development. Giguere et al. (12) and Petkovich et al. (13) showed that cell nuclei contain four receptors for retinoic acid, termed RAR-alpha to gamma. Retinoic acid is thought to be transported to the nucleus on cellular retinoic acid binding protein (CRABP), where it interacts with one or more of the RARs. The activated RAR in turn interacts with the different hormone responses of appropriate genes to influence transcription.

In both phototopic (day and color) and scotopic (night) vision, the aldehyde form of vitamin A, retinal in its *cis* configuration, 11-*cis*-retinal, binds to the rod or cone opsins to form rhodospin or porphyropsins, respectively. Light causes retinal to change its configuration to *trans* form, which initiates a series of complex reactions leading to a decrease in sodium ion entry to sodium channels and a change in membrane potential that is transmitted to the brain. Only a part of the light energy is dissipated in the nerve impulse, the remainder being used to release opsin and regenerate *cis*-retinal from *trans*-retinal in the visual cycle (Fig. 2) (14). The rod cells are more sensitive to vitamin A deficiency than the cone cells, resulting in night blindness. Olson (4) has recently reviewed the role of retinoids in vision.

Apart from vision, other important physiological functions of vitamin A include its role in fetal development, the immune response (particularly cell-mediated immunity), spermatogenesis, appetite, hearing, physical growth, and hematopoiesis, the latter possibly through interactions with iron (15). Underwood (16) suggested that the fundamental role of vitamin A in cellular development may be implicated in most of these functions.

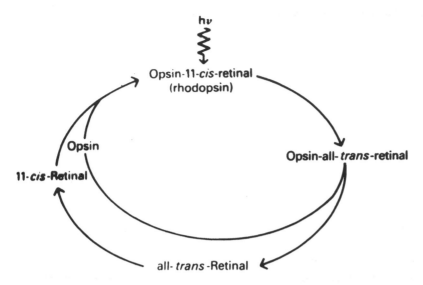

Figure 2 Visual cycle of vitamin A showing involvement of 11-*cis*-retinal, opsins, and rhodopsin. (From Ref. 3.)

3. Vitamin A Status and Deficiency

The vitamin A status of population groups can be assessed by knowing the capacity of the body to store amounts of vitamin A, especially in the liver. The state of these stores and other factors influencing them are used to categorize status. As is the case for all nutritional indices, individual values must be interpreted with caution.

Based on experimental animal and human studies, the lower limit of liver vitamin A concentration in humans of both sexes is considered to be 0.07 µmol/g (20 mg/g) (17). The relative dose response (RDR) and modified relative dose response (MRDR) tests have been found to be promising in the indirect assessment of liver reserves made from a plasma assay (18,19). The observation that in the presence of vitamin A deficiency with diminished liver stores, apo RBP accumulates in the liver to several times its normal concentration forms the basis of RDR and MRDR tests. In the RDR, 450 micrograms of retinyl palmitate is given orally, after the measurement of base line serum retinol. Some of the retinyl palmitate is taken up by the liver and combines with some of the excess apo RBP there. The holo RBP is then released into circulation and in proportion to the preexisting deficiency causes a rise in serum retinol, which is sampled again after about 5 hours. The difference between the two serum retinol values divided by the final value expressed as a percentage serves to assess vitamin A status. Values of 50% to 20% indicate marginal liver stores, and those exceeding 50% indicate vitamin A deficiency (3).

Serum or plasma levels of vitamin A can be measured readily, and standards are available to assess vitamin A status in certain population groups, though serum levels fail to truly reflect vitamin A status, because of the liver's capacity to store vitamin A, barring extreme stages of deficiency and toxicity accompanied by the clinical signs (20). The standards set by WHO for plasma vitamin A levels for assessing vitamin A status are given in Table 1.

With the increasing severity of vitamin A deficiency, ocular manifestations in the form of xerophthalmia, broadly classified, indicate vitamin A status (21). Serum retinol levels are depressed significantly by the time human subjects begin to show evidence of night blindness.

Before this stage, dark adaptometry may be performed to obtain objective evidence of impaired dark adaptation in positive cases (22). The occurrence and epidemiology of xerophthalmia are dealt with in Chapter 21.

4. Hypervitaminosis A

Ingestion of several hundred thousand units of vitamin A has been shown to cause a rise in intracranial pressure, especially in young children, with symptoms of vomiting, headache, and papilledema. Drowsiness, repeated vomiting, and skin exfoliation occur with very large doses of vitamin A (23). Spontaneous recovery without residual damage may follow on stopping the vitamin. Bush and Dahms (24) attributed the death of a one-month-old baby to the administration of one million units of vitamin A over 11 days. Arctic explorers and Eskimos have died by eating polar bear or seal liver because of their extremely high vitamin A content (Table 2).

Chronic vitamin A ingestion of doses exceeding 10 times the RNI (reference nutrient intake), taken over period of months or years, is accompanied by the syndrome of headache, loss of hair, dry and itchy skin, hepatosplenomegaly, and bone and joint pains. Cessation of the vitamin often leads to complete recovery gradually, with persistence of liver damage, bone and muscle pain, and impaired vision in some cases (3).

Table 2 Typical Values of Dietary Sources of Provitamin and Preformed Vitamin A (Micrograms Retinol/100 g Edible Portion)

Dietary source	Provitamin A
Vegetables/Fruits	
Mango (golden)	307
Papaya (solo)	124
Cucurbita (mature pulp)	862
Buriti palm (pulp)	3000
Red palm oil	30000
Carrot	2000
Dark green leafy vegetables	685
Tomato	100
Apricot	250
Sweet potato (red and yellow)	670
Animal products	
Fatty fish liver oils	
Halibut	900000
Cod	18000
Shark	180000
Herring and mackerel	50
Dairy products	
Butter	830
Margarine (vitaminized)	900
Eggs	140
Milk	40
Cheese, fatty type	320
Meats	
Liver, sheep and ox	15000
Beef, mutton, pork	0–4

Source: Ref. 3.

Congenital malformation in the offspring of mothers receiving large doses of vitamin A during the organogenetic period in utero have been reported in animals. The retionids accutane (13-*cis*-retinoic acid and an aromatic analogue of the ethyl ester of all-*trans*-retinoic acid), used in the treatment of severe acne and other skin disorders, have been reported to produce a set of characteristic birth defects in the offspring of women treated with them (25).

Prolonged ingestion of large amounts of carotenoids in green and yellow leafy vegetables, carrot juices, citrus fruit, and tomatoes may result in hypervitaminosis A, with a rise in blood carotenoid levels of over 250 micrograms/100 ml, as in cases of hypothyroidism, diabetes mellitus, and anorexia nervosa, either from excessive ingestion or defective metabolism.

B.   Vitamin D (Calciferols)

Though the condition called rickets was known earlier, this disease was given rigorous scientific basis in the early twentieth century (26,27). Funk (28) had earlier advanced the concept of "vital amines" coining the term *vitamin* for the nutritionally vital organic substances. McCollum and Davis (29) discovered a factor in butterfat and cod liver oil that was essential for the growth of animals and termed it vitamin A. Because Mellanby was able to cure a rachitic disorder produced in dogs by giving them cod liver oil, it was logically assumed that 'vitamin A' that was found in cod liver oil prevented or cured rickets. However McCollum et al. (30) demonstrated that even when the vitamin A activity of cod liver oil was destroyed by oxidation, the oil could still prevent the onset of rickets, suggesting the presence of a different factor, which was called vitamin D. Clinical studies further showed that the exposure of rachitic children to sunlight or ultraviolet light also prevented or cured the disease. The cure of rickets thus appeared to be related both to sunlight exposure and a factor associated with cod liver oil.

Vitamin D is the generic term used to designate two molecules: ergocalciferol (vitamin D_2), obtained by irradiating the plant sterol ergosterol, which served for many years as the major form of vitamin D for the prevention and treatment of rickets; and cholecalciferol (vitamin D_3), the principal form of natural vitamin D, which can be made by irradiating 7-dehydrocholesterol. Vitamin D_3 is more effective in preventing and curing rickets in chicks than vitamin D_2. Vitamin D must be hydroxylated at the C-25 position in the liver (31) and further at the C-1 position in the kidney (32) to produce biologically active vitamin D.

Provitamin D_3 (7-dehydrocholesterol) is first converted in the light to previtamin D_3 within the skin (33,34), the amount of photoconversion depending on both the quantity and the quality of the radiation reaching the basal and spinosum layers of the epidermis. Wavelengths of 280 to 320 nm are required, with the maximum conversion taking place at 295 nm. Previtamin D_3 is then further photoconverted to tachysterol and lumisterol, or by heat-induced isomerization to vitamin D_3; around 50% of this isomerization takes place within 28 hours at normal body temperatures. Thus, production of vitamin D_3 within the skin can take several days.

Vitamin D is stored in various fat depots throughout the body. The lipid nature of vitamin D and its metabolites limits their transport in blood circulation, which is facilitated by the presence of a specific vitamin D transport protein, an alpha 2 globulin. According to Norman (35), there are at least 37 metabolites of vitamin D, but only three (viz., 25-hydroxyvitamin D_3 [25(OH)D_3], 1,25-dihydroxy vitamin D [1,25(OH)$_2D_3$], and 24,25-dihydroxyvitamin D [24,25(OH$_2$)D_3]) have higher biological activity, the role of the last being controversial. The other metabolites of vitamin D appear to represent pathways of inactivation of the active forms of the molecule (3).

Vitamin D_3 is coverted to 25(OH)$_2D_3$ in the liver by the microsomal 25-hydroxylase, requiring NADPH, molecular oxygen, Mg^{++}, and a cytosolic component (33). The circulating 25(OH)$_2D_3$ is further hydroxylated by 1-alpha hydroxylase, a cytochrome P-450 enzyme, requiring NADPH and an adrenodoxin component that incorporates molecular oxygen into the 1-alpha position of $25(OH)_2D_3$, thus converting it into $1,25(OH)_2D_3$.

The circulating concentration of $1,25(OH)_2D_3$ is tightly controlled, it being the most active biological form of cholecalciferol. The kidney produces both the dihydroxylated forms of the vitamin ($1,25(OH)_2D_3$ and $24,25(OH)_2D_3$), the dominant form being determined by the level of circulating parathyroid hormone (PTH) and the body's vitamin D status. In the vitamin D–deficient state, the production of $1,25(OH)_2D_3$ is higher and that of $24,25(OH)_2D_3$ is low because the former has its own negative feedback control of suppressing 1-alpha hydroxylase enzyme. In the adequate vitamin D status, more of $24,25(OH)_2D_3$ is produced. A fall in plasma calcium stimulates PTH production, which in turn increases the kidney's 1-alpha hydroxylase activity to stimulate the production of $1,25(OH)_2D_3$ when the body's vitamin D status is low. Enhanced $1,25(OH)_2D_3$ directly reduces PTH production to regulate the vitamin D status in the body.

Vitamin D [$1,25(OH)_2D_3$] can be regarded as a hormone because it is produced solely by the kidney and is carried in the circulation by its binding protein to the target cells located elsewhere in the small intestine and bone tissue (33). During pregnancy the placenta also secretes significant amounts of $1,25(OH)_2D_3$ derived from the stimulation of 1-alpha hydroxylase activity in macrophases (36).

1. Sources and Requirements

The natural human diet is only a trivial source of vitamin D, though certain foods such as egg yolk, fish oils, and milk are good sources of this vitamin (Table 3). Vitamin D in its natural or added form is stable, and cooking, processing, and storage do not decrease its activity. Major amounts of vitamin D can be derived from exposure to sunlight. Its production in the skin is related to latitude: the farther the distance from the equator, the lower the synthesis of vitamin D, because at higher latitudes the angle of the sun's rays will be greater, with shorter UV wavelengths of light necessary for the photoconversion of 7-dehydrocholesterol (34).

It is difficult to establish allowances or requirements for vitamin D, its major source being skin exposed to sunlight. Also, careful judging of oral dose is important because vitamin D toxicity can occur when its levels are only around five times higher than normal. Fraser (37) questioned the effectiveness of dietary supplementation of vitamin D, based on the studies on addition of vitamin D to the diet of submariners or astronauts (who are not exposed to sunlight) at 2.5 micrograms/day (equal to UK requirements), showing that a fall in plasma $25(OH)D_3$ levels could not be prevented by the dose.

Policies regarding dietary allowances of vitamin D vary in different countries, which have different levels of sunlight exposure. In the United States, where cow's milk (10 micrograms or 400 IU/quart) and margarine are supplemented, the RDAs for adults (24 years and above) are set at 5 micrograms (200 IU)/day, despite the estimated dietary intake of about 1.25 to 1.75 micrograms/day and rare clinical nutritional osteomalacia in the country. In Australia, with higher levels of natural sunlight and also an increased toxicity risk, vitamin D deficiency is restricted only to the housebound (38). In the United Kingdom, where the levels of sunlight are low and margarine is the only food fortified with vitamin D, the average dietary intake ranges from 0.5 to 8 micrograms/day (average 3 micrograms/day). A recent report has not set dietary reference value (DRV) for people between 4 and 50 years of age, barring those confined to indoors, for whom intake is set at 10 micrograms/day (39).

Because of the heavy demand for calcium during pregnancy and lactation, US RDAs have been doubled to 10 micrograms (400 IU) per day in women over 24 years of age. UK recommendations are 10 micrograms of vitamin D/day during pregnancy and lactation, but in Australia supplementation is not considered necessary, provided there is reasonable exposure to sunlight.

Table 3 Vitamin D Content of Some Foods (Micrograms/100 g)

Foods	Vitamin D
Cereals	
Grains, flours, starches	0
Milk and dairy products	
Cow's milk	0.01–0.03
Human milk	0.04
Dried milk	0.21
Cream	0.01–0.28
Cheese	0.03–0.5
Yoghurt	Trace–0.04
Eggs	
Whole	1.75
Yolk	4.94
Fats and oils	
Butter	0.76
Cod-liver oil	210
Margarine and spreads[a]	5.8–8.0
Meat and meat products	
Beef, lamb, pork, veal	Trace
Poultry	Trace
Liver	0.2–1.1
Fish and fish products	
White fish	Trace
Fatty fish	Trace–25
Crustacea and molluscs	Trace
Vegetables	0

[a] Added during production (vitamin D_2).
Source: Ref. 179.

The U.S. RDAs for breast-fed infants under 6 months are set at 5 to 7.5 micrograms (300 IU)/day, whereas for the ages from 6 months to 24 years they are 10 micrograms (400 IU)/day, considering the increased demand of calcium for the growing skeleton and attainment of the peak bone mass until the third decade. The same intake level has been set for babies and young children up to age of 3 years in the United Kingdom; no supplements are recommended in Australia for this age group. However, a dose of 10 micrograms/day has been recommended for elderly persons in Australia. In the United States, only 5 micrograms/day are recommended for adults; in the United Kingdom, an intake of 10 micrograms/day is recommended for all adults over the age of 65.

2. *Physiological and Biochemical Functions*

The fat-soluble vitamin D and its metabolites readily pass through the cellular membranes and interact with a specific receptor molecule, similar to other steroid hormone receptors (40). This receptor binds $1,25(OH)_2D_3$ more readily and avidly than $24,25(OH)_2D_3$, the $25(OH)D_3$ being least actively bound; in the blood, however, the last two forms of the vitamin bind more avidly than $1,25(OH)_2D_3$, so that it is readily concentrated within the cell. The receptor-bound-$1,25(OH)_2D_3$ is then translocated to the nucleus (Fig. 3), where it binds to the DNA of specific responsive genes. Special loops in the receptor, known as "zinc fingers" (because of their zinc

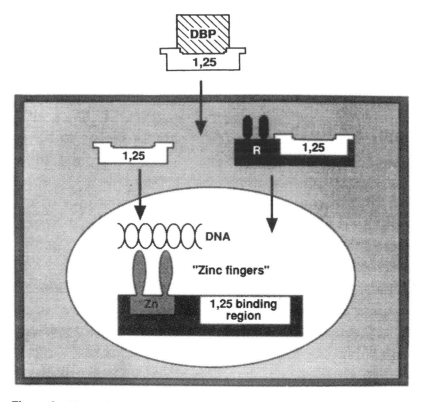

Figure 3 Mechanism of action of 1,25 $(OH)_2D_3$. The biologically active form of vitamin D, 1,25 $(OH)_2D_3$ is carried in the circulation by a vitamin D binding protein (DBP). At the target cell, the 1,25 $(OH)_2D_3$ is released and enters the cell, where it binds to a specific receptor (R), which then translocates to the nucleus, or passes directly to the nucleus before associating with the receptor. 1,25 $(OH)_2D_3$ bound to the carboxy-terminal portion contains structures known as "zinc fingers," which interdigitate with the double helix of DNA, leading to the initiation of the transcription and translation of specific genes and the production of specific proteins involved in the action of 1,25 $(OH)_2D_3$. (From Ref. 3.)

content), which are common to all steroid hormone receptors, enable the receptor to interdigitate with the helical structure of DNA. After binding to the DNA, the receptor induces m-RNA production for the specific protein (or peptide) that is controlled by $1,25(OH)_2D_3$. This process of protein synthesis, including transcription and translation, takes a lag period of about 10 to 12 hours and accounts for the majority of the actions of $1,25(OH)_2D_3$. However, the $1,25(OH)_2D_3$–induced calcium uptake by the small intestine takes place within a matter of minutes, indicating that part of the vitamin D effect does not involve the conventional genomic action on the nucleus (36).

Vitamin D acts to maintain of plasma calcium by stimulating intestinal calcium absorption by the small intestine and by increasing the resorption of calcium from the bone (Fig. 4). The hormone $1,25(OH)_2D_3$ stimulates calcium transport across the intestinal cells by inducing the production of a calcium-binding protein (CBP) within the villi, through the normal process of receptor binding, DNA interaction and production of m-RNA. The resulting CBP maintains the usual extremely low concentration of cytosolic calcium within the cell. The calcium may diffuse into the villi passively, but its transfer into blood appears to involve active transport mechanism, such

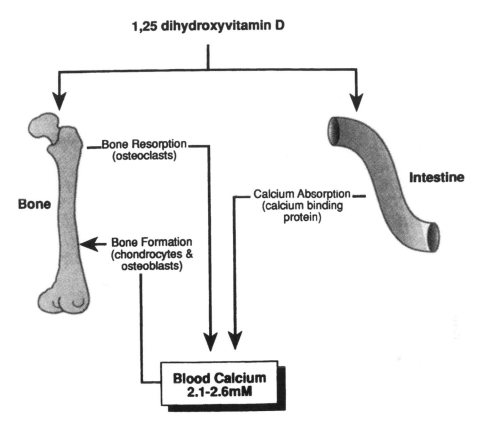

Figure 4 1,25 $(OH)_2D_3$ and calcium homeostasis. Plasma calcium is maintained within tight limits by stimulation of calcium absorption in the small intestine by the hormone 1,25 $(OH)_2D_3$, which activates production of an intracellular calcium-binding protein. The hormone 1,25 $(OH)_2D_3$ also affects bone metabolism, stimulating both resorption and formation of bones. (From Ref. 3.)

as calcium-activated adenosine triphosphatases; $1,25(OH)_2D_3$ also promotes cell maturation within the intestine (41).

Calcium may be sacrificed from the skeleton through bone resorption into the blood plasma to maintain its appropriate concentration for the vital functions such as nerve and muscle activity. A demand for excess supply of calcium in a mature adult with normal calcium balance is met by the skeletal calcium. A decrease in plasma calcium raises parathyroid hormone (PTH), which in turn increases $1,25(OH)_2D_3$ synthesis. The latter acts on the bone-forming cells—the osteoblasts—which produce factors that stimulate the activity of the bone-removing cells, the osteoclasts. The active vitamin D ($1,25(OH)_2D_3$) also promotes bone resorption by increasing the synthesis of new osteoclasts (41), thus increasing both the number and activity of osteoclasts within the bone and removing the bone matrix to release the bound calcium (Fig. 5).

Bone formation is stimulated by $1,25(OH)_2D_3$ by providing sufficient calcium within the body, allowing calcification. Growing children with vitamin D deficiency fail to absorb enough calcium and will have poorly mineralized skeletons. $1,25(OH)_2D_3$ also stimulates the synthesis of osteocalcin protein formed by osteoblasts, which binds up to four calcium ions, and is found exclusively in bone (Fig. 6). $1,25(OH)_2D_3$ also influences bone formation processes, including induction of alkaline phosphatase activity and collagen synthesis. The chondrocytes proliferate, differentiate, and finally are calcified to form bone, the process resulting in the longitudinal bone

OSTEOCLAST ACTIVATION

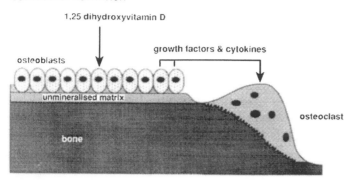

OSTEOCLAST ACTIVATION

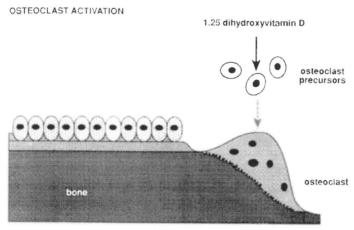

Figure 5   1,25 (OH)$_2$D$_3$ and bone resorption. The hormone 1,25 (OH)$_2$D$_3$ increases bone resorption by stimulating both the activity and the number of osteoclasts that remove bone matrix. The stimulation of osteoclastic activity is indirect, relying on the initial stimulation of the bone-forming cells, osteoblasts, which release cytokines and growth factors that stimulate osteoclastic activity. (From Ref. 3.)

growth (Fig. 6). As the bones mature, the chondrocytes release matrix vesicles, the sites of beginning of calcification. The vitamin D metabolites may influence bone mineralization by altering chondrocyte differenciation, though the need for both 24,25(OH)$_2$D$_3$ and 1,25(OH)$_2$D$_3$ in bone calcification has been disputed (3,42).

Some other metabolic actions of 1,25(OH)$_2$D$_3$ in the process of cellular proliferation and maturation include correction of certain abnormalities associated with the immunohematopoitic system, characterized by increased frequency of infections, impaired neutrophil phagocytosis, anemia, and decreased bone marrow function. 1,25(OH)$_2$D$_3$ receptors being found inactivated (not quiescent) lymphocytes, the hormone 1,25(OH)$_2$D$_3$ stimulates cell proliferation, which partly explains the susceptibility to infection of the rachitic patient. Neonatal skin cells responsible for keratin synthesis produce 1,25(OH)$_2$D$_3$ under experimental conditions that do not occur

GROWTH PLATE MINERALISATION

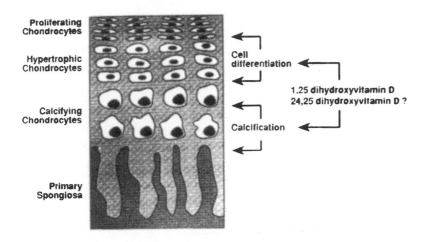

OSTEOBLAST ACTIVITY

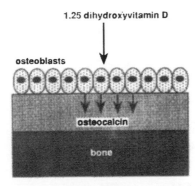

Figure 6   Vitamin D metabolites and growth plate mineralization and bone formation. Longitudinal growth depends on the proliferation, maturation, and calcification of chondrocytes within the ends of the long bones. Both maturation and calcification involve the action of 1,25 $(OH)_2D_3$. A vitamin D metabolite, 24,25 $(OH)_2D_3$, may also play a role in calcification. Bone formation within the skeleton is controlled by osteoblasts, for which 1,25 $(OH)_2D_3$ is required to control formation of certain proteins and enzymes, such as osteocalcin and alkaline phosphatase.

in adults. According to McLaren et al. (3), 1,25$(OH)_2D_3$ may also have a role in the treatment of cancers of blood, lungs, and colon, by inhibiting cellular proliferation.

Typical vitamin D deficiency symptoms include skeletal deformity with bone pain or tenderness and muscle weakness; delayed tooth eruption; and low plasma calcium (in florid rickets). Patients are anemic and prone to respiratory infections.

Adult rickets (osteomalacia) is characterized by a wide seam of unmineralized matrix (osteoid) lining the bone surfaces; it is usually accompanied by bone pain and tenderness in the shoulders, hip, or spine. Hypocalcemia and hypophosphatemia with low plasma levels of 25$(OH)D_3$ are other clinical features (see Chapter 27).

C. Vitamin E (Tocopherols)

A fat-soluble dietary factor, essential for the prevention of sterility and death in rats was identified in 1922 and was called "antisterility factor" or "Factor X." Later named vitamin E, it was isolated from wheatgerm oil in 1936, and called 'tocopherols' (Greek *tocos* and *pherein*, meaning to bring forth children). Several forms of tocopherols are now known to exist naturally, the term, vitamin E being used to denote any mixture of these biologically active tocopherols (43). Animals cannot synthesize tocopherols, which as such are the dietary essential factors to prevent many deficiency syndromes.

Pure vitamin E is a colorless, odorless compound soluble in most organic solvents. Eight naturally occurring tocopherols have been identified and known to be synthesized by plants from homogenistic acid, all derived from 6-chromanol. They differ in the number and position of the methyl groups on the ring structure (Fig. 7). The four tocopherol homologues (alpha, beta, gamma, and delta) have a saturated 16-carbon phytol side chain; in tocotrienols, the side chain has three double bonds. The structural differences are reflected in their biological activity as vitamin E. A synthetic vitamin E (dl-alpha-tocopherol), consisting of a mixture of eight stereoisomers in equal amounts, is often used to fortify animal feeds and available in capsules as a nutritional

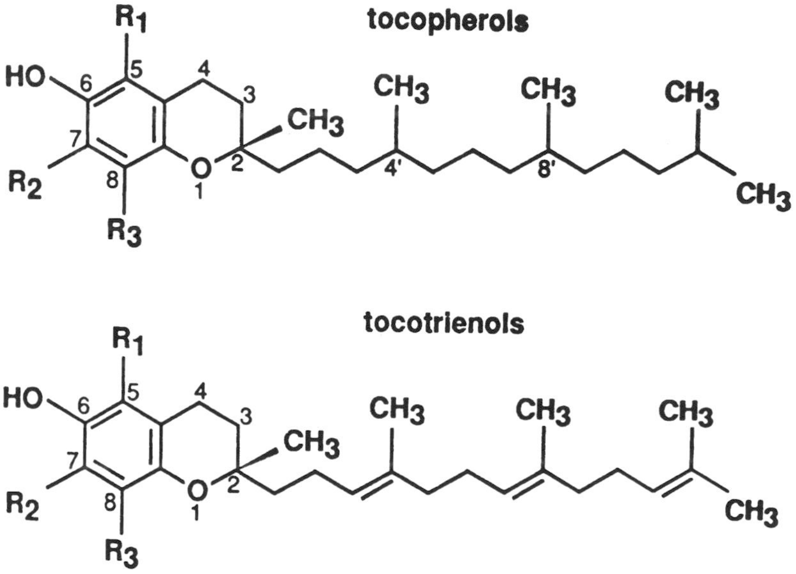

Homologue	Formula	R1	R2	R3
-(alpha)	5,7,8-trimethyl	CH_3	CH_3	CH_3
-(beta)	5,8-dimethyl	CH_3	H	CH_3
-(gamma)	7,8-dimethyl	H	CH_3	CH_3
-(delta)	8-methyl	H	H	CH_3

From Ref. 3.

Figure 7 Structures of naturally occurring tocopherols and tocotrienols. In tocotrienols, the 16-carbon phytol chain has three double bonds, unlike in tocopherols. The number and position of the methyl groups on the chromanol ring denotes different homologues (see table).

supplement. Both tocopherols and tocotrienols are unstable and readily oxidized to quinones, dimers, and trimers by light, alkali, and divalent metal ions such a copper and iron. Commercial vitamin E preparations therefore need to be protected by acetylation and succinylation (3).

1. Sources and Requirements

The relative abundance of the tocopherol homologues in plant oils and fats varies according to species and extraction method used. Gamma-tocopherol, for example, constitutes about 60% of the total tocopherols in soya oil, whereas alpha-tocopherol predominates in safflower and olive oils. Palm oil has significant quantities of alpha and gamma-tocotrienols (44) (Table 4). The nutritional significance of tocotrienols remains to be established. Other major food sources of vitamin E are most vegetables, poultry, fish, fortified breakfast cereals, and wholegrain bread (45) (Table 5).

Vitamin E deficiency has been found to be associated with a variety of disease syndromes related to cell-membrane damage and leakage of cell contents to external fluids in different animals. The most common disorders include myopathies, neuropathies, and liver necrosis. Early clinical features of vitamin E deficiency are leakage of muscle enzymes (creatine kinase) into plasma, increased plasma levels of lipid peroxidation products, and enhanced erythrocyte hemolysis, leading to microcytic anemia.

Infrequent occurrence of clinical signs of vitamin E deficiency, which often develop only in premature infants or in adults with fat malabsorption, pose difficulty in the assessment of vitamin E requirements for humans. Epidemiological evidence suggests that intakes of vitamin E and other antioxidants are inversely correlated with the risk of intestinal, breast, and lung cancer and coronary heart disease (46,47). According to McLaren et al. (3), it is necessary to distinguish between the amount of vitamin E required to avoid overt deficiency and the optimum intake needed to reduce the risk of the development of these diseases.

In addition to infrequent clinical symptoms of vitamin E deficiency, the estimations of the dietary requirements of vitamin E are further complicated by the variation in the composition of the diet and differential biological activities of the homologues. The high dietary intakes of polyunsaturated fatty acids often tend to increase the requirements of vitamin E, because of the increased susceptibility of the tissues to peroxidation. The studies carried out of fetal resorption in pregnancy, and of the susceptibility of red cells to hemolysis and ability to prevent muscular dystrophy, have indicated that the homologues of tocopherol may differ in their biological activity by more than 30-fold. These tests also showed that the d-alpha-tocopherol has the greatest

Table 4 Total and Individual Isomers of Tocopherols in Some Vegetable Oils

Vegetable oil	Total tocopherol (mg/100 g)	Tocopherols				Tocopherols			
		Alpha-	Beta-	Gamma-	Delta-	Alpha-	Beta-	Gamma-	Delta-
Soya	56–160	4–18	—	58–69	24–37	—	—	—	—
Cottonseed	30–81	51–67	—	33–49	—	—	—	—	—
Corn	53–162	11–24	—	76–89	—	—	—	—	—
Coconut	1–4	14–67	—	—	<17	<14	<3	<53	—
Peanut	20–32	48–61	—	39–52	—	—	—	—	—
Palm	33–73	28–50	—	—	<9	16–19	4	34–39	—
Safflower	25–49	80–94	—	6–20	—	—	—	—	—
Olive	5–15	65–85	—	15–35	—	—	—	—	—

Source: Ref. 180.

Table 5 Concentrations of Alpha- and Gamma-Tocopherols in Some
Common Foods

Foods	(mg/100 g edible portion)	
	Alpla-tocopherol	Gamma-tocopherol
Cereals	0.88	0.77
Pulses	0.27	5.66
Nuts and seeds	9.92	10.97
Vegetables	0.81	0.14
Fruits	0.27	No data
Meat	0.31	0.21[a]
Eggs	1.07	0.35
Milk	0.34	No data
Lard	1.37	0.70
Butter	1.95	0.14
Hard margarine	9.09	19.38
Soft margarine	18.92	26.02

[a] Value obtained from third revised version of German Food Composition and Nutrition
  Tables, 1986/87.
Source: Ref. 3.

biopotency of the naturally occurring isomers. The biological activity of vitamin E is expressed
in International Units (IU); 1IU of vitamin E is equivalent to 1 mg of synthetic d-alpha-tocopherol
acetate. The biological activities of d-alpha- and d-gamma-tocopherols are 1.49 and 0.15 IU/mg,
respectively. Vitamin E activity is also expressed alternatively as tocopherol equivalents (TE), 1
mg TE having vitamin E activity equivalent to 1 mg d-alpha-tocopherol, which is in turn equal to
1.49 IU.

Based on the inverse correlations between plasma vitamin E concentrations and mortality
from heart disease and certain cancers, it has been suggested that the dietary requirements of vitamin E should be increased for optimal health, rather than prevention of chronic deficiency; i.e.,
the US RDA value of 10 mg TE/day should be increased fourfold (46). The present mean vitamin
E intake in the U.S. diet is close to the RDA, one-fifth of it coming from fats and oils. The general nutritional advice to reduce total fat intake and increase the proportion of unsaturated fat in
the diet may decrease dietary intake of vitamin E, as opposed to increasing requirements for vitamin E. Also, the high consumption of soya oil in the United States of America accounts for over
50% of total tocopherol intake in the form of the less biologically active gamma-tocopherol present in soya oil (58–69%). Horwitt (48) therefore proposed a basal daily requirement of $5 \cdot 96$ IU
of vitamin E plus a factor for the polyunsaturated fatty acid component of the diet as follows:

Vitamin E requirement (IU) = 5.96 + 0.25 (% PUFA kcal + 9 PUFAs)

The Nutrition Working Group of the International Life Sciences Institute Europe (NWG/ILSIE,
1990) also suggested that until optimum intakes of vitamin E are established by long-term intervention studies, the RDA should be calculated assuming a daily intake of 14 g of polyunsaturated
fatty acid (5% of energy intake) and an energy intake of 2400 kcal/day, with 40% of the energy
derived from fat with a P:S (PUFA: saturated fatty acid) ratio of 0.33 to 0.40. This gives a vitamin E requirement of 18 IU/day or 12 TE/day.

The dietary reference values (DRVs) in the United Kingdom have recently superseded the
US/RDAs, by taking into consideration the practical difficulties of setting the vitamin E require-

ment. The dietary requirement in the United Kingdom is that needed to maintain a serum toco-pherol:cholesterol value above 2.25 micromol/mmol; the DRVs are 3.5 to 19.5 and 2.5 to 15.2 mg alpha-tocopherol/day for men and women, respectively.

Duthie et al. (49) suggested that supplementation with vitamin E reduces free radical activity and possibly the risk of developing heart disease and lung cancer in smokers. Tobacco smoke contains vast quantities of reactive free radicals. The alveolar fluid in smokers is often deficient in vitamin E, and they exhibit signs of increased lipid peroxidation, such as pentane expiration, erythrocyte lipid peroxidation, and high plasma concentrations of conjugated dienes.

2.   Assessment of Vitamin E Status

Plasma concentrations of vitamin E can be used to estimate an individual's vitamin E status. The current European guidelines have sugested the following categories:

Category	Vitamin E (micrograms/ml)
Deficient	Less than 6.5
Marginally deficient	6.5–8.6
Normal	8.6–10.8
Optimum	More than 10.8

McLaren et al. (3) have cautioned against the use of such system, because plasma vitamin E concentrations may not accurately reflect intakes or tissue reserves of vitamin E. According to Lehmann et al. (50), platelet and red cell vitamin E contents may be more valid predictors of nutritional status in humans than the plasma concentrations; Thurham et al. (51) indicate that in the clinical environment, the ratio in serum of tocopherol to total lipid or to cholesterol plus triglyceride may be useful in judging vitamin E status.

3.   Physiological and Biochemical Functions

Vitamin E is a highly effective antioxidant, readily donating its hydrogen from the hydroxyl group on the ring structure to free radicals, which are reactive and potentially damaging molecules with an unpaired electron; the latter on receiving hydrogen becomes unreactive and harmless. Vitamin E has a major biochemical role in protecting polyunsaturated fats and other membrane components from oxidation by free radicals. Vitamin E is therefore primarily located within the phospholipid bilayer of cell membranes.

The damaging free radicals arise during normal aerobic metabolism. Activated oxygen species are formed during stepwise reduction of oxygen to water and through secondary reactions with protons and divalent cations such as copper and iron. The superoxide anion (O^-_2) is produced in many cellular redox systems involving xanthine oxidase, aldehyde oxidase, membrane-associated NADPH oxidases, and cytochrome P-450 system. About 1% to 4% of the total oxygen taken up by mitochondria may be used to produce O^- radicals, and about 20% of this may be ejected into the cell. O^-_2, not being particularly reactive, diffuses through the cell and is then converted in a metal-catalyzed reaction into more reactive and potentially injurious hydroxyl radical (OH*). Free radicals can also come from pollutants, halogenated anesthetics, and cigarette smoke.

Polyunsaturated fatty acids (PUFAs), which are the major constituents of cell membranes, are particularly susceptible to free radical–mediated oxidation, because of their methylene-interrupted double-bond structure. The lipid peroxidation thus leads to disturbances in membrane structure and function (52). The process is briefly initiated by a free radical such as OH*, extracting a hydrogen from PUFA:H, with the formation of a PUFA radical (PUFA*). The double bond is then rearranged to form a conjugated diene, which combines with oxygen to produce a peroxyl radical (PUFAOO*), which in turn reacts with more PUFA:H to form a hydroperoxide (PUFA:OOH) and another PUFA*, leading to a self-propagating reaction (3):

$$PUFA:H \longrightarrow PUFA*$$
$$PUFA* + O_2 \longrightarrow PUFA:OO*$$
$$PUFA:OO* + PUFA:H \longrightarrow PUFA:OOH + PUFA*$$

In the presence of copper or iron, PUFA:OOH can undergo a fission of the double bonds and one electron reduction to form more free radicals, including the highly reactive OH*.

$$PUFA:OOH \xrightarrow[\quad Cu^{++}, Fe^{++} \quad]{} PUFA:O* + OH*$$

Such autoxidation continues until all the free radicals are scavenged by antioxidants. Vitamin E breaks the chain of events leading to the formation of PUFA:OOH by donating hydrogen atom of the hydroxyl group on its chromanol ring to the free radical to form a stable species. The resulting vitamin E radical, being fairly stable, contributes little to the propagation of the chain reactions.

If vitamin E fails to prevent the formation of PUFA:OOH in the cell membrane, as a second line of defense, the PUFA:OOH is released from phospholipids by phospholipase A_2 and is then degraded by selenium-containing glutathione peroxidase in the cytoplasm. The antioxidant activities of vitamin E and selenium through glutathione peroxidase are thus closely related. Other important enzymes having antioxidant roles are superoxide dismutase, catalase, glucose-6-phosphate dehydrogenase and compounds like carotenoids, ubiquinone, uric acid, glutathione, carnosine, and ascorbic acid.

Vitamin E is regenerated in vivo by vitamin C (also in vitro) and by an unidentified reductase that reduces vitamin E radical back to its native state.

Other than its antioxidant function, vitamin E has several other important roles in biological processes (3):

1. Structural maintenance of cell-membrane integrity
2. DNA synthesis
3. Stimulation of immune response,
4. Anti-inflammatory effects by direct and regulatory interaction of vitamin E with the prostaglandin synthetase enzyme complex participating in the arachidonic acid metabolism.

Tocopherols are turned into micelles by bile salts and pancreatic lipase before they can be absorbed from the gut, like lipids. Vitamin E deficiency often occurs in patients with fat malabsorption. Maximum absorption of tocopherols occurs in the upper and middle thirds of the small intestine. The tocopherol uptake is probably enhanced by long-chain polyunsaturated fatty acids. Tocopherol micelles may passively diffuse through the brush border; its further transport across the intestinal epithelial cells has not been resolved. The vitamin is released from enterocyte into the lymphatic system within chylomicrons, which are subsequently degraded in the circulation by lipoprotein lipase (53). The chylomicron remnants are then absorbed by the liver, which preferentially secretes the alpha form of the vitamin E into the plasma in newly formed very-low-density lipoproteins (VLDL), but excretes most of the gamma-tocopherol into the bile (54). The gamma-homologue, therefore, although taken up, constitutes only about 10% of the plasma toco-pherol. The paradoxical discrimination of the organism against gamma-tocopherol, which is abundant in the diet and is also the most effective antioxidant in vitro, has not been resolved.

Tocopherols incorporated within plasma lipoproteins are taken up by the LDL receptors on peripheral cells and are then transported within the cell and incorporated into the cell membranes by an unknown mechanism. Available evidence indicates that cytosolic binding proteins (mol.wt.32,000) and membrane receptors that favor the d-alpha-form of the vitamin are involved in this incorporation (55,56). The tocopherols then accumulate at those sites in the cell where they are needed most, i.e., where the production of O^-_2 radicals is greatest, such as in heavy and light mitochondria, and endoplasmic reticulum (3).

4. *Hyper Vitaminosis E*

Cases of acute and chronic toxicities of oral vitamin E are rare, vitamin E being well tolerated by animals even in pharmacological doses. Animal studies have shown that high doses of vitamin E do not produce mutagenic, carcinogenic, or teratogenic effects. Relatively few side effects have been observed in humans, even at doses as high as 3200 IU/day, although some case reports have indicated that vitamin E may cause breast soreness, muscular weakness, gastrointestinal and emo-tional disorders in some individuals.

A study conducted by Bendich and Machlin (57) showed that a daily intake of 600 IU of vitamin E for 28 days significantly decreased serum thryroid hormone levels, and administration of vitamin E to vitamin K–deficient human subjects could exacerbate coagulation effects. Data are not available to indicate either beneficial or detrimental effects of long-term consumption of pharmacological levels of vitamin E, but daily intakes of 200 to 700 mg of TE appear to be with-out any side effects (3).

Because vitamin E functions as an effective antioxidant against free radicals—and the lat-ter have been implicated in many human diseases—vitamin E supplements have often been used as a therapeutic agent. Diplock et al. (58) suggested that high doses of vitamin E slow down the progression of Parkinson's disease, reduce the severity of neurological disorders such as tardive dyskinesia, prevent periventricular hemorrhage in preterm babies, decrease tissue injury arising from ischemia and reperfusion during surgery, ameliorate malignant hyperthermia syndrome, delay cataract development, and improve mobility arthritis. More research is needed to confirm the possible important uses of vitamin E in preventing, delaying, or curing many human diseases.

D. Vitamin K

An essential blood coagulation factor in the diet was first described by Dam and Schonheyder in Denmark (59). A bleeding disorder in chicken could be cured by feeding a variety of foods, espe-cially lucerne (alfalfa) or putrid fish meal. The active factor identified was called Koagulation-vitamin, which was later isolated by Swiss chemists (Karrer and associates) as a new fat-soluble vitamin, K, in 1939. Shortly thereafter, it was synthesized in America by several groups.

Vitamin K exists in two forms: vitamin K_1 (phylloquinone) and vitamin K_2 (menaquinone); both have 2-methylnaphthoquinone rings with phytyl side chains at position three (Fig. 8). Mena-dione (vitamin K_3) is a synthetic form of vitamin K, with a naphthoquinone ring without a side chain; it is water soluble and becomes biologically active only after alkylation in vivo. Vitamin K_1 occurs only in plants, whereas vitamin K_2 is a group of compounds synthesized by bacteria (some of which occur naturally in animal intestines). The menaquinones (MK) have side chains consisting of a number of isoprene units, varying from 1 to 14 (Fig. 8). Vitamin K is progressively destroyed on exposure to ultraviolet light.

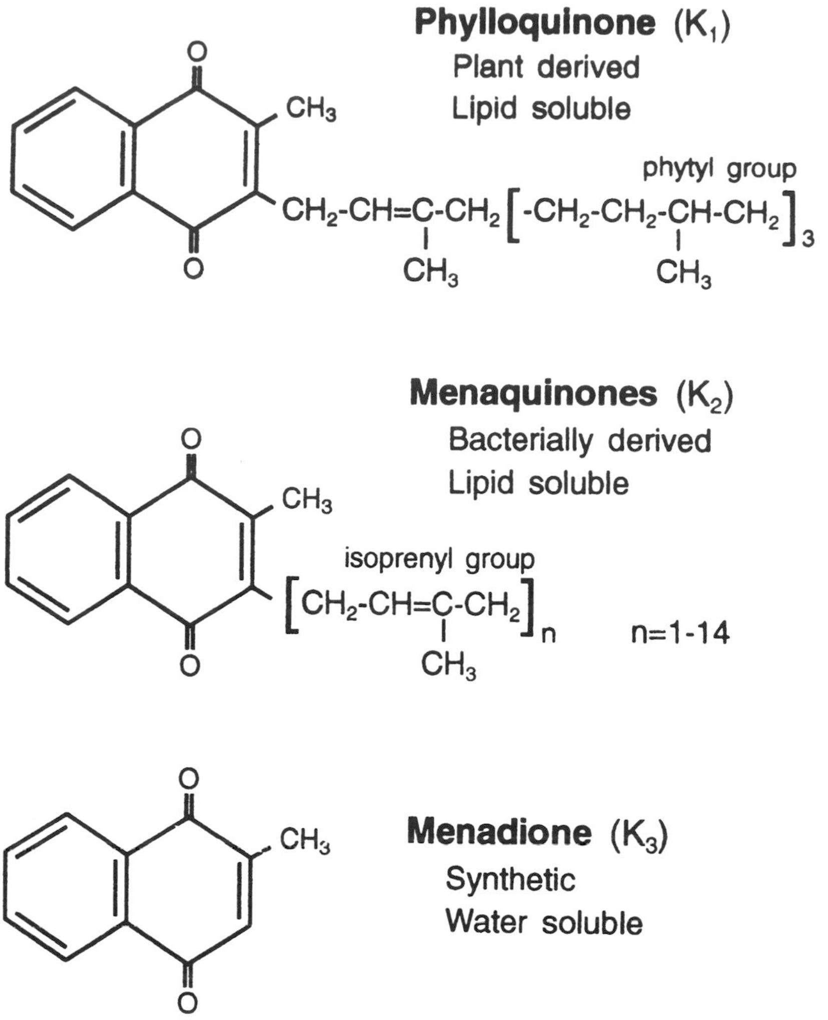

Phylloquinone (K$_1$)
Plant derived
Lipid soluble

$$\text{CH}_2\text{-CH=C-CH}_2 \left[\text{-CH}_2\text{-CH}_2\text{-CH-CH}_2 \right]_3$$

phytyl group

Menaquinones (K$_2$)
Bacterially derived
Lipid soluble

isoprenyl group

$$\left[\text{CH}_2\text{-CH=C-CH}_2 \right]_n \quad n=1\text{-}14$$

Menadione (K$_3$)
Synthetic
Water soluble

Figure 8   Structures of vitamin K. (From Ref. 3.)

1.   Dietary Sources and Requirements

Vitamin K, is ubiquitous in plants and is especially abundant in leafy green vegetables, such as broccoli (150–200 µg/100g) spinach (300–400 µg/100 g), parsley (500–600 µg/100 g), and cabbage. The greener the leaves, the higher the content of vitamin K; the outer, greener cabbage leaves have higher vitamin K content (200 µg/100 g) than the paler inner leaves (50 µg/100 g). Margarines (20–150 µg/100 g) and vegetable oils such as soya oil (around 130 µg/100 g) are also good sources of vitamin K$_1$. Fresh oils are richer sources of vitamin K; exposure to light destroys vitamin K content of foods. Other foods, such as vegetables, fruits, cow's milk, and tea leaves, contain varying smaller amounts of vitamin K (0.4 µg/cup of tea). Certain fermented foods, such as milk products and cheeses, contain bacterially derived vitamin K$_2$, contributing to vitamin K intake. Vitamin K is primarily stored in the liver of animals, constituting a dietary source of vitamin K. Intestinal and colon bacteria synthesize menaquinones K$_2$ and contribute to the physiologically available pool of vitamin K in the body.

According to CMAFP (39), the dietary requirement of vitamin K for adult humans is around 1 μg/kg body weight, and the average daily dietary intake of adults in the United Kingdom varies from 50 to 100 μg, meeting the recommended value. For infants, a higher level of vitamin K, 2 μg/kg body weight (10 μg/day) has been recommended, in view of their lower liver stores and poorly developed gut microflora.

Nearly 50 to 80% of the vitamin K in the small intestine is absorbed, aided by bile salts and pancreatic lipase, like other fat-soluble vitamins. It is then transported to the liver in chylomicrons via the lymphatic and plasma circulation, predominantly in the form of triacylglycerol-rich VLDLs. The liver stores about 90% of menaquinones. The fasting plasma levels of vitamin K in healthy adults and infants range from 0.2 to 0.7 ng/ml and 16 pg/ml to undetectable levels, respectively, but hypertriglyceridemia conditions result in higher circulating vitamin K, up to 13 ng/ml (60). According to Barkhan and Shearer (61), vitamin K is metabolized in to a variety of water-soluble, bile-acid conjugated products that are finally excreted in the urine and feces.

2. Vitamin K Status and Deficiency

Diet, drugs, and surgical interventions are the major factors that influence the vitamin K status of the body. Vitamin K–deficient diets in humans have been shown to elevate levels of prothrombin while depressing the vitamin K levels; these effects are reversed on vitamin K supplementation (62). The diets that enhance colonic fermentation (high in soluble nonstarch polysaccharides and resistant starch) are thought to increase menaquinone (K_2) production. The latter is possibly absorbed from the colon and lower ileum by passive uptake. The gut menaquinones are unlikely to meet the human requirements of vitamin K in the absence of dietary intake of vitamin K.

Dicoumarins (e.g., warfarin), the classic anticoagulant drugs, block the recycling of vitamin K, resulting in bleeding, Warfarin poisoning in rats can be overcome by large oral or intramuscular doses of vitamin K (10–20 mg/8 hr).

Broad-spectrum antibiotics destroy menaquinone-producing intestinal bacteria, and drugs containing N-methylthiotetrazole derivatives may inhibit vitamin K function. Overt vitamin K deficiency in adult humans is rare, barring patients with fat-malabsorption syndromes or post-intestinal surgery who are taking antibiotics. The combination of inadequate absorption of dietary vitamin K, with decreased menaquinone production in the gut can predispose to severe vitamin K deficiency.

3. Physiological and Biochemical Functions

The biochemical function of vitamin K is associated with its ability to change its forms in redox reactions, i.e., quinone and epoxide in the oxidized state and quinol in the reduced form during the vitamin K cycle. The quinol is converted to epoxide by enzyme(s) with epoxidase and carboxylase activity. The latter converts glutamate (glu) residues of proteins to gamma-carboxyglutamate (gla) residues, the proteins then being termed "vitamin K–dependent" or "gla-proteins." The enzymes of vitamin K cycle are located in rough endoplasmic reticular membranes of liver and bone and to a lesser extent in other tissues. The gla-proteins can readily bind to calcium ions, giving them the biological activity of vitamin K (63).

Vitamin K–dependent plasma proteins (gla-proteins) were the first established coagulation proteins, Factors II (prothrombin), VII, IX, and X (64). The calcium-binding properties of these proteins enable them to associate specifically with the acidic phospholipids on cell and platelet membranes, an essential step in the coagulation cascade. Recently, two plasma vitamin K–dependent proteins, C and S, have been identified, which inhibit coagulation by blocking the activation of factors V and VIII. A small amount of bone gla-protein, osteocalcin, found in the plasma may be a useful marker of osteoblast activity and bone function. The osteocalcin is the main gla-protein of mineralized tissue, bone, and dentine, produced by osteoblast and odontoblast cells, respectively, in addition to matrix gla-protein found in both mineralized tissue and cartilaginous tissue. Both osteocalcin and matrix gla-protein bind hydroxyapatite and are thought to be involved in bone mineralization (3,65).

Levels of vitamin K in human milk vary and may be inadequate for some babies who are solely breast-fed. The syndrome, termed hemorrhagic disease of the newborn (HDN), or idiopathic late-onset HDN, occurring between 3 and 8 weeks of life, is characterized by spontaneous bruising/bleeding, or intracranial hemorrhage that may lead to death. This vitamin K deficiency disease is not common in countries such as United Kingdom where vitamin K is given as prophylaxis (66). An oral dose (1 mg) to the infants at birth or 20 mg doses to the mother for several days before parturition have been recommended forms of prophylaxis to meet vitamin K requirements of the babies. The vitamin K deficiency may result either from poor maternal nutrition, inadequate placental transfer, or intestinal malabsorption. HDN detection has been complicated by the normal hypoprothrombinemic state of the newborns.

Thrombosis-associated diseases of vitamin K deficiency include coronary heart disease (CHD) and veno-occlusive diseases (VOD). The hypercoagulable state that predisposes to CHD and VOD is throught to result from high levels of the functional vitamin K–dependent proteins (Factors II, VII, IX and X). Oral anticoagulant therapy reduces the risk of secondary myocardinal infarction, though moderate bleeding may continue as a side effect. More research is required to establish whether low-dose oral anticoagulation regiments are definitely beneficial for the prevention of thrombosis and CHD (67).

Evidence also indicates that lower vitamin K status may prevail in patients with osteoporosis (68). However, owing to the uncertain physiological role of osteocalcin and bone matrix gla-protein, it is not known whether vitamin K in any way is involved in the development of osteoporosis (3).

III.　WATER-SOLUBLE VITAMINS

There are nine water-soluble vitamins, a vitamin C (ascorbic acid) and eight vitamins belonging to a B complex group, viz., thiamin (B_1), riboflavin (B_2), niacin, biotin, pantothenic acid, folacin (folic acid), cyanocobalamin (B_{12}), and pyridoxine (B_6). The function of all these vitamins depends on their chemical structure, and these chemical vitamins are equally effective whether they are derived from natural sources, such as bacteria or yeast, or by synthesis in the laboratory.

The water-soluble vitamins are not normally stored to any extent in the body, and thus vitamins consumed in excess of the body's requirements are excreted through the kidneys. Also, the daily supply of these vitamins is necessary for the body to carry out its normal functions. These vitamins are extensively lost by leaching during cooking and food processing operations. Some of the B group vitamins are derived from the bacterial activity in the small intestine; most others are obtained from sources such as liver, yeast, and bran of cereal grains. Many water-soluble vitamins are synthesized in the laboratory and used as food additives. B vitamins have been grouped together because all of them occur together naturally. Thus, a diet lacking in one B complex vitamin often lacks in other vitamins of the group; as a result, single discretary deficiency diseases involving these vitamins are mostly multiple in nature, though the deficiency symptoms of a specific vitamin of the group may predominate. Most of the vitamins of the B complex group are essential components (coenzymes) of the essential enzymes playing vital roles in the metabolic processes of all living cells.

A. Thiamin (Vitamin B₁)

Thiamin is an anti-beriberi factor isolated first from rice polishings by Funk (28), who used the term *vitamin* to describe this "amine" essential for life. Jansen and Donath (69) isolated thiamin in the crystalline form and tested it in deficient small birds. The structure of thiamin was elucidated and its synthesis accomplished by Williams and Cline (70).

1. Sources and Requirements

Thiamin occurs ubiquitously in all natural foods, plant seeds being the most important sources of thiamin, e.g., whole grain cereals, organ meats, pork flesh, nuts, and legumes. Being water-soluble, it is not present in animal fats and vegetable oils. It is removed easily from cereals by refining and other processing methods. Much of the thiamin in the diet of the Western countries is obtained by eating fortified cereals and breads.

Owing to thiamin's vital role in carbohydrate metabolism, dietary intake is often expressed on the basis of energy intake. According to Sauberlich et al. (71), clinical symptoms of thiamin deficiency are evident at less than 0.12 mg/1000 kcal, and intakes higher than 0.3 mg/1000 kcal are compatible with good health. The British recommendations rely on both urinary thiamin excretion and transketolase activities, and are 0.4 mg/1000 kcal. An additional 0.4 mg/day is recommended in U.S. RDAs to accommodate the higher energy needs of pregnancy and demands of the growing fetus, but no extra allowance is made by the UK. Lactating mothers in the United States of America are advised to consume a total of 0.5 mg/day above the adult requirement to meet secretory losses, whereas the United Kingdom presupposes increased food intake at the RNI of 0.4 mg/1000 kcal (72).

Human subjects with wet beriberi respond dramatically to intramuscular doses of 25 mg of thiamin, followed by three daily oral doses of 10 mg, with an improvement in cardiac function. Dry beriberi (peripheral neuropathy) is more resistant to thiamin treatment. Thiamin injections (50 mg daily for 2–3 days) have been found to cure ocular disturbance of Wernicke disease. Oral doses of 50 mg/day are prescribed for patients with other manifestations of Wernicke-Korsakoff syndrome.

Although no known toxicity is associated with oral thiamin administration, parenteral doses exceeding 400 times the RDA have been reported to cause nausea and mild ataxia (73).

2. Physiological and Biochemical Functions

Thiamin has a pyrimidine ring joined to a thiazole ring (Fig. 9). Thiamin pyrophosphate (TPP) serves as a coenzyme for many enzymes of carbohydrate metabolism, e.g., pyruvate dehydroge-

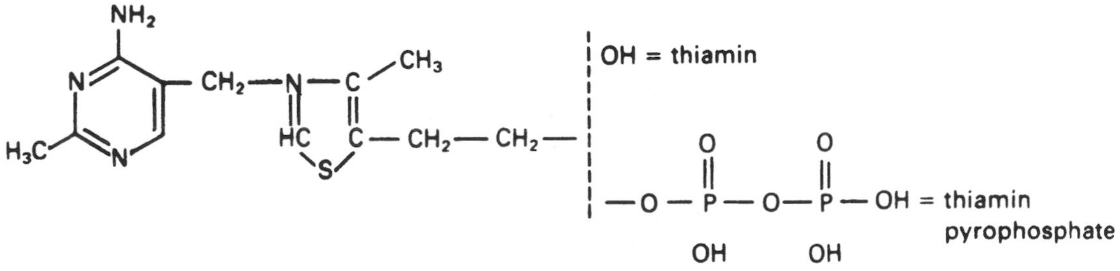

Figure 9   Structure of thiamin. (From Ref. 72.)

nase reaction in the mitochondria. The acetyl-CoA produced by this enzyme is an important substrate for the TCA cycle as well as a precursor for lipids and acetylcholine, providing a biochemical link between TPP and the normal functioning of the nervous system. Even within the TCA (Kreb's) cycle, TPP is a cofactor for the oxidative decarboxylation of alpha-ketoglutarate to succinyl-CoA, and is also required for decarboxylation of the ketoacids of the branched-chain amino acids and for many cytosolic transketolase reactions in the hexose monophosphate pathway (HMP) of glucose oxidation. The latter provides reduced pyridine nucleotides (nicotinamide adenine dinucleotide phosphate, NADPH) for the lipid biosynthesis (72).

Peters (74) noted that the essentiality of TPP for carbohydrate metabolism accounted for the development of brain anoxia and lactic acidosis in thiamin-deficient pigeons. Williams et al. (75) earlier also had observed that lactic acidosis followed excessive carbohydrate administration to severely malnourished patients.

Thiamin is absorbed in the small intestine by an active process involving sodium-dependent adenosine triphosphatase (ATPase). It may also be absorbed passively at plasma thiamin concentrations of more than 1 μmol or at oral intakes of over 5 mg/day. Hoyumpa et al. (76) observed that ethanol inhibited the active, but not the passive intake of thiamin. Around 30 mg of the absorbed thiamin is phosphorylated and stored as TPP in different proportions in heart (2.7 μg/g), brain (1.2 μg/g), liver (1.0 μg/g), and skeletal muscle (0.7 μg/g) (77). Free thiamin circulates in the blood and is excreted in the urine intact, with small amounts of its metabolites as thiamin diphosphate and disulfide. Urinary thiamin excretion decreases rapidly in thiamin deficiency, indicating a renal conservation mechanism (73).

3. Assessment of Thiamin Status and Deficiency

The thiamin status of the body can best be ascertained by an erythrocyte transketolase (ETKA) assay, which measures the availability of TPP for generating hexoses required for HMP pathway (78). Specific values of ETKA can be obtained before and after the in vitro addition of TPP. Thus, more than a 20% increase in ETKA activity after the addition of TPP is taken as an indication of thiamin deficiency, whereas a rise of 0 to 15% denotes thiamin sufficiency.

The old microbiological assay of serum thiamin has now been replaced by the more sophisticated HPLC method (79). Urinary excretion of thiamin and its metabolites before and after oral loading reflects tissue depletion and retention. This method is time consuming, however, and may not detect marginal deficiencies (78).

Thiamin deficiency may set in due to inadequate intake, poor absorption or enhanced metabolic demand. Clinical symptoms of thiamin deficiency are evident in poor malnourished subjects in several parts of Asia and Africa and in patients with intestinal malabsorption, in chronic anorexia and alcoholism as well as in states with increased demand for thiamin during excessive carbohydrate therapy used to cure malnourished patients. Acute symptoms with peripheral neuropathy and lactic acidosis may also occur.

Two types of beriberi occur: wet and dry. Wet beriberi is associated with the development of progressive dyspnea and edema after several years of progressive weakness. Physical symptoms include cardiac failure with a wide pulse rate, tachycardia, enlarged heart, vasodilation, pulmonary congestion, venous distension, and peripheral edema. ECGs and echocardiograms reveal low voltages and a large dilated heart. Dry beriberi is often superimposed on wet beriberi, and shows extreme muscle weakness, with progressive polyneuropathy and intervenal features of Wernicke-Korsakoff disease. In the developing Asian and African countries, the edema in protein-calorie malnutrition, associated with disorders such as marasmus and kwashiorkor, is not accompanied by cardiac failure and other vitamin deficiencies of peripheral neuropathy. In alcoholics, cardiomyopathy results from the toxicity caused by prolonged exposure to alcohol in the absence of thiamin deficiency. Wet beriberi can be diagnosed by rapid cardiac response to thiamin therapy and other laboratory tests for thiamin deficiency.

Thiamin deficiency is commonly seen in chronic alcoholics with liver damage. More than one-third of such patients show low circulating levels of erythrocyte TPP and 50% decrease in hepatic thiamin concentration (in alcoholic hapatitis).

Wernicke-Korsakoff disease is characterized by a horizontal nystagmus of the eyes, paralysis of one or more ocular muscles, a wide-based gait, and a global confusion state (80). Untreated patients develop Korsakoff psychosis, with amnesia for the recent past and the inability to memorize new information. Blass and Gibson (81) suggested a genetic predisposition to Wernicke disease by decreased transketolase activity, with the presence of different isoenzymes (82).

Ocular changes in Wernicke disease often respond dramatically to one or more injections of thiamin, whereas cerebellar gait may require thiamin treatment for months. Korsakoff psychosis, however, is often irreversible (72).

Halsted and Heise (83) showed that thiamin deficiency in humans can be multifactorial. Malabsorption of thiamin is caused by ethanol through acute inhibition of the thiamin-transporting enzyme, Na^+-dependent ATPase and decreased active transport of thiamin across the enterocyte membrane. Folic acid deficiency may also cause inhibition of thiamin absorption in chronic alcoholism. Decreased liver thiamin in alcoholics with liver disease is mainly due to years of poor intake and absorption, with the added effects of acute hepatic inflammation (see Chapter 30).

B. Riboflavin (Vitamin B_2)

Riboflavin is an orange-yellow pigment, changing to a colorless form on reduction. It is less soluble in water than thiamin but is more stable to heat in acid and neutral media, though it is destroyed by heating in alkaline solution. Owing to its heat stability and limited water solubility, very little vitamin is lost during cooking and processing of food. Baking soda used in cooking destroys riboflavin content of the food. Also, on exposure to light, riboflavin readily loses its vitamin activity as the result of photochemical cleavage of the ribitol moiety, forming lumiflavin, which is a stronger oxidant than riboflavin and can destroy a number of other vitamins, such as ascorbic acid.

1. Sources and Requirements

Riboflavin is widely distributed in plant foods and, to a lesser extent, in animal foods. Leafy vegetables, dried yeast, milk, cheese, liver, and eggs are good sources of riboflavin. Pulses and lean meats contain appreciable amounts of riboflavin.

The U.S. RDAs for adults are 1.6 mg/day for males and 1.2 mg/day for females, with an additional 0.3 mg/day during pregnancy and 0.5 mg/day during lactation. Women using oral contraceptives may have increased riboflavin requirements (84).

2. Physiological and Biochemical Functions

Free riboflavin, such as is found in some foods, must be phosphorylated in the intestinal tract before it can be absorbed. On combining with phosphoric acid, riboflavin becomes part of the structure of two flavin coenzymes, flavin mononucleotide (FMN) and flavin adenine dinucleotide (FAD), essential for the activities of flavoproteins, catalyzing oxidation-reduction reactions.

The fused ring structure of flavin nucleotides (the isoalloxazine ring) undergoes reversible reduction, accepting either one or two electrons in the form of hydrogen atoms (electron plus proton) from a reduced substrate ($FMNH_2$ and $FADH_2$). The reduction of flavin nucleotides is accompanied by a change in a major absorption band, which serves as an assay reaction involving a flavoprotein. Some flavoprotein enzymes that employ flavin coenzymes are FMN-requiring NADH dehydrogenase and glycolate dehydrogenase and FAD-requiring succinic dehydrogenase, fatty acyl-CoA dehydrogenase, dihydrolipoyl dehydrogenase, and alpha-glycerophosphate dehydrogenase, which take part in the redox reactions of cells.

Riboflavin is thus essential for growth and has multiple physiological/biochemical functions in the production of corticosteroids, formation of erythrocytes, synthesis of glucose from noncarbohydrate substrates (gluconeogenesis), and thyroid enzyme regulation. Its deficiency in humans results in reddened, denuded areas on the lips, with cracks at the corners of the mouth (cheilosis), swollen and reddened tongue (glossitis), and scaly, greasy dermatitis of the face, ears, and other body parts. Some other deficiency symptoms include eye disorders such as itching, burning, lacrimation, dimness of vision and cataract, general debility, and changes in behavior (84).

C. Niacin

Roe (85) described pellagra as a disease of malnutrition occurring among corn eaters, who developed a particular red rash in sun-exposed areas of the skin, and glossitis. Pellagra has been recognized as three D's disease—with dermatitis, diarrhea, and dementia as its prominent symptoms; it killed many prisoners during the American Civil War of 1861–1865 (85). Goldberger (86) showed that feeding convicts diets devoid of animal protein caused pellagra, which could be treated by substituting a diet of mixed grains for corn. Goldberger established black tongue in dogs as an experimental model, in which a pellagra-like syndrome could be cured by feeding animal protein or a boiled extract of yeast that was almost devoid of protein.

Both nicotinic acid and its amide, nicotinamide, have vitamin niacin activity, and occur naturally in foods in their original forms or as their coenzyme forms, nicotinamide adenine dinucleotide (NAD) and its phosphate derivative, nicotinamide adenine dinucleotide phosphate (NADP), known as pyridine nucleotides. The latter are the essential constituents of the enzymes involved in the energy-yielding reactions of carbohydrate, fat, and protein metabolism. Reduced pyridine nucleotides ($NADH_2$ and $NADPH_2$) can also reduce the riboflavin-containing coenzymes in the electron transport reactions for the release of biological energy.

1. Sources and Requirements

Niacin occurs abundantly in both plant and animal foods, such as lean meat, yeast, fish, poultry, peanuts, pulses, and whole grain cereals. Vegetables and fruits are relatively poor sources of niacin. Bacteria synthesize niacin in the intestine. The tryptophan content of dairy products is more than 1% of protein, thus 60 g of milk or egg protein equals 10 niacin equivalents (NE) or 600 mg niacin; i.e., about 60 mg of tryptophan in the diet are equal to 1 mg of niacin. Meat, being rich in both tryptophan and niacin, supplies large amounts of niacin whereas cereals such as oat meals, rice, or wheat provide moderate amounts. Niacin bioavailability of cereals increases by treatment with lime (72).

Owing to the niacin-sparing effect of tryptophan, the body's niacin requirements are often expressed as niacin equivalents (NE). Niacin requirement and allowances are based on human experimental studies involving measurement of blood and urinary niacin metabolites as an index of tissue saturation, after the subjects have eaten varied amounts of dietary tryptophan and niacin. Jacob et al. (87) recently measured dietary effects on blood and urinary metabolites of niacin. The recommended daily allowance of niacin is 16 to 20 mg for men and 13 to 16 mg for women. An additional 2 NE have been recommended during pregnancy in the United States of America, but not in the United Kingdom, where enhanced tryptophan conversion to niacin during pregnancy has been deemed sufficient.

Halsted et al. (88) noted that the classic disorder pellagra responded dramatically to 100 mg niacin at 4-hour intervals or more slowly in the form of dietary animal protein. A treatment of 40 to 200 mg niacin/day cured pellagra symptoms in Hartnup's disease or in the carcinoid syndrome. Doses up to 1 to 2 g/day are used to treat patients with hypertriglyceridemia and/or hypercholesterolemia. Niacin administration in such large doses, however, results in significant side effects of flushing and stimulates gastric acid secretion, with an enhanced risk of peptic ulcers (89).

2.. *Physiological and Biochemical Functions*

Niacin is the generic name for the specific vitamin nicotinic acid and its amide, nicotinamide (or niacin amide), which is a constituent of the structure of NAD and NADP, the coenzymes of numerous oxidoreductases of the glycolytic pathway, fatty acid metabolism, tissue respiration, and detoxification. In the diet it is present as a protein-bound coenzyme and is hydrolyzed and absorbed as nicotinic acid, nicotinamide, and nicotinamide mononucleotide (NMN).

Nicotinamide has been isolated from both NAD and NADP. The relationship of dietary tryptophan to niacin was isolated through human experiments, by monitoring niacin metabolism, after the administration of tryptophan in different doses. Goldsmith et al. (90) demonstrated that 60 mg of tryptophan in the diet of humans produced the same metabolic effect as 1 mg of niacin, tryptophan being converted to nicotinic acid as follows:

Tryptophan

    ↓   Tryptophan 3,2 dioxygenase

Kynurenine

    ↓

3-OH-Kynurenine

    ↓   Kynureninase, vitamin B_6

3-OH-anthranilic acid

    ↓   (several intermediate steps)

Nicotinic acid

3. *Assessment of Status and Deficiency*

Blood niacin content cannot be measured by any specific method directly. Urinary excretion of its metabolite, 1-methylnicotinamide, is decreased in subjects with niacin deficiency to less than 0.5 mg/g creatinine (78).

Deficiency of niacin is common in the form of pellagra in parts of Asia and Africa and is found in malnourished alcoholic patients, and also in patients with Hartnup's disease, an autosomal recessive disorder marked by impaired absorption of certain amino acids like tryptophan. Pellagrous symptoms are also seen in carcinoid syndrome, in which endogenous tryptophan is diverted into excessive production of serotonin and away from the niacin pathway (72).

D. Pyridoxine (Vitamin B_6)

Gyorgy (91) first identified and isolated a heat-labile factor that cured a scaly dermatitis in rats fed purified diets. This factor was later known to be pyridoxine or vitamin B_6, whose structure and synthesis was established in 1939, followed by definition of its active form as pyridoxal phosphate.

Vitamin B_6 naturally occurs in three forms: pyridoxine, pyridoxal, and pyridoxamine (Fig. 10). Synthetic pyridoxine hydrochloride with vitamin B_6 activity is also available for pharmaceutical uses. All three natural forms of vitamin B_6 are phosphorylated in the 5-position and oxidized to the active coenzyme form, pyridoxal phosphate. Drugs such as penicillamine that bind

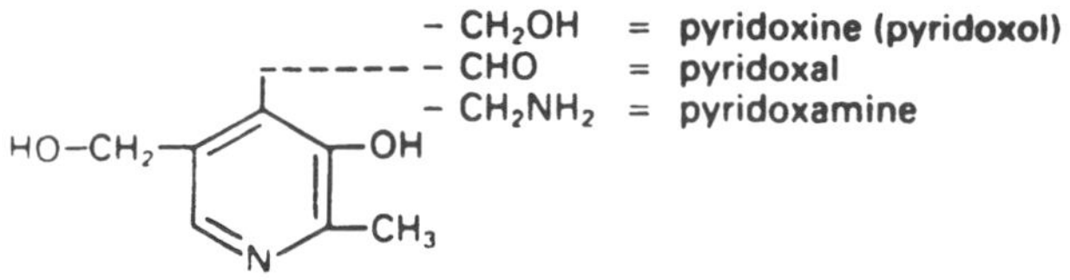

Figure 10 Structure of pyridoxine (Vitamin B$_6$). (From Ref. 72.)

pyridoxal phosphate can produce vitamin B$_6$ deficiency, in addition to a number of natural phosphorylation-inhibiting molds and fungi (92).

1. Sources and Requirements

Animal foods, such as poultry, fish, pork, eggs, liver, and kidney, are rich sources of pyridoxine. Vitamin B$_6$ is also present in plant foods such as soybeans, oats, peanuts, walnuts, and whole grain cereals in fairly good amounts. The availability of pyridoxine from different foods varies greatly, about 60 to 80% of the vitamin being absorbed from the pure product (93). A considerable amount of the vitamin may be lost due to freezing and thawing of foods (94).

The amount of vitamin B$_6$ required in the human diet is directly proportional to the amount of protein in the diet. The requirements of vitamin B$_6$ for both men and women are 1.6 to 2.0 mg/day, with supplementation of 2.5 mg/day for pregnant and lactating women.

Higher doses of pyridoxine in doses of 2 to 10 mg/day are used only in cases of suspected or proven deficiency. Larger doses (up to 100 mg/day) have been used to treat peripheral neuropathy, associated with chronic alcoholism or when drugs like penicillamine are used. Oral vitamin B$_6$ is often given routinely with these drugs.

Attempts to treat menstrual syndrome with chronic doses of 100 to 200 mg of pyridoxine was found to result in severe toxicity in the form of sensory neuropathy of hands and feet (95).

2. Physiological and Biochemical Functions

Pyridoxal phosphate is a coenzyme for numerous biochemical reactions related to protein metabolism, e.g. aminotransferases and decarboxylases. Pyridoxal phosphate-dependent decarboxylation is a central reaction for the synthesis of several amines, including epinephrine, norepinephrine, and serotonin. The coenzyme is also required for aminolevulinic acid synthetase activity, catalyzing reaction in the synthesis of heme from glycine and succinyl coenzyme A. Vitamin B$_6$ also plays an important role in glycogen metabolism and in sphingolipid synthesis in the nervous system (92). It is also intimately involved in the synthesis of niacin from tryptophan.

The phosphorylated forms of dietary vitamin B$_6$ are hydrolyzed by the intestinal alkaline phosphatases, before being absorbed. They are rephosphorylated in the liver, kidney, and brain to form pyridoxal phosphate by an oxidase. The latter reaction can also occur in erythrocytes, where pyridoxal phosphate is bound to hemoglobin. An alkaline phosphatase converts vitamin B$_6$ to free pyridoxal, and hepatic and renal aldehyde oxidase converts unbound pyridoxal phosphate to pyridoxic acid, which is excreted by the kidney (92).

3. Assessment of Status and Deficiency

Different forms of vitamin B$_6$ can be directly measured in serum and urine by microbiological methods. The plasma pyridoxal phosphate can be measured using labeled tyrosine. The normal plasma values are 5 to 23 mg/ml. Pyridoxine metabolites may be measured indirectly in the tryptophan-niacin pathway. Urine tests carried out after tryptophan loading are time consuming.

Pyridoxine deficiency may result from drug antagonism, congenital disorders, certain chronic diseases, intestinal malabsorption, and alcoholism. Clinical symptoms of vitamin B_6 deficiency include inflammation of tongue, lesions of the lips and corners of the mouth, and peripheral neuropathy. The deficiency often sets in clinically with other water-soluble vitamin deficiencies. Infants fed formula diets deficient in vitamin B_6 may have seizures with decreased activity of pyridoxal phosphate-dependent glutamate decarboxylase (96). Deficient pyridoxine-dependent aminolevulinic acid synthetase results into sideroblastic anemia, expressed as unincorporated iron granules in the red-cell precursors of the bone marrow (97).

Biochemical B_6 deficiency symptoms are seen within 2 weeks on a B_6-free diet, with abnormal excretion of xanthurenic acid following tryptophan loading due to decreased activity of pyridoxal phosphate–dependent kynurinase. The plasma pyridoxal phosphate and urinary excretion of pyridoxic acid are also decreased (98).

Several drugs (e.g., isoniazid, used to treat tuberculosis, and penicillamine, for treating Wilson's disease) act as antagonists complexing pyridoxine (99). Women taking oral contraceptive agents have been reported to develop abnormalities of tryptophan metabolism, consistent with vitamin B_6 deficiency (100). Pharmacological doses of vitamin B_6 may help to suppress some symptoms induced by contraceptive drugs, though the latter do not increase B_6 requirements.

Based on the involvement of pyridoxal phosphate in the synthesis of neurotransmitters and sphingolipid, deficiency of vitamin B_6 has been suggested in neurological disorders, such as Down's syndrome (101) and epilepsy (102), and in patients with Parkinson's disease who are receiving levodopa treatment (99). McCully (103) observed that homocystinuria, a congenital disorder in the conversion of homocysteine to methionine, can result from vitamin B_6 deficiency, with a possibility of accelerated development of atherosclerosis.

Pyridoxine deficiency has also been reported in patients undergoing dialysis for chronic renal failure due to accelerated loss of pyridoxal phosphate (104), in celiac disease (105), in patients with biliary obstruction and/or cirrhosis (106), in which loss of pyridoxal phosphate is enhanced by the increased hepatic levels of alkaline phosphatase, as in many chronic alcoholic patients.

Halsted and Heise (83) noted low serum levels of pyridoxal phosphate in 50 to 80% of alcoholics, depending on the presence of liver disease, multiple vitamin deficiencies being more common. Vitamin B_6 deficiency changes the pattern of serum amino transferases, with a 2 to 1 ratio of aspartate to alanine aminotransferase in alcoholics with liver damage. This enzyme depends on pyridoxal phosphate and its routine measurement aids diagnosis of vitamin B_6 deficiency in alcoholism, though the latter is a multifactorial syndrome including poor diet, decreased release of the vitamin from bound food proteins, and enhanced degradation and excretion of the vitamin from the body (72).

E. Folic Acid (Folacin)

Folic acid (Latin, *folium* or leaf) was first isolated from spinach leaves and is widely distributed in green leafy vegetables and other plants. Nutritionists use the term folacin to include a number of related compounds exhibiting the biological properties of folic acid.

British physician Lucy Wills (107) induced macrocytic anemia in rats and monkeys by feeding them a purified diet and cured it with yeast or liver extract. These remedies also cured anemic human subjects. The specific effects of folic acid on the macrocytic anemia of poverty have been demonstrated (108,109).

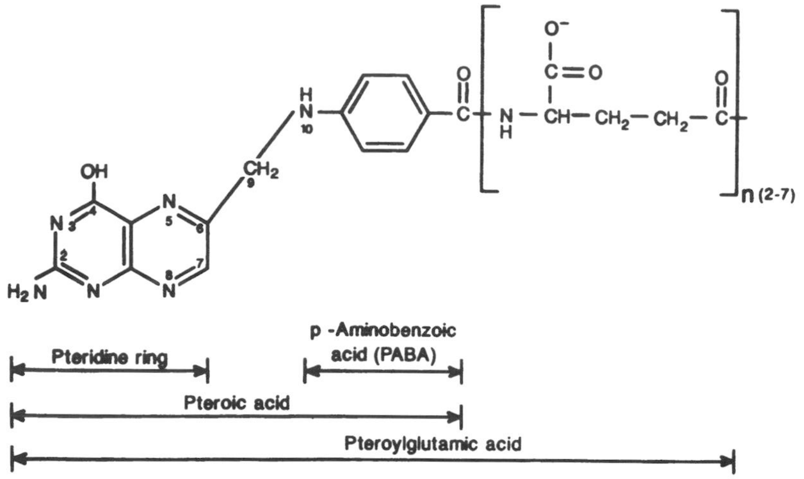

Figure 11 Structure of folate. Monoglutamyl folate (pteroylglutamic acid) is reduced at the 5-, 6-, 7-, and 8- positions of the pteridine ring to form H_4 folate, and substituted at the 5-position to form 5-methyl-H_4 folate, the circulating form of the vitamin. Addition of 2–7 glutamates in the gamma linkage results in polyglutamyl folate (pteroylpolyglutamate), the major dietary and intracellular form of the vitamin. (From Refs. 72 and 135.)

Folacin belongs to a group of compounds known as pterins, consisting of three components: a pteridine ring attached to p-aminobenzoic acid, (PABA) which is coupled with glutamic acid. Thus, folacin is chemically pteroyl glutamic acid (Fig. 11). In many foods, folic acid contains more than one glutamic moity, with glutamates linked in peptide bonds. In addition, 5, 6, 7, and 8 positions of the pteridine ring may be reduced in various forms to yield a range of di- or tetrahydro folates (110).

1. Sources and Requirements

Leafy green vegetables, nuts, whole grains, and liver and yeast are rich sources of folates. About three-fourths of dietary folic acid occurs in the form of polyglutamates. Boiling and cooking during food preparation cause loss of folates (111). Endogenous inhibitors of folate hydrolase and other factors limit the availability of folacin from different food sources. Tamura and Stockstad (112) studied changes in urinary folate excretion as an index of absorption, by following intakes of different foods of known folate content. The availability of folate from lettuce, eggs, oranges, and wheat germ was about one-half that from lima beans, liver, yeast, and bananas.

It is assumed that about 50% of polyglutamyl dietary folate is absorbed, for the purposes of estimating requirements. Based on metabolic ward studies, daily intakes of 200 to 250 µg of dietary folate were found to be sufficient to sustain normal red-cell folate levels. In Canada, folate dosages of 150 to 200 µg/day resulted in a folate content of 3µg/g, in liver autopsy samples with only 8 to 10% of the population's red-cell folate falling below 150 µg/ml. On this basis, the RNIs in the UK have been set at 200 pg of folate per day, the US RDAs are 3 pg/kg body weight for adults of all ages. During pregnancy, the needs for folacin are enhanced substantially to meet the demands of the growing fetus. Unsupplemented pregnant women are at risk for premature birth (113) or bearing small-for-dates babies (114). Red-cell folate levels can be maintained at normal by supplements of 100 µg/day (115). Human milk contains about 50 µg of folate/1 providing 40 to 45 µg of folate/day, so there is an increased drain on folate stores of lactating mothers. Assuming a minimal 50% absorption of dietary folate, the US RDA for pregnancy and for the first 6 months of lactation is set at 400 µg/day and 280 µg/day, respectively, whereas the UK RNI are 300 and 260 µg/day, respectively. Zinc supplements must be considered while providing folate supplements given before and during pregnancy, because oral folate supplements may reduce zinc absorption (116).

Unborn children are at risk for megaloblastic anemia because small folate stores in them are rapidly used for growth. Infants fed human milk grow well on about 40 µg folate/day, without anemia. Since formula feeds result in red-cell folate levels lower than those in breast-fed babies, despite providing a higher folate intake, the UK RNIs have been set at 50 µg/day in boiled milk or goat's milk, which contains substantially less folate than human or cow's milk (117).

Folacin supplements of 1 mg/day are used in chronic diseases associated with deficiency risks. Klipstein (118) noted that patients with malabsorption, anemia and intestinal pathology responded to a folacin dose of 5 mg/day, together with the tetracycline antibiotic.

Folacin toxicities are extremely rare. Drugs such as diphenylhydantoin given for epilepsy, being folate-antagonists, produce convulsions on excessive doses. Whereas folic acid decreases the drug's concentration in the cerebrospinal fluid and increases excitatory effects, the drug itself produces folate deficiency anemia (119).

2. Physiological and Biochemical Functions

Folic acid is pteroyl glutamate (PteGlu), a monoglutamyl form of the vitamin. Reductions and substitutes in the pteridine ring constitute 5-methyl-H_4 folate, the circulating form of the vitamin. The addition of up to 7 glutamates in gamma-carboxyl linkages enhances folate-dependent reactions by producing polyglutamyl folate, the major form in which both dietary and intracellular folates occur.

The major biochemical function of folate coenzymes is the transfer of single-carbon atoms in reactions essential to the metabolism of several amino acids and nucleic acid synthesis (110). The folacin interacts with vitamin B_{12} in the action of methionine synthetase. The H_4-folate is in turn required for polyglutamation and to make 5,10-methylene-H_4 folate, a cofactor of thymidylate synthetase reaction in the DNA synthesis. Lack of either folate or vitamin B_{12} decreases supply of H_4 folate, limiting the production of both polyglutamyl folate and DNA (72).

Folic acid in the diet exists in the form of polyglutamated, reduced, and substituted pteroylglutamate, which are hydrolyzed to the monoglutamyls that are actively transported and absorbed by enterocytes. In humans, there are two folate hydrolases in the intestinal mucosa, one in the brush-border membrane and the other in the intracellular lysosomes.

Zinc is essential for polyglutamyl folate hydrolysis. The hydrolyzed monoglutamyl folate derivative binds to a specific folate receptor on the brush border of the enterocyte, which probably transports the vitamin (120).

The liver is the major storage site for folate, containing about 7 pg folate/g; total body folate is about 7.5 ± 2.5 mg in healthy adults (111,121). In the liver, 5-methyl-H_4 folate is converted to H_4 folate, by donating its methyl group to methionine. H_4 folate then reacts with polyglutamate synthetase to reestablish polyglutamyl folate, which is bound to several enzymes, serving the metabolic functions of the vitamin. Hydrolyzed folate leaves the liver to circulate in both plasma and bile as 5-methyl-H_4 folate, and is taken up and utilized by bone marrow, circulating as polyglutamates in the red-cell-pool. 5-methyl-H_4 folate is concentrated in the bile and may be conserved through intestinal reabsorption (122). Folic acid is finally excreted in both urine and feces in the form of 5-methyl-H_4 folate (72).

3. Assessment of Status and Deficiency

Microbiological methods using *Lactobacillus casei* or radioassays are commonly employed to measure serum folate levels, more than 5 ng/ml being considered normal. Tissue folate deficiency is directly reflected in the red cell levels; over 160 ng/ml is taken as normal. Megaloblastic bone marrow with anemia may occur due to the development of hypersegmentation of neutrophil nuclei, with identical symptoms of vitamin B_{12} deficiency and pernicious anemia (low red cell folate) (123).

Experimental nutritional folate deficiency in man was reported by progressively measuring serum folate levels, after subjects ate a monotonous diet of thrice-boiled and extracted food (124). Serum folate levels fell by 3 weeks, with tissue depletion by 7 weeks. Hypersegmented nuclei in circulating neutrophils and a fall in red-cell folate were evident by 17 weeks, followed by megaloblastic anemia in 20 weeks.

Essentiality of folate for DNA synthesis enables expression of clinical deficiency of folate in tissues with high cell turnover rates. In addition to megaloblastic anemia, jejunal biopsy in folate-deficient alcoholics indicates megaloblastosis of the absorbing intestinal enterocytes (125) and in tropical sprue (118).

Halsted (72) grouped etiology of folate deficiency into five categories: (a) decreased dietary intake (inadequate or improper diets), (b) decreased intestinal absorption (patients with celiac disease or tropical sprue), (c) increased requirements (multiple pregnancies, unsupplemented lactation, hemolytic anemia, and leukemia), (d) drug effect (salicylazosulfapyridine in patients with inflammatory bowel), and (e) chronic alcoholism (decreased folate availability to the bone marrow and lower liver storage).

F. Cobalamin (Vitamin B$_{12}$)

Being found as a co-ordination complex with cobalt, vitamin B_{12} is also known as cobalamin or cyanocobalamin, the commercial and therapeutic product. Several cobalamin compounds show vitamin B_{12} activity. Minot and Murphy (126) reported that pernicious anemia (PA) was a nutritional disorder that could be cured by a diet containing 100 to 200 g of whole calf liver. A water-soluble liver extract given by injection was also found to be effective in treating PA. Castle (127) cured PA by orally giving beef muscle (extrinsic factor), together with normal human gastric juice (intrinsic factor). The extrinsic factor, vitamin B_{12} was later isolated from the liver (128,129). An intrinsic factor described by Castle (127) was found to be a glycoprotein secreted by perietal cells of stomach, required for the absorption of vitamin B_{12} (130).

1. Sources and Requirements

Vitamin B_{12} is present in animal food proteins, liver and kidney being excellent sources. Milk, muscle, meat, cheese, eggs, and seafood are also good sources of vitamin B_{12}. Because plant foods do not contain vitamin B_{12}, vegetarians may not obtain sufficient vitamin B_{12} from their diet. However, human requirements of this vitamin are very low and are generally met by intestinal bacterial synthesis. Vitamin B_{12} is water-soluble and fairly heat-stable, though most of the vitamin may be lost by heating in alkaline solutions or in the presence of reducing agents such as ascorbic acid and sulfite.

All vitamin B_{12} is synthesized by bacteria, fungi, or algae and reaches the human diet after it is incorporated into animal protein, following intestinal bacterial synthesis, including the human's (131).

The forms of vitamin B_{12} in the diet include mainly 5-deoxyadenosyl and hydroxocobalamin, with lesser amounts of methylcobalamin in dairy products, and little or no cyanocobalamin.

Current recommendations of vitamin B_{12} are based on body-pool size and turnover studies, and the minimal amounts needed to maintain normal health or to treat PA, i.e., 0.5 to 1.0 µg/day (132). Vegetarians may develop vitamin B_{12} deficiency on diets containing 0.5 µg/day or less (133). The US RDAs and UK RNIs have been set at 2 µg/day and 1.25 µg/day, respectively; an additional quantity, 0.5 µg/day, is recommended for pregnant and lactating women.

Whereas vegetarians may be advised to take multivitamin supplements containing vitamin B_{12} routinely, patients with intrinsic factor (IF) deficiency can be treated with oral vitamin B_{12} doses exceeding 300 µg/day, because only about 1% of the vitamin is absorbed without IF binding (123). According to Herbert and Colman (123), a practice of administering 100 to 1000 µg of vitamin B_{12} through i.m. injections each month is more reliable. There is no known toxicity of vitamin B_{12} in single doses upto 1000 µg (72).

2. Physiological and Biochemical Functions

Vitamin B_{12} has a porphyrin-like ring structure with cobalt linked to ribose and phosphoric acid (Fig. 12).. Dietary forms of vitamin B_{12} analogues include 5-deoxyadenosyl cobalamin, methyl-cobalamin, and hydroxocobalamin. Vitamin B_{12} is a coenzyme factor in only two known human enzymes, viz., methionine synthetase and methyl-malonyl-CoA mutase (134).

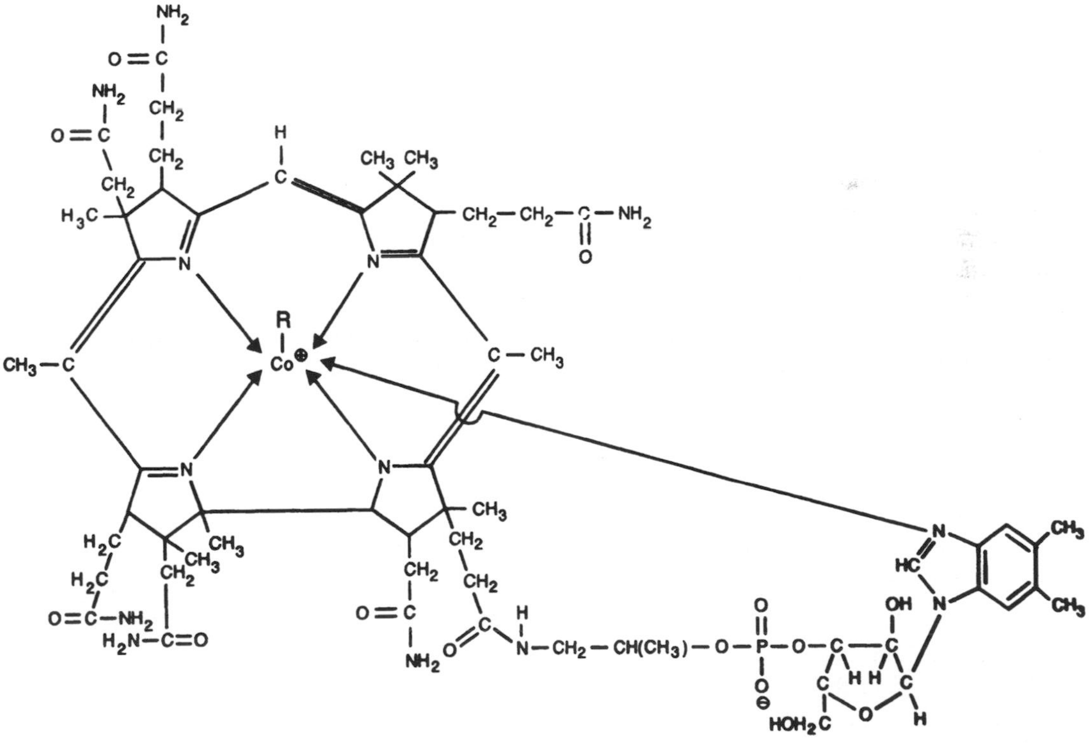

Figure 12   Structure of vitamin B_{12}. Substitutions at R-position include CN (cyanocobalamin), OH-(hydroxocobalamin), 5′-deoxyadenosyl (5′-deoxyadenosylcobalamin), and CH_3 (methylcobalamin). (From Ref. 72.)

Methionine synthesis takes place in the cytoplasm and involves folate. The methyl group of 5-methyltetrahydrofolate (5-methyl H_4 folate) is transferred to cobalamin to form methylcobalamin, which in turn donates the methyl group to homocysteine. The end products of this reaction are methionine, cobalamin B_{12}, and H_4 folate; the latter is required for the synthesis of polyglutamyl folates and 5,10-methylene-H_4 folate, the cofactor for thymidylate synthetase required for DNA synthesis. The essentiality of vitamin B_{12} in the methionine biosynthesis thus accounts for the development of megaloblastic anemia when both vitamin B_{12} and folacin are deficient (135).

Methylmalonyl CoA mutase reaction taking place in mitochondria requires deoxyadenosylcobalamin as a cofactor, to convert methylmalonyl CoA to succinyl-CoA. This reaction is essential for the degradation of propionate and odd-chain fatty acids, especially in the nervous system. When vitamin B_{12} is deficient, methylmalonate accumulates with acidosis and high serum glycine and glucose concentrations (134). Reduction in the activity of methylmalonyl CoA mutase probably accounts for the neurological changes, though this concept has been challenged based on animal studies of nitrous oxide–induced vitamin B_{12} deficiency (136).

Approximately 70% of vitamin B_{12} is absorbed at normal intake levels, which may decrease to less than 10% at intakes greater than 5 times the RDA (117). Dietary vitamin B_{12} is released from its bound protein by gastric acid and pepsin and rebound immediately to R (rapid electrophoretic mobility) proteins in the stomach. The latter are secreted in saliva, gastric juice, and bile. Pancreatic trypsin releases vitamin B_{12} from the R proteins in the duodenum and it is bound immediately to intrinsic factor (IF). The vitamin B_{12} IF complex binds to a specific receptor on the brush border membrane of the terminal ileum, where it is taken up and split within the enterocyte (137,138). The vitamin is then transferred to another protein (transcobalamin II) (139,140), and transported to the liver, taking about 8 to 12 hours from ingestion of the vitamin to its appearance in the portal vein (138). The transcobalamin-II–bound vitamin B_{12} is transported to various tissues by specific receptors. The R factors, TC-1, TC-3, and haptocorrin, are the glycosylated binding proteins found in plasma and other secretions and have a role in vitamin B_{12} absorption, transportation and their disposal in the bile (141). Over 95% of the intracellular vitamin B_{12} appears to be bound to either cytoplasmic methionine synthetase or to mitochondrial methylmalonyl CoA mutase (72,134).

3. Assessment of Status and Deficiency

Out of the body pool of 2 to 3 mg of vitamin B_{12}, daily about 1.2 to 1.3 µg is excreted in the urine and feces (142). Lack of intrinsic factor can interrupt intestinal absorption of vitamin B_{12}, leading to development of deficiency within 4 to 10 years (117). Endogenous vitamin B_{12} is more efficiently absorbed by the ileum than its other analogues (143). Thus, vitamin B_{12} deficiency develops very rapidly through its interruption in the enterohepatic circulation caused by ileal disease or surgery.

Herbert (144) noted that functional changes in vitamin B_{12}–related metabolism occur as tissue B_{12} levels fall, followed by decrease in serum B_{12} levels below 200 pg/ml. The latter can be measured by microbiological methods, aided recently by the radioassay.

Functional vitamin B_{12} deficiency can be diagnosed by appearance of hypersegmented polymorphonuclear neutrophills in the circulation, with an increased "lobe average" (123). At this time, the red-cell folate levels fall below 140 mg/ml. The need of vitamin B_{12} for the conversion of circulating 5-methyl-H_4 folate to metabolically active H_4 folate results in a normal or elevated serum folate but a decreased red-cell folate level. In the final stage of deficiency (anemia), enlarged red blood cells appear with an enhanced mean corpuscular volume, low hemoglobin level, and megaloblastic red-cell precursors in the bone marrow.

Because both vitamin B_{12} and folate interact in the synthesis of methionine, a deficiency of either is associated with elevated serum levels of the precursor, homocysteine (145).

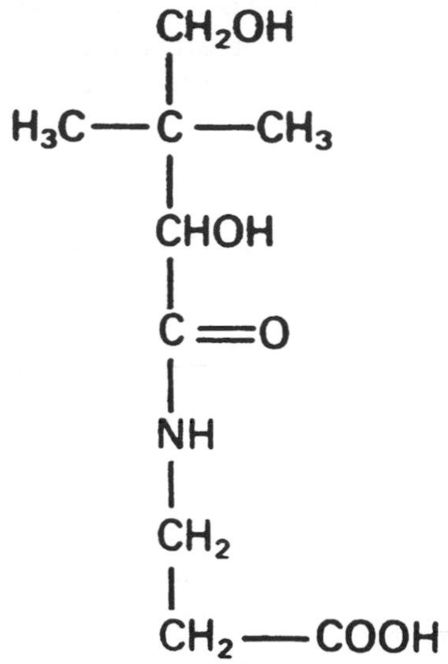

$$
\begin{array}{c}
CH_2OH \\
| \\
H_3C - C - CH_3 \\
| \\
CHOH \\
| \\
C = O \\
| \\
NH \\
| \\
CH_2 \\
| \\
CH_2 - COOH
\end{array}
$$

Figure 13   Structure of pantothenic acid. (From Ref. 72.)

G.   Pantothenic Acid

Pantothenic acid was discovered as a vitamin during investigations of an antidermatitis growth factor from yeast. It is a dimethyl derivative of butyric acid linked to beta-alanine (Fig. 13). The vitamin is linked through phosphate to form 4′—phosphopantetheine and CoA, the primary active form. As a constituent of CoA and its esters, the vitamin is essential for several biochemical reactions of carbohydrate and lipid metabolism, including fatty acid synthesis and degradation, gluconeogenesis, and synthesis of steroid hormones.

1.   Sources and Requirements

As its name indicates, pantothenic acid is widely distributed in nature, especially in animal products, whole grain cereals and legumes. Intestinal bacteria may synthesize some amount of this vitamin. It is more stable in solutions, at pH range 4 to 7, than in the dry form, and is decomposed by alkali and dry heat. Being very widely distributed in a variety of foods, pantothenic acid deficiency is not common in humans. However, its deficiency can be induced by administering metabolic antagonists, such as omega-methyl pantothenic acid, with symptoms like pain in arms and legs, loss of appetite, nausea, indigestion, and increased susceptibility to infection.

Experimental data are not enough for RDAs or RNIs, though intakes of 3 to 7 mg/day are thought to be safe for adults, and more than 5 mg/day is adequate during pregnancy and lactation, and 2 to 3 mg/day is adequate for children up to 11 years. There are no specific therapeutic uses of pantothenic acid and no reports of serious toxicity with excessive intakes of up to 10 g/day.

2.   Physiological and Biochemical Functions

The 4′-phosphopantetheinyl moiety binds to acyl carrier protein, which functions in acyl-group transfer reactions (146). The primary physiological role of pantothenic acid is that as a component of coenzyme A, it is involved in acetylation and other acylation reactions concerned with the release of energy from carbohydrates, glucose synthesis, fatty acid metabolism, and syntheses of steroids and steroid hormones.

Pantothenic acid ingested as a part of CoA is hydrolysed by intestinal phosphatases to yield 4-phosphopantetheine and pantothenic acid, the absorbable form of the vitamin (147). CoA is resynthesized in liver cells, and after it is used is finally excreted in the urine, mainly as a metabolic product of CoA.

3. Assessment of Status and Deficiency

The blood and urine status of pantothenic acid can be measured by microbiological or radioimmunoassay (148). Normal blood values of pantothenic acid are more than 100 µg/dl; urinary excretion ranges between 1 and 15 mg/day (149). The urinary values of pantothenic acid are considered a sensitive indicator of dietary intake. According to McCormick (146), red blood cell CoA levels do not precisely indicate pantothenic acid status of the body.

A clinical deficiency syndrome of pantothenic acid has not been clearly established. Glusman (150) described a syndrome of "burning feet" paresthesias, observed in starving prisoners of war. Deficient diets produce dermatitis and myelin degeneration in chickens, with more profound deficiencies producing adrenal insufficiency (146). Deficiency symptoms in two human experiments, involving a vitamin antagonist or a deficient diet, included paresthesias with burning feet, postural hypotension, and impaired eosinophilic response to ACTH (adrenocorticotropic hormone) (151,152).

H. Biotin

Biotin is a water-soluble, sulfur-containing vitamin (Fig. 14), essential for the health of many animal species, including man. It is stable to heat and light at pH 5 to 8, but is destroyed with strong acids and alkalis. It is also susceptible to oxidation by air.

1. Sources and Requirements

Biotin is widely distributed in nature, especially in animal foods. Liver, kidney, egg yolk, nuts, and certain vegetables are good sources of biotin. However, cereals, fruits, and meat are comparatively poor in biotin. The availability of biotin-bound vitamin varies widely: wheareas biotin of maize and soybean meal is completely available to test animals, that of wheat is almost unavailable. Biotin is synthesized by intestinal bacteria.

Dietary requirements of biotin for humans have not been established. However, 0.4 mg of biotin for adult humans is thought to be adequate, with additional supplements of 0.4 mg and 0.2 mg/day during pregnancy and lactation, respectively.

2. Physiological and Biochemical Functions

Biocytin is a coenzyme required by several carboxylating enzymes, with a function of adding or removing one-carbon groups such as carbon dioxide. Carboxylases have vital roles in carbohy-

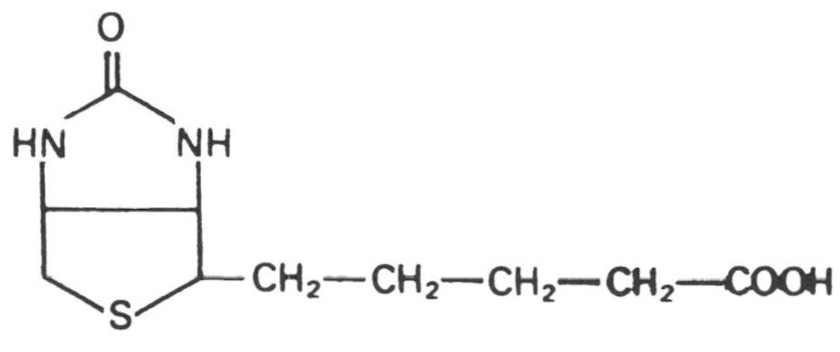

Figure 14   Structure of biotin (From Ref. 72.)

drate and lipid metabolism. Biocytin is a specialized carrier of one-carbon compounds in their most oxidized forms, such as CO_2, the transfer of one carbon groups in more reduced forms being mediated by other CO-enzymes, notably H_4-folates and S-adenosyl methionine. Carboxyl groups are attached to biotin at the ureido group within the biotin ring system.

Pyruvate carboxylase of carbohydrate metabolism contains four identical subunits, each with a molecule of biotin covalently bound through an amide linkage between its valerate side chain and the amino group of a specific lysine residue in the enzyme active site; this biotinyllysine is called biocytin.

Deficiency of biotin in man is rare and observed only when large quantities of raw eggs are consumed. Egg whites contain a large amount of the protein avidin, which binds to biotin very tightly, preventing its absorption by the intestine. The presence of avidin in egg whites may be a defense mechanism to inhibit bacterial growth. Avidin is denatured by heat (cooking) along with all other egg white proteins.

I. Ascorbic Acid (Vitamin C)

Ascorbic acid is a highly soluble antiscorbutic substance, having both acidic and strong reducing properties. It is the most unstable of all known vitamins and is easily oxidized in solution, especially on exposure to heat; the process is accelerated in the presence of metal ions such as copper and in alkaline pH. It is reversibly oxidized to dehydroascorbic acid without losing its vitamin activity. Dehydroascorbic acid treated with weak acid is irreversibly converted into diketogulonic acid, with no vitamin activity. Being readily soluble in water and susceptible to oxidation, ascorbic acid is lost during cooking and food processing through leaching. Prolonged cooking at high temperature and exposure to oxygen, copper, and iron result in a significant loss of vitamin C. In addition to temperature, oxygen, and metal ions, other factors influencing degradation of ascorbic acid include pH, enzymes, amino acids, oxidants or reductants, salt and sugar concentration, initial vitamin concentration, and ratio of ascorbic acid to dehydroascorbic acid.

The early seamen and explorers forced to subsist on a diet devoid of fresh foods (dried beef, biscuits) suffered from weakness, followed by bleeding gums, tissue hemorrhage, edema, and ulcerations, and death. Lind (153) published a treatise on scurvy, describing feeding trials of British seamen given daily supplements of vinegar, seawater, or two oranges and one lemon. The citrus group was rapidly cured of scurvy. Holst and Frolich (154) induced scurvy in guinea pigs by feeding them cereal diets. Zilva (155) extracted the antiscorbutic factor from lemons, which was later isolated from diverse sources and characterized simultaneously by Svirbely and Szent-Gyorgyi (156) and King and Waugh (157). Following its synthesis the next year (158), it was established that the tissue-extracted antiscorbutic factor, vitamin C, ascorbic acid, and hexuronic acid were all the same (72).

1. Sources and Requirements

Vegetables and fruits, especially fresh spinach, tomato, potato, broccoli, strawberries, oranges, limes, lemons, and other citrus fruit are rich sources of vitamin C. Certain tropical fruits like the West Indian cherry (acerola) (1300 mg/100 g), rose hips (1000 mg/100 g), and amla (onla) are the richest sources of ascorbic acid. Meat and dairy products contain little vitamin C, none being found in unfortified cereals. The U.S. (NRC) RDAs for vitamin C are 60 mg/day for adults of all ages, on the basis of early turnover studies, an estimated absorption of 85% of dietary intake, and variable losses during food preparation. The RDAs for smokers are 100 mg/day, and an additional 10 mg/day and 35 mg/day have been recommended for pregnant and lactating women, respectively. Infants should receive 30 mg/day of vitamin C. The UK RDIs are slightly less than the U.S. RDAs, viz., 40 mg/day for adults, with similar additional supplements recommended during pregnancy and lactation.

Vitamin C has been claimed to have wide-ranging effects. Nobel Laureate Linus Pauling (159) claimed that large daily doses of vitamin C decrease susceptibility to the common cold. This concept prompted several clinical trials that failed to show the claimed effect (160), yet large segments of the population believe that daily intake of vitamin C in amounts far exceeding the RDAs is essential to maintain good health (161).

Vitamin C is known to play a role in neutrophil migration, owing to its antioxidant effect on free-radical metabolism. Ascorbic acid improves neutrophil migration in chronic granulomatous disease in vitro and reduces the frequency of bacterial infection when used clinically (162), although the effects of vitamin C on immune functions remain to be proved in other clinical conditions (163). ACTH hormone of the adrenal gland stimulates release of ascorbic acid and the latter serves as a reductant in hydroxylation reactions in the formation of adrenaline and noradrenaline. The role of ascorbic acid in cortisone metabolism has not been established (163).

Ascorbic acid in large doses decreases the raised serum triglyceride levels in some individuals (164), but this effect has not been proved clinically. Cameron et al. (165) suggested a potential role of ascorbic acid in cancer therapy based on its in vitro effect in inhibiting nitrosamine formation from nitrates, though this effect is different from claims that ascorbic acid may prolong the survival of terminal cancer patients.

Vitamin C has an absorption threshold value at intakes of 2 to 3 g/day; therefore, massive oral doses are likely to produce diarrhea from the osmotic effects of the unabsorbed vitamin in the intestinal lumen. The body pool size of the vitamin is about 200 mg/kg body weight, so the rise in intake is likely to increase urinary output of ascorbic acid as a kidney's safeguard measure (166).

The potential toxic effects of excessive doses of ascorbic acid are linked to intraintestinal events and to effects of metabolites in the urinary system. The permissive effect of ascorbic acid on iron absorption may accentuate the iron overload within the intestine (167). Hyperoxaluria and an enhanced risk of kidney stones are the likely effects of excessive daily intakes of ascorbic acid; oxalate is the major metabolite of ascorbic acid, accounting for most of the catabolism of the vitamin C. Schmidt et al. (168) reported a modest increase in urinary oxalate excretion with an increase in the oral intake of ascorbic acid from 5 to 10 g/day, indicating the lower risk of oxalate stones with excessive vitamin C intake—a risk that may become significant in subjects with a higher tendency to stone formation (169).

2. *Physiological and Biochemical Functions*

Ascorbic acid is synthesized either from D-glucose or D-galactose in most organisms, except primates, guinea pigs, an Indian fruit-eating bat, and certain birds. Ascorbic acid is a strong reducing agent and serves as an antioxidant and as a cofactor in hydroxylation reactions. Ascorbic acid appears to influence several biological processes that remain to be quantified. It helps absorption of non-heme iron (see Chapter 7).

Many aspects of vitamin C deficiency and scurvy appear to be closely related to impaired collagen synthesis or deposition. Ascorbic acid is required for the hydroxylation of proline and lysine to constitute hydroxyproline backbone and the hydroxylysine cross-linkage needed for the formation of collagen fiber. According to Hornig et al. (163), this action of ascorbic acid may be secondary to its reducing effect on iron cofactor of prolyl hydroxylase. Defective hydroxylation increases the intracellular degradation of collagen fiber precursors and the synthesis of various cross-linking amino acids in collagen is disturbed.

Ascorbic acid is required for the synthesis of carnitine and noradrenaline. Carnitine is necessary for the transport of long-chain fatty acids into mitochondria for oxidation, and depletion of carnitine precedes the development of clinical symptoms of scurvy in experimental pigs (170). Also, the carnitine depletion with weakness and fatigue may be an early symption of vitamin C deficiency (163). In vitamin C–deficient guinea pigs, the ascorbate-dependent conversion of dopamine to noradrenaline is impaired, but human responses are not known (171).

Vitamin C is absorbed by an active, Na^+-dependent process (172). The absorbed ascorbate circulates freely in plasma, leukocytes, and red blood cells. Tissue concentrations of about 1.2–1.5 mg/dl are achieved with oral intakes of 90 to 150 mg/day (166), the highest concentrations being found in the adrenal and pituitary glands and retina. Excess vitamin C is excreted by the kidney, conserving the plasma levels up to 0.8 to 1.5 mg/dl (173). Ascorbic acid is metabolized principally to oxalates, appearing in the urine at all levels of intake, including the unchanged ascorbate whose concentration increases when intakes exceed 80 to 200 mg/day. The body ascorbate level may reach a maximum of 20 mg/kg body weight, with a total body pool size of about 1.5 g at 30 to 180 mg/day intakes, above which the vitamin is excreted in the urine rapidly (174).

Hodges et al. (175) investigated metabolic turnover in healthy adult humans on a diet with less than 10 mg/day of ascorbic acid. The plasma and urinary excretion of ascorbate decreased rapidly in the first week, reaching deficient levels by 40 days. The body ascorbate content declined by 3% a day until it reached 300 mg on day 55, when clinical signs of scurvy appeared with skin bruises from defective capillary basement membranes, perifollicular hemorrhages, and bleeding gums, followed by more severe changes occurring by day 80, such as joint pains and effusions. The body pool at this stage was less than 100 mg. Thus, 100 mg/day of vitamin C was the minimal dose to produce clinical improvement (175).

Scurvy impairs the collagen formation needed for wound healing and the defective extracellular bone matrix impairs osteoblast function, resulting in pathological bone fractures. Plasma ascorbate levels of less than 0.10 mg/dl and leukocyte levels of less than 7 mg/dl help to confirm scurvy (176).

Symptoms of scurvy are seen with other nutrient deficiencies, in intestinal malabsorption syndromes such as celiac sprue and in chronic alcoholics, because alcohol depresses absorption of ascorbic acid (177). Cigarette smoking increases ascorbate turnover by more than 40% because of free-radical scavenging (178).

3. Assessment of Status and Deficiency

Plasma or leukocyte levels of ascorbic acid are measured colorimetrically, using dinitrophenylhydrazine reagent. Plasma levels in general reflect the daily intake of ascorbic acid, whereas leukocyte levels are a better index of tissue stores (176). The normal plasma values of vitamin C should be more than 0.2 mg/dl and the levels below 0.1 mg/dl indicate deficiency (175). Fatigue and depression with a plasma level between 0.1 and 0.2 mg/dl may reflect a clinical condition other than vitamin C deficiency in itself (72).

REFERENCES

1. McCollum, E. V., and M. Davis, The necessity of certain lipids in the diet during growth, *J. Biol. Chem. 15*: 167 (1913).
2. McLaren, D. S., Pathogenesis of vitamin A deficiency, *Vitamin A Deficiency and Its Control*, (J. C. Bavernfeind, ed.), Academic Press, Orlando, 1980, p. 153.
3. McLaren, D. S., N. Loveridge, G. Duthie, and C. Bolton-Smith, Fat-soluble vitamins, *Human Nutrition and Dietetics*, 9th ed. (J. S. Garrow and W. P. T. James, eds.), Churchill Livingstone, London, 1993, p. 208.
4. Olson, J. A., Vitamin A., *Present Knowledge in Nutrition*, 6th ed. (M. L. Brown, ed.), Nutrition Foundation, Washington, D.C., 1990, p. 96.
5. F. A. O., Requirements of vitamin A, iron, folate and vitamin B_{12}, Report of a Joint FAO/WHO Expert Committee, FAO Food and Nutrition Series No. 23, Food and Agriculture Organiztion, Rome, 1989.

6. Olson, J. A., The provitamin A function of carotenoids, *J. Nutr. 119*: 105 (1989).

7. Blomhoff, R., M. H. Green, T. Berg, and K. R. Norum, Transport and storage of vitamin A, *Science. 250*: 399 (1990).

8. Sauberlich, H. E., R. E. Hodges, and D. L. Wallace et al., Vitamin A metabolism and requirements in the human studies with the use of labelled retinol, *Vitam Horm 32*: 251 (1974).

9. Goodman, D. S., Plasma retinol-binding protein, *The Retinoids*, Vol. 2 (M. B. Sporn, A. B. Roberts, D. S. Goodman, eds.), Academic Press, Orlando, 1984, p. 41.

10. Bhat, P. V., P. Poissant, P. Falardeau, and A. La Croix, Enzymatic oxidation of all *trans* retinol to retinoic acid in rat tissues, *Biochem. Cell. Biol. 66*: 735 (1988).

11. Bernstein, P. S., W. C. Law, and R. R. Rando, Isomerization of all-*trans* retinoids to 11-*cis* retinoids in vitro, *Proc. Natl. Acad. Sci. USA*, 84: 1849 (1987).

12. Giguere, V., E. S. Ong, P. Segiu, and R. M. Evans, Identification of a receptor for the morphogen retinoic acid, *Nature 330*: 624 (1987).

13. Petkovich, M., N. J. Brand, A. Krust, and P. Chambon, A human retinoic acid receptor which belongs to the family of nuclear receptors, *Nature 330*: 444 (1987).

14. Wald, G., Photoreceptor function of carotenoids and vitamin A, *Vitamins and Hormones 1*: 195 (1943).

15. Mejia, L. A., R. E. Hodges, and R. B. Rucker, Clinical signs of anemia in vitamin A–deficient rats, *Am. J. Clin. Nutr. 32*: 1439 (1979).

16. Underwood, B. A., Vitamin A in animal and human nutrition, *The Retinoids* Vol.I. (M. B. Sporn, A. B. Roberts, and D. S. Goodman, eds.), Academic Press, Orlando, 1984, p. 281.

17. Olsen, J. A., Recommended dietary intakes (RDI) of vitamin A in humans, *Am. J. Clin. Nutr. 45*: 704 (1987).

18. Flores, H., F. Campos, C. R. C. Araujo, and B. A. Underwood, Assessment of marginal vitamin A deficiency in Brazilian children using the relative dose response, *Am. J. Clin. Nutr. 40*: 1281 (1984).

19. Tanumihardjo, S. A., P. G. Koellner, and J. A. Olson, Application of the modified relative dose response (MRDR) assay as an indicator of vitamin A status in a population of well-nourished American children, *Am. J. Clin. Nutr. 52*: 1068 (1990).

20. Pilch, S. M., Analysis of vitamin A data from the Health and Nutrition Examination Surveys, *J. Nutr., 117*: 636 (1987).

21. WHO/UNICEF/IV ACG Task Force, Vitamin A Supplements, World Health Organization, Geneva, 1988.

22. McLaren, D. S., *Nutritional Ophthalmology*, Academic Press, London, 1980b.

23. Bendich, A., and L. Langseth, Safety of vitamin A, *Am. J. Clin. Nutr. 49*: 358 (1989).

24. Bush, M. E., and B. B. Dahms, Fatal hypervitaminosis in a neonate, *Arch. Pathol. Lab. Med. 108*: 838 (1984).

25. Rosa, F. W., A. L. Wilk, and F. O. Kelsey, Teratogen update: vitamin A congeners, *Teratology 33*: 355 (1986).

26. Mellanby, E., A further determination of the part played by accessory food factors in the aetiology of rickets, *J. Physiol. 52*: 1 (1919).

27. Mellanby, E., An experimental investigation on rickets, *Lancet 1*: 407 (1919).

28. Funk, C., The chemical nature of the substance which cures polyneuritis in birds induced by a diet of polished rice, *J. Physiol. 43*: 395 (1911).

29. McCollumn, E. V., and M. Davis, The necessity of certain lipids in the diet during growth. *J. Biol. Chem. 15*: 167 (1913).

30. McCollumn, E. V., N. Simmonds, J. E. Becker, and P. G. Shipley, Studies on experimental rickets. XXI. An experimental demonstration of the existence of a vitamin which promotes calcium deposition, *J. Biol. Chem. 53*: 293 (1922).

31. Blunt, J. W., H. F. DeLuca, and H. K. Schnoes, 25-hydroxy cholecalciferol. A biologically active metabolite of vitamin D_3, *Biochemistry 7*: 3317 (1968).

32. Fraser, D. R., and E. Kodicek, Unique biosynthesis by kidney of a biologically active metabolite of vitamin D, *Nature 228*: 764 (1970).

33. DeLuca, H. F., Vitamin D: metabolism and function, *Monographs on Endocrinology* Vol. 13 (F. Gross, M. M. Grumbach and A Labhart et al., eds.), Springer-Verlag, Berlin, 1979.

34. Webb, A. R., and M. F. Holick, The role of sunlight in the cutaneous production of vitamin D$_3$, *Annu. Rev. Nutr. 8*: 375 (1988).

35. Norman, A. W., The vitamin D endocrine system and bone, *Bone regulatory factors: morphology, biochemistry, physiology and pharmacology*, Nato ASI series, Vol. 184, (A. Pecile and B. de Barnard, eds.), Plenum, New York, 1990, p. 1993.

36. Reichel, H., H. P. Koffler, and A. W. Norman, The role of the vitamin D endocrine system in health and disease, *N. Engl. J. Med. 320*: 980 (1989).

37. Fraser, D. R., The physiological economy of vitamin D, *Lancet 1*: 969 (1983).

38. Fraser, D. R., Vitamin D, *J. Food Nutr. 44*: 3 (1987).

39. CMAFP, Dietary reference values for food energy and nutrients for the United Kingdom, Committee on the Medical Aspects of Food Policy, HMSO, London, 1991.

40. Haussler, M. R., D. J. Mangelsdorf, and B. S. Komm, et al., The molecular biology of the vitamin D hormone. *Recent Prog. Horm. Res. 44*: 263 (1988).

41. Suda, T., T. Shinki, and N. Takahashi, The role of vitamin D in bone and intestinal cell differentiation, *Ann. R. Nutr., 10*: 195 (1990).

42. DeLuca, H. F., The vitamin D story: a collaborative effort of basic science and clinical medicine: *FASEB J. 2*: 224 (1988).

43. Mason, K. E., The first two decades of vitamin E history, *Federation Proc. 36*: 235 (1977).

44. Jacobsberg, B. P. Delmide, and A. Gapor, Tocopherols and tocotrienols in palm oil, *Oleagineax 33*: 239 (1978).

45. Murphy, S. P., A. F. Subar, and G. Block, Vitamin E intakes and sources in the United States, *Am. J. Clin. Nutr. 52*: 361 (1990).

46. Diplock, A. T., Dietary supplementation with antioxidants. Is there a case for exceeding the recommended dietary allowance? *Free Radical Biol. Med., 3*: 199 (1987).

47. Duthie, G. G., K. W. J. Wahle, and W. P. T. James, Oxidants, antioxidants and coronary heart disease, *Nutrition Res. Rev. 2*: 51 (1989).

48. Horwitt, M. K., Supplementation with vitamin E, *Am. J. Clin. Nutr. 47*: 1088 (1988).

49. Duthie, G. G., J. R. Arthur, and W. P. T. James, Effects of smoking and vitamin E on blood antioxidant status, *Am. J. Clin. Nutr. 53*: 1061(s) (1991).

50. Lehmann, M. S., D. D. Rao, J. J. Canary, and J. T. Judd, Vitamin E and relationships among tocopherols in human plasma, platelets, lymphocytes and red blood cells, *Am. J. Clin. Nutr. 47*: 470 (1988).

51. Thurham, D. I., J. A. Davies, B. J. Crump, and M. Davis, The use of different lipids to express serum tocopherol: lipid ratios for the measurement of vitamin E status, *Ann. Clin. Biochem. 23*: 514 (1986).

52. Halliwell, B., Oxidants and human diseases: some new concepts, *FASEB J. 1*: 358 (1987).

53. Bjorneboe, A., G. A. Bjorneboe, and C. A. Drevon, Absorption, transport and distribution of vitamin E, *J. Nutr. 120*: 233 (1990).

54. Traber, M. G., and H. J. Kayden, Preferential uptake of alpha-tocopherol vs gamma-tocopherol in human lipoproteins, *Am. J. Clin. Nutr. 49*: 517 (1989).

55. Behrens, W. A., and L. T. Madere, Transfer of alpha-tocopherol to microsomes mediated by a partially purified liver alpha-tocopherol-binding protein, *Nutrition Res. 2*: 611 (1982).

56. Kitabchi, A. E., and J. Wimalasena, Specific binding sites for d-alpha-tocopherol on human erythrocytes, *Biochim. Biophys. Acta 684*: 200 (1982).

57. Bendich, A., and L. J. Machlin, Safety of oral intake of vitamin E, *Am. J. Clin. Nutr. 48*: 612 (1988).

58. Diplock, A. T., L. J. Machlin, L. Packer, and W. A. Pryor, Vitamin E: Biochemistry and health implications, *Ann. N. Y. Acad. Sci. USA 570*: 555 (1989).

59. Dam, H., The antihaemorrhagic factor of the chick, *Biochem. J. 29*: 1273 (1935).

60. Shearer, M. J., P. T. McCarthy, O. E. Crampton, and M. B. Mattock, The assessment of human vitamin K status from tissue measurements, *Current Advances in Vitamin K Research* (J. W. Suttie, ed.), Elsevier, New York, 1988, p. 437.

61. Barkhan, P., and M. J. Shearer, Metabolism of vitamin K (phylloquinone) in man, *Proc. Royal Soc. Med. 70*: 93 (1977).

62. Suttie, J. W., L. L. Mummah-Schendel, D. V. Shah, B. J. Lyle, and J. L. Greger, Development of human vitamin K deficiency by dietary vitamin K restriction, *Am. J. Clin. Nutr. 47*: 475 (1988).

63. Vermeer, C., Gamma-carboxyglutamate-containing proteins and the vitamin K-dependent carboxy-lase, *Biochem J. 266*: 625 (1990).

64. Senflo, J., P. Fernlund, W. Egan, and P. Roepstorff, Vitamin K-dependent modifications of glutamic acid residues in prothrombin, *Proc. Nat., Acad. Sci. USA, 71*: 2730 (1974).

65. Price, P. A., Role of vitamin K-dependent proteins in bone metabolism, *Annu. R. Nutr. 8*: 565 (1988).

66. McNinch, A. W., and J. H. Tripp, Haemorrhagic disease of the newborn in the British Isles: two-year prospective study, *Br. Med. J. 303*: 1105 (1991).

67. Poller, L., P. K. MacCallum, J. M. Thomson, and W. Kerns, Reductions of factor VII coagulant activity (VII C), a risk factor for ischaemic heart disease by fixed-dose warfarin: a double-bind crossover study, *British Heart J. 63*: 231 (1990).

68. Knapen, M. H. J., K. Hamulyak, and C. Vermeer, The effect of vitamin K supplementation on circulating osteocalcin (bone gla-protein) and urinary calcium excretion, *Ann. Intern. Med. 111*: 1001 (1989).

69. Jansen, B. C. P., and W. F. Donath, Proceedings of KoninKlijke Nederlandse Akademie van Wetenschappen (Amsterdam). *29*: 1390 (1926).

70. Williams, R. R., and J. K. Cline, Synthesis of vitamin B_1, *J. Am. Chem. Soc. 58*: 1504 (1936).

71. Sauberlich, H. E., Y. F. Herman, C. O. Stevens, and R. H. Herman, Thiamin requirement of the adult human, *Am. J. Clin. Nutr. 32*: 2237 (1979).

72. Halsted, C. H., Water-soluble vitamins, *Human Nutrition and Dietetics*, 9th ed. (J. S. Garrow and W. P. T. James, eds.), Churchill Livingstone, London, 1993, p. 235.

73. McCormick, D. B., Thiamin, *Modern Nutrition in Health and Disease*, 7th ed. (M. E. Shils and V. R. Young, eds.), Lea & Febiger, Philadelphia, 1988, p. 355.

74. Peters, R. A., Significance of biochemical lesions in the pyruvate oxidase system, *Br. Med. Bull. 9*: 116 (1953).

75. Williams, R. D., H. L. Mason, B. F. Smith, and R. M. Wilder, Induced thiamine (vitamin B_1 deficiency and the thiamin requirement of man, *Arch. Intern. Med. 60*: 721 (1942).

76. Hoyumpa, A. M., Jr., S. G. Nichols, F. A. Wilson, and S. Schenker, Effect of ethanol on intestinal (Na, K) ATPase and intestinal thiamin transport in rats, *J. Lab. Clin. Med. 90*: 1086 (1977).

77. Ferrebee, J. W., N. Weissman, D. Parker, and P. S. Owen, Tissue thiamin concentrations and urinary thiamin excretion, *J. Clin. Invest. 21*: 401 (1942).

78. Sauberlich, H. E., R. P. Dowdy, and J. H. Scala, Laboratory tests for the assessment of nutritional status, CRC Press, Cleveland, 1974.

79. Kawasaki, T., Determination of thiamin and its phosphate esters by high-performance liquid chromatography, *Methods Enzymol. 122*: 15 (1986).

80. Reuler, B., D. E. Girard, and T. G. Cooney, Wernicke's encephalopathy, *N. Engl. J. Med. 312*: 1035 (1985).

81. Blass, J. P., and G. E. Gibson, Abnormality of a thiamin-requiring enzyme in patients with Wernicke-Korsakoff Syndrome, *N. Engl. J. Med. 297*: 1367 (1977).

82. Nixon, P. F., M. J. Kaczmarek, J. Tate, R. A. Kerr, and J. Price, An erythrocyte transketolase isoenzyme pattern associated with the Wernicke-Korsakoff syndrome, *Eur. J. Clin. Invest. 14*: 278 (1984).

83. Halsted, C. H., and C. Heise, Ethanol and vitamin metabolism, *Pharmacol. Ther. 34*: 453 (1987).

84. Manay, N. S., and M. Shadaksharaswamy, *Foods: Facts and Principles*, Wiley Eastern Ltd., New Delhi, 1987, p. 59.

85. Roe, D. A., *A Plague of Corn: The Social History of Pellegra*, Cornell University Press, Ithaca, New York, 1973.

86. Goldberger, J., The relation of diet to pellagra, *J. Am. Med. Assoc. 78*: 1676 (1922).

87. Jacob, R. A., M. E. Swendseid, R. W. McKee, C. S. Fu, and R. A. Clemens, Biochemical markers for assessment of niacin status in young men: urinary and blood levels of niacin metabolites, *J. Nutr. 119*: 591 (1989).

88. Halsted, C. H., S. Sheir, N. Sourial, and U. N. Patwardhan, Small intestinal structure and absorption in Egypt: influence of parasitism and pellagra, *Am. J. Clin. Nutr. 22*: 744 (1969).

89. Wooliscroff, J. O., Megavitamins: factor fancy, *Disease-A-Month 29*: 7 (1983).

90. Goldsmith, G. A., O. N. Miller, and W. G. Unglaub, Efficiency of tryptophan as a niacin precursor in man, *J. Nutr. 73*: 172 (1961).

91. Gyorgy, P., Vitamin B_2 and pellagra-like dermatitis in rats, *Nature 133*: 498 (1934).
92. McCormick, D. H., Vitamin B_6, *Modern Nutrition in Health and Disease*, 7th ed. (M. E. Shils and V. R. Young, eds.), Lea & Febiger, Philadelphia, 1988, p. 376.
93. Tarr, J. B., T. Tamura, and E. L. R. Stokstad, Availability of vitamin B_6 and pantothenate in an average American diet in man, *Am. J. Clin. Nutr. 34*: 1328 (1981).
94. Schroeder, H. A., Losses of vitamins and trace elements resulting from processing and preservation of foods, *Am. J. Clin. Nutr. 24*: 562 (1971).
95. Dalton, K., and M. J. T. Dalton, Characteristics of pyridoxine overdose neuropathy syndrome, *Acta Neurol. Scand. 76*: 8 (1987).
96. Henderson, L. M., Vitamin B_6, *Present Knowledge in Nutrition*, 5th ed. Nutrition Foundation, Washington, D.C., 1984, p. 303.
97. Lindenbaum, J., Hematologic complications of alcohol abuse, *Semin. Liver Dis. 7*: 169 (1987).
98. Baker, E. M., J. E. Canham, W. T. Nunes, H. E. Sauberlich, and M. E. McDowell, Vitamin B_6 requirement for adult men, *Am. J. Clin. Nutr. 15*: 59 (1964).
99. Rivlin, R. S., Disorders of vitamin metabolism: deficiencies, metabolic abnormalities, and excesses, *Cecil Textbook of Medicine* 17th ed. (J. B. Wyngaarden and L. H. Smith, eds.) Saunders, Phildelphia, 1985, p. 1197.
100. Leklem, J. E., R. R. Brown, D. P. Rose, and H. M. Linkswiler, Vitamin B_6 requirements of women using oral contraceptives, *Am. J. Clin. Nutr. 28*: 535 (1975).
101. McCoy, E. E., C. Colombini, and M. E. Badi, The metabolism of vitamin B_6 in Down's syndrome, *Ann. N. Y. Acad. Sci. 166*: 116 (1969).
102. Ebadi, M., M. Itoh, J. Bifano, K. Wendt, and A. Earle, The role of Zn^{2+} in pyridoxal phosphate mediated regulation of glutamic acid decarboxylase in brain, *Int. J. Biochem. 13*: 1107 (1981).
103. McCully, K. S., Vascular pathology of homecysteinemia: implications for the development of atherosclerosis, *Am. J. Pathol. 56*: 111 (1969).
104. Kopple, J. D., K. Mercurio, M. J. Blumenkrantz, et al., Daily requirement for pyridoxine supplements in chronic renal failure, *Kidney Int. 19*: 694 (1981).
105. Reinkin, L., and H. Zieglauer, Vitamin B_6 absorption in children with acute celiac disease and in control subjects, *J. Nutr. 108*: 1562 (1978).
106. Mitchell, D. C. Wagner, W. J. Stone, G. R. Wilkinson, and S. Schenker, Abnormal regulation of plasma pyridoxal-5'-phosphate in patients with liver disease, *Gastroenterology 71*: 1043 (1976).
107. Wills, L., The nature of the haemopoietic factor in Marmite, *Lancet 1*: 1283 (1933).
108. Spies, T. D., C. F. Vilter, M. B. Koch, and M. H. Caldwell, Observations of the anti-anaemic properties of synthetic folic acid, *South. Med. J. 38*: 707 (1945).
109. Roe, D. A., Lucy Wills (1988–1964): a biographical sketch, *J. Nutr. 108*: 1379 (1978).
110. Shane, B., and E. L. R. Stockstad, Vitamin B_{12}–folate interrelationships, *Annu. R. Nutr. 5*: 115 (1985).
111. Herbert, V., Recommended dietary intakes (RDI) of folate in humans, *Am. J. Clin. Nutr., 45*: 661 (1987).
112. Tamura, T., and E. L. R. Stockstad, The availability of food folate in man, *Br. J. Haematol. 25*: 513 (1973).
113. Baumslag, N., T. Edelstein, and J. Metz, Reduction of incidence of prematurity of folic acid supplementation in pregnancy, *Br. Med. J., 1*: 16 (1970).
114. Iyengar, L., and K. Rajalakshmi, Effect of folic acid supplement on birth weight of infants, *Am. J. Obtet. Gynecol. 122*: 332 (1975).
115. Chanarin, I. D., Rothman, A. Ward, and J. Perry, Folate status and requirements in pregnancy, *Br. Med. J. 2*: 390 (1968).
116. Simmer, K., C. A. Iles, C. James, and R. P. H. Thompson. Are iron-folate supplements harmful? *Am. J. Clin. Nutr. 45*: 122 (1987).
117. Herbert, V., Recommended dietary intakes of vitamin B_{12} in human, *Am. J. Clin. Nutr. 45*: 671 (1987).
118. Klipstein, F. A., Tropical spruce, *Gastrointestinal Disease*: Pathophysiology, Dignosis, Management, 3rd ed. Vol. 2 (M. H. Sleisennger and J. S. Fordtran, eds.), W. B. Sauders, Philadelphia, 1983, p. 1040.
119. Reynold, E. H., Mental effects of anticonvulsants, and folic acid metabolism, *Brain 91*: 197 (1968).
120. Mason, J. B., Intestinal transport of monoglutamyl folates in mammalian system, *Folic acid Metabo-*

lism in Health and Disease: *Contempory Issues in Clinical Nutrition* (M. F. Picciano, E. L. R. Stockstad, and J. F. Gregory, eds.), Alan R Liss, New York, 1990, p. 47.

121. Hopper, K., and B. Lampi, Folate levels in human liver from autopsies in Canada, *Am. J. Clin. Nutr. 33*: 862 (1980).

122. Steinberg, S., Mechanisms of folate homeostasis, *Am. J. Physiol. 246*: G319 (1984).

123. Herbert, V., and N. Colman, Folic acid and vitamin B_{12} *Modern Nutrition in Health and Disease*. 7th ed. (M. E. Shils and V. R. Young, eds.), Lea & Febiger, Philadelphia, 1988, p. 388.

124. Herbert, V. Experimental nutritional folate deficiency in man, *Trans. Assoc. Am. Physicians 75*: 307 (1962).

125. Hermos, J. A., W. H. Adams, Y. C. Lin, and J. Tries, Mucosa of the small intestine in folate-deficient alcoholics, *Ann. Intern. Med. 76*: 957 (1972).

126. Minot, G. R., and W. P. Murphy, Treatment of pernicious anemia by a special diet, *J. Am. Med. Assoc. 87*: 470 (1926).

127. Castle, W. B., Observations on the etiologic relationship of achylia gastrica to pernicious anemia. I. The effect of the administration to patients with pernicious anemia of the contents of the normal human stomach recovered after the ingestion of beef muscle, *Am. J. Med. Sci. 178*: 748 (1929).

128. Rickes, E. L., N. G. Brink, F. R. Koniuszy, T. R. Wood, and K. Folkers, Crystalline vitamin B_{12}, *Science 107*: 396 (1946).

129. Smith, E. L., and L. F. J. Parker, Purification of antipernicious anemia factor, *Proc. Biochem. Soc. 43*: 8 (1948).

130. Grasbeck, R., K. Simons, and I. Sinkkonen, Isolation of intrinsic factor and its probable degradation product as their vitamin B_{12} complexes from human gastric juice, *Biochim. Biophys. Acta 127*: 47 (1966).

131. Herbert, V., G. Drivas, C. Manusselis, M. Mackler, J. Eng, and E. Schwartz, Are colon bacteria a major source of cobalamin analogues in human tissues? 24-h human stool contains only about 5 µg of cobalamin but about 100 µg of apparent analogue (and 200 µg folate)., *Trans. Assoc. Am. Physicians 97*: 161 (1984).

132. Sullivan, L. W., and V. Herbert, Studies on the minimum daily requirement for vitamin B_{12}. Hematopoietic responses to 0.1 µg of cyanocobalamin or coenzyme B_{12} and comparison of their relative potency, *N. Engl. J. Med. 272*: 340 (1965).

133. Stewart, J. S., P. D. Roberts, and A. V. Hoffbrand, Response of dietary vitamin B_{12} deficiency to physiological oral doses of cyanocobalamin, *Lancet 2*: 542 (1970).

134. Cooper, B. A., and D. S. Rosenblatt, Inherited defects of vitamin B_{12} metabolism, *Annu. Rev. Nutr. 7*: 291 (1987).

135. Shane, B., and E. L. R. Stockstad, Vitamin B_{12} folate interrelationships, *Annu. Rev. Nutr. 5*: 115 (1985).

136. Weir, D. G., S. Keating, A. Molly, et al., Methylation deficiency causes vitamin B_{12}-associated neuropathy in the pig, *J. Neurochem. 51*: 1949 (1988).

137. Kapadia, C. R., D. Serfilippi, K. Voloshin, and R. M. Donaldson, Jr., Intrinsic factor-mediated absorption of cobalamin by guinea-pig ileal cells, *J. Clin. Invest. 71*: 440 (1983).

138. Cooper, B. A., Complex of the intrinsic factor and B_{12} in human ileum during vitamin B_{12} absorption, *Am. J. Physiol. 214*: 832 (1968).

139. Chanarin, I., M. Muir, A. Hughes and A. V. Hoffbrand, Evidence for an intestinal origin of transcobalamin II during vitamin B_{12} absorbtion, *Br. Med. J. 1*: 1453 (1978).

140. Rothenberg, S. P., J. P. Weiss, and R. Cotter, Formation of transcobalamin II–vitamin B_{12} complex by guinea-pig ileal mucosa in organ culture after in vivo incubation with intrinsic factor-vitamin B_{12}, *Br. J. Haematol. 40*: 410 (1978).

141. Kanazawa, S., V. Herbert, B. Herzlich, G. Drivas, and C. Manusselis, Removal of cobalamin analogue in bile by enterohepatic circulation of vitamin B_{12}, *Lancet. 1*: 707 (1983).

142. Hall, C. A., Long term excretion of ^{57}Co vitamin B_{12} and turnover within the plasma, *Am. J. Clin. Nutr. 14*: 156 (1964).

143. Kanazawa, S., and V. Herbert, Mechanism of enterohapatic circulation of vitamin B_{12}: movement of vitamin B_{12} from pancreatic trypsin, *Trans. Assoc. Am. Physicians 96*: 336 (1983).

144. Herbert, V., Pathogenesis of megaloblastic anaemias, *Nutrition and the Origins of Disease* (C. H. Halsted and R. B. Rucker, eds.), Academic Press, San Diego, 1989, p. 47.

145. Stabler, S. P., P. D. Marcell, E. R. Podell, R. H. Allen, D. G. Savage, and J. Lindenbaum, Elevation of total homocysteine in the serum of patients with cobalamin or folate deficiency detected by capillary gas chromatography–mass spectrometry, *J. Clin. Invest. 81*: 466 (1988).

146. McCormick, D. B., Pantothenic acid, *Modern Nutrition in Health and Disease*, 7th ed. (M. E. Shils and V. R. Young, eds), Lea & Febiger, Philadelphia, 1988, p. 383.

147. Rose, R. C., A. M. Hoyumpa, R. H. Allen, H. M. Middleton, L. M. Henderson, and I. H. Rosenberg, Transport and metabolism of water-soluble vitamins in intestine and kidney, *Federation Proc. 43*: 2423 (1984).

148. Wyse, B. W., C. Wittwer, and R. G. Hansen, Radioimmunoassay for pantothenic acid in blood and other tissues, *Clin. Chem. 25*: 108 (1979).

149. Sauberlich, H. E., R. P. Dowdy, and J. H. Scala, *Laboratory Tests for the Assessment of Nutritional Status*, CRC Press, Cleveland, 1974.

150. Glusman, M., The syndrome of 'burning feet' (nutritional melalgia) as a manifestation of nutritional deficiency, *Am. J. Med. 3*: 211 (1947).

151. Hodges, R. E., W. B. Bean, M. A. Ohlson, and R. Bleiler, Human pantothenic acid deficiency produced by omega-methyl pantothenic acid, *J. Clin. Invest. 38*: 1421 (1959).

152. Fry, P. C., H. M. Fox, and H. G. Tao, Metabolic response to a pantothenic acid deficient diet in humans, *J. Nutr. Sci. Vitaminol. 22*: 339 (1976).

153. Lind, J., *A treatise on the scurvy in three parts*, Crowder, London, 1972, p. 149, 177.

154. Holst, A., and T. Frolich, Experimental studies relating to ship beri-beri and scurvy, *J. Hygiene* (London) *7*: 634 (1907).

155. Zilva, S. S. The influence of aeration on the stability of antiscorbutic factor, *Lancet 1*: 478 (1921).

156. Svirbely, J. L., and A. Szent-Gyorgyi, The chemical nature of vitamin C, *Biochem. J. 26*: 865 (1932).

157. King, C. G., and W. A. Waugh, The chemical nature of vitamin C, *Science 75*: 357 (1932).

158. Haworth, W. N., and E. L. Hirst, Synthesis of vitamin C, *J. Soc. Chem. Industry 52*: 645 (1933).

159. Pauling, L., *Vitamin C and Common Cold*, W. H. Freeman, San Francisco, 1970.

160. Chalmers, T. C., Effects of ascorbic acid on the common cold: an evaluation of the evidence, *Am. J. Med. 58*: 532 (1975).

161. CSA/AMA, Vitamin preparations as dietary supplements and therapeutic agents, *J. Am. Med. Assoc. 257*: 1929 (1987).

162. Anderson, R., Ascorbate-mediated stimulation of neutrophil motility and lymphocyte transformation by inhibition of the peroxidase/(H_2O_2) halide system in vitro and in vivo, *Am. J. Clin. Nutr. 34*: 1906 (1981).

163. Hornig, D. H., U. Moser, and B. E. Glatthaar, Ascorbic acid, *Modern Nutrition in Health and Disease*, 7th ed. (M. E. Shils and V. R. Young eds.), Lea & Febiger, Philadelphia, 1988, p. 417.

164. Ginter, E., O. Cerna, J. Budlovsky, et al., Effect of ascorbic acid on plasma cholesterol in humans in a long-term experiment, *Int. J. Vitamin Nutr. Res. 47*: 123 (1977).

165. Cameron, E., L. Pauling, and B. Leibovitz, Ascorbic acid and cancer: a review, *Cancer Res. 39*: 663 (1979).

166. Olson, J. A., and R. E. Hodges, Recommended dietary intakes (RDI) of vitamin C in humans, *Am. J. Clin. Nutr. 45*: 693 (1987).

167. Cook, J. D., and E. R. Monsen, Vitamin C, the common cold and iron absorption. *Am. J. Clin. Nutr. 30*: 235 (1977).

168. Schmidt, K. H., V. Hagmaier, D. H. Hornig, J. P. Vuilleumier, and G. Rutishauer, Urinary oxalate excretion after large intakes of ascorbic acid in man, *Am. J. Clin. Nutr. 34*: 305 (1981).

169. Chalmers, A. H., D. M. Cowley, and J. M. Brown, A possible etiological role for ascorbate in calculi formation, *Clin. Chemistry 32*: 333 (1986).

170. Nelson, P. J., R. E. Pruitt, L. L. Henderson, R. Jenness, and P. M. Henderson, Effect of ascorbic acid deficiency on the in vivo synthesis of carnitine, *Biochim. Biophys. Acta 672*: 123 (1981).

171. Deana, R., B. S. Bharaj, Z. H. Verjee, and L. Galzigna, Changes relevant to catecholamine metabolism in liver and brain of ascorbic acid–deficient guinea-pigs, *Int. J. Vitamin Nutr. Res. 45*: 175 (1975).

172. Stevenson, N. R., Active transport of l-ascorbic acid in the human ileum, *Gastroenterology 67*: 952 (1974).

173. Ralli, E. P., G. J. Friedman, and S. H. Rubin, The mechanism of excretion of vitamin C by the kidney, *J. Clin. Invest. 17*: 765 (1938).

174. Kallner, A., D. Hartman, and D. Hornig, Steady-state turnover and body pool of ascorbic acid in man, *Am. J. Clin. Nutr. 32*: 530 (1979).

175. Hodges, R. E., J. Hood, J. E. Canham, H. E. Sauberlich, and E. M. Baker, Clinical manifestations of ascorbic acid deficiency in man, *Am. J. Clin. Nutr. 24*: 432 (1971).

176. Sauberlich, H. E., R. P. Dowdy, and J. H. Scala, *Laboratory Tests for the Assessment of Nutritional Status*, CRC Press, Cleveland, 1974.

177. Fazio, V., D. M. Flint, and M. L. Wahlqvist, Acute effects of alcohol on plasma ascorbic acid in healthy subjects, *Am. J. Clin. Nutr. 34*: 2394 (1981).

178. Kallner, A. B., D. Hartmann, and D. H. Hornig, On the requirements of ascorbic acid in man: steady-state turnover and body pool in smokers, *Am. J. Clin. Nutr. 34*: 1347 (1981).

179. Holland B., A. A. Welch, I. D. Unwin, D. H. Buss, A. A. Paul, and D. A. T. Southgate (eds), *The Composition of Foods*, 5th ed., Royal Society of Chemistry, and Ministry of Agriculture, Fisheries and Food, London, 1991.

180. Chow, C. K., Vitamin E and blood, *World Rev. Nutr. Diet 45*: 133 (1985).

7
Minerals

I. INTRODUCTION

Minerals, like vitamins, are required by the body in small amounts for the maintenance of health and life. However, unlike the vitamins and all other nutrients, they are not organic compounds. These are the essential inorganic minerals present in the soil and obtained by all organisms primarily through plant foods. There are 21 minerals recognized as being essential for humans and several more that occur in the body, but their function and essentiality are yet to be known.

The minerals are generally classified into two groups, depending on their amounts in the adult body (Table 1): (1) the macro nutrients (*macro* = large) which exist in the body at levels greater than 0.005% of body weight and are required at levels of 100 mg or more per day, and (2) the micro nutrients (*micro* = small), the minerals that are in the body at levels less than 0.005% of the body weight and are essential at levels of only a few milligrams or less per day. Minerals, like vitamins, are involved in enzyme reactions as cofactors but also have several other functions (1):

1. Act as cofactors for enzymes.
2. Constitute a part of essential compounds such as vitamin B_{12} and amino acids.
3. Regulate and balance fluids in the body.
4. Effect transfer of nerve impulses.
5. Control transfers across membranes.
6. Serve as buffers to regulate acid levels in the body.
7. Constitute major structural components of the body such as in bone and teeth.
8. Are necessary for blood formation.
9. Are essential for growth and reproduction.

The minerals are a complex group of compounds and are very reactive chemically. They exist with positive or negative charges, affecting their ability to be absorbed into the body. The minerals can combine with other compounds in food. Some of these compounds aid in their absorption into the blood and are said to increase the mineral's availability or "bioavailability." Certain other compounds inhibit mineral absorption and thus decrease their bioavailability. Certain foods such as flour and cereals are fortified with some of the minerals to increase their nutritive value.

Minerals can become toxic compounds in higher doses: the difference between the amount required for good health and that which can produce toxicity may only be factor of 5 or 10, depending on the mineral. This is a good reason to limit intake of minerals to their RDAs and avoid self-dosing. Also, the absorption of certain minerals is some times competitive; e.g., an excess of iron might prevent the absorption of zinc, and vice versa. Thus, if one consumes too much of a single mineral, it might inhibit the absorption and availability of the other mineral, cre-

Table 1 Macro and Micro Nutrients (Minerals) in the Body

Type	Minerals
1. Macronutrients (More than 0.005% of body weight; 100 mg or more needed per day)	Calcium Phosphorus Sulfur Sodium Potassium Chlorine Magnesium
2. Micronutrients (Less than 0.005% of body weight; a few mg or less needed per day)	Iron Copper Zinc Fluorine Iodine Chromium Cobalt Selenium Manganese Molybdenum Tin Silicon Nickel Vanadium

Source: Ref. 1.

ating its deficiency in the body. The body, however, seems to protect itself against overdoses of some minerals by absorbing less from the diet when there is more in the body and vice versa.

According to Mertz (2), by definition, every essential trace element must have a range of intakes safe from toxicity but adequate enough to meet nutritional needs. That range is part of the total dose response curve and its lower and upper limits are delineated on the basis of nutrition and toxicity data, respectively. Close coordination of activities to set these limits is necessary to avoid recommendations that are either impractical (narrow zones of safe and adequate intakes) or contradictory (overlapping limits, i.e., no zones of safe and adequate intakes).

The conference "Risk Assessment of Essential Elements" was organized by the Risk Science Institute of the International Life Science Institute, and sponsored by the Office of Science Planning and Regulatory Evaluation of the Environmental Protection Agency and the Agency for Toxic Substances and Disease Registry of the U.S. Public Health Service held at Herdon, VA, March 10–12, 1992. This meeting produced "unanimous agreement that there is a range of exposures to essential elements that is both safe and compatible with good health. All elements known to be nutritionally essential are associated with adverse health outcomes at both the deficiency and excess ends of the spectrum" (3). This agreement has emphasized the need to define the total dose-response curves and their ranges of safe and adequate intakes. Evidence indicates that this need can be met only by closer collaboration between experts in toxicology and nutrition.

Not all experts agree on one universal definition of essentiality, especially for the "new" trace elements and their biochemical mechanisms of action. Further research should produce the information to resolve present uncertainities. Although there is no scientific contradiction between essentiality and toxicity of an element, its practical importance depends on geochemistry, industrial emissions, and the lifestyle of the inhabitants in an area. An experience in China has shown that selenium exposure is toxic in one area and life-saving in another (2).

The so-called new elements comprise a group of 11 for which animal experiments during the past three decades have postulated nutrition essentiality: aluminum (4,5), arsenic (6), boron (6) bromine (7), cadmium (8), lithium (9), nickel (6), lead (10), rubidium (11), silicon (6), and vanadium (6). Independent investigations have confirmed the original reports, often in more than one species, and human studies have confirmed the effects of boron first reported in animals (12).

II. BONE MINERALS: CALCIUM, PHOSPHORUS, AND MAGNESIUM

The minerals present in the skeleton influence the normal physiology and metabolism of bone. The skeleton is not an inert material; in addition to minerals, it has an important organic component. Also, the skeleton is continually being removed and replaced by the action of the bone cells within it, which are controlled by mechanical and hormonal factors. The skeleton has both mechanical and biochemical functions and cannot be regarded just as a repository for calcium and phosphorus (13).

A. Physiological Composition of Skeleton

Calcium, phosphorus, and magnesium are the major minerals of bone with minor quantities of copper, aluminium, and fluorine. Strontium in much smaller amounts is often associated with foods that are rich in calcium, and its radioactive form, ^{90}Sr, may be incorporated into the skeleton through contamination and pollution (13). About 1 kg of calcium is present in the adult human skeleton complexed with phosphate in the form of hydroxyapatite. Calcium is laid down in the organic matrix composed mainly of collagen, along with some non-collagen proteins.

The calcium present in fully mineralized bone as hydroxyapatite is preceded by other crystal forms, and during mineralization a small fraction of mineral is present in an amorphous form. According to Smith (14), mineralization occurs in two separate ways that may overlap each other. The first involves formation of crystals within matrix or mineralizing vesicles, derived from osteoblasts. In the second process, mineral is laid down in a orderly fashion, beginning in the hole zones of collagen fibrils (15).

The skeleton contains more than one-half of the body's collagen, whose numerous genetic types are known. The component of this extracellular protein is the fibrillar collagens, of which adult bone contains only type I, a heteropolymer containing two similar (alpha-1) and one different (alpha-2) chains—wound helically around each other. Each chain has a glycine residue in every third position, i.e., it is a repeating polymer of (Gly. XY) 338, where X is often proline and Y is hydroxyproline. The three dimensional-overlap structure (quarter stagger array) provides gaps (hole zones) in which mineralization first begins (16).

A wide variety of non-collagen substances and factors promoting cartilage formation occur in the organic matrix (17). The non-collagen fraction has been provisionally classified into sialoproteins; the proteins containing carboxyglutamic acid (Gla-proteins); phosphoproteins, including osteonectin; bone proteoglycans; and plasma proteins.

The bone cells, osteoblasts, osteoclasts, and osteocytes, are actively involved in bone metabolic turnover (18). Osteoclasts, which are derived from hemopoietic cells, are responsible for the resorption of bone, and osteoblasts belonging to the stromal cell system are involved in bone formations. Osteocytes derived from osteoblasts lie within the mineralized bone matrix, communicating with each other through the bone canaliculi.

The ways in which various bone cells communicate with each other are very complex and have been reviewed by Krane et al. (19). The skeleton is constantly being resorbed and replaced, the osteoblasts having a central role in this process The osteoblasts respond to a large number of endocrine and mechanical signals. They also seem to control the mineralization process and modify the activity of the major bone-resorbing cells (osteoclasts) (20).

B. Calcium

The most important and predominant mineral of the skeleton is calcium; it has a large number of vital functions within the body, including the muscular, neurological, and endocrine systems (21). The adult skeleton calcium (about 1 kg) is in equilibrium with the plasma calcium at about 2.23–3.60 mmlo/1 (9.0–10.4 mg/100 ml). A number of factors control calcium balance (Fig. 1). The amount of calcium within the skeleton changes with age, body size, and composition, increasing during growth and declining in parallel with the bone loss during aging (22). Figure 1 also shows that the external balance of calcium (i.e., the difference between intake and output) is determined by exchange between the skeleton, the intestine, and the kidney. These fluxes are regulated by the calcitropic hormones, PTH, 1,25-dihydroxycholecalciferol, and calcitonin (CT)

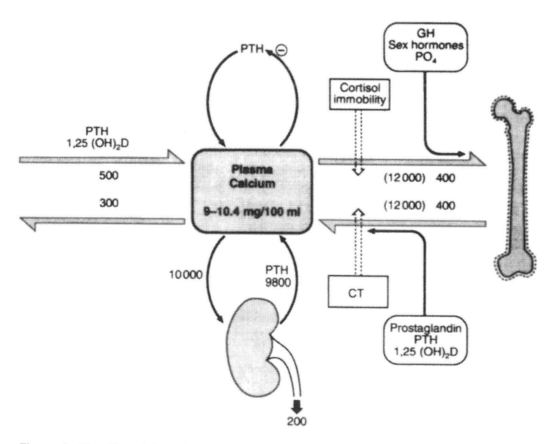

Figure 1 The effect of the major hormones on calcium balance in the normal adult. The figures in exchange of calcium through the cellular barrier of bone. Units are in mg/day (divided by 40 = mmol). CT = Calcitonin, GH = Growth hormone. Note that PTH (parathyroid hormone) is suppressed by an increase in plasma calcium. (From Ref. 14.)

(23). They are also influenced by sex hormones, growth hormones, corticosteroids and a range of locally acting hormones. Significant physiological changes in calcium balance occur during growth, pregnancy, lactation, and aging (14). The hormones that have major effects on calcium metabolism (calcitropic hormones) are active vitamin D, $1,25(OH)_2D_3$, PTH, and CT. The effects of these hormones are not restricted to those on calcium metabolism, and there are several other locally active hormones (cytokines) with effects on calcium metabolism. Thus, the classification of calcitropic hormones is not very rigid.

Vitamin D is synthesized in the skin under the action of ultraviolet light, all actions of vitamin D being mediated through its active metabolite, $1,25(OH)_2D_3$, which may be more appropriately called a hormone. Advances have been made in the understanding of the mechanisms of formation of vitamin D in the skin, the metabolic steps it undergoes, and the action of $1,25(OH)_2D_3$.

The action of $1,25(OH)_2D_3$ directly concerns calcium uptake and transport and is important in the control of plasma calcium, by controlling the intestinal absorption of calcium and the osteoclastic resorption of bone, probably via osteoclasts. However, it has been shown that the calcitropic function is only one aspect of $1,25(OH)_2D_3$ metabolism. The identification of the specific cellular receptor of this metabolite has led to its discovery in a wide range of tissues (24). The hormone $1,25(OH)_2D_3$ also has an important role to play in cellular differentiation and the immune system (25).

As the result of the better understanding of vitamin D metabolism, it has been possible to treat many of the causes of rickets and osteomalacia (see Chapter 27). This knowledge has also provided an insight into the cause of renal glomerular osteodystrophy and vitamin D–dependent rickets.

The PTH regulates plasma by its indirect action on intestinal calcium asborption, by controlling 1-alpha 25(OH)D, and its direct effect on the renal reabsorption of calcium and on bone resorption. The last effect probably takes place through the osteoblasts containing PTH receptors (not present in osteoclasts). The PTH directly acts on the cells of renal tubule and bone by the classic activation of adenyl cyclase, or via phosphokinase C and inositol triphosphate pathway (26).

The plasma concentration of calcium regulates the secretion and synthesis of PTH at its various stages of metabolism. The parathyroid hormones have a unique property of being stimulated by a decline rather than an increase in calcium concentration. The activity and size of thyroid glands is often increased in diseased states by hyperplasia secondary to prolonged hypocalcemia. The latter condition is caused by vitamin D deficiency and disturbances of its metabolism as well as by hypoparathyroidism. The plasma calcium concentration may be increased abnormally (hypercalcemia) due to one or another of the following causes (13): (a) malignant disease, (b) primary hyperthyroidism, (c) sarcoidosis and other granulomas, (d) vitamin D overdosage, (e) milk alkali syndrome, (f) immobilization, (g) thyrotoxicosis. (h) hypercalcemia of infancy, and (i) familial hypocalciuric hypercalcemia.

The physiological role of calcitonin has not been established (27). Evidence available suggests that it has a role in protection of the skeleton during times of stress such as growth and pregnancy.

The skeleton is also affected by several other hormones, such as growth hormones, sex hormones, thyroxine, corticosteroids, and, to a smaller extent, by insulin (28). An excess of growth hormone during childhood and before the closure of the epiphyses causes gigantism; its lack results in proportionate short stature. Hypopituitarism leads to osteoporosis. Similarly, lack of estrogen after oophorectomy or occurring naturally after menopause is an important cause of accelerated bone loss. Also, lack of male testosterone associated with cryptorchidism is thought to cause osteoporosis in men. An excess of corticosteroids, resulting from Cushing's syndrome, produces severe osteoporosis with excessive callus, which may also be caused by high doses of glucocorticoids used treating asthma or temporal arteritis. Thyrotoxicosis has been known to produce excessive bone turnover (with an increase in resorption more than an increase in bone formation), leading to osteoporosis, associated with hypercalcemia (13).

Changes in calcium metabolism are also caused by locally active hormones, especially in cases of hypercalcemia associated with malignancy (29). Among various factors that stimulate bone resorption are tumor necrosis factors (alpha and beta), transforming growth factors (alpha and beta), epidermal growth factors, platelet-derived growth factor, and metabolites of arachidonic acids such as prostaglandins and leukotrienes.

According to Kanis and Passmore (22), during growth the skeleton increases in size, in calcium content, and in calcium requirements, and even after growth stops, the amount of bone and its calcium content together (bone mass) may continue to rise. The age of about 30 years has often been quoted as the peak time of bone mass formation. Before this age, osteoblastic new bone formation exceeds osteoclastic new bone resorption (reverse osteoporosis). The peak bone mass is greater in men than in women, having important determinants. The amount of bone declines after the age of peak bone mass and is primarily brought about by an imbalance between formation and resorption, always in favor of the latter.

Osteoporosis is a condition in which the amount of bone per unit volume decreases significantly, the bone composition remaining more or less the same (30,31). The imbalance in formation and resorption leads to the bones becoming porous, the loss of bone being sufficient to predispose them to fracture. The reduction in the amount of bone is more than 2 SD from the mean value for the young adult. Osteoporosis predisposes bones to fractures, the most common ones being vertebral, the forearm, and the femoral neck (30). The most important fracture associated with osteoporosis is the femoral neck fracture, because of its high frequency and because it leads to immediate disability, early and late mortality, and considerable morbidity. The most important determinats of osteoporosis are the peak bone mass and its subsequent rate of loss.

The amount of bone present in the young adult (peak bone mass) is determined by genetic factors, gender, the use of the skeleton, the nutritional status and intake, especially that of calcium (32), and endocrine factors. The effect of calcium on the peak bone mass is normally associated with that of energy and protein, which occur together in the diet. Excessive alcohol intake, cigarette smoking, and self-imposed starvation may decrease bone mass to a certain extent (33).

Smith (13) categorized factors determining peak bone mass into the following four categories: (a) genetic (race, family, and gender), (b) nutritional (calcium and protein energy), (c) endocrine factors (growth hormone, sex hormones, and calcitropic hormones), and (d) mechanical factors. The risk factors for bone loss include immobility, early menopause, positive family history, low calcium intake, underweight, alcohol, and smoking.

The bone mass varies from one race to another, being highest in blacks and lowest in whites and Asians. Within races, peak bone mass appears to be familial and controlled by single genes (or a set of them). The inherited disorders of collagen can lead to osteogenesis imperfecta (34). Also, failure to use the skeleton during growth leads to overall bone loss with bizarre changes in the limbs (e.g., in poliomyelitis, muscular dystrophy, and osteogenesis imperfecta). Lanyon and Rubin (35) noted that continual use of the growing skeleton increased bone mass in the experimental animals.

Starvation in childhood, associated with protein energy malnutrition, leads to temporary cessation of growth and eventual short stature. In humans, it is not possible to produce bone disease by restricting calcium alone, and in children any bone disease produced resembles rickets (22).

The relationship of bone loss to calcium deficiency has been extensively reviewed (22, 36–38). The form of calcium given, the efficiency of its absorption, and the reommended requirements are the most important factors in calcium nutrition (39). The rate of bone loss appears to be unrelated to prevailing calcium intake (40,41). Also, the addition of calcium alone to the diet does not reduce the rate of postmenopausal bone loss (41,42). Increasing calcium intake, however, may have beneficial effects in cortical bone (43). The most effective treatment for preventing postmenopausal bone loss is the therapeutic use of naturally occurring estrogen and progesterone, which have no side effects. Physical activity, calcium intake, and estrogen therapy are all important in preventing proximal femoral fractures (44–46).

C. Phosphorus

Phosphorus in the human body is found both in its organic and inorganic forms, and is distributed throughout the body, though a majority (85%) is present in the skeleton. The effects of phosphorus deficiency are widespread, and disorders of phosphorus metabolism are closely related to important bone diseases. The distribution, function, and control of phosphorus within the body differs from that of calcium, and phosphorus appears to have a secondary role in bone metabolism. The phosphorus deficiency has been known to cause osteomalacia, myopathy, defects in leukocyte function, and growth failure. Most biochemical reactions require adenosine triphosphate (ATP), for which phosphate is necessary. Phosphorus is also an integral part of phospholipids, phosphoproteins, and sugar phosphates.

Many factors control phosphorus balance in the body, the most important being the amount of phosphorus reabsorbed by the renal tubules. Hormones appear to influence phosphorus balance in various ways that are not fully understood. Administration of vitamin D to vitamin D–deficient subjects increases intestinal phosphate absorption. Whereas PTH decreases renal reabsorption of phosphate, leading to hypophosphatemia, calcitonin increases phosphate excretion by the kidney. Plasma phosphate levels are often higher in children than in adults. The renal handling of phosphorus is usually expressed in terms of the maximum tubular reabsorption of phosphate (TmP) as related to the glomerular filtration rate (GFR). Whereas TmP is decreased in hyperparathyroidism, it is increased above normal in tumoral calcinosis, with hyperphosphatemia (13).

Smith (13) divided the causes of abnormal plasma phosphate into the following categories:

---

1. Hypophosphatemia

  a. Inherited: Vitamin D–resistant rickets
  b. Acquired: Hyperparathyroidism
                 Aludrox overdosage
                 Vitamin D deficiency
                 Prolonged parenteral nutrition

2. Hyperphosphatemia

  a. Inherited: Tumoral calcinosis
                 Pseudohypoparathyroidism
  b. Acquired: Hypoparathyroidism
                 Renal glomerular failure

A shift in the TmP/GFR ratio is observed in vitamin D–resistant rickets (inherited hypophosphatemia), tumoral calcinosis (inherited hyperphosphatemia) as well as in hyper-and hypothyroidism. In contrast, the major determinant of hypophosphatemias in vitamin D deficiency and aluminium hydroxide overdosage is a reduction in intestinal phosphate absorption. Hyperphosphatemia in renal glomerular failure, on the contrary, result from the continuing intestinal absorption of phosphate with declining renal clearance (13).

D. Magnesium

Human skeleton contains up to 70% of total body magnesium, which is distributed widely in the soft tissues and skeleton. Magnesium is the most abundant intracellular divalent cation involved in a large number of metabolic processes. Plasma magnesium levels are maintained remarkably constant by rapid adaptation by the kidney; a fall in magnesium intake is rapidly followed by a fall in the urinary output, and only later by hypomagnesemia. Like calcium, magnesium is not mobilized selectively in the tissues through homeostatic mechanisms. The body appears to protect against magnesium loss by reducing urinary excretion, losing magnesium significantly only under the conditions of very low intake for a prolonged time, and high intestinal losses. Certain inherited disorders may lead to selective malabsorption of magnesium, resulting in hypomagnesemia and hypocalcemia (13).

Total plasma magnesium (1.7–2.3 mg/100) is distributed into an ionized fraction (1.3 mg %), a small complexed fraction (0.3 mg %), and the rest in the protein-bound form, which can be measured by the difference between total and ultrafilterable magnesium.

Like phosphorus, the absorption of magnesium can occur at very low intakes. In humans, magnesium is primarily absorbed through the small intestine and it is increased by both vitamin D and PTH through unknown machanisms.

The magnesium balance of the body is influenced by several factors, the most common cause of hypomagnesemia being malabsorption, especially when this results from small-bowel resection. Other causes include dietary deficiency, protein calorie malnutrition, and prolonged intravenous feeding; excessive renal loss, as with diuretics and alcohol; and diabetes, in which there is both an increase in the renal loss of magnesium and its increased transport into soft tissues after insulin administration.

Hypermagnesemia is very common in patients with renal glomerular failure; as with phosphorus, the bones of these patients show an increase in magnesium content. The latter is thought to delay the transition of bone mineral from amorphous to crystalline form, affecting the normal formation of bone matrix collagen (13).

E. Sulfur

1. Biochemical Function

Sulfur is primarily required by humans and other animals in the form of sulfur-containing amino acids, methionine and cysteine. Sulfur is present in all proteins but is more prevalent in the keratin of skin and hair. Sulfur is also a component of glutathione. Sulfur exists in the reduced form (SH), as in the cysteine, having vital functions in the specific configuration and structural conformation of some proteins and activities of enzymes. Sulfur is also a constituent of vitamins such as thiamin and biotin.

III. MONOVALENT ELECTROLYTES: SODIUM, POTASSIUM, AND CHLORIDE

The monovalent electrolytes, sodium (Na^+), potassium (K^+), and chloride (Cl^-) are conveniently considered together, in association with body water (see Chapter 2), because these ions are responsible for almost the entire osmolality of body fluids, and their deposition within the body determines the volumes of extracellular and intracellular fluids. Whereas K^+ is predominantly confined intracellularly, accompanied by magnesium phosphate (largely the orgnic fraction) and proteinate anion, Na^+ and Cl^- are associated mainly with the extracellular fluid. These ions in the body are usually measured by isotope dilution method, by whole-carcass analysis, and by neu-

Table 2 Total Body Na$^+$, K$^+$, and Cl$^-$ by Neutron Activation Analysis

Electrolyte		Average (mmol)	Average (mmol/kg)
Na$^+$	Men	3540	47
	Women	2620	43
K$^+$	Men	3190	26
	Women	2030	25
Cl$^-$	Men	2110	28
	Women	1720	28

Source: Refs. 47 and 48.

tron activation analysis. The values of total body Na$^+$, K$^+$, and Cl$^-$ by the latter method are shown in Table 2. (47,48).

The total concentration of ions in mEq is greater in intracellular than in extracellular fluid because of the greater electrical charge of the polyvalent intracellular ions such as proteinates, but the osmolality (number of molecules in solution per kg of water) of both the fluids is indentical. Plasma has slightly lower concentration of Cl$^-$ and bicarbonate and a slightly higher Na$^+$ concentration (5%) than extracellular fluid.

Active cellular extrusion of Na$^+$ at the cell membrane, involving Na$^+$/K$^+$-linked ATPase, is responsible for the predomination of Na$^+$ in the extracellular fluid, and that of K$^+$ in the intracellular position (49). The Na$^+$ concentration of the cells actively involved in secreting or absorbing Na$^+$ is higher, e.g. the renal tubules, sweat glands, and alimentary tract. Approximately one-half of the body Na$^+$ is immobilized in bone, as an integral part of the mineral lattice. This bone Na$^+$ is not fully exchangeable with the Na$^+$ in extracellular fluid, and it does not support extracellular fluid volume or osmolality in clinical states of Na$^+$ depletion or hyponatremia.

The asymmetric distribution of diffusible ions between extra- and intracellular fluid (ICF) produces an electric charge across the cell membrane (average about 80 mV), negative on the cell interior. This membrane potential contributes to many cell functions as well as to the normal behavior of muscle and nerve. The ratio of extracellular fluid (ECF) concentration determines the contribution of each electrolyte to the membrane potential. The clinical significance of ECF concentration of K$^+$ has been well recognized, and its normally very low concentrations have a much more marked effect on ECF/ICF ratio than the much larger changes in ICF concentration of the ions.

Like Na$^+$, Cl$^-$ also predominates as an extracellular ion, but it is not sequestered in bone. The ICF Cl$^-$ concentrations vary from about 3 mmol/1 in skeletal muscle to 90 mmol/1 in red cells and neuroglia, with intermediate levels in the ICF of the secreting and absorbing cells of the renal tubule and gastrointestinal (G.I.) tract. In red cells, Cl$^-$ has an important function in the transport of carbon dioxide through the exchange of erythrocyte bicarbonate with plasma Cl$^-$ during blood deoxygenation (the chloride shift) to assist the venous transport of carbon dioxide to the lungs and transport of oxygen from lungs to the peripheral tissue in the reverse process. The gastric juice of the stomach has high acidity—pH around 1.0—contributed by higher concentrations of H$^+$ and Cl$^-$ (140 mmol/l).

Unlike some other nutrients, water and monovalent ions have no storage depots in the body. The amounts of these electrolytes present in the body are regulated at a very constant level by a precise balance between their intake and output, through urinary excretion and to a certain extent by sweating.

The balances of Na$^+$, K$^+$, and Cl$^-$ in the body can be measured precisely by determining their dietary intake, either by the use of food tables or more accurately by analysis of a duplicate diet, and by knowing the amounts lost in urine, feces, or any abnormal body secretions (e.g., vomit, intestinal secretion, and fistulas). Losses of Na^+, K^+, and Cl^- through sweat are negligible, especially in the temperature regions, and often disregarded. The electrolyte balance of these ions, however, has little clinical significance, except for knowing electrolyte deficiencies.

Correction of abnormal Na^+, Cl^-, and K^+ balances by the body is precise but takes 2 to 5 days to complete or even longer, if the initial disturbance is greater. The dietary intakes of Na^+ and K^+ are very similar to their daily urinary outputs, viz., 75 to 350 (mean 180) and 30 to 100 (mean 65) mmol, respectively. Dietary Na^+ and Cl^- are also ingested through other minor sources, such as sodium sulfite in preservatives and monosodium glutamate used as a flavoring agent.

Because the excretion of either Na^+ or Cl^- by routes other than urine is negligible, both their intake and output are almost identical. Most natural foods such as cereals, fruits, and vegetables contain little Na^+ and Cl^-, though meats contain larger amounts (Table 3) (50). The details of the electrolyte balance of Na^+, Cl^-, and K^+, including their intake, output, and body deficits and excesses, have been dealt with in Chapter 2.

IV. THE TRACE ELEMENTS (Fe, Zn, Cu, Se, Mn, Mo, F, AND Cr)

A. Iron

Iron (Fe) is a constituent of vital proteins of the body such as myoglobin and hemoglobin, which serve as carriers of oxygen to the tissues, heme and non-heme enzymes (cytochromes, catalases, peroxidases, and many others), ferritin, and hemosiderin, as storage forms of iron (51–54).

Table 3 Na^+, K^+, and Cl^- Contents of Some Common Foods (mmols/100 g)

Foods	Na^+	K^+	Cl^-
Natural foods			
Wheat flour	0.1	9	1
Beef, lean	3	9	2
Cod, frozen steaks	3	8	3
Eggs, boiled	4	4	5
Cow's milk, fresh	2	4	3
Lettuce, raw	0.4	6	1
Cabbage, raw	0.3	7	1
Carrots, raw	4	6	2
Potatoes, raw	0.3	15	2
Oranges	0.1	5	0.1
Bananas	0.1	10	0.2
Apples, eating	0.1	0.3	0.03
Processed foods			
White bread	23	3	25
Bacon, raw lean	81	9	79
Kippers, baked	23	7	23
Cheese, cheddar	27	3	30
Salted butter	38	0.5	38
Beans, canned in tomato sauce	21	7	23
Tomato ketchup	49	15	51

Source: Ref. 50.

A majority of the body's iron is present in RBCs as hemoglobin—2400 and 1600 mg in men (75 kg wt.) and women (55 kg body wt.), respectively—followed by that present in myoglobin (350 mg in men and 230 mg in women). The total functional iron content of men and women is around 2900 and 1940 mg, respectively. The iron stored in the form of ferritin and hemosiderin varies from 500 to 1500 and 0 to 300 mg in men and women, the total iron content of the body being around 4000 and 2100 mg, respectively (55). Several vital enzymes, such as cytochromes and others, have one heme group and a polypeptide (protein) chain, whose structures do not permit a reversible loading and unloading of oxygen (as in hemoglobin), but act as electron carriers within the cell. Iron thus has an important function in oxidative metabolism: transferring energy within the cell and the mitochondria. In addition to oxygen and electron transport, a large number of iron-containing enzymes play key roles as signal-controlling substances in neurotransmitter systems in the brain (e.g., the dopamine and serotonin systems). Certain Fe-containing enzymes (e.g., cytochrome P-450) have important functions in the synthesis of steroid hormones and bile acids (hydroxylation), as well as detoxification of various foreign substances in the liver. The Fe-bound transferrins are involved in the transport of iron between various body compartments. Transferrin carries iron from the intestinal mucosal cells to the red cell precursors in the bone marrow and to other cells in the body during growth and development.

Hallberg et al. (55) divided iron metabolism into two categories: internal loop and external loop. The internal iron metabolism constitutes the synthesis and degradation of RBCs. When RBCs die, after about 120 days, the iron is released and delivered to the transferrin molecules in the plasma, by the macrophages of the reticular-endothelial system. The iron is brought back to the red cell precursors in the bone marrow and to other cells for its reutilization. The internal Fe metabolism can be monitored by labeling the transferrin-bound iron with a radioactive iron tracer. Thus the total iron turnover in plasma and its appearance in RBCs can be measured to quantify erythropoiesis. The external Fe metabolism is represented by the loss of Fe from the body from cellular losses, including bleeding and the absorption of dietary iron.

1. Iron Requirements

The body uses the following three mechanisms for maintaining iron balance and preventing iron deficiency (55):

    a.   Continuous reutilization of iron from catabolized RBCs.

    b.   Regulation of the iron absorption from the intestine, i.e., an increase in Fe absorption when Fe is deficient and vice versa, and

    c.   Access to ferritin (storage Fe protein), which stores and releases iron bank of the body.

The iron requirements of the body are determined by several factors, including the basal iron losses, growth, pregnancy, and lactation, menstrual iron losses, iron absorption, and others.

Certain amounts of iron are lost from the skin cells and the interior surfaces of body (intestines, urinary tract, and airways); the total amount of iron lost is estimated at 14 mg/kg body weight/day. The amount of iron lost through sweating is negligible (56).

The newborn infant has an iron content of around 200 to 300 mg (75 mg/kg wt.). During the first 2 months, the hemoglobin concentration of the newborn infant decreases slightly due to the improved oxygen supply. The latter results in the redistribution of iron from catabolized RBCs to iron stores that meet the requirements for iron during the first 4 to 6 months of life. The iron requirements during this period thus can be met from breast milk alone, which contains very little iron. Owing to the marked supply of iron to the fetus during the last trimester of pregnancy, the iron status of premature babies and low-birth-weight infants is much less favorable than those of the full-term babies. An extra supply of iron is needed in these infants even during the first 6 months.

Table 4 Basis for Calculation of Absorbed Iron Requirements for Growth

| Age (years) and Sex | Weight gain (kg) | mg iron/kg body wt. | | | | Mean iron required for growth (mg/day) |
		Hemoglobin	Myoglobin	Enzymes	Total	
0.25–1.0	4.2	32	3	2	37	0.65
1–2	2.4	32	3	2	37	0.24
2–6	7.9	32	6	2	40	0.22
6–12	20.2	33	6	2	41	0.38
Boys 12–16	26.2	37	7	2	46	0.66
Girls 12–16	15.2	34	7	2	43	0.36
Adult men	—	39	7	2	48	—
Adult women	—	34	7	2	43	—

Source: Refs. 55 and 57.

The basis of iron requirements for growth have been reviewed by an expert group for FAO/WHO (1988) (Table 4). For the full-term infant, iron requirement rises markedly after the age of 4 to 6 months, amounting to about 0.5 to 0.8 mg/day during the remaining part of the first year. These are very high iron requirements in relation to the body size and energy intake (55).

The full-term normal-weight baby must double its total iron content and triple its body weight within the first year of its life. The iron content of the body during this period changes mainly between 6 to 12 months of age. The body iron content is again doubled during 1 to 6 years of age. The iron requirement of the infant and child are of the same magnitude as that of an adult human. The absorbed iron requirements of infants and children are very high in relation to their energy requirements, (about 1.5 mg/1000 kcal), and about one-half of this amount is required up to the age of 4 years.

The rapidly growing weaning infant has no iron stores in the body and must rely on dietary iron. During the weaning period, the iron requirements as related to energy intake are the highest of a human's life span, barring the last trimester of pregnancy, when the iron requirements are to be met primarily from the iron stores of the mother. The high requirements of weaning infants can be met if the diet has a high content of meat and ascorbic acid–rich foods. In developing countries where cereals constitute the main staple food, it is important that cereal products are fortified with iron and ascorbic acid.

The iron requirements of the body are also high in adolescents, especially during periods of rapid growth. There requirements may be considerably higher than the calculated mean values shown in Table 4, because of marked variation in the growth rates of some individuals. Girls often have their growth spurt before the menarche (though growth does not stop at this stage), increasing their total iron requirements (57).

Considerable variation exists in menstrual blood and iron loss from one individual to other and losses are also influenced by geography and genetics. The mean menstrual iron loss, averaged over the entire menstrual cycle of 28 days, is around 0.56 mg/day. By adding the average basal iron loss (0.8 mg), the mean total iron requirements in adult women comes to around 1.36 mg/day, which may exceed the value 2.27 mg/day in 10% of women, to as high as 2.84 mg/day; and in 5% of these girls, requirements are 3.2 mg/day, considering individual variations. The FAO/WHO recommendations for girls are slightly lower and have been reexamined (58).

In postmenopausal women and in physically active elderly people, the iron requirements are about the same as in men, which decrease with reduction in physical activity due to aging, owing to reduction in the blood volume and hemoglobin mass.

2. *Absorption of Heme and Non-Heme Iron*

Hallberg (59) distinguished two kinds of iron in the diet, with respect to their mechanism of absorption: heme iron and non-heme iron, which utilize two separate receptors on the mucosal cells (60). According to Baynes and Bothwell (60), the absorption of heme iron is influenced by factors such as amount of heme present in meat, the calcium content of the meal, and food preparation (time, temperature, etc), whereas absorption of non-heme iron is influenced by factors such as iron status of subjects, amount of bioavailable non-heme iron and balance between dietary factors enhancing and inhibiting iron absorption. Iron absorption in general is enhanced by the presence of ascorbic acid, meat, fish, seafood, and certain organic acids in the diet, whereas the presence of phytates, iron-binding phenolics, calcium, and soy protein usually inhibit iron absorption.

The porphyrin ring of heme iron is split by hemoxynase enzyme after heme iron is taken up by the mucosal cells, releasing the iron. Both the heme and non-heme iron are then transported similarly to the serosal side of the mucosal cells, using a common transfer system. The iron is most probably absorbed into the cells and passes through the mucosal membrane in its ferrous (Fe^{++}) form, and reducing substances such as ascorbic acid therefore enhance iron absorption.

Meat and meat products contain about 1 to 2 mg of heme iron, constituting about 5 to 10% of the daily iron intake in the Western countries. Approximately 25% of the heme iron present in the meat is absorbed (61). Unlike that of non-heme iron, the absorption of heme iron is very little influenced by the iron status of the subject. The presence of meat in the diet appears to enhance absorption of heme iron (55).

Non-heme iron is the main form of dietary iron present in cereals, vegetables, fruits, beans, and peas. Unlike that of heme iron, the absorption of non-heme iron is influenced significantly by individual iron status, more iron being absorbed by iron-deficient subjects and vice versa. Also, the absorption of non-heme iron is influenced by several other dietary factors, such as presence of phytates, phenolics, calcium, and soy protein.

Phytates (salts of inositol hexaphosphates) strongly inhibit iron absorption in a dose-dependent fashion, even smaller amounts of phytate having a marked effect. Ascorbic acid in sufficient amounts partly counteracts this inhibition (62).

Bran has a very high phytate content, and in bread, phytate is degraded to inositol phosphates during the fermentation of the dough by the phytase present in flour. These inositol phosphates also inhibit iron absorption. However, prolonged fermentation for a couple of days (sourdough fermentation) almost completely degrades the phytate, increasing iron absorption (63). Oats, because of their high phytate content and destruction of native phytase by heat treatment, strongly inhibit iron absorption.

Fiber content of the diet per se does not influence the iron absorption. Fiber-rich cereal foods, however, are rich in phytates. High-extraction flours and oats with high fiber content will lead to a reduction of total iron absorption. Thus any advantage of high-fiber intake in the diet, which increases fecal bulk and counteracts constipation, must be carefully balanced against the disadvantage of markedly reducing absorption of iron and other micronutrients such as calcium and zinc.

Phenolic compounds are present in most plant foods in varying amounts and have a role in defending plants against insects and other pests. Out of thousands of known phenolics, only some seem to inhibit iron absorption. It is mainly the galloyl group in the phenolics that specifically binds iron (64). Foods containing much iron-binding polyphenols include tea, coffee, cocoa, vegetables such as spinach, and several herbs and spices (e.g. oregano), which contain appreciable amounts of galloyl groups. This type of inhibition is also partly counteracted by ascorbic acid and meat (55).

Consumed in the form of salt or as dairy products such as milk or cheese, calcium significantly reduces iron absorption (65,66). The inhibition is equally strong for both heme and non-heme iron. One glass of milk containing about 165 mg of calcium can reduce iron absorption by more than half. The inhibition is probably not localized to the gastrointestinal lumen but to the mucosal cells and to the final transfer step. Calcium being an essential nutrient, its inhibition cannot be considered in the same sense as that of phytates or phenolics. Higher calcium content of meals, however, markedly inhibits bioavailability of iron, and epidemiological studies have shown an association between the intake of milk and prevalence of iron deficiency. These findings may either lead to an avoidance of excess dietary calcium, or increased dietary iron in groups with a high calcium intake.

Addition of soybean protein to a meal has been found to decrease iron absorption, which may be attributed to the high phytate content of soy protein. However, because of the high iron content of soy proteins, the iron availability may be a positive one. The inhibitory effect of soy proteins in the infant foods can be overcome by addition of ascorbic acid.

Ascorbate is the most potent enhancer of non-heme iron absorption, both natural and synthetic vitamin C having the same effect. Hallberg et al. (67) noted a strong exponential dose-related effect of ascorbic acid on non-heme iron absorption, probably by reducing ferric iron to ferrous state. Ferric ions bind more strongly to various ligands than the ferrous iron. The dietary iron in the duodenum, in its normal alkaline pH range, can be converted into ferric hydroxide and be precipited in a nonabsorbable form. Ascorbate increases iron absorption by converting ferric iron to its ferrous state or by forming soluble iron-ascorbate complexes. It has been suggested that the requirements of ascorbic acid for iron absorption should be taken into account while calculating the requirements of vitamin C.

Meat, fish, and seafoods promote absorption of non-heme iron, through some unknown mechanism. Meat also increases the absorption of heme iron. Certain organic acids like citric acid also have been found to enhance the asorption of non-heme iron. Similarly, sauerkraut and other fermented vegetables and fermented soy sauces have an enhancing effect on iron absorption.

3. *Iron Balance*

Iron balance can be defined as the presence of a steady state when the absorption of iron from the diet covers both the actual losses of iron from the body and the requirements of growth and/or pregnancy (also a kind of growth). The amount of iron lost with menstruation is influenced by the hemoglobin level. Menstrual iron losses decrease successively with diminishing hemoglobin levels, prior to the development of an iron deficiency anemia. Skin iron losses also decrease in a state of iron deficiency, and increase if the subject is given an iron dose overload. This is followed by a state in which iron losses equal the amount absorbed from the diet, achieving iron balance. Hallberg et al. (55) cited the following hypothetical example to show that there are an infinite number of iron balance states of the human body when absorption equals loss: in a population of menstruating women with varying iron requirements, consuming the same diet, the iron status may vary from anemia of different degrees to iron stores of different magnitudes. This variation in iron status influences the 'setting' ability of the mucosal cells to absorb iron. Thus, iron balance is maintained by regulating the iron absorption in relation to the iron status. This regulation can only partially counteract the variation in iron requirements. Any measures taken to change the iron losses or its absorption in a population will move the existing point of balance, affecting the prevalence and severity of iron deficiency in that population. Thus, iron fortification of foods will increase absorption, leading to a reduction in prevalence of iron deficiency and an increase of iron stores of the population. The increase in iron stores, however, will decrease the iron absorption. This feedback system enables the body to establish new states of iron balance, with more iron available for absorption. In a state of positive iron balance, the amount of iron in stores will at certain new balance levels flatten out to new steady states (55).

There is no risk of developing iron overload in otherwise healthy subjects. The normal iron stores of healthy adults (30 years) in the Western countries vary from 500 to 1000 mg with a high bioavailability iron diet. The iron stores in women seldom reach 500 mg; about 20 to 30% of women have no iron stores at all, the average level of iron stores being estimated around 150 mg.

4. Iron Deficiency and Anemia

Iron deficiency in terms of the absence of iron stores can be detected when no stainable iron in the reticular endothelial cells of bone marrow smears is seen. Also, serum ferritin concentration decreases to less than 15 g/1. The absence of iron stores, though not associated with immediate negative effects, is a reliable and good indicator of an increased risk of probable iron deficiency.

Iron deficiency syndrome with a negative iron balance is a commonly experienced phenomenon in iron-replete women using intrauterine contraceptive devices. Menstrual iron losses in such women are doubled, with progressive increases in iron absorption that cannot balance the higher iron losses. The iron stores are then successively emptied. Negative iron balance during this phase is indicated by lesser and lesser stainable iron seen in bone marrow smears, and plasma ferritin reaches a value of about 15 g/1.

With immobilization of iron from the stores, sufficient iron is not supplied to transferrin, the circulating iron transport protein. A reduction of the transferrin saturation (TS) is indicated by lesser iron bound on the binding sites of transferrin. With a reduction in TS to a critical level (16%), red cell precursors get an insufficient supply of the iron, accompanied by impaired supply of iron to other tissues by transferrin. High-turnover cells with a short life span (e.g., intestinal mucosal cells) are the first to be affected, with iron deficiency in growing tissues. Hemoglobin (Hb) synthesis is impaired rather early in the development of iron deficiency, with Hb level falling below the normal value. Severe and long-lasting negative iron balance and prolonged impairment in hemoglobin synthesis lead to an anemic condition. The prevalence of iron-deficiency anemia (a Hb level below the 2.5th perceptible value of the population) is less frequent than iron deficiency defined as an absence of iron stores.

Iron deficiency anemia can be suspected if anemia is present in subjects who are iron deficient and the diagnosis can be fully established by seeing the positive response of the subjects to iron treatment. An iron-deficient erythropoiesis is recognized by low TS, high content of transferrin receptors in plasma, high protoporphyrin in the red cells, and a microcytic hypochromic anemia (55).

Nutritional iron deficiency implies that the diet does not meet the physiological requirements of the body's iron needs. Infestation with hookworms that leads to blood losses and poor diets are among common causes of iron deficiency in many tropical countries of Asia, Africa, and South America. The average blood loss in hookworm infestation can be estimated by examination of stool for egg counts. Other pathological causes of blood loss include tumors in tract of uterus; achlorhydria, with 50% reduction in the absorption of dietary iron; and extensive gastric surgery leading to impaired iron absorption.

Nutritional factors are important in vegetarian people. Chanarian et al. (68) reported that about 63% of 138 Hindu Indian vegetarians in the affluent society of London, who had cobalamin deficiency, showed overt iron deficiency also (53 women and 38 men), and marrow iron stores were absent in 71%.

Around 600 to 700 million of the world's population suffer from iron deficiency anemia (69). In the industrialized countries, the prevalence is much lower (2–8%); however, the absence of iron stores or subnormal serum ferritin values are found in around 20 to 30% of women of childbearing age in these countries. Worldwide, the highest rates of iron deficiency are found in infants, children, teenagers, and child-bearing women.

Lozoff (70) and Youdim (71) established the relation between iron deficiency and brain function. Several structures in the brain have a high iron content—about the same magnitude as that found in the liver. There is an active transferrin-receptor mediated transport of iron into the brain. The iron content of human brain increases continuously during development and up through the teenage period. Approximately 10% of brain iron is present at birth, and at age 10, the human brain reaches only one-half of its normal iron content; optimal amount is reached at the age of 20 to 30 years. The lower iron content of the brain in iron-deficient growing rats could not be restituted by providing iron later on, suggesting the importance of the supply of iron of the brain cells during the early phase of brain development. The early iron deficiency in animals may lead to irreparable damage. Youdim (71) has shown that brain functions related to the neurotransmitter systems are adversely affected by iron deficiency. The iron deficiency leads to a decreased sensitivity of the dopamine-D2 receptor of the brain's dopamine system. This is associated with an impaired catabolism of biogenic amines such as serotonin and endogenous opiopeptides. The iron deficiency also has been shown to cause an impairment in memory and learning, an increase in the pain threshold, reduction in the release of thyrotropin release hormone (TRH), resulting in body's decreased thyroid function and thermoregulation.

Iron deficiency has been found to negatively influence the body's normal defense system and immune function. The cell-mediated immunological response by the action of T-lymphocytes is impaired, because of their reduced synthesis, for want of normal DNA synthesis, which depends on iron-requiring ribonucleotide reductase.

Iron deficiency also impairs the function of neutrophil leukocytes in the defense mechanism. The iron-sulfur enzyme, NADPH-oxidase and cytochrome B (a heme enzyme) must be activated for the synthesis of free OH radicals required for killing of bacteria (phagocytosis). Myeloperoxidase, another important and much-studied enzyme involved in the defense system, is also adversely affected by iron deficiency. Owing to significant impairment of defense system against infection, iron-deficient human subjects are more prone to infection, with marked severity, than are control subjects.

Iron deficiency has been shown to be closely related to human behavior; attention, memory, and learning are adversely affected in iron-deficient infants and children, and up through the period of adolescence into early adulthood (55).

The translation of the absorbed iron requirements into dietary iron requirements must take into consideration the following two facts: (a) the iron status of the body desired to be maintained in a fraction of a population group, and (b) the bioavailability of the iron in differents diets. About twice as much iron is absorbed from a certain diet by borderline iron-deficient subjects with no iron stores, compared to those having about 300 mg of stored iron. Thus, in order to maintain such a level of stored iron, twice as much iron would be required in the diet to cover the physiological demands of the body.

The diets of different population groups vary considerably in the bioavailability of iron, owing to variation in the content of meat, fish, ascorbic acid–rich foods, milk products, and phytates, which influence iron absorption. Thus, the bioavailability of iron in the diets of the population of many developing countries (with low meat and fish and high phytate-containing cereals) may be very low, compared to those of the industrialized nations. In borderline iron-deficient subjects, the bioavailability of iron may be around 14% to 16% (58).

The marked physiological changes occurring during pregnancy significantly influence the iron requirements. The pregnant woman has to rely on her iron stores, if present. The iron requirements during pregnancy are well established, based on gross loss of iron as follows: fetus (300 mg), placenta (50 mg), expansion of maternal cell mass (450 mg), and basal iron loss (240 mg), amounting a total of 1040 mg of iron loss. Assuming a gain of 450 mg for the maternal red cell mass at the time of delivery and a loss of 200 mg as maternal blood loss, there would be a net gain of 200 mg iron at delivery. Deducting this value from the gross loss of 1040 mg, the net total loss of iron during pregnancy would be 840 mg (55). Most of this iron is required to increase the hemoglobin mass of the mother, which occurs in healthy pregnant women who have sufficiently large iron stores, as well as in those who are adequately supplemented with iron. The increase in the iron requirement is directly proportional to the increased need for oxygen transport during pregnancy, which is one of the important physiological adaptations occurring during pregnancy (72).

The iron requirements in pregnancy are not equally distributed over its duration. The exponential growth of the fetus suggests that the iron needs are comparatively very low or almost negligible in the first trimester, increasing to more than 80% during the last trimester. The total daily iron requirements, including the basal iron losses (0.8 mg), increase during pregnancy to about 10 mg during the last 6 weeks.

The amount of iron absorbed during pregnancy depends on the amount of iron in the diet, its bioavailability (meal composition), and changes in iron absorption occurring during pregnancy. In the first trimester there is a marked decrease in iron absorption that is related to the reduction in iron requirements during this period. In the second trimester, iron absorption increases by about 50%, and in the last trimester it increases about fourfold. Despite the marked increase in iron absorption, it is not possible for the pregnant woman to cover her very high iron requirements from the diet alone. It has been estimated that even with the diets prevailing in the industrially developed countries, there will be a deficit of about 400 to 500 mg of iron between total iron requirements and the amounts of iron absorbed during pregnancy (55).

Iron deficiency can be prevented by (a) iron supplementation—i.e., providing iron tablets to specific target groups such as pregnant women and preschool children, (b) iron fortification of certain foods, and (c) nutrition education to improve iron absorption from the diet (55).

5. Effects of Iron Overload

The amount of iron in the human body seldom exceeds 2000 mg; in fact, in women it is often below 400 to 500 mg and in men less than 1500 mg. Increased amounts of iron occur either by increased absorption from intestine or by increased parenteral administration of iron or through blood transfusions. In healthy subjects, a high dietary iron intake does not lead to any organ damage due to pathological accumulation of iron. A nutritional iron overload condition has been described in Bantu populations consuming large amounts of a special beer with very high iron content brewed in iron containers, and in alcoholics taking large amounts of wines with high iron content. Iron overload may also occur in patients with chronic anemias with an increased, ineffective erythropoiesis, which induces an increase in the absorption of dietary iron, e.g., in thalassemia major.

B. Zinc

Although the essentiality of zinc in animal nutrition has been known for more than 100 years, McCance and Widdowson in the early 1940s first reported studies on zinc metabolism, including its balance and absorption (73,74). Sandstead et al. (75) and Halstead et al. (76) reported zinc-responsive growth failures in adolescent boys in Egypt and Iran. With the advances in the analytical techniques made in the measurement of zinc in foods and tissues, such as atomic absorption spectroscopy, the biochemical role of zinc in human nutrition has been elucidated extensively, including the clinical manifestations of severe zinc deficiency in man. However, the metabolic origin of the pathological changes in zinc deficiency, diagnostic criteria for marginal zinc deficiency, and a sound scientific basis for setting RDAs for zinc remain to be investigated.

1. Biochemical Function and Metabolism

Zinc is a constituent of more than 200 metallo-enzymes, including carbonic anhydrase, alcohol dehydrogenase, superoxide dismutase, DNA-polymerase, RNA-polymerase, alkaline phosphatase, and carboxy-peptidases. Thus, zinc is involved in the biosynthesis of nucleic acids, protein metabolism (synthesis and digestion), bone metabolism, oxygen transport, dark adaptation, defense system, and many others. Whereas in some metallo-enzymes, zinc is present at the active site (e.g., acting as electron-acceptor), in others and in non-enzyme proteins it has a structural role, such as disulfide linkages or cross-links between thiolates and imidazoles.

Zinc has an important biochemical role in the stabilization of structure of organic components and membranes. Bound zinc stabilizes the structures of RNA, DNA, and ribosomes. Chesters (77) suggested that zinc influences normal chromatin restructuring and gene expression. Zinc has an important biochemical role in the structure and function of membranes (78).

Zinc is also essential for the immune function and defense system of the body. Zinc deficiency in experimental animals has been reported to cause marked atrophy of the thymus, a reduction in leukocytes and in antibody-mediated, cell-mediated, and delayed-type hypersensitivity responses (55).

Zinc is thought to be released from the food matrix by the action of enzymes and gastric juices during digestion and is associated with low-molecular-weight legands, such as amino acids, peptides, organic acids, and phosphates. Much higher absorption of zinc has been reported from aqueous solutions during the fasting state (60% to 80%) than in the presence of food (5% to 40%) (79–81). Coppen and Davis (82) suggested that the mucosal uptake of zinc in rats is carrier-mediated and occurs via several processes that can be both saturable and non-saturable.

All tissues and fluids of the body contain zinc. An adult human body contains a total of 2 to 3 g zinc, of which about 60% is in the skeletal muscle and 30% in the bones. Zinc is primarily intracellular; very low amounts are present in extracellular fluids. Plasma zinc is only about 0.1% of the total body content and it has a rapid turnover-transport vehicle. Choroid of eye and prostatic fluids have high concentrations of zinc.

The hormonal balance and stress conditions influence the distribution of zinc between extracellular fluids, tissues, and organs, the liver playing an important role in this distribution. The body appears to depend on a small pool of "active" zinc, and there is no "store" of zinc in a conventional sense. Zinc present in bone has a low turnover rate but can be mobilized in extreme cases, such as zinc deficiency during pregnancy (83). It has been suggested that higher zinc intakes lead to synthesis of a sulfur-containing protein, metallo-thioneine, that binds zinc and probably serves as an intracellular storage form of zinc and is invloved in the "fine-tuning" of the intracellular levels of active zinc (84).

Zinc is lost from the body through the kidneys, the skin, and the intestine, the intestine being the major route of zinc excretion. Zinc is lost via the digestive juices and in shed intestinal cells. The endogenous intestinal losses of zinc can be as high as 2 to 4 mg/day (85–90).

About 0.5 mg/day of zinc is lost in the urine of healthy subjects. The majority of the primarily filtered zinc in the kidneys is reabsorbed; urinary excretion is unaffected by normal day-to-day variations in zinc intake. Jackson and Edwards (91) noticed that starvation and muscle catabolism increased zinc losses in the urine and feces. About 0.5 mg of zinc is thought to be lost daily through the desquamation of skin, growth of hair, and sweating.

Significant quantities of zinc are lost through prostatic fluids—e.g., a semen ejaculation can contain up to 1 mg of zinc (92); zinc is lost through menstruation only to the extent of 0.01 mg/day (93). Certain diseases, such as inflammatory bowel disease substantially enhance intestinal zinc losses (94), as they do in kidney diseases and alcoholism (95).

The tissue content of zinc is maintained constant over a wide range of dietary zinc intakes, by altering both absorption and excretion rates. The fractional absorption decreases and intestinal secretion increases with an increase in zinc uptake (87,90). Chronic low zinc intakes seem to increase zinc absorption efficiency to as high as 59% to 84% (85), accompanied by a decrease in urinary losses and losses via skin (96,97).

Thus, the role of zinc in cell replication and growth and its stabilizing function in organic compounds and membranes makes it a key nutrient for optimum health and growth of humans and animals. A number of organs and functions are affected by severe zinc deficiency, but the functional consequences of marginal deficiency are little understood.

2. Assessment of Status and Deficiency

Assessment of zinc status of the body is difficult, owing to the homeostatic regulation of zinc distribution and tissue concentration and its intracellular location. A poor zinc status, however, can be ascertained by giving a zinc supplement and finding a resultant biochemical or functional improvement or the disappearance of a clinical symptom. Plasma or serum levels of zinc in the circulation are the most widely used indices of zinc status. In addition to severe zinc deficiency, the plasma zinc level is also influenced by infection, fever, or intake of a protein-rich meal that lowers the plasma zinc. In contrast, long-term fasting and hemolysis tend to increase plasma zinc levels. The levels of zinc in leukocytes, erythrocytes, and hair, as well as urinary zinc excretion are also used as biochemical indices of zinc status. Functional indices, such as the zinc tolerance test (98), taste acuity (99), and dark adaptation (100) have been tested to assess the zinc status. According to Hallberg et. al. (55), none of these biochemical and functional measures has been proved to be useful in dignosing marginal zinc deficiency in humans. This is probably because overt symptoms can occur with almost no reduction in the tissue concentration of zinc (101), and because zinc supplementation rapidly improves the symptoms before any change in the tissue content. Milder zinc deficiency at present cannot be detected for want of a reliable, sensitive index of zinc status. Bremner et al. (102) correlated the circulating levels of metallothionine in plasma and the erythrocytes with the tissue levels and zinc status, and noted that the circulating metallothionine levels were less sensitive than plasma zinc to infection and trauma and might be useful for population surveys of zinc status.

Symptoms of severe zinc deficiency include circumoral and acral dermatitis, diarrhea, alopecia, and neuropsychiatric disorders. Zinc-responsive night blindness is seen in alcoholism and Crohn's disease (103). Growth retardation, immune defects, delayed sexual maturation, and failure to thrive are also regarded as clinical symptoms of zinc deficiency. These clinical manifestations of zinc deficiency are seen in certain inborn errors of zinc metabolism, such as acrodermatitis enteropathica (104) and Crohn's disease (105), in patients fed incomplete parenteral solution (106), and occasionally in infants (107).

Nutritional zinc deficiency (malnutrition) may show as skin ulcerations, decreased immunity for infection, and growth failures. Golden and Golden (108) observed that zinc status in Jamaican children recovering from malnutrition affected not only the growth rate but composition of the synthesized tissue, lean tissue synthesis being positively and closely related to dietary zinc intake.

An early sign of zinc deficiency in animals is a reduced feed intake leading to a decreased growth rate, which could be regarded as a useful adaptation to an inadequate zinc supply. Animal studies have shown that vitamin A metabolism, immune function, and skeletal maturation are especially sensitive to an insufficient zinc intake (109–111).

Healthy human subjects with intake of an almost zinc-free diet for 5 weeks showed signs of dermatitis, sore throat, and immune defects (112,113). Wada and King (114) also noticed changes in energy metabolism and decreased blood plasma proteins in subjects fed experimental diets with a low zinc content (5.5 mg/day), though these values were still within the normal range. The study of infants and children in Colorado, fed with a controlled zinc-supplemented diet, showed a significantly greater weight increment in male infants after zinc supplementation (115,116), which also increases energy and protein intake (117).

Wells et al. (118) suggested that maternal leukocyte zinc at the beginning of the third trimester could be used as an indicator of fetal growth retardation. Low maternal serum zinc levels in pregnant women have been found to be associated with pregnancy complications (119–121). Thus, pregnancy complications have not correlated well either with the body's zinc status or with dietary zinc intake, which may be partly because of the decreased plasma zinc levels owing to plasma expansion. The zinc plasma levels required for normal pregnancy are not known (55).

3. Food Sources and Requirements

Food sources vary widely in their zinc content. The zinc content of some common foods and the relation between zinc and energy and protein contents are shown in Table 5. Significant variations can occur in zinc intakes when foods are selected on the basis of energy needs, e.g. higher energy sources like fats, oils, sugar, and alcohol are rather poor sources of zinc. In animal foods such as beef and pork, the fat tissue contains much less zinc than the muscle tissue. Dark red meat generally has a higher zinc content than white meat and fish muscle tissue has a lower zinc content than meat.

Cereals are the major source of both energy and zinc in most parts of the world. Zinc is located in the outer layer of grain, so the supply of zinc from cereals depends on the degree of grain polishing and refinement. Zinc content of vegetable foods varies greatly with variety, species, and growing location (122). Because of their high water content, green leafy vegetables and fruits are only modest sources of zinc.

Food processing and preparation affect the zinc content of foods significantly. Galvanized cooking utensils and waterpipes are important additional sources of zinc. Leakages of about 10% to 12% of the zinc content of food into cooking water or canning media can occur (123).

The 'true' physiological requirement of zinc is the amount of zinc that has to be absorbed to replace endogenous losses to provide zinc for tissue synthesis and for growth and milk secretion. These requirements vary according to age and physiological status of the subject. The physiological requirement of zinc is quite different from the dietary requirement of zinc which takes into account the composition of the diet that influences both absorption and utilization.

The endogenous losses of zinc have been measured, using zinc-free diets and diets of normal zinc intake, by the use of stable zinc isotopes (89,90,124). In healthy adults consuming a typical industrial refined diet providing 10 to 12 mg of zinc, the endogenous zinc losses are about 2.5 mg/day, and in elderly people about 1.5 mg/day. The intake of phytate increases intestinal losses of zinc, and persons who consume vegetarian diets need about 4 mg of absorbed zinc per day.

Swanson and King (125) estimated that the total zinc requirement for gestation, for fetal placental tissue, aminotic fluid, uterine and mammary tissues, and maternal blood is about 100 mg, and the daily requirement of zinc during the last part of pregnancy is approximately 0.7 mg.

Table 5 Zinc Contents of Some Foods Expressed on a Raw Wet Weight Basis and in Relation to Their Protein and Energy Contents

Foods	Raw wet weight (mg/g)	Protein (mg/g)	Energy (mg/MJ)
Beef			
Lean	43	0.21	8.3
Fat	10	0.11	0.4
Pork			
Lean	24	0.12	3.9
Fat	4	0.06	0.1
Chicken			
Light meat	7	0.03	1.4
Dark meat	16	0.08	3.0
Fish, cod	4	0.02	1.2
Milk	3.5	0.11	1.3
Cheese (Cheddar)	40	0.15	2.4
Butter	1.5	—	0.05
Lentils	31	0.13	2.4
Wheat			
Whole meal	30	0.23	2.2
White	9	0.08	0.6
Maize (sweet corn)	12	0.29	2.2
Rice (polished)	13	0.20	0.8
Potatoes	3	0.14	0.8
Yam	4	0.20	0.7
Coconut	5	0.16	0.3

Source: Ref. 81.

Assuming the same endogenous losses during pregnancy, the total requirement for tissue growth and replacement of losses is 3.2 mg/day toward the end of pregnancy.

Human milk contains 2.5 µg/ml zinc in the first month of lactation, the zinc level drops to 1.0 µg/ml after 3 months. Assuming a total milk volume of 750 ml/day, an additional 2 mg/day zinc would be required in early lactation and about 0.7 mg/day after 3 months (126).

Krebs and Hambidge (127) estimated zinc requirement for growth to be about 175 µg/kg body weight/day in the first month of infant growth, which decreases to about 30 µg/day at 9 to 12 months of age. The endogenous losses of zinc as related to body size and the total zinc requirements for infants have been estimated at 1 to 1.2 mg/day in males and 0.9 to 1.05 mg/day in females.

It has been estimated that from a refined diet typical for industrialized countries, about 20% to 40% of zinc is absorbed depending on its concentration in the diet; about 10% to 15% is absorbed from whole-grain cereal–based diets. Thus, in modern society, the typical refined diet with a high content of fat, sugar, and alcohol provides a low zinc intake, especially in subjects with low energy requirement. In other parts of the world, the diet may contain larger amounts of zinc but because of the presence of complexing agents such as phytate and a reduced zinc availability, the intake can be insufficient for periods of high requirement, such as during adolescent growth (55).

The dietary recommendations for zinc intakes in adults vary from 8 mg/day in Czechoslovakia to 12 to 16 mg/day in Australia (128). In many countries, the U.S. RDA values (129) of 15 mg/day are used, which were based on results from zinc balance studies and on a calculated turnover rate of body zinc at 6 mg/day, allowing for 40% absorption from the diet. The U.S. RDAs published in 1989 use the factorial approach: assuming an average requirement for absorbed zinc of 2.5 mg/day and 20% efficiency of absorption results in recommending an intake of 15 mg/day for men and 12 mg/day for women. Assuming slightly lower obligatory endogenous losses at 2.2 mg for men and 1.6 mg for women and a higher absorption efficiency of 30%, the UK panel of 1991 have given RNIs of 9.5 mg/day for men and 7.0 mg/day for women (55).

4. Zinc Toxicity

Zinc has a relatively low order of toxicity compared to most other trace elements, only a few cases of acute zinc poisoning having been reported thus far. Symptoms of zinc toxicity include nausea, vomiting, diarrhea, and fever, which were observed after intake of food and beverages contaminated with zinc from galvanized containers, and lethargy was observed after the ingestion of 4 to 8 g of zinc (130–132).

Prolonged zinc intakes higher than the body's requirements may interact with the metabolism of other trace elements. Copper seems to be especially sensitive to high zinc doses. Low copper and ceruloplasmin levels and anemia were noticed after high doses of zinc (133,134). Also an intake of 50 mg/day of zinc had antagonistic effects on both copper and iron (135). Chandra (136) reported impaired immune responses after excessive zinc intakes.

C.   Copper

Copper (Cu) is widely distributed in the body and is incorporated into organic complexes, such as various metalloproteins and enzymes. The adult human body has on average about 80 mg (50–120 mg range) of Cu, of which 40% is located in the muscle, 15% in the liver, 10% in the brain, and 6% in the blood. Most of the red cell Cu is in the metalloenzyme superoxide dismutase (SOD), involved in the free radical scavenging. About 60% of the plasma Cu is bound to ceruloplasmin, 30% to transcuprein, and the remainder to albumin and amino acids (137).

1.   Biochemical Function

As a constituent of metalloenzymes, Cu is involved in such fundamental functions as the cytochrome chain of mitochondrial oxidation, the synthesis of complex proteins of collagenous tissues in the skeleton and blood vessels, and in the synthesis of neurotransmitters (e.g., noradrenaline) and neuropeptides (e.g., encephalins). Some important Cu-containing enzymes in the human body are listed in Table 6 (137).

2.   Assessment of Status and Deficiency

Cu status is usually assessed by measuring plasma Cu concentrations. Plasma or serum Cu levels vary from 0.8 to 1.2 µg/ml; female levels are 10% higher than male. Plasma Cu is increased threefold in late pregnancy and in women taking estrogen-based oral contraceptives, as well as during the acute-phase response to stress when ceruloplasmin concentrations increase. A level of less than 0.8 µg/ml of Cu is considered below normal; low levels of ceruloplasmin (180–400 mg/l), urinary Cu (32–64 µg/24 h), and hair (10–20 µg/g) are found in very deficient subjects. A fall in the concentration of erythrocyte SOD (0.47–0.067 mg/mg hemoglobin) is a more sensitive test of mild Cu deficiency. A fall in the neutrophil count is also an indicator of a marginally low Cu status. In chronic Cu toxicity, plasma levels of Cu and ceruloplasmin exceed the normal levels (55).

Danks (138) summarized typical symptoms and signs of Cu deficiency (Table 7). Clinical Cu deficiency symptoms that can be experimentally demonstrated include decreased metabolic

Table 6 The Principal Mammalian Cuproenzymes

Enzymes	Activities/Functions
Cytochrome c oxidase	Mitochondrial oxidation, requires iron, oxidative phosphorylation
Superoxide dismutase (SOD)	Cytosolic antioxidant: $2O_2 + H_2O$ SOD $H_2O_2 + O_2$
Dopamine-beta-hydroxylase	Synthesis of adrenaline and noradrenaline
Tyrosinase	Tyrosine $\rightarrow$ dope $\rightarrow$ dopaquinone, synthesis of pigment in choroid and epidermis
Uricase	Renal and hepatic metabolism of uric acid
Lysyl oxidases	Condensation of amino acids, cross links of elastin and collagen
Amine oxidases	Plasma and connective tissues
Ceruloplasmin	Multiple oxidase activities
Thiol oxidase	Formation of disulfide linkages

Source: Ref. 137.

activity of the brain and heart, as seen by cardiac slowing and altered conduction of neuromuscular control of heart rhythms, and heart muscular hypertrophy. Other effects not necessarily found in humans include degeneration of exocrine pancreas and a defective thyroxine secretion in response to TSH stimulation.

Castillo-Duran et al. (139) reported Cu deficiency in preterm infants, in full-term infants fed inappropriately on unmodified cow's milk, and in children with protracted diarrhea. Supplementation of 1.25 µmol (80 µg) Cu/kg body weight daily to children recovering from malnutrition resulted in decreased infection rates, maintaining plasma concentration of Cu (140). Parenteral nutrition with solutions that provide inadequate amounts of Cu can create its deficiency in children and adults (141).

Menkes' syndrome is an autosomal defect in the intracellular metabolism of copper that is manifested by features of copper deficiency, despite the presence of excess copper in the system. The symptoms include abnormal hair, failure to thrive, progressive cerebral degeneration, loss of skin and hair pigmenttion, thrombosis and arterial rupture, and hypothermia that is evident soon after birth, followed by growth retardation, with poor mental development and convulsions, occurring from 3 months of age onwards (see Chapter 29).

The occurrence of dietary Cu deficiency in human adults is rare. Turnland et al. (142) noticed no observed changes in plasma lipids, cardiac rhythm or electrical conductivity, or ceruloplasmin changes in adult men on customary diets with intakes of 0.79 Cu/day for 42 days, whereas Shike et al. (141) found that for adults on parenteral nutrition, 0.3 mg of Cu/day is ade-

Table 7 Some Clinical Features of Copper Deficiency

1. Babies fail to thrive, feed poorly
2. Edema with low serum albumin
3. Anemia with altered iron metabolism and bone marrow changes
4. Impaired immunity with low neutrophil count
5. Skeletal changes numerous, with fractures and generalized osteoporosis
6. Herniae and tortuous dilated blood vessels from collagen and elastin cross-linking defects
7. Hair and skin depigmentation, with steely, uncrimped hair

Source: Ref. 138.

quate. It has been suggested that low Cu intakes in humans may be atherogenic, may impair cardiac function, and may cause abnormal heart rhythms.

3. Sources and Requirements

Good dietary sources of copper are shellfish, legumes, whole grain cereals, nuts, and liver. Pig's liver is a rich source of copper, owing to the practice of adding high concentrations of Cu to pig feed to alter intestinal microflora and to improve animal growth. Copper pipes used for drinking water can add 0.1 µg/day to intakes in hard water areas and 10 times this amount in acid and soft water conditions.

According to Mills (143), adult women need about 0.6 mg Cu/day and men need 0.7 mg/day or 13 mg/kg body weight. The UK/RNIs have been set on this basis of 17 µg/kg/day. The US/RDAs for Cu are 1.5 to 3.0 mg/day, which is considered a safe and adequate range of Cu intake for adults. The livers of full-term babies can store about 8 mg Cu, which is probably adequate for first 1 to 2 months of life. Adaptive changes in Cu homeostasis are presumed to be capable of accommodating the needs of pregnancy, but 0.38 mg/day was added for lactating mothers who secrete about 0.22 mg of Cu/day in their milk (55).

4. Copper Toxicity

Toxicity of Cu can arise from the deliberate ingestion of copper salts, or accidently from contamination of water and drinks. Acute Cu toxicity may affect the gastrointestinal tract with diarrhea and vomiting, followed by variable degrees of intravascular hemolysis, hepato-cellular necrosis, and renal tubular necrosis leading to death.

With chronic exposure, Cu accumulates in the liver, resulting in hepatic necrosis or cirrhosis and liver failure. Infants and children are particularly vulnerable to Cu toxicity. Bhave et al. (144) described Indian childhood cirrhosis, at 1 to 3 years of age, possibly caused by the ingestion of milks that have been stored or heated in copper or brass utensils. A similar syndrome in infants may arise by eating foods prepared with acidic well water that has leached Cu from pipes (145).

Wilson's disease (hepatolenticular degeneration) is an autosomal recessive defect in Cu metabolism with excessive accumulation of hepatic copper. Copper accumulating in the liver, eyes, brain, and kidneys accounts for most of the pathological changes, leading to liver failure with cirrhosis and gallstones in children and adolescents. Cerebeller changes begin between 12 and 30 years, with deteriorating mental function and splasticity, accompanied by psychosis and behavioral changes. Oxidative stress induced in the erythrocytes by the excess Cu produces chronic hemosis. Due to excessive excretion of amino acids, glucose, uric acid, phosphte, calcium, and proteins, abnormalities occur in proximal renal tubular function. Bone abnormalities with osteoporosis, fractures, bone cysts, and rickets are common in children who have Wilson's disease.

C. Selenium

1. Biochemical Function

Selenium (Se) occurs as a selenocysteine residue in certain mammalian oxidases. The cytosolic antioxidant enzyme, glutathione peroxidase, uses glutathione to reduce a range of organic hydroperoxides, such as hydrogen peroxide, hydroperoxides of sterol, steroids, prostaglandins, free fatty acids, proteins, and nucleic acids, to corresponding alcohols (146,147). The reduced glutathione provides protons (H+) to convert hydrogen peroxide to water by the glutathione peroxidase. The glutathione reductase and NADPH produced by the hexose monophosphate shunt regenerate the reduced glutathione in the cell for reuse. The enzyme peroxidase is present in all body cells and its concentration in erythrocytes is readily monitored. Without this enzyme, the ability of cells to cope with oxidative stress would be impaired, despite a range of other antioxidants present in the cell. The presence of hepatic microsomal type 1 iodothyronine 5′-deiodinase in rats (148,149) has raised the possibility that Se deprivation may influence systemic responses to marginal iodine intakes in humans.

The total body content of Se varies from 3 to 30 mg, depending on the geochemical environment and dietary intakes. Two Se pools exist in tissues: the biologically active pool depends on selenocysteine, which is synthesized endogenously from inorganic Se and serine. The second pool is selenomethionine in protein and is subject to factors influencing methionine metabolism. When methionine intake is limited, selenomethionine is used as methionine, even if concomitant Se is released from degraded selenomethionine and contributes to the active Se pool (55).

Selenoamino acids are systemically degraded to yield amino acid residues and selenite. The inorganic Se ions are sequentially reduced from selenate via selenite to selenide by glutathione reductase. The Se homeostasis is mediated by adjusting Se catabolism with the excretion of various reduced and methylated derivatives (e.g., trimethylselenium) in the urine. At excessive intakes, dimethylselenide is produced, which when exhaled has a characteristic garlic odor (146,147).

2. Sources and Requirements

Cereal grains, meat, and fish are good sources of Se (146). Daily intakes of Se vary between 20 and 300 µg according to the Se content of the soil from which the foods are derived. In China, dietary intakes range from 11 to 5000 µg/day, causing extreme deficiency and toxicity syndromes (150). Se is present in foods mainly as selenomethionine and selenocysteine. The seleno amino acids are probably absorbed by similar energy-dependent mechanisms as those of their sulfur analogues. All the usual dietary forms of Se, including organic and inorganic, are absorbed efficiently.

Se adapts well metabolically to changing intakes, making balance studies of little value in assessing Se requirements (146). Graded supplementation studies of Chinese men on low Se intakes have been employed in conjunction with glutathione peroxidase measurements to assess the dietary intakes for achieving plateau activities. Based on adjustments for body weight and individual variation, the US/RDAs are set at 70 and 55 µg/day for male and female adults, respectively, whereas the British RNIs are slightly higher (75 and 60 µg). The US/RDAs call for an extra 10 µg of Se/day during pregnancy whereas UK RNIs do not because of the adaptive changes in pregnancy. Infant RNIs are set at 0.2 µg Se/kg body weight taking growth factor into the account.

3. Assessment of Status and Deficiency

With a decrease in the intake of Se, the plasma and red cell levels of Se fall, but the plasma concentrations, which change more rapidly, do not necessarily reflect tissue Se concentrations (146). The red cell glutathione peroxidase activity is a more valid index of detecting Se deficiency in populations with low Se intakes and is easier to measure than Se itself. At higher Se intakes, 55% to 65% of dietary Se continues to be absorbed, but urinary Se output rises and blood and tissue Se levels, as well as glutathione peroxidase activities, reach a plateau (151).

The most striking Se-responsive syndrome in humans is Keshan disease, which is a Se-responsive cardiomyopathy, predominantly affecting children, young adolescents, and young women in China with low Se intakes; people with intakes of less than 12 µg/day are at risk, whereas those with 19 µg/day intakes are not (152,153). Keshan disease is noticed particularly in areas with low Se levels in the soil, leading to low Se levels in staple cereals as well as in samples of blood, hair, and other tissues in the people living in these areas.

A virus infection may promote the Se deficiency syndrome, as may low intakes of vitamin E, proteins, methionine, and other trace elements. According to severity, Keshan disease may be of four types; acute, subacute, chronic, and insidious. The heart muscle gets damaged extensively (especially the mitochondria) and there is a clear evidence of cardiac and skeletal muscular damage as the plasma creatine kinase increases. Congestive cardiomyopathy with low Se levels has also been reported in patients receiving total parenteral nutrition. Patients with less severe Se deficiency show skeletal myopathy with enhanced plasma creatinine kinase activity, macrocytosis, and lightening of the skin and hair pigmentation. An increased degree of hemolytic sensitivity to peroxide of red cells in vitro, is the clear evidence of the metabolic effects of reduced glutathione peroxidase activity. Kashin-Bek disease, which is an osteoarthritic disorder involving severe joint deformity, afflicts children 5 to 13 years of age living in areas of the former Soviet Union and China. This disease is characterized by prominent cartilaginous degeneration and is thought to be another form of Se deficiency (153).

Kukreja and Khan (154) measured selenium levels and activity of selenoenzyme, glutathione peroxidase in whole blood in order to assess the selenium status. Delayed-type hypersensitivity (DTH) reaction was suppressed significantly in selenium-deficient rats, indicating the decrease in cellular immunity. The B cell function was impaired in selenium-deficient rats, as evidenced from the decrease in the number of plaque-forming cells and antibody titer. Selenium supplementation for 30 days recovered the DTH response and B cell function markedly.

According to Reilly (155), dietary intake of the essential trace element selenium is decreasing in the United Kingdom and several other European countries with possible health consequences. Evidence available indicates that Se deficiency may be related to a variety of degenerative diseases, including cancer, and that protection against such conditions can be conferred by increasing Se intake. Health authorities in the United Kingdom are considering whether intervention is required to bring this about, either by food fortification or other means. In addition, industry has begun to look at how Se can be used as a health-promoting ingredient in foods. Reilly (155) has reviewed recent information on the nature and biological role of Se levels in the diet, and the pros and cons of its use in functional foods.

Human diseases and conditions that are associated with Se deficiency include (155) aging, arthritis, cancer, cardiovascular disease, cataracts, cholestasis, Crohn's disease, crib death, cystic fibrosis, diabetes, goiter, immunodeficiency, Kashin-Bek disease, Keshan disease, lymphoblastic anemia, macular degeneration of the retina, muscular dystrophy, stroke, and ulcerative colitis. Selenium content of some selected foods and food groups and the dietary selenium intakes in different countries are given in Tables 8 and 9, respectively. Levels usually found in foods in parts

Table 8 Selenium Content of Some Selected Foods and Food Groups

	Se content (micrograms/g fr. wt.)
Food groups	
Cereals, cereal products	0.01–0.55
Meat, fish, eggs	0.01–0.36
Milk, dairy products	<0.001–0.17
Vegetables, fruit	<0.001–0.022
Selected high-Se foods	
Beef kidney	0.78–1.45
Brazil nuts	0.85–53
Broccoli	<0.001–0.46
Crab	0.028–1.26
Lobster roe	0.08–4.43
Mushrooms	0.01–1.40

Source: Ref. 156.

Table 9 Dietary Selenium Intakes in Selected Countries

Country	Se intake (range µg/d)
Australia	57–87
Bangladesh	63–112
Canada	98–224
China (low soil Se area)	3–11
China (high soil Se area)	3200–6690
Finland (1974)	25–60
Finland (1992)	90 (Mean)
Germany	38–48
Greece	110–220
Mexico	10–223
New Zealand	6–70
Portugal	10–100
Russia	60–80
UK (1978)	60–80
UK (1995)	60 (Mean)
USA	62–216
Venezuela	86–500

Source: Ref. 157.

per billion range between 10 and 500. Certain plants such as Brazil nuts can contain more than 50 mg/kg, i.e., 105 times the levels found in most other foods. Variations in levels of Se in foods produced in different countries are reflected in the ranges of dietary intakes reported worldwide (Table 9) (156,157).

4. Selenium Toxicity

Severe selenosis can occur at dietary intakes of 3.2 to 6.7 mg/day, with a malodorous breath, an erythematous bullous and intensely itchy dermatitis, dystrophic nails, dry brittle hair, alopecia, and neurological abnormalities involving neuropathies with paraesthesia, paralysis, and hemiplegia (153). Also, mottled tooth enamel and dental caries are endemic disorders in the affected areas.

D. Manganese

1. Biochemical Function

Manganese (Mn) was reported to be an essential factor for the growth of rats in 1931 and its deficiency later was found to be a practical problem in the poultry and pig industry. Mn deficiency in man is very rare. The human body contains about 10 to 20 mg of Mn; one-fourth of it is present in bones. Mn cannot be stored in the body.

Manganese (Mn) is a key constituent of metalloenzymes and functions as an enzyme activator IV. It is a component of arginase, pyruvate carboxylase, and mitochondrial superoxide dismutase. Various hydrolases, kinases, decarboxylases, and phosphotransferases and glutamine synthetase also require Mn for their activities. Phosphoenol pyruvate carboxylase, prolidase, and glycosyl transferases specifically require Mn, otherwise their in vivo activation may depend more on magnesium (158).

2. Sources and Dietary Intakes

Vegetable foods and beverages such as tea are abundant sources of Mn. Daily dietary intakes of Mn are about 2 to 3 mg/day and may be higher in some individuals (8.3 mg/day). Only about 10% of dietary Mn is absorbed through the small intestine. The absorption of Mn increases at low intakes, along with renal conservation. High dietary levels of calcium, phosphorus, and phytate may impair intestinal absorption of Mn, though no human Mn deficiency has been demonstrated. Neonatal absorption of Mn is higher than adult and special transport mechanisms controlling Mn uptake have been envisaged that probably involve variations in biliary excretion of the metal. Mn is also found in intestinal and pancreatic secretions.

3. Mn Deficiency

Mn deficiency produces several abnormalities in the offspring of Mn-deprived animals, including congenital irreversible ataxia, which is a prominent feature. This arises from the development of the calcified otoliths in the inner ear, thought to be responsible for maintaining balance. Other signs of Mn deficiency include growth retardation and impaired skeletal development, with bowed shorter long bones and many cartilaginous problems leading to joint abnormalities and displaced tendons. Pancreatic damage impairs insulin secretion, leading to glucose intolerance. Fat accumulates in the liver and kidneys, with a low serum cholesterol (HDL) (158).

Young men fed a low-Mn diet (0.01 mg/day) were found to develop an evanescent skin rash and hypocholesterolemia, though neither of these two features responded unequivocally to Mn repletion (159). Reports of Mn deprivation in humans include Mn-responsive glucose intolerance; reduced Mn concentrations in the hair of some mothers whose babies had congenital abnormalities or in the blood or hair (or both) of children with skeletal abnormalities; osteoporosis; and non-traumatic epilepsy (160).

4. Mn Toxicity

Mineworkers in Chile exposed to Mn ore dust develop (possibly by inhaling, rather than ingesting) a disorder called manganic madness, which is characterized by psychosis, hallucinations, and extrapyramidal damage with features of Parkinson's disease. Kondakis et al. (161) described an increased incidence of parkinsonian syndrome in an area of Greece where well waters have a high Mn content.

F. Molybdenum

1. Biochemical Function

Molybdenum (Mo) is a cofactor bound to a pterin in three important enzymes of tissues in man and animals: xanthine oxidase, sulfite oxidase, and aldehyde oxidase, and is essential for their activities. Thus, Mo is involved in the metabolism of purines, pyrimidines, quinolines, sulfite, and bisulfite (162,163).

Wadman et al. (164) described an autosomal defect, with distinctive fatal syndrome in infants, involving severe developmental retardation, neurological abnormalities, ectopic eye lenses, and an impaired metabolism of sulfur amino acids and nucleotides, as related to an absence of hepatic molybdenum cofactor. Abumrad et al. (165) reported an analogous metabolic syndrome in a patient on prolonged intravenous feeding who developed hypermethionemia, low urinary excretion of sulfate but increased thiosulfaturia, an intolerance of intravenous sulfur amino acids, manifested as an encephalopathy, and low urinary and plasma uric acid concentrations; all these features responded to Mo supplementation.

2. Metabolism and Intakes

About 80% of dietary Mo is absorbed by the intestinal tissue. Mo is metabolized as molybdate anion, and its renal excretion is influenced in response to changes in Mo absorption. Daily intakes of Mo vary from 44 to 460 µg, according to geography. Human adults experimentally fed 25 µg Mo daily have shown Mo-responsive defects. The tissue concentration of Mo also varies markedly depending on geographical area, populations living in regions with a high soil Mo content showing higher tissue Mo contents.

Kovalsky et al. (166) suggested a possibility that disturbed copper metabolism may occur in people living in a Mo-rich geochemical environment. This possibility has been emphasized by the successful management of Wilson's disease by tetrathiomolybdate (167). Sulfur and Mo have been known to interact to interfere with Cu absorption in ruminants (162). Owing to meager evidence of Mo deficiency and limited studies on its metabolism, only provisional RDAs for Mo have been set.

G. Iodine

Iodine is an integral part of the thyroid hormones, thyroxine and triiodothyronine, which have important metabolic roles in the body. It is required by all animals, including man.

1. Assessment of Status and Deficiency

The human body contains about 20 to 30 mg of iodine, about 60% of which is present in the thyroid gland; the remainder is distributed in other tissues. Iodine deficiency, among other causes, leads to the enlargement of the thyroid gland and a disease condition known as goiter.

2. Food Sources and Requirements

All seafoods, including fishes such as shellfish, shrimp, oysters, clams, crabs, and lobsters, are excellent sources of iodine. In the absence of food containing iodine, use of iodized salt can readily rectify iodine deficiency.

Dietary intakes of 150 µg/day have been recommended for adolescents and adults of both sexes, and an additional quantity of 25 to 30 µg/day is required by pregnant and lactating women.

3. Iodine Toxicity

Iodine toxicity in humans has not been established.

H. Fluoride

1. Biochemical Function

Fluoride plays an important role in bone mineralization and in the hardening of tooth enamel, though its essentiality remains to be proved unequivocally (55). Also, low fluoride intakes are associated with an increased incidence of dental caries, which can be treated with addition of 1 mg/l of fluoride to drinking waters. The body fluoride load is regulated by renal excretion.

2. Metabolism and Intakes

Leverett (168) reported that children with fluoride in excess of 0.1 mg/kg body weight daily had mottled teeth, indicating mild fluorosis. Krishnamachari (169) also stated that chronic high intakes of fluoride can cause bone disease and joint abnormalities. This fluorosis is especially common in Tanzania, South Africa, India, China, and Senegal, where subsoil water with a high fluoride content enters the food chain either directly or via plants. In arid and tropical climates, large intakes of fluorine may arise from drinking large volumes of water, though its fluorine content may be within the acceptable range (170). Fluorosis is also common in people eating sorghum as a staple food, because sorghum retains this element.

3. Excess of Fluoride

Severe fluorosis may appear as early as 6 years of age; men are afflicted more than women. Earliest features include dark mottling of the tooth enamel. Radiological evidence of focal areas of osteoclerosis and osteoporosis, with calcification of ligaments and tendons, are seen in otherwise asymptomatic cases. In the advanced stages, patients develop stiffness, joint pains, and deformities of the spine and of the legs—bent tibias and fibulas. Low calcium intakes and high Mo intakes may exacerbate the syndrome. High fluoride intakes have been known to interfere with iodine metabolism, causing hypothyroidism (55).

I. Chromium

1. Biochemical Function

Chromium (Cr^{3+}) is thought to enhance the potential action of insulin, possibly by optimizing the number of membrane insulin receptors, or their interaction with insulin, or both (171,172). Chromium has been found to be beneficial in the management of both hypo- and hyperglycemic responses to glucose loads. A glucose tolerance factor has been proposed that comprises chromium, niacin, cysteine, and glycine but remains to be characterized. Patients with chromium-responsive defects were found to benefit from parenteral supplements of inorganic chromium. However, experiments with Cr^{3+} in the management of diabetes mellitus have shown inconsistent results. Some of the effects of chromium may arise from a nonspecific effect on phosphoglucomutase (173). In addition, chromium may have a direct or indirect role in the metabolism of lipids, perhaps via insulin action. Okada et al. (174) suggested that chromium may participate in RNA synthesis from the DNA template.

Absorption of chromium is low, about 0.5% to 2.0% of dietary intakes. Though the organic form of chromium is absorbed more efficiently, it is also excreted rapidly in the urine.

2. Food Sources and Requirements

Meat, whole grains, nuts, legumes, spices, cheese, and brewer's yeast are good sources of chromium; processed products are poor sources. Only tentative recommendations have been developed for chromium requirements. A chromium intake of 50 to 200 µg/day has been recommended for adults.

3. Chromium Status and Deficiency

Tissue chromium stores do not readily equilibrate with the blood chromium levels, the latter being poor indicators of the chromium status of the body. High urinary chromium levels may serve as good indicator of excessive intakes. Prolonged parenteral nutrition can induce chromium deficiency in children and in adults (173,175). The features of chromium deficiency include an insulin-resistant hyperglycemia, elevated serum lipids, weight loss, ataxia, peripheral neuropathy, and encephalopathy. Adult patients respond to intravenous injections of chromium chloride, but responses in children are less conclusive (55).

4. Chromium Toxicity

Trivalent chromium (Cr^{3+}) has a low level of toxicity, but its hexavalent form (Cr^{6+}) was found to be more toxic in animal experiments, at intakes of 50 µg/g diet. Higher doses of chromium cause renal and hepatic necrosis and growth retardation.

J. Cobalt

1. Biochemical Function

Cobalt (Co) is a constituent of vitamin B_{12} (cobalamin), and inorganic cobalt is required for the synthesis of this vitamin. It is also required for the microbial synthesis of cobalamin in the gut of animals.

2. Deficiency

Cobalt deficiency has not been demonstrated in humans. In the absence of cobalt, ruminant animals develop anemia and muscular atrophy, and eventually die.

K. Other Trace Elements

Several other trace elements essential for humans are present in the body, e.g., silicon, vanadium, tin, and nickel. The amounts of these elements required by humans have not been fully established.

REFERENCES

1. Clydesdale, F. M., and F. J. Francis, *Food, Nutrition and Health* AVI Publishing Co. Westport, Conn, 1985.
2. Mertz, W., Risk assessment of essential trace elements: New approaches to setting recommended dietary allowances and safety limits, *Nutr. Rev. 53*: 179 (1995).
3. Mertz, W., C. O. Abernathy, and S. S. Olin (eds.) *Risk Assessment of Essential Elements*, ILSI Press, Washington, DC, 1994.
4. Carlisle, E. M., and M. J. Curran, Aluminum: an essential element for the chick, *Trace Elements in Man and Animals-8* (M. Anke, D. Meissner, and C. F. Mills, eds.), Media Touristik, Gersdorf, Germany, 1993, p. 695.
5. Angelow, L., M. Anke, B. Groppel, M. Glei, and M. Muller, Aluminum: an essential element for goats, *Trace Elements in Man and Animals-8* (M. Anke, D. Meissner, and C. F. Mills, eds.), Media Touristik, Gersdorf, Germany, 1993, p. 699.
6. Nielsen, F. H., Other trace elements, *Present Knowledge in Nutrition* (M. L. Brown, ed.), 6th ed., ILSI Press, Washington, DC, 1990, p. 294.
7. Anke, M., B. Groppel, L. Angelow, W. Dorn, and S. Drusch, Bromine: an essential element for goats, *Trace Elements in Man and Animals-8* (M. Anke, D. Meissner, and C. F. Mills, eds.), Media Touristik, Gersdorf, Germany, 1993a, p. 737.
8. Schwarz, K. Essentiality versus toxicity of metals, *Clinical Chemistry and Chemical Toxicity of Metals* (S. S. Brown, ed.), Elsevier, Amsterdam, The Netherlands, 1977, p. 3.
9. Anke, M., B. Groppel, H. Kronemann, and M. Gru, Evidence for the essentiality of lithium in goats, *Lithium 4. Spuren element symposium* (M. Anke, W. Baumann, H. Braunlich, and C. Bruckner, eds.), Friendrich Schiller Universitat, Jena, 1983, p. 58.

10. Reichlmayr-Lais, A. M., and M. Kirchgessner, Lead—an essential trace element, *Trace Elements in Man and Animals—7* (B. Momcilovic, ed.), Institute for Medical Research, Zagreb, Yugoslavia, 1991, p. 35.

11. Anke, M., L. Angelow, A. Schmidt, and H. Gurtler, Rubidium: an essential element for animals and man? *Trace Elements in Man and Animals—8*, Media Touristik, Gersdorf, Germany, 1993, p. 719.

12. Nielsen, F. H., C. D. Hunt, L. M. Mullen, and J. R. Hunt, Effect of boron on mineral estrogen and testosterone metabolism in post menopausal women, *FASEB J. 1*: 394 (1987).

13. Smith, R., Bone minerals, *Human Nutrition and Dietetics*, 9th ed. (J. S. Garrow and W. P. T. James, eds.) Churchill Livingstone, London, 1993, p. 162.

14. Smith, R., Recent advances in the metabolism and physiology of bone, *Recent Advances in Physiology*, Vol. 10 (P. F. Baker, ed.), Churchill Livingstone, Edinburgh, London, 1984, p. 317.

15. Arsenault, A. L., Crystal-collagen relationships in calcified turkey leg tendons visualised by selected-area dark-field electron microscopy, *Calcified Tissue Intl. 43*: 202 (1988).

16. Smith, R., The molecular genetics of collagen disorders, *Clin. Science 71*: 129 (1986).

17. Wozney, J. M., V. Rosen, and A. J. Celeste, Novel regulations of bone formation: molecular clones and activities, *Science: 242*: 1528 (1988).

18. Owen, M., and A. J. Friedenstein, Stromal stem cells, marrow-derived osteogenic precursors, *Cell and Molecular Biology of Vertebrate Hard Tissues*, Ciba Foundation Symp., No. 136, Wiley, Chinchester, 1988, p. 42.

19. Krane, S. M., M. B. Goldring, and S. R. Goldring, Cytokines, *Cell and Molecular Biology of Vertebrate Hard Tissues*, Ciba Foundation Symp., 136, Wiley, Chinchester, 1988, p. 239.

20. Chambers, T. J., The regulation of osteoclastic development and function, *Cell and Molecular Biology of Vertebrate Hard Tissues*, Ciba Foundation Symp., 136, Wiley, Chinchester, 1988, p. 92.

21. Evered, D., and S. Harnett, Calcium and the cell, Ciba Foundation Symp. 122, Wiley, Chinchester, 1986.

22. Kanis, J. A., and R. Passmore, Calcium supplementation of diet, *Br. Med. J. 298*: 137 (1989).

23. MacIntyre, I., The hormonal regulation of extracellular calcium, *Br. Med. J. 42*: 343 (1986).

24. Haussler, M. R., D. J. Mangelsdorf, and B. S. Komm, Molecular biology of vitamin D hormone, *Recent Prog. Horm. Res. 44*: 263 (1988).

25. Reichel, H., and A. W. Norman, Systemic effects of vitamin D, *Annu. Rev. Med. 40*: 71 (1989).

26. Farndate, R. W., J. R. Sandy, S. J. Atkinson, S. R. Pennington, S. Meghji, and M. C. Meikle, Parathyroid hormone and prostaglandin E_2 stimulate bone inositol phosphates and cyclic AMP accumulation in mouse osteoblast cultures, *Biochem. J. 252*: 263 (1988).

27. MacIntyre, I., The hormonal regulation of extracellular calcium, *Br. Med. Bull. 42*: 343 (1986).

28. Raisz, L. G., Local and systemic factors in the pathogenesis of osteoporosis, *N. Engl. J. Med. 318*: 818 (1988).

29. Mundy, G. R., Hypercalcaemia of malignancy revisited, *J. Clin. Invest. 82*: 1 (1988).

30. Riggs, B. L., and L. J. Melton, Evolutional osteoporosis, *N. Engl. J. Med. 314*: 1671 (1986).

31. Smith, R., Osteoporosis: cause and management, *Br. Med. J. 294*: 329 (1987).

32. Heaney, R. P., Calcium, bone health and osteoporosis, *Bone and Mineral Research*, Vol. 4 (W. A. Peck, ed.), Elsevier Science Publishers, 1986, p. 255.

33. Stevenson, J. C., B. Lees, M. Devenport, M. P. Cust, and K. F. Ganger, Determinants of bone density in normal women: risk factors for future osteoporosis, *Br. Med. J. 298*: 924 (1989).

34. Cole, W. G., R. Jaenisch, and K. F. Bateman, New insights into the molecular pathology of osteogenesis imperfecta, *Quart. J. Med. 70*: 1 (1989).

35. Lanyon, L. E., and C. T. Rubin, Regulation of bone mass in response to physical activity, *Osteoporosis, A Multidisciplinary Problem* (Ast J. Dixon, R. G. G. Russell, and T. C. B. Stamp, eds.), Royal Society of Medicine, Int. Congress Series No. 55, 1983, p. 51.

36. Nordin, B. E. C., The calcium deficiency model for osteoporosis, *Nutr. Rev. 47*: 65 (1989).

37. Nordin, B. E. C., The calcium debate, *Med. J. Aust. 148*: 608 (1988).

38. Barrett-Conner, E., The RDA for calcium in the elderly: too little, too late, *Calcified Tissue Intl. 44*: 303 (1989).

39. Blanchard, J., Calcium and osteoporosis: some caveats and pleas, *Calcified Tissue Intl. 44*: 67 (1989).

40. Riggs, B. L., H. W. Waller, L. J. Melton, L. S. Richelson, H. L. Judd, and W. M. O'Fallen, Dietary calcium intake and the rate of bone loss in women, *J. Clin. Invest. 80*: 979 (1987).
41. Stevenson, J. L., M. I. Whitehead, and M. Padwick, Dietary intake of calcium and post menopausal bone loss, *Br. Med. J. 297*: 15 (1988).
42. Selby, P. L., C. E. Davidson, R. M. Francis, and C. G. Robinson, Calcium and postmenopausal bone loss, *Br. Med. J. 297*: 481 (1988).
43. Riis, B., K. Thomsen, and C. Christiansen, Does calcium supplementation prevent postmenopausal bone loss? *N. Engl. J. Med. 316*: 173 (1987).
44. Cooper, C., D. J. P. Barker, and C. Wickham, Physical activity, muscle strength and calcium intake in fractures of the proximal femur in Britain, *Br. Med. J. 297*: 1443 (1988).
45. Holbrook, T. L., E. Barrett-Connor, and D. Wingard, Dietary calcium and the risk of hip fracture: 14-year prospective population study, *Lancet 2*: 1046 (1988).
46. Lau, E., S. Donnan, D. J. P. Barker, and C. Cooper, Physical activity and calcium intake in fracture of the proximal femur in Hong Kong, *Br. Med. J. 297*: 1441 (1988).
47. Cohn, S. H., A. Vaswani, I. Zanzi, J. F. Aloia, M. S. Roginsky, and K. J. Ellis, Changes in body chemical composition with age measured by total-body neutron activation, *Metabolism 25*: 85 (1976).
48. Ellis, K. J., A. Vaswani, I. Zanzi, and S. H. Cohn, Total body sodium and chlorine in normal adults, *Metabolism 25*: 645 (1976).
49. Wrong, O., Water and monovalent electrolytes, *Human Nutrition and Dietetics*, 9th ed. (J. S. Garrow and W. P. T. James, eds.), Churchill Livingstone, Edinburgh, London, 1993, p. 146.
50. Paul, A. A., and D. A. T. Southgate, *McCance and Widdowson's The Composition of Foods*, 4th ed. HMSO, London, Elsevier, Amsterdam, 1978.
51. Bothwell, T. H., R. W. Charlson, J. D. Cook, and C. A. Finch, *Iron Metabolism in Man*, Blackwell Scientific Publications, Oxford, 1979.
52. Hallberg, L., Iron Absorption and Iron Deficiency, *Human Nutr. Clin. Nutr. 36C*: 259 (1982).
53. Hallberg, L., Iron, *Present Knowledge in Nutrition* (M. L. Brown, ed.), 5th ed., The Nutrition Foundation Inc., Washington, D.C., 1984, p. 459.
54. Dallman, P. R., Biochemical basis for the manifestations of iron deficiency, *Annu. Rev. Nutr. 6*: 13 (1986).
55. Hallberg, L., B. Sandstrom, and P. J. Aggett, Iron, zinc and other trace elements, *Human Nutrition and Dieteties*, 9th ed. (J. S. Garrow and W. P. T. James, eds.), Churchill Livingstone, Edinburgh, London, 1993, p. 174.
56. Brune, M., B. Magnusson, H. Persson, and L. Hallberg, Iron losses in sweat, *Am. J. Clin. Nutr. 43*: 438 (1986).
57. FAO/WHO, Report of a Joint Expert Group: Requirements of vitamin A, iron, folate and vitamin B_{12}, FAO Food and Nutrition Series No. 23, Food and Agriculture Organization of United Nations, Rome, 1988.
58. Hallberg, L., and L. Rossander-Hulten, Iron requirements in menstruating women, *Am. J. Clin. Nutr. 54*: 1047 (1991).
59. Hallberg, L., Bioavailability of dietary iron in man, *Annu. Rev. Nutr. 1*: 123 (1981).
60. Baynes, R. D., and T. H. Bothwell, Iron deficiency, *Annu. Rev. Nutr. 10*: 133 (1990).
61. Hallberg, L., W. Bjorn-Rasmussen, L. Howard, and L. Rossander, Dietary haem iron absorption. A discussion of possible mechanisms for the absorption-promoting effect of meat and for the regulation of iron absorption, *Scand. J. Gastroenterol. 14*: 769 (1979).
62. Hallberg, L., M. Brune, and L. Rossander, Iron absorption in man: ascorbic acid and dose-dependent inhibition by phytate, *Am. J. Clin. Nutr. 49*: 140 (1989).
63. Brune, M., L. Rossander-Hulten, L. Hallberg, M. Erlandsson, and A-S, Sandberg, Iron absorption from bread. Inhibiting effect of cereal fiber, phytate and inositol phosphates with different number of phosphate groups, *J. Nutr. 122*: 442 (1992).
64. Brune, M., L. Rossander-Hulten, and L. Hallberg, Iron absorption and phenolic compounds: importance of different phenolic structures, *Eur. J. Clin. Nutr. 43*: 547 (1989).
65. Hallberg, L., L. Rossander-Hulten, M. Brune, and A. Gleerup, Calcium and iron absorption—mechanism of action and nutritional importance, *Eur. J. Clin. Nutr. 46*: 317 (1992).

66. Hallberg, L., M. Brune, M. Erlandsson, A-S, Sandberg, and L. Rossander-Hulten, Calcium: effect of different amounts of non-heme and heme iron absorption in man, *Am. J. Clin. Nutr. 53*: 112 (1991).

67. Hallberg, L., M. Brune, and L. Rossander, Effect of ascorbic acid on iron absorption from different types of meals, *Human Nutrition Appl. Nutrition. 40A*: 97 (1986).

68. Chanarian, I., V. Malkouska, A. M. O'Hea, M. G. Rinsler, and A. B. Price, Megaloblastic anaemia in a vegetarian Hindu community, *Lancet 2*: 1168 (1983).

69. DeMaeyer, E., and M. Adiels-Tegman, The prevalence of anaemia in the world, *World Health Stat. Q. 38*: 302 (1985).

70. Lozoff, B., Behavioural alterations in iron deficiency, *Adv. Pediatr. 35*: 331 (1988).

71. Youdim, M. B. H. (ed.), *Brain Iron: Neurochemical and Behavioural Aspects*, Taylor and Francis, London, 1988.

72. Hallberg, L., Iron balance in pregnancy, *Vitamins and Minerals in Pregnancy and Lactation* (H. Berger, ed.), Nestle Nutrition Workshop Series, Vol. 16, Nestec Ltd., Veveyl Raven Press Ltd., New York, 1988, p. 115.

73. McCance, R. A., and E. M. Widdowson, Mineral metabolism of healthy adults on white and brown bread dietaries, *J. Physiol. 101*: 44 (1942).

74. McCance, R. A., and E. M. Widdowson, The absorption and excretion of zinc, *Biochem. J. 36*: 692 (1942).

75. Sandstead, H. H., A. S. Prasad, and A. R. Schulert, Human zinc deficiency, endocrine manifestations and response to treatment, *Am. J. Clin. Nutr. 20*: 422 (1967).

76. Halstead, J. A., H. A. Ronaghy, and P. Abadi, Zinc deficiency in man: the Shiraz experiment, *Am. J. Med. 53*: 277 (1972).

77. Chesters, J. K., Biochemistry of zinc in cell division and tissue growth, *Zinc in Human Biology* (C. F. Mills, ed.), Springer-Verlag, Berlin, 1989, p. 109.

78. Bettger, W. J., and B. L. O'Dell, A critical physiological role of zinc in the structure and function of biomembranes, *Life Sci. 28*: 1425 (1981).

79. Sandstrom B., L. Davidsson, A. Cederblad, and B. Lonnerdal, Oral iron, dietary legands and zinc absorption, *J. Nutr. 115*: 411 (1985).

80. Sandstrom, B., and A. Cederblad, Effect of ascorbic acid on the absorption of zinc and calcium in man, *Int. J. Vitam. Nutr. Res. 57*: 87 (1987).

81. Sandstrom, B., Dietary pattern and zinc supply, *Zinc in Human Biology* (C. F. Mills, ed.), Springer Verlag, Berlin, 1989, p. 351.

82. Coppen, D. E., and N. T. Davies, Studies on the effects of dietary dose of ^{65}Zn absorption and body loss in young rats, *Br. J. Nutr. 57*: 35 (1987).

83. Hurley, L. S., and S. Tao, Alleviation of teratogenic effects of zinc deficiency by simultaneous lack of calcium, *Am. J. Physiol. 222*: 322 (1972).

84. Richards, M. P., and R. J. Cousins, Metallothionein and its relationship to the metabolism of dietary zinc in rats, *J. Nutr. 106*: 1591 (1976).

85. Jackson, M. J., R. Giugliano, L. G. Giugliano, E. F. Oliveira, R. Shrimpton, and I. G. Swainbank, Stable isotope metabolic studies of zinc nutrition in slum-dwelling lactating women in the Amazon valley, *Br. J. Nutr. 59*: 193 (1988).

86. Jackson, M. J., D. A. Jones, R. H. T. Edwards, I. G. Swainbank, and M. L. Coleman, Zinc homeostasis in man: studies using a new stable isotope-dilution technique, *Br. J. Nutr. 51*: 199 (1984).

87. Turnlund, J. R., J. C. King, W. R. Keyes, B. Gong, and M. C. Michel, A stable isotope study of zinc absorption in young men: effects of phytate and alpha-cellulose, *Am. J. Clin. Nutr. 40*: 1071 (1984).

88. Turnlund, J. R., N. Durkin, F. Costa, and S. Margen, Stable isotope studies of zinc absorption and retention in young and elderly men, *J. Nutr. 116*: 1239 (1986).

89. Turnlund, J. R., A. A. Betschart, W. R. Keyes, and L. L. Acord, A stable isotope study of zinc bioavailability in young men from diets with white vs whole wheat bread or beef vs soy, *Federation Proc. 46*: 879 (1987).

90. Wada, L., J. R. Turnlund, and J. C. King, Zinc utilization in young men fed adequate and low zinc intakes, *J. Nutr. 115*: 1345 (1985).

91. Jackson, M. J., and R. H. T. Edwards, Zinc excretion in patients with muscle disorders, *Muscle Nerve 5*: 661 (1982).

92. Baer, M. J., and J. C. King, Tissue zinc levels and zinc excretion during experimental zinc depletion in young men, *Am. J. Clin. Nutr. 39*: 556 (1984).

93. Greger, J. L., and S. Buckley, Menstrual blood loss of zinc, copper, magnesium and iron by adolescent girls, *Nutrition Rep. Int. 16*: 639 (1977).

94. Wolman, S. L., G. H. Anderson, E. B. Marliss, and K. N. Jeejeebhoy, Zinc in total parenteral nutrition: requirements and metabolic effects, *Gastroenterology 76*: 458 (1979).

95. Linderman, R. D., D. J. Baxter, A. A. Yunice, and S. Kraikitpanitch, Serum concentrations and urinary excretion of zinc in cirrhosis, nephrotic syndrome and renal insufficiency, *Am. J. Med. Sci. 275*: 17 (1978).

96. Hess, F. M., J. C. King, and S. Margen, Zinc excretion in young women on low zinc intakes and oral contraceptive agents, *J. Nutr. 107*: 1610 (1977).

97. Milne, D. B., W. K. Canfield, J. R. Mahalko, and H. H. Sandstead, Effect of dietary zinc on whole-body surface loss of zinc: impact on estimation of zinc retention by balance method, *Am. J. Clin. Nutr. 38*: 181 (1983).

98. Fickel, J. J., J. H. Freeland-Graves, and M. J. Roby, Zinc tolerance tests in zinc-deficient and zinc-supplemented diets, *Am. J. Clin. Nutr. 43*: 47 (1986).

99. Bales, G. W., L. C. Steinman, J. H. Freeland-Graves, J. M. Stone, and R. K. Young, The effect of age on plasma zinc uptake and taste acuity, *Am. J. Clin. Nutr. 44*: 664 (1986).

100. Sandstrom, B., L. Davidsson, L. Lundell, and L. Olbe, Zinc status and dark adaptation in patients subjected to total gastrectomy: effect of zinc supplementation; *Human Nutr. Clin. Nutr. 41C*: 235 (1987).

101. Aggett, P. J., R. W. Crofton, M. Chapman, W. R. Humphries, and C. F. Mills, Plasma leucocytes and tissue zinc concentrations in young zinc deficient pigs, *Pediatr. Res. 17*: 433 (1983).

102. Bremner, I., J. N. Morrison, A. M. Wood, and J. R. Arthur, Effects of changes in dietary zinc, copper and selenium supply and of endotoxin administration on metallothionine. I Concentration in blood cells and urine in the rat, *J. Nutr. 117*: 1595 (1987).

103. Morrison, S. A., R. M. Russell, E. A. Carney, and E. V. Oaks, Zinc deficiency: a case of abnormal dark adaptation in cirrhosis, *Am. J. Clin. Nutr. 31*: 276 (1978).

104. Moynahan, E. J., Acrodermatitis enteropathica; a lethal inherited human zinc deficiency disorder, *Lancet 2*: 399 (1974).

105. McClain, G., C. Soutor, and L. Zieve, Zinc deficiency: a complication of Crohn's disease, *Gastroenterology 78*: 272 (1980).

106. Kay, R. G., C. Tasman-Jones, J. Pybus, R. Whiting, and H. Black, A syndrome of acute zinc deficiency during total parenteral alimentation in man, *Ann. Surg. 183*: 331 (1976).

107. Kuramoto, Y., Y. Igarashi, S. Kato, and H. Tagami, Acquired zinc deficiency in two breast-fed mature infants, *Acta Derm. Venereol. 66*: 359 (1986).

108. Golden, B. E., and M. H. N. Golden, Effect of zinc supplementation on the composition of newly synthesized tissue in children recovering from malnutrition, *Proc. Nutr. Soc. 44*: 110 (1985).

109. Golub, M. S., M. E. Gershwin, L. Hurley, D. L. Baly, and A. G. Hendrickx, Studies of marginal zinc deprivation in Rhesus monkeys. II. Pregnancy outcome, *Am. J. Clin. Nutr. 39*: 879 (1984).

110. Baly, D. L., M. S. Golub, M. E. Gershwin, and L. S. Hurley, Studies on marginal zinc deprivation in Rhesus monkeys. III. Effects on vitamin A metabolism, *Am. J. Clin. Nutr. 40*: 199 (1984).

111. Leek, J. C., C. L. Keen, and J. B. Vogler, Long-term marginal zinc deprivation in Rhesus monkeys. IV. Effects on skeletal growth and mineralization, *Am. J. Clin. Nutr. 47*: 889 (1988).

112. Baer, M. J., and J. C. King, Tissue zinc levels and zinc excretion during experimental zinc depletion in young men, *Am. J. Clin. Nutr. 39*: 556 (1984).

113. Baer, M. J., J. C. King, and T. Tamura, Nitrogen utilization, enzyme activity, glucose intolerance and leucocyte chemotaxis in human experimental zinc depletion, *Am. J. Clin. Nutr. 41*: 1220 (1985).

114. Wada, L., and C. King, Effect of low zinc intakes on basal metabolic rate, thyroid hormones and protein utilization in adult men, *J. Nutr. 116*: 1045 (1986).

115. Walravens, P. A., and K. M. Hambidge, Growth of infants fed a zinc supplemented formula, *Am. J. Clin. Nutr. 29*: 1114 (1976).

116. Walravens, P. A., N. F. Krebs, and K. M. Hambidge, Linear growth of low-income preschool children receiving a zinc supplement, *Am. J. Clin. Nutr. 38*: 195 (1983).

117. Krebs, F., K. M. Hambidge, and P. A. Walravens, Increased food intake of young children receiving a zinc supplement, *Am. J. Dis. Children 138*: 270 (1984).

118. Wells, J. L., D. K. James, R. Luxton, and C. A. Pennock, Maternal leucocyte zinc deficiency at start of third trimester as a predictor of fetal growth retardation, *Br. Med. J. 294*: 1054 (1987).

119. Jameson, S., Effects zinc deficiency in human reproduction, *Acta Med. Scand.* 593 (Suppl.): 1 (1976).

120. Simmer, K., C. A. Iles, B. Slavin, P. W. N. Keeling, and R. P. H. Thompson, Maternal nutrition and intrauterine growth retardation, *Human Nutrition Clin. Nutr. 41C*: 193 (1987).

121. Lazebnik, N., B. R. Kuhnert, P. M. Kuhnert, and K. L. Thompson, Zinc status, pregnancy complication and labor abnormalities, *Am. J. Obstet. Gynecol. 158*: 161 (1988).

122. Davis, K. R., L. J. Peters, R. F. Cain, D. Le Tourneau, and J. McGinnis, Evaluation of the nutrient composition of wheat. III. Minerals, *Cereals Foods World, 29*: 246 (1984).

123. Schmitt, H. A., and C. M. Weaver, Effects of laboratory-scale processing on chromium and zinc in vegetables, *J. Food Sci. 47*: 1693 (1982).

124. Swanson, C. A., J. R. Turnlund, and J. C. King, Effect of dietary zinc sources and pregnancy on zinc utilization in adult women fed controlled diets, *J. Nutr. 113*: 2557 (1983).

125. Swanson, C. A., and J. C. King, Zinc and pregnancy outcome, *Am. J. Clin. Nutr. 46*: 763 (1987).

126. Krebs, N. F., K. M. Hambidge, M. A. Jacobs, and J. O. Rasbach, The effects of a dietary zinc supplement during lactation on longitudinal changes in maternal zinc status and milk zinc concentrations, *Am. J. Clin. Nutr. 41*: 560 (1985).

127. Krebs, N. F., and K. M. Hambidge, Zinc requirements and zinc intakes of breast fed infants, *Am. J. Clin. Nutr. 43*: 288 (1986).

128. IUNS, Recommended dietary intakes around the world, Part 2, *Nutr. Abstr. Rev. 53*: 1076 (1983).

129. NRC, Zinc, *Recommended Dietary Allowances*, 9th ed, National Academy of Sciences, National Research Council (Committee on Dietary Allowances, Food and Nutrition Board) Washington, DC, 1980, p. 144.

130. Brown, M. A., J. V. Thom, G. L. Orth, P. Cova, and J. Juarez, Food poisoning involving zinc contamination, *Arch. Environ. Health 8*: 657 (1964).

131. Gallery, E. D. M., J. Bloomfield, and S. R. Dixon, Acute zinc toxicity in haemodialysis, *Br. Med. J. 4*: 331 (1972).

132. Murphy, J. V., Intoxication following ingestion of elemental zinc, *J. Am. Med. Assoc. 212*: 2119 (1970).

133. Porter, K. G., D. McMaster, M. E. Elmes, and A. H. G. Love, Anaemia and low serum copper during zinc therapy, *Lancet 2*: 774 (1977).

134. Patterson, W. P., M. Winkelmann, and M. C. Perry, Zinc-induced copper deficiency: megamineral sideroblastic anaemia, *Ann. Intern. Med. 103*: 385 (1985).

135. Yadrick, M. K., M. A. Kenney, and E. A. Winterfeldt, Iron, copper and zinc status: response to supplementation with zinc or zinc and iron in adult females, *Am. J. Clin. Nutr. 49*: 145 (1989).

136. Chandra, R. K., Excessive intake of zinc impairs immune responses, *J. Am. Med. Assoc. 252*: 1443 (1984).

137. O'Dell, B. L., Copper, *Present Knowledge in Nutrition* 6th ed. (M. L. Brown, ed.), International Life Sciences Institute Nutrition Foundation, Washington, D.C., 1990, p. 261.

138. Danks, D. M., Copper deficiency in humans, *Annu. Rev. Nutr. 8*: 235 (1988).

139. Castillo-Duran, C., P. Vial, and R Uauy, Trace mineral balance during acute diarrhoea in infants, *J. Pediatr. 113*: 452 (1988).

140. Castillo-Duran, C., M. Fishberg, A. Valenzuela, J. I. Egana, and R. Uauy, Controlled trial of copper supplementation during the recovery from marasmus, *Am. J. Clin. Nutr. 37*: 898 (1983).

141. Shike, M., M. Roulet, R. Kurian, J. Whitewell, S. Stewart, and K. N. Jeejibhoy, Copper metabolism and requirements in total parenteral nutrition, *Gastroenterology 81*: 290 (1981).

142. Turnland, J. R., W. R. Keys, H. L. Anderson, and L. L. Acord, Copper absorption and retention in young men at three levels of dietary copper by use of the stable isotope ^{65}Cu, *Am. J. Clin. Nutr. 49*: 870 (1989).

143. Mills, C. F., The significance of copper deficiency in human nutrition and health. *Trace Elements in Man and Animals* (B. Momcilovic, ed.), IMI, Zagreb, 1991, p. 1.

144. Bhave, S. A., A. N. Pandit, S. Singh, B. N. S. Walia, and M. S. Tanner, The prevention of Indian childhood cirrhosis, *Ann. Trop. Paediatrics* (in Press) 1992.

145. Muller-Hocker, J., U. Meyer, and B. Wiebecke, Copper storage disease of the liver and chronic dietary copper intoxication in two further German infants mimicking Indian childhood cirrhosis, *Pathol. Res. Pract. 183*: 39 (1988).

146. Levander, O. A., A global view of human selenium nutrition, *Annu. Rev Nutr. 7*: 227 (1987).

147. Sunde, R. A., Molecular biology of selenoproteins, *Annu. Rev. Nutr. 10*: 451 (1990).

148. Arthur, J. R., F. Nicol, and G. J. Beckett, Hepatic iodothyronine 5-deiodinase: the role of selenium, *Biochem. J. 272*: 537 (1990).

149. Benne, D., A. Kyriakopoulos, H. Meinhold, and J. Kohrle, Identification of Type I iodothyronine 5'-deiodinase as a selenoenzyme, *Biochem Biophys. Res. Commun. 173*: 1143 (1990).

150. Yang, G., K. Ge, J. Chen, and X. Chen, Selenium-related endemic disases and the daily selenium requirement of humans, *World Rev. Nutr. Diet 3*: 98 (1988).

151. Diplock, A. T., and F. A. Chaudhry, The relationship of selenium biochemistry of selenium-responsive disease in man, *Essential and Toxic Trace Elements in Human Health and Disease.* (A. Prasad, ed.), Alan R Liss, New York, 1981, p. 211.

152. Chen, X., G. Yang, J. Chen, Z. Wen, and K. Ge, Studies on the relations of selenium and Keshan disease, *Biol. Trace Elem. Res. 2*: 91 (1980).

153. Yang, G., K. Ge, J. Chen, and X. Chen, Selenium related endemic diseases and the daily selenium requirement of humans, *World Rev. Diet 3*: 98 (1988).

154. Kukreja, R., and A. Khan, Effect of selenium deficiency and its supplementation on DTH response, antibody forming cells and antibody titre, *Indian J. Exp. Biol. 36*: 203 (1998).

155. Reilly, C., Selenium: A new entrant into the functional food arena, *Trends Food Sci. Technol. 9*: 114 (1998).

156. Reilly, C., *Selenium in Food and Health*, Blackie Academic and Professional, London, 1996.

157. Barclay, M. N. I., A MacPherson, and J. Dixon, Selenium content of a range of UK foods, *J. Food Comp. Ana. 8*: 307 (1995).

158. Hurley, L. S., and C. L. Keen, Manganese, *Trace Elements in Human and Animal Nutrition* (W. Mertz, ed.), Vol. I, Academic Press, San Diego, 1987, p. 185.

159. Friedman, B. J., J. H. Freeland-Graves, and C. W. Bales, Manganese balance and clinical observations in young men fed a manganese-deficient diet, *J. Nutr. 117*: 133 (1987).

160. Anonymous, Manganese deficiency in humans: fact or fiction? *Nutr. Rev. 46*: 348 (1988).

161. Kondakis, X. G., N. Makris, M. Leotsinidis, M., Prinou, and T. Papapetropoulos, Possible health effects of high manganese concentrations in drinking water, *Arch. Environ. Health 44*: 175 (1989).

162. Mills, C. F., and G. K. Davis, Molybdenum, *Trace Elements in Human and Animal Nutrition* (W. Mertz, ed.), Vol. I., Academic Press, New York, 1986, p. 429.

163. Rajagopalan, K. V., Molybdenum: an essential trace element in human nutrition, *Annu. Rev. Nutr. 8*: 401 (1988).

164. Wadman, S. K., M. Duran, and F. A. Beemer, Absence of hepatic molybdenum cofactor: an inborn error of metabolism leading to a combined deficiency of sulphite oxidase and xanthine dehydrogenase. *J. Inherit. Metab. Dis. 6* (Suppl.): 78 (1983).

165. Abumrud, N. N., A. J. Schneider, D. Steel, and L. S. Rogers, Amino acid intolerance during prolonged total parenteral nutrition reversed by molybdate therapy, *Am. J. Clin. Nutr. 34*: 2551 (1981).

166. Kovalsky, V. V., G. A. Jaravaja, and D. M. Smavonjan, Changes in purine metabolism in man and animals in various molybdenum-rich biogeochemical provinces, *Zhurnal Obshcheiviologii 22*: 179 (1961).

167. Brewer, G. J., R. D. Dick, V. Yuzbasiyan Gurkin, R. Tankanow, A. B. Young, and K. J. Kluin, Initial therapy of patients with Wilson's disease with tetrathiomolybdate, *Arch. Neurol. 48*: 42 (1991).

168. Leverett, D. H., Fluorides and the changing prevalence of dental caries, *Science 217*: 26 (1982).

169. Krishnamachari, K. A. V. R., Skeletal fluorosis in human: a review of recent progress in the understanding of the disease, *Progress Food Nutr. Sci. 10*: 279 (1986).

170. Brouwer, I. D., A De Bruin, O. Backer Dirks, and J. G. A. J. Hautvast, Unsuitability of World Health Organization guidelines for fluoride concentrations in drinking water in Senegal, *Lancet 1*: 223 (1988).

171. Stoecker, B. H., Chromium, *Present Knowledge in Nutrition*, 6th ed. (M. L. Brown, ed), International Life Sciences Institute, Nutrition Foundation, Washington, D.C. 1990, p. 287.
172. Offenbacher, E. G., and F. X. Pi-Sunyer, Chromium in human nutrition, *Annu. Rev. Nutr. 8*: 543 (1988).
173. Anonymous, Is chromium essential for humans? *Nutr. Rev. 46*: 17 (1988).
174. Okada, S., H. Ohba, and M. Taniyama, Alterations in ribonucleic acid synthesis by chromium (III), *J. Inorg. Biochem. 15*: 223 (1981).
175. Brown, R. O., S. Forloines-Lynn, R. E. Cross, and W. D. Heizer, Chromium deficiency after long-term total parenteral nutrition, *Dig. Dis. Sci. 31*: 661 (1986).

8
Energy

I. INTRODUCTION

All living organisms must perform work to stay alive, to grow, and to reproduce themselves. Living organisms are able to harness energy from various sources and to channel it into different types of biological work. Organisms carry out a remarkable variety of energy transductions, i.e., conversion of one form of energy to another; e.g., animals use chemical energy in the form of food (fuels) to synthesize complex molecules from simple precursors, producing macromolecules with highly ordered structures. They also convert the chemical energy of various fuels into concentration gradients and electrical gradients, motion, heat, and even light (as in fireflies). Photosynthetic organisms and higher plants transduce the sun's (light) energy into all other forms of energy.

Antoine Lavoisier in the 18th century recognized that animals somehow transform chemical fuels (foods) into heat and that this process of respiration is essential to life. He stated that "respiration is a slow process of combustion of carbon and hydrogen which is entirely similar to that occurring in a lighted lamp or candle, and from this point of view, animals that respire are true combustible bodies that burn and consume themselves. This analogy between combustion and respiration has not escaped the notice of the poets and philosophers who mentioned phrases like *'this fire stolen from heaven,'* *'this torch of Prometheus,'* to represent faithful picture of the operatures of nature. At least for the animals that breathe, one may therefore say that the torch of life lights itself at the moment the infant breathes for the first time, and it does not extinguish it self except at death."

Early efforts to build a large human respiration chamber by Reynault and Reiset in Paris in the 1940s were not successful. Pattenkoffe and Voit constructed a chamber in Munich in the late 19th century in which a man could live for several days and have all the respiratory changes measured. After 24-hour measurements of a fasting man, the protein "burned" was computed from the urinary nitrogen and the fat combustion from the respiratory carbon dioxide, after deducting the carbon burned in the protein, and assuming no change in the carbohydrate store of the body. A difference of only 6.2% was noticed between the measured oxygen absorption and that calculated as necessary for the combustion of the body materials metabolized, indicating the experimental skill and soundness of the basic assumptions used.

It was Atwater, a student of Voit, who later established the essential quantitative physiological knowledge on which all assessments of human energy needs are based. Atwater returned to the United States from Germany in 1892, and constructed a human calorimeter to measure the heat produced by man, with an accuracy of 0.1%. The walls of this chamber are insulated and heat produced in it is absorbed by water passing in and out. The temperatures of entering and leaving water are recorded by thermometers. Also, the volume of water that has flowed through the cooling system is measured in the vessel. The human subject can be observed through the glass window, and food is introduced and excreta removed through the porthole. Air leaving the chamber passes through a blower and over sulfuric acid and soda-lime to absorb water and carbon dioxide. The oxygen measured by a gas meter is added to the system before the air passes into the chamber (1). The Atwater chamber incorporated the respiration apparatus of Pottenkofer and Voit. The data presented in Table 1 show how accurately Atwater was able to measure human energy exchange by using the chamber. Despite the increase in our knowledge of the biochemical pathways underlying energy utilization, the understanding of the respiratory process from the whole body perspective is essentially unchanged (2).

II. PHYSIOLOGY OF ENERGY EXCHANGE

Lusk (3) has described the detailed experimentation that laid the foundations for our current understanding of energy exchange and measurement of energy expenditure in humans.

A. Forms and Units of Energy

Various forms of energy, such as solar (light), chemical (foods), mechanical, electrical, and thermal are exchanged in the biological systems. According to the first law of thermodynamics, energy can neither be created nor destroyed, it can only be changed between its different forms. All living organisms, including plants and animals, obey this law. Plants differ from animals in that they can use solar (light) energy to make complex organic molecules such as carbohydrates, proteins, and lipids, whereas animals have to depend on the synthetic ability of plants to derive their source of chemical (food) energy, to perform mechanical (muscular contraction, movement), electrical (maintenance of ionic gradients across membranes), and biochemical work (synthesis of new macromolecules). The conversion of food energy to these other forms of energy in man and animals is not a very efficient process; only about 75% of the original food energy may be dissipated as heat during the oxidation of food in the body. The human body, however, is much more efficient in this respect than most steam engines and is roughly equivalent to a good internal combustion engine. Barring very low temperatures, the heat generated as a by-product of the combustion process is sufficient to maintain the body temperature of organisms, especially if the body in insulated by proper clothing. When energy utilization increases substantially, the extra heat generated in the body is often in excess of that required to maintain body temperature and must be dissipated to the environment by means of sweating.

The SI (System International) unit of energy is the joule (J), which is the energy used when 1 kilogram (kg) is moved 1 meter (M) by a force of 1 newton (N); 1 joule being a very small amount of energy in the nutritional studies, the kilojoule (kJ) (i.e., 10^3 J) or the megajoule (MJ)

Table 1   A Four-Day Experiment of Atwater and Benedict in 1899

a. Gross energy of food	10.31 MJ/day
b. Gross energy of feces	0.32 MJ/day
c. Gross energy of urine	0.56 MJ/day
d. Gross energy of alcohol excreted	0.09 MJ/day
e. Energy content of net protein oxidation	0.29 MJ/day
f. Energy content of fat stores oxidized	0.56 MJ/day
g. Energy of nutrients oxidized [a–(b+c+d)+e+f]	10.19 MJ/day
h. Heat produced (by direct calorimetry)	10.02 MJ/day

Difference between (g) and (h) = –1.6%
Source: Ref. 2.

(i.e., 10^6 J) are used more conveniently. In the SI system, the rates of energy are expressed either in J per unit time (e.g., kJ/min or MJ/24 h), or in watts (W), where 1 W = 1 J/S or 1 kW = 1 kJ/S. Watts can be converted to kJ/min and kJ/24 h by multiplying by 0.06 and 86.4, respectively.

In many old textbooks, energy has been expressed in kilocalories (kcal or Cal). The calorie has been defined in relation to SI units; e.g., the 15°C calories is the energy required to raise the temperature of 1g of water from 14.5° to 15.5° and is equivalent to 4.1855 J, whereas the thermochemical calorie is the heat liberated on the total combustion of 1 g of pure benzoic acid and is equivalent to 4.184J. The Royal Society of London recommends the use of the thermochemical calorie conversion factor, so that 1 kcal = 4.184 J or 1J = 0.239 kcal (or roughly, 4.2 J = 1 kcal). The energy values in cals can be obtained by dividing by 4.184 (kJ) or 4.184×10^{-3} (MJ).

B. Chemical Energy of Foods

A bomb calorimeter is used to measure the chemical energy content of the food. The bomb is placed inside a vessel of water, the temperature of which can be measured accurately. The foodstuff is placed in a small crucible. The bomb is filled with oxygen at high pressure and the foodstuff is ignited electrically. The material in the bomb burns and the heat produced leads to a rise in temperature of the surrounding water.

Bomb calorimetry determined the gross energy (GE) of a food, representing the total chemical energy present in the food. All of this gross energy, however, is not available to the animal that eats the food for two reasons. First, not all food eaten by an animal is absorbed from the digestive tract. Atwater's experiment with human subjects showed that young men on typical American diets of the time absorbed 99% of the ingested carbohydrate, 95% of the fat, and 92% of the protein. The second reason is that the nitrogen-containing compounds (notably proteins) are not completely oxidized in the body to nitrogen oxides (which would be toxic) but are instead converted to less toxic urea to be excreted in the urine. The urea still has around a quarter of the chemical energy of the original protein, equivalent to 5.23 kJ/g protein (2).

The energy that is lost through feces and urine has to be subtracted from the gross energy of a food to estimate the energy available to the body, known as the metabolizable energy (ME) of the food. Man's ME intake on a mixed diet can be determined by performing bomb calorimetry on the food, feces, and urine over a given period of time (Table 2). Atwater estimated the ME content of protein, fat, carbohydrate, and alcohol separately, so as to predict the ME content of a food or diet from the knowledge of the amounts of each of these major nutrients. The ME values for the major nutrients, as calculated by Atwater (Table 3) are referred to as "Atwater factors," which provide an excellent approximation to the true ME content of most foods and mixed diets (4).

Table 2   Calculation of Metabolizable Energy Intake[a]

a. Gross energy of diet	9279 (SD 1125) kJ/day
b. Fecal energy loss	647 (SD 154) kJ/day
c. Urinary energy loss	318 (SD 70) kJ/day
Metabolizable energy (ME) intake [a–(b+c)]	8314 (SD 1137) kJ/day
ME as a % of gross energy	89.5 (SD 1.7)%
ME as a % of food table ME	100.5 (SD 2.0)%

[a]Ten women on a diet in which 55% of energy was in the form of carbohydrate and which contained 30 g fiber (Southgate method) per 8 MJ measured over 7 days.
Source: Ref. 2.

Table 3 Metabolizable Energy of Major Nutrients

Nutrients	GE[a] (kJ/g)	Percentage absorbed (Atwater's values)	Digestible energy (kJ/g)	Urinary loss (kJ/g)	ME[b] (kJ/g)	Atwater factor (kcal/g)
Starch	17.5	99	17.3	—	17.3	4
Glucose	15.6	99	15.4	—	15.4	4
Fat	39.1	95	37.1	—	37.1	9
Protein	22.9	92	21.1	5.2	15.9	4
Alcohol	29.8	100	29.8	Trace	29.8	7

[a]GE = Gross energy.
[b]ME = Metabolizable energy.
Source: Ref. 2.

It should be noted that the exact values for ME for each major nutrient may vary with the type of the food; e.g., the values assume that 6.25 g of protein contains 1 g of nitrogen, while for cereal and milk proteins, these values are closer to 5.7 and 6.4, respectively. Also, starch has a higher energy content than the same weight of simple sugars. This problem can be solved by expressing the carbohydrate content of foods in terms of their constituent monosaccharides, and using the ME value of 15.7 kJ/g monosaccharide. Food composition tables can be used to calculate ME of the various components of the diet (5,6).

According to McNeill (2), variations in the exact values used to estimate the ME content of foods may in practice introduce negligible error in the estimation of energy intake than differences in the energy content of different samples of the same food. Animal foods like meats, poultry, and fish vary considerably in their fat content, and fruits and vegetables differ in their water content, leading to significant variations in their energy content per unit weight of food. The ME values from food tables may also be misleading when diets are based on certain unusual proteins and fats, or with a high proportion of non-digestible carbohydrates such as cellulose. The fecal and urinary losses of energy may increase abnormally under disease conditions. In these unusual situations, ME intakes can be reliably estimated only by direct bomb calorimetry of food, feces, and urine.

III. ENERGY EXPENDITURE

A. Components of Energy Expenditure

Human energy expenditure is usually divided into the following three components:

1. The basal metabolic rate (BMR)
2. Physical activity
3. Postprandial thermogenesis (PPT)

The basal metabolic rate (BMR) is the single largest component of 24-hour energy expenditure in the individual. This is the energy expended by an individual lying at physical and mental rest in a thermoneutral environment at least 12 hours after the previous meal. The MBRs are often measured early in the morning, before the subject has engaged in any significant physical activity, and with no ingestion of tea, coffee, or even inhalation of nicotine for at least 12 hours before the measurement. Heavy physical exercise on the day before the measurement may also alter the BMR values. If all the conditions of BMR are not met, the energy expended should be termed the resting metabolic rate (RMR), rather than BMR.

The BMR of a subject is influenced by several factors, such as age, sex, body size, body composition, nutritional and physiological state and so forth (see below). Nevertheless BMR indicates energy expended under standardized conditions and can be compared within and between individuals. BMR is not necessarily the minimum metabolic rate of a subject, and estimates of sleeping metabolic rate have been found to vary from 90% to 100% of the BMR of the same subjects (2).

Physical activity accounts for about 20% to 40% of total daily energy expenditure in most individuals. The energy expended in physical activity depends both on the nature and duration of different activities carried out. Activities that involve little muscular work, but that are carried out for a longer duration of time, such as sitting or standing, may contribute more to the total daily energy expenditure than the more strenuous activities carried out for shorter times.

The energy spent on any particular activity varies considerably between individuals, because the size of the subject, and the speed and dexterity with which the activity is carried out, influence the energy expended (7). Heavy physical exercise may increase the RMR by a small amount over the following day (8). This effect is referred to as excess post-exercise oxygen consumption (EPOC). Some examples of the energy expenditure on different physical activities carried out by men and women expressed in terms of BMR multiples are given in Table 4. James and Schofield (9) have presented a comprehensive account of the energy cost of various physical activities. The accurate values for a particular individual or a group can be obtained only by direct measurements (2).

The postprandial thermogenesis (PPT), referred to earlier as specific dynamic action or diet-induced thermogenesis (DIT), includes the effect of food intake, drugs, cold, and hormonal state of the body on the thermogenic processes. The diet-induced thermogenesis includes the body's response to recent food ingestion as well as the longer-term effects of food intake on energy expenditure; e.g., when BMR increases in overfeeding, PPT is a result of energy expended in the digestion, absorption, and transport of the ingested nutrients, as well as the physical activity required for ingestion and any increase in mental arousal due to sensory stimuli from food. It is usually assumed to amount to around 10% of the energy content of a normal diet. Cold-induced thermogenesis involves shivering and non-shivering components, which increase energy expenditure to maintain body temperature when heat loss into the environment increases due to cold, air movement, or lack of shelter and insulation.

Table 4 Estimates of the Energy Costs of Selected Activities[a]

Activity	Men	Activity	Women
Sitting	1.2	Sitting	1.2
Standing	1.4	Standing	1.5
Walking (normal pace)	3.2	Walking (normal pace)	3.4
Carpentry	3.5	Light—cleaning	2.7
Mining with pick	6.0	Hard—threshing grain	5.0

[a]All values are expressed as a multiple of basal metabolic rate.
Source: Ref. 9.

B. Factors Influencing Energy Expenditure

McNeill (2) described the following factors that influence energy expenditure by the human body:

1. *Body Size*: This is one of the major determinants of energy expenditure in humans, accounting for more than one-half of the variability in BMR between individuals. Larger people with bigger body size have higher BMR. A difference in body weight of 10 kg may account for a variation in BMR of about 500 kJ/day in adults, or a difference in daily energy expenditure of around 800 kJ/day in subjects with light physical activity.

2. *Body Composition*: Another major determinant of energy expenditure. At rest, adipose tissue has a lower BMR than other (fat-free or lean) tissue. Due to this, BMRs are often expressed per kilogram of fat-free mass. Adipose tissue contributes significantly to the energy expended in a physical activity involving body movements.

3. *Age*: The energy expended per unit weight of the human body declines rapidly from birth to old age. The energy expenditure in children is increased by the energy cost of growth, and in very young infants, by the energy required to maintain body temperature. In adulthood, the fat-free mass of the body declines with an increase in the adipose (fat) tissue, which accounts for a large part of the decline in metabolic rate during the aging process.

4. *Sex*: The variations in the energy expenditure due to sex are largely governed by differences in the body size and body composition of males and females; e.g., a 65 kg adult man has a BMR of around 1 MJ/day higher than a woman of the same age and weight.

5. *Diet*: Food consumption influences energy expenditure, both immediately after a meal (PPT effect) and over longer periods (DIT effect). The PPT effect is greater in response to protein ingestion than to the same energy intake in the form of carbohydrate or fat (10). The energy intakes above or below energy requirements lead to either an increase or decrease in BMR, over and above that expected from the change in body weight and composition. These "adaptive" changes in energy act to offset the energy surplus or deficit; they are usually around 5% to 15% of the difference between energy intake and expenditure and thus slightly diminish the weight change produced by the energy imbalance.

6. *Climate*: Climate influences energy expenditure due to the need to maintain body temperature. The important parameters contributing to climatic factor are air temperature, wind speed, and the radiant temperature of the surrounding materials; e.g., in lightly clothed adults in an indoor environment, air temperatures below 25°C will increase energy expenditure, and at air temperatures above 30°C, energy expenditure may increase due to the additional work of sweating.

7. *Genetic Variation*: The BMRs measured under standardized conditions vary by up to ±10% between the subjects of the same age, sex, body weight, and fat content. This variation is attributed to genetic factors. It has been demonstrated that the RMR and energy cost of activities in Asian and African subjects were lower than in Causasian subjects of similar body weight and composition. Some other studies, however, reported no significant differences in energy expenditure between subjects of different ethnic groups (2).

8. *Hormonal State*: Energy expenditure is notably changed in endocrine disorders, such as hypo- or hyperthyroidism, either decreasing or increasing the energy expenditure, respectively. The effects of physiological hormones are seen especially during preg-

nancy and lactation. BMR appears to decrease during the early stages of pregnancy (11), whereas toward the end of gestation, the increased body weight accounts for an overall increase in BMR. The early fall in BMR is larger in women with low energy intakes, such as those in poor rural communities of developing countries. In lactation, there may be a reduction in energy expenditure, due to decreased BMR, physical activity, and other thermogenic processes (12).

9. *Psychological State*: Acute anxiety is a potent stimulant of energy expenditure. It is not known whether chronic psychological stress also influences energy expenditure.

10. *Drugs and Beverages*: Several pharmacological agents influence metabolic rate, such as nicotine (13), caffeine, and theophylline (14), all of which increase expenditure by small but measurable amounts. Therapeutic agents such as amphetamines and experimental drugs used to treat obesity also increase energy expenditure. Other drugs used to treat high blood pressure, including beta-blockers, may on the contrary decrease energy expenditure and lead to slight weight gain.

11. *Diseases*: A disease condition of the body may increase BMR, especially infections with fever, tumors, and skin burns, probably by involving intracellular signalling agents like cytokines (2).

C.　Measurement of Energy Expenditure

1.　Direct and Indirect Calorimetric Methods

Direct calorimetry involves measurement of the energy expended by a subject over a given period of time by measuring the heat generated by the body. A number of room-sized chambers have been designed to determine the heat loss by the human body. In practice, the construction and operation of such chambers is technically difficult for a number of reasons. Every part of the walls, floor, and roof need to be sensitive to heat, and anything that produces heat other than the subject (e.g., the operating staff or any electrical equipment) has to be excluded from the vicinity of the chamber. A water-cooled garment in which the human subject can move more freely has recently been developed. Also, direct calorimetry requires several hours for each measurement, because the technique assumes that no heat is stored in or lost from the body. Owing to these disadvantages and the fact that both direct and indirect calorimetry agree well, indirect calorimetry in humans has become a more practical and convenient method of measurement of energy expenditure than direct calorimetry.

Indirect calorimetry is based on the fact that as foods are oxidized to produce heat in the body, the oxygen consumed and carbon dioxide released in the process are in proportion to the heat generated, as per the following stoichiometric relation of the oxidation of one mole of glucose:

$$C_6H_{12}O_6 + 6O_2 \text{ -------- } 6\,CO_2 + 6\,H_2O + Heat$$
$$(18 \text{ g}) \, (6 \times 22.41) \, (6 \times 22.41) \, (6 \times 18 \text{ g}) \, (2.78 \text{ MJ})$$

It can be seen from the above equation that the energy released on oxidation of 1 g of glucose is 2780/180 = 15.4 kJ, and that each liter of oxygen consumed is equivalent to the production of 2780/6 × 22.4 = 20.7 kJ of heat. Thus, from this relationship of the oxygen consumed and the heat produced (energy expenditure), the latter can readily be calculated (2).

Similar equations can be written for protein and fat that show that each liter of oxygen consumed is equivalent to an energy expenditure of around 19.3 kJ, when either fat or protein is oxidized (Table 5) (15). The data in Table 5 show the value for oxygen consumed, carbon dioxide released, and heat produced per gram of each major food nutrient, along with its respiratory quotient (RQ). The RQ is the ratio of the moles of carbon dioxide produced to the moles of oxygen consumed on oxidation of a unit amount of each nutrient. The RQ values are close to 0.7 for fat and alcohol and 1.0 for carbohydrates, the protein having an intermediate value.

The data in Table 5 further indicate that the energy expended per liter of oxygen consumed is very similar for all three major nutrients. Thus, if the mixture of nutrients being oxidized is close to the mixture of nutrients in a normal diet, a value of 20.3 kJ per liter of oxygen consumed would be a good approximation of the energy expenditure for all three nutrients together.

Indirect calorimetry can be made more accurate by measuring carbon dioxide produced, and in experiments of sufficient duration, the urinary nitrogen excreted. Weir (16) has developed the following formulas that are widely used in human indirect calorimetry:

$$EE \ (kJ) = 16.489 \ V \ O_2 \ (1) = 4.628 \ V \ CO_2 \ (1) - 9.079 \ N(g)$$

If nitrogen excretion is not measured, it is assumed that protein accounts for about 15% of total energy expenditure, to approximate the same formula as:

$$EE \ (kJ) = 16.3/8 \ VO_2 \ (1) + 4.602 \ V \ CO_2 \ (1)$$

Other researchers have developed similar formulas with minor differences, arising from differences in the assumptions regarding the composition of carbohydrate, fat, and protein in the diet, leading to about 3% variation in the estimated energy expenditure under most normal dietary conditions (15).

By measuring nitrogen excreted along with O_2 consumed and CO_2 released, it is possible to calculate the proportions of energy derived from the three major nutrients. The following equations are based on the values for glucose, fat, and protein given in Table 5 and assuming that 6.25 g of protein contain 1 g of nitrogen:

Carbohydrate oxidation (g)

$$= 4.706 \ V \ CO_2 \ (1) - 3.340 \ V \ O_2 \ (1) - 2.714 \ N \ (g)$$

Fat oxidation (g)

$$= 1.768 \ V \ O_2 \ (1) - 1.778 \ V \ CO_2 \ (1) - 2.021 \ N \ (g)$$

Protein oxidation = 6.25 N (g)

This approach remains valid even when there is net synthesis of lipid from carbohydrate in the body. The results are very sensitive to the accuracy of the measurements of O_2 consumed and CO_2 produced. In unusual nutritional situations, such as during elemental feeding, the underlying

Table 5 Values for Oxidation of Major Nutrients

Nutrients	O_2 Consumed (l/g)	CO_2 Produced[a] (l/g)	RQ[b]	Energy Released	
				kJ/g	kJ/CO_2
Starch	0.829	0.824	0.994	17.49	21.10
Glucose	0.746	0.742	0.995	15.44	20.70
Fat	1.975	1.402	0.710	39.12	19.81
Protein	0.962	0.775	0.806	18.52	19.25
Alcohol	1.429	0.966	0.663	29.75	20.40

[a]CO_2 is not an ideal gas: 1 mole at STP occupies 22.26, not 22.4 liter.
[b]Volumetric RQ.
Source: Ref. 15.

assumptions of stoichiometry of oxidation of the different nutrients may require alteration to increase the accuracy of the results (17).

2. *Equipment Used in Indirect Calorimetry*

The equipment required for the measurement of energy expenditure by indirect calorimetry ranges from simple equipment designed to operate under rugged field conditions to technically sophisticated whole body chambers (18).

The Douglas bag technique is the most widely used system to measure energy expenditure. The subject breathes through a valve that separates inspired air from expired, directing all the expired air into a plastic bag of about 150 liter capacity. After becoming accostomed to breathing through the valve, all the expired air is collected over a measured period of time. The volume of expired air is then measured and adjusted to the volume at STP, with no humidity. The concentration of oxygen (and sometimes CO_2) is measured in a sample of expired air from the bag, using either a chemical apparatus (Haldane apparatus) or a specially designed gas analyzer that depends on the paramagnetic properties of oxygen and the infrared absorbance of CO_2. Assuming the O_2 and CO_2 contents of atmospheric (i.e., inspired) air in a well-ventilated surrounding to be 20.95% and 0.03%, respectively, the amount of oxygen consumed and CO_2 produced and hence the energy expenditure of the subject can be computed.

The Douglas bag has been used to measure energy expenditure, both at rest and during exercise, although for the latter it is not very ideal, since the bag fills quickly during heavy activity. Under such situations, the Kofrani-Michaelis (KM) respirometer (Max Planck respirometer) are more widely used. This apparatus measures the volume of the expired air as it is collected, requiring only a small of the expired air for gas analysis. A portable equipment called the Oxylog has taken the place of the KM respirometer, which is no longer manufactured. The Oxylog (2.2 kg weight) incorporates both a volume meter and oxygen sensors for O_2 analysis. The electronic components are powered by rechargeable batteries to calculate the oxygen consumed, providing a digital display of result on a minute-to-minute basis. Another successor to the KM, the Cosmed K_2 has been produced most recently. The Cosmed K_2 (400 g weight) incorporates an oxygen sensor and a device to transmit data to a radio receiver remote from the subject. The ventilated hood systems introduced in respirometers avoid the need for a face mask in respirometers or a one-way breathing valve and nose-clips (that cause discomfort to the subject) by maintaining a high rate of air flow through the restricted space in which the subject breathes. The system has more accurate gas analyzers and is best suited to situations in which the subject can lie at rest for periods of 30 minutes to 6 hours.

The whole-body indirect calometer chambers operate on the same principle as the ventilated hood, and range in size from 5 to 25 m^3. Both O_2 and CO_2 can be monitored; subjects follow a fixed schedule of activity with meals, sleep, and exercise. Thus, a value for the 24-hour energy expenditure for the standardized activities can be obtained (2).

3. *Non-Calorimetric Methods*

Measurement of heart rate over a 24-hour period has been used by some workers as an alternative to the measurement of energy expenditure by indirect calorimetry. This method requires the establishment of the relationship between heart rate and energy expenditure in individual subjects, monitoring both the heart rate and energy expenditure by indirect calorimetry, simultaneously. The method is not as accurate as indirect calorimetry, but it is inexpensive and doesn't restrict the subject, and it provides information on the energy expenditure pattern at different times of day. Thus, it can be used in large numbers of subjects and in children, in whom 24-hour calorimetry would be difficult to use to estimate energy expenditure under free-living conditions.

Schoeller and Van Santen (19) recently developed the doubly labeled water technique to provide information on the total energy expenditure of a non-restricted subject, over a period of up to 3 weeks, thus reflecting the true energy requirements of the subject. The subject takes an oral dose of water containing stable isotopes, deuterium (^2H) and ^{18}O, which mix with the normal hydrogen and oxygen in the body water within a few hours. As the energy is expended in the body, carbon dioxide and water are produced. The CO_2 is lost from the body through the breath, skin, and urine. The isotope ^{18}O is present in both CO_2 and water and will be lost from the body faster than ^2H, which is present only in water. The difference between the rate of loss of the two isotopes is used to calculate the CO_2 production of the subject, from which energy expenditure can be computed by the traditional formulas for indirect calorimetry (16).

The rates of loss of the stable isotopes (^{18}O and ^2H) are known by measuring the decline in the concentration of the isotopes in any body fluid (e.g., urine) over 10 to 21 days of the experiment. Several other variables need to be accounted for while calculating the results, viz., the diet composition, to give an estimate of RQ and hence oxygen consumption; the amount of evaporative water loss; and the extent of incorporation of the isotopes into the body tissue, especially during growth. The comparisons of the doubly labeled water method with whole body indirect calorimetry have shown an accuracy of better than 5% under carefully controlled experimental conditions.

The doubly labeled water technique has the advantage that the subject is completely free to follow his or her normal life style during the measurement, and therefore it can be used for ill, young, elderly, or exceptionally active subjects for whom other methods are not practical. However, the method involves the high cost of doubly labeled water and the mass spectrometer required to measure the concentrations of the isotopes in the body fluid samples. Also, this technique does not provide information on energy expenditure at different times of the day or on different days of a study. The combination of both methods produces a complete picture of total energy expenditure and its components (2).

IV. ENERGY REQUIREMENTS

The energy requirement of a human subject can be defined as "the energy intake which will balance the energy expenditure when the individual has a body size and composition and level of physical activity consistant with long-term good health, and that will allow for the maintenance of economically necessary and socially desirable physical activity" (20). In children and pregnant or lactating woman, the energy requirement includes the energy needs associated with the deposition of tissues or the secretion of milk at rates consistent with good health (2).

For an individual who is neither gaining nor losing weight, energy intake and energy expenditure must be equal. Thus, the energy requirements of healthy adults are often estimated from the estimates of energy intake. In infants and children up to 10 years of age, in whom measurements of energy expenditure are difficult to obtain, the current estimates of energy requirements are based on estimates of energy intake, in subjects gaining weight at an acceptable rate. This is done by estimating breast milk and supplementary food intake at different ages. However, it is difficult to determine the energy content of breast milk with accuracy. Prentice et al. (21) estimated energy expenditure using deuterated water in infants and suggested that the intake method may overestimate energy requirement in young children. The energy requirements of children from birth to 10 years as estimated by the Department of Health (1991) are given in Table 6 (22).

In a group of normal-weight healthy adults, energy intake, measured over 7 days or more by the weighted food inventory technique (23), has been found to agree well with eatimates of energy expenditure over the same period, though the agreement for each individual is usually less than for the mean values of intakes and expenditure for any one group. It should be noted that

Table 6 Estimated Energy Requirements of Children, 1–10 years

	Average weight (kg)		Energy Requirements			
			(kJ/kg/day)		(kJ/day)	
Age	Boys	Girls	Boys	Girls	Boys	Girls
1 month	4.15	4.00	480	480	1990	1920
2 months	6.12	5.70	420	420	2570	2390
6 months	8.00	7.44	400	400	6200	2980
12 months	10.04	9.50	400	400	4020	3800
2 years (yr)	12.39	11.80	400	400	4960	4720
3 yr	14.40	13.85	400	400	5760	5540
4 yr	17.0	16.8	395	365	6730	6120
5 yr	19.3	18.9	370	345	7190	6480
6 yr	21.7	21.3	350	320	7570	6770
7 yr	24.2	23.8	325	290	7920	7050
8 yr	26.8	26.6	305	275	8240	7280
9 yr	29.7	29.7	290	255	8550	7510

Source: Ref. 22.

even the most careful records of food intake may be subject to bias due to under-recording or changes in food habits, or due to random errors caused by unrepresentative samples. Studies conducted by Prentice et al. (24) and Livingstone et al. (25) have shown that energy intake estimates are often lower than energy expenditure when measured by the doubly labeled water technique. Thus, even the most careful estimates of energy intake in adults may not reflect habitual energy expenditure, unless there is reasonable agreement between the mean energy intake and the predicted energy requirement of the group (2).

Energy requirements are also determined from energy expenditures, which are estimated in a number of ways: the common approach is the factorial method in which the different components of energy expenditure are determined separately. The BMR can be measured by indirect calorimetry or can be predicted from tables based on measurements in large numbers of similar subjects. FAO/WHO have compiled an extensive BMR data based on a world-wide survey of about 11,000 technically acceptable measurements of individuals of all ages and both sexes in the 1980s. This included all the measurements on which earlier equations for predicted BMR were based, i.e., the Harris-Benedict and Aub-du Bois formulas. The statistically analyzed data showed that simple linear equations can be used to predict BMR from data on weight for different age and sex groups, as well as those including height, or based on more complex mathematical relations. The equations used to predict BMR from body weight are given in Table 7 (22).

After predicting the BMR, the energy required for physical activity and other thermogenic processes are added to obtain total energy requirements. The energy spent on physical activity can be measured directly by indirect calorimetry. It is difficult to measure energy spent on all major activities of each subject; therefore, this can be alternatively estimated from tables. James and Schofield (9) have provided the most comprehensive set of tables of the energy cost of various activities for adults (Table 4). In these tables the energy cost of activities are given as BMR multiples for men and women, allowing one value to be given for each activity that is applicable to all individuals of any body weight and age group. By knowing the duration of each activity, its energy cost can be readily determined by multiplying it with the measured or predicted BMR value of the subject. Thus, the subject is taken into account while estimating energy cost of physical activity. The earlier tables provided a single figure for the total energy expended in each activ-

Table 7 Equations for Predicting Basal Metabolic Rate from Body Weights

	Age range (years)	Prediction equation[a]	95% confidence limits
Men	10–17	BMR (MJ/day) = 0.074 (wt.) + 2.754	±0.88 MJ/day
	18–29	BMR (MJ/day) = 0.063 (wt.) + 2.896	±1.28 MJ/day
	30–59	BMR (MJ/day) = 0.048 (wt.) + 3.653	±1.40 MJ/day
	60–74	BMR (MJ/day) = 0.0499 (wt.) + 2.930	(N/A)[b]
	75+	BMR (MJ/day) = 0.0350 (wt.) + 3.434	(N/A)[b]
Women	10–17	BMR (MJ/day) = 0.056 (wt.) + 2.898	±0.94 MJ/day
	18–29	BMR (MJ/day) = 0.062 (wt.) + 2.036	±1.00 MJ/day
	30–59	BMR (MJ/day) = 0.034 (wt.) + 3.538	±0.94 MJ/day
	60–74	BMR (MJ/day) = 0.0386 (wt.) + 2.875	(N/A)[b]
	75+	BMR (MJ/day) = 0.0410 (wt.) + 2.610	(N/A)[b]

[a]Body weight in kg.
[b](N/A) = Not available.
Source: Ref. 22.

ity, regardless of the body size of the subject. Also, the measurements are made in subjects without standardization of the time of meals and the influence of other thermogenic stimuli, so that the value obtained by multiplying the BMR by the value for each physical activity is assumed to include the energy expended in other thermogenic processes (See Table 4).

The duration of various physical activities can be estimated either by respective recall by the subject or by keeping an activity diary or by time-and-motion records kept by unobstructive observers. In the absence of such detailed information, a crude estimate can be made from knowledge of the subjects' lifestyles. A recent UK report has used three activity categories for both work and leisure. The multiples of BMR for man and women in each of these categories is shown in Table 8. McNeill (2) cited the following two examples of the estimation of energy requirements of a male office clerk and a rural woman in a developing country:

a. A male office clerk, age 25 yr, weight 65 kg: predicted BMR = 6078 kJ/day

Activity	Multiple of BMR	Duration of activity (Hr)	Energy expended (kJ)
In bed	1.0	8	2340
At work	1.7	6	2970
Discretionary			
Household tasks	3.0	2	1760
Fitness training	6.0	0.33	580
Remainder	1.4	7.67	3140
Total	1.54	24	10780

b. A rural woman in a developing country, age 35 yr, weight 50 kg; predicted BMR = 5290 kJ/day

In bed	1.0	8	1780
Domestic work	2.7	3	1800
Agricultural work	2.8	4	2490
Discretionary	2.5	2	1110
Residual	1.4	7	2180
Total	1.76	24	9360

Table 8   BMR Multiples for Light, Moderate, and Heavy Activity

Non-occupational activity level	Occupational activity level					
	Light		Moderate		Heavy	
	Male	Female	Male	Female	Male	Female
Non-active	1.4	1.4	1.6	1.5	1.7	1.5
Moderately active	1.5	1.5	1.7	1.6	1.8	1.6
Very active	1.6	1.6	1.8	1.7	1.9	1.7

Source: Ref. 22.

The definition of energy requirement advanced by WHO allows for energy expenditure in desirable physical activities such as physical training. In subjects who are below the desirable weight or in whom the existing energy level of expenditure departs from the optimum value for any reason, a correction factor may be used while estimating the energy requirement, depending on whether the estimate of energy requirement is designed to maintain or to improve the status quo.

The estimates of energy requirements of adolescents and of pregnant and lactating women should include an allowance for the energy cost of tissue deposition or breast milk secretion. The weight gain during normal growth is thought to require 21 kJ per gram of tissue deposited (20). By assuming appropriate rates of weight gain and standard patterns of physical activity, the energy requirements of adolescents are estimated to be around $1.65 \times BMR$ for boys and $1.57 \times BMR$ for girls.

Hytten and Leitch (26) suggested that during pregnancy additional energy requirements are required for development of the fetus and the supporting tissues (placenta, uterus, breasts, and adipose tissue depots), which amount to 1200 kJ per day throughout the pregnancy. This allowance does not take into account any possible reduction in BMR or the energy expended in physical activity, and therefore may be regarded as generous. There may be some increase in energy intake during the last few months of pregnancy. The current UK recommendations have therefore suggested an increase of 800 kJ/day in the last trimester of pregnancy (22).

During lactation some of the energy cost of breast milk secretion may be met by the adipose tissue stores laid down in pregnancy (4 kg of 11 kg gained theoretically during gestation). Assuming secretion of breast milk containing 3 MJ per day for 6 months and an estimated efficiency of production of 80%, and depletion of adipose tissue stores laid down in pregnancy, the net increase in energy requirement during lactation would be around 2.1 MJ per day over the 6-month period. This allowance would be too large for women who bottle-feed or who breast-feed for periods less than 6 months. Goldberg et al. (27) estimated an energy intake of lactating women in the United Kingdom of around 1.5 MJ/day, suggesting that a decrease in physical activity and/or alterations in the thermogenic processes observed in lactation may operate to reduce the additional energy requirements of lactation in many women.

The energy requirement estimates thus appear to be imprecise, but they are necessary to roughly indicate the food needs of individuals and group of populations. According to McNeill (2), the final test regarding the correctness of the energy requirement estimate depends on whether a subject fed his or her estimated energy requirement over a period of time changes weight by the amount intended. Newer methods of measuring energy expenditure, such as the doubly labeled water technique, are expected to improve the process of estimating energy requirements in times to come: the suitability of subjects' energy intake is validated by simple observation of body weight.

REFERENCES

1. Bell, G. H., J. N. Davidson, and H. Scarborough, *Textbook of Physiology and Biochemistry*, 7th ed., Livingstone, Edinburgh, London, 1968.
2. McNeill, G., Energy, *Human Nutrition and Dietetics*, 9th ed. (J. S. Garrow and W. P. T. James, eds.), Churchill Livingstone, Edinburgh, London, 1993, p. 24.
3. Lusk, G., *The Elements of the Science of Nutrition*, 4th ed., Johnson Reprint Corp. New York, 1928 (Reprinted in 1976).
4. Southgate, D. A. T., and J. V. G. A. Durnin, Calorie conversion factors. An experimental reassessment of the factors used in the calculation of the energy value of human diets. *Br. J. Nutr. 24*: 517 (1970).
5. Widdowson, E. M., Assessing of the energy value of human foods, *Proc. Nutrition Soc. 14*: 142 (1955).
6. McCance, R. A., and E. Widdowson, *The Composition of Foods*, 5th ed., HMSO, London, 1991.
7. Mahadeva, K., R. Passmore, and B. Woolf, Individual variation in the metabolic cost of standardized exercises: the effect of food, age, sex, and race, *J. Physiol. 121*: 225 (1953).
8. Maehlum, S. M. Grandmontagne, E. A. Newsholme, and O. M. Sejersted, Magnitude and duration of excess of postexercise oxygen consumption in healthy young subjects, *Metabolism 35*: 425 (1986).
9. James, W. P. T., and C. Schofield, *Human Energy Requirements*, Oxford University Press, 1990.
10. Nair., K. S., J. S. Garrow, and D. Halliday, Thermic response to isoenergetic protein, carbohydrate or fat meals in lean and obese subjects, *Clin. Sci. 62*: 43 (1981).
11. Durmin, J. U. G. A., et al., The energy requirements of human pregnancy, *Lancet 1*: 895, 953, 1010, 1072, 1029 (1987).
12. Illingworth, P. J., R. T. Jung, P. W. Howie, P. Leslie, and T. Isles, Diminution in energy expenditure during lactation, *Br. Med. J. 292*: 437 (1986).
13. Dulloso, H. M., and W. P. T. James, The role of smoking in the regulation of energy balance, *Int. J. Obesity 8*: 365 (1984).
14. Dulloo, A. G., C. A. Geissler, T. Horton, A. Collins, and D. S. Miller, Normal caffeine consumption: influence on thermogenesis and daily energy expenditure in lean and post-obese-human volunteers, *Am. J. Clin. Nutr. 49*: 44 (1989).
15. Brockway, J. M., Derivation of formulae used to calculate energy expenditure in man, *Human Nutrition: Clin. Nutr. 41C*: 463 (1987).
16. Weir, J. B. de V., New methods for calculating metabolic rate with special reference to protein metabolism, *J. Physiol. 109*: 1 (1949).
17. Licesey, G., and M. Elia, Estimation of energy expenditure, net carbohydrate utilization and net fat oxidation and synthesis by indirect calorimetry: evaluation of errors with special reference to the detailed composition of fuels, *Am. J. Clin. Nutr. 47*: 608 (1988).
18. Mclean, J. A., and G. Tobin, *Animal and Human Calorimetry*, Cambridge University Press, Cambridge, 1987.
19. Schoeller, D. A., and E. van Santen, Measurement of energy expenditure in humans by doubly labelled water method, *J. Appl. Physiol. 53*: 955 (1982).
20. FAO/WHO/UNO, Energy and Protein Requirements, WHO Tech. Report Series No. 224, World Health Organization, Geneva, 1985.
21. Prentice, A. M., A. E. Black, and W. A. Coward, High levels of energy expenditure in obese women, *Br. Med. J. 292*: 983 (1986).
22. Department of Health, Dietary Reference Values for Food, Energy and Nutrients for the United Kingdom, HMSO, London, 1991.
23. Ralph, A., Appendix 1: Methods for dietary assessment, *Human Nutrition and Dietetics*, 9th ed. (J. S. Garrow and W. P. T. James, eds.), Churchill Livingstone, Edinburgh, London, 1993, p. 777.
24. Prentice, A. M., A. Lucas, L. Vasquez-Velasqueez, P. W. S. Davies, and R. G. Whitehead, Are current dietary guidelines for young children a prescription of overfeeding? *Lancet 2*: 1066 (1988).

25. Livingstone, M. B. E., A. M. Prentice, and J. J. Strain, Accuracy of weighed dietary records in studies of diet and health, *Br. Med. J. 300*: 708 (1990).
26. Hytten, F. E., and I. Leitch, *The Physiology of Human Pregnancy*, 2nd ed., Blackwell, Oxford, 1971.
27. Goldberg, G. R., A. M. Prentice, and W. A. Coward, Longitudinal assessment of the components of energy balance in well-nourished lactating women, *Am. J. Clin. Nutr. 54*: 788 (1991).

9

Health and Dietetic Foods

I. INTRODUCTION

Food is a basic requirement of daily human life, more essential and, to some, more comforting than religion, love, or sex. The emotional and social resonances connected with food have long been explored by writers in prose and poetry (1). Human attitudes to food are as various as food itself. Moral attitudes have changed over the history of the world, along with the religious, economic, social, and sexual behavior of human beings. Food, like sleep, however, has remained a basic daily human requirement—more necessary in most climates than either clothing or shelter.

Man's food has several dimensions, the most obvious being the quantitative dimension: the insufficiency of food leads progressively from mild discomfort to severe hunger and ultimately to dealth. But food also has a qualitative aspect; e.g., improper diets lead to malnutrition, obesity, or disease. Food thus affects health, life span, physical fitness, body size, and mental development. Food also has a cultural dimension. Food habits are part of our cultural and emotional life. Human beings cling to their food habits, which have become rituals and patterns in the daily routine. Satisfactory dining soothes both body and soul and is a major factor in quality of human life.

Scientists in the field of aging, cancer, diabetes, cardiovascular diseases, and many of the diseases related to aging are becoming aware of the value of preventive therapies. Terms like functional foods, medical or health foods, designer foods, therapeutic foods, nutraceuticals, and the like are being used by the media. However, information that is currently available is not sufficient to address all unsolved health problems. There is a need to investigate plant products in a more systematic way. Effects that have been observed in the laboratory with animal experiments need to be interpreted carefully, and documented with more in vivo evidence. Traditional foods that have been used for several generations are likely to be the subject of in-depth research in the near future. According to Ramarathnam et al. (2), new types of plant antioxidants and novel biofactors may be developed and it is very likely that the increased consumption of plant foods will become the trend of the next decade.

Hillium (3) has described functional foods from the Western consumer viewpoint, considering how increasing consumer awareness of health tissues and functional ingredients may lead to the development of a functional foods market in Europe. Based on several European consumer and market studies carried out by the Leatherhead Food Research Association (LFRA) between 1990 and 1995, Hillium (3) concluded that consumer interest in health and awareness of the potential benefits of functional foods is on the increase in the West, and this increase is reflected in the growing number of products appearing on the market. Interest in functional foods has yet, however, to have a major impact on the food and drinks markets of countries outside Asia. Europe and the United States of America appear to have just begun to take the idea seriously. The manufacturers have reformulated and repositioned existing products to emphasize their health benefits, in addition to launching new products.

The inclusion in food products of ingredients claimed or perceived to be beneficial is likely to continue. However, full development of a potentially enormous functional food market may await resolution of the legislative problems surrounding health claims on food products. Until these problems are satisfactorily resolved, or until consumer health education reaches a point at which health claims are not required, mainstream market development will not be able to really begin. According to Hillium (3), functional foods are difficult to define because of the diverse nature of the products that the term encompasses and the fact that functional ingredients can be added to almost any food or drink. The LFRA reports have however used a common definition— that functional food is food and/or drink derived from naturally occurring substances that is consumed as part of the daily diet and possesses particular physiological benefit(s) when ingested.

Ohigashi et al. (4) suggested cancer preventive potential of vegetables and fruits and their active constituents as an approach to functional food. These authors indicated that the high cancer preventive potential of tropical Southeast dietary plants and several anti-tumor-promoting food phytochemicals found in nonnutritionally consumed dietary plants may lead to the development of important functional foods. Among several compounds identified, [1′,S]-1′-acetoxychavicol acetate (ACA) and 1,2-di-alpha-linolenoyl-3-O-beta-galactopyranosyl-sn-glycerol (DLGG) have shown to be promising cancer preventive agents. According to Ohigashi et al. (4), before functional food and medicine can have a practical application, however, several hurdles must be cleared: the mechanism of action, acute and chronic toxicity, metabolic and degradative pathways in the body, agent availability, and cost. Nevertheless, this area of research is expected to greatly contribute to the reevaluation of our daily dietary habits and effective prevention of diseases.

II. MEDICAL/HEALTH FOODS

A large and varied range of products are often referred to as "medical" or "health" foods and as such they cannot be adequately defined. These are not strictly scientific terms. Also, various marketing and legislating bodies use different definitions. Even within one country, many such products are called foods, while others can legally be either foods or drugs, quite apart from differing legislation between countries. Sometimes they are described as food products for which claims are made regarding the prevention, alleviation, or cure of certain diseases, although it is illegal in most countries to make such claims except for licensed medical products. The following products are generally included among medical/health foods (5):

1. Dietary supplements prepared from natural sources, including traditional remedies such as ginseng, garlic, aloe vera extract, and honey, as well as modern products like royal bee jelly, evening primrose oil, the alga *Spirulina*, and long-chain fish oils. The basis for claiming benefits for these products may be ancient usage—e.g., ginseng has a history of about 5000 years—or more recent discoveries such as with evening primrose oil. Thus, reputation of these dietary supplements rest on a variety of materials ranging from those that can only be described as old wives' tales, to unverified indications of potential benefits reported in recent scientific literature.
2. Individual nutrients, such as amino acids, purified proteins, vitamins, and mineral salts (with emphasis on zinc, magnesium, selenium, and calcium), designed to make good a real or perceived dietary deficiency.
3. Pseudoscientific remedies, including nonexistent vitamins and chemicals that are routinely made in the body from ordinary foods, which may be a vital component(s) of the metabolic pathways in the tissues (e.g., lecithin, carnitine, DNA and RNA, and enzymes.

In addition to these supplements, the term 'health foods' may also include the following foods grown or prepared under specific conditions:

1. Organically grown foods, i.e., those grown without the use of synthetic agricultural chemicals, such as fertilizers and chemical pesticides (insecticides, fungicides, herbicides, etc.) and growth regulators.
2. Whole, unprocessed foods with all the nutrients intact or foods that have been lightly processed to avoid nutrient losses—whole grain products such as whole wheat meal bread and brown rice contain more vitamins and minerals than milled white flour, white bread, and white rice.
3. Common foods and their extracts are claimed to offer protection from numerous disorders such as rheumatism and arthritis (e.g. cherry, lettuce) and herbal remedies such as comfrey sassafras, and several herbal teas.
4. Foods that are unusual in one country but are common elsewhere, e.g., buckwheat, sesame, carob beans, kelp (seaweed), ginger, aniseed, quinoa (a high-protein cereal), capsicum, etc.
5. Nutritionally enriched foods.

The health food business lays emphasis on foods termed natural, some of which are described as "ecologically friendly" foods (e.g., jaggery or black sugar), because their production causes less damage to the land and environment and requires less energy for its production, preparation, and waste disposal. The health food business is often associated with vegetarian, vegan, and macrobiotic diets, and linked with alternative or complementary medicine.

The health food manufacturers (UK Association and European Federation) have forwarded the following definitions of health foods:

1. The food products are prepared primarily with the specific intention of maintaining and/or improving health.
2. The products are as far as possible naturally based.
3. The products are to be provided with consumer information regarding their health benefits and are thus sold in specialist stores by a trained staff.
4. Health foods are supplied with their full information on nutritional composition.
5. Food suplements are selected to supply nutrients lacking in the diet to prevent their deficiency.
6. In addition to the health foods, there also may be appropriate literature and equipment to assist maintenance and development of good health.

Food ingredients are carefully selected from high-quality raw food materials, with a minimum of synthetic pesticides and other harmful substances. Artificial additives and preservatives are used only to comply with the necessary technical and qualitative standards. Thus, several manufacturers and retail outlets and many shopkeepers are involved, causing an enormous degree of variation in the application of these standards.

The first health food stores were started in Germany (Reform Haus) in 1890, followed by similar stores in the United Kingdom in 1894. An estimated 20% to 25% of consumers in the European Economic Community (EEC) today buy some of these food products, representing about 70 to 80 million customers. The rapid growth in the sales of these products in recent years has led to pharmacies and supermarkets stocking some of such health foods, e.g., vitamin and mineral supplements, ginseng, bees' royal jelly, garlic extracts and tablets, and fish oils.

A. Health Food Claims

Direct claims on leaflets, on labels, and in the media for the proprietary brands of any of these products are illegal in most countries, but apart from the fact that governmental regulations are not always very strictly enforced, it is not illegal to make claims for the benefits of generic products in the media. The claims made frequently include lists of health disorders that may be prevented, alleviated, or cured by the product or claims that it confers special physiological powers such as increased physical and mental capacity, improved memory, beauty and longevity, restored hair growth and increased vitality and virility. It is often not possible to verify any of these claims and indeed many of them are not even verifiable, most such claims resting on testimonials from satisfied customers.

Claims made for nutritional supplements range from the undoubted fact that they help to ensure adequacy of an individual's diet in respect of all the needed nutrients, to rather unacceptable claims based on the presumption that the greater part of a given population is deficient in the nutrients involved, and that extra nutrients will confer special benefits.

Macrae et al. (5) described the following health foods having one or other claims of improving human health:

1. Lecithin

Lecithin is the name given to a mixture of fats that have phosphate in their molecule and are chemically phosphoglycerides. Pure lecithins are phosphatidyl cholines and are found to differ in their fatty acid content. Commercially made lecithin is an impure mixture extracted from vegetable oils such as peanut oil, soybean oil, and eggs. Soybean oil contains 2% to 3% lecithin. Commercial lecithin is used in food processing to assist emulsification in the manufacture of candies, ice cream, margarine, and bakery products. It is added to "instant" powers to assist wetting and to frying oils to prevent spattering when wet foods are added to hot fat. Lecithins thus may be regarded as "functional foods," because they improve the quality of the processed foods.

Lecithin, however, is not a dietary essential, for it is made in the body from the basic materials provided in the normal diet. Moreover, it is often ingested ready-made, present in milk, nuts, fish, liver, eggs and vegetable oils. Lecithins are part of the cell's structure and are involved in the fat metabolism in the liver and aid in the absorption of fat from the intestine and its transport in the blood. This last function of lecithin has led to incorrect claims that lecithin supplements assist in slimming because they help to remove fat from the fat deposits. Lecithins are also claimed to help prevent heart attacks, to decrease insulin needs of diabetics and to improve the memory, concentration, and appetite of children, for which scientific evidence is lacking.

Any additional lecithin in the diet has no effect other than to provide extra energy (9 kcal or 36 kJ per g)—it is not a dietary essential. It is also naturally present in many foods and certain processed foods may contain additional amounts. Lecithin is a good example of the use of pseudoscience in health foods, because it is possible to describe the importance of its role in biochemical and physiological functions of the body, so as to imply, if not state directly, that it is a valuable dietary supplement.

Lecithin deficiency is most unlikely to occur, except possibly among a few food faddists. Thus, supplementation of a normal diet with lecithin tablets will be without any beneficial effects. Despite this, unfounded claims have been made that added lecithin, generally in the form of soybean extracts, counters obesity or slows the changes leading to atherosclerosis. Occasionally, it has been used as a source of chlorine in the hope of treating dementia or extrapyramidal disorders. These claims also appear to be superfluous, since the quantities used are much smaller than those present in the diet.

2. *Kelp (Seaweed)*

Seaweed is a common food in Japan; small amounts are eaten in other countries, e.g., Irish moss, or carrageen (*Chondrus crispus*), and laver bread made from *Porphyra* sp. Kelp is a large, greenish-brown seaweed and is found in several species. Most of the commercial kelp tablets are prepared from *Fucus vesiculosis* or bladder wrack.

It is claimed that kelp cures a number of physiological disorders such as arthritis, hypertension, eczema, and migraine, without substantial evidence for these claims, only a statement that kelp is a source of many amino acids, carbohydrates, vitamins, and minerals (as is any other living tissue). One kelp tablet contains about 300 mg and thus may provide very small amounts of these nutrients. However, kelp may be an important source of iodine. Kelp probably acquired a reputation as a health aid because of its iodine content, and like many such beliefs, its reputation has gone beyond the scientific evidence. Kelp tablets prepared from various seaweeds vary in their contents of sodium, potassium, phosphorus, and iodine, together with a small amount of protein and fat. The sodium content can be sufficient to render the use of kelp tablets undesirable or even harmful in patients on a salt-restricted diet. In cases of iodine deficiency, also, kelp tablets cannot be considered a reliable or adequate source of supplementary iodine. The amounts of other nutrients are negligible compared with those in a normal human diet.

3. *Pollen*

Pollen contains protein, fat, carbohydrate, minerals, and vitamins in relatively higher proportion than other foods. This is because pollen is dryer than protein-rich foods such as beef (50 to 60% water), eggs (75%), fish (80%), and milk (88%). Thus, pollen has about five times more protein than eggs, cheese, or beef. This claim, however, is misleading because the amount of pollen consumed is insignificantly small, compared to other foods consumed in larger quantities at a meal.

Many different products are sold under one name, for there is no particular standard for any generic product, and products sold differ in composition. Pollen products are rarely provided with any compositional data and depend on testimonials of its benefits by the users, especially athletes, which could be due to the placebo effect. Tablets containing pollen are purported to benefit one's general condition and physical performance, reflecting a popular misconception that genetic material from other species must contain a high concentration of life-giving materials of value to humans. The claims made generally refer only to the content of protein, vitamin B and trace elements, with a veiled reference to a large number of other valuable constituents. However, there is no scientific evidence to show that pollen is of any value to humans.

4. *Ginseng*

The roots of several (but not all varieties) of the ginseng shrub (*Panax* sp.) have historical repute as a tonic or stimulant in China and other Asian countries. Ginseng has been used to sustain armies on long marches or in battle. The commercial ginseng products available all over the world are claimed or thought to promote alertness, sexual powers, general good health, and long life. These health properties of ginseng are often attributed to its supposedly high nutrient content. However, the literature concerning the manner in which ginseng should be harvested, prepared, and consumed is so contradictory that there is a wide variation in what is finally ingested. Both European and American laboratories examining ginseng products, supposedly backed by government guarantees in their country of origin, found that many products contained no materials derived from ginseng at all—e.g., a so-called ginseng wine consisted of plain turnips in Italian table wine (6).

Very little satisfactory pharmacological or clinical studies on ginseng have been reported. Some Bulgarian and other researchers have claimed that ginseng extracts sustain mice during exhausting exercise, but this work is methodologically deficient. Some Japanese workers noted stimulant effects of ginseng extracts on some rats but depressant effects on others when the extractant was given parenterally. Chemical analysis has identified the presence of various surfactants (ginsenosides), the pharmacological effects of which are not clear. In active quantities, ginseng might act as a laxative. Some ginseng preparations have been found to contain female sex hormones; symptoms of ginseng "abuse syndrome" may be nostalgia in women and euphoria. It is possible that ginseng root samples have wild stimulatory effects on the central nervous system, reflecting the root's reputed effects, but there is no evidence that ginseng preparations have any beneficial effects on human health (6). A 'Russian root' reputed to be similar to ginseng is derived from *Eleutherococcus* sp.

5. *Royal Jelly*

This thick, white, salivary secretion of the worker bee is necessary for the development of the queen bee. Certain preparations of royal jelly, supplied in the form of drinking ampules, have reputed claims of prolonging life and delaying the appearance of degenerative diseases. Chemical analysis shows that the jelly contains small quantities of various vitamins and minerals and a number of organic substances whose pharmacological effects have not been established. There is no scientific evidence to show that royal jelly has any effects on human physiology.

6. *Evening Primrose Oil*

The seeds of the evening primrose (*Oenithera biennis*) and related plants provide an oil containing linoleic acid and a small quantity of gamma-linolenic acid, both of which are precursors of prostaglandins, previously misnamed vitamin F. The oil has been claimed to have a wide range of beneficial effects on malignant neoplasms, multiple sclerosis, premenstrual tension, atopic eczema, and diabetic neuropathy. Barring responses to the placebo therapy, no effect has been found, though theoretically a preparation containing linoleic acid might have effect in some cases of infantile atopic eczema (5).

7. *Garlic*

The reputation of garlic as a health food seems to rest on its pungent odor, which suggests some particular potency, thus explaining its use as an expectorant (to loosen mucus in bronchitis). Garlic's antifungal and antimicrobial effects are probably insufficient to be of any therapeutic value. A belief that garlic may delay the onset of atherosclerotic disorders has led to some research on its antihyperlipidemic effects, and the results obtained do suggest that a garlic powder can potentiate the lipid-lowering effects of diet. However these effects of garlic are less marked than those of other lipid-lowering agents, and it is not known whether garlic is beneficial in the long run (see Chapters 24 and 25).

8. *Cider Vinegar*

Vinegar prepared by refermenting cider or wine is often preferred in food preparation, owing to its retention of a wine flavor. Chemically, however, it is just like unbrewed vinegar, a solution of acetic acid with insignificant content of potassium. The alleged therapeutic or prophylactic value of cider vinegar can be traced back to unscientific work of a Vermont physician who had reportedly found that inhabitats of the state had unusually long life expectancy, which was attributed to a local habit of drinking cider vinegar. Since then a wide range of medical claims have been made for the product but none of these have been supported with any scientific basis or theoretical credibility.

9. Laetrile

Laetrile (amygdalin), misnamed vitamin B_{17}, also has no nutrient value. It is an extract of apricot kernels, occasionally modified during processing, and contains cyanide combined with carbohydrate. It has been widely claimed to cure cancer when taken either orally or parenterally, based on the theory that the released cyanide will kill the cancer cells without affecting healthy tissue. An alternative, unfounded claim was that cancer was caused by a deficiency of vitamin B_{17}, which would be alleviated by giving laetrile. Although both the parenteral administration and oral ingestion of a small quantity of laetrile has no effect, oral use of higher doses may lead to release of dangerous quantities of cyanide with fatal effects. A study by the U.S. National Cancer Institute showed that laetrile had no therapeutic value in cancer.

10. Fish Oils

A finding that Greenland Eskimos had a much lower incidence of ischemic heart disease than Danish people has led to various studies on the effects of dietary fish oils on serum lipids and cardiovascular disease (7,8). These studies indicated that there is a case for providing low levels of n-3 fatty acids to patients at an increased risk for coronary heart disease, especially those who cannot further increase their fish intake. However, it is possible that the supposed beneficial effects of n-3 fatty acids on cardiovascular disease might in fact be attributable to another cause. Evidence that fish oils supplements might help to prevent restenosis after coronary angioplasty also needs further evidence (7) (see Chapter 24).

11. Vitamin and Mineral Supplementation

There are very few specific situations in which the daily diet is deficient in certain vitamins and/or minerals. These include the case of old people living in isolation who have become indifferent to their food intake and population groups with little access to fresh fruits, and vegetables or to sunlight, as well as some food faddists. In the higher latitudes, infants and small children may need vitamin D supplementation, in addition to that obtained from breast milk or infant formula. There also may be an individual case for providing either a broad range of vitamins and minerals at a level approaching the RDA intake or specific vitamins (e.g., A, D, or C) which are likely to be deficient. However, individuals who are not eating well are often not likely to purchase such supplements, the cost of which would possibly be either equal to or more than that of simple dietary adjustment. The vast majority of the vitamin and mineral supplements consumed yearly in the industrially developed countries are undoubtedly wasted, for they are purchased and consumed by families already enjoying nutritionally adequate diets. Food fortification with specific vitamins and minerals, such as vitamins A or D, iodine, and iron, would be more efficient where deficiencies are likely to affect a large group of population. Reasonably formulated vitamin and minerals should remain on sale in order to meet popular demand, but the claims made for them must be rigidly restricted because they are of so little value when the normal diet is quite adequate (5).

Megavitamin therapy and beliefs have primarily centered around claims that high doses of vitamin C can cure the common cold or have a favorable effect on malignant disease. Equivocal evidence on these scores indicates that megavitamin C is probably no more than a convenient form of placebo therapy. Physicians commonly administer elevated doses of mixed vitamins from the B group, along with vitamin C, on the basis of very uncertain evidence that this may favorably influence neurological disorders.

B.   The Placebo Effect (Placebo Therapy)

A placebo is an inactive substance given for the gratification of the patient, and a placebo effect is observed when the patient actually benefits from an inactive substance because he or she expects it. Many patients recover from disorders without any treatment because of the body's own curing mechanism. Thus, the placebo effect may be basis for testimonials obtained from the satisfied customers of these so-called health foods.

The British Food Standards Committee in its *1980 Report on Claims and Misleading Descriptions* has stated that "In a general sense all foods can be considered health-giving in that a lack of the right amounts of a sufficient variety eventually results in bad health. To this extent the term 'health' applied to any food is a superfluous and misleading description, but it is generally used to imply an extra health-giving quality which an ordinary food may not possess. Some of the claims made for this extra quality stray into areas of nutrition about which there may still be insufficient knowledge and yet others may be pure fantasy."

The consumers association magazine *Which?* in its June 1978 issue states that "We could find no clear difference between most 'health food' brands and other comparable brands of beans, peas, lentils, seeds, sugars, drinks, nuts, yeast extracts, yogurts, herbs, honey and spices." This article also denied the curative properties of so-called wonder foods such as bees' royal jelly, pollen, cider vinegar, wheat germ, molasses, honey, brewers' yeast and kelp. The magazine further stated that "We know of no scientifically acceptable evidence of miracle cures by these wonder foods."

III.   DIETETIC FOODS

Dietetic foods are the special foods used for particular nutritional purposes and dietary management of people suffering from certain metabolic disorders (e.g., diabetics), those who are unable to digest or absorb nutrients from a normal diet, those having special dietary requirements (e.g., sportsmen and athletes), and those whose food intake requires special compositional standards (e.g., babies). Macrae et al. (9) have described various types and uses of dietetic foods, on which the following discussion is mainly based.

A.   Legislatory Controls and Claims

The Food and Agricultural Organization (FAO) and World Health Organization (WHO) of the United Nations Organization are jointly working through the Codex Alimentarius Commission to define standards for various types of dietetic foods (10–12). In addition to these, local regulations and recommendations apply in many countries. In the United States of America, the Code of Federal Regulations (CFR) defines standards for foods for special dietary uses, including foods for infants, diabetics, weight reduction or control and hypoallergenic and low sodium foods (13). The European Society of Pediatric Gastroenterology and Nutrition (ESPGAN) is setting compositional standards for foods for infants and young children. Since May 1991, dietetic foods have been controlled by an EEC council directive relating to foodstuffs for particular nutritional uses (14) on the provision that they fall into one of the following:

1.   of certain categories of persons whose digestive processes or metabolism are disturbed
2.   of certain categories of persons who are in a physiological condition and who are, therefore, unable to obtain special benefit from controlled consumption of certain substance(s) in food stuffs
3.   of infants or young children in good health.

This directive has laid down general guidelines for the complete category of foods, their labeling, and the introduction of new groups of foods on the markets. In regard to the labeling, presentation, and advertising, manufacturers of these dietetic foods must not attribute properties for the prevention, treatment, or cure of human disease to such products, or imply such properties. The directive has further classified groups of foods for which provisions will be laid down by specific directives. The food groups include:

1. Infant formulas and follow-on foods
2. Baby foods
3. Low-energy and energy-reduced foods intended for weight control
4. Dietary foods for special medical purposes
5. Low-sodium foods, including low-sodium or sodium-free dietary salts
6. Gluten-free foods
7. Foods intended to meet expenditure of intense muscular effort, especially for sports persons
8. Foods intended for persons suffering from carbohydrate metabolic disorders (diabetics)
9. Food supplements.

In addition to the general directive relating to foodstuffs for particular nutritional uses (PARNUTS) and specific directives contained within it, other EEC directives cover provisions such as nutrient substances used in their manufacture, additives for technological purposes, flavors, and colors as well as purity criteria for all these substances. As with other foods, dietetic food products are controlled by general claims, weights and measures, hygiene standards and so on, except where these are overridden, either by the PARNUTS and/or a specific directive (9). Examples of some therapeutic diets that alleviate disease symptoms, and those used to correct disturbances in certain physiological or metabolic function, are given in Tables 1 and 2, respectively.

B. Infant and Baby Foods

Infant formulas are intended for infants below one year of age, whose mothers are either unable or unwilling to breast-fed them; these may be replaced, partially or totally, by follow-on formulas from 4 months onwards, or after solids are introduced. Because infant formulas constitute the only source of nutrition, the compositional standard is defined, as are the ingredients used to supply nutrients and technological additives. Purity criteria regarding microbiological quality and levels of chemical contaminants are strictly adhered to. EEC legislation defines a clear code for

Table 1 Examples of Therapeutic Diets that Alleviate Disease Symptoms

Symptoms	Condition	Diet
Nausea	Gall bladder disease	Low-fat
	Renal disease	Low-protein
Dysphagia	Disease of mouth or esophagus	Semisolid
Weight loss	Trauma, carcinoma, severe burns	High-energy
Constipation	Diverticular disease and others	High-fiber
Diarrhea	Pancreatic insufficiency	Low-fat
	Lactose intolerance	Lactose-free

Source: Ref. 9.

Table 2 Examples of Therapeutic Diets Used to Correct Disturbances in Physiological or Metabolic Function

Condition	Cause	Diet
Uremia	Renal failure	Low-protein, low-phosphate
Edema	Heart failure, liver or renal diseases	Low-salt or low-sodium
Failure of absorption	Pancreatic disease, gall bladder disease	Low-fat and medium chain triglyceride
Reduced glucose tolerance	Diabetes mellitus	Control energy, low-fat, high-carbohydrate
Villous atrophy	Celiac disease	Gluten-free

Source: Ref. 9.

labeling, advertising, and any claims made for the product. The follow-on foods that are formulated to complement weaning foods also have strict compositional standards and purity criteria.

The infant formula foods available include milk and soya-protein based products as dry powders to be reconstituted with water, or in a liquid, ready-to-feed form. These may contain only lactose as a carbohydrate source or may be lactose free. Other claims may be made for adapted-protein, low-sodium, added-iron, and sucrose-free formulas.

Babies are usually weaned between 4 and 6 months of their age, as their feeding behavior progresses from sucking to biting and chewing. An EEC working party draft directive proposes dividing weaning foods into two categories for setting compositional standards. These reflect the types of foods that are currently available in the EEC market and include the following:

1. Processed cereal-based products which are subdivided into simple cereals, cereals with an added high-protein food, pasta, and rusks and biscuits.
2. Baby foods which are primarily intended for use during the usual infant weaning period and for progressive adaptation of infants and young children to ordinary food. Baby foods constitute a diverse group of food products, comprising complete or incomplete meals, soups, desserts, puddings, vegetable juices, fruit juices, and nectars, presented either as ready to use in jars or cans, or in a dried form, requiring reconstitution.

Baby foods are formulated to meet the particular needs of infants at different stages of weaning. Those recommended for early introduction are of smooth texture and bland flavor, more or less similar to milk. As weaning progresses, stronger and more varied flavors with a wider range of textures to encourage chewing are available. Strict in-house compositional standards of these foods are imposed. Babies are not exposed to unsuitable levels of sodium or refined sugars, and they should receive a balanced diet with respect to vitamin and mineral content. In addition, the microbiological standards set are also very high.

The European Commission intends to detail compositional standards with respect to protein, carbohydrate, fat, and some vitamins and minerals, as well as labeling standards.

C. Medical/Functional Foods

According to Stephen (15), the increasing interest in natural products seen since the late 1980s will undoubtedly continue to grow in the next century. The recognition by consumers that they must take some responsibility for their own health has led to the explosion of interest in functional foods, nutraceuticals, dietary supplements, herbal products, and botanicals. Along with consumer interest, the food and pharmaceutical industries also have seen an enormous market potential for these health products. However, the health of consumers depends on such products being safe and having the effects they are said to have. Health agencies within governments must ensure that population is not put at risk by the sale of unsafe products or the promotion of products for actions they do not have. Consumers should not self-diagnose their illness or make decisions about medication for existing conditions without consulting health professionals. Those who are developing and promoting health products must be responsible for the health claims of their products in relation to health and disease. Because this is often not the case, government agencies have been compelled to institute regulations that limit what can and cannot be said on packaging and in advertising. There is a need for dialogue between manufacturers and government health agencies so that the potential benefit of new products and new scientific findings can be promoted to improve the health of the population, while at the same time limiting the sale and promotion of unsafe products and those making inappropriate claims. Most countries are working to create an environment of collaboration, drawing on each other's experience to develop workable regulations. Stephen (15) envisages that by the beginning of the new century, the confusion that currently surrounds the regulation of natural health products will be diminished.

1. Nutritionally Complete or Incomplete Foods

The unique nutritional requirements for certain specific medical conditions have resulted in the formulation of foods either by specialized industries or within the hospitals in consultation with medical profession. There are two distinct types recognized:

1. Enteral nutrition in which foods are administered through the gastrointestinal (G.I.) tract, either orally or by means of a tube into the stomach or intestine, and,
2. Parenteral nutrition in which foods are administered intravenously. This is used to provide nutritional support in situations where enteral feeding is not possible, e.g., when the G.I. tract is unable to absorb nutrients, or complete bowel rest is required. It is more expensive and complicated than enteral feeding and requires skill and equipment to administer. Enteral nutrition may be adopted with benefits in the following cases:

    a. Patients who have an intact G.I. tract but who are not able to maintain a satisfactory nutritional status on a normal diet. This may include postoperative patients, those with central nervous system or psychiatric disorders, burns or stroke victims, and comatose patients,
    b. Patients with a disease or abnormality of the G.I. tract that impedes digestion and absorption of nutrients.
    c. Patients with limited oral access to the G.I. tract, as the result of facial or esophageal injuries, diseases, or obstruction of the upper G.I. tract,
    d. Persons having specific nutritional requirements either because of an inborn metabolic disorder such as phenylketonuria (disorder of phenylalanine metabolism), or because of individual organ failures.

The medical foods recommended by the medical profession are often categorized into two classes: nutritionally complete foods and nutritionally incomplete foods. The nutritionally complete foods are generally available either in powder or ready-to use liquid forms. These may be general purpose formulas manufactured from common food ingredients or defined formulas manufactured from more specialized ingredients; e.g., proteins may be hydrolyzed to various degrees to reduce their chain length and aid digestibility, or simple sugars may replace complex carbohydrates. Conversely, the nutritionally incomplete foods may be modules or supplemental formulas, often in the form of a single source of a particular nutrient (protein, fat, or carbohydrate), used to supplement the patient's diet when specialized nutritional needs are recognized by the health care professional. These food products also may be formulated for specific metabolic conditions or diseases, or for the patients with specific organ failure or nutritional requirements. These are not nutritionally complete for the general population but are often appropriately balanced for the specific medical situation of the patient.

In addition to patients receiving complete nutritional formulas under medical supervision, there are groups of otherwise healthy persons who may temporarily lose the desire to eat regular foods, e.g. the elderly or those convalescing from minor illness. These people may use nutritionally complete foods that are freely available in markets.

Subhan et al. (16) reported that citrus fruits containing 50 mg of ascorbic acid per 100 g fresh fruit were used in 207 patients to enhance male fertility potential by eliminating sperm agglutination in 183 (88.4%) patients. It was postulated that a continuous use of citrus fruits can improve the state of human male fertility.

Steiner et al. (17) in a double-blind crossover study with a group of moderately hypercholesterolemic (220–290 mg/dl) men gave 7.2 g of aged garlic (*Alluim sativum*) extract (AGE) in divided doses or an equal number of placebos for 4 to 6 months. The total and LDL cholesterol showed a significant reduction compared to baseline, as well as to placebo; HDL cholesterol and triglyceride levels were unaffected. The aggregation of platelets was decreased, but the degree of inhibition varied with the inducer. AGE also decreased systolic blood pressure. Thus, AGE effectively decreased several of the risk factors responsible for thromboembolic diseases of heart and brain. The results suggested that AGE is a very convenient dietary supplement to lessen the risk of thromboembolic disease in susceptible individuals.

Krishnaswamy (18) described turmeric (*Curcuma longa*) as a functional food with a broad spectrum of action as an anti-initiator and antipromoter of cancer. The amount of turmeric required to prevent cancer appears to be well within cultural norms and safety limits. Toxicological studies on turmeric conducted in India in several animal experiments (rats, monkeys, guinea pigs, and rabbits) have shown that curcumin taken orally in doses of 40 to 1800 mg/day for periods ranging from 1 to 3 months was free from toxic side effects (19) and growth, behavioral, biochemical, and histopathological indexes were essentially normal (20). Extrapolated doses from studies of mutagenicity and the formation of carcinogen DNA adducts were also within safe limits. Turmeric in daily amounts of 0.5 to 1.0 g can be consumed without any adverse effects (21), whereas population surveys indicate that consumption of spices in general ranges from 10 to 30 g/day (22).

2. *Low-Sodium Foods*

Processed foods with a low, or reduced sodium content were originally developed for patients with kidney disorders, hypertension, and other disease conditions requiring reduced sodium intake. Experiments have shown that the average salt intake is about 10 times that required for physiological needs to maintain optimum muscle and nerve activity and normal blood pressure. Sodium chloride has been traditionally used as a food preserving agent and as flavor enhancer. The latter property, which increases food palatability, can also be achieved by using sodium-free salt substitutes, herbs, and spices. The EEC draft directive has recommended two categories of low-sodium foods:

1. Very-low sodium foods in which the sodium content should not exceed 40 mg per 100 g or 100 ml in the ready-to-eat product, and
2. Low-sodium foods in which the sodium content should not exceed 120 mg per 100 g or 100 ml of the ready-to-eat product.

The directive has also listed salt substitutes with maximum addition levels where applicable, and these must be given on the food label.

3. Diabetic Foods

In a healthy person, the blood glucose level rises immediately after meals and returns to a fasting level at about 0.8 g per liter of blood at the end of the postprandial period. In an untreated diabetic person, blood glucose level remains chronically higher than normal.

In cases of low or no insulin secretion or insulin-dependent diabetes, patients are under medical supervision aimed at controlling insulin supply, so that the diet is not a major concern as long as carbohydrates are supplied at a regular level. Another type of diabetes is characterized by normal or exaggerated secretion of insulin, accompanied by a resistance of tissues to insulin that is controlled by the diet and not by insulin. Foods formulated for persons with this type of diabetes allow them to receive a normal daily supply of carbohydrates (50–60% of the energy intake) which requires as little insulin as possible in order to limit the effects of insulin in sufficiency.

EEC directive has discussed the following two options on nutritional requirements and compositional standards for diabetic foods.

1. Controlling carbohydrate to limit the addition of D-glucose, invert sugar, disaccharides, maltodextrins, or glucose syrup to 6% in ready-to-use products, and only if needed for technical reasons or if from natural sources.
2. Declaring glycemic index to allow the consumer to evaluate the effects of a food on the blood glucose level in comparison to a reference product to quality; the glycemic index of the food must be reduced by one-third in comparison to that of the corresponding normal food, with at least 20% of the energy provided by carbohydrates.

For both the above options, the total energy and fat content should not be more than those of comparable normal foods. The wide choice in this regard includes confectionery, bakery products, dairy products, desserts and puddings, fruit juices, soft drinks and beer, sauces and salad dressings, sweeteners and tablets and pills rich in soluble fiber for diet supplementation.

The EEC has considered including food suplements in the group of generally recognized dietetic foods, provided that these are not marketed with a medical claim and are thus convered by the normal pharmaceutical product legislation, e.g. single vitamin and mineral supplements, multivitamin and/or mineral supplements.

To support the diverse needs of the diabetic food industry, many raw material suppliers manufacture certain speical ingredients that include basic nutrients such as single minerals, vitamins, amino acids, fatty acids, and sugars, as well as specially treated food ingredients. The latter group may consist of proteins, hydrolyzed to varying degrees to aid digestibility or reduce allergenicity; or products tailored to a specific amino acid profile; tailored fats with a specific fatty acid profile, with a balanced blend of fats, a special fraction such as medium-chain triglycerides, or randomized or co-randomized at blend; and carbohydrates, which may be simple or complex oligosaccharides and may or may not be partially hydrolyzed.

The formulation of diabetic foods also needs special technological processing and use of additives as process aids, thickening and emulsifying agents, stabilizers, and so on to improve the shelf-life and palatability of the diabetic foods (9).

Upadhyaya et al. (23) made a detailed survey of different regions of India to find antidiabetic plants used in folklore and by tribal people. A literature survey on these plants was undertaken for their distribution, chemical composition, and uses. Clinical study was conducted on potent hypoglycemic plants. It was found that *Pterocarpus marsupium* and *Monmordica charan-*

tia are useful for treating non-obese diabetics, while *Saussurea ilappa* and *Eugenia jambolana* have been most effective for obese diabetics.

4. Gluten-Free Foods

Gluten-free foods are needed for the dietary management of people with celiac disease in which the causative agent is the gluten of cereals such as wheat, rye, barley, and oats. Most symptoms result from malabsorption of nutrients from the intestine caused by damage to the cell wall. The sufferers of celiac disease need to avoid all foods containing cereals, and in order to maintain dietary choice, they require reliable gluten-free raw materials. The food industry is particularly suited to manufacture foods for gluten-free diets, which are substitutes for cereal-based foods, utilizing rice and corn flour. Vitamins and minerals are often added to the equivalent level with regard to the foods they replace. The food products available include bakery products and raw materials for baking, and pasta as well as foods that are naturally free from gluten. Freedom from gluten is also a requirement for infant foods; some manufacturers provide gluten-free foods even for babies and young children.

For the purpose of labeling, "gluten-free" means that the total nitrogen content of the gluten-containing cereal grain ingredient does not exceed 0.05% (i.e., 0.3% protein) of the food product. A food may be labeled "gluten-free by nature" to indicate that it is naturally free from gluten and is suitable for use in a gluten-free diet.

5. Slimming Foods

A range of slimming foods available on the market include the following types:

1. Portion control foods for which the manufacturer calculates and declares the energy content of a complete food as a convenience to the consumer.
2. Energy-reduced foods, with a maximum of 25% energy reduction of the normal food, or low-calorie foods, with a maximum of 50 kcal (210kJ) per 100g or 100 ml of product.
3. Products with a sole source of nutrition, classified as very-low-calorie diets (VLCD) at 400–800 kcal (1680–3360 kJ) per day, and low-calorie diet (LCD), containing 800–1200 kcal (3360–5040 kJ) per day. Complete diets below 400 kcal per day are not classified as foodstuffs, and may be taken only under strict medical supervision.

Enegy-reduced or low-energy foods should be nutritionally equivalent in terms of vitamins and minerals to "normal" food. The proposed compositional standards for LCDs are as follows:

1. Proteins, minimum 20–50g at 100% of the WHO/FAO quality reference.
2. Lipids, maximum 30% of total energy.
3. Linolenic acid, minimum 4.5g.
4. Vitamins and minerals, to 100% of the RDA, as detailed in the EEC labling directive.

D. Junk Foods or Junk Diets

The term "junk food" is meaningless to nutritionists, because there is no food that is totally worthless, anymore than there is a perfect food that meets all nutritional needs. Obviously, some foods contribute more nutrients than do others, but almost any food has some redeeming value under the right circumstances. The problem arises when foods that contribute more calories than nutrients become so important in one's diet that foods of higher nutrient(s) value are excluded. It is equally possible to make an unbalanced selection from among the most sacred nutritious foods (e.g., milk and apples) and wind up with a diet overabundant in some nutrients yet deficient in others. In both cases, the result can be labled junk food.

In terms of nutrient density—roughly defined as the nutrients derived per kcalorie—foods with low values seldom carry much nutritional weight, e.g. most calories in some cakes and cookies come from fat and sugar and relatively few from nutrient-rich milk, flour, and eggs. However, if eating a cookie means that a child also drinks milk or fruit juice, then cookie and milk or cookie-and-beverage can be considered a unit, judging them together, rather than condemning one and applauding the other. While for an 8-year-old, milk and one or two cookies makes a nutritious combination, milk and 5 cookies may create an imbalance between calories and nutrients—and thus must be considered lower in nutrition. Similarly, potato chips can form a valuable food in the right context. Eaten alone, potato chips have insufficient vitamin C, pyridoxine, and copper to make them a meaningful source. Eaten with a sandwich, potato chips become part of a balanced diet, but if one eats so many potato chips that one is too full to eat dinner, then they are being misused. Pizza is frequently seen as a junk food, high in calories, cholesterol, and fat, but with essentially the same ingredients, pizza has nutritional merits comparable to a meat-and-cheese sandwich served with tomato, providing valuable amounts of protein, calcium, iron, and many vitamins.

Even the classic health foods such as milk, chicken, orange juice, and oatmeal are not always desirable. Non-fat milk has an impressive nutrient profile, but it is not perfect. Although high in calcium, protein, and riboflavin, it is low in iron and vitamin C. In contrast, oranges are high in iron and vitamin C, but low in calcium, protein, and riboflavin.

When a food does not meet an immediate nutritional need, its nutritional value becomes limited. Extra milk (lacking in vitamin C) that displaces a fruit juice (rich in vitamin C) would be "junk" food. So foods cannot be judged in isolation, but in relation to the total diet and the individual's needs. Thus, if the daily nutrient needs are met, except for calories, technically one can obtain the rest of the calories from any food. In selecting food, moderation is a virtue, and so is avoidance of excess amount of fat, sodium, and calories, all of which are essential in controlled amounts. In choosing nutrious foods, cost per nutrient is also important. Special medical consideration aside, a healthful diet can include at least small amounts of any food one enjoys as long as his/her overall diet is moderate in calories and balanced to provide essential nutrients.

E. Sports Foods (for Intense Performance)

Sportspersons and athletes have special nutritional requirements beyond those adequate for normal levels of activity to maintain enhanced physical fitness, coupled with intense physical performance, and stresses that such activity places on the body. Initially food products were designed for body building and weight training, but with an appreciation for different needs for the nature of the sport, food products have been formulated for activities such as track and field athletics.

The EEC legislation has classified sports foods as follows:

1. Food products specially formulated to supply energy, with an emphasis being placed on the type and amount of the carbohydrate used, which has a significant effect on the storage and utilization of glycogen in the body. These products are also required to supply other energy-producing nutrients, such as fat and protein in the appropriate ratio. In addition to direct meal replacements, supplements are also available as carbohydrate concentrates, sold in powder form, often with added vitamins and minerals, energy bars, and instant-energy drinks.

2. Food products, tablets, capsules, and hydration beverages with a defined content of minerals, trace elements, vitamins, and other nutrients or their combination, to support physiological performance.

3. Food products with a defined content of protein and/or amino acids, especially formulated for intense muscular effort, which include high-protein powders, concentrates, protein-enriched foods such as bars, muesli, or special beverages, and single or multiple amino acid supplements available in tablet or capsule form.
4. A combination of the products described above.

IV. ROLE OF NUTRITION IN DISEASE RESISTANCE AND IMMUNE FUNCTION

Many infectious diseases and cancers exacerbate nutritional stresses. Cancer, trauma, and infectious diseases can alter intakes and requirements for different nutrients, e.g., hyperalimentation or renutrition is being accepted in nutritional treatment to maintain optimum immune functions of hospitalized adults, including cancer patients. Immune functions are known to be altered by both nutrition and disease.

Supplementary levels of vitamin E, 3 to 6 times over the levels that are considered nutritionally adequate, contribute to the optimal functioning of immune responses and other host defense mechanisms, thereby enhancing humoral immunity and disease resistance (24). It is likely that vitamin E exerts this optimizing effect partially by an antioxidant function, through interference with oxidative metabolism of key cellular regulators, such as prostaglandins, ubiquinones, and vitamin A, and partially by a membrane-stabilizing and regulatory function that facilitates optimal functions and cellular cooperation.

Adlercreutz and Mazur (25) stated that lignans and isoflavonoids are converted by intestinal bacteria to hormone-like compounds that exhibit weak estrogenic activity. The precursors of the biologically active compounds detected in men are found in soybean products, whole-grain cereals, seeds, and berries. These compounds also reduce hot flushes and vaginal dryness in postmenopausal women and may inhibit osteoporosis. Lignans and isoflavonoids may have significant inhibitory role in cancer development. However, no definite recommendations have been made as the dietary amount needed for prevention of diseases. Plants rich in lignans and isoflavonoids are soybeans, oatmeal, carrots, garlic, peanuts, and black and green teas. Among these, flax seeds are the richest source.

Saroja et al (26) tested several food materials such as vegetable flowers (cooked drumstick, neem, onion, plantain), green leafy vegetables (cooked curry leaves, drumstick, fenugeek), fruits (amla, gooseberry, jack fruit, pomegranate) and found that they provided optimum nutrition and protection against cancer. Among beverages (coffee, green tea, black tea), drinking of coffee was linked with cancer of bowel, pancreas, and bladder. Pickled foods should be eaten in small quantities. Thus, by consuming the right kind of protective foods, the risk of cancer can be lowered.

Oku (27) recently classified several newly developed oligosaccharides (sucrose substitutes) with beneficial health effects as follows:

1. Those providing less available energy (about 2 kcal/g) than that produced by sucrose.
2. Those having no effect on insulin secretion from the pancreas—e.g., nondigestible oligosaccharides do not increase blood glucose level.
3. Those improving intestinal microflora. The beneficial bacteria increase and the harmful microbes decrease. As a result, putrefactive products decrease, and the production of carcinogens declines.
4. Those preventing dental caries. *Streptococcus* mutants cannot use nondigestible oligosaccharides, and these oligosaccharides do not produce insoluble glucans.

Oligosaccharides such as Neosugar[R], xylooligosaccharides, soybean oligosaccharides, isomaltooligosaccharides, galactosyl-sucrose, maltitol and palatinose have been reported to improve the colonic environment and prevent dental caries (26).

Delaquis and Mazza (28) have reviewed work on many vegetables, including crucifers and alliums, which contain a variety of biologically active phytochemicals thought to have a role in the prevention of diseases such as cancer. Despite recent advances, however, much remains to be learned about the role of these compounds in human health and disease.

The impact of food handling and processing on nutrients such as vitamins and minerals is well known, although the stability and fate of phytochemicals such as sulfur-containing compounds in processed foods have not been investigated fully. Despite this paucity of data, there is a widespread but unsubstantiated belief that beneficial phytochemicals or bioactive compounds derived from them are depleted by processing, particularly by thermal processing. It is possible to develop, through biotechnological and classical plant breeding methods, new cultivars of Cruciferae, Alliums, and other vegetables with new or elevated levels of beneficial phytochemicals. Many of these compounds are highly odoriferous and many impart undesirable sensory characteristics to the plant. Delaquis and Mazza (28) suggested that current cabbage cultivars are largely the result of early attempts to reduce sulfurous odors in cooked cabbage. Several sulfur-containing compounds have been shown to exert toxic effects at higher concentrations. The dietary contributions of individual vitamins differ significantly among the species of cruciferous vegetables (Table 3). Certain bioactive compounds isolated and characterized for biological activity include (28): allicin (antimicrobial), allin (hypolipidemic, antimicrobial, hypoglycemic); ajoene (antithrombotic); diallyl sulfide (chemopreventive, insecticidal); thiosulfinates (antiinflammatory, antiasthmatic); cepaenes (antiphlogistic, antiasthmatic); saponin (antihyperlipemic); ascor-

Table 3 Water soluble Vitamins in Various Raw and Processed Cole Crops

Source	Vitamin A (RE[a])	Vitamin C (mg)	Thiamin (mg)	Niacin (NE[b])	Riboflavin (mg)
Cabbage, fresh	13.51	56.8	0.06	0.54	0.03
Cabbage, boiled and drained	8.86	24.0	0.06	0.38	0.06
Sauerkraut, canned	2.01	14.9	0.02	0.32	0.02
Cauliflower, fresh	1.9	71.6	0.08	1.06	0.06
Cauliflower, boiled and drained	0.8	51.1	0.06	0.99	0.05
Rutabaga, fresh	0	25.0	0.09	0.95	0.04
Rutabag, boiled and drained	0	21.7	0.07	0.83	0.04
Radish, fresh	Trace	22.2	0.29	0.44	0.04
Turnip, fresh	0	21.2	0.04	0.58	0.03
Turnip, boiled and drained	0	9.1	0.03	0.41	0.02
Broccoli, fresh	154.3	93.4	0.07	1.13	0.12
Broccoli, boiled and fresh	140.8	62.8	0.08	1.28	0.21

[a]Retinol equivalents.
[b]Niacin equivalents.
Source: Ref. 39.

bic acid (antioxidant); caffeic acid (antitumor, antimutogenic, antioxidant, antiviral); linoleic acid (immunomodulation), and S-methyl methane thiosulfonate (antimutogenic). Various disorders for which both garlic and onion have been used include asthma, arthritis, arteriosclerosis, chicken pox, the common cold, diabetes, malaria, tumors, and heart problems (30). Thus, modern science has shown that alliums and their constituents have several therapeutic effects, such as antiplatelet aggregation activity, fibrinolytic activity, anticarcinogenic effects, antimicrobial activity, and anti-inflammatory and antiasthmatic efects (30–33). However, further research is needed on the physiological properties, stability, and safety of these seemingly beneficial phytochemicals occurring in vegetables, fruits, and other plant products. Meydani (34) has recently pointed out that among the nutrients, marine-derived (n-3) PUFA and vitamin E, at present, appear to be the most prominent nutrients with positive effects on the reduction of risk of cardiovascular disease. This conclusion has been mainly derived from compelling evidence that has emerged from epidemiologic, clinical, and experimental studies linking the observed beneficial effects of the nutrients to their mechanisms of action at tissue, cellular, and molecular levels.

Newmann (35) has presented recommendations at a conference on "Nutrition and Immunity." Increasing interest among researchers in understanding the complex relationships between nutrition, immunity, and health has led to several studies on the influence of diet and nutrition on immunity and the relationship of both to health. There is a need to examine the effects of various nutrients on the specific immune response, especially on responses to pathogens. The question of whether and how essential nutrients change with age, and identification of possible age-related optimal nutrient intake requirements that correlate with effective immunological function, and whether nutrient intake modulation can alter the pathogenesis of disease need to be resolved.

Woodware (36) reviewed the influence of dietary protein and energy on immune defenses, and pointed out that immunologic influences of dietary protein and energy must be understood as components of a larger, systemic attempt to adapt to diet or to dietary change. According to Hoffman-Goetz (37), the significance of exercise and physical activity–associated changes in innate immunity in modifying disease risk, pathogenesis, and outcome has become the subject of active research. Physical activity and aerobic exercise are associated with a transient increase, followed by a decrease in natural killer (NK) cell number and activity. Chronic exercise or training enhances innate immune functions in athletes sampled at rest. The majority of studies have shown that moderate exercise augments the activity and number of NK cells. The clinical relevance of these in innate immunity is not known, though animal data suggest a protective role in tumor metastases (37). Fernandes and Jolly (38) have recently reviewed the influence of nutrition on autoimmune diseases and disorders in human and animal models.

Recent advances in understanding the effects of nutritional stresses on immune development have led to increasing use of immunological measures to assess nutritional status. Although this is often applied to identify severe or moderate deficiency problems, adequacy of immune function can help to determine optimal diet. Also, chemoprevention of cancers is being studied with intakes well above the RDAs for vitamins A, C, and E. Such high intakes of vitamins are not related to well-characterized deficiency diseases but instead are based on observations of improved immune function and cancer resistance with intakes that are currently accepted as very high. Thus, the broad potential effects of nutrition offer readily available tools to manipulate immune function and hence, health and longevity (29).

REFERENCES

1. Allen, B. (ed.), *Food*: An Oxford Anthology, Oxford University Press, Oxford, New York, 1994, p. 1.
2. Ramarathnam, N., T. Osawa, H. Ochi, and S. Kawakishi, The contribution of plant food antioxidants to human health, *Trends Food Sci. Technol. 6*: 75 (1995).

3. Hilliam, M., Functional foods: The Western consumer view point, *Nutr. Rev. 54*: (S): 189 (1996).

4. Ohigashi, H., A. Murakami, and K. Koshimizu, An approach to functional food: cancer preventive potential of vegetable and fruits and their active constituents, *Nutr. Rev. 54*: 524 (1996).

5. Macrae, R., P.K. Robinson, and M.J. Sadler (eds.), *Encyclopaedia of Food Science and Technology and Nutrition*, Vol. 4, Academic Press, London, 1993a, p. 2293.

6. Liberti, L.E., and A. der Marderosia, Evaluation of commercial ginseng products, *J. Pharmaceut. Sci. 67*: 1487 (1978).

7. Van Houwelingen, R., H. Zevenbergen, P., Groot, S. Kester and G. Hornstra, Dietary fish effects on serum lipids and apolipo proteins, a controlled study, *Am. J. Clin. Nutr. 51*: 393 (1990).

8. Harris, W.S., Fish oils and plasma lipid and lipoprotein metabolism in humans: a critical review, *J. Lipid Res. 30*: 785 (1989).

9. Macrae, R.P.K. Robinson, and M.J. Sadler (eds.), *Encyclopaedia of Food Science and Technology and Nutrition*, Vol. 2, Academic Press, London, 1993b, p. 1412.

10. CAC, joint FAO/WHO Food Standards, Programme, Infant, formula, CAC 72, 1981. Canned Baby Foods 1981, Processed Cereal Based Foods, CAC 118, 1981, Foods With Low Sodium Content, CAC 53, 1981, FAO/WHO, 1981.

11. CAC, Labelling of and Claims for Pre-packaged Foods for Special Dietary Uses, CAC 146, FAO/WHO, 1985.

12. CAC, Follow-up formula, CAC, 156, 1987, *Codex Alimentarius Commission*, Food and Agriculture Organization, Rome, World Health Organization, Geneva, 1987.

13. CFR, Code of Federal Regulations (Parts 100–169), Office of the Federal Register of National Archives and Records Administration, Washington, DC, 1990.

14. EEC Council, Directive on the Approximation of the Laws of Member States Relating to Foodstuffs Intended for Particular Nutritional Uses, *Official J. Eur. Communities*. 50: (127, 186) 1989.

15. Stephen, A.M., Regulatory aspects of functional products, *Functional Foods: Biochemical and Processing Aspects* (G. Mazza, ed.), Technomic Publishing Co., Lancaster, 1998, p. 403.

16. Subhan, F., F. Tahir, W. Alam, and I. Fayyaz, Enhancement of male fertility potential through citrus fruits, *Hamdard Medicus 40*: 53 (1997).

17. Steiner, M., A.H. Khan, D. Holbert, and R.I. Lin, A double blind crossover study in moderately hypercholesteremic men comparing the effect of aged garlic extract and placebo administration on blood lipids and platelet function, *Phytomedicine 3*: 141 (1997).

18. Krishnaswamy, K., Indian functional foods: Role in prevention of cancer, *Nutr. Rev. 54* (S): 127 (1996).

19. CDRI, Report on the toxicity state of curcumin, Central Drug Research Institute, Lucknow, India, 1977.

20. NTP, Toxicology and carcinogenesis studies of turmeric oleoresin, CAS No. 8024-37-1, National Toxicology Program, National Institutes of Health, Bethesda, MD, 1993. NIH Pub. No. 93-3158, Tech.Rep. Ser. No. 427, 1993.

21. Krishnaswamy, K., Antimutagens and anticarcinogens in Indian diets, *Recent Trends in Nutrition* (C. Gopalan, ed.), Oxford University Press, New Delhi, (1993), p. 125.

22. NNMB, Annual Diet and Nutrition Survey Report, 1991–92, National Nutrition Monitoring Bureau, Indian Council of Medical Research, Hyderabad, India, 1993.

23. Upadhyay, O.P., R.H. Singh, and S.K. Dutta, Studies on antidiabetic medicinal plants used in Indian folk-lore, *Sachitra Ayurveda 48*: 949 (1996).

24. Tengerdy, R.P., M.M. Methias, and C.E. Nokels, Vitamin E, immunity and disease resistance, *Diet and Resistance to Disease: Advances in Experimental Medicine and Biology*, Vol. 135 (M.Phillips and A. Baetz, eds.), Plenum Press, New York, 1981, p. 27.

25. Aldercreutz, H., and W. Mazur, Phytoestrogens and Western diseases, *Ann. Med. 29*: 95 (1997).

26. Saroja, S., A. Jayasree, and S. Annapurani, Screening of foods for the presence of mutagens, co-mutagens and anti-mutagens, *Indian J. Nutr. Diet. 32*: 165 (1995).

27. Oku, T., Oligosaccharides with beneficial health effects: A Japanese perspective, *Nutr. Rev. 54* (S): 59 (1996).

28. Delaquis, P., G. Mazza, Functional vegetable products, *Functional Foods: Biochemical and Processing Aspects* (G. Mazza, ed.), Technomic Publishing Co., Lancaster, 1998, p. 193.

29. Watson, R.R. (ed.), *Nutrition, Disease Resistance and Immune Function*, Marcel Dekker, New York, 1984.
30. Fenwick G.R., and A.B. Hanley, The genus Allium Part 1, *CRC Crit. Rev. Food Sci. Nutr. 22*: 199 (1985).
31. Block, E., The chemistry of garlic and onions, *Sci. Am. 252*: 111 (1985).
32. Hanley, A.B., and G.R. Fenwick, Cultivated alliums, *J. Plant Foods 6*: 211 (1985).
33. Breu, W., and W. Dorsch, Allium cepa L. (onion): Chemistry, analysis and pharmacology, *Econ. Med. Plant. Res. 6*: 116 (1994).
34. Meydani, M., Nutrition, immune cells and atherosclerosis, *Nutr. Rev. 56* (IIS): 177, 1998.
35. Neumann, D.A., Nutrition and immunity: Conference recommendations, *Nutr. Rev. 56* (IIS): 183, 1998.
36. Woodward, B., Protein calories and immune defenses, *Nutr. Rev. 56* (IIS): 84 (1998).
37. Hoffman-Goetz, L., Influence of physical activity and exercise on innate immunity, *Nutr. Rev. 56* (IIS): 126 (1998).
38. Fernandes G., and C.A. Jolly, Nutrition and autoimmune disease, *Nutr. Rev. 56* (IIS):161 (1998).
39. HWC, Nutrient value of some common foods, *Health and Welfare of Canada*, Canadian Government Publishing Services, Ottawa, 1988.

10
Foods of Plant Origin

I. INTRODUCTION

Sunlight is the ultimate source of energy for all living organisms, which derive their energy, directly or indirectly, from the radiant energy of the sun arising from the thermonuclear fusion reactions. Plants evolved as photosynthetic organisms, absorbing the sun's radiant energy and using it to drive electrons from water to carbon dioxide, thus forming energy-rich carbon compounds such as sucrose, starches, and cellulose. The molecular oxygen released by the photosynthetic organisms into the early atmosphere has paved the way for the existence of non-photosynthetic organisms, which in turn depend on plants as the source of energy. The latter obtain their energy needs by oxidizing the energy-rich carbon compounds of photosynthesis, by passing electrons to atmospheric oxygen to form water, carbon dioxide and other end products. Plants are thus the forerunners of energy source for most heterotrophs.

Cereals, pulses, oilseeds, fruits, nuts, vegetables, sugar crops, and spices form the major categories of foods originating from the plant world. Although humankind has developed a range of crop plants to meet the demand for food, considering the long history of domestication, the number of crop species involved is rather limited. Over 80% of the edible dry weight of food is derived from only eleven crop species, two-thirds of which are cereals (1). Even though only a few species of cereals predominate, several others play an important role in sustaining human life. Pulses (legumes) provide nearly a quarter of the world's dietary protein requirements, and over 50% in the developing countries. Though pulses have traditionally been described as poor man's meat, the ever-increasing costs and unfavorable energy balance of animal food production may well force us to place a greater reliance on these plants in the times ahead. Potatoes do not occupy a large proportion of the total cultivated area of the world, yet their productivity per unit area is very high. Fruits and vegetables enrich and improve our diet both esthetically and nutritionally. Several other crops do not serve as food directly, but find their way into our diet after processing; e.g., sugar cane and sugar beet provide sweeteners, oil seed crops such as peanut, sunflower, and soybean yield oils and fats. Crops such as barleys, potatoes, grapes, spices, and condiments constitute an important place in the human diet.

A. Plant Foods Are Vital to Human Survival

On a global basis, over 65% of food protein and more than 80% of food energy is derived from plants. In terms of gross tonnage, around 98% of the total world food production is harvested from land sources and only 2% from the ocean and inland waters (Table 1) (2–4). Again, of the total world food harvest, plant products contribute more than 82% of the gross tonnage, whereas animal and marine products together contribute only 17% (2). According to Deshpande and

Table 1 World Food Production, 1994

Source	Production (MMT)	Proportion[a] (% grand total)
Land		
Total cereals	1950	42.3
Wheat	528	
Rice	535	
Maize	570	
Barley	161	
Other	156	
Total root crops	583	13.8
Potatoes	265	
Other	318	
Total pulses	58	1.3
Vegetables and melons	485	10.3
Total fruits	388	8.0
Total nuts	4.6	0.1
Oil crops (oil equiv.)	88	1.6
Sugar	110	2.5
Coffee, tea, cocoa	10.6	0.2
Meat	195	4.0
Milk	527	12.7
Eggs	39	0.8
Total food from land	4438.2	97.8
Water		
Total catch from ocean and inland waters[a]	93	2.2
Total food from land and waters	4531.2	100.0

[a]*Sources*: Refs. 2 through 4.

Damodaran (5), the average production of plant protein potentially edible by humans has been estimated to be 196.8 million metric tons (MMT), compared to 49.1 MMT of animal protein.

Of about 350,000 plant species documented in the annals of botany and plant sciences, only 3000 plant species have been utilized to feed human beings (6). Approximately 150 different plant species are being grown in sufficient quantities to have entered world trade. Human population primarily depends upon the following 24 (in approximate order of importance) plant crops (1): rice, wheat, maize, potato, barley, sweet potato, cassava, soybean, oats, sorghum, millets, sugarcane, sugar beet, rye, peanut, field bean, chick-pea; pigeon pea, mung bean, cowpea, broad bean, yam, banana, and coconut. Of these, cereal grains constitute the largest and the most important single group of foods (Table 1). Owing to their high-yielding ability, cereals are expected to play a more dominant role in the total world food supply in years to come.

The world food production is partially offset by severe problems of wastage (Table 2) (7). These food losses occur throughout production, harvesting, threshing, drying, storage, processing, marketing, and distribution. Under the best possible circumstances of human management, global crop losses have been estimated to be over 2 MMT, representing over 140 billion U.S. dollars; the potential for such losses is even greater. Insect pests, deceases, and weeds (biotic factors) alone account for about 70% of these food losses. According to Salunkhe and Desphande (1), the magnitude of food losses (Table 2) would be even greater if we consider all other losses currently

Table 2 Annual World Crop Losses

Commodity	Tonnage (value)[a]		Crop loss cause			
	Actual	Potential	Insects	Disease	Weeds	Total
Cereals	161.1	1467.5	203.7	135.3	167.4	506.4
	(63.9)	(98.0)	(14.4)	(8.7)	(11.0)	(34.1)
Potatoes	270.8	400.00	23.8	88.9	16.5	129.2
	(10.6)	(15.6)	(1.0)	(3.4)	(0.6)	(5.0)
Sugarcane/sugarbeet	694.6	1330.4	228.4	232.3	175.1	635.8
	(7.6)	(13.9)	(2.3)	(2.3)	(1.7)	(6.8)
Vegetables	207.7	279.9	23.4	31.3	23.7	78.2
	(16.7)	(23.1)	(2.0)	(2.3)	(2.0)	(6.3)
Fruits	141.7	197.2	11.3	32.6	11.6	55.5
	(14.3)	(20.1)	(1.2)	(3.3)	(1.2)	(5.7)
Stimulants	10.2	16.5	1.9	2.6	1.8	6.3
	(7.2)	(11.4)	(1.3)	(1.7)	(1.2)	(4.2)
Oils	94.7	137.0	14.5	13.5	14.3	42.3
	(10.6)	(15.7)	(1.8)	(1.6)	(1.7)	(5.1)
Fibers and rubber	18.3	26.2	3.1	3.1	1.7	7.9
	(8.6)	(12.7)	(1.8)	(1.5)	(0.8)	(4.1)
All crops	2393.1	3854.7	510.1	539.6	412.1	1461.6
	(139.7)	(210.5)	(25.8)	(24.8)	(20.2)	(70.8)

[a]Tonnage in million metric tons (MMT), value in 10^9 U.S. dollars (in parenthesis).
Source: Ref. 7.

occurring in agriculture and the food system that will have long-term ramifications on our global food supply (7).

Improved pre- and postharvest technologies can increase the global food supplies by at least 30% to 40%, without bringing any additional area under cultivation or incurring expensive inputs on various intensive crop-management practices (8–13). Thus, loss-prevention technology should receive at least as much attention as increasing production. Four major plant food groups—viz., cereals, legumes, fruits and vegetables, and sugar crops, which make sizable contributions to the caloric and protein intake of humans—have been dealt with in detail by Salunkhe and Deshpande (1), who describe the major problems in the global food production system, the crop production technology, options and methods for processing individual food groups, their modes of utilization, and nutritional contributions to the human diet.

II. CEREALS

The human race depends for its food almost wholly on cereal grains. In most of the developing countries of the world in Asia, Africa, and Latin America, rice, maize (corn), and sorghum have been recognized as the staple foods on whose yields famine or feast depends. Cereals provide more than two-thirds of the dietary calories to the population of these countries. Even among the developed countries, there are many (e.g., Russia and Japan) in which cereals still provide more than half the dietary calories. Although cereals make a smaller direct contribution to the diet of people in such developed countries as the United States and Canada, total use per person is extremely high; however, most of the cereal grain is fed to livestock and becomes an indirect component of human diets (14).

A. Production and Distribution

The world production of cereals over the past 3 to 4 decades has increased more rapidly than the world population, the increase in yield per unit area having contributed much more than the increase in the area under cereal crops (2). This is particularly so in the developed countries. In the less developed countries, however, rather smaller increases in grain production have been due about equally to increases in yield and area.

The world average yield of cereal grains is approximately 2.5 metric tons per hectare (MT/ha) which is 2 to 3 times greater than that of legume crops and oilseeds. Because of their higher yielding ability and greater economic returns, especially under subsistence farming, cereals are displacing pulses and oilseeds in many developing countries, even though they complement one another both agronomically and nutritionally. Because the rate of increase in yield, on a global scale, is much greater in the major cereals than in the food legumes, cereals are becoming a progressively more predominant component of the total world food supply.

Frey (15) divided the total world cereal production roughly into four groups: The first three are wheat, rice, and maize; the fourth includes barley, oats, rye, sorghum, buckwheat, and various millets. The world cereal production in the recent past has shown variable trends (Table 3). The total production increased up to 1986 and then decreased slightly during 1987–88. In 1988, although rice production in the tropics increased, production of wheat, barley, and other coarse grains declined. This could be attributed to a decrease in cereal production in the United States of America and Canada, the two largest cereal-producing countries having recently experienced drought conditions (Table 4). However, there was a substantial increase in the production of maize, wheat, rice, and barley from 1960 to 1980, varying from a 75% increase in rice production to 92% for barley (15). Sorghum and millet production in Africa and Asia also increased nearly by 66% and 100%, respectively; there was a spectacular sixfold increase in millet production in the Latin America. The total cereal grain production was around 1800 MMT during 1986–88. The average yield for 1961–79 was highest for maize, followed by rice, barley, wheat, rye, oats, sorghum, and millets. The yield trend of cereals varies considerably depending on the cultivars and the year of introduction of the crop; e.g., barley cultivars showed a large variation in grain yield from 1960 to 1980 (Table 5) (16).

Table 3 Global Production Trends of Cereals, Coarse Grains, Pulses and Oil Crops (MMT), 1989–1994

Crops	1989	1990	1991	1992	1993	1994
Total cereals	1868.8	1946.6	1876.3	1960.2	1891.6	1950.6
Wheat	538.3	592.6	546.8	564.8	564.0	528.0
Rice (paddy)	515.5	519.5	517.3	526.6	527.1	534.7
Coarse grains	815.0	834.6	812.2	868.7	800.4	887.9
Maize	473.0	477.1	488.0	528.0	470.3	569.6
Barley	164.0	177.6	168.2	164.6	169.1	160.8
Total pulses	54.1	57.8	56.0	54.3	57.1	58.6
Oil crops						
Oil equiv.	72.3	75.7	77.4	78.7	79.7	87.7
Cake equiv.	144.0	149.0	148.7	153.8	153.3	176.7

Source: Ref. 4.

Table 4 Production of Total Cereals in Different Regions of the World

Region	Production (10^6 MT)		
	1979–81	1988	% Change
World	1590.3	1743.0	+9.6
Africa	72.6	89.2	+22.9
North America	369.5	269.3	−27.1
United States of America	301.3	206.5	−31.5
South America	66.8	80.2	+20.0
Asia	640.0	797.2	+24.6
China	286.6	352.3	+22.9
India	138.2	175.6	+27.1
Europe	248.9	296.9	+19.3
Oceania	219.6	230.4	+4.9

Source: Ref. 2.

The United States of America, Canada, Argentina, Australia, New Zealand, South Africa, and Thailand are the major exporters of cereal grains (17), nearly 80% of the total export coming from the United States of America and Canada alone, despite the fact that their share of total world cereal grain production is only around 25%.

The world cereal production is not related geographically to the food needs of the people. Total per capita grain consumption varies from less than 200 kg per year in Pakistan, Philippines, Indonesia, and Nigeria to over 700 kg in the United States of America. Of the 700 kg consumed per person in the United States, only about 100 kg is consumed directly as bread, pastries, and breakfast foods; the remaining 600 kg is fed to livestock (17). The total world production of the eight major cereals at present would be sufficient to provide around 370 to 390 kg of cereal grains per person per annum, if shared equally among the entire world population. However, the present average human consumption of cereals is only around one-third of this figure. According to Deshpande et al. (14), this is largely due to a major proportion of cereal production being used for purposes other than human food—mainly as animal feed, industrial processing, and seed. In addi-

Table 5 Grain Yield of Some Barley Cultivars Released During 1960–1980, Grown at the Plant Breeding Institute, Cambridge, England

Cultivars	Year of introduction	Grain yield (kg/ha)
Vada	1960	5700
Zephyr	1966	5960
Golden Promise	1966	5510
Julia	1968	6200
Maris Mink	1973	5930
Sundance	1976	6320
Georgie	1976	6300
Ark Royal	1976	6350
Egmont	1980	6930
Koru	1980	6740
Triumph	1980	6680

Source: Ref. 16.

tion, there is considerable wastage of grains during storage, postharvest handling, and processing of cereals.

B. Botany and Origin

The term *cereal* is derived from *Cerealia munera*, meaning the gifts of the goddess Ceres. It is commonly used to refer to the grain itself and to the cultivated grass plants yielding the grain—wheat, rice, maize, barley, oats, sorghum, rye, and millets. All these crops belong to the large monocotyledonous family Gramineae (Fig. 1). Two other species belonging to Gramineae are economically important sources of food: sugarcane (*Saccharum* spp., tribe Andropogoneae), the major source of common sugar, and bamboo (*Arundinaria* spp., tribe Bambuseae), whose young tender shoots are consumed as vegetables in many East and Southeast Asian countries (14).

Certain "pseudocereals" that are botanically different plants are also grouped with the cultivated grasses (cereals) because of their similarity of use. Many of these were perhaps used as human food long before the grasses were successfully cultivated. Some pseudocereals, such as buckwheat, were cultivated in China and by the Native Americans. The true cereals represent the world's most important source of food, and a failure of the major cereals may bring starvation and malnutrition to most parts of the world.

Barring maize, which originated in America, all other cereals are native to the Old World (14). The cultivation of cereal crops, together with the domestication of animals and the invention of pottery, marked the beginning of the Neolithic period (18,19). Table 6 summarizes the chromosome numbers and primary and secondary centers of diversity of the commonly cultivated cereal crops (20,21).

1. Wheat (Triticum *sp.*)

The wild diploid progenitor of wheat occurs throughout the Fertile Cresent of the Middle East, where it was first domesticated about 10,000 years ago, along with barley and some pulses, by selecting nonshattering larger-seeded types. Tetraploid wheats were also developed in this area, at about the same time. Finally the hexaploid bread wheat (2n = 42), *Triticum aestivum. A. squarrosa* was evolved by the hybridization of the tetraploids with *Aegilops squarrosa*, conferring on wheat the protein characteristics required for bread making as well as increased adaptive range (22). Thus, wheat was spread through Central Europe to higher altitudes and more humid regions.

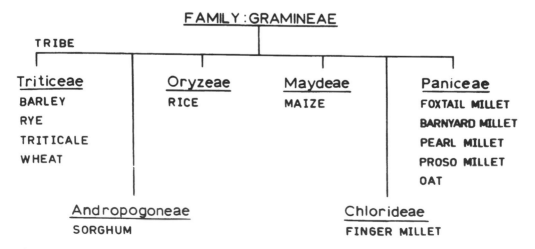

Figure 1   Botanical classification of cereals. (From Ref. 14.)

Table 6 Chromosome Numbers and Centers of Diversity of Commonly Grown Cereal Crops

Cereals	Chromosome	Centers of diversity
Wheat	14	NE
Einkorn	28	NE, ES
Emmer	42	CJ, HI, CE
Bread wheat	42	CJ, HI, CE
Club wheat	42	ES, NE, CE
Rice	24	CJ, II, HI
Wild rice	30	NA
Maize	20	MA, SA, CJ
Barley	14, 28	NE, ME, CJ
Oats	42, 48, 63	ME, NE, CJ
Sorghum	20	CJ, HI, ME
Rye	14–29	CE, NE, CJ
Millets		
Finger millet	36	HI, AF
Italian millet	18	CJ
Pearl millet	14	AF
Proso millet	36, 54, 72	CJ
Triticale	42, 56	NA, ES
Buckwheat	16, 32	NE

[a]The possible center of origin is listed first.

Abbreviations: AF, Africa; CE, Central Asia; CJ, China, Japan; ES, Euro-Siberian; HI, Hindustani (India), II, Indochina, Indonesia; MA, Middle America; ME, Mediterranean; NA, North America; NE, Near East; SA, South America.

Source: Refs. 20 and 21.

The tetraploid wheat *T. durum* grows best in warmer regions and is important source of semolina flour used to make pasta products. The hexaploid wheat *T. aestivum vulgare*, which is the choice wheat for bread making, has most widely spread throughout the world.

From the bakers' point of view, wheat can be classified into hard and soft types, respectively yielding the strong and weak flours (23). The strong flour from hard wheat has a coarse texture and is suitable for bread making, whereas the weak flour from soft wheat has a fine powdery texture and is preferred for cookie manufacture. Various grades of flours can be obtained from different kinds of wheats or by blending strong and weak flours together.

2. Rice (Oryza *sp.*)

Rice (*Oryza* sp.) species and varieties (Tribe Oryzeae, Fig. 1) are the main cereals consumed in Far East and Southeast Asian countries. Rice was grown in China about 5000 years ago and was first brought to Europe by Alexander the Great; its cultivation began in the eighth century A. D. The wild perennial, *Oryza glaberrima*, was domesticated in West Africa; the cultivated annual, *O. sativa*, was developed in Asia (22). It is predominantly a rain-fed crop, the flooded fields of the tropics being its most characteristic environment. Most wild forms and tropical cultivars of rice are short-day plants and exhibit strong photoperiodism.

The commonest rice species, *O. sativa* varieties, are divided into three subspecies: japonica (short-grained), javanica (intermediate types), and indica (long-grained). Japonica species are better adapted to cooler temperatures and longer days than the indica rices.

3.   *Maize* (Zea mays)

Maize (corn) is native to tropical Central America. It is intolerant to both shade and drought. The spikelets of maize are unisexual, forming separate male and female inflorescences on the individual plant. The staminate flowers form the terminal panicle (tassel) and the pistillate flowers on spikelets form the spadix (cob), from which the grains develop.

 Zea mays var. saccharata is the common sweet corn used mostly as "corn on the cob" in the United States. *Zea mays*; var. everta is a special variety from which popcorn is produced. Other varieties of maize include dent corn, *Zea mays*, var. americana, characterized by indentation or depression on the top of the grain, caused by shrinkage of the soft endosperm. This is the typical maize of the American corn belt. Flint corn, *Zea mays*, var. praecox (=indurata), with a hard endosperm and no indentation is normally cultivated in Europe. Flour or soft maize, *Zea mays*, var. amylacea, having no horny endosperm, is grown almost exclusively by Native Americans for their own use. Waxy corn is valuable for its starch (amylopectin) content.

4.   *Sorghum* (S. vulgare, S. bicolor)

Sorghum belongs to the tribe Andropogoneae (Fig. 1) and was a known cereal crop in ancient Egypt by 2200 B. C. It was probably domesticated in Africa, about 5000 years ago, in the savanna belt stretching from Lake Chad to the Sudan (24); from here it spread through Africa and India to China. Many tropical sorghums are strict short-day plants and locally adapted to day-length response. Initially confined to the Southern United States (owing to short-day requirement), the selection of early maturing varieties and hybrids has led to its cultivation in higher lattitudes (25). Sorghum is not so well adapted to cooler climates as is maize, but it is more drought tolerant. Major cultivated varieties of the most common species, *S. vulgare*, include var. durra (durra sorghum), var. caffrorum (kaffir sorghum of Africa), var. rexburgil (Indian sorghum, also known as *Shallu*), and var. nervosum (Chinese sorghum, kaoliang).

5.   *Barley* (Hordeum *sp.*)

Brouk (18) dated the origin of barley as far back as 8000 B. C. It was known to the Greeks and Romans, and was cultivated in ancient China, from where it was introduced to Japan about 100 B. C. Barley was probably domesticated at the same time and placc as wheat, and may have been even more important than wheat in the early stages of domestication. It is a wholly diploid crop and not so well adapted to extreme cold. The bulk of the barley produced today is used for brewing. *H. distichum* (six-rowed type), in which only the central spikelet is fertile and awned, and *H. vulgare* (=hexastichum), a (six-rowed type) in which all three spikelets are fertile and awned, are the most common barley species. The cultivated barley varieties were probably derived from the wild two-rowed barley, *H. spontaneum* of southwest Asia. However, the more recent discovery of a wild six-rowed barley, *H. agriocrithon*, growing in Tibet has led to a reexamination of the origin of cultivated barley (18,19). According to Deshpande et al. (14), it is more likely that either *H. agriocrithon* gave rise to the cultivated species, *H. vulgare*, and that *H. spontantum* was the parent of *H. distichum*, or that a cross between *H. agriocrithon* and *H. spontaneum* produced the ancestors of both cultivated varieties.

6.   *Oats* (Avena *sp.*)

The origin of oats is uncertain, though it is believed to be native to Asia. Oats may have appeared as weeds in wheat and barley fields in the Middle East. Oat crops achieved importance as the temperate cereals spread to higher latitudes and cooler, wetter climates (22). Oats are derived from a polyploid series like wheat. The most common cultivated species, *A. sativa* (hexaploid) was derived from wild oats, *A. fatua*, whereas the cultivated red oat, *A byzantina*, was descended from the wild red oat, *A. sterilis*. According to Brouk (18), however, *A. sativa* is more likely to have been derived directly from *A. byzantina*. Hence, *A. sterilis* is probably the progenitor of all other species of oats. Though oats are a highly nutritious cereal food, they are widely grown as fodder for horses and other animals in the temperate regions. Oat bran and fiber have recently been popularized and are used in breakfast foods because of their possible cholesterol-lowering effects in human beings.

7. Rye (Secale cereale)

Rye is thought to have originated in Afghanistan and Turkey, where its wild ancestor, *S. montanum* is still noticed (26). Another wild form of rye, *S. anatolicum*, is also seen in Syria and Iraq. Like oats, rye also may have appeared as a weed in the wheat and barley fields of the Middle East. Similar to barley, rye is a diploid with a notable winter hardiness and is able to grow on light acidic soils (22). Rye is mainly cultivated in Europe (90% of world production), where rye bread is preferred in countries such as Germany, Austria, Czechoslovakia, Poland, and Russia.

8. Triticale

Triticale is the first man-made cereal, produced from a cross between the genera *Triticum* and *Secale*. The F_1 hybrids between the hexaploid wheat (*T. aestivum*) and diploid rye (*S. cereale*) were very vigorous but sterile. Many years later, in Russia, spontaneous chromosome doubling apparently occurred in some wheat × rye F_1 hybrids, resulting in the first true-breeding diploid triticale. Spring triticale is currently grown in Australia, Argentina, and Canada; winter triticale is largely produced in Russia, United States, France, and China.

9. Millets

Finger millet (*Eleusine coracana*) is the only millet belonging to the tribe Chlorideae; all others belong to the tribe Piniceae. Finger millet, also known as bird's-foot millet or African millet, probably originated in India (*ragi, nagli*) and is grown in India, Malaya, China, and parts of Central Africa.

   Foxtail millet (*Setaria italica*), depending on its country of origin, is also known as Italian, German, Hungarian, or Siberian millet. In Europe it was used for human food, but at present it is mainly cultivated for fodder. Foxtail millet probably originated in Asia and was cultivated in China in the year 2700 B.C. (18). Japanese barnyard millet (*Echinochloa crusgalli*, var. frumentqaceae), also known as samwa millet is grown in Japan and Korea as human food, mostly used in the form of a porridge. In the United States, it is cultivated for fodder.

   Pearl millet (*Pennisetum typhoideum, p. glaucum*) or bulrush millet possibly originated in tropical Africa. It is mainly grown in India and Africa, where it is used in the form of bread or porridge.

   Proso millet (*Panicum milaceum*), also known as hog or broom millet, is the true millet of the ancient Romans who called it milium. Proso is a Russian word for millet. It probably originated in Egypt or Arabia, and from there it spread to the former Soviet Union, India, China, and Japan.

C. Nutritional Composition and Quality

Cereal grains differ widely in their proximate composition (Table 7) (27). Starch is the major constituent of cereal endosperm, making up 58% to 70% of the total kernel weight. The total carbo-

Table 7 Proximate Composition of Cereal Grains (% Dry Weight)

Cereal	Nitrogen	Protein[a]	Fat	Fiber	Ash	NEF[b]
Wheat						
Bread	1.4–2.6	12	1.9	2.5	1.4	71.7
Durum	2.1–2.4	13	—	—	1.5	70.0
Rice						
Brown	1.4–1.7	8	2.4	1.8	1.5	77.4
Milled	—	—	0.8	0.4	0.8	—
Wild	2.3–2.5	14	0.7	1.5	1.2	74.4
Maize	1.4–1.9	10	4.7	2.4	1.5	72.2
Barley						
Grain	1.2–2.2	11	2.1	6.0	3.1	—
Kernel	1.2–2.5	9	2.1	2.1	2.3	78.8
Oats						
Grain	1.5–2.5	14	5.5	11.8	3.7	—
Kernel	1.7–3.9	16	7.7	1.6	2.0	68.2
Sorghum	1.5–2.3	10	3.6	2.2	1.6	73.0
Rye	1.2–2.4	10	1.8	2.6	2.1	73.4
Millets	1.7–2.0	11	3.3	8.1	3.4	72.9
Triticale	2.0–2.8	14	1.5	3.1	2.0	71.0

[a]Typical or average figure.
[b]NEF = Nitrogen-free extract (an approximate measure of total carbohydrates other than fiber).
Source: Ref. 27.

hydrates may account for as much as 68 to 90% of the seed weight (Table 8). Whereas endosperm contains most of the starchy carbohydrates, the nonstarchy polysaccharides are primarily concentrated in the bran fractions which contain 9 to 12% of the dietary fiber (Table 8) (28,29).

Cereal bran and germ portions are often richer in proteins than the endosperm. Cereal grains vary in their protein content from 5.6% to 21.0% (wheat) and from 8% to 18.2% in maize kernel (30,31). According to Deshpande and Damodaran (5), cereal grains supply over 70% of the total dietary intake of proteins worldwide, despite the fact that the protein content of cereal grains is only one-half that of most food legumes.

The amino acid composition of different cereal proteins (Table 9) indicates that lysine and tryptophan are the first and second limiting amino acids in cereals. These proteins, however, appear to be rich in the sulfur-containing amino acids, viz., methionine and cysteine, and thus complement well the lysine-rich, sulfur-amino acid–deficient legume proteins. Prolamines and glutelins are the major storage proteins of cereal grains, with the exception of oats, which have globulin as their predominant protein fraction (32).

Because of their lysine deficiency, cereal proteins have poor protein quality, their protein efficiency ratios (PER) ranging from 0.8 to 2.0, as compared to 2.5 of the milk casein (Table 10). Among different cereals, rice and oat proteins have higher PER values, and sorghum and maize proteins have comparatively lower PER values. Some of the good-quality protein is perhaps lost during the processing of the cereal grains.

It has been reported that consumption of sorghum is associated with poor absorption and retention of nitrogen, and with higher fecal losses of energy and nitrogen than with other cereals. It was also found to be inferior to wheat or maize in promoting growth of weaning rats (1).

The comparison of true digestibility of various cereal proteins (Table 11) indicates that the digestibility of wheat gluten is by far the highest, closely followed by that of white wheat flour.

Table 8 Carbohydrate Contents of Cereal Grains and Their Products

Cereal	Product	Total carbohydrates (g/100 g)	Fiber (g/100 g)
Wheat	Durum	70.1	1.8
	Hard red spring	69.1	2.3
	Hard red winter	71.7	2.3
	Bulgur soft red winter	72.1	1.9
	Club wheat	79.5	1.7
	Hard red winter	75.7	1.7
	White wheat	78.1	1.3
	Wheat flour		
	80% extraction	74.1	0.5
	Patent, all purpose	76.1	0.3
	Straight, hard wheat	74.5	0.4
	Straight, soft wheat	76.9	0.4
	Wheat bran	61.9	9.1
	Wheat germ	46.7	2.5
Rice	Brown	77.4	0.9
	Bran	50.8	11.5
	Polished	57.7	2.4
	White	80.4	0.3
Maize	Field corn	72.2	2.0
	Sweet corn, raw	22.1	0.7
	Pop corn		
	Unpopped	72.1	2.1
	Popped, plain	76.7	2.2
	Corn flour	76.8	0.7
Barley	Pearled	78.8	0.5
	Malt, dry	77.4	5.7
	Malt extract, dried	89.2	trace
Oats	Dry oatmeal	68.2	1.2
Sorghum	Grain	73.0	1.7
Rye		73.4	2.0
	Rye flour		
	Light	77.9	0.4
	Medium	74.8	1.0
	Dark	68.1	2.4
Millet	Proso	72.9	3.2
Buckwheat	Whole grain	72.9	9.9
	Flour		
	Dark	72.0	1.6
	Red	79.5	0.5

Source: Refs. 28 and 29.

The digestibility of proteins in whole maize, rice, and wheat flour, though comparable, decreases considerably due to processing; e.g., the true digestibility of the ready-to-eat wheat, maize, and rice was 77%, 70%, and 72%, respectively (Table 11) (33).

Protein availability primarily depends upon digestibility, and incomplete digestion significantly decreases the absorption and utilization of protein by the body. Oats have high levels of utilizable protein, whereas sorghum has the lowest value (Table 12) (34).

Table 9 Amino Acid Composition of Cereals (% by Weight)

Amino acids	Wheat (HRS)	Rice (brown)	Maize (field)	Barley	Oats	Sorghum	Rye	Pearl millet	Triticale
Alanine	3.50	3.56	9.95	4.60	6.11	—[a]	5.13	—	3.53
Arginine	4.79	5.76	3.52	5.15	6.58	3.79	4.88	4.60	4.99
Aspartic acid	5.46	4.72	12.42	5.56	4.13	—	7.16	—	5.00
Cysteine	2.19	1.36	1.30	2.01	2.18	1.66	1.99	1.33	1.55
Glutamic acid	31.25	13.69	17.65	22.35	20.14	21.92	21.26	—	31.80
Glycine	6.11	6.84	3.39	4.55	4.55	—	4.79	—	4.05
Histidine	2.04	1.68	2.06	1.87	1.84	1.92	2.28	2.11	2.48
Isoleucine	4.34	4.69	4.62	4.26	5.16	5.44	4.26	5.57	3.71
Leucine	6.71	8.61	12.96	6.95	7.50	16.06	6.72	15.32	6.87
Lysine	2.82	3.95	2.88	3.38	3.67	2.72	4.08	3.36	2.77
Methionine	1.29	1.80	1.86	1.44	1.47	1.73	1.58	2.37	1.44
Phenylalanine	4.94	5.03	4.54	5.16	5.34	4.97	4.72	4.44	5.26
Proline	10.44	4.84	8.35	9.02	5.70	—	5.20	—	12.06
Serine	4.61	5.08	5.65	4.65	4.00	5.05	4.13	—	4.70
Threonine	2.88	3.92	3.98	3.38	3.31	3.58	3.70	4.00	3.11
Tryptophan	1.24	1.08	0.61	1.25	1.29	1.12	1.13	2.18	1.08
Tyrosine	3.74	4.57	6.11	3.64	3.69	2.75	3.22	—	2.14
Valine	4.63	6.99	5.10	5.02	5.95	5.71	5.21	5.98	4.39

[a]Not estimated.
Source: Ref. 27.

Table 10 Protein Quality of Cereal Grains (PER)

Cereal	Actual	Estimate[a]	Cereal	Actual	Estimate[a]
Wheat			Maize (corn)		
Whole	1.5	1.3	Normal	1.2	1.2
Germ	2.5	2.5	Opaque-2	2.3	1.9
Gluten	—	0.7	Barley	—	1.6
Flour			Oats	1.9	1.7
80–90%	—	1.1	Sorghum	1.8	0.9
			Rye	1.6	1.6
70–80%	—	1.0	Millets		
60–70%	—	0.8	Finger millet	0.8	—
Bulgar	—	1.2	Fortail millet	—	1.0
Rice			Pearl millet	1.8	2.6
Brown	1.9	1.8	Proso millet	—	1.4
Polished	1.7	1.7	Triticale	1.6	1.4
Buckwheat	—	1.8			

[a]Estimated from the amino acid content assuming availability of amino acids the same as the amino acids in casein.
Source: Ref. 27.

Table 11 True Digestibility by Adults of Protein in Some Cereal Protein Sources

Protein source	Processed version	No. of reports	Digestibility % Mean	Range
Wheat	Whole	6	87	90–93
	Flour (white)	2	96	96–97
	Bread (white)	5	97	95–101
	Bread (coarse, brown, or whole wheat)	2	92	91–92
	Gluten	4	99	96–104
	Ready-to-eat cereal	9	77	53–88
Rice	Polished	4	89	82–91
	Ready-to-eat cereal	3	75	77–85
Maize	Whole	4	87	84–92
	Ready-to-eat cereal	5	70	62–78
Oats	Ready-to-eat cereal	4	72	63–89
Animal Protein		41	96	90–106

Source: Ref. 33.

Table 12 Utilizable Protein and Growth of Weaning Rats on Cereals Fed Alone (100%) and from 90% Cereal + 10% Bean Mixtures

Protein source	Protein in diet (%)	Utilizable protein (%)	Average weight gain (4 weeks)	PER
Wheat	11.0	4.28	19	1.05
+ bean	12.0	5.94	41	1.73
Rice	6.9	4.01	43	2.15
+ bean	7.9	4.96	56	2.32
Maize	8.5	2.41	13	0.87
+ bean	10.3	4.10	32	1.40
Oats	13.8	8.22	34	1.60
+ bean	14.6	8.73	75	2.37
Sorghum	7.7	2.23	12	0.88
+ bean	8.6	3.93	30	1.39
Casein	10.7	8.02	75	2.37

Source: Ref. 34.

The data on the mineral and vitamin contents of cereal grains (Table 13 and 14, respectively) indicate that cereals are rich sources of both phosphorus and potassium and provide fairly good amounts of calcium, iron, and magnesium. However, around 70% to 80% of the total phosphorus in cereals is present as phytic acid (35). Cereals supply fair amounts of thiamin, niacin and, pyridoxine, but are poor sources of fat-soluble vitamins. More than 80% of the total minerals and vitamins in cereal grains is present in aleurone layers that are often removed during processing operations such as polishing, pearling, or milling. The whole-grain cereals are therefore more nutritious than their processed products (14).

In comparison to pulses and other food legumes, cereals do not contain appreciable quantities of antinutritional factors, such as enzyme inhibitors and lectins. Phytic acid (myoinositol 1,2,3,5/4,6- hexa cis (dihydrogen phosphate), which chelates dietary minerals such as iron, calcium, and zinc and lowers their bioavailability, is the predominant antinutritional compound in

Table 13 Mineral Contents (mg/100 g Dry Wt.) of Cereal Grains and Cereal Products

Cereal	Ca	Fe	Mg	P	K	Na	Cu	Mn	Zn
Wheat									
Grain	50	10	160	360	520	3	0.72	4.88	3.40
Bran	140	70	555	1170	1240	9	1.23	11.57	9.80
Rice									
Brown	40	3	60	230	150	9	0.33	1.76	1.80
White	30	1	20	120	130	5	0.29	1.09	1.30
Maize									
Grain	30	2	120	270	280	1	0.21	0.51	1.69
Bran	30	—	260	190	730	—	—	1.61	—
Germ	90	90	280	560	130	—	1.10	0.90	—
Barley	80	10	120	420	560	3	0.76	1.63	1.53
Oats	100	10	170	350	370	2	0.59	3.82	3.40
Sorghum	40	4	170	310	340	—	0.96	1.45	1.37
Rye	60	10	120	340	460	1	0.78	6.69	3.05
Proso millet	50	10	160	280	430	—	2.16	2.91	1.39
Triticale	20	4	—	—	385	—	0.52	4.26	0.02
Buckwheat	110	4	390	330	450	—	0.95	3.37	0.87

Source: Ref. 29.

Table 14 Vitamin Contents[a] of Cereal Grains and Cereal Products

Cereal	Thiamin	Riboflavin	Niacin	Vitamin B_6	Folic acid	Pantothenic acid	Biotin	Vitamin E
Wheat								
Grain	0.57	0.12	7.4	0.35	78	1	6	1
Germ	2.01	0.68	4.2	0.92	328	2	—	—
Bran	0.72	0.35	21.0	1.38	223	3	14	—
Patent flour	0.13	0.04	2.1	0.05	25	1	1	—
Rice								
Brown	0.34	0.05	4.7	0.62	20	2	12	2
Polished	0.07	0.03	1.6	0.04	16	1	5	1
Maize	0.37	0.12	2.2	0.47	26	1	21	2
Barley	0.23	0.13	4.52	0.26	67	0	6	1
Oats	0.67	0.11	0.8	0.21	104	1	13	3
Sorghum	0.38	0.15	3.9	—	—	—	—	—
Rye	0.44	0.18	1.5	0.33	34	1	—	2
Millet	0.73	0.38	2.3	—	—	—	—	1
Buckwheat	0.60	—	4.4	—	—	1	—	—

[a]Vitamin contents are expressed in mg/100 g, expect for folic acid and biotin (μg/100 g) and vitamin E (IU/100g).
Source: Ref. 29.

cereals. Reddy et al. (35) regarded phytic acid as the primary storage form of both phosphorus and inositol in cereal grains.

Phytic acid is located in the aleurone layer as globoid particles, which are rich on phytate (25–70%) as well as in potassium (2–20%) and magnesium (1.5–12%). Phytate in cereals thus probably occurs as K-Mg salt (14).

Nelson et al. (36) reported that phytate accounts for over 81% of the total phosphorus in brown rice, 60 to 80% in wheat, 18 to 53% in triticale, 83 to 88% in maize, 66 to 70% in barley, 59 to 66% in oats and 72% and 89% in low- and high-tannin sorghum cultivars, respectively. The phytate content of some cereals and morphological distribution of phytic acid in different parts of the cereal grains is shown in Tables 15 and 16, respectively. These data indicate that phytic acid is primarily concentrated in the aleurone layer and to a lesser extent in the germ portion (Table 16). Lasztity and Lasztity (37) reviewed the chemistry, biochemistry, and nutritional and processing aspects of phytate in various cereals.

In addition to phytates, tannins are also present in significant amounts in some cereals, such as sorghum and millets (38). The normal levels of tannins in sorghum range from 1 to 3%, whereas some red-pigmented, high-tannin cultivars may contain as much as 7 to 8% tannins (39). The latter varieties thrive well under drought conditions and are resistant to attack. Deshpande et al. (38) reviewed the various deleterious effects of tannins in human nutrition. In animal studies, when fed at levels commonly occurring in cereals (1 to 2%), tannins were found to depress the growth rate and result in poor feed efficiency ratio and an increase in the amount of feed required per unit weight grain. Some other deleterious effects of tannins include damage to the mucosal lining of the gastrointestinal tract, alteration in the exceretion of certain cations, and increased excretion of proteins and essential amino acids. Such deleterious effects of tannins in the diet are often related to their interactions with dietary proteins (5,14).

Table 15 Phytate Content (% Dry wt.) of Various Cereals

Cereal	McCance and Widdowson (Ref. 105)	Averill and King (Ref. 106)	Oke (Ref. 107)	Lolas et al. (Ref. 108)	Other researchers
Wheat (whole grain)	0.596	1.230	—	0.62–1.35	—
Rice (unpolished)	0.851		0.284		
Maize (corn)			0.532		0.89[a]
Barley		1.130		0.97–1.16	
Oats	0.770			0.79–1.01	
Sorghum					0.57–0.96[b]
Rye		1.340			0.97[c]
Millet		1.120	0.532		0.17–0.47[d]
Triticale					0.50–1.89[c]

[a]DeBoland et al. (Ref. 109).
[b]Radhakrishnan and Sivaprasad (Ref. 110).
[c]Singh and Ready (Ref. 111).
[d]Lorenz (Ref. 112).
Source: Ref. 37.

Table 16 Phytate Content (%) in Morphological Parts of Some Cereals

Cereal	Type	Morphological part	O'Dell et al. (Ref. 113)	Lorenz (Ref. 112)	Laszity (Ref. 114)
Wheat	Hard winter	Endosperm			0.001–0.01
		Germ			0.86–1.35
		Aleurone			0.91–1.42
	Soft	Endosperm	0.001		
		Germ	1.10		
		Aleurone	1.16		
Rice	Brown	Endosperm	0.004		
		Germ	0.98		
		Pericarp	0.95		
Maize (corn)	Yellow dent	Endosperm			0.01–0.03
		Germ			0.72–1.78
		Hull			0.05–0.19
	High lysine	Endosperm	0.01		
		Germ	1.61		
		Hull	0.07		
Millet	Proso	Hull		0.51–1.60	
		Dehulled grain		0.18–0.27	

Source: Ref. 37.

III. PULSES AND OILSEEDS

Food legumes, including soybeans and peanuts, are ranked fifth in terms of annual world grain production (around 170 MMT) after wheat, rice, maize, and barley. Over 50% of the total land area under food legumes is used for soybeans and peanuts alone (2).

A. Production and Distribution

The data on world legume production (Table 17) indicate that over 50% of the total land area under food legumes is used to grow soybeans and peanuts alone (2,40,41). The American subcontinent produces more than 70% of the world's soybeans, the United States of America alone contributing to about 50%; the countries of tropical Asia together produce the bulk of the remaining food legumes. Barring soybeans, over 60% of pulses and nearly all peanuts are produced by the developing nations. However, the mean yields of food legumes in these countries are approximately one-half those of the developed countries, with mean yields ranging from 0.5 to 2.0 t/ha.

Well-defined preferences for food legumes are noticed in different regions of the world. Significant variations also exist in the types and amounts of legumes produced. India produces nearly a quarter of total dry beans grown, and about 80% of the chickpeas, whereas China is the major producer of broad beans. Both India and Africa produce a diverse varieties of pulses, but Central America almost exclusively produces cultivars of dry beans (42).

The availability of pulses and oilseeds in different regions of the world also shows distinct patterns and preferences. For example, in Latin America, availability ranges from very low in Argentina to very high in Mexico (43). The legume consumption in North America and most parts of Europe is also very low. In contrast, the Indian subcontinent depends on pulses to a great extent. Though the per capita availability of legumes in India is only about 50 g/day, the daily intake of pulses in different regions varies from 14 to 140 g/day/person (44). Barring peanuts and

Table 17 World Acreage, Production, and Protein and Lysine Yields of the Major Food Legumes Compared with Cereals, 1988

Crops	Protein		Area (10^6ha)	Production (1000 metric tons)		
	% Amount	% Lysine		Crop	Protein	Lysine
Legumes						
Total pulses	25[a]	7.0[b]	68.5	54,652	13,663	956
Dry beans	22		27.3	15,533		
Peas	22		9.9	15,505		
Chickpeas	21		8.7	5,803		
Soybeans	40	7.0	54.7	92,333	36,933	2,585
Peanuts	27	4.1	19.5	22,752[c]	3,003	123
Total				169,737	53,599	3,664
Cereals						
Wheat	12	1.8	220	4,509,952	61,194	1,101
Rice	7	3.9	145	6,483,466	33,843	1,320
Maize	8	3.0	126	6,405,460	32,437	973
Total					1,27,474	3,394

[a]From Refs. 40 and 41.
[b]From Ref. 40.
[c]In-shell basis.
Source: Ref. 2.

to some extent dry beans (legumes of the New World), pulses gown in India predominantly belong to the Old World (green gram, black gram, chickpea, pigeon pea, lentil, and *kesari dhal*). The legume utilization in the Far East (China and Japan) is also high, most of it soybeans. Japan is a rare example of a technologically advanced country with a high level of pulse utilization. The African continent is characterized by moderate to intensive use of food legumes. Smartt (45) noted that in some parts of Africa, the intake of beans is as high as 65% of the caloric intake, only about 35% of the energy coming from other food sources. Cowpea, which is the indigenous legume of Africa, is widely grown and consumed throughout the continent. Other pulses used to a lesser extent in these areas include dry beans, broad beans, chickpeas, and lentils (42).

A. Botany and Origin

Despite the successful use of radiocarbon dating to determine the approximate ages of materials found in archaeological sites, it has been difficult to reconstruct the chronology of origin and domestication of food legumes. The species of the Leguminosae are thought to have originated in the late Jurassic period, having expanded and diversified in the Cretaceous (46). Grain legumes appear to have originated both in the Old and New Worlds. The Old World grain legumes possibly belong to one or more of the following regions: the Mediterranean, Central Asia, Asia Minor, Africa, India and the Sino-Japanese region. In the New World, Central and South America are the most important centers, though domestication of a single legume species could have occurred in more than one gene center. Smartt and Hymowitz (47) considered the Mediterranean and Asia Minor gene centers more important in the evolution of the major Old World temperate grain legumes. The tropical grain legumes of the Old World probably originated in the Asian and African gene centers, whereas those of the New World evolved in Central and South America. Indonesia, Australia, and North America are probably involved only as secondary centers of origin. Barring peanuts, other grain legumes have possibly been domesticated from the wild by prehistoric planters who both cultivated these species and made selections within them to suit their evolving environment (42).

Some grain legumes such as soybean and peanut spread so widely to have been far removed from the centers of their origin. Such migration to new areas tends to accentuate changes that occur as a result of domestication, e.g., partial or complete failure of nodulation. Hutchinson (48) noted the following obvious effects of pulse domestication in modifying the growth habit: thickening of stems, leaves turn larger, branches fewer, node number lower, and internode length shorter. This process may culminate in the evolution of self-supporting plants well adapted to mono-crop-farming systems (45). Other changes associated with domestication include an alteration from perennial to annual life form, earlier flowering, increasing self-pollination, loss of seed dormancy and pod dehiscence mechanisms, and increased seed size at the expense of seed number per pod, leading to an increase in yield potential. Also, following domestication, seed coats have become more readily permeable to water (a consequence of selection), thus decreasing their dormancy and leading to uniform germination as well as ease and speed of cooking.

Adams and Pipoly (49) and Isely (50) reviewed the distinguishing characteristic features of the origin and distribution of food legumes. According to these authors, though the Asian Near East has been cited as the region of primary diversity more frequently than any other centers of the world, useful legume species appear to have originated on every continent. Many legume species have possibly experienced typically rapid increases in variability at some stage during their evolution. Some legume species (e.g., cowpeas and broad beans) are probably still actively evolving. In several cases, wild ancestors have been identified and genetic bridges to domesticated forms are available. The present patterns of genetic diversity are not closely correlated with geographical diversity. Legumes, though unique in certain morphological characteristics that distinguish them taxonomically and in some physiological and architectural traits, are not significantly different from other plant groups in respect to their breeding systems as well as in their origin, distribution, and patterns of diversity (49,50). Food legumes are unusually rich in their genetic potential for increases (from the wild types) in seed size. They have a unique capacity of fixing nitrogen symbiotically with rhizobia, resulting in larger concentrations of protein in the seed than cereals. Humankind, in seeking to exploit legume species rich in genetic potential for meeting its nutritional needs, appears to have played a significant role in influencing the present-day distribution and usage patterns of the economic species of pulses and oilseeds (42).

After Compositae and Orchidaceae, Leguminosae (or Fabaceae) is the third largest family of flowering plants in economic importance and is second only to the grasses (Graminae). The human food they supply is of three kinds: edible tubers; leaves, green pods, and unripe seeds (vegetable legumes); and ripe dry seeds (pulses). The domesticated legumes or pulses are all members of the Papilionoideae. This subfamily is divided into 10 botanical tribes, three of which together contain the major vegetable and grain legumes; the oilseed crop, peanuts belonging to the tribe Hedysareae (Fig. 2). The tribe Vicieae (or Fabeae) includes lentils, peas, chickpeas, *kesari dhal*, broad beans, and horse beans. Another tribe, Phaseolaeae, includes soybeans, lablab beans, common beans, grams, cowpeas, pigeon peas, and sword and jack beans.

In addition to peanut and soybean, cottonseed and sunflower constitute the major oilseed crops of the world. Rapeseed, coconut, olive, palm, safflower, sesame, and castor also constitute economically important oilseed crops grown all over the world. The detailed botany and origin of all important oilseed crops has been described by Salunkhe and Desai (10). Only 12 species of food legumes are grown widely, which constitute the bulk of the legumes grown and consumed all over the world. These include common beans, green peas, chickpeas, cowpeas, pigeon peas, lentils, green and black grams, broad and lima beans, and the two oilseed crops, viz, soybeans and peanut.

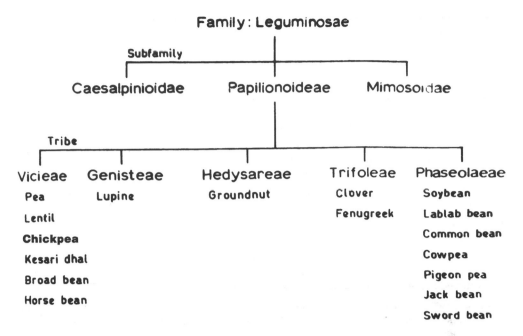

Figure 2   Botanical classification of food legumes. (From Ref. 42.)

B. Nutritional Composition and Quality

Pulses and oilseeds have a special place in the human diet because they contain nearly 2 to 3 times higher levels of protein than cereals. The oilseeds are also rich source of both oil and protein. Although the total protein production from cereals in 1988 was about 2.5 times that from food legumes, the yield of lysine was greater from the pulses (Table 17). Because lysine (essential amino acid) is the principal amino acid deficient in most plant proteins, the importance of legumes in human nutrition may be vastly underestimated. Although cereals supply nearly 50% of the dietary protein worldwide, their unfavorable balance of amino acids requires that these proteins must be complemented nutritionally. In the diets of the people of Western developed countries, the poor quality of cereal proteins is of minor importance, because their diets comprise of a substantial quantities of animal proteins (meat, fish, poultry, eggs, and milk). In the developing countries, however, proteins are either too expensive (e.g., in Latin America and Africa) or not readily accepted (e.g., in India). Food legumes and oilseeds serve as main sources of both protein and calories in many of the tropical and subtropical countries. Dry pulses and their products constitute the richest source of protein from plants (5). Although pulses also provide calories and are important sources of several B-complex vitamins, minerals and fiber, their major importance lies in their actual and potential value as a source of plant protein for human nutrition. Legume proteins alone, however, are of poor quality; it is when they are consumed with cereals that their complementary effect is exemplified. The mutually supplementary effect of combining cereals with pulses in the human diet is due to the fact that the sulfur-containing amino acids (methionine and cysteine) are the first limiting amino acids in food legumes, whereas lysine is the limiting amino acid in cereals. According to Hellendoorn (43), the maximum complementary effect often occurs near a 50:50 ratio of the two proteins. The maximum increase in the nutritive value can be obtained for cereals such as maize and sorghum, which have poor protein quality, followed by wheat, rice, and oats (42).

III. FRUITS, NUTS, AND VEGETABLES

Fruits and vegetables are, soft, fleshy, edible plant products and, because of their high moisture content (varying from about 75% in banana to around 93% in watermelon), are relatively perishable in the freshly harvested state. A nut is a dry, indehiscent fruit usually shed as a one-seeded unit. Although it forms more than one carpel, only one seed develops, the rest getting aborted. The pericarp in nuts is usually lignified and is often partially or completely surrounded by a cum-shaped structure of cupule. True nuts include the acorn, hazelnut, and beechnut. However, the word "nut" is often loosely applied to any woody fruit or seed such as the walnut and almond (which are drupes) or Brazilnut, which is a seed (51).

A. Production and Distribution

Based on the size of production, Samson (52) distinguished four groups of fruit crops of the world: (1) those having a production of more than 10 million metric tons (MMT) per year, viz., grape, citrus, banana, apple, plantain, and mango; (2) those having 1 to 10 MMT production, viz., pear, avocado, papaya, peach, plum, pineapple, date, fig, and strawberry; (3) those with production figures of 100,000 to 1 MMT, such as cashew nut; and (4) the rest, for which there are no reliable production statistics, e.g., guava, Brazil nut, litchi, soursop, and macadamia.

The production figures for major fruits, vegetables, and nuts and their leading producing countries are shown in Tables 18 and 19, respectively. The production of major fruits—grapes, citrus, bananas, and apples—as well as of vegetables and nuts has remained more or less stationary in recent years or increased slightly (Table 18).

Samson (52) postulated that an increase in fruit production is not always accompanied by a rise in consumption; if consumption continues to lag for many years, the resultant overproduc-

Table 18 Global Production Trends of Fruits, Vegetables (Plus Melons), and Total Nuts (MMT), 1989–1994

Crops	1989	1990	1991	1992	1993	1994
Fruits	354.6	354.2	353.7	380.7	384.3	388.0
Grapes	59.0	60.4	57.3	62.4	57.0	56.4
Citrus	79.2	76.4	80.7	83.7	85.8	85.3
Bananas	46.7	48.8	49.8	51.3	52.2	52.6
Apples	42.4	41.1	36.5	44.6	47.5	49.0
Vegetables and melons	449.6	460.4	464.3	470.2	474.0	485.6
Root crops	579.5	574.5	568.3	590.6	608.2	582.7
Potatoes	276.5	267.2	257.4	277.2	291.5	264.4
Total nuts	4.6	4.5	4.7	5.0	4.7	4.7

Source: Ref. 4.

Table 19 Major Producers of Fruits (Excluding Melons) (in MMT)

Country	1979–81	1992	1993	1994
Brazil	18.6	32.7	32.0	32.5
India	20.4	31.2	32.4	33.2
Italy	20.7	20.7	19.0	18.0
Spain	12.6	15.2	13.0	11.6
United States	26.5	26.9	28.9	28.9
Mexico	7.3	10.0	10.8	9.5
World	300.8	380.7	38,403.0	388.0

Source: Ref. 4.

tion leads to diminishing production. Though fruit growing is a long-term process, and changes only gradually, the twofold increase in the production of grapes, pomes, and stone fruits (drupes), threefold increase in the production of bananas and citrus, and sixfold increase in pineapple in three decades since 1950 appears to have slowed down in the 1990s and onwards.

The present production of vegetables (including melons) and that of total nuts, according to FAO statistics, is around 485 and 4.7 MMT per annum, respectively; China and India together produce around one-third of the world's vegetables (Table 20). The world production of vegetables and melons is much higher than the total production of fruits and nuts, but is much lower than that of root and tuber crops, including potatoes (Table 18). Roots and tubers (cassava, potato, sweet potato, yam, and aroid root) constitute most of the total vegetables produced in the tropical countries, providing staple food for over 500 million people. According to Pantastico and

Table 20 Major Producers of Vegetables and Melons (in MMT)

Country	1979–81	1992	1993	1994
China	83.2	123.1	125.5	128.8
India	43.9	64.2	63.8	65.1
USSR	30.9	—	—	—
United States	25.5	33.4	33.2	36.4
Japan	15.2	14.3	13.7	13.9
Italy	13.4	14.5	14.1	13.6
Korea (Rep.)	9.0	10.1	10.3	10.5
Spain	8.5	10.5	10.2	10.7
Egypt	7.3	9.7	9.7	9.4
France	7.0	7.1	7.1	7.2
Brazil	4.1	5.4	5.8	6.2
Mexico	3.9	5.5	6.3	6.1
United Kingdom	3.8	5.5	6.3	3.8
World	363.6	470.1	474.0	485.6

Source: Ref 4.

Bautista (53), the total vegetable growing area of the developing countries was around sixfold larger than that of the developed countries but the mean yield per hectare was only one-half. The export of vegetables by developing countries has also been low, and there is lack of uniformity in vegetable quality. The higher production of vegetables in most developing countries can be attributed to increases in area under cultivation. Yet, despite these increases, fruit, nuts, and vegetables constitute a largely neglected group of agricultural crops in the developing countries. Apart from poor production statistics and deficiencies in data related to fruits, vegetables, and nuts, their production also suffers from severe handicaps, including uncertain prices received by the growers, and the extreme volatility in prices at the consumer level, mitigating the interests of both the producers and consumers. Also, owing to poor pre-harvest crop production and improper harvesting, handling, storage, transportation, processing, and marketing of these perishable commodities, very high pre- and post-harvest losses occur in the tropical and subtropical countries, varying widely according to commodity and areas (8,9).

Like fruit crops, vegetables also suffer from poor production statistics. Production data are not available for many countries, and available estimates refer only to crops grown in fields and market gardens for sale, excluding those cultivated in kitchen and small family gardens and meant for household consumption.

B.   Botany and Origin

Botanically, the word "fruit" refers to the mature seed-bearing structures of the flowering plants, covering a very wide and heterogenous group of plant products such as cereals, pulses, oilseeds, spices, and fleshy fruits. The edible fleshy fruits, however, represent a well-defined class on their own and exhibit a wide variety of plant products. They have much in common from a culinary point of view with the soft, edible structures developed from other parts of the plant body commonly referred to as vegetables. Although botanically the line between fruits, nuts, and vegetables cannot be clearly drawn, these plant products have been differentiated based on common verbal usage and the way in which they are consumed. Popularly, the term "fruit" has been restricted in its use to those botanical plant parts that have fragrant, aromatic flavors, and are either naturally sweet or normally sweetened with sugar before eating; that is, fruits are essentially consumed as dessert items. The term *vegetable*, in contrast, is applied to all other soft, edible plant products that are usually eaten with meat, fish, or other savory dish, either fresh or cooked. Both fruits and vegetables are utilized in different ways in different parts of the world and in some instances, even within a given community; e.g., banana and plantain, the fruits of two very closely related plant species, are utilized distinctively: whereas banana is an important dessert fruit, the starchy plantain is usually consumed as a vegetable after cooking.

Botanically, fruit is the structure that develops from the ovary wall (pericarp) as the enclosed seed(s) matures. Although fruit is often an important feature in the diagnosis of family or genus, its classification is somewhat arbitrarily, based on gross morphology rather than mode or origin. Thus, fruits may be classified as succulent or dry, depending on whether or not the middle layer (the mesocarp) of the pericarp develops into a fleshy covering. It may be further classified as dehiscent or indehiscent based on whether the fruit wall splits open to release the seed. Fruits that develop from the gynoecium of a single flower are termed simple or true fruits; those derived from a single ovary are termed monocarpellary, and those incorporating a number of fused ovaries are called polycarpellary. An aggregate fruit may develop from an apocarpous gynoecium (e.g., pomes and strawberries); others may develop from a complete inflorescence (e.g. pineapples, mulberries, and figs). Certain fruits may develop even though the ovule has not been fertilized (e.g. parthenocarpic fruits such as melons, figs, cucumbers, and bananas).

Duckworth (54) pointed out the probable original centers of distribution of the ancestors of some of the modern cultivated fruit and vegetable species as follows:

Center	Species
Central Asia	Apple, broad bean, cherry, lentil, mulberry, olive, onion, pea, pear, plum, pomegranate, quince, radish, spinach
Mediterranean	Carrot, celery, cucumber, date, eggplant, lettuce, melon, mustard, turnip
Mediterranea and Southeast Asia	Artichoke, asparagus, cabbage, cauliflower, fig, horseradish parsley, parsnip
Southeast Asia	Banana, breadfruit, peach, persimmon, orange, yam
Central America	Avocado, cassava, maize (sweet corn), cranberry, kidney bean, lima bean, pineapple, potato, pumpkin, squash, sweet potato, tomato

The wild ancestors of all the important fruits and vegetables grown today were originally confined to one or another of four main centers of distribution. The ancient Greek and Roman civilizations were familiar with many edible plant species, including fruits, nuts, and vegetables, that were indigenous to Central and Southeast Asia and the Mediterranean region. The Greeks and Roman probably cultivated quite a wide range of fruits, nuts, and vegetables and lived largely on a vegetarian diet. The solar drying of fruits such as grapes and plums was widely practiced during these times, and the trade in dried fruit products flourished around the Mediterranean (54).

Having realized the nutritional value of fruits and vegetables in the human diet and as a good source of income, their cultivation on a commercial scale reached a high level of development in Europe during the Middle Ages. A majority of tropical and subtropical fruits gradually spread from their original centers of distribution to other areas where the climate was suitable for their cultivation. Bananas, for example, have been grown in Malaysia since the second millennium B.C., and were introduced to tropical America at the beginning of the 16th century; the orange, another native of Southeast Asia, also probably reached America about the same time. Greenhouse culture, introduced in the 17th century, enabled the small-scale cultivation of exotic species such as vines, peaches, and citrus. In the 18th century, medical science was positively affirming the essentiality of fruits and vegetables in the human diet for normal well-being. As the consumption of these products increased worldwide during the 19th century, foundations were laid for the subsequent exploitation of such modern methods of food preservation as cold storage, canning, and artificial drying of fruits, and commercial production of jams, jellies, sauces, and fruit juices. Per capita supplies of starchy vegetables worldwide have increased about 20% since World War II.

C. Nutritional Composition and Quality

Fruits are highly remarkable sources of wholesome food and are valued for their flavor, aroma, and texture. Fresh fruits appeal to all the senses: smell, taste, touch, sight, and even sound (crunchy apple). Nutritionally, they play a vital role in supplying significant amounts of vitamins and minerals. The percentage of nutrients contributed by fruits and vegetables as a group, according to the amount consumed per year in the United States are as follows (8,9): Vitamin C (91%), vitamin A (beta carotene) (48%), vitamin B_6 (27%), magnesium (26%), iron (19%), thiamin (17%), niacin (15%), and calories (9%).

Some fruits are a fairly rich source of energy, and may contribute notable amount of fat (e.g., avocados, nuts), sugars (dates, figs, bananas), protein (tucuma) (55,56) and dietary fiber

(57). Fruits play an especially important role in human health by providing low-sodium diets to people with health problems such as hypertension and kidney disorders (58). One of the greatest health problems of the more affluent societies of the Western world is malnutrition and obesity, and fresh fruits and vegetables can supply a large portion of a diet while contributing very few calories (57). Because of their higher nutrient ratios, a normal serving of fruits can supply the recommended daily dietary allowances for most nutrients without concomitantly supplying excess calories (59).

Barring high-protein nuts and fat-rich avocados, fruits are neither good nor economic sources of protein, fat, and calories, but are indispensable as sources of vitamins and minerals. Most fruits contain more than 80% water, this value varying considerably based on the availability of water to the crop, especially at the time of harvest (Table 21) (60,61). To maintain their crisp texture and freshness after harvest, fruits are often harvested when their moisture content is at a maximum. Carbohydrates, the next most abundant group of nutrient constituents, are present as low-molecular-weight sugars (glucose, fructose, and sucrose) or their high-molecular weight polymers, such as starch, hemicellulose, cellulose, and pectins. Most ripe fruits are characterized by the presence of water-soluble sugars, whereas starch is the predominant constituent of unripe fleshy fruits such as bananas. Cellulose, hemicellulose, pectins, and lignin (a polymer of aromatic alcohols linked by propyl units), which together constitute the dietary fiber, are essential components of the human diet. The incidence of such disorders as constipation, diverticulosis, and colon cancer has been attributed to lack of fiber in the human diet.

The protein content of most fruits varies from 0.5 to 1% (Table 21). These are mostly the functional proteins (e.g. globular proteins such as enzymes), rather than storage proteins. Barring olives and avocados, fruits generally have less than 1% of lipids, which are mostly associated with the protective cuticle layers of the fruit surface and the cell wall. Citrus fruits contain more than 3% of organic acids (citrate and malate as predominant acids). Tartaric and isocitric acids predominate in grapes and blackberry, respectively (8).

Ascorbic acid (vitamin C) is one of the most important essential constituents of the human diet, a deficiency of which causes scurvy. Dietary vitamin C (about 90%) is essentially obtained from fruits and vegetables. Many fruits such as citrus, cherries, berries, guava, and *aonla* provide the recommended dietary allowance of about 50 mg of vitamin C in less than 100 g of the fruit tissue. Papaya and mango are rich in vitamin A (beta-carotene), and nuts are excellent sources of thiamin. The human body converts beta-carotene into retinol, an active vitamin A compound required to maintain visual processes. Fruits are also important sources of calcium, iron, and other minerals, but generally their contibution to total dietary requirement is of less importance. Recent research in human nutrition suggests that sodium is responsible for blood pressure–related disorders, and that potassium acts antagonistically. Since fruits have higher K:Na ratios (Table 21), nutritionists advise a daily intake of at least 100 g of fruits and as much variety as the season permits. Some fruits may be nutritionally harmful and even poisonous (e.g., in the akee, the unripe aril and the pink vein that attaches it to the seed are highly poisonous (62). Carambola and bilimbi contain 1% to 6% oxalic acid which can cause calcium deficiency and kidney stones. Plantains contain serotonin, which when consumed in large quantities may cause high blood pressures.

The nutritional composition and quality of the fruit varies considerably throughout its growth and maturation periods. Some fruits reach their highest nutritive value while still immature, others when physiologically mature, and some when fully mature or overmature. Even within a given species, some cultivars differ significantly from others on their nutrient contents. Okuse and Ryugo (63) noted an increase in the ascorbic acid content of kiwi fruit with maturation. Papaya also showed an increase in ascorbic acid with maturation (64), but mangoes (65), bananas (66), 'Maracuya' passion fruit (67), and acerola (68) showed a decrease. Harding and Sunday (69) demonstrated that the immature tangerines had the highest vitamin C concentration,

Table 21 Nutritional Composition of Some Fruits (Values per 100g Edible Portion)

Fruits	Water (g)	Energy (Cal)	Protein (g)	Fat (g)	Carbohydrates (g)	Minerals (mg)						Vitamin A (IU)	Thiamin (mg)	Riboflavin (mg)	Niacin (mg)	Vitamin C (mg)
						Ca	P	Fe	Na	K	Mg					
Apricot	85.3	51	1.0	0.2	12.8	17	23	0.5	1	281	12	2700	0.03	0.04	0.6	10
Peach	89.1	38	0.6	0.1	9.7	9	18	0.5	1	202	10	1300	0.02	0.05	1.0	7
Orange	86.0	49	1.0	0.2	12.2	41	20	0.4	1	200	11	200	0.10	0.04	0.4	50
Grapefruit	88.4	41	0.5	0.1	10.6	16	16	0.4	1	135	12	80	0.04	0.02	0.2	38
Plum	81.1	66	0.5	0.2[a]	17.8	18	17	0.5	2	299	9	300	0.08	0.03	0.5	5[a]
Grape	81.6	69	1.3	1.0	15.7	16	12	0.4	3	158	13	100	0.05	0.03	0.3	4
Sour cherry	83.7	58	1.2	0.3	14.3	22	19	0.4	2	191	14	1000	0.05	0.06	0.4	10
Apple	84.4	58	0.2	0.6	14.5	7	10	0.3	1	110	8	90	0.03	0.02	0.1	4
Strawberry	89.9	37	0.7	0.5	8.4	21	21	1.0	1	164	12	60	0.03	0.07	0.6	59
Watermelon	92.6	26	0.5	0.2	6.4	7	10	0.5	1	100	8	590	0.03	0.03	0.2	7
Pear	83.2	61	0.7	0.4	15.3	8	11	0.3	2	130	7	20	0.02	0.04	0.1	4
Banana	75.7	85	1.1	0.2	22.2	8	26	0.7	1	370	33	190	0.05	0.06	0.7	10

[a]From Heinz (Ref. 61).
Source: Ref. 60.

whereas the ripe fruits had the least. Although there was a decrease during ripening, the total vitamin C content per fruit tended to increase with increased juice volume and fruit size.

Jone et al. (70) noted a significant increase in total carotenoids and beta-carotene both in the peel and the pulp during the maturation of mangoes. There was an increase in thiamin content of citrus fruits also with maturity (71). Compared with many other fruits, grapes and black currants had the highest level of thiamin, and that of grapes also increased during ripening (72).

Folic acid (folacin) is chemically pteroylmonoglutamic acid. Several compounds exhibiting folacin activity may differ only in the number of glutamate residues they contain. Barring citrus, most other fruits contain low amounts of folic acid whereas citrus fruit juice contained about 20 to 50 µg folacin/100 ml (74), its concentration increasing with fruit maturation. The folic acid content of some other fruits was found to be as follows:

Fruits	Folic acid content	Ref.
Fig	39 µg/100g dried fruit	Hall et al. (75)
Mango	36 µg/100g pulp	Ghosh (76)
Avocado	10–60 µg/100g pulp	Hall et al. (77)
Grape	1–2 µg/100ml juice	Peynaud and Ribereau-Gayon. (72)

The contents of pantothenic acid, riboflavin, niacin, vitamin B_6 (pyridoxine), vitamin B_{12}, and tocopherols in many fruits are found at levels below 10% of the U.S. RDA (78). Apricots, gooseberries, black currants, figs, and citrus fruits contain moderate amounts of patothenic acid (79); mangos, pineapples, papayas, acerolas, and passion fruit are fairly good sources of riboflavin; and tamarinds, guavas and passion fruit provide niacin (80). Among the 26 fruits tested by Polansky and Murphy (81), bananas (5.4 µg/g) and avocados (4.5 µg/g) had the highest amount of vitamin B_6.

In addition to a large quantity of water, the major chemical constituents of fresh vegetables are carbohydrates, proteins, fats, vitamins, minerals, and dietary fiber. Beta-carotene (provitamin A), thiamin (B_1), riboflavin (B_2), pyridoxine (B_6), niacin, pantothenic acid, folacin, ascorbic acid (vitamin C), and vitamins E and K have been reported to be present in different vegetable products. Among the minerals present in significant amounts are Mg, Cu, Co, S, Zn, and F. Salunkhe and Desai (82) have reviewed the effects of agricultural practices, handling, processing, and storage on the quality and nutritional composition of vegetables. Salunkhe et al. (83) described the major functions of nutrients in the human body. Fruits and vegetables are often bought and consumed for their characteristic flavor and variety in taste rather than for their nutritive values. The nutritional contribution of major fruits and vegetables compared to percentage of total food supply is shown in Fig. 3. Because the extent to which a food contributes nutrients to the human diet is governed by the amount of food consumed, vegetables are generally not regarded as economic sources of energy, protein, fat, calcium, or riboflavin (84). A vegetable may be rich in minerals and vitamins, but the consumer will need another source of food if only a small quantity of that vegetable is eaten; e.g., although the concentration of ascorbic acid in green peppers is about 7 times higher than that in potatoes, the average consumer obtains more of this vitamin from potatoes than from peppers because of higher potato consumption. Rick (85) showed the relative concentration of 10 major vitamins and minerals in some fruits and vegetables and their importance in the typical U.S. diet. This ranking indicated that while tomatoes and oranges are relatively low in nutrient concentration, they contribute greatly to the U.S. diet because they are consumed in large quantities. Vegetables supply only negligible amounts of fat and protein (7% and 8% of the body's requirements of energy and protein, respectively); other foods such as cereals, meat, milk,

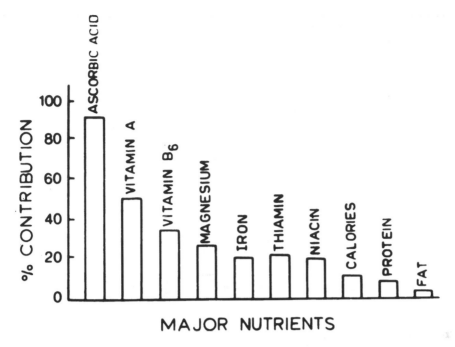

Figure 3 Nutritional contribution of some important fruits and vegetables. (From Ref. 83.)

and eggs are more efficient sources of these nutrients. Vegetables, however, contribute significantly to a well-balanced diet in that they are major sources of beta-carotene and ascorbic acid, and good sources of thiamin, niacin, and iron (Table 22) (86–89).

Tindall and Proctor (88) summarized the nutritive values of some selected typical vegetables and concluded that vegetables contribute significantly to human dietary requirements of essential minerals, vitamins, proteins, and carbohydrates, especially in areas of low animal protein availability, and where cereals comprise most of the human diet. Vegetables also furnish bulk (dietary fiber) which helps in the proper function of the human digestive system. According to Wills et al. (90), several human diseases such as appendicitis, colon cancer, constipation, deep vein thrombosis, diabetes, diverticulosis, gallstones, hemorrhoids, hiatus hernia, ischemic heart disease, obesity, rectal tumors, and varicose veins have been claimed to be due to lack of fiber in the diet. Most vegetables, especially such leafy greens as spinach, lettuce, celery, cabbage, and fenugreek, are characterized by a high percentage of cellulose (crude fiber). Owing to their succulence (high water content) and large bulk (roughage), leafy greens and root vegetables aid in the digestion and utilization of concentrated foods.

The nutritional composition of 12 cruciferous and 18 other vegetables (83) indicates that most vegetables are low in calories, fats and carbohydrates, but rich in vitamins and minerals (Table 23) (91). In general, the cruciferous vegetables appear to be more efficient in synthesizing high concentrations of proteins, amino acids, minerals, and vitamins, and they are low in caloric content.

Gopala Rao et al. (92) analyzed several leafy green vegetables including amaranth (*A. tricolor* and *A. spinosus*), drumstick leaves (*Moringa oleifera*), coriander (*Coriandrum sativum*), mint (*Mentha spicata*) and green sorrel (*Rumex acetosa*) for beta-carotene, B vitamins (B$_1$, B$_2$, B$_6$, niacin), reducing and non-reducing sugars, starch, protein, soluble protein, and total nitrogen,

Table 22 Nutritional, Mineral, and Vitamin Content of Some Important Vegetables[a]

Vegetables	Nutrients					Minerals					Vitamins			
	Water (g)	Energy (g)	Protein (g)	Fat (g)	Carbohydrates (g)	Ca (mg)	P (mg)	Fe (mg)	Na (mg)	K (mg)	Thiamin (mg)	Riboflavin (mg)	Niacin (mg)	Vitamin (mg)
Roots/tubers														
Cassava	60(ml)	153	0.7	0.2	37.0	25	—	1.0	—	—	0.07	0.03	—	30
Yam	73.0	131	2.0	0.2	32.4	10	(40)	0.3	—	(500)	0.10	0.03	0.4	10
Sweet potato	70.0	91	1.2	0.6	21.5	(22)	(47)	(0.7)	(19)	(320)	0.10	0.16	0.8	25
Irish potato	75.8	87	0.1	0.1	20.8	8	40	0.5	7	520	0.11	0.04	1.2	8
Other vegetables														
Onion	92.8	23	0.9	Trace	5.2	31	30	0.3	10	140	0.03	0.05	0.2	10
Tomato	93.4	14	0.9	Trace	2.8	13	21	0.4	3	290	0.06	0.04	0.7	20
Melons														
Pumpkin	94.7	15	0.6	Trace	3.4	39	19	0.4	1	310	0.04	0.04	0.4	5
Cantaloupe	93.6	24	1.0	Trace	5.3	19	30	0.8	14	320	0.05	0.03	0.5	25
Water melon	94.0	21	0.4	Trace	5.3	5	8	0.3	4	120	0.02	0.02	0.2	5
Leaves (Carotene level[b])														
Low	93 (ml)	23	1.5	0.2	4.0	40	—	0.5	—	—	0.05	0.05	—	40
Medium	91 (ml)	28	2.0	0.3	4.0	80	—	2.5	—	—	0.08	0.20	—	50
High	85 (ml)	48	5.0	0.7	5.0	250	—	4.0	—	—	2.10	0.30	—	100

[a]Per 100g edible portion. Figures in parentheses are estimated from related foods or more rarely, are tentative values based on a limited number of published sources (87).

[b]Low-carotene (pale green) leaves = cabbage, kohlrabi, Chinese cabbage; medium-carotene leaves = New Zealand spinach, cassava leaves, watercress, squash, pumpkin; high-carotene leaves = spinach, sweet potato, tops of kale.

Source: Refs. 86–89.

calcium, and iron contents. These authors recommended *Trtianthema portulacastrum* as a nutritionally rich new vegetable crop.

Like fruits, vegetables also may contain certain toxic factors. Cruciferous vegetables in general, and those belonging to the genus *Brassica* in particular, contain goitrogens that cause enlargment of the thyroid glands. Natural thioglucosides (glucosinolates) are sources of goitrogens; however, these compounds, with their associated enzymes, also impart the desirable culinary flavor of cabbage, broccoli, and cauliflower. A thioglucoside, allylthioglucoside (sinigrin), is present in cabbage, kale, Brussels sprouts, broccoli, cauliflower, and mustard. When these vegetables are chopped, a specific enzyme, thioglucosidase (myrosinase) hydrolyses it into glucose, potassium bisulfate, and allylthiocyanate, a goitrogenic compound. Similarly, progoitrin or epiprogoitrin is responsible for the typical flavor of kale, rape, turnip, rutabaga, and kohlrabi. It is hydrolyzed by thioglucosidase to yield glucose, potassium bisulfate, and highly unstable intermediate compounds such as thiocyanate, nitrite plus sulfur, and goitrin. Goitrin (5-vinyl-oxazolidine-2-thione) is a potent thyrotoxin and is formed through cyclization of an unstable isothiocyanate containing the hydroxyl group. The thyroid-inhibiting effect of goitrins is due to the irreversible inhibition of organic binding of iodine. However, thiocyanate, isothiocyanate, and nitrite ions act as goitrogens only when the iodine content of the diet is low. In such regions, benign goiter may be accentuated by eating excessive amounts of brassica vegetables (51,83). Most of the goitrogenic properties of vegetables are however, lost during cooking.

Crosby (93) noted that ethylacetate extracts from leaves of broccoli, cabbage, rutabaga, turnip, and radish inhibit human plasma choline esterase. The flatulence distress syndrome experienced after eating cooked cruciferous vegetables is not as chronic and offensive as that produced after the consumption of beans, sweet potatoes, and onions. Other naturally occurring toxicants of vegetables include oxalates, salicylates, arsenic, nitrite, and alkaloids, such as solanine. Potatoes contain solanine, arsenic, and nitrite, and some green leafy vegetables contain toxic oxalates. The anthraquinones of rhubarb are mainly in the root, but human poisoning generally occurs from eating rhubarb leaves. Though leaf poison is commonly thought to be oxalates, other factors, possibly quinones, are also involved (94).

Sreeja and Leelamma (95) recently reported a hyperglycemic effect of low-protein cassava diet. Cyanogenic plants, such as cassava (*Manihot esculenta*), which are major components of many human diets, contain cyanide poison, leading to pathological conditions. Linamarin (hydroxyisobutyronitrile beta-D-glucose) is the main cyanogenic glucoside in cassava, which liberates hydrocyanic acid (HCN) on hydrolysis. Sreeja and Leelamma (95) showed that rats fed a low-protein, high-cyanide diet had an increased level of blood glucose and decrease in liver glycogen. The activity of glycogen phosphorylase, glucose-6-phosphatase, and phasphoglucomutase showed higher levels in the livers of the low-protein, high-cyanide group compared with the control group. It was suggested that a cassava diet with low protein can induce hyperglycemia.

In terms of human lives lost due to plant phenols, the salicylate aspirin ($C_9H_8O_4$) is probably the most dangerous (four deaths per one million people every year). Low-molecular-weight salicylates are associated with hyperactivity. Feingold (96) recommended omitting 21 fruits and vegetables containing natural salicylates for the dietary treatment of this disorder. According to Robertson and Kermode (97), the concentration of salicylates in fresh vegetables ranged from 0.01 mg/kg in cabbage to 0.1 mg/kg in whole-kernel sweet corn. Canned sweet corn and some tomato products contained higher levels of salicylic acid than the fresh vegetables.

The distribution of oxalates in vegetables varies with species and families. Leaves, in general, contain higher amounts of oxalates than stalks. The ratio of oxalates to calcium also varies greatly. Fassett (98) divided vegetables into three classes, based on oxalate:calcium ratio:

1. those with a ratio of more than 2.0 (e.g., spinach, beet leaves, and rhubarb)

Table 23 Nutritional Composition of Some Cruciferous and Other Vegetables[a]

Vegetables	Macro-Nutrients					Minerals						Vitamins				
	Water (%)	Energy (Cal)	Protin (%)	Fat (%)	Carbohydrates (%)	Ca (mg)	P (mg)	Fe (mg)	Na (mg)	K (mg)	Mg (mg)	Vit. A (I.U.)	Thiamin (mg)	Riboflavin (mg)	Niacin (mg)	Vit. C (mg)
1	2	3	4	5	6	7	8	9	10	11	12	13	14	15	16	17
Cruciferous																
Cabbage	92.2	24	1.3	0.2	5.4	49	29	0.4	20	233	13	130	0.05	0.05	0.3	47
Broccoli	89.1	32	3.6	0.3	5.9	103	78	1.1	15	382	24	2500	0.10	0.23	0.9	113
Brussels sprout	85.2	45	4.9	0.4	8.3	36	80	1.5	14	390	29	550	0.10	0.16	0.9	102
Cauliflower	91.0	27	2.7	0.2	5.2	25	56	1.1	13	295	24	60	0.11	0.10	0.7	78
Kale	82.7	53	6.0	0.8	9.0	249	93	2.7	75	238	37	10000	0.16	0.26	2.1	186
Watercress	93.3	19	2.2	0.3	3.0	151	54	1.7	52	282	20	4900	0.08	0.16	0.9	79
Mustard green	89.5	31	3.0	0.5	5.6	183	50	3.0	32	377	27	7000	0.11	0.22	0.8	97
Turnip green	90.3	28	3.0	0.3	5.0	246	58	1.8	40[b]	250[b]	58	7600	0.21	0.39	0.8	139
Chinese cabbage	95.0	14	1.2	0.1	3.0	43	40	0.6	23	253	14	150	0.05	0.04	0.06	25
Rutabaga	87.0	46	1.1	0.1	11.0	66	39	0.4	5	239	15	580	0.07	0.07	1.1	43
Collard	85.3	45	4.8	0.8	7.5	250	82	1.5	40[b]	450	57	9300	0.16	0.31	1.7	152
Kohlrabi	90.3	29	2.0	0.1	6.6	41	51	0.5	8	372	37	20	0.06	0.04	0.3	66
Noncruciferous																
Carrot	88.2	42	1.1	0.2	9.7	37	36	0.7	47	341	23	11000	0.06	0.05	0.6	8
Sweet potato	70.6	114	1.7	0.4	26.3	32	47	0.7	10	243	31	8800	0.10	0.06	0.06	21
Tomato	93.5	22	1.1	0.2	4.7	13	27	0.5	3	244	14	900	0.06	0.04	0.7	23
Sweet corn	72.7	96	3.5	1.0	22.1	3	111	0.7	10[b]	280	48	400	0.15	0.12	1.7	12
Pepper	93.4	22	1.2	0.2	4.8	9	22	0.7	13	213	18	420	0.08	0.08	0.5	128

Lettuce	95.1	14	1.2	0.2	2.5	35	26	2.0	9	264	11	900	0.06	0.06	0.3	8
Potato	79.8	76	2.1	0.1	17.1	7	53	0.6	3	407	34	20[c]	0.10	0.04	1.5	20
Squash	94.0	19	1.1	0.1	4.2	28	29	0.4	1	202	17	410	0.05	0.09	1.0	22
Onion	89.1	38	1.5	0.1	8.7	27	36	0.5	10	157	12	40	0.03	0.04	0.2	10
Cucumber	95.1	15	0.9	0.1	3.4	25	27	1.1	6	160	11	250	0.03	0.04	0.2	11
Spinach	90.7	26	3.2	0.3	4.3	93	51	3.1	71	470	88	8100	0.10	0.20	0.6	51
Limabean	67.5	123	8.4	0.5	22.1	52	142	2.8	2	650	67	290	0.24	0.12	1.4	29
Pea	78.0	84	6.3	0.4	14.4	26	116	1.9	2	316	35	640	0.35	0.14	2.9	27
Asparagus	91.7	26	2.5	0.2	5.0	22	62	1.0	2	278	20	900	0.18	0.20	1.5	33
Cantaloupe	91.2	30	0.7	0.1	7.5	14	16	0.4	12	251	17[b]	3400	0.04	0.03	0.6	19
Snap bean	90.1	32	1.9	0.2	7.1	56	44	0.8	7	243	32	600	0.08	0.11	0.5	19
Beet	87.3	43	1.6	0.1	9.3	16	33	0.7	60	335	25	20	0.03	0.05	0.4	10
Celery	94.1	7	0.9	0.1	3.9	39	28	0.3	126	341	22	240	0.03	0.03	0.3	9

[a]Values per 100 g edible portion.
[b]Nutritional Composition of fresh California-grown vegetabes (1962). California Exp. Sta. Bull No. 788.
[c]Ref. 51.
Source: Ref. 91.

2. those with a ratio 1–2 (e.g., potatoes),
3. those with a ratio less than 1 (e.g., lettuce, cabbage, and peas)

Several types of mushroom also may contain oxalates and other toxic factors (82).

IV. SUGAR AND BEVERAGE CROPS

A. Sugar Crops

Sugar or sucrose is a commercially important substance because of its versatile use in foods and in a variety of industrial products. It plays a unique role in varied aspects of human chemistry, biology, nutrition, physiology, and clinical medicine. Both sugars and beverages are of interest to a wide range of specialists, including chemists, biochemists, physiologists, nutritionists, clinicians, sociologists, and food scientists.

1. Production and Distribution

The total production of world sugar (sucrose) and beverage crops (coffee, tea, cocoa) is around 110 and 111 million metric tons currently (Table 1). About 55% of the sugar comes from cane and roughly 45% from beet. Sucrose from all other sources (sugar palm, sweet sorghum, and maple tree) amounts to about 1% of the total (Table 24).

The world production of raw sugar has increased more than seven- to eightfold since the year 1900. During this period, per capita sugar consumption also increased about threefold, despite a substantial increase in population. This increase has been greatest (about 200%–300%) in the developing countries of Latin America, the Near East, and Africa. The average sugar consumption is around 15 kg/person/year but varies widely from one country to another; about 50 kg/person/year in Canada, UK, Australia and Sweden, and less than 5 kg/person/year in India, Pakistan, and China. The major sugar-producing countries are Cuba, Brazil, the United States, India, and the former Soviet Union (Table 25).

2. Botany and Origin

Sugarcane (*Saccharum officinarum* L.) belongs to the family Gramineae of the order Glumaceae and class Monocotyledon. It is closely related to grasses of which it is a giant member. Stems or stalks develop from the bud of another stem following vegetative propagation by cuttings (setts, points, or seeds). Unlike most grasses, sugarcane does not have a hollow stem, but one that is filled, as in maize and sorghum. It is a short-day plant and its photoperiodic flowering conditions can be attained only in the tropics. Flowering is not desirable in agricultural cane production, for

Table 24 Botanical Sources of Sugar (sucrose)

Source	Scientific name	Family	Percent of production
Sugarcane	*Saccharum officinarum*	Gramineae	55
Sugar beet	*Beta vulgaris*	Chenopodiaccac	44
Sugar palm	*Phoenix dactylifera*	Palmaceae	1
Sorghum	*Sorghum vulgare* var. *durra*	Gramineae	0.1
Maple	*Acer saccharum*	Aceraceae	0.05

Source: Ref. 4. (Approximate total annual sugar production in 1994 was 110 MMT).

Table 25 Major Sugar-Producing Countries (MMT)

Country	1979–81	1992	1993	1994
Centrifugal (raw) sugar				
USSR	7.02	—	—	—
Cuba	7.51	7.10	4.20	4.00
Brazil	7.99	9.99	10.04	11.65
India	5.38	14.34	11.35	10.59
USA	5.34	7.04	6.96	7.37
China	3.86	8.92	8.53	6.79
France	4.72	4.69	5.04	4.99
Germany	3.94	4.40	4.35	3.94
Australia	3.24	4.26	4.30	5.10
World	88.78	117.25	111.10	109.96
Noncentrifugal sugar				
India	8.11	7.96	8.76	9.50
Pakistan	1.76	0.82	0.63	0.53
Colombia	0.92	0.84	0.87	0.88
China	0.35	0.45	0.37	0.50
Thailand	0.16	0.33	0.35	0.35
World	12.85	11.77	12.42	13.20

Source: Ref. 4.

it reduces cane yields. Desai et al. (99) have recently described the botany and origin of all sugar crops, including sugarcane.

The earliest Western reference to sugar was written in 325 B.C. by an officer of Alexander's invading army in India, where sugarcane may already have been cultivated for several centuries. New data seem to place the origin of sugarcane in the South Pacific about 8000 year ago. Probably a native of New Guinea, the plant moved northward to southeast Asia and India. Sugarcane cultivation and refining spread east to China about 100 B.C., but reached Mediterranean Europe relatively late, probably as a result of Arab conquests after A.D. 636 (100). Sugar was probably introduced to the Western world in the 13th century, Venice becoming the sugar capital of the world in the year 1300.

Sugar beet (*Beta vulgaris* L.) is a herbaceous, long-day dicotyledon belonging to the Chenopodiaceae family. Sugar beet is a biennial plant that stores a reserve food supply in a large fleshy root forming in the first growing season. The plant then overwinters, producing flower, stems, and the seed the following year. The seed of multigerm varieties of sugar beet is actually a fruit consisting of a cluster of seeds enclosed on the woody outer casing (husk). The life cycle of sugar beet is interrupted by harvesting the fleshy roots during the first autumn when the amount of sugar in the root is at its peak. The crop is adapted to cooler regions of the world.

3. Nutritional Composition and Quality

Sugar is one of the important constituents of the human diet. Much of the sucrose in the diets of the high-consumption countries is found in manufactured foods—confectionery, soft drinks, cakes, ice creams, and bakery products. In the United Kingdom, about one-half of the sugar is consumed in the form of manufactured foods, the remaining half being used in tea and coffee, on cereals and pudding, and in cooking and baking.

Dietary sucrose is a mixed blessing (101). On the one hand, it is credited with making food more attractive and appetizing; on the other hand, it is claimed to leave in its trail (especially on excessive consumption), various pathological conditions, including dental caries, coronary thrombosis, diabetes, obesity, and certain disorders of the skin, the digestive tract, and the joints.

Sugar is available in a variety of types or forms: granulated, cubed, confectioner's, and so forth. The sugar refiner thus supplies the food manufacturer with a variety of sucrose products tailored for specific uses. Some basic grades of industrial sugars, their characteristics and uses, are as follows (102):

Sugar grade	Characteristics	Some uses
Mineral water	Pure white, low ash	Preserves, drinks, high-quality foods, and medicines
Standard, granulated	High purity, consistent quality	Manufacturing
Canners	Low bacterial count	Canning
Manufacturing	White, off-white, yellow, brown, various crystal sizes	Baking, confectionery
Liquid sugars	Equivalent grades to above	As above

The sweetness of 1 lb of sucrose can be matched with that 1g of saccharin or 10 g of cyclamate. Sugar thus provides bulk to the human diet in addition to sweetness. Brook (102) stated the following valuable characteristics of sucrose besides its sweetness. It:

1. increases sweetness, osmotic pressure, viscosity, boiling point, moisture retention
2. enhances flavor, appearance (improved by clarity, lustre, and gloss)
3. imparts plasticity
4. assists emulsification and color development
5. provides calories, bulk (or body) to the diet
6. affects solubility of other ingredients
7. penetrates other ingredients (e.g. fruits and vegetables)
8. depresses freezing point (hence its use in ice cream); can be fermented, crystallized, and the crystal size controlled

Sucrose has many possible nonfood uses (103): fuels, explosives, elastomers, lubricants, solvents, soil conditioners, fibers, adhesives, paper, pesticides, plasticizers, plastics, surface coatings, and surfactants. Foods, however, constitute the greatest preponderance of the current market for sugar.

B. Beverage Crops

Beverages include many liquids or liquorous foods, such as coffee, tea, cocoa, soft drinks and alcohol-containing drinks. These may contain stimulants or flavoring agents. Soft drinks are non-alcoholic beverages containing syrup, essences or fruit concentrates mixed with water or carbonated water. The world production of sugar and beverage crops is shown in Table 26.

1. Botany and Origin

Coffee (*Coffea* spp.) is an evergreen shrub indigenous to central Africa and Asia. Three species of coffee are of commercial importance (104): *Coffea arabica*, which supplies the largest and best quality coffee beans; *Coffea robusta* (=*canephora*), which yields beans of lower quality, and *Cof-*

Table 26 Total World Production of Sugar and Beverage Crops (MMT)

Crops	1989	1990	1991	1992	1993	1994
Sugar (centrifuge, raw)	106.1	111.3	112.6	117.2	111.1	110.0
Cocoa beans	2.5	2.5	2.3	2.3	2.5	2.6
Coffee, green	6.0	6.1	6.1	6.0	6.0	5.4
Tea	2.4	2.5	3.0	2.4	2.6	2.6

Source: Ref. 4.

fea liberica, whose beans are of still lower quality. *Coffea arabica* is indigenous to Ethiopia and was introduced to India through Arabia. It is cultivated in southern parts of India. It is also grown in the American tropics, Brazil being the largest producer and exporter of Arabica coffee.

Tea (*Camellia sinensis*) is also an evergreen shrub growing wild in India and China. There are about 45 species of Camellia, of which *C. sinensis* is considered native to India and is commercially important. Commercial tea is obtained from plants propagated by seed sown in a nursery or through cuttings. Trees for plucking are pruned regularly to obtain a bush shape for maximum leaf production.

Cocoa (*Theobroma cocoa*) is a small tree native to the American tropics, but now grown in all tropical parts of the world. Like the jackfruit tree, the cocoa tree bears its flowers and subsequently its pods on the main trunk, as well as on the branches. Cocoa pods when mature are yellow or red in color. The pods (10–18 cm diameter) inside their thick leathery rinds contain 20 to 50 beans in rows. The seeds are embeded in white or pinkish pulp. The seeds are the principal source of cocoa or cocoa powder, highly prized as a nutritious beverage and chocolate used as food.

2. Production and Distribution

Whereas the world production of green coffee decreased from 1989–90 to 1994, that of cocoa beans and tea remained steady or increased slightly during this period (Table 27). These three beverage crops together had a production of around 10.6 MMT during 1994 on the global scale (Table 1). The chief cocoa-producing countries of the world are Ghana, Nigeria, Ivory Coast, and Brazil, whereas India and China are the major producers of tea and coffee.

3. Nutritional Composition and Quality

The flavor and bitter substances, and caffeine are primarily responsible to impart quality in making a good beverage. Caffeine in coffee beans is present both in the free and combined states. Its

Table 27 The World Production of Cocoa Beans, Coffee Green, and Tea from 1989 to 1994 (Figs. in 1000 MT)

Crop	1989	1990	1991	1992	1993	1994
Cocoa beans	2546	2538	2348	2373	2493	2564
Coffee green	5977	6125	6107	6032	5890	5430
Tea	2446	2543	2591	2439	2645	2623

Source: Ref. 4.

content in *C. arabica* varies from 1.0 to 1.2%. The caffeine content of a cup of coffee (150 ml) is about 100 mg. Caffeine is a stimulant, and its excess use causes undesirable effects on mind and physique. Symptoms of caffeinism may include sleep disturbance, frequent urination, muscular tension, jitteriness, and anxiety. The average nutritional composition of green and roasted *C. arabica* coffee beans, as reported in Wealth of India, Vol. II (1950), and compiled by Munay and Shadaksharaswamy (104) are as follows:

Nutritional constituent	*C. arabica* (green)	*C. arabica* (roasted)
Moisture	9.98[a]	0.63
Protein	9.87	11.23
Fat	12.60	13.59
Sugar	9.55	0.43
Dextrose	0.87	1.24
Ash	3.74	4.56
Caffeine	1.08	0.82
Chlorogenic acid	8.46	4.74

[a]Values in g per 100 g.

Several organic acids are present in the aqueous extract from green coffee beans, the predominant being chlorogenic acid and the least, acetic acid. During roasting, formic and acetic acids are increased and chlorogenic and others (citric, malic) are partially destroyed. The pH and acidity influence coffee flavor; the more acid-tasting the coffee, the better are its flavor and aroma. More than 600 volatile compounds have been identified in roasted coffee. Chlorogenic acid contributes to the body and astringency of the coffee beverage, and its decomposition products contribute to the aroma and flavor of coffee. Sucrose decomposition products are responsible for the color of the beverage and also to some extent the aroma, bitterness, and sourness. Protein decomposition compounds are the major precursors of coffee aroma. The phenolics (tannins) contribute to the bitterness of coffee.

The important chemical constituents of tea contributing to its flavor are caffeine, polyphenols, and essential oils. Munay and Shadaksharaswamy (104) stated the following values of fresh tea leaves: polyphenols, 22.2%; protein, 17.2%; caffeine, 4.3%; crude fiber, 27.0%; starch, 0.5%; and ash, 5.6%. Fresh tea leaves also contain carotenes, B vitamins, and ascorbic acid, which is lost during the manufacture of black tea.

Caffeine is mainly present in the bud and the first two leaves. Other compounds related to caffeine, viz., theophylline, theobromine, xanthine and hypoxanthine are also present in small quantities. Catechins and gallocatechins constitute the important polyphenols of tea leaves. These undergo changes during fermentation to black tea by polyphenol oxidases. Tea leaves contain a volatile oil, consisting of alcohols, aldehydes, phenols, and some fatty acids. These impart characteristic aroma and flavor to tea. Like coffee, tea also has no nutritive value. The proteins present in tea leaves are rendered insoluble in the processing. Whatever little nutritive value of tea the beverage has, comes from added milk and sugar. Tea as a beverage is consumed mainly for its stimulating value.

Processed cocoa beans have the following analysis (104): moisture, 2.13%; fat, 54.68%; total N, 2.16%; starch, 6.14%; pentosans, 11.19%; and tannins, 6.15%. The total nitrogen is from proteins, theobromine, and other related alkaloids. The theobromine content of cocoa is about 2.8%. Cocoa also contains about 0.6% caffeine. The proteins of cocoa are present in combination with polyphenols.

Unlike coffee and tea, which are strained forms of beverage, cocoa and chocolate remain in the beverage and contribute to the nutritive value of the beverage. Because of their high fat content, cocoa products are a rich source of energy. Milk, a usual constituent of cocoa and chocolate drinks, adds to the nutritive value of the beverage. Both theobromine and caffeine contribute to the stimulating effect of cocoa beverages.

C. Fruit Beverages

The beverage industry is the largest outlet for fruit juices and concentrates, absorbing about 80% of the production. Different types of beverages, such as fruit juices, fruit drinks, squashes, cardinals, and fruit punches are used. *Fruit juice* is a natural juice pressed out of a fruit and is unaltered in its composition during its preparation and preservation. *Fruit drinks* are made by liquefying the whole fruit and at least 10% of the volume of undiluted drink must be the whole fruit. It may be diluted before being served. *Fruit squash* consists essentially of strained juice containing moderate amount of fruit pulp to which sugar is added for sweetening (e.g., orange squash, lemon squash, mango squash, etc.). *Fruit cordial* is a fruit squash from which all suspended material is completely removed and is a clear liquid (e.g., lime juice cordial). *Fruit punches* are made by mixing the desired fruit juices at the time of serving. *Fruit juice concentrate* is the fruit juice that has been concentrated by removing water, either by heat or freeze drying. *Sherbets* are cooled drinks of sweetened diluted fruit juices.

Fruit juices are highly nutritive beverages and are rich in vitamins, minerals, and other nutrients. Besides, they are delicious and have a universal appeal for their taste, aroma, flavor, and color, when freshly expressed.

D. Soft Drinks

These constitute one of the largest food industries in the world. The flavored components of most of the renowned soft drink brands are well-guarded trade secrets. The most popular soft drinks sold today are "cola" (an extract from the tree cola), orange, root beer, ginger, lemon, and lime. The soft drinks are grouped into three classes: carbonated, fruit flavored (still), and sparkling (soda water). The carbonated beverages in turn are of two types: those with artificial flavor, and those with natural fruit juice.

The major ingredients of soft drinks are sweeteners, flavor emulsion and cloudifiers, coloring agents, acids and preservatives, water, and carbon dioxide. The quality of a soft drink depends on a balanced blend of flavor at the proper intensity, leaving a clean mouth taste with no lingering flavor or unpleasant aftertaste. It should have proper carbonation to impart zest and sparkle to the drink.

E. Alcoholic Beverages

Alcoholic beverages have been known to humankind since antiquity. They are judged in terms of flavor and stimulating effects, rather than as sources of calories, though alcohol gives about 7 kcal/g. The distilled liquors, such as whisky, brandy, gin, and rum have their caloric value only due to alcohol, whereas beers and wines contain some nutrients present in the original malted barley and the fruit juice used to make wine. Thus the energy value of beers and wines is higher than the distilled liquors.

Though alcohol is absorbed without prior digestion, the body has limited capacity to oxidize it. The effects of alcohol vary from mild stimulation to loss of coordination and even death, when consumed in large amounts.

Alcohol beverages may be divided into three types: wines, malted beverages (beer), and distilled liquors. Different starting materials and methods are used in the manufacture of these beverages. However, they are all made by the process of fermentation, whereby glucose is converted into alcohol by the yeast enzyme.

V. SPICE CROPS

Spices play an important role in the human diet. A diet containing all the nutritive components required by the body may be quite insipid without spices. To make a diet palatable, food should have flavor: It has to be seasoned by adding flavoring agents, which include spices and condiments. The spices and condiments have not been classified clearly, according to the International Organization of Standardization. The term *spice* or *condiment* applies to "such natural plant or vegetable products or mixtures thereof, in whole or ground form, as are used to impart flavor, aroma and piquancy to and for seasoning food."

Of about 70 species of spices and condiments grown in different parts of the world, many varieties of spices are grown in India. India has been "home land of spices" for many centuries and spices constitute an important place in its national economy. Manay and Shadaksharaswamy (104) classified spices based on the origin and presence of active principle as follows:

1. Pungent spices—pepper, ginger, mustard, and chilies
2. Aromatic fruits—cardamom, nutmeg and mace, fenugreek, anise, fennel, caraway, dill, celery, cumin, and coriander.
3. Aromatic barks—cinnamon, cassia
4. Phenolic spices containing eugenol—clove, allspice (pimento)
5. Colored spices—paprika, saffron, and turmeric

Spices are used as flavoring agents in a number of foods such as curries, soups, bakery products, pickles, processed meats, beverages, and liqueurs. Spices may enhance or vary food flavors. They are also used as flavor disguisers, i.e., they help to mask the off-flavor of certain foods. Some spices have antioxidant properties, while others are used as preservatives in foods such as pickles and *chutney*. Spices such as cloves and mustard possess strong antimicrobial property, thus preventing food spoilage. Spices have been used to preserve highly perishable fish and meat products for long periods. Many spices also possess vital physiological and medicinal properties.

Of the various spices available, only nine species, viz., pepper, ginger, cloves, cinnamon, cassia, mace, nutmeg, pimento, and cardamom, together contribute to over 90% of the total world trade in spices. The major spices of India include pepper, cardamom, ginger, turmeric and chilies, forming about 85% of the total export of spices. The important minor spices grown in India are ajowan, aniseed, caraway, coriander, cumin, dill seeds, fennel, fenugreek, garlic, onion, saffron, and vanilla.

A. Pepper (Black, White, and Green)

Black pepper, *Piper nigrum* or *kali mirch*, is the dried, mature but unripe fruit (berry) of a perennial climbing vine cultivated as a plantation crop. It is considered as "king of spices," because it is the largest used spice in the domestic and industrial sectors. Pepper is obtained by harvesting the spikes when the fruits are fully mature and start becoming yellowish. The berries are removed from the spikes by rubbing, threshing, or trampling and are sun-dried for a few days. When dry, the outer skin of the berries turns dark brown to black and gets shrivelled. Before drying, if the berries are heat-treated (boiling water for 2 min.), a glossy uniform black product is obtained after drying, because the heat treatment arrests enzyme activity and the dried product has better keeping quality and a fresher aroma.

Indian black pepper has the following nutritional composition (104): moisture, 8.7–14.0%; total nitrogen, 1.55–2.6%; ether extract (volatile plus non volatile), 4.2–16.7%; carbohydrates (starch), 28.0–49.0%; crude fiber, 8.7–14.0%; and ash, 3.5–5.7%. A major portion of the nitrogen in pepper is nonprotein nitrogen in the form of alkaloids. The spice value of pepper is primarily due to the presence of about 4 to 5% of a group of alkaloids, piperine and related compounds (chavicine, piperidine, and piperettine). In addition to the pungent constituents, pepper also contains about 2.5% volatile oil (pepper oil), having approximately 95% terpene hydrocarbons and about 4% oxygenated terpenes, which are responsible for the oil color.

White pepper is also obtained from *P. nigrum* by harvesting ripe berries, yellowish red or red in colour. White pepper is prepared by removing the outer coating of seeds either before or after drying. White pepper has less flavor and pungency than black pepper.

Green pepper is obtained by harvesting immature berries and canning them in brine or vinegar. Dehydrated green pepper is also produced for export purposes. Bottled green pepper is used to garnish meat dishes in the Western countries.

Long pepper (*Piper longum*) is derived from wild plants grown in northern parts of India. It contains alkaloids with a pungent taste and an essential oil with a spicy odor resembling that of pepper and ginger oils. Long pepper is used as a spice in pickles and preserves. It is also used to relieve certain bodily ailments.

B. Cardamom (*Elettaria cardamomum*)

These are dried ripe fruits of *E. cardamomum*. Two distinct varieties, based on fruit size, are recognized: *E. cardamomum*, var. *major*, comprising wild, indigenous cardamom of Sri Lanka, and *E. cardamomum*, var. *minor*, indigenous to India, cultivated in southern parts of India. The Indian cardamom seeds have the following nutritional composition (104): moisture, 7.0–10.0%; ether extract, 7.5–15.0%; protein, 7.0–14.0%; carbohydrates, 39.0–49.0%; ash, 3.8–6.9%; calcium, 0.3%; phosphorus, 0.4%; thiamin, 1.8 mg/100 g; riboflavin, 0.23 mg/100 g; niacin, 2.3 mg/100 g; and vitamin A, 175 I.U.

The spice value of cardamom depends on the volatile oils (2–10%) present in the seeds. Cardamom oil of commerce is obtained by distilling seeds or whole fruits. The major constituents of cardamom oil are the terpenes—cineol, terpenoil, terpinene, limonene, sabinine, and terpinyl acetate, which determines the quality of cardamom oil.

Cardamom seeds have a pleasant aroma and characteristic pungent taste. They are used as a spice and in medicine. Cardamom seeds are common ingredients of curry powder, cakes, and several confectioneries.

C. Ginger (*Zinger officinate*)

Ginger is the dried underground stem or rhizome of the zingiberous herbaceous plant. The irregular rhizomes are formed at a shallow depth in the soil. Major ginger-producing countries are India, Taiwan, Jamaica, Nigeria, and Malaysia. The tender rhizome, sold as green ginger, is used in preserves and pickles. Dry ginger is made by treating rhizomes with lime and sulfur dioxide after drying.

The nutritional composition of Indian dry ginger is as follows (104): moisture, 6.9%; protein, 8.6%; fat, 6.4%; fiber, 5.9%; carbohydrates, 66.5%; and ash, 5.7%. Ginger contains 1 to 3% essential oil (oil of ginger) with a characteristic pleasant odor. The major constituents of ginger oil are monoterpenes (4%), sesquiterpenes (65%), and oxygenated terpenes (17%). The pungent principles of ginger are nonvolatile and can be extracted from ground, dried spice with organic solvents. The ginger oleoresin, known as 'gingerine', contains essential oils and the non-pungent matter includes carbohydrates and palmitic and other fatty acids. The pungent substances are oxymethyl phenols, such as gingerol, shagaol and related compounds.

Ginger is used in dried, preserved and green forms as a flavoring agent in curry powders, confectioneries, pickles, soft drinks and carbonated drinks (gingerella, ginger beer). It is also used to make oleoresin and essential oils.

D. Chilies (*Capsicum annum*)

Chilies (red pepper) are fruits of the plant species belonging to the genus *Capsicum*. Chilies are a common and indispensable ingredient of Indian food. Chili crop was introduced to India from its native home, Brazil and South America. *Capsicum annum* and *C. fruitescens* are the main two species. The former is an annual, growing flowers singly in the leaf axils. The ripe fruits are generally red but also may be yellow or orange. The long and thin to round or oblong varieties having thin, smooth pericarp are highly pungent and used as spice in the preparation of hot foods. The larger bell-shaped fruits with thick pericarp (bell pepper) are less or non-pungent and used as vegetables in salads and pickles (e.g., paprika).

The nutritional composition of Indian red chilies is as follows (104): moisture, 10.0%; protein, 15.0%; fat, 6.2%; fiber, 30.2%; carbohydrates, 31.6%; ash, 6.1%; calcium, 0.16%; phosphorus, 0.37%; and iron, 0.23%. The chili powder, on extraction with an organic solvent, gives a fatty oil (9–13%) which is viscous and red with a sharp pungent taste. Volatile oil (0.16–0.39%), is obtained on steam distillation. Chili seeds have about 26% oil, and the protein content of fat- and moisture-free seeds is around 29%.

The pungent principle of chilies is an alkaloid, capsaicin, which retains its pungency even in dilution. Chilies contain high amounts of vitamin C, which varies with the variety, locality, and stage of fruit maturity. Dry chili is used as a spice in different curried dishes and in curry powder made by grinding roasted dry chilies with other spices such as coriander, cumin, and turmeric.

Chili helps digestion and stimulates the taste buds, resulting in increased flow of salivary amylase. Paprika and green chili are good sources of vitamins A and C. Chilies are also used in medicines.

E. Turmeric (*Curcuma longa*)

Turmeric belongs to the ginger family. Of about 70 turmeric species, *C. longa* is the most important cultivated variety (96% of the cultivated area), whereas *C. aromatica* accounts for 4% of the area under cultivation (kasturi turmeric). The cured turmeric has a sweet fragrance and is largely used to make bathing powders, bathing oils, and toilet soaps.

The turmeric rhizomes, like ginger, are cured for the development of color and aroma. The rhizomes are cooked in water, limewater, or soda bicarbonate solution, and the soft, cooked rhizomes are sun-dried, cleaned, and polished mechanically in rotary drums. The cured and finished product is brittle and has a striking yellow color.

The nutritional composition of Indian turmeric has the following values (104): moisture, 5.8%; protein, 8.6%; fat, 8.9%; carbohydrates 63.0%; fiber, 6.9%; ash, 6.8%; calcium, 0.2%; phosphorus, 0.26%; and iron, 0.05%. The vitamin content of turmeric (mg/100 g) is thiamin, 0.09; riboflavin, 0.19, niacin, 4.9, and vitamin A, 175 IU/100g.

Turmeric gives 1.5% essential oil on steam distillation. It consists of 56% of sesquiterpene ketones (termerones) and 9% tertiary alcohol. An oleoresin containing all the aroma and flavor of turmeric can be obtained on solvent extraction, followed by removal of solvent. It has a great value in food and pharmaceutical industries. Curcumin pigment gives turmeric its yellow color.

Turmeric powder is used as a flavoring agent and a colorant in many foods to give them agreeable flavor and color. It is a constituent of curry powder and prepared mustards. It is also used for dyeing wool, silk, and cotton. Turmeric is an antioxidant and has germicidal properties. Thus, it finds a use in cosmetics and medicines.

F. Minor Herbs and Spices

1. *Garlic and Onion* (Allium *sp.*)

Garlic is a bulb made up of several cloves enclosed within white or pink skin of the parent bulb. Garlic (*Allium sativum*) and onion (*A. cepa*) are grown virtually all over the world for flavoring various dishes and used in various food preparations such as *chutneys*, pickles, curry powders, curried vegetables, meat preparations, and so forth. Garlic and onion flavors are less appreciated by some people. Both garlic and onion have a strong flavor due to sulfur-containing allicin, which is formed from the odorless alliin, viz., S-2-propenyl (allyl) cysteine sulfoxide (in garlic) and S-1-propenyl cysteine sulfoxide (in onion) by the action of the enzyme allinase. The allicin undergoes nonenzymatic decomposition to disulfide and thiosulfinate. The disulfide further decomposes to give a mixture of mono- and tri-sulfide in garlic. In onion. the precursor, S-1-propenyl cysteine sulfoxide, is cleaved to form unstable propenyl-sulfenic acid which rearranges to synthesize thiopropanal-S-oxide, the lachrymatory factor.

Garlic has antibacterial and anti-insecticide activity and is a remedy for a number of ailments and physiological disorders. It has been reported to decrease serum cholesterol and reduce hypertension (see Chapters 24 and 25).

Onions of different varieties (white, yellow, red of various sizes and shapes) differ in their pungency. They are eaten raw, fried, boiled or roasted, in soups, curries and a variety of other savory dishes as well as in pickles and *chutneys*. The dehydrated garlic and onions (powder, flakes) are also used as flavoring agents.

2. *Fenugreek* (Trigonella foenum-graecum)

Fenugreek (*methi*) is a dried ripe fruit of an annual herb, native of south east Europe and West Asia. Fresh tender leaves and shoots of fenugreek are rich in minerals (Ca, P, and Fe) and vitamins A and C, and are eaten as vegetables. Fenugreek seeds are small, hard, smooth and oblong and yellowish brown in color, and contain protein, starch, sugars, mucilage, volatile oil, nonvolatile oil, vitamins, enzymes, and minerals. In addition to flavor, fenugreek thus adds to the nutritive value of foods. It is a constituent of curry powder. The seeds possess medicinal properties.

3. *Mustard* (Brassica nigra)

The spice value of mustard seeds is the result of the thiocyanates present in them as glycosides, which are released by an enzyme in presence of water under suitable conditions. The dried whole seeds of mustard are used in pickles and preserves and for seasoning vegetables.

4. *Cinnamon* (Cinnamomum zelanicum)

Cinnamon (*dalchini*) is the inner bark of the young shoots of cinnamon tree. The quality of cinnamon depends upon the length, breadth, and thickness of the bark. The bark has 0.5 to 1.0% volatile oil and is used as a spice in the form of small pieces or powder. It is aromatic, astringent, and stimulatory and used for flavoring confectionery, liquors, pharmaceuticals, soaps, and dental preparations.

5.   Mace and Nutmeg (Myristica fragrance)

Mace and nutmeg (*Jaipatri* and *Jaiphal*) are two species of the same tree, *M. fragrance*, which is native to Indonesia. The ripe, fleshy fruit splits to expose the mace as a scarlet fleshy covering, the aril enclosing in a network the seed (nutmeg). This mace is carefully removed, flattened and dried; it turns brown during drying. The nutmeg is also dried. Both the mace and nutmeg contain the volatile oil (4–15% in mace and 7–16% in nutmeg), which in turn contains 93% terpenes and 7% aromatics (mace), and 84% terpenes and 11% aromatics (nutmeg). Nutmeg yields 24 to 30% nonvolatile oil (nutmeg butter). Both mace and nutmeg are used as flavoring agents in foods (savory and sweet dishes). The volatile oil is also used for flavoring foods, and in dental preparations, essences, confectionery, vegetables dishes, and beverages. Both have medicinal properties and are used as drugs.

6.   Saffron (Crocus sativus)

Saffron (*kesar*) consists of the rich gold or yellowish red stigmas of the flower of *C. sativus* plant. Spain and France produce saffron in large quantities, followed by India. Saffron is used as a spice or dye (saffron yellow), a cosmetic, and a medicine. It contains a glycoside, crocin, which is its coloring principle. The flavor and spice value of saffron are due to its content of volatile (1.4%) and nonvolatile (13.4%) oils, respectively.

7.   Mint (Mentho arvensis)

Mint (*pudina*) is an aromatic herb. It is an important source of peppermint oil and menthol. Leaves are steam-distilled to obtain a golden yellow volatile oil. On cooling, about 50% of menthol gets separated. After removing menthol, the remaining oil is used as peppermint oil for flavoring mouthwashes and toothpastes, and in pharmaceuticals and medicines. Mint in India is also popularly used in the preparation of *chutneys*.

8.   Cloves (Eugenia caryophyllus)

Cloves (*lavang*) are flower buds of the clove tree. When the base of the flower buds turns reddish, they are harvested and dried. Clove is the second most important spice crop of the world from the commercial point of view, after the pepper. Tanzania alone produces over 80% of the world crop.
       Clove buds contain 16 to 17% essential oil, of which about 90 to 95% is eugenol. The spice value of clove is the result of its volatile oil. Both whole and ground clove powder are ingredients of spice mixtures. Clove oil has medicinal properties and is used in toothpastes.

9.   Vanilla (Vanilla flagrans)

Vanilla is native to eastern Mexico and Brazil. The fruit (pods) is a long bean containing small, hard, black seeds. The pods are cured by dipping them in boiling water, followed by long, slow drying process. During drying, the enzyme beta-glucosidase hydrolyzes the glycoside, vanillin, to form vanilla with a strong aromatic flavor. The beans are cut into small pieces and extracted with dilute alcohol to produce vanilla essence. Vanilla is used to flavor various confectioneries, puddings, ice creams, and salads. Natural vanilla contains other useful aromatic substances in addition to vanilla.

10.   Asafoetida (Ferula asafoetida)

Asafoetida (*hing*) is a gum resin exuded from the rhizome of several species of *Ferula*. It contains gum, resin, and essential oil in varying proportions that are together responsible for the strong flavor. Therefore, in trade, compounded asafoetida is marketed using flour of corn, wheat, barley, and gum as diluent. The steam volatile organic sulfur compounds predominantly contribute to the characteristic odor of asafoetida. It is popularly used to flavor curries, sauces, and pickles in combination with other spices. Asafoetida also has several medicinal properties and is used in Ayurvedic and allopathic medicines.

11. Ajowan, Coriander, and Cumin

Ajowan or bishop's weed or *omum* (*Trachy-spermum ammi*), aniseed or *vilaiti saunf (Pimpinella anisum)*, carawy or *shia jira (Carum carvi)*, celery (*Apium guaveolens*), coriander (*dhania*) (*Coriandrum sativum*), cumin (*jira*) (*Cuminium cymimum*), dill (*Anethum sowa*), and fennel (*saunf*) (*Faeniculum vulgare*) are the minor herbs and spices of India, all belonging to the family *Umbelliferae*. The seeds of all these herbs are used as spices for culinary purposes. They contain essential oils that are used as flavoring material in medicines and in toilet soaps. Celery leaves and stalks are also used as salads, in soups and appetizers. The stem, leaves, and fruits of coriander give a pleasant aromatic odor. The entire plant, when young, may be used for flavoring curries and soups. Coriander seeds are a constituent of curry powder, pickling spices, sausages, and seasonings. Young dill leaves are used to flavor soups and sauces.

12. Allspice or Pimento

Allspice consists of dried, unripe berries, reddish brown in color. Allspice is said to possess the characteristic flavor and aroma of cloves, nutmeg, cinnamon, and black pepper, all combined in one spice, hence the name allspice.

The allspice tree is indigenous to the West Indies and tropical Central America. The characteristic odor of allspice is due to its essential oil (3.3–4.5%). It also contains an acid, responsible for the astringency, a soft resin with a burning taste, nonvolatile oil (5–8%), proteins (5–8%), starch (20%), and traces of alkaloids.

The berries are used as a flavoring ingredient in ketchup, soups, sauces, pickles, and meat. It is also an important ingredient of spice mixtures of curry powders and mincemeat spice. The berry oil is rich in eugenol (65–80%) and is used for flavoring a variety of food products and in perfumery.

REFERENCES

1. Salunke, D.K., and S.S. Deshpande, eds. *Foods of Plant Origin: Production Technology and Human Nutrition*, New York, Van Nostrand Reinhold, 1991, p. 1.
2. FAO, Production Yearbook, Rome: Food and Agriculture Organization, 1988.
3. FAO, Yearbook of Fishery Statistics, Rome: Food and Agriculture Organization, 1988.
4. FAO, Production Yearbook, Rome: Food and Agriculture Organization, 1994.
5. Deshpande, S.S., and S. Damodaran, Food legumes: Chemistry and technology, *Adv. Cereal Sci. Technol. 10*: 147 (1990).
6. Borlaug, N.E., Using plants to meet world food needs, *Future Dimensions of World Food and Population*, R. G. Woods, ed., Boulder, Westview Press, 1981, p. 101.
7. Cramer, H.H., *Plant Protection and World Crop Production*, Bayer Pflanzenschutz, Leverkusen (West Germany), 1967.
8. Salunkhe, D.K., and B.B. Desai, *Postharvest Biotechnology of Fruits*, Vol. 1 and 2, CRC Press, Boca Raton, Florida, 1984a.
9. Salunkhe, D.K. and B.B. Desai, *Postharvest Biotechnology of Vegetables*, Vol. 1 and 2, CRC Press, Boca Raton, Florida, 1984b.

10. Salunkhe, D.K., and B.B. Desai, *Postharvest Biotechnology of Oilseeds*, CRC Press, Boca Raton, Florida, 1986.

11. Salunkhe, D.K., and B.B. Desai, *Postharvest Biotechnology of Sugar Crops*, CRC Press Boca Raton, Florida, 1988.

12. Salunkhe, D.K., J.K. Chavan, and S.S. Kadam, *Postharvest Biotechnology of Cereals*, CRC Press, Boca Raton, Florida, 1985a.

13. Salunkhe, D.K., S.S. Kadam, and J.K. Chavan, *Postharvest Biotechnology of Food Legumes*, CRC Press, Boca Raton, Florida (USA), 1985b.

14. Deshpande, S.S., B.B. Singh, and U. Singh, Cereals, *Foods of Plant Origin: Production, Technology and Human Nutrition*, Van Nostrand Reinhold, New York, 1991, p. 6.

15. Frey, K.J., Breeding approaches for increasing crop yields, *Cereal Production* (E.J. Gallagher, ed.) Butterworths, London, 1984, p. 47.

16 Riggs, T.J., P.R. Hanson, N.D. Start, D.M. Miles, C.L. Morgan and M.A. Ford, Comparison of spring barley varieties grown in England and Wales between 1960 and 1980, *J. Agric. Sci.* (Cambridge) *97*: 599 (1981).

17. USDA, *Agricultural Statistics*, Washington, D.C. U.S.G.P.O., 1989.

18. Brouk, B., *Plants Consumed by Man*, Academic Press, London, 1975.

19. Langer, R.H.M., and G.D. Hill, *Agricultural Plants*, Cambridge Univ. Press, Cambridge, 1982.

20. Jung, G.A., *Crop Tolerance to Suboptimal Land Conditions*, Am. Soc. Agron. Madison, 1978.

21. Hanson, A.A., *Practical Handbook of Agricultural Science*, CRC Press, Boca Raton, 1990.

22. Evans, L.T., I.F. Wardlaw, Aspects of the comparative physiology of grain yield in cereals, *Adv. Agron. 28*: 301 (1976).

23. Pomeranz, Y., *Modern Cereal Science and Technology*, VCH Publishers, New York, 1987.

24. Harlan, J.R., Agricultural origins: Centers and noncenters, *Science 174*: 468 (1971).

25. Ross, W., and J.D. Eastin, Grain sorghum in the USA, *Field Crop Abstr. 25*: 169 (1972).

26. Lorenz, K., Rye: Utilization and processing, *Handbook of Processing and Utilization in Agriculture*, Vol.II pt.II: *Plant Products* (A. Wolff, ed.), CRC Press, Boca Raton, 1982, p. 243.

27. Simmonds, D.H., Structure, composition and biochemistry of cereal grains, *Cereals '78: Better Nutrition for the World's Millions* (Y. Pomeranz, ed.), Am. Assoc. Cereal Chem., St. Paul, 1978, p. 105.

28. Watt, B.K. and A.L. Merrill, *Composition of Foods: Raw, Processed and Prepared*, Agric. Handbook No. 8, USDA, Washington, D.C. 1963.

29. Lockhart, H.B., and R.O. Nesheim, Nutritional quality of cereal grains, *Cereals '78: Better Nutrition for the World's Millions* (Y. Pomeranz, ed.) Am. Assoc. Cereal Chem., St. Paul, 1978, p. 201.

30. Mattern, P.J., J.W. Schmidt, and V.A. Johnson, Screening for high-lysine content in wheat, *Cereal Sci. Today. 15*: 409 (1970).

31. Bressani, R., and E.T. Mertz, Studies on corn proteins. Protein and amino acid content of different corn varieties, *Cereal Chem. 35*: 227 (1958).

32. Croy, R.R.D., and J.A. Gatehouse, Genetic engineering of seed proteins: Current and potential applications, *Plant Genetic Engineering* (J.H. Dodds, ed.), Cambridge Univ. Press, Cambridge, 1985, p. 143.

33. Hopkins, D.T., *Protein Quality in Humans: Assessment and Evaluation*, AVI Publ. Co., Westport, 1981.

34. Bressani, R. Legumes in human diets and how they might be improved, *Nutritional Improvement of Food Legumes by Breeding* (M. Milner, ed.), Wiley, New York, 1975, p. 15.

35. Reddy, N.R., S.K. Sathe, and D.K. Salunkhe, Phytates in legumes and cereals, *Adv. Food Res. 28*: 1 (1982).

36. Nelson, T.S., L.W. Ferrara, and N.L. Storer, Phytate phosphorus content of feed ingredients derived from plants, *Poultry Sci. 47*: 1372 (1968).

37. Lasztity, R., and L. Lasztity, Phytic acid in cereal technology, *Adv. Cereal Sci. Technol. 10*: 309 (1990).

38. Deshpande, S.S., S.K. Sathe, and D.K. Salunkhe, Chemistry and safety of plant polyphenols, *Nutritional and Metabolic Aspects of Food Safety* (M. Friedman, ed.), Plenum, New York, 1984, p. 457.

39. Deshpande, S.S., M. Cheryan, and D.K. Salunkhe, Tannin analysis of food products, *CRC Crit. Rev. Food Sci. Nutr. 24*: 401 (1986).

40. Rockland, L.B., and D.M. Hahn, Quick-cooking grain legumes: An alternative food processing technology, Paper presented at FAO/UN Expert Consultation of Grain Legume Processing, 14–18 Nov, 1977, Central Food Technol. Res. Inst. Mysore, India, 1977.

41. Powel, A.A., S. Matthews, and M. de A. Oliveira, Seed quality in grain legumes, *Adv. Appl. Biol. 10*: 217 (1984).

42. Deshpande, U.S., and S.S. Deshpande, Legumes, *Foods of Plant Origin: Production, Technology, and Human Nutrition* (D.K. Salunkhe and S.S. Deshpande, eds.), Van Nostrand Reinhold, New York, 1991, p. 137.

43. Hellendoorn, E.W., Beneficial physiological activity of leguminous seeds, *Qual. Plant. Plant Foods Hum. Nutr.*, *29*: 227 (1979).

44. Salunkhe, D.K., Legumes in human nutrition: Current status and future research needs, *Curr. Sci.* (Bangalore), *51*: 387 (1983).

45. Smartt, J., *Tropical Pulses*, Longman, London, 1976.

46. Delwiche, C.C., Legumes: Past present and future, *Bioscience 28*: 565 (1978).

47. Smartt, J., and T. Hymowitz, Domestication and evaluation of grain legumes, *Grain Legume Crops* (R.J. Summerfield and E.N. Roberts, eds.), Collins, London, 1985, p. 37.

48. Hutchinson, J.B., The evolutionary diversity of the pulses, *Proc. Nutr. Soc. 29*: 49 (1969).

49. Adams, M.W., and J.J. Pipoly, Biological structure, classification and distribution of economic legumes, *Advances in Legume Science* (R.J. Summerfield and A.H. Bunting, eds.), Royal Botanic Gardens, Kew, 1980, p. 1.

50. Isely, D., Leguminosae and *Homo Sapiens*, *Econ. Bot. 36*: 46 (1982).

51. Desai, B.B., and D.K. Salunkhe, Fruits and vegetables, *Foods of Plant Origin: Production, Technology and Human Nutrition* (D.K. Salunkhe and S.S. Deshpande, eds.) Van Nostrand Reinhold, New York, 1991, p. 301.

52. Samson, J.A., *Tropical Fruits*, 2nd ed., Tropical Agric. Series, Longman, London, 1986.

53. Pantastico, E.B., and O.K. Bautista, Postharvest handling of tropical vegetable crops, *Horti. Science. 11*: 22 (1976).

54. Duckworth, R.B., *Fruits and Vegetables*, Pergamon Press, Oxford, 1966.

55. Hall, N.T., J.M. Smoot, R.J. Knight, and S. Nagy, Protein and amino acid compositions of ten tropical fruits by gas-liquid chromatography, *J. Agric. Food Chem. 28*: 1217 (1980).

56. Nagy, S., and P.E. Shaw, *Tropical and Subtropical Fruits*, AVI Publ. Co., Westport, 1980.

57. White, P.L., Challenge for the future: Nutritional quality of fruits and vegetables, *Hort. Science. 14*: 257 (1979).

58. Goddard, M.S., and R.H. Matthews, Contribution of fruits and vegetables to human nutrition, *Hort. Science 14*: 245 (1979).

59. Hansen, R.G., B.W. Wyse, and A.W. Sorenson, *Nutritional Quality Index of Foods*, AVI Publ. Co., Westport, 1979.

60. Pao, S.K., and G.G. Dull, Assessment of nutritive value, quality and stability of cruciferous vegetables during storage and subsequent processing, *Storage, Processing and Nutritional Quality of Fruits and Vegetables* (D.K. Salunkhe, ed.), CRC Press, Boca Raton, 1974, p. 1.

61. Heinz, M., *Handbook of Nutrition*, McGraw-Hill, New York, 1959.

62. Purseglove, J.W., *Tropical Crops: Dicotyledons, Monocotyledons*, Longman, London, 1968.

63. Okuse, I., and K. Ryugo, Compositional changes in the developing 'Hayword' kiwi fruit in California, *J. Amer. Soc. Hortic. Sci. 106*: 73 (1981).

64. Arriola, M.C. de, J.F. Calzada, J.F. Menchu, C. Rolz, and R. Garcia, Papaya, *Tropical and Subtropical Fruits* (S. Nagy and P.E. Shaw, eds.). AVI Pub. Co., Westport, 1980, p. 316.

65. Askar, A., A. El-Tamini and M. Raouf, Constituents of mango fruits and their behavior during growth and ripening, *Mitt. Rebe Wein, Fruchteverwert. 22*: 120 (1972).

66. Thornton, N.C., CO_2 storage. XIV. Influence of CO_2, O_2 and ethylene on the vitamin C content of ripening bananas, *Contrib. Boyce Thompson Inst. 13*: 201 (1943).

67. Arriola, M.C. de, J.F. Menchu, and C. Rolz, *Characterization, Handling and Storage of Some Tropical Fruits*, Central Amer. Res. Inst. For Industry (ICAITI), Guatemala (Spanish), 1976.

68. Asenjo, C.F., and C.G. Moscoso, Ascorbic acid content and other characteristics of the West Indian Cherry, *Food Res. 15*: 103 (1950).

69. Harding, P.L., and M.P. Sunday, Seasonal changes in Florida tangerines, *USDA Tech. Bull. No. 753.* USDA, Washington, D.C. 1949.

70. John, C.J., C. Subbarayan, and H.R. Cama, Carotenoids in mango (*Mangifera indica*) fruit, *Indian J. Chem. 1*: 36 (1963).

71. Hsu, J.W., Seasonal variations of thiamin in citrus juices, Florida Dept. of Citrus (Unpublished), 1974.

72. Peynaud, E., and P. Ribereau-Gayon, The grape, *The Biochemistry of Fruits and Their Products.* Vol. 2, (A.C. Hulme, ed.), Academic Press, New York, 1971, p. 172.

73. Ting, S.V., J.A. Attaway, E.J. Deszyck and W.F. Newhall, Nutrient assay of Florida frozen concentrated orange juice for nutrition labeling, *Proc. Fla State Hortic. Soc. 87*: 206 (1974).

74. Varsel, C., Citrus juice processing as related to quality and nutrition, *Citrus Nutrition and Quality*, Am. Chem. Soc. Symp. Ser. No. 143, American Chemical Society, Washington DC, 1980, p. 225.

75. Hall, A.P., A.F. Morgan and P. Wheeler, The amount of six B-vitamins in fruits and dried figs, *Food Res. 18*: 206 (1953).

76. Ghosh, S., The content of folic acid and its conjugates in some common Indian fruits, *Sci. Cult. 26*: 287 (1960).

77. Hall, A.P., J.F. More, and A.F. Morgan, B-vitamin content of California grown avocados, *J. Agric. Food Chem. 3*: 250 (1955).

78. Hulme, A.C. (ed.), *The Biochemistry of Fruits and Their Products.* Vol. 2, Academic Press, New York, 1971.

79. Mapson, L.W., Vitamins in fruits, *The Biochemistry of Fruits and Their Products.* Vol. 1 (A.C. Hulme, ed.), Academic Press, New York, 1971, p. 369.

80. Nagy, S., and P.E. Shaw, *Tropical and Subtropical Fruits*, AVI Publ. Co., Westport, 1980.

81. Polansky, M.M., and E.W. Murphy, Vitamin B_6 components in fruits and nuts, *J. Am. Diet. Assoc. 48*: 109 (1966).

82. Salunkhe, D.K., and B.B. Desai, Effects of agricultural practices, handling, processing and storage on vegetables, *Nutritional Evaluation of Food Processing* 3rd ed. (E. Karmas and R.S. Harris, eds.), AVI/Van Nostrand Reinhold, New York, 1988, p. 23.

83. Salunkhe, D.K., S.K. Pao, and G.G. Dull, Assessment of nutritive value, quality and stability of cruciferous vegetables during storage and subsequent processing, *Storage, Processing and Nutritional Quality of Fruits and Vegetables* (D.K. Salunkhe, ed.), CRC Press, Boca Raton, 1974, p. 1.

84. Vittum, M.T., Effects of fertilizers on the quality of vegetables, *Agron. J. 55*: 425 (1963).

85. Rick, C.M., The tomato, *Sci. Amer. 239*: 66 (1978).

86. Platt, B.S., *Table of Representative Values of Foods Commonly Used in Tropical Countries*, Medical Research Council, Special Rep. Ser. No. 302, HMSO, London, 1962.

87. Paul, A.A. and D.A.T. Southgate, Dietary fiber, *The Composition of Foods.* 4th ed. (R.A. McCance and E.M. Widdowson, eds.), HMSO, London, 1978, p. 162.

88. Tindall, H.D., and F.J. Proctor, Loss prevention of horticultural crops in the tropics, *Progr. Food Nutr. Sci. 4*: 25 (1980).

89. FAO, *Food Composition Table for Use in East Asia*, U.S. Dept. of Health, Education and Welfare, Washington, D.C. and F.A.O., Rome, 1972.

90. Wills, R.B.H., T.H. Lee, D. Graham, W.B. McGlasson, and E.G. Hall, *Postharvest: An Introduction to the Physiology and Handling of Fruits and Vegetables*, Granada, London, 1981.

91. USDA, *Agriculture Handbook No. 8*, United States Dept. Agriculture, Washington, D.C. 1963.

92. Gopala Rao, P.I., K. Mallikarjuna, and G. Gururaja Rao, Nutritional evaluation of some green leafy vegetables, *Indian J. Nutr. Diet. 17*: 9 (1980).

93. Crosby, D.G., Natural choline storage inhibitors in food, *Toxicants Occurring Naturally in Foods*, National Academy of Sciences, National Research Council, Washington, D.C., 1966, p. 112.

94. Singleton, V.L., and F.H. Kratzer, Plant Phenolics, *Toxicants Occurring Naturally in Foods*, 2nd ed., National Academy of Sciences, National Research Council, Washington, DC, 1973, p. 309.

95. Sreeja, V.G., and S. Leelamma, Hyperglycemic effect of low protein cassava diet, *Indian J. Exp. Biol. 38*: 308 (1998).

96. Feingold, B.I., *Why Your Child is Hyperactive?* Random House, New York, 1975.

97. Robertson, G.L., and W.J. Kermode, Salicylic acid in fresh and canned fruits and vegetables, *J. Sci. Food Agric. 32*: 833 (1981).

98. Fassett, D.W., Oxalates, *Toxicants Occurring Naturally in Foods*, 2nd ed., National Academy of Sciences, National Research Council, Washington, DC, 1973, p. 346.

99. Desai, B.B., P.M. Kotecha, and D.K. Salunkhe, *Seeds Handbook: Biology, Production, Processing and Storage*, Marcel Dekker, Inc., New York, 1997, p. 397.

100. A Fact Sheet, A Summary of Basic Information About Sugar and Its Uses, Sugar Association, Inc, New York, 1975.

101. Watson, R.H.J., The psychology of sweetness, *Sweetness and Sweeteners* (C.G. Birch, L.F. Green, and C.B. Coulson, eds.), Applied Science, London, 1971, p. 1.

102. Brook, M., Sucrose and food manufacture, *Sugar* (J. Yudkin, J. Edelman, and L. Hough, eds.), Butterworths, London, 1971, p. 32.

103 Hickson, J.L., Utilization of sucrose by the chemist, *Sugar* (J. Yudkin, J. Edelman, and L. Hough, eds.), Butterworths, London, 1971, p. 60.

104. Manay, N.S., and M. Shadaksharaswamy, *Foods: Facts and Principles*, Wiley Eastern Ltd., New Delhi, 1987, p. 153.

105. McCance, R.A., and E.M. Widdowson, Phytin in human nutrition, *Biochem J. 298* (1935).

106. Averill, H.P., and C.G. King, The phytin content of food stuffs, *J. Amer. Chem. Soc. 48*: 724 (1926).

107. Oke, O.L., Phytic acid phosphorus content of Nigerian foodstuffs, *Indian J. Med. Res. 53*: 417 (1965).

108. Lolas, G.M., N. Palamidis, and P. Markakis, The phytic acid-total phosphorus relationship in barley, oats, soybeans and wheat, *Cereal Chem. 53*: 867 (1976).

109. DeBoland, A., G.B. Garner, and B.L. O'Dell, Identification and properties of phytate in cereal grains and oilseed products, *J. Agric. Food Chem. 23*: 1186 (1975).

110. Radhakrishnan, M.R., and J. Sivaprasad, Tannin content of sorghum varieties and their role in iron bioavailability, *J. Agric. Food Chem. 28*: 55 (1980).

111. Singh, B., and N.R. Reddy, Phytic acid and mineral composition of triticales, *J. Food Sci. 42*: 1077 (1977).

112. Lorenz, K., Tannins and phytate content of prosomillets (*Panicum milliaceum*), *Cereal Chem. 53*: 867 (1983).

113. O'Dell, B.L.A.R. DeBoland, and S.R. Koirtyohann, Distribution of phytate and nutritionally important elements among the morphological components of cereal grains, *J. Agric. Food Chem. 20*: 718 (1972).

114. Lasztity, L., Phytic acid in foods, D.Sc. thesis, Academy of Sciences, Budapest, Hungary, 1988.

11

Foods of Animal Origin

I. INTRODUCTION

Humankind is omnivorous and obtains its food either directly from plants or indirectly from them by consuming a variety of products such as meat, poultry, eggs, fish, milk, and their products made by animals that derive their sustenance from plants. In this sense, all flesh is grass, and the sun is the ultimate source of all food energy. Thus, efficiency of food production is closely linked to the proximity of our foods to the source of solar energy. The efficiency of conversion of sun's energy into the chemical energy stored by plants in the form of carbohydrates, fats, and proteins is around 1% or 2%. Each time this energy is transferred to another organism, significant loss in energy occurs. The flow of energy through a succession of living organisms (a food chain or web: plants-animals-humans) means that the further a person's diet gets away from plants, the higher will be the cost of food. Therefore, when food gets scarce humans must be a direct rather than an indirect consumer of plants.

Animal proteins are more complete than plant proteins because they supply 8 to 10 amino acids humans require in a proportion close to their needs. To get an even approximate nutritive equivalent from plant protein, we must mix a number of sources and consume larger bulk because the essential amino acids must be consumed simultaneously, and the concentration of proteins in plants, and that of the essential amino acids in plant proteins, is lower. Also, animal protein is a food source found more palatable by majority of the human population.

Human civilization depends on the complex relationship between humans and a few other life forms, viz., crop plants and domestic animals. After the Neolithic Revolution, agriculture has ensured a dependable food supply and buildup of food reserves.

As humans moved from food gathering to cultivation, hunting also gave way to husbandry. Cattle proved to be a reliable source of food, providing both meat and milk (and in some cultures, blood). Cattle also proved to be beasts of burden, long before horsepower was harnessed. The inedible parts of the animal (hide, bones, and fat) served a number of other valuable uses. Animal manure was found to be a good supplement in farming, and a convenient fuel supply in some parts of the world. Animal products, today, are a valuable source of drugs and pharmaceuticals (hormones, enzymes).

Milk production has played a dominant role in the domestication of cattle. This product of female mammal is the only food provided by nature for the purpose of nurturing young. The lactating mammary cell is second only to the photosynthetic plant cell as a factor in maintaining mammalian life (1)

Animal breeds have been developed to adapt to specific environments—from frigid north to hot tropics. Cattle have been selected for their efficiency in meat and milk production. Crossbreeding and genetic improvement of cattle, coupled with advances in animal nutrition, have revolutionized animal husbandry and dairying. Other warm-blooded animals, such as hogs, goats, and sheep are also used as sources of food and fiber. Hogs are more efficient converters of grain to meat protein than goats, sheep, and even cattle. However, pigs, being non-ruminants, are direct competitors of man for high-energy foods.

Domestic fowl (chicken, geese, ducks, turkey, and quail) are raised in many parts of the world, mostly on a small-scale cottage-industry level. Poultry farming in the United States has been adapted to mechanization and mass production, bringing down the prices of these products.

Fish and other forms of ocean life constitute an important source of protein and food to man and his domestic animals. Fishing, an aquatic equivalent of hunting, yields several millions of metric tons of fish per year, about one-tenth that of animal agriculture. About one-half of the yields of the ocean are used as protein supplements for animal feed. Because fishing is a mining operation (there is no "planting"), enormous investments have gone into the extractive mechinery, with profitable results, though with little consideration given to guaranted continued productivity. Ocean management is complicated by the "Law of Commons," the decisions of individual nations not compatible with optimum total productivity. Thus, an individual decision to add a vessel to the whaling fleet, though marginally productive to the individual, may decrease the future total yields because of excessive exploitation of the ocean. The problems of attaining and maintaining maximum productivity from the seas are both political and technical, adding a new dimension to food production. The overall efficiency of fisheries can be increased merely by reducing the size of the fishing fleet or by increasing the mesh size of nets (leaving smaller fish free to grow and breed). However, international agreements to adopt, much less to comply with, these commonsense concepts have been difficult to obtain. Management of our ocean resources thus requires emphasis on biological realities rather than political expediencies. Like that of land agriculture, the objective of marine agriculture must also be sustained yield. Overexploitation and pollution may reverse the trend toward greater productivity permanently.

II. MEAT AND MEAT PRODUCTS

Cattle stand first among the animals serving mankind. Though they are outnumbered by sheep, they render a variety of services to human well-being. To the American and European consumer, cattle represent beef, veal, milk, butter, cheese, and leather.

The term meat refers to muscle of warm-blooded terrestrial four-legged animals, mainly cattle, sheep, and pigs. Meat also includes the glands and organs of these animals. Meat products constitute by-products from animal slaughter, e.g. animal gut used for sausage casings or fat from meat used to make lard, gelatin, and other products.

The annual consumption of meat varies greatly from one country to another. The average per capita consumption of meat in the developed countries such as the United States is over 65 kg per annum, compared to less than 1.5 kg in India. The world production of meat, milk, and hen eggs during 1989 to 1994 is shown in Table 1 (2).

Table 1 The World Production of Meat, Milk, and Hen Eggs (MMT)

	1989	1990	1991	1992	1993	1994
Meat	171.8	177.5	181.3	184.3	188.4	194.7
Milk	535.7	543.8	537.8	528.0	528.0	526.6
Hen eggs	34.3	35.3	36.6	37.1	38.4	39.4

Source: Ref. 2.

A. Nutritional Composition and Quality

Meat is rich nutritionally, supplying most of the nutrients required by humans. This is to be expected, because the tissues and body fluids of the human being are very similar to those of animals.

The protein content of lean meat is around 20 to 22%. Of the total nitrogen content of the meat, approximately 95% is protein, and 5% is in the form of small peptides and amino acids. The quality of meat protein in terms of amino acid composition is very good, as required for the growth and maintenance of human tissue.

The fat content of meat varies from 5% to 40% with the type, breed, feed, and age of the animal. In well-fed animals, fat deposits subcutaneously as a protective layer around the organs, then accumulating around and between muscles. Finally, fat penetrates between the muscle fiber bundles (marbling). The marbling is desirable in some meats like beef, as the fat in such meats increases the water-holding capacity and juiciness of the meat. Meat fats, being rich in saturated fatty acids, may cause certain forms of atherosclerosis. The cholesterol content of meat is around 75 mg/100 g. The lean portion of meat contains greater proportions of phospholipids (0.5–1.0%) which are located in cell membranes. Carbohydrates are present in very small quantities in meat as glycogen and glucose.

Meat color is primarily due to myoglobin, color variation depending on the chemical state of myoglobin. Meats cured with nitrates remain pink, because nitric oxide myoglobin is stable. Hemoglobin also contributes to the color of meat to a lesser extent.

The nutritional composition and quality of meats depends on the ratio of fat to lean portion of the meat, which also determines its energy value and the concentrations of all other nutrients. There is an increasing demand for leaner meats and leaner carcases, owing to the lesser commercial value of meat fat. Carcases are often graded based on their composition and fat content to determine payments to producer. Using the results of breeding and selection, attempts are being made to reduce the fat content in carcases, with a significant decrease in fat to lean ratio in times to come (3,4). Thus, the nutritional composition and quality of meat cannot be determined precisely unless the fat to lean ratio is estimated.

The composition of lean and fat portions of some important meats in the United Kingdom (Table 2) indicates that the lean of three major carcase meats is similar in gross composition, which is expected because they are all mammalian muscles. The poultry muscle has less fat, most of the fat being associated with the skin. The ratio of lean to fat is also influenced by the variation in retail cuts of meat, depending on the anatomical position of the cut and the extent of trimming the joint (5).

Meager information is available on the composition of less common meats and of those eaten in the developing countries. The proximate composition of some such meats is shown in Table 2. The water content in these meats declines as the fat increases. The protein content of most meats is around 20%. Also, the fat content of wild animals is usually lower than that of the domestic species (Table 3). According to Southgate (6), the fat content of a retail joint is an important factor in the development of flavor during cooking and adequate fat levels are required to produce acceptable eating quality of meat.

The organs, such as heart, kidney and liver (collectively known as offal) vary less in their chemical composition. The protein content of heart, kidney, and liver vary from 15.2–17.1, 15.7–16.5, and 19.1–21.3%, respectively. The corresponding values for the water and fat contents of these organs in percent are 73.6–79.2, 78.8–79.8, 67.3–72.9 and 2.6–9.3, 2.6–2.7, and 6.3–10.3, respectively. The liver is richer in its energy content (153–179 kcal), than either heart (86–150 kcal), or kidney (86–90 kcal).

A wide range of meat products is available, especially in the more developed countries. Many of these products contain substantial concentrations of fat, but this is very variable. There

Table 2   Typical Composition of Some Raw Meats (Values per 100 g edible material)

Meat	Separable components[a]	Water (g)	Protein[b] (g)	Fat (g)	Energy (kcal)
Beef	Lean	74.0	20.3	4.6	123
	Fat	24.0	8.8	66.9	637
Lamb	Lean	70.0	20.8	8.8	162
	Fat	21.2	6.2	71.8	671
Pork	Lean	71.5	20.7	7.1	147
	Fat	21.1	6.8	71.4	670
Veal fillet		74.9	21.1	2.7	109
Chicken meat		74.4	20.5	4.3	121
Meat and skin		64.4	17.6	17.7	230
Turkey meat		75.5	21.9	2.2	107
Meat and skin		72.0	20.6	6.9	145

[a]By usual 'domestic' procedure, not rigorous dissection.
[b]Nx6.25
Source: Ref. 13.

Table 3   Composition of Meats of Some Other Animals (per 100 g edible matter)

Species	Energy (kcal)	(kJ)	Water (g)	Protein (g)	Fat (g)
Dog	274	1146	60.8	14.5	23.5
Camel	267	1117	59.1	19.6	20.3
Frog	68	285	83.6	15.3	0.3
Goat					
Lean	179	749	69.2	18.0	11.3
Medium	357	1494	51.6	15.2	32.4
Hare	115	480	75.0	21.5	3.1
Horse	170	713	70.0	19.0	10.0
Moose (lean)	111	420	76.0	22.0	1.2
Rabbit	126	529	74.6	22.2	4.0
Reindeer	117	490	74.0	21.0	3.6
Roe deer	120	500	74.0	21.0	4.0
Snake	94	393	75.0	14.4	3.3
Squirrel	110	460	72.2	26.3	0.4
Venison	120	500	74.0	21.0	4.0
Water buffalo	120	502	76.5	17.7	4.6

Source: Ref. 6.

is a tendency for the cheaper products to contain more fat and connective tissue, these being cheaper ingredients than steak.

Meats and meat products are the conventional protein foods, which is true for the lean meat; it has substantial amounts of a protein with a high biological value. Its balance of amino acids is very close to the reference protein. However, the major proteins of connective tissue, collagen and elastin, have rather imbalanced and inadequate amino acid composition and do not support growth. Thus, meat products prepared from joints (with high connective tissue) have lower biological value, though this may be of little nutritional significance in the context of the whole diet.

Meats are a rich source of fat and energy. Different lipids present in meat include triglycerides of adipose tissues in subcutaneous fat and abdominal fats surrounding kidney and intestines and marbling fats between the muscle blocks; phospholipids of the cell membranes and nervous tissues; glycolipids of brain and other neural tissues and lipoproteins present in many tissues. The fat in meat is predominantly triglyceride (adipose tissue), though lean tissues contain a higher proportion of phospholipids (7).

The ruminant character of an animal determines the fatty acid composition of the fat in meats. Whereas the fat in non-ruminants depends on the composition of fats in the animal's diet, that of the ruminant is influenced by the activities of microflora in the rumen. The latter hydrogenate much of the ingested fat, making it highly saturated fat (Table 4). These data indicate that liver lipids are less saturated than the whole animal fat, because they contain phospholipids in their cell membranes. Also, fats in wild ruminants are less saturated, because the fat contents are lower and phospholipids consequently form a greater proportion of the total lipid (8).

Meats are relatively low in Na and Ca, and high in K, P and Mg. Meats have high bioavailability of the micronutrients they contain, especially Fe, Zn, Cu, and several other trace elements. Meat contains most of the B complex vitamins and is an important source of vitamin B_{12}. Retinol

Table 4 Fatty Acid Composition of Some Meats (Lean Plus Fat Portion of Meat)

Fatty acid[a]	Meats						
	Beef	Lamb	Pork	Chicken[a]	Turkey	Calf liver	Lamb liver
Saturated							
14:0	3.2	5.4	1.6	1.3	1.3	0.8	1.3
15:0	0.6	0.6	Tr	Tr	Tr	Tr	0.5
16:0	26.9	24.2	27.1	26.7	25.0	16.5	20.4
17:0	1.2	1.0	Tr	Tr	0.5	0.6	1.0
18:0	13.0	20.9	13.8	7.1	10.0	23.3	18.3
%	44.9	52.1	42.5	35.1	36.5	41.2	41.5
Monounsaturated							
16:1	6.3	1.3	3.4	7.2	5.0	1.9	3.5
17:1	1.0	1.0	Tr	Tr	Tr	0.7	1.6
18:1	42.0	38.2	43.8	39.8	21.5	20.8	29.7
20:1	Tr	Tr	0.7	0.6	0.4	Tr	0
%	49.3	40.5	47.9	47.6	26.9	23.4	34.8
Polyunsaturated							
18:2	2.0	2.5	7.4	13.5	20.0	15.0	5.0
18:3	1.3	2.5	0.9	0.7	1.0	1.4	3.8
20:3	Tr	0	0	Tr	Tr	2.1	0.6
20:4	1.0	0	Tr	0.7	5.0	9.0	5.1
20:5	Tr	Tr	Tr	Tr	1.5	0.3	0
22:5	Tr	Tr	Tr	Tr	2.0	4.0	3.0
%	4.3	5.0	8.3	14.9	29.5	16.8	17.5

[a]Composition depends on diet being fed.

Tr = Trace

Source: Ref. 13.

is mainly stored in liver. Thiamin, riboflavin, and niacin occur in significant amounts in all types of meat.

B. Meat Types

Major carcase meats in Europe and the United States are produced from cattle, sheep, and pigs, whereas in the Middle East, Africa, and India other animals, such as goats, camels, and water buffalo, are also used.

1. Beef

Meat from different types of cattle are designated with various terms. Veal is the meat from cattle slaughtered 3 to 4 weeks after birth. Beef is the meat of cattle more than one year old. Beef carcass is classified according to sex, age, and sexual conditions of the animals as follows:

Stear	a bovine male castrated at very young age
Heifer	a bovine female that has not yet borne a calf
Cow	a bovine female, that has borne a calf
Stag	a bovine male that is castrated after maturity
Calf	a male or female bovine animal of up to 12 months age (3–8 months).

The quality of meat from stear and heifer is the same, if animals are of the same grade. The quality of meat from cow and bull depends upon maturity, but is generally inferior to that of stear or heifer. The meat quality of stag varies according to the age at which it is castrated.

Beef production systems range from extensive ranging of cattle to very intensive "feed-lots" in the United States. The animals are usually raised initially on grass, which may be grazed or fed as conserved hay or silage, with cereal-based concentrates fed during the finishing stages. Veal is produced from calves under semi-intensive systems, using milk-based concentrated rations to produce very light-colored meats.

Horsemeat is mainly used for animal food in United Kingdom, but it is widely consumed in continental Europe by human beings. Goats and camels are major meat animals in the Arab countries. Since mature camels produce rather tough meat, young animals are preferred for meat. Water buffalo are important in the Middle East and Asia and are usually farmed extensively in traditional ways.

Acceptance of animals or their parts as foods varies considerably with national preferences and religious beliefs. While the consumption of horsemeat, dogmeat, and guinea pigs is not considered normal in the United Kingdom, these foods are eaten elsewhere. The Jewish food laws proscribe a number of animals whose flesh is regarded as unclean, for example those who chew the cud, but do not have cloven feet (e.g., coney or rock hyrax, hare, camel) and those with cloven feet, but do not chew the cud (pigs). The rules also prohibited consumption of many other animals such as birds of prey or carrion eaters, waterfowl, snakes, and marine mammals (6). Islam has proscribed the pig as unclean. Both Islam and Judaism have prescribed a ritual protocol for the slaughter of animals for human consumption.

In the United States, careful management of wildlife provides an important source of meat, and in Sweden deer and reindeer are important meat animals. Wild animals often flourish on poor forages and the composition of their meat is attractive to many consumers.

The Normans introduced rabbits to England, which were farmed in warrens as a source of meat. Much of the venison produced in Scotland is exported and it contributes little to total meat consumption in the United Kingdom.

2. Mutton

Sheep carcasses may be classified, based on the age of animal, into (a) lamb, (b) yearling mutton, and (c) mature mutton. Lamb carcasses as a group are distinguished from mutton carcasses by their smaller and tender bones, lighter colored flesh, and softer and whiter external and internal fats (the age of ovine animals of both sexes is less than one year). The carcasses of young sheep, from 12 to 20 months old, are usually termed yearling mutton, with harder and whiter bones, darker and coarser flesh, and thicker external and internal fat. The flesh of both males (castrated and uncastrated) and females of ovine species that are 20 months in age at the time of slaugher is termed mature mutton. It has light to dark red color. The break joint fails to break due to the hardening of bones. Mature mutton has a strong characteristic odor, different from the delicate flavor of lamb.

3. Pork

Pork is a pigmeat. A good quality pork is obtained from swines between ages of 3 to 12 months, before the amount of fat becomes excessive. Pork is not differentiated according to the age and size of the pig. Pork generally has more fat than other meats. Bacon is the cut from the belly portion of hog carcass and has a high fat content.

4. Sausages

These are made of ground or minced meat, using mostly the cured meats. A variety of sausages are marketed under different classes depending on whether the ground meat is fresh or cured and whether the sausage is cooked or uncooked, smoked or unsmoked, and dried or not during manufacture. The cooked and smoked sausages are known as table-ready meats. The sausages are enclosed in natural casings made from animal intenstine or of plastic films.

5. Organ Meats (Offal)

These include liver, kidney, heart, sweetbread (thymus and pancreas), brain, lung, tripe (first and second stomach of the ruminants), head and tail of the animal. The organ meats are less expensive and more nutritious. The cooking methods vary according to their tenderness.

Though muscles form the bulk of the carcass meat, animal production and slaughter produces a wide range of by-products. Some of these products are edible and considered delicacies in many cultures, whereas other religious traditions restrict the consumption of offals as unclean (e.g., blood and blood products). Liver, kidneys, brain, and pancreas (sweetbreads) are often consumed, but other organs (intestine, tripe, pigs' trotters and cow heel) are delicacies with restricted consumption.

The organs can form the foci of infection in an animal. Most developed countries therefore have veterinary inspections at slaughterhouses to eliminate this possibility.

C. Meat Processing

In developed countries, animals are slaughtered for meat production under closely regulated conditions. Cattle and sheep are often killed humanely with a captive bolt, and pigs and lambs are usually stunned electrically. The animal is then strung up and bled. The abdominal cavity is opened and the viscera are removed. Pigs are often scalded in hot water to remove the bristles before cleaning. The carcasses are then split longitudinally and chilled. The meat may be separated from the bone before chilling (hot boning). Rapid chilling tends to toughen the meat but is usually employed to improve throughput. Electrical stimulation is widely used to reduce the cold-shortening that accompanies very rapid chilling.

The carcass is often divided into primal cuts, which are distributed to the retail meat trade. The carcass may be trimmed to remove some fat at this stage, but trimming is usually carried out when the carcass or primal cuts are further butchered.

Whereas in the United Kingdom and United States of America, the cuts divide the carcass into anatomical regions, in Europe, butchering follows the muscle boundaries (muscle seaming). Thus, it is often not possible to compare the composition of meat cuts in different countries or regions on the basis of their nomenclature alone.

The division of the carcass almost invariably leaves relatively large amounts of fat, both subcutaneously and deep-body, and muscle on and off the bone, which cannot be sold in its unprocessed state. This includes parts of the animal that are unattractive to the consumer (heads, feet, and intestines). These by-products constitute important sources for a wide range of meat products such as sausages, where meat is ground finely into an emulsion and mixed with cereal or soya rusk (U.K.). Continental sausages are made without such additions (6). The emulsion is then extruded into a case of gelatin or cellulose to manufacture the conventional sausage. Whereas Continental sausages are usually cooked before sale and eaten cold, in the United Kingdom they are cooked before consumption. Meat pies are made by chopping or mincing meat and encasing it in pastry and baking. The tougher meats from mature animals are often made into canned meats.

Because the conventional knife trimming of the bony residual carcass leaves considerable amounts of muscle and connective tissue on the bone, newer mechanical techniques are being employed to recover this material. The latter involves massive maceration of the residual carcasse, followed by extrusion through an equipment separating bone fragments. The mechanically recovered meat emerges as an emulsion which is used in various meat products. Other techniques of using small pieces of meat include a process involving "tumbling" meat pieces in a hot phosphate buffer to solubilize the actomycin. The latter acts as an adhesive when the meat is cooled and compressed. This re-formed meat is difficult to distinguish visually from steak or ham.

1. Effect of Aging and Cooking

When the meat is held cold for some time after it has gone into rigor mortis, the muscle again turns soft and pliable with improved flavor and juiciness. The aging or ripening changes include progressive tenderization of meat owing to the denaturation of the muscle protein and mild hydrolysis of denatured proteins by the intracellular proteolytic enzymes (cathepsins). The latter slowly break down the connective tissues between muscle fibers and the muscle fibers themselves.

Meat aging or ripening is performed by holding meat at 0.5° to −2°C in a cold room for 1 to 4 weeks. The best flavor and the greatest tenderness develop in meat aged from 2 to 4 weeks. The humidity of the cold room must be controlled, and meat is re-covered with wrapping to minimize drying and weight loss. Meat aging can also be effected by holding it at higher temperatures for shorter times, often at 20°C for 48 hours. Ultraviolet light is used to suppress the surface bacterial growth. Beef is the only kind of meat that is commercially aged; lamb and mutton are only occasionally aged, but pork is never aged because of its high fat content (9).

In addition to natural aging (ripening) of meat, tenderizing it with the meat's natural enzymes, several artificial methods are used to increase tenderness of meats. These include mechanical methods and use of enzymes and salts.

The mechanical methods include pounding, cutting, grinding, needling, or pinning and use of ultrasonic vibrations to cut or break the muscle fibers and connective tissues. Whereas the pounding process merely breaks and tears only surface meat fibers, grinding cuts all the muscle fibers and connective tissues, increasing the tenderness.

Papain from papaya is often used to tenderize the meat, e.g., by wrapping meat in papaya leaves before cooking. Papain is now commercially available and used extensively in meat tenderization. Other enzymes used for this purpose are bromelin from pineapple, ficin from figs, and trypsin from pancreas and fungal enzymes. These enzymes hydrolyze proteins (elastin) of the connective tissues to different degrees. Papain is often injected into the veins of animals about 10 min. before slaughter. This results in uniform distribution of the enzyme throughout the animal body and increases tenderness of the cooked meat. Freeze-drying the meat and rehydrating it in water containing proteolytic enzymes also has been found to be effective. Papain remains active from 55° to 82°C. Over-tenderization is not desirable as it changes meat texture, resulting in the loss of flavor and juiciness.

Meats may also be tenderized using lower concentrations of salts. Salts increase the water-holding capacity of the muscle fibers and thus increase juiciness and tenderness of the meat. Salts also solubilize the meat proteins. Tenderness of meat is improved when freeze-dried meat is rehydrated in a weak salt solution instead of water. Sodium chloride, sodium bicarbonate, and sodium or potassium phosphate salts are often used for tenderization of meats. The latter can also be achieved by change of pH. Decreasing or increasing pH of meat increases hydration and its tenderness. Soaking beef for 48 hours in concentrated vinegar, for example, increases its tenderness and juiciness.

2.   Effects of Curing

The curing of meat brings about modification in meats, affecting their keeping quality (preservation), flavor, color, and tenderness. Curing was practiced as a means of preservation before the days of refrigeration. With the availability of modern methods of preservation, curing is currently used to produce the unique flavored meat products and to preserve the red color of meat. The cured beef (corned beef) and cured pork (ham) remain red on cooking; the uncured meat turns brown.

The most commonly used curing agents are common salt (NaCl), sodium nitrate or nitrite, sugar, and spices. The salt retards microbial growth and gives flavor to the meat. Nitrite fixes the red color of myoglobin, increases flavor of the cured meat, and inhibits *Clostridium botulinum*; sugar helps to stabilize color, counteract saltiness, and add to the flavor. Spices are used mainly as flavoring agents.

During salt curing, the high osmotic pressure of the external fluid initially draws water and soluble proteins out of the meat. Then, salt diffuses into the meat and binds to the proteins, causing swelling of the meat.

Curing also has some detrimental effects during storage. The pink color of nitrite-cured meat changes to brown in the presence of oxygen. The cured meat, therefore, must be packed in containers to exclude oxygen. The salts of cured meat enhance oxidation of lipids in meats, reducing their shelf life. The carcinogenic effects of nitrite are also of great health concern.

3.   Effects of Smoking

The cured meat may be dried and smoked. Smoking was also originally used as a method of preservation. However, today smoking is mostly used to enhance flavor and coagulation of proteins in meat. Ham is often processed by smoking. The sawdust from hardwoods is used as a fuel for smoking. Slow smoking over an extended period of time enables more uniform drying, enhancing keeping quality. The smoke contains compounds having antiseptic properties that destroy microorganisms present in meat. It also prevents development of fat rancidity in meat (9).

4.   Effects of Cooking

Cooking may render meat more or less tender than the original raw cut. An increase in tenderness is due to the melting of fat, dissolution of collagen in hot liquid to become soft gelatin, and softening of tissue along with separation of muscle fibers. Heating, however, may also have toughening effects on meat. Overheating causes muscle fibers to contract and meat to shrink and become tougher.

Both the dry and moist heat methods are employed to cook meats. The choice of the method for a meat cut depends on its tenderness. Less tender cuts become more tender when prepared by moist heat methods, during which collagen is converted to gelatin. Moist heat methods comprise braising, stewing (cooking in simmering water), and pressure cooking. The tender cuts that do not require conversion of connective tissue are often cooked by dry heat methods, such as roasting, broiling, pan broiling, and frying.

Lower cooking temperatures for longer periods of time are preferred to higher temperatures for shorter time. This results in decreased drip, less shrinkage, increased juiciness, and more uniform color throughout the cut.

Meat thermometers are used to test the degree of doneness of cooking. The recommended temperatures in the center of cut for rare, medium, and well-done stages for lamb are 77°, 79°, and 82°C, respectively and the corresponding values for beef are 60°, 71°, and 77°C. Fresh pork is heated to a well-done stage (77°C) to destroy *Trichinella spiralis*. Moist heat methods do not require use of thermometers.

In addition to the destruction of microorganisms, heat also brings about changes in color, flavor, and tenderness, owing to changes taking place in meat fiber and connective tissue. The nutritional value of cooked meat generally remains high. Proteins and minerals are not lost by heat. Some minerals may be lost in meat drippings, but cooking also dissolves some calcium from bone. Some B complex vitamins are lost during cooking; most of the cooked meats, however, retain more than 50% of the vitamins of the B complex group present in the uncooked meats.

D. Meat Products

1. Gelatin and Gels

Gelatin is a partially degraded collagen. If the collagen molecule is completely unstructured, glue is produced instead of gelatin. Gelatin is prepared from the collagen of connective tissues and bones of animals. The bones are first demineralized to remove calcium and phosphorus by soaking bones in acid. The demineralized bone (ossein) is then hydrolyzed with alkali or acid. The alakline hydrolysis is often carried out with lime.

Gelatin preparations, such as jellied fruits and vegetables, sponges, and creams are very popular products. Gelatin gel is prepared by completely dispersing the gelatin to form a sol and chilling it to form the desired gel. Different grades of gelatin, modified gelatins, and gels are used in various industrial products such as canned foods, semipreserves, confectionery, marshmallows, ice cream, and gelatin desserts. Gelatin is also used in the form of jellies such as jelled desserts, sponges, and cream salads as well as in pharmaceutical preparations (capsules).

III. POULTRY AND EGGS AND THEIR PRODUCTS

The term poultry refers to domestic fowls reared for their flesh, eggs, or feathers, and includes chicken, ducks, geese, turkey, guineas, and pigeons. Among these, chicken and turkey are most commonly used for their meat.

A. Poultry

Chicken may be grouped into different classes, depending on the fowl's ability to produce a product of commercial value; e.g., egg type, meat type, dual purpose, and miscellaneous ones. Meat types are usually large in size with plenty of flesh, but they are often not good layers. Dual-purpose types yield meat of excellent quality and lay a good number of eggs. Each of these types is classified on the basis of age, which influences tenderness and fat content of meat and determines the method of cooking. In India, chickens are classified as follows (9).

1. *Broiler or fryer*: Chicken of 8 to 10 weeks of age of either sex, tender-meated with soft, pliable, smooth-textured skin and flexible breastbone cartilage.
2. *Rooster*: A young chicken (3 to 5 months of age) of either sex, tender-meated with soft, pliable, smooth-textured skin and breastbone cartilage that is somewhat less flexible than that of the broiler or fryer.
3. *Stag*: a male chicken, under 10 months of age, with coarse skin, somewhat toughened and darkened flesh and a considerable hardening of the breastbone cartilage.
4. *Stewing chicken or fowl*: A mature chicken, usually more than 10 months of age, with meat less tender than that of a roaster and nonflexible breastbone tip.
5. *Cock*: A mature male chicken, usually over 10 months of age, with coarse skin, toughened and darkened meat, and hardened breastbone tip.

Poultry were domesticated many centuries ago, probably in China, and were reared under free-range foraging conditions, as a source of eggs and meat. In the Western countries, their consumption has increased significantly, with the development of intensive systems to produce "broiler chickens." Under these conditions, growth is rapid and the feed conversion ratio is high, making possible large-scale production at low prices.

1. Nutritional Composition and Quality

Typical nutritional composition of chicken and turkey meat is shown in Table 2. Poultry meat has a quality and nutritive value comparable to other meats. Its protein (about 21%) contains all the essential amino acids required for the growth of body tissues. There is little fat in the meat of young birds, but the fat content varies greatly with age and species of poultry. Chicken fat has higher proportion of unsaturated fatty acids than that of red meat. Like other meats, poultry flesh is also a good source of B vitamins and minerals. The dark meat of chicken in richer is riboflavin, but the light meat is richer in niacin. Because of its higher protein to fat ratio, poultry meat is beneficial for persons with restricted fat intakes.

    a.　Processing of Poultry.　Poultry is marketed in ready-to-cook form, i.e., the head, feet, and entrails removed (dressed chicken). Birds are generally not fed for 12 hours before slaughter to ensure that their crops are empty, to help cleaner operations. The birds are killed by stunning (electrical) or making them unconscious with a blow on the head. The jugular vein is cut to facilitate complete bleeding in order to obtain high quality meat. The bird is then scalded by dipping in hot water briefly (60°C for 45 sec or more or at 52°C for 2 min). Scalding loosens the feathers. After defeathering, the abdominal cavity is opened by transverse cut, and after inspection, the entrails are removed, followed by removal of head, feet, and oil glands. The eviscerated birds are thoroughly washed and chilled rapidly at 1.7°C to control growth of contaminating bacteria. Rapid cooling helps to retain tenderness of the meat by avoiding toughening of the muscle due to lowering of pH by accumulation of lactic acid. Like other meats, poultry also goes into and out of rigor, but more rapidly than others. Dressed chicken is graded for marketing, depending on the condition of the bird prior to the slaughter, during evisceration and packing. The graded poultry is packed in low-moisture and low-oxygen transmission films or bags and sealed after expelling the air from the bag. The sealed bags are stored under refrigeration or frozen.

    b.　Poultry Cooking.　The flavor develops during cooking. The method of cooking depends on the tenderness of the poultry and its fat content, which are mainly influenced by the age of the bird. Whereas the moist-heat methods are applied to older and tougher meats, dry heat methods are used for the more tender meats. Low to moderate heat is employed to obtain tender, juicy, and uniformly cooked poultry.

Young tender poultry is cooked by broiling, frying, baking, or roasting. The whole bird or halves may be broiled at temperatures of 177°C, till the internal temperature of the breast muscle reaches 95°C (45–60 min). Frying and deep fat frying are suitable for cooking low-fat, young, tender poultry and are used more commonly than broiling. The poultry may be roasted, stuffed or unstuffed. When the whole bird is roasted, its tender parts (breast) may be overcooked before the legs and thighs are cooked to the desired state. For stuffed birds, roasting may be continued till the internal temperature of the stuffing reaches 74°C. The unstuffed poultry may be cooked at an oven temperature of 163°C, till the internal temperature of the thigh muscle reaches 85°C.

The older tougher birds are cooked by braising and stewing. Disjointed chicken pieces are usually braised. They are first browned by frying, after which water is added and the bird is simmered until it is tender. Whole bird or cut pieces may be used for stewing. They are cooked in water with seasonings and vegetables, till they are rendered tender.

Tandoor chicken is a popular delicious barbecued chicken dish in India. The cooking is carried out in a clay oven, *tandoor*. Charcoal is put inside and the oven is made red hot. Whole or cut tender chicken is used. The skin is removed and the flesh pricked with a fork and sprinkled with salt. Tandoor sauce is then smeared on the chicken and is left aside for 6–8 hours and cooked in the tandoor. Half way through the cooking time, it is removed from the oven and brushed all over nicely with butter and oil and cooked again until the chicken is fork tender.

B. Eggs and Their Products

The eggs of a range of species are eaten by many human cultures and constitute an important source of nutritious food supplying high-quality protein and other nutrients. In most parts of the world, hen's eggs are of commercial importance, with minor usage of duck, goose, and quail eggs. In the developed countries, hen eggs are normally produced intensively under battery conditions. The eggs are also produced under less intensive systems, such as deep-litter, where the hens are enclosed in a controlled environment ('barn' eggs) or range eggs, where the hens have access to open space to forage, though they are fed specially formulated rations. True free-range production, where hens range freely in search of food, though seen as ideal, is not common. The comparison of the composition of eggs produced by different systems, however, have shown no significant differences in their nutritional quality (10,11). The world production of hen eggs during 1989–94 is shown in Table 1.

1. Nutritional Composition and Quality

The comparison of the nutritional composition of eggs indicates a remarkable similarity between the eggs of different species (Table 5). The egg proteins contain essential amino acids for the development of the embryo. For this reason, egg protein was regarded as ideal with perfect amino acid composition and used as a reference standard for biological evaluation of other proteins for a long period. It is now known that though it is perfect for the chicken, it is not so for other species. Other amino acid compositions are therefore seen as ideal for humans (6).

Egg lipids are rich in phospholipids and the fatty acid composition has a high polyunsaturated/saturated (P/S) fatty acids ratio. Cholesterol present in the egg lipid forms a key precursor for membrane synthesis in the chick. The cholesterol content of the egg can be manipulated by dietary means, but it is not known whether this is a useful or stable change. Eggs also contain the range of vitamins and minerals required for the development of the chick and thus are a valuable food. Egg iron has a high bioavailability, possibly because it is bound to egg proteins. The avidin

Table 5 Nutritional Composition of Eggs of Different Species (Values per 100 g)

Nutrients	Hen	Duck	Pigeon	Quail	Goose	Turkey	Turtle
Water (g)	74.8	70.6	79.8	73.7	70.4	72.2	75.6
Energy (kcal)	147	188	116	161	185	171	148
(kJ)	615	787	485	674	774	715	619
Protein (g)	11.8	13.2	10.7	13.1	13.9	13.1	12.0
Fat (g)	9.6	14.2	7.0	12.1	13.9	12.1	10.0
Calcium (mg)	52	64	62	49	56	49	84
Iron (mg)	2.0	3.6	3.5	4.1	2.8	4.1	1.3
Retinol (µg)	140	370	95	—	—	—	445
Vitamin D (µg)	1.75	—	—	—	—	—	—
Thiamin (mg)	0.09	0.16	0.13	—	0.18	0.11	0.11
Riboflavin (mg)	0.47	0.40	0.65	—	0.36	0.47	0.46

Source: Ref. 6.

(protein) of egg white binds to biotin, making it unavailable to humans, though cooking denatures the avidin, abolishing the effect.

Eggs provide a versatile food of high biological value. They are currently produced efficiently and relatively cheaply, even in many developing countries, where they constitute an important source of protein. In the developed countries, egg consumption is decreasing because of concerns about the effects of dietary cholesterol in the diet as a potential risk factor for coronary heart disease. In the UK, average consumption of eggs is 3 per person per week (20–24 g/day). Eggs are consumed through processed foods in significant quantities.

Eggs are an excellent source of vitamin A, present in the yolk (Table 5), which is also a good source of vitamin D. Egg yolk is second only to fish oil in this respect. The quantity of vitamin D depends upon the extent of direct sunlight the layers are exposed to.

Egg-white proteins, frequently referred to as albumins, are ovalalbumin (55% of the egg white proteins), conalbumin (13%), ovomucoid (10%), ovomucin, lysozyme, avidin, and ovoglobulin. Egg-yolk proteins contain phosvitin (proteins rich in phosphorus), lipovitellins (high-density lipoproteins), livetin, and low-density lipoprotein. The pale yellow to brilliant orange color of the yolk is due to the presence of carotenoids and xanthophylls.

2. Egg Processing

Eggs, in addition to storage in the shell, may be preserved by freezing or by drying of their contents. The egg cannot be frozen in the shell. Therefore, the whole of the liquid contents of the egg is frozen, or is frozen after separation into yolk and white portions. The shells are washed before the eggs are broken from the shell to reduce microbial contamination, followed by rapid freezing. Prevalence of *Salmonella* pathogenic bacteria can be avoided by pasteurizing the product. Frozen egg white retains its quality fairly well but, the yolk and whole egg cannot be frozen satisfactorily, because they turn viscous and gummy (gelation), with altered functional properties, which can be maintained by treating the yolk with pepsin.

Eggs can be dried to prepare egg-powder, which is used in the preparation of several commercial egg products. The white, yolk, or whole egg, after pasteurization, may be dried. Of several methods of drying, spray-drying is most commonly employed. The liquid egg is forced through an atomizer as a fine spray into a drying chamber through which hot air is blown. The product is cooled and packaged.

When the white or whole egg is stored much above freezing, the glucose present in the white combines with egg proteins, resulting in browning, which can be prevented by removing glucose with glucose oxidase or by fermenting with yeast prior to drying.

3. Egg Products

The eggs may be cooked without adding any ingredients or may be included in various recipes. The color, flavor, texture, binding, emulsifying, and foaming properties of eggs have been used in many egg products. The egg yolk contributes to color of the products such as meringues and various cream pie fillings. The emulsifying property of eggs is used in salad dressings and different baked products; the binding properties of eggs are accomplished as a result of the coagulation of proteins during heating. The foaming of egg white is an important property in the development of light structure and good volume in bakery products such as cakes.

a. In Shell Eggs. Eggs may be soft or hard-cooked in the shell. In a soft-cooked egg, the white should be firm but tender, and the yolk a thick liquid. In hard-boiled eggs, the white becomes an opaque tender gel and the yolk is completely coagulated. Eggs are simmered in boiling water for 3 to 5 min (soft-cooked) or for 15 to 20 min (hard-cooked).

b. Out-of-Shell Eggs. Poached egg is prepared by sliding the contents of a good quality egg carefully into a pan of water heated to simmering temperature. The egg is removed from water quickly when the white is coagulated completely.

Fried-egg is prepared by frying it in just enough fat to prevent it sticking to the pan. The temperature should be sufficient to coagulate the egg-white, but not to toughen it or to decompose the fat. The yolk should be unbroken and covered with a layer of coagulated white.

Scrambled egg is prepared by blending both the yolk and white until an uniform mixture is formed. A small amount (one tablespoon per egg) of milk, cream or water may be added to the mix, along with salt and seasonings. The mix is then heated slowly and the egg is scraped as it coagulates, to make the product moist, tender, and fluffy.

French omelet or plain omelet is prepared by beating the whole egg, with or without a small amount of liquid and flavoring agent. The mixture is cooked in a greased pan until it is coagulated. The omelet is then folded or rolled. A variety of omelets are prepared by using various fillings and sauces.

c. Egg Products as Thickening Agents. The thickening property of eggs (coagulation of proteins) is used in a number of egg products such as custards and cream pie fillings. Proper control of coagulation temperature determines the product quality.

Two types of custards are made: the soft or stirred custard, which gives a product of creamy consistency, and baked custard, which is coagulated without stirring.

The ingredients of custard are eggs, sugar, milk, salt, and flavorings. The egg is blended and strained, to which milk and sugar are added with stirring. The use of scalded milk to about 85°C shortens the cooking time and improves the flavor and texture of the product. The custard mixture is heated over hot water (just below the boiling point). A slow heating rate is essential to prepare a smooth, viscous stirred custard. The stirring breaks up the gel as it forms. After reaching desired thickness, it is poured into a shallow dish, placed in cold or ice water to cool the custard rapidly. Excessive coagulation may result in curdling. The product should have the viscosity of a heavy cream and be very smooth, with no signs of curdling. This custard is nutritious and a pleasing dessert sauce served over cakes, fruits, and various baked desserts.

A baked custard is made similarly as the stirred custard. The stirred homogeneous mixture of custard ingredients is placed in a pan of hot water in an oven at 170°C. The water allows slow rate of heat penetration to keep the outside of the custard from being overbaked before the interior is set. An overheated baked custard becomes porous, the pores filled with watery serum. A baked custard should be firm, yet tender, with a smooth and uniform texture and without porosity.

Cream puddings and pie fillings are made by boiling the cornstarch, sugar, salt, and water together until the mixture becomes thick. The mixture is removed from the heat and part of it is stirred carefully into beaten egg yolk. The yolk mixture is then blended with the starch mixture, and the pudding is heated over simmering water until the protein coagulates. Slow stirring promotes uniform coagulation of yolk, avoiding lumps. The cream puddings and pie fillings should be smooth, without gumminess or stickiness.

d. Egg Foam Products. *Meringues* are egg-white foams into which some acid and sugar are incorporated. Soft meringues are used as toppings for cream pies and hard ones as confections in combinations with fruits, ice creams, or syrups. The soft meringues are made by beating the egg white to the foam stage. About 25 g sugar per egg white is then added gradually and beaten until the peaks just bend over. The fine-structured meringue is spread on soft pie fillings. Soft meringues are baked at 177°C to a pleasing, medium brown color on the ridges. The hard meringues contain twice as much sugar as the soft ones. The large amount of sugar delays foam formation. The product is baked at a lower temperature and for a longer time than the soft meringue. The hard meringues should be dry, crisp, and tender, with a delicate color and a fluffy look.

Fluffy omelets are prepared by beating egg white and yolk separately and folding them together, and then baking. Souffles are made similarly, but they contain white sauce and other flavoring agents, such as grated cheese, meats, poultry, fish, pureed vegetables, and so forth. Foam cakes, like angel, chiffon, and sponge cakes are prepared using the foaming property of the egg white.

e. Egg Products as Emulsifying Agent. Egg yolk is a good emulsifying agent, yolk itself being an emulsion. Salad dressings that are emulsions of oil-in-water are stabilized, with either whole egg or egg yolk. These emulsifiers are used in various baked products such as cheese souffles, cream puffs, and shortened cakes (9).

IV. MILK AND DAIRY PRODUCTS

Milk and its products have become a part of the normal human diet, right from the beginning of civilization itself. Milk of many species of animals is used as a food and a source of a range of dairy products. Liquid milk being an unstable commodity, many fermented products were developed that could be stored and transported, extending their market value.

The selection of high-yielding breeds of cattle and their genetic improvement, using modern techniques such as artificial insemination from bulls of proven productivity and embryo transfer, have led to significant developments in dairy industry during the past three to four decades, especially in Western countries such as the United States of America, and New Zealand. These developments were accompanied by close attention to hygiene during the production and distribution of milk. The introduction of pasteurization and animal health programs to eliminate milk as a vector for the transmission of bacterial diseases have contributed greatly to the present place of dairy industry in the agricultural economy of several countries, including India. The world production of milk during 1989–94 is shown in Table 1.

A. Nutritional Composition and Quality

Milk is secreted by the mammary gland and is the staple food of all young mammals, including human infants. The composition of the milk secreted by each species has been adapted to the specific needs of the species. Thus, there are distinct differences in different milks used as human foods. These differences may be related to the variation in the rates of animal growth, and the ways in which maternal immunity is transferred to the young animal (12).

Table 6 Nutritional Composition of Milks of Different Species (Values per 100 g)

Nutrient	Cow	Goat	Sheep	Camel	Buffalo	Human
Water (g)	87.8	88.9	83.0	88.8	83.3	88.2
Energy (kcal)	66	60	95	63	92	69
(kJ)	276	253	396	264	385	289
Protein (g)	3.2	3.1	5.4	2.0	4.1	1.3
Fat (g)	3.9	3.5	6.0	4.1	5.9	4.1
Lactose (g)	3.9	4.4	5.1	4.7	5.9	7.2
Calcium (mg)	115	100	170	94	175	34

Source: Refs. 11 and 13.

The comparison of the nutritional composition of milks of different animal species (Table 6) shows that milks differ significantly in their fat, protein, and calcium contents. Human milk is sweeter, with higher lactose content (13). The differences in the composition of some milk products, including different types of cheeses, is illustrated in Table 7. The creams and cheeses are rich in their fat and energy contents; the protein content of cheeses is much higher than those of milks and creams. Ruminant milks such as cow's milk contain a higher proportion of short-chain volatile fatty acids, which are derived from the fermentation of carbohydrates in the rumen (Table 8). This anaerobic fermentation also leads to the saturation of fatty acids, so that the milk fat con-

Table 7 Nutritional Composition of Some Milk Products (Values per 100 g)

Products	Water (g)	Energy (kcal)	(kJ)	Protein (g)	Fat (g)	Lactose (g)	Sucrose (g)
Milks							
Semi-skimmed	89.8	46	194	3.3	1.6	4.7	
Skimmed	91.1	33	140	3.3	0.1	4.8	
Dried skimmed	3.0	350	1491	36.0	1.0	50.1	
Evaporated whole	69.1	159	664	8.2	9.0	12.0	
Condensed, sweetened							
whole	25.9	329	1390	8.5	9.0	12.3	43.2
Creams							
Single	74.0	188	776	2.6	18.0	3.9	
Double	48.0	449	1849	1.7	48.0	2.6	
Cheeses							
Camembert	50.7	297	1232	20.9	23.7		
Cheddar	36.0	412	1708	25.5	34.4		
Danish blue	45.3	347	1437	20.1	29.6		
Edam	43.8	333	1382	26.0	25.4		
Parmesan	18.4	462	1880	39.4	32.7		
Cottage	79.1	98	413	13.8	40		
Processed	45.7	330	1367	20.8	27.0		

Source: Ref. 11.

Table 8 Fatty Acid Composition of Cow's and Human Milk (Values in % of Total Fatty Acids)

Fatty acids	Cow's milk	Human milk
4:0	3.2	0
6:0	2.0	0
8:0	1.2	Tr
10:0	2.8	1.4
12:0	3.5	5.4
14:0	11.2	7.3
16:0	26.0	26.5
18:0	11.2	9.5
14:1	1.4	Tr
16:1	2.7	4.0
18:1	27.8	35.4
18:2	1.4	7.2[a]
18:3	1.5	0.88

Tr = Trace
[a]Value varies widely depending on maternal diet
Source: Ref. 13.

Table 9 Inorganic Constituents of Some Milks and Milk Products (Values in mg/100 g)

Products	Na	K	Ca	Mg	P	Fe	Zn	Protein (g)
				(mg)				
Milks								
Cow	55	140	115	11	92	0.06	0.4	3.2
Goat	42	170	100	13	90	0.12	0.5	
Sheep	44	120	170	18	150	0.03	0.7	
Human	15	58	34	3	15	0.07	0.3	
Milk products								
Skimmed milk	54	150	120	12	94	0.06	0.4	3.33
Dried skimmed milk	550	1590	1280	130	970	0.27	4.0	36.1
Yogurt, whole	80	280	200	19	170	0.1	0.7	5.7
Cottage cheese	380	89	73	9	160	0.1	0.6	13.8
Cheddar cheese	670	77	720	25	490	0.3	2.3	25.5
Parmasan cheese	1090	110	1200	45	810	1.1	5.3	39.4

Source: Ref. 12.

tains low levels of unsaturated fatty acids. In non-ruminants, the saturation of fat can be altered by dietary means (12).

The data on inorganic constituents of some milks and their products (Table 9) show that human milk contains lower levels of Na, K, Ca, Mg, and especially P (16% of that in cow's milk). The mineral concentrations in the milk products are in proportion to the protein or solids-no-fat (SNF) contents, because the inorganic nutrients are primarily associated with the aqueous phase.

Thus, skimmed milk products have higher levels of mineral matter. In cheese, addition of common salt (NaCl) produces substantial increases in the Na level.

The fat-soluble vitamins (retinol, carotene, vitamins D and E) of milks and their products (Table 10) are broadly in proportion to their fat content. The latter in turn depends on the type of feed given to the animal. The values of fat-soluble vitamins are usually higher in the summer months, when the animals are grazing, and lower in the winter, when they are fed concentrates (12). Milks are also a good source of water-soluble vitamins of the B group, although the riboflavin levels decline on storage, if the milk is exposed to sunlight or fluorescent lighting. Pasteurization and sterilization increase losses of thiamin, vitamin B_6, B_{12} and folic acid contents of milk. Substantial losses in the vitamin C content of milk also occur on storage and heat processing.

Milk and milk products are excellent sources of several macro and micro nutrients. Milk proteins are of high quality (high biological value), with high lysine content. Thus, milk and milk products can supplement well the cereals, which are generally low in lysine content. Milk fat is low in unsaturated fatty acids. This has led to a decline in the consumption of dairy products in the more developed countries, with an increase in the consumption of skimmed milk and its products. The major role of milk in the provision of nutrients such as calcium and riboflavin should not be disregarded by the improper interpretation of nutritional guidance, which recommends a modest reduction in fat intake, not total abstinence (14). Milk and its products are particularly valuable in the nutrition of young children (15).

Milk and its products, however, may have certain adverse effects in some individuals. Allergic reactions to milk proteins, including inherited disorders such as galactosemia and lactose intolerance, are common in some people. Infants with such disorders cannot metabolize galactose effectively, and because their consumption of galactose will lead to cataract formation, all lactose-containing foods must be replaced with other foods such as soya milk products.

The production of cheese leads to the release of free amino acids into the product, and the conversion of some of these to amines. The presence of tyramine in the diet can stimulate the sympathetic nervous system and is thought to be associated with migraine in susceptible persons. Patients receiving monoamine oxidase inhibitory drugs should avoid the consumption of tyramine and therefore cheese (12).

Table 10 Vitamin Content of Some Milks and Milk Products (Values per 100 g)

Vitamins	Milks			Creams		Cheeses	
	Whole	Skimmed	Channel island	Single	Double	Edam	Cheddar
Fat (g)	3.9	0.1	5.1	18.0	48.0	26.0	34.4
Retinol (µg)	52	1	65(s) 27(w)	315	600	175	325
Carotene (µg)	21	Tr	115(s) 27(w)	125	325	150	225
Vitamin D (µg)	0.03	Tr	0.03	0.14	0.27	—	0.26
Vitamin E (mg)	0.09	Tr	0.09	0.40	1.10	0.48	0.53
Thiamin (mg)	0.03	0.04	0.04	0.04	0.02	0.03	0.03
Riboflavin (mg)	0.17	0.17	0.19	0.17	0.18	0.35	0.40
Vitamin B_6 (mg)	0.06	0.06	0.06	0.05	0.03	0.09	0.10
Vitamin B_{12} (mg)	0.4	0.4	0.4	0.3	0.2	2.1	1.1
Folic acid (µg)	6	5	7	7	7	40	33

(s) = Summer; (w) = Winter
Source: Ref. 11.

B. Milk Processing

Fresh milk is required to be processed to ensure safe milk free from disease-producing bacteria, other toxic substances, and foreign odors. Processed milk has a good flavor and satisfactory keeping quality and a low bacterial count.

Milk is first clarified using a centrifugal clarifier to remove all dirt, impurities, and some bacteria. Milk is then pasteurized, either by holding it at $61.7°C$ (sometimes $62.8°C$) for 30 min, followed by rapid cooling (batch process) or by the HTST method, in which milk is held at $71.7°C$ for 15 sec. (continuous process). Ultra-high temperature treatments at $93.4°C$ for 3 sec or $149.5°C$ for 1 sec are also employed. Because pasteurized milk is not sterile, it must be cooled quickly to prevent multiplication of surviving bacteria. The pasteurizing temperatures do not normally alter the constituents or properties of milk. Pasteurization does not produce any objectionable cooked flavor and retains the nutritive value of the milk, except for slight decrease in the heat-labile vitamins (thiamin and vitamin C). Pasteurization increases the shelf life of milk considerably.

Homogenization is a process of making a stable emulsion of milk fat and serum mechanically. This is achieved by passing warm milk or cream through a small aperture under high pressure and velocity. High-pressure homogenizers, low-pressure rotary-type homogenizers and sonic vibrators are employed for this purpose. The homogenized milk has a creamier structure, bland flavor, and whiter appearance. A soft curd is formed when homogenized milk is coagulated.

C. Milk Products

Milk is processed into a range of stable dairy products:

1. Vitamin D Milk

The vitamin D content of milk can be increased by irradiating milk with ultraviolet light, which converts milk sterol (7 dehydrosterol) into vitamin D. A vitamin D concentrate may also be added alternatively to raise the vitamin D content of the milk.

To meet the specific nutritional requirement of certain communities, milk is fortified with multivitamins and minerals. Low-sodium milk is prepared by passing it through ion exchange resins, to meet the specific diet requirements of some people. Also, milk may be treated with lactase to produce low lactose milk for persons suffering from lactose intolerance disorder.

2. Skimmed Milk

The removal of fat from whole milk by centrifugation produces skim milk. It contains all other milk nutrients, except vitamin A and D, but can be fortified by adding these vitamins. By varying the amount of milk fat removed from whole milk, low-fat milk (0.5–2.0% fat) can be prepared for consumers advocated low fat intake. Skimmed and condensed milk is used extensively in the manufacture of several bakery and confectionery products.

3. Concentrated Milks

The large water content of the milk makes it a bulky food, leading to problems of storage and refrigeration. A considerable part of water or all of it can be removed in evaporated (condensed milk) or dry milk powders, respectively.

Evaporated milk is whole milk from which more than half the water is removed by evaporation. Generally, raw whole milk is clarified and concentrated in a vacuum pan at $74°$ to $77°C$, followed by fortification with vitamin D, homogenization, filling into sterilized cans, and cooling. The heat treatment gives evaporated milk a light brown color (due to sugar-protein reaction) and a characteristic flavor.

Sweetened condensed milk, unlike evaporated milk, is not sterile, but microbial multiplication in this product is prevented by the preservative action of sugar. Pasteurized whole milk is concentrated and sweetened with sucrose, followed by canning.

4. Dry Milk or Milk Powders

Whole milk can be dehydrated to about 97% by spray-drying and vacuum-drying. Skim milk and low-fat milk are also dehydrated to make milk powder. Nonfat dry milk has vitamin A and D added to enhance its nutritive value. It is a low-cost product with a good shelf life and does not need refrigeration for storage. Dry milk can be reconstituted into fluid milk by mixing the recommended quantity of water. Dry milks must be sealed in airtight, moisture-free containers.

5. Cream

Cream is a milk fat concentrated into a fraction of the original milk. In unhomogenized milk, fat globules rise to the top to form a layer of cream, which can be separated by centrifugation. Creams with varying amount of fat are made. A mixture of milk and milk fat of 10 to 12% is known as half-and-half, whereas table cream (coffee cream) contains about 18% fat and whipping cream has 30 to 36% milk fat. The high fat content gives a more stable foam when whipped. Cream used for butter making may contain 25% to 40% fat. Sour cream is used in various baked products.

6. Butter

Butter is about 80% milk fat, though farm butter may contain only 60% to 65% fat. The nonfat components of butter are water, solids not fat, and salt, if added. Butter is made from sweet or sour cream. The cream is pasteurized at 62.8°C for 30 min or by HTST method and cooled quickly. A culture of desirable microorganisms (starter) is then added and cream is ripened at 21.1°C for the fermentation to take place. The acidity of curd determines the yield, quality, and keeping quality of butter. The ripened cream (*dahi*) is churned to bring about denaturation of the fat-globule surface, the membranes being eliminated in buttermilk. The fat globules clump together to form a water-in-oil-emulsion from an oil-in-water emulsion. The buttermilk is drained off and the butter is washed with water. Salt may be added to butter and worked to bring it into a compact mass. Butter is then cut to size, wrapped, and packed.

7. Cheese

Processing milk to make cheese is an excellent method of preserving milk nutrients. It is manufactured on a commercial scale in the Western countries, where it is a popular food. It is consumed as such or in cookery.

Cheeses are known after their place of origin. Cheddar cheese originated in Cheddar (England); Camembert and Roquefort cheeses originated in France. Cheese varieties are differentiated according to their flavor, body, and texture, which depend on the type of milk used, manufacturing method adopted, salts and seasonings added, and type of bacteria and mold species used for ripening. Cheeses are classified as hard, semihard, and soft cheeses based on their moisture content and whether they are ripened (by bacteria or molds) or unripened. Cheeses made directly from milk are "natural" cheeses, whereas "processed" cheeses are essentially melted or blended forms of the natural cheeses. Whey cheese is made from the whey remaining after coagulation and removal of casein. The composition of cheese varies according to manufacturing method, the protein content varying from about 20% to 40% (Table 7) and fat content varying from 4% to 35%. Cheeses also contain appreciable quantities of Ca, P, and vitamins. About 150 g of cheese is considered equivalent in food value to one liter of whole milk (9).

Cheese is made by coagulating or curdling milk with acid or rennin or both, drawing off the whey and processing the curd. Desirable flavor and texture of cheese are obtained by curing or ripening, i.e., by holding it at the specified temperature and humidity for a specified time. Pasteurized whole milk is brought to 31°C and lactic acid starter culture is added. The required coloring matter may also be added at this stage. After 30 min, rennin solution is added to the mildly acidic milk with stirring and allowed to set. The milk forms a firm curd within about 30 min. The curd is then cut into cubes of different sizes (for different types of cheese) to facilitate removal of whey from the cubes. The cut curd is heated slowly to 38°C in 30 min, and is held at this temperature for about 45 min, during which the curd is stirred to prevent matting. Heating squeezes out whey from the curd cubes and increases the rate of acid production, which makes the curd cubes shrink. The whey is then drained off and the curd is allowed to mat. The matted curd is cut into blocks, which are turned at 15 min intervals, and they are piled on one another (2 or 3 deep) (cheddaring process). The cheddared curd is then passed through a curd mill, which cuts the slabs of curd into strips. The whey is eliminated during this process. The milled pieces are sprinkled with salt and stirred for its uniform distribution. The added salt draws the whey out of curd by osmosis and acts as a preservative, holding down spoilage organisms, and adds flavor to the final product. The milled and salted pieces are placed in a hydraulic press overnight to remove moisture. The pressing determines the final moisture content of the finished product. The cheese is placed in a cool dry room to permit surface drying. It is dipped in hot paraffin to prevent mold growth and excessive drying during the long period of ripening. The waxed cheese is packaged and cured at 2.2°C and 85% RH for at least 60 days, which may be continued for 12 months or longer for maximum flavor. Rennet enzymes and microbes used for souring bring about a number of changes during ripening, giving the product desirable texture and flavor.

8. Yogurt

Yogurt is a coagulated milk product with a curd-like consistensy. It is made from partially skimmed or whole milk. The milk is heated to 82° to 85°C, homogenized, and cooled. It is then inoculated with a mixed culture containing *Lactobacillus bulgaricus* and *Streptococcus thermophilus* and held at 40° to 42°C for several hours. The nutritive value of yogurt (*dahi*) is similar to that of milk, except that yogurt has a small amount of lactic acid formed from the lactose of milk.

9. Cultured Buttermilk (Lassi)

Lassi is made from skim milk or partially skimmed milk by mildly coagulating it with lactic acid culture containing *Leuconostoc* species for flavor; it is consumed as a beverage. *Lassi* (buttermilk) is the liquid obtained after separation of butter from *dahi*.

10. Ghee

Ghee (or butter oil) is a stable milk product with a highly desirable flavor and aroma. It is 99.5% milk fat, and contains some fat-soluble vitamins and essential fatty acids. In India it is made exclusively by fermenting whole milk into curd (*dahi*), churning the curd into butter, and boiling the latter to *ghee*. Industrially it is made by separating the cream from milk mechanically, fermenting it and churning it into butter, followed by its conversion to *ghee*. The curd-butter route produces excellent-quality *ghee*, with proper care and control.

11. Ice Cream

Ice cream is a popular milk product in nations of the Western world and many other countries. It is frozen dairy product containing a variety of ingredients, including milk, skim milk, cream, butter, butter oil, condensed milk, and dried milk products. Milk fat and milk solids-not-fat constitute about 60% of the total solids in the ice cream. These components give ice cream a rich flavor and improve body and texture. In addition to these dairy products, ice cream contains sugar, stabilizer, emulsifier, water, air, and flavoring agents. The mixture of all these ingredients, before the air is incorporated and the mixture is frozen, is known as ice cream mix.

The sugar used in ice cream may be sucrose, corn syrup, dextrose, or fructose syrups. In addition to the sweetness, sugar imparts smoothness to the ice cream and lowers the freezing point of the ice cream mix. Stabilizers prevent the formation of ice crystals during freezing. They form a gel with the water in the formula, thereby improving the body and texture of the product. Gums, gelatin, sea wood, and cellulose (carboxymethyl cellulose) derivatives are often used as stabilizers. The emulsifiers help to disperse the fat globules throughout the mix, thus preventing them from clumping together during freezing-mixing operation. Emulsifiers also help to make the ice cream dry and stiff. Egg-yolk may be used as a natural emulsifier, whereas mono and diglycerides are the commercial emulsifiers used. Vanilla is the most common flavoring agent; others include strawberry, chocolate, and coffee. A large number of fruits and nuts are added in quantities to enhance the taste.

Some indigenous milk products made in India include *dahi* (yogurt), *khoa* (a semi-solid obtained by evaporating milk), *rabbri* (a sweetened milk product made by heating milk in a wide pan), and *mallai* (made by simmering milk until a thick layer of milk fat and coagulated protein forms on the surface).

V. FISH, OTHER SEAFOODS, AND THEIR PRODUCTS

Fish and a range of other foods from the ocean constitute an important source of highly nutritious food for humans and animals. The development of refrigerated transport and on-board refrigeration on fishing vessels have greatly enhanced the shelf life and quality of fish and other seafoods. The development of attractive processed products of these foods has further widened fish consumption to populations distant from the sea. Though fish catches on the global scale have increased in recent years, fish stocks in some waters are falling due to overfishing. Much of the fish caught is manufactured into animal feeds.

With the exception of farmed trout and salmon, fish are wild creatures that have to be located and taken from their natural environment. A very large number of fish species are consumed as food by the world human population. Most fishing is done from deep-sea trawlers, with on-board processing and refrigeration facilities, and/or accompanied by factory ships that process fish at sea. The fish are cooled as quickly as possible after the catch to minimize postmortem deterioration. Fish are a highly perishable commodity. Trimethylamine and ammonia are some of the early products of their spoilage, reducing consumer acceptability of the fish. The netted fish struggle and usually die from asphyxiation, which may produce certain metabolic changes that are rather disadvantageous to the shelf life of the fish as food (6).

A. Nutritional Composition and Quality

Southgate (6) classified fish used as foods into the following:

1. The bony fish—the Teleosts fall into two compositional groups: (a) white fish such as cod, haddock, halibut, lemon sole, plaice (and most other flat fish), saithe, and whiting and (b) fatty fish, such as eels, herring, pilchards, salmon, sardines, sprats, trout, tuna, and whitebait
2. The cartilaginous Elasmobranch fish, such as dogfish, shark, and skate

1. White Fish

The white fish are very low in fat and have muscle blocks surrounded by thin sheets of connective tissue. They have lower concentrations of most of the B group vitamins than mammalian muscle, except perhaps vitamin B_6. The mineral matter content of white fish is similar to that of mammalian muscle. The consumption of very fine bones of these fish with the flesh may raise the calcium content. Like most other marine organisms, the fish accumulate trace elements from seawater, and thus are a rich source of iodine. They may, however, be contaminated with certain toxic metals taken from heavily polluted waters (16). White fish accumulate fats (oils) in their livers which are a rich source of vitamin A (retinol) and vitamin D, as well as long-chain polyunsaturated fatty acids in their triglycerides.

2. Fatty Fish

These fish have high fat content in their flesh, which is much darker, with similar blocks of muscle interspersed with connective tissue. The fat content changes according to the breeding cycle of fish; i.e., after breeding the fat content decreases significantly. Herring, for example, have only 5% fat from February to April, and fat increases to 20% from July to October. Herring are therefore fished when they have higher fat content. The flesh of the fatty fish is normally richer in the B complex vitamins than the white fish, with significant amounts of vitamin A and D. The minerological composition is similar to that of the white fish. The fat has a higher proportion of very long chain polyunsaturated fatty acids, making the fat very prone to develop oxidative rancidity. Therefore, fatty fish are often smoked or pickled to preserve them.

3. Cartilagious Fish

These are the marine fish, such as sharks and rays. The flesh has low fat content, though their livers are rich in oil content, the content of vitamins and minerals being similar to that of the white fish. They remarkably maintain the osmolality of their extracellular fluids by increasing the urea content, thus giving an overestimate of the protein values based on total nitrogen content (6). The nutritional composition of some fish, molluscs, and crustaceans given in Table 11 shows that within the major groups of these marine species, there is a considerable similarity with respect to their fat and protein content.

The muscle of fish, molluscs, and crustacea is a good source of protein, providing similar amounts of lean meats. The protein quality in terms of amino acid composition is very similar in most fishes (Table 12), though the molluscan and crustacean proteins appear to be rich sources of essential amino acids (Table 11) (13). Their low fat content, however, has a high proportion of long-chain polyunsaturated fatty acids (Table 13). The mineral matter content of fish and the concentration of inorganic nutrients is comparable with other meats, with the exception of calcium content of fine bones in fish like herring. The levels of Na and intercellular elements, K and P, are higher than in meats, but the Fe and Zn levels tend to be lower, except in shellfish. Oysters are particularly rich sources of Zn, with levels as high as 100 mg/100 g. Fish are also a major source of iodine.

4. Invertebrate Seafoods

The popular shellfish species include two major phyla, the Mollusca (true shellfish) and the Arthropoda, Order Crustacea which include species such as crabs, shrimps, prawns, and lobsters.

a. Molluscs. The variety of molluscs eaten by humans include bivalves such as mussels, oysters, and scallops, gastropods such as winkles and whelks, and other molluscs who have lost their external shells, retaining an inner pen, the squids and octopuses. The true shelled molluscs may be eaten whole after boiling or occasionally raw. The muscular flesh has low fat and vitamin

Table 11   Composition of Some Fish, Molluscs, and Crustaceans (Values per 100 g Edible Matter)

Species	Energy (kcal)	(kJ)	Water (g)	Protein (g)	Fat (g)
White fish					
Cod	76	322	82.0	17.4	0.7
Haddock	73	308	81.3	16.8	0.6
Halibut	92	390	78.1	17.7	2.4
Lemon sole	81	343	81.2	17.1	1.4
Plaice	91	386	79.5	17.9	2.2
Catfish	90	376	78.1	16.1	2.7
Carp	115	481	77.8	18.0	4.2
Bream	103	430	78.0	16.7	4.3
Perch	84	355	81.0	18.1	1.3
Pike	81	343	80.0	18.4	0.7
Fatty fish					
Eel	168	700	71.3	16.6	11.3
Herring	234	970	63.9	16.8	18.5
Mackerel	223	926	64.0	19.0	16.3
Salmon	182	761	65.4	18.8	12.0
Trout, rainbow	160	670	71.0	18.6	9.6
Tuna	185	770	65.0	24.2	9.9
Cartilaginous fish					
Dogfish	156	653	72.3	17.6	9.9
Shark	100	418	77.0	20.6	1.3
Skate	98	410	77.8	21.5	0.7
Molluscs					
Abalone	98	410	75.8	18.7	0.5
Clam	82	343	80.8	14.0	1.9
Cockle	81	339	79.9	16.8	1.0
Mussel	95	397	78.6	14.4	2.2
Oyster	73	276	84.6	8.4	1.8
Scallop	81	339	79.8	15.3	0.2
Whelk	69	289	83.6	11.6	0.6
Cuttlefish	81	339	81.0	16.1	0.9
Octopus	73	305	82.2	15.3	0.8
Squid	75	314	82.0	15.3	0.8
Crustaceans					
Crab	100	418	76.8	17.9	2.0
Crayfish	69	285	82.0	14.6	0.5
Lobster	87	365	79.0	16.9	1.9
Shrimp	87	365	79.0	18.1	0.8

Source: Ref. 6.

content, but the mineral levels are generally higher than in true fish. Being filter feeders, they often accumulate trace elements, both essential and contaminant, from the seawater. They are also rather prone to contamination from aqueous pathogenic organisms, necessitating stringent regulations regarding the sites of their catch. Some rules require that these animals should be "rested" in unpolluted water for a period before they are sold. The muscular squids and octopuses are generally eaten after cooking.

Table 12 Amino Acid Composition of Some Fish Protein Compared with Other Protein (mg/g Total N)

Amino acid	Fish	Crustacea	Molluscs	Beef	Milk	Egg	Wheat
Essential							
Histidine	180	120	150	230	190	150	130
Isoleucine	330	290	300	320	350	350	210
Leucine	530	540	480	500	640	520	420
Lysine	610	490	500	570	510	390	150
Methionine	180	180	170	170	180	200	100
Phenylalanine	260	250	260	80	340	320	280
Threonine	300	290	290	290	310	320	170
Tryptophan	70	70	80	80	90	110	70
Valine	360	300	390	330	460	470	280
Non-essential							
Arginine	400	520	470	420	250	380	290
Alanine	430	420	350	440	240	340	230
Aspartic acid	650	680	700	600	530	670	310
Cystine	70	80	100	80	60	110	160
Glutamic acid	950	980	880	1080	1440	750	1710
Glycine	290	410	320	350	140	190	250
Proline	260	270	260	320	590	240	660
Serine	310	320	320	280	370	490	330
Tyrosine	220	230	260	240	280	250	190

Source: Ref. 6.

Table 13 Fatty Acid Composition of the Lipids of Some Fish Compared with Other Foods (% of Total Fatty Acid Content, Approx.)

Fatty acids	Cod	Herring	Beef	Milk	Maize
Saturated					
C16:0	21.5	13.7	26.9	26.0	14.0
C18:0	3.5	1.2	13.0	11.2	2.3
Others	1.1	7.4	5.0	26.0	0.9
Monounsaturated					
C16:1	2.3	10.0	6.3	2.7	0.3
C18:1	11.0	15.2	42.0	27.8	30.0
C20:1	1.8	13.2	—	—	0.2
C22:1	0.8	17.4	—	—	0.2
Others	—	—	2.5	3.2	—
Polyunsaturated					
C18:2	0.5	1.4	2.0	1.4	50.0
C18:3	0.1	1.2	1.3	1.5	1.6
C18:4	0.2	1.8	—	—	—
C20:4	3.9	0.6	1.0	—	—
C20:5	17.2	7.0	—	—	—
C22:5	1.5	1.1	—	—	—
C22:6	33.4	6.5	—	—	—

Source: Ref. 6.

b. Crustacea. Both freshwater (crayfish) and marine species (crabs, shrimps, prawns, and lobsters) constitute the phylum crustacea. They are characterized by tough exoskeletons made of chitin and protein. Only the muscular parts of the thorax and the specialized appendage muscles (the claws of crabs and lobsters) are eaten. In addition to their trapping from the wild ocean, they are being farmed because of their high gastronomic value in some communities. The crustaceans' flesh is especially low in fat, but higher in minerals such as sodium than most other marine species. These animals tend to accumulate trace elements from the water, their vitamin levels being similar to those of white fish (6).

The average consumption of fish in the United Kingdom in 1991 was about 29 g/person/day, of which about 18% was frozen convenience products (17), shellfish accounting for 2.5% of the total fish consumption. The consumption of fish in other European countries such as Spain, Portugal, and Italy is much higher than in the United Kingdom, probably because of their access to a wider range of species used as fresh foods. Thus the contribution of fish and other ocean foods to the nutrient intakes in a country such as the United Kingdom is relatively minor, providing only about 1% of energy, 4.7% of protein, and 1.3% of fat (3.2% of polyunsaturated fatty acid intakes). The only vitamin provided in significant quantity is vitamin D (14% of the total by the fish).

B. Processing of Fish and Seafoods

Fish being a highly perishable product, various processing methods have been developed to preserve them. First they are washed with a clean water to remove slime, blood stains, and so on. Larger fish may be gutted (i.e., all the internal organs or viscera are removed and the body cavity is washed). The fish are often processed by drying, salting, smoking, freezing, and canning.

1. Drying

Fish are sun-dried to remove moisture from the tissues and to arrest bacterial and enzymatic putrefaction. In India, about 35% to 40% of the total sea catch is cured in the sun. This method is not hygienic and there are significant losses due to spoilage. Also, the dried fish develop a peculiar odor.

2. Salting

Salting or pickling is widely followed in countries such as India; both dry-salting and wet-salting methods are adopted. For dry-salting, fish are first rubbed with salt powder, and then packed in tubs with dry salt powder sprinkled in between layers of fishes. After a period of about 10 to 20 hours, the fish are removed, washed in brine, and dried in the sun for 2 to 3 days. In wet-salting, cleaned fish are packed in large vats containing concentrated salt solution, and stirred daily till properly pickled. Large-sized fish may be cut longitudinally to produce slits to facilitate penetration of salt. After 7 to 10 days of pickling, the salty water oozing out from the fish is drained off and fish is sold without drying. This fish does not keep long and must be disposed of within 2 to 3 months. The fishes soaked in salt solution may be taken out and smoked.

The products of sun-drying and salting are unattractive; these methods are often associated with case-hardening, development of rancidity, color changes, mold growth and attack of insects and mites. Preservatives, such as acids, sodium benzoate, ethylene oxide or an antibiotics like aureomycin can help to prolong shelf-life of fish. However, many countries do not permit the use of these preservatives. Irradiation of fish with gamma-radiation prolongs the shelf life of fish by 20 to 25 days.

3. Freezing and Canning

These are the current methods of preserving high-quality fish, greatly extending the storage life and maintaining freshness. If the fish is gutted and frozen down to −29°C within 2 hours of its catch, its storage life can be extended as long as 2 years. In some cases, clean whole fish is frozen. Fin fish are usually frozen as fillets (lengthwise cuts), steaks (cross-cut section), or sticks (lengthwise or crosswise cut from fillet or steaks). Large fish are frozen by the sharp freeze, a comparatively slow freeze, and small fish, fillets, and steaks are quick frozen. Slow freezing can result in protein denaturation, if proper care is not taken. Freezing may also result in desiccation or drying caused by the transfer of moisture from fish surface to the cold surface of freezing equipment. Frozen fatty fish may undergo oxidative rancidity more quickly than lean ones. Desiccation and oxidation can be prevented by properly protecting fish with suitable wrappers prior to freezing.

The fat fish are more suitable for canning (e.g., salmon, tuna, sardine, herring, lobster, shrimp). In the cases of salmon, tuna, sardine, and mackerel, an additional quantity of fish or vegetable oil is usually added to the fish prior to its canning, whereas shrimps are often canned in brine. Canning retains the natural flavor of the fish. Shellfish, however, can turn dark or discolored during canned storage, owing to the release of hydrogen sulfide from its sulfur compounds. The latter reacts with the iron of the can to produce black iron sulfide. This can be prevented by using an enamel containing zinc, because zinc sulfide is white in color.

C.   Fish Products

A range of products made from fish and other seafoods include fish meal used as animal feed, fish flour used for protein enrichment of human food, fish oil used for feeding and industrial purposes, fish glue (isinglass), and a high-grade fish collagen used to clarify wines, beer, and vinegar.

1.   Fish Meal

Fish meal is prepared from parts of fish not used as human food and sometimes the whole fish is of low quality. The material is ground, usually with removal of some oil followed by dehydration. Fish meal contains about 55 to 70% protein, 2 to 5% fat, 10 to 12% ash, and 6 to 12% moisture. It is used as animal and poultry feed. A low-grade fish meal can also be used as a manure for plantation crops.

2.   Fish Flour

After the solvent extraction of oil and fatty substances from the ground fish tissues to remove all the fishy odor, the tissue is dehydrated and milled to produce a bland nutritious powder rich in protein and mineral matter. Fish flour produced under appropriate bacteriological and sanitary control can be utilized in human food, as fish flour or fish protein concentrate. It can be incorporated at 3 to 10% level into a variety of dishes without altering their acceptability. Fish flour has about 85 to 90% of high quality protein.

3.   Fish Oils

Two kinds of fish oils, viz., liver oils and fish body oils, are produced. Liver oil is the principal natural source of vitamin A and, to a lesser extent, vitamin D. Fish species such as cod, halibut, tuna, and shark are good sources of fish liver oils. Both the oil and vitamin A contents vary in different fishes. Body oil is obtained from fishes such as sardine, herring, and salmon, which are fatty fishes (Table 11).

Liver oil can be obtained by cooking good quality minced fish liver at 85°–95°C which results in disintegration of liver cells and release of oil. The oil floating on the steam condensate can then be skimmed off or separated by centrifugation.

Fish body oils are produced along with the fish meal by first grinding fishes to a pulp and steaming. The oil and water become separated from the protein. The cooked flesh is then pressed to produce oil and presscake. The latter is used for fish meal. The press liquor (or stick water) is concentrated and the oil is recovered (9).

REFERENCES

1. Patton, S., S., Milk, *Food*: *Sci. Am.*, W.H. Freeman & Co., 1973, p. 115.
2. FAO, *Production Yearbook*, Food and Agriculture Organization, Rome, 1994.
3. Wood, J.D., P.J. Buxton, F.M. Whittington, and M. Enser, The chemical composition of fat tissues in the pig: the effects of castration and feeding treatment, *Livestock Prod. Sci. 15*: 73 (1986).
4. Greenfield, H. (ed.), Composition of Meat in Australia, *Food Technology in Australia*, *39*: 1 (1987).
5. Paul, A.A., and D.A.T. Southgate, A study on the composition of retail meats: dissection into lean, separable fat and inedible portions, *J. Human Nutr.*, *31*: 259 (1977).
6. Southgate, D.A.T., Meat, fish, eggs and novel proteins, *Human Nutrition and Dietetics*, 9th ed. (J.S. Garrow and W.P.T. James, eds.), Churchill Livingstone (Longman), London, 1993, p. 305.
7. Sinclair, A.J., and K. O'Dea, The lipid levels and fatty acid compositions of the lean portions of Australian beef and lamb, *Food Technol. in Australia*, *39*: 229 (1987).
8. BNF, Nutritional aspects of meat, BNF Briefing Paper No. 18, British Nutrition Foundation, London, 1988.
9. Manay, N.S., and M. Shadaksharswamy, *Foods*: *Facts and Principles*, Wiley Eastern, New Delhi, 1987, p. 375.
10. Tolan, A., J. Robertson, and C.R. Orton. The chemical composition of eggs produced under battery, deep litter and free range conditions, *British J. Nutr. 31*: 1985 (1974).
11. Holland, B., I.D. Unwin, and D.H. Buss, Milk products and egg, 4th Suppl., *McCance and Widdowson's "The Composition of Foods"*, Royal Society of Chemistry, London, 1989.
12. Southgate, D.A.T., Milk and milk products, fats and oils, *Human Nutrition and Dietetics*, 9th ed. (J.S. Garrow and W.P.T. James, eds.), Churchill Livingstone, (Longman Group), London, 1993, p. 317.
13. Paul, A.A., and D.A.T. Southgate, *McCance and Widdowson's The Composition of Food*, 4th ed., HMSO, London, 1978.
14. HEC, Proposals for nutritional guidance for health education in Britain, National Advisory Committee on Nutrition Education, Health Education Council, London, 1983.
15. DHSS, Diet and cardiovascular disease, Report on Health and Social Subjects No. 28, Dept. of Health and Social Security, HMSO, London, 1984.
16. MAFF, Steering Group of Food Surveillance, Series of Reports Published at Irregular Intervals, Ministry of Agriculture, Fisheries and Food, HMSO, London, 1980.
17. MAFF, Household food consumption and expenditure, Annual (1991) Report of the National Food Survey Committee, Ministry of Agriculture, Fisheries and Food, HMSO, London, 1992.

12

Potential Proteins, Fats, and Oils

I. INTRODUCTION

Proteins are usually considered the most important of all the known substances present in living matter, without which life would be impossible on our planet. The proteins are one of the three principal organic constituents of living organisms (the other two are fats and carbohydrates), but in importance and diversity of their biological functions they stand alone. Proteins represent nearly one-half of the body's dry matter (about 70% of the body is water). Of the total body protein, more than a third is found in the muscles. These are the myosin fibers, which are the fundamental contractile elements in muscular movement. The bones and cartilages account for another 20%, where the protein collagen contributes to the structural stability of the skeleton. The skin has about 10% of the body protein, the keratin serving to protect the interior tissues against attack from the external environment.

Enzymes are by far the most important of all proteins. These are present in only minute amounts in comparison with myosin, collagen, or keratin, but they are indispensable for the promotion and direction of the body's myriad biochemical (metabolic) reactions. The food consumed by man is digested in the stomach and intestine by the activity of protein enzymes like pepsin or trypsin. The use of oxygen by the body to oxidize carbon and hydrogen in food as well as to eliminate waste products is brought about through the synchronized action of a series of proteins, including hemoglobin and enzymes, thereby providing the chemical energy (ATP) for several vital functions; for example, movement, reproduction, repair of wear and tear of living tissues by the continuous regeneration of body constituents, including proteins, fats, and carbohydrates, under specific directive influence of a host of enzyme proteins.

Several hormones are also proteins that are secreted by the endocrine organs and are carried by the blood in infinitesimal amounts to the tissues, where they play a remarkable, decisive role in the regulation of the pace and direction of various anabolic and catabolic reactions. Other proteins, such as the antibodies of blood, help to defend the organism against viruses (proteins) and the harmful substances produced by pathogenic bacteria. The genes, the basic units of heredity, also contain a type of protein called nucleoprotein.

The proteins obviously have a diverse chemical structure to enable them to carry out such varied functions in the body. The number of identified proteins in living organisms is extremely large and growing rapidly. Each cell of the bacterium *Escherichia coli* contains more than 6000 different kinds of organic compounds, including about 3000 different proteins and a similar number of different nucleic acid molecules.

The fats and oils used almost universally as stored forms of energy in living organisms are highly reduced organic compounds derived from fatty acids. The latter are in turn derived from the hydrocarbons (4 to 36 carbon chains). In some fatty acids, the hydrocarbon chain is fully saturated with no double bonds and unbranched, whereas in others one or more double bonds occur (mono- or polyunsaturated fatty acids). Triglycerides are fatty acid esters of glycerol, also referred to as oils, fats, or neutral fats and provide stored energy and insulation. Most natural fats such as vegetable oils, dairy products, and animal fat are complex mixtures of simple and mixed triacylglycerols, containing a variety of fatty acids differing in chain length and degree of saturation. Vegetable oils such as corn and olive oils are composed largely of triacylglycerols with unsaturated fatty acids, and thus are liquids at room temperature, whereas triacylglycerols containing only saturated fatty acids like tristearin (the major component of beef fat) are white, greasy solids at room temperature and are usually referred to as fats. The liquid oils are converted industrially into solid fats by catalytic hydrogenation to enhance their keeping quality. When lipid-rich foods are exposed too long to oxygen in air, they may spoil and become rancid. The unpleasant taste and odor associated with rancidity result from the oxidative cleavage of the double bonds in unsaturated fatty acids to produce aldehydes and carboxyacids of shorter chain length and therefore higher volatility.

The world nutrition problem is essentially a question of providing proteins and energy to the increasing global population. At present, roughly one-half of the people in the world have a poorly balanced diet that retards normal growth. The main lack in their diet is animal protein; they live principally on cereal grains and tubers that contain inferior proteins lacking in certain essential amino acids that are present only in animal proteins. Kwashiorkor, protein-calorie deficiency disease, is on the increase among the children of many tropical countries of Asia, Africa, and Latin America. Protein poverty is one of the principal factors holding back the underdeveloped countries. The widespread prevalance of protein-energy malnutrition and undernutrition in the developing world has created a considerable interest in the development of protein supplements for use in weaning foods. The search for the development of alternative protein sources from plants, animals and microbes has begun in many countries of the world. Increasing production of animal protein, in general, has resulted in an inefficient use of plant protein. Thus, two lines of research have been developed: (a) to produce isolates of plant proteins, and (b) to explore the production of protein microbiologically using bacteria, yeast, and other fungi.

II. PLANT PROTEIN ISOLATES, CONCENTRATES, AND LEAF PROTEINS

Proteins present in plants constitute the primary source. Plants utilize the carbon in the carbon dioxide of the air to manufacture a range of organic substances, including proteins. The proteins of the most common vegetable foods, however, lack some of the essential amino acids. The cereal grains, for example, generally lack the amino acid lysine and are frequently poor in methionine and tryptophan. It is the missing essential amino acids that make most vegetable proteins inferior in quality from the standpoint of human nutrition. Of about 20 amino acids required by the human body, humans must obtain 11 from food because the body does not synthesize them. There are some plant products that contain well-balanced proteins with most of the essential amino acids, e.g., soybeans, chickpeas and oilseed meals of certain plants. These are important potential staples for protein nutrition but have not yet been developed into major foods.

A. Proteins from Groundnuts

Seed legumes, which are rich sources of both proteins and oils, have been considered as potential sources of proteins. From both of these sources, proteins are extracted with alkali to solubilize the protein, which is filtered off the structural plant material. The pH of the filtrate is adjusted to the isoelectric point of the protein to precipitate the protein curd. The latter is then washed and dried. The leaf protein concentrates retain the plant pigments and are therefore green in color. This has been regarded as a disadvantage precluding the use of leaf proteins in many foods. The concentrates can be produced with simple equipment, a low-technology approach being considered better for the developing countries.

The protein isolates from legumes are amorphous, lightly colored powders. The soya protein isolates in particular have wide use as food ingredients in this form. The plant protein isolates have been used to produce meat analogues, but the main technological problems have been the introduction of the essential sensory properties of proteins, mainly the texture and flavor. Suitable textures are being developed by spinning fibers (using textile machinery). The alterations in the alignment of the fibers can produce a range of textures, simulating different types of meat. The flavors can be added easily; their retention in the simulated meat when it is chewed is the major problem. The simulated stewing-steak type products have now been well accepted.

The protein isolates and concentrates from legumes have lower biological values than meat proteins with the sulfur amino acids, methionine and cysteine, being limiting; though in a mixed diet, however, this is of little nutritional significance. However, the levels of B vitamins, especially B_{12} are very low, needing fortification (1). The levels of iron and zinc are also low in these isolates and the presence of phytates decreases the bioavailabilty of these minerals (2).

In addition to serving as potential sources of oils, food legumes such as peanuts are rich sources of protein. Oil extraction produces a protein-rich co-product that can be utilized for human consumption if the products are processed for edible-grade products. Soybean and peanut products are available in the form of flakes, grits, or flours that can be further processed into a variety of protein-rich concentrates, isolates, and co-isolates (3). The production technology of edible protein products of peanuts has been reviewed extensively (4–6).

Protein concentrates from peanut, with 60% to 70% protein content, can be produced through process variations, such as water leaching at the isoelectric point, aqueous alcohol leaching, air classification, liquid cycline fractionation, moist heat denaturation followed by water leaching, and aqueous extraction (Fig. 1). All these processes, with the exception of aqueous extraction method, use defatted flours or flakes to begin with. The aqueous extract of comminuted full-fat seed at pH 4.0 is simultaneously separated into oil, solid, and aqueous phases in the aqueous extraction method. The acid-soluble proteins, carbohydrates, oil and other constituents are extracted, leaving the fiber and acid-insoluble substances in the protein; sugars and salts that are not precipitated are recovered from the whey by ultracentrifugation and reverse osmosis, removing about 90% of the oil (7).

Peanut isolates with 90% or more protein can be prepared by extracting the water-insoluble polysaccharides, water-soluble sugars, and other minor constituents such as minerals, in addition to those constituents that are necessary to make concentrates. Various factors influencing the yield and extractability during the preparation of protein isolates include particle size of the flour, flour to water ratio, pH, and time and temperature of extraction (6,8–13).

The method of making protein isolates basically involves extraction of protein from defatted peanut seed flour with aqueous alkaline solution, followed by removal of insoluble material by centrifugation and/or filtration. The proteins are then precipitated at their isoelectric pH 4.5 and the protein curd thus precipitated is collected through centrifugation or filtration. The protein isolates are dried by spray-drying or by lyophilization (freeze-drying). Fig. 2 shows the steps involved in the processing of protein isolates from peanut seeds. The aqueous alkaline extraction is carried out at pH below 9.0 to minimize protein denaturation. The protein isolates are often neutralized before drying to make them water dispersible. The methods using techniques to minimize protein denaturation have been found to produce maximum yields of isolates having high solubility properties. Peanut seed protein isolates are separated from the oil component by an aqueous extraction method (Fig. 2) similar to that used for peanut protein concentrates (Fig. 1). The major difference in these two methods is the use of an alkaline (pH 8.0) extraction and a filtration

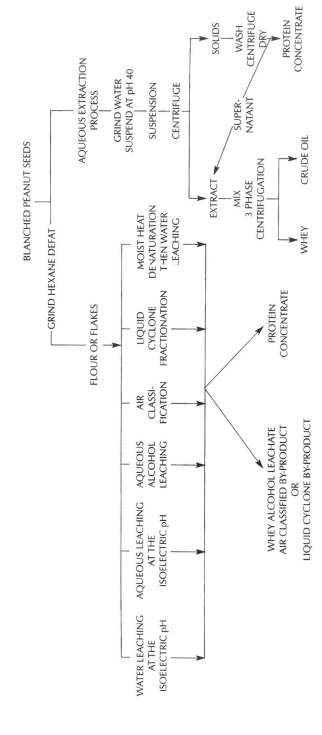

Figure 1 Processing of peanut seed protein concentrates. (From Refs. 4 and 12.)

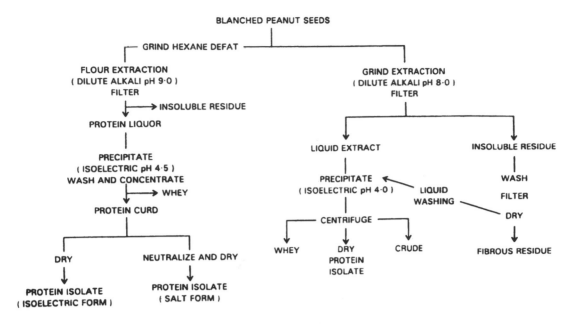

Figure 2 Processing of peanut seed protein isolates. (From Refs. 4, 11, and 14.)

step to separate protein isolates from the fibrous fraction of the peanut seed (Fig. 2) (14,15). The peanut protein isolates can also be precipitated from alkaline extracts by heating in the presence of Ca^{2+} ions. This assists the elimination of the beany flavor and aflatoxins (16).

Co-precipitated isolates (or protein co-isolates) with 95% protein may be prepared by combining different quantities of peanut seed, cotton seed, and soybean flours (17–19). Protein isolates can also be made from these flours by this method. The co-isolate method, however, requires protein extraction with dilute aqueous sodium hydroxide, acidification of protein extract to pH 5.0 to precipitate protein curds (Fig. 3) (20). The disc-gel electrophoresis of these product showed that some of the proteins in the combined extracts dissociated into their subunits at pH 2.5, then reassociated into their original or new protein forms, or both as the pH was raised to 7.0, these co-isolates were found to possess better amino acid composition and functional and nutritional properties than their corresponding isolates (3,4).

B. Protein from Soybeans (Soy Proteins)

Soy proteins have been considered equivalent to animal proteins and possible replacements for animal proteins in times to come. A gradual switch to plant proteins would be necessary for economic reasons, if nothing else. Soybean products are traditionally associated with Asia, however the United States of America has dominated the soybean market in recent years. In 1994, the world production of soybean was 136.7 million metric tons (MMT) (21), of which the United States of America contributed to 69.9 MMT, Brazil, 24.9 MMT and China, 16.3 MMT. In the United States of America, soybeans are second only to corn in importance. Soy oil completely dominates the American edible oil industry, and soy proteins have become the mainstay of the meat and poultry industries. They also constitute the major component of high-protein animal

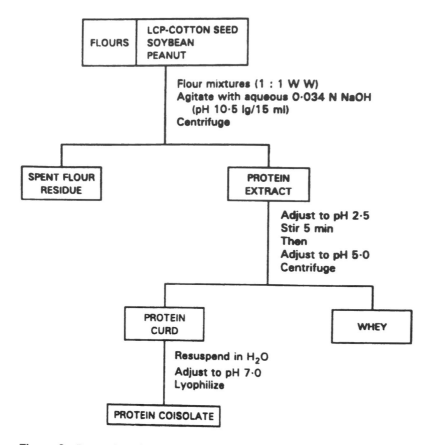

Figure 3   Processing of peanut seed protein co-isolates. (From Refs. 4 and 20.)

rations. The number of soy products introduced into the human food chain also have increased considerably in recent decades.

Clydesdale and Francis (22) divided food-grade soy products into four categories: whole beans, flours, concentrates, and isolates.

1.   Whole Beans

The whole beans are canned in the immature stage as green beans in the pods like conventional green beans. The mature beans may also be canned in tomato sauce or ground with water to make a milk-like beverage. A number of soy-based beverages are sold as formulas for infants allergic to cow's milk (patients with lactose intolerance and galactosemia).

A large portion of the soybeans produced is used to make traditional oriental seasonings and high-protein foods. Soy sauce is made in Asia by mixing cooked defatted soy flakes with wheat, inoculating this mixture with *Aspergillus oryzae*, followed by salting and fermentation for 8 to 12 months. In the USA, soy sauce is usually made by acid hydrolysis (22).

Tofu is made by precipitating the curd from soy milk, whereas *tempeh* is made from cooked soybeans inoculated with *Rhizopus oligospores* and fermented for 24 hours, the resulting cake-like mass being sliced and fried. Other soybean-based popular foods in Asia include dried *tofu*, *kinako, miso, and natto.*

2. Soy Flours

Soy flours and grits are usually incorporated into other food products. The grits and flours differ in their particle size, the latter being ground finer. Both are made in a defatted form, a full-fat form, and combination of both forms. Full-fat flour is made by cleaning the soybeans, hulling, and heating them to minimize their beany flavor and inactivate the enzymes, followed by drying and grinding. Defatted flour is made by solvent-extracting the dehulled and crushed flour to remove fat. A defatted flour has about 51% protein, 34% carbohydrate and 1.5% fat, whereas a full-fat flour has 41% protein, 25% carbohydrate, and 21% fat.

3. Protein Concentrations and Isolates from Soybeans

Protein concentrates are made by removing the water-soluble sugars, ash, and other minor low-mol.wt. components from defatted soy flakes. These components are usually removed by extracting them with water or alcohol. The resulting product has 66% to 70% protein content.

Protein isolates are prepared from defatted soy flour in two steps. First the flour is treated with dilute alkali to dissolve the protein (mixture has pH 7–9). The insoluble residues are removed and the liquid is acidified to bring its pH to 4.5. The protein is precipitated and filtered off as a curd. In the second step, the protein can be redissolved and extruded in any shape or passed through fine nozzles to produce threads like nylon. A dried bundle of soy isolate threads looks like blond hair. The threads are bundled together, colored, flavored, and packaged to stimulate chicken ham, beef and other foods. A typical soy isolate has a protein content of 93% to 95%.

Soy proteins have been used as "functional" or "filler" proteins in other foods to give them additional protein content; they have some functional value for emulsification (in ground meat products like sausages and wieners), fat absorption (in hamburgers and sausages), water absorption (in baked products, simulated meats, and pet foods), and desirable texture (for thickening soups and gravies in many foods).

C. Leaf Protein Concentrates (LPC)

Green leaves of plants are the novel sources of potential proteins. The technology of leaf protein concentrate (LPC) has been slow to develop; it was started in Hungary (Europe) in the 1930s and pursued by N. Pirie in England. Many types of plants have been tested for their ability to produce protein under different horticultural and agricultural conditions, and suitable plants were chosen for processing (23).

The basic procedure involves pulping and pressing of plants in one operation to separate the fibrous matter from the green slurry containing the protein. The latter is heat-treated to coagulate the protein, which is then pressed. The final product is a green curd that can be dried and added to other food products. The product has about 40% high-quality protein, with a good biological value. It has been mainly used in animal feeds. Unfortunately, for human consumption, the green crude protein has a bitter taste and unattractive color. Dr. Pirie has developed a series of food dishes for human consumption, such as soups and baked products, using LPC. They are required to be highly flavored and are very dark in color.

Attempts have been made to purify the protein and to remove the dark green color and bitter taste of the green crude protein. Alfalfa leaves have been used in the United States as a source of yellow pigment for poultry. At the USDA laboratories, fresh alfalfa leaves are ground and pressed. The resulting green liquid is heated to 60°C to coagulate chloroplast proteins, which are filtered off as a green curd. The liquid is then heated to 80°C to coagulate the cytoplasmic proteins, which are filtered off as a gray curd. The resulting liquid, known as 'alfalfa solubles' are dried and together with the original press cake sold as animal feed. The protein curd resulting from both pressings is rich in protein and has been developed as a feed for nonruminant animals. The protein concentrate can be further purified to produce a source of protein for human consumption, especially in the developed countries like United States of America. In countries like India with predominant vegetarian diets, many foods are greenish brown in color and are often highly spiced. Neither the green color nor the bitter taste of LPC would be very disadvantageous with these types of foods.

D. Protein from Algae

As a source of single-cell protein (SCP), algae (chlorella) has received considerable publicity in the press and scientific community as another "factory" for protein. Algae require carbon dioxide from air, sunlight as a source of energy, and a simple inorganic source of minerals for their growth. Algae give out oxygen and remove minerals from sewage effluents. Thus algae can also be used to clean up the effluent from sewage and other waste disposal plants before this liquid is released into rivers, thus controlling environmental pollution. Ponds of 10 feet wide, 6 inches deep, and hundreds of yards long are employed for this purpose and have been found to be very effective. Sewage is an excellent source of nutrients for algae, with plentiful supply.

The production of SCP from algae is uneconomical at present time, because of its cost of recovery and purification. However, with changing economics, SCP from algae may be available in large quantities in the future (22).

Algae have been used as human foods by many cultures. The Chinese and Japanese, for example, have eaten algae in the form of seaweed (*Porphyra*, *Chondrus*, and others) for centuries. The natives around Lake Chad in Africa have consumed *Spirulina maxima* since ancient times, and it is produced in large quantities in Lake Texcoco (Mexico).

According to Clydesdale and Francis (22), the ocean produces around 20 trillion tons of algae annually—more than 5 tons for each person on the earth. However, the concentration of algae in seawater is only about 3 mg/liter, and the minimum considered feasible for harvesting is around 250 mg/liter. Also, some algae are toxic to human beings, e.g. red tide (*Gonyaulax*), which causes large fish kills periodically on the Atlantic coast. Currently there is no more efficient technology of harvesting algae economically from seawater than through fishes.

III. PROTEINS FROM PETROLEUM AND CARBOHYDRATES (SCP)

A. Yeasts

Production of proteins by microorganisms, such as yeasts (fungi), bacteria, and algae, is not a new idea. The growing of yeast fungi on carbohydrates such as molasses to produce animal and human foods has been practiced for a long time. The yeast fungi can produce vitamins and proteins comparable to those of animals. This method of obtaining proteins from microorganisms has the following major advances:

1. The microorganisms grow very rapidly, doubling their weight every 5 hours or less, which is several thousand times faster than the rate of protein synthesis by farm animals.
2. The microorganisms can be grown in tanks; they do not require soil, sunlight, or rainfall or any assistance from human labor.
3. The fungi belong to the plant kingdom, hence their meat (protein) is not outlawed by religious or traditional taboos (24).

The researchers at the Massachusetts Institute of Technology have coined the term "single cell protein" (SCP) as a general term for all proteins produced by microorganisms.

It has been known that molds often grow on petroleum products; they are found in the bottom of oil tanks, in refineries, in oil-impregnated soils, and even under tarry road surfaces. In 1952, a German scientist, Felix Just noticed that yeasts could be grown successfully in the laboratory on pure hydrocarbons (waxy paraffins). This report launched a search for efficient microorganisms that can grow on petroleum to make proteins.

The production of single-cell protein (SCP) from yeasts grown on carbohydrates is a major industry in the world today. Nearly all of the SCP produced in this way is used in the animal feed industry, barring small quantities incorporated into the human food chain. Three major sources of materials used to grow yeasts are molasses, spent sulfite liquor, and whey. The SCP produced from molasses using the yeast, *Saccharomyces cereviseae*, is the largest of the three types. Both cane- and beet-sugar molasses are used, though the latter contains more nutrients. The conventional fermentation in large tanks is optimized for the growth of yeast cells rather than encouraging production of alcohol from molasses. The product is called *primary dried yeast*.

The SCP can also be produced from spent sulfite liquor from the pulp and paper industries. The composition of liquor varies with the source of wood and the type of process used, but it contains 2 to 3% sugar. These sugars are fermented by the yeast *Candida utilis*, which is recovered as SCP. Huge quantity of sulfite liquor remains unused and can become a source of pollution. It can be utilized to produce SCP. The yeast from this source is called *torula dried yeast*.

SCP can also be made by utilizing whey, a by-product of the cheese industry. The lactose sugar present in the whey can be fermented by the yeast *Saccharomyces fragilis*, making a product called *dried fragilis yeast*. Like sulfite liquor, much of the whey currently remains unutilized, forming a source of pollution. Efforts have been made to treat whey to recover high-quality milk proteins present in low concentrations in the whey and to use lactose for fermentation. The major problem faced by large-scale yeast plants is collection of whey from the small and scattered cheese plants, only about one half of the available whey being utilized at present. Brewer's yeast is another potential source of SCP from carbohydrates. It has been estimated that 25,000 tons of dry brewer's yeast can be recovered as a by-product of brewing 100 million barrels of beer (22). Obviously, the product of SCP from yeast alone by fermentation could be very large if all the available existing raw materials were used.

When the yeast is grown on sugar, the fermentation medium usually consists of the carbohydrate in a water solution, soluble mineral and organic compounds containing N, P, and K, with certain trace elements and vitamins. The air is bubbled through the liquid to provide oxygen and to maintain a good mixture of the materials in the fermentation vessel. The temperature and pH of the medium are controlled carefully for maximal production of yeast cells, which are harvested by centrifugation or filteration. They are further washed, then dried to solid food stock containing about 50% protein. With flavors added, this stock can be used to prepare a variety of protein-rich foods, from soups to ice cream.

The prospect of producing protein by growing microorganisms on petroleum products instead of carbohydrates has been a fascinating idea during the past two decades. The prospect of obtaining high-quality protein from a factory rather than through animals has captured the attention of researchers, this being one of the most promising ideas of obtaining the needed protein.

However, growing yeasts on petroleum instead of sugar presents certain problems. First is the insolubility of hydrocarbons in water. The waxy hyrocarbons can be mixed in the watery medium only in suspension, and the mixture must be stirred strongly to keep the oil droplets well dispersed throughout the medium. This is particularly a formidable task to perform on a large scale. The second major difficulty is the greater need for oxygen. The hydrocarbons have no oxygen, whereas sugar has about 50% oxygen. Consequently, the oxygen supplied to the organisms growing on petroleum must be at least three times greater than those grown on sugar substrate. Also, this results in a threefold increase in the cells' output of heat, necessitating a cooling system to control the temperature of the growth medium. These disadvantages are offset, however, by the doubled rate of production of yeast cells grown on petroleum. Under favorable conditions, one kg of hydrocarbon can produce one kg of yeast, compared to 0.5 kg produced when sugar substrate is used.

Almost any source of carbon can be used as a substrate for growing microorganisms. A substrate with nutrients, water, and oxygen from the air is pumped into a vertical tube (fermenter), the output is drawn off from the top; it consists of cells, metabolites produced during the fermentation, carbon dioxide, and heat. The choice of a substrate depends on the cost availability, safety, ease of purification of the cells, viscosity, and so forth.

Exploiting the possibility of producing SCP from petroleum, the British Petroleum Co. built a 4000-ton-per-year pilot plant in Grangemouth, Scotland, in 1970. This plant used specially purified C-10 to C-18 alkane hydrocarbons from petroleum. Similarly a 20,000-ton-per-year plant was built in Lavera, France, which was designed to use a portion of the distillate from the petroleum refineries. The yeast used the hydrocarbon as a source of carbon for energy, and what was not used was sent back to the refinery. Both the plants used *Candida lipolytica* yeast.

The SCP produced by these two plants was used in feeding trials carried out on a variety of animals. Protocols for testing SCP for both animal and human food uses were established by the Protein Advisory Group of the WHO-FAO. The safety tests alone involved multigeneration feeding trials with rats, dogs, and other species for 2 years. Economic and acceptance studies on various animals took about 6 years. After providing the required data on safety, acceptance, supply, economics, and so forth, a stage was set for the commercial production of SCP on a large scale. Eight members of the EEC (Belgium, Denmark, France, West Germany, Iceland, Luxemberg, the Netherlands and Great Britain) approved the use of SCP for animal feed.

British petroleum teamed up with Anic, the petrochemical wing of the Italian state-owned hydrocarbon company, to build a plant in Sardinia; and another Italian company, Liquichemica, built a plant in Calabria. Both plants used purified hydrocarbons and had an annual capacity to produce 100,000 tons of SCP. After the completion of construction in 1976, both the plants applied for an operating permit and they were refused by the Italian health authorities for the reason that the plants produced too much dust, and that about 70 ppm of waxes were found in the fat of pigs fed Torpina (the trade name of BP product). The American FDA allows 950 ppm waxes in meats and 1500 ppm in breads. Eventually both the plants were sold for scrap in 1978 and British Petroleum withdrew from the SCP business. The efforts made to produce SCP in other countries such as Saudi Arabia, Venezuela, and Japan have also failed on similar grounds.

The Imperial Chemical Industries (ICI) in England built a plant at Billingham to produce 110,000 metric tons of SCP per year since 1980. The plant uses the bacterium *Methylophilus methylotriphus*. The product is sold under the trade name "Pruteen" directed toward animal feed.

In Germany, Hoechst started a 1000-ton-per-year pilot plant in 1978. Their product is being sold under the trade name Probion. The process is based on growing bacteria, *Methylomonas clara*, using methanol. They have also developed processes to decrease the nucleic acid content in the protein to make it suitable for human consumption. Nucleic acids consumed in amounts exceeding 2 g/day may cause gout, a painful disease caused by precipitation of uric acid crystals in the joints. Hoechst has plans to pursue the development of SCP for both animal and human use.

In the United States of America, the American Oil Company has developed a process to grow *Torula* yeast on ethanol. They built a 5000 ton-per-year plant at Hutchinson, Illinois, using ethanol from petroleum. Though ethanol is more expensive than methanol, it is more acceptable to the public than methanol. The product "Temptein" is currently being marketed as a flavor adjunct, i.e. as a functional rather than a filler protein.

In the former Soviet Union, a plant to produce protein from purified petroleum waxes using yeast has been built at Gorky and is the only plant in the world using petroleum products to make protein. The proteins from microorganisms will certainly become much more important in the future. It will be first introduced as a major animal feed source and later as a human food. According to Clydesdale and Francis (22), the market for protein concentrates is estimated at up to 2 million tons, a major part of which is currently being supplied by soy meal. SCP is not subject to the vagaries of nature, and thus has a great potential to increase the world production of protein.

B. Other Fungi

Fungi are normally not considered as a source of protein. In the U.S. food industry, mushrooms, for example, provide only about 0.05% of the required protein. The fungi are primarily used as flavor enhancers in cheese and condiments. In Asia, however, a range of fermented products such as soybeans, wheat, rice, copra, peanuts, fish, and dairy products are made by inoculation with fungi. Fungi considerably increase the nutritive value of the high-carbohydrate foods, in addition to increasing the protein content. The protein content of rice can be doubled by inoculation with a fungus, *Trichoderma* sp. Similarly, the protein content of the starch-containing foods like cassava or tapioca can be increased from about 0.7% to 5.7% by inoculation with fungus within 4 days. Some strains of sugarcane can produce more protein per unit of land than soybeans (22); the carbohydrate in the cane can be the substrate for a fungus that is capable of producing about 3 tons of protein compared with the 800 pounds produced by one acre of soybeans. Other carbohydrate foods such as white and sweet potatoes, maize, sorghum, millets also can be employed to enhance their protein content by this method. According to Gray (25), the world protein supply can be greatly increased by combining the carbohydrate-synthesizing capacity of nongreen plants like fungi. The Western world, however, is not used to eating fungi, except in the form of mushrooms and in cheese. The problem of contamination with fungi producing toxins must also be solved. The use of fungi to produce proteins on a large scale remains one of the exciting methods, yet to be harnessed fully.

IV. PROTEINS FROM FISH AND OTHER MINOR SOURCES

A. Fish Protein Concentrate

Fish protein concentrate (FPC) has been considered as an important source of high-quality protein to enrich both animal and human food products. Fishes are apparently available in unlimited quantities and can be made into a bland grayish powder with a high nutritive value that can be incorporated in a range of foods, such as soups, gruels, breads, noodles, and others. Most of peoples have consumed a form of food in which FPC could be utilized.

In the 1950s, several methods of making FPC were known; most of these methods used solvent extraction, treatment with acids or alkalis, or mechanical procedures. Dichloroethane and isopropanol were the common solvents used. In the Halifax method, the whole fish are ground and the slurry is washed with acidified water. The mixture is then treated with isopropanol in countercurrent fashion, the slurry and isopropanol moving in the opposite direction. The solvent removes oil, water, and some nitrogenous compounds from the mixture. After removing the isopropanol from the mixture, a tasteless creamy-colored powder with a faint fishy odor is produced. It is possible to make a range of products depending upon variation in the fish type, degree of purity required, and use of flavors, and so forth.

The Astra Nutrition Development Corporation of Sweden teamed up with Nabisco Inc. of the United States in 1970 to make a high-quality FPC that was intended to be used in bakery products and in the American school lunch program. This venture, however, was not successful.

FPC appeared to be a real panacea for the world protein shortage, especially to provide proteinous food to the hungry developing nations but this has not proved to be the reality for several reasons, including fish shortages and the need for sophisticated technology (where it is needed) to produce, package, and distribute the product. Also, the product could not be consumed alone; it had to be added to something to increase its consumer acceptability. For these reasons, there has not been any appreciable production of FPC in the world at present time.

Efforts to produce FPC in the USA also have failed. Research on FPC in the U.S. Bureau of Commercial Fisheries, Department of the Interior, started in 1961. The FDA, in 1962, ruled that FPC could not be made from fish containing viscera (intestinal matter) or heads, on the premise that unwholesome material could not be added to food. The production of FPC from whole fish was thought to be economical; thus, the FDA ruling was a major deterrent for the development of FPC in the USA. The Committee on Marine Protein Resource Development, appointed to study the situation, reported that FPC prepared from whole hake fish was safe, nutritious, and wholesome. In 1967, the FDA ruled that FPC could be made from whole hake, if it contained 75% protein, equivalent in quality to milk protein. A further regulation permitted its domestic distribution only for household use in package weight of not more than one pound. The bulk use of FPC was not permitted unless preceded by the presentation of data to show that the proposed use of FPC would not be deceptive to the customers. The Agency for International Development to Alpine Geophysical Corporation proposed to produce 970 tons of FPC for Biafra and Chile, for which a plant was to be constructed by Ezra Levin in New Bedford, Massachusetts. Winter storms, shortage of hake, and technological problems prevented delivery of FPC, except for 70 of the 265 tons delivered to meet the specifications. The contract was required to be cancelled.

B.   Miscellaneous Sources

Other miscellaneous sources for protein production include cottonseed meal, which contains a high-quality protein. However, it contains a toxic yellow pigment, gossypol. The heat treatment required to degrade gossypol lowers the protein quality. Cottonseed meal is mainly used at present as a cattlefeed, but nonruminant animals are fed the heat-treated meal. Some newer varieties of cotton contain little or no gossypol in their seeds. The USDA laboratories have developed the "liquid cyclone process" to remove the pigment glands that contain gossypol. The final cottonseed flour contains about 65% protein of high biological value. The potential of producing high-quality proteins from oilseed crops such as cottonseed, peanuts, and soybeans (see section II,A & B) is very large, because the current world production of cottonseed alone is more than about 330 million tons.

Animal protein from herds of antelope-like animals in Africa remain underutilized. Several insects have been used as a source of food for human beings. The giant African snail (8 inches long) has been found to be a good source of delicious edible protein. Several animal and insect species, such as termites, caterpillars, ants, rats, lizards, locusts, bird nests, and many others can be utilized as a source of edible protein. Most people, however, do not yet seem to be ready or hungry for them.

All these novel protein foods, including leaf protein isolates, fish-protein concentrates, and proteins from microorganisms require sophisticated technology to produce them and do not provide the ideal solution to the need for protein-rich weaning foods in the developing countries. They can, however, play an important role in the diet of people in the developed countries, where they can form attractive alternatives to meat. The nutritional composition of these novel proteins must be regulated to protect the consumer from possible toxic factors.

V. FATS AND OILS

A variety of fats and oils derived both from animal and plant sources are consumed by the humans, especially in the technologically developed countries. In the developing countries, the consumption of separated fats is comparatively lower.

Fats and oils are mainly triglycerides—esters of fatty acids with glycerol—and can be distinguished based on their physical state; oils are fluid at ambient temperatures, whereas fats are solid. In addition to the triglycerides, fats and oils also contain minor quantities of non-saponifiable matter, with traces of mono- and diglycerides. During their utilization, some triglycerides are hydrolyzed to form free fatty acids, but their levels in fresh products are very low. Even at low concentrations, the presence of free fatty acids can cause production of rancidity and off-flavors. The lipids isolated from animal sources are solid fats, whereas those from plant seeds are usually oils. This distinction, however, is related to the fatty acid composition of the triglyceride, rather than the source of origin.

A. Plant Oils

Seeds of many plants contain storage lipids, and those that are rich in oil (oilseeds) are used to produce plant oils commercially. The flesh of certain fruits (avocado) also can be a good source of oils and fats. Based on the principal fatty acid present, vegetable oils and fats can be subdivided into the following six groups (26):

1. *Lauric*—coconut, palm kernel, and babassu
2. *Palmitic*—palm
3. *Oleic*—olive and peanut
4. *Medium linoleic*—soybean, cottonseed, sesame, and maize
5. *High linoleic*—sunflower and safflower seed
6. *Erucic*—rapeseed

1. Lauric Oils

The lauric oils are characterized by a high (more than 40%) amount of C12 saturated fatty acid, and a relatively low unsaturation. Coconut oil has the highest lauric acid content of the three oils in this group, and the lowest melting point (24°C as compared to 26° and 28°C for babassu and palm kernel oils, respectively). Coconut oil contains about 8% to 10% unsaturated fatty acids, mostly oleic acid, whereas palm kernel oil has about 17% unsaturated acids, mostly oleic. Owing to their natural low unsaturation, lauric oils are very resistant to the development of rancidity or reversion flavors. However, free fatty acids from the lauric oils are very noticeable even in low concentrations, as they are sufficiently volatile and soluble to contribute a definite odor and flavor (27).

2. Palm Oil

Palm oil is characterized by its high palmitic acid (C16) content (35% to 45%). This combined with rather low unsaturation confers on palm oil an elevated melting point, and a relatively flat dilatation line. Palm oils contain high amounts of carotenes and thus have deep orange-red color. Palm fruits have high lipase activity during harvesting and their subsequent handling often results in the formation of free fatty acids. Palm fruits are therefore sterilized on plantations soon after their harvesting to improve palm oil quality, by decreasing the free fatty acid content.

3. Oleic Oils

Oleic oil is a stable oil of excellent quality, widely used as a table and cooking oil. It contains around 10% to 12% unsaturated fatty acids, largely oleic acid. Peanut oil contains about 17% to 20% saturated and 80% to 83% unsaturated fatty acids. The saturated part consists mainly of palmitate, with significant amounts of stearic acid, arachidic acid, and higher fatty acids. West African peanut oils contain about 60% oleic and 20% linoleic acids, whereas the peanut oils from other parts of the world have around 40% oleic and 40% linoleic acids. The oils from African peanut varieties have good keeping quality and excellent deep-frying property. Owing to their appreciable odor and flavor, they have high demand as a salad oil.

4. Medium Linoleic Oils

Soybean oil has high proportion (up to 2.5%) of phosphatides, which are separated during refining and are made into a valuable product, lecithin. Soybean oil contains 12% to 15% saturated acids, most palmitic, and 85% to 88% unsaturated acids, 25% to 30% of which are oleic, 50% to 55% linoleic, and 5% to 10% linolenic. The characteristic flavor of soybean oil is due to the relatively high proportion of linolenic acid, which tends to restrict its use in margarines and also as cooking oil. Soybean oil is partially hardened to improve its taste and stability by reducing linolenic acid content, which also reduces the content of linoleic acid, thus somewhat limiting the value of soybean oil as a source of linoleic acid. Langstraat (27) showed that newer specific hardening catalysts can be used to improve this situation.

Cottonseed oil requires drastic refining treatment to remove the strong flavor and dark color that are associated with the crude oil. It contains about 25% saturated and 75% unsaturated fatty acids. The saturated part is nearly all palmitic acid, whereas the unsaturated portion consists of about 45% linoleic acid and the remainder is nearly all oleic acid.

Sesame oil is characterized by its content of strong antioxidants, viz., sesamol and tocopherol. Thus, sesame oil is particularly resistant to oxidative rancidity. The phenolic antioxidant, sesamol, gives a strong red color in the Bauduin test with furfuraldehyde. In some countries, the use of 2% to 10% sesame oil is compulsory as an indicator substance of margarine blends. Total saturated acids, with the predominance of palmitic and stearic acids, constitute between 13% and 17% of cottonseed oil, the unsaturated part consisting of around 35% to 45% of oleic and linoleic acids.

Corn (maize) oil is a by-product of maize starch production, manufactured mainly in the United States. It is primarily utilized as cooking and salad oil and is considered too expensive for margarine, outside the producing countries. Corn oil has a fatty acid composition similar to that of sesame oil, though the former has slightly higher linoleic acid. Owing to its relatively high tocopherol content, corn oil has better stability against oxidative deterioration, despite its high degree of unsaturation.

5. High Linoleic Oils

Sunflower oil has a high (about 60% to 72%) linoleic acid. The amount of this essential fatty acid in the sunflower is influenced by the climate, especially the temperature to which the plant is exposed during growth. Low-temperature conditions generally tend to increase the linoleic acid content of sunflower seed. Sunflower oil is fairly stable against oxidative rancidity, despite its high linoleic acid (around 75%) content, the rest being mainly oleic acid. It is thus a important source of linoleic acid.

6. High Erucic Oils

Rapeseed oil is characterized by high erucic acid content, in addition to its high linoleic acid content, compared to that of soybean oil. Oils from *Brassica napus* and *B. campestris* contain around 40% to 50% and 25% to 30% eurucic acid, respectively. Erucic acid has possible physiopathological harmful effects on human health. Newer low erucic acid varieties of rapeseed, containing less than 5% erucic acid, have now been developed. The fatty acid composition of low erucic acid rapeseed is approximately between that of peanut and soybean oils.

An important feature common to most finished vegetable oils is the high percentages of unsaturated fatty acids in the triglyceride molecules. The iodine value of an oil or fat is a more meaningful indicator of the total chemical unsaturation of a vegetable oil (28).

Two groups of phospholipids, viz., lecithins and cephalins, occur in oilseeds. These are substituted fats in which one fatty acid is displaced by phosphoric acid to which a nitrogen base— choline (in lecithins) or amino ethanol (in cephalins)—is attached. Rewald (29) reported the following proportions of lecithins and cephalins in the phospholipids of the following oilseeds:

Oilseed	Lecithins (%)	Cephalins (%)
Groundnut	35.7	64.3
Sesame	52.2	40.6
Cottonseed	28.8	71.2
Linseed	36.2	63.8
Sunflower	38.5	61.5

The unsaponifiable fraction in the vegetable oils may vary from a fraction of a percent to a few percent of the oil, whether the oils are pressed out or extracted with solvents (30).

Langstraat (27) presented a detailed survey of the commercially most important oilseeds and sketched their place in the nutrition of the world population, both as a source of fat and as a potential source of proteins. More than 100 varieties of plants are known to have oil-bearing seeds, but only about a dozen or so are important commercially. Fruits and nuts from trees include coconut, palm fruit, palm kernel, olive, and babassu, while the beans, seeds, and plant nuts include soybean, sunflower, peanut, cottonseed, rapeseed, sesame, safflower, and corn. The oil-bearing trees are generally more confined to a certain locality and climate than the other oilseed crops.

The oil content of vegetable oil-bearing materials varies from 15% to 70% of the total weight of the seed or fruit meat. They all share the glycerol part (triglycerides), so the differences in their properties are largely determined by the content of fatty acids. Three aspects have an important bearing on oil or fat quality: chain length, number, and position of fatty acids with regard to the glycerol. Barring minor quantities of higher and lower fatty acids, the length of the carbon chain in vegetable oils varies between C12 and C22 (only even numbers occur) with up to three double bonds. The most important saturated fatty acids occurring in vegetable oils are lauric (C12), myristic (C14), palmitic(C16), stearic(C18), arachidic (C20), and behenic(C20), whereas the important mono-unsaturated fatty acids are oleic (C18:1) and erucic (C22:1). The important di- and tri-unsaturated fatty acids are linoleic (C18:2) and linolenic (C18:3), respectively. The *cis* and *trans* configurations of unsaturated fatty acid chains have different physical and physiological properties, the fatty acid composition primarily determining the quality of the oil or fat.

The processes used to produce seed oils differ for differant oils. In general, the seeds are brought to a suitable moisture content and then crushed. The oil is expressed using hydrolic pressure or a continuous expeller. The presses require a heated meal (hot-pressed oil). The expeller can press unheated meal, though precooking the meal gives higher yields. The solid particles present in the expressed oils are separated, followed by their treatment with alkali to neutralize any free fatty acids formed during extraction. Some oils may require decolorization and deodorization treatments with charcoal and steam.

B. Animal Fats

The most important fat from animal sources is butter, which is obtained by churning cream or milk vigorously enough to break the emulsion and to separate the fat as a mass. The butter milk is drained off and the mass is washed with cold water and may be salted and worked to distribute the salt. It is molded prior to its division into packs for retail sale.

Lard is the fat from adipose tissues of pork (swine meat) and is rendered by heating, liquifying, and straining. *Ghee*, used mainly in Asian cultures, is made by heating and clarifying butter. *Suet* is obtained from the shredded adipose tissue of cattle or other ruminents, and it contains a little protein.

C. Oil and Fat Products

Oil-bearing seeds, fruits, and nuts are processed for the manufacture of salad and cooking oils, refined finished oils, speciality fats, hard butters, hydrogenated fats, margarine oils, shortenings, *vanaspati* emulsifiers such as lecithin, protein concentrates, isolates, a range of confectionery products, oilseed flours, oil cakes and meals, and other poultry and livestock feeds as well as numerous industrial products from nonedible oils. Galloway (31) described the techniques and equipment for cleaning, cracking, dehulling, decorticating, and flaking of oilseeds and discussed the particular methods and cautions for unusual oil-bearing materials.

1. Salad and Cooking Oils

About 45% of the edible oils and fats produced in the world are consumed as salad and cooking oils, and around 66% of the raw materials used for these purposes is of vegetable origin, soybean oil taking the first place among them. According to Lesier (32), the criteria for choosing salad and cooking oils vary from the points of view of the consumer, the nutritionists, and the industrial manufacturer. Whereas the price, taste, odor, tendency to solidify, cloud point, foaming resistance, consistency of quality and stability, presentation, packing, and nutritional aspects are the prime considerations from the consumer point of view, the nutritionists' criteria include adequate polyunsaturated fatty acid content, maximum saturated fatty acid content, good heat resistance to minimize the formation of new compounds (free oxidation radicals, polymers and cyclic compounds), and vitamin content. The polyunsaturated fatty acid content of cooking oil used for deep frying should not be high in order to avoid its tendency to oxidize. It is therefore advisable to eliminate linolenic acid and restrict the content of linoleic acid to 40%. Soybean and rapeseed oils, being more highly polyunsaturated (linolenic), have been recommended for use in cold applications (salad oils), owing to their low heat stability and objectionable taste and odors when used in deep frying (32). Burkhalter (33) described the methods of handling and storage of crude vegetable oils, which are often overcooked in the production of good quality salad and cooking oils. The effects of temperature, time, tank size, agitation, and blending on oil quality have been discussed.

2. Finished (Refined) Oils

Crude vegetable oils are refined by degumming, neutralization, water washing, drying, bleaching, filtration, and deodorization. They are further polished, cooled, and stored as finished edible oils.

The methods of handling and storage of finished oils have been described (34,35). In the United States, finished oils are normally stored in closed vessels in atmosphere that excludes oxygen and moisture and where temperatures are controlled at minimum levels. The effects of factors such as temperature, oxygen, heavy metals, and antioxidants on quality of the deodorized oils have been described (35). The fat must be protected against oxidative deterioration, contact with water and dirt and other unwanted fats, absorption of foreign odors and taste, thermal decomposition, microbial contamination, hydrolysis, and contamination from packaging materials.

The contamination of finished oils with heavy metals, especially Cu, Mn, and Fe, must be avoided as they increase oxidation rate. Fats requiring storage for a long period, such as mayonnaise, caviar, and chocolate products, do not tolerate contamination by other fats like coconut and palm kernel, which give short chain (C4 to C12) products after hydrolysis. Contamination of deodorized oils with microorganisms (yeasts, molds, and bacteria) results into the lipolytic hydrolysis of oils. Contamination from packaging materials, especially by vinyl chloride monomers emanating from PVC packaging material, must be avoided.

3. Margarines, Shortenings, and Vanaspati

The flavor, texture and functional properties of margarine, shortening and vanaspati initially had to be as similar as possible to their natural prototypes—butter, lard, and *ghee*. Later, it was possible to feature specific plus points in newer, vegetable fat–type products. The processing technology of margarine production has not changed significantly during the past 3 to 4 decades, although a great number of technological modifications for quality improvement and adaptation to market requirements have been achieved. The latter include tailor-made refining procedures for more flexible blend formulations, careful exclusion of oxygen in closed systems (refining, dosing, emulsification, and cooling), and development of soft margarine, rich in linoleic acid and mostly packed in tubes. Margarine processing today is fully mechanized and partly automated. The processing of *vanaspati* needs a slow crystallization phase that is not compatible with mechanization and automation. Several flexible blend formulations of both margarine and *vanaspati* with improved flavor and texture are available in the market.

Shortening is a highly processed fat, a natural fat that has been treated to give it useful properties. It is a creamy white, homogeneous mass, nearly odorless and tasteless, which melts into a clear, almost colorless, oily liquid when warmed slightly. Some of the fatty parts of shortening are rather resistant to oxidation by air, which makes them stand for long periods without development of rancidity. Both shortenings and salad oils are obtained from oil and fats extracted from oilseeds, oil-fruits, and nuts.

4. Oilseed Flours, Grits, Protein Concentrates, Isolates, and Textured Protein Products

Bastiaens (36) described the methods of producing oilseed flours, primarily from soybeans for human consumption. Pretreatment involves bean handling, drying, cleaning and dehulling, followed by solvent extraction, desolventization, stripping (removal of residual hexane), and cooling. In developing countries such as India, edible oilseed proteins for use as food ingredients are formulated in various types or grades, whose standards are based on the levels of protein, fiber content, and antinutrients. Proteins from various sources may enter products such as protein mixes, weaning and toddler foods, biscuits, vegetable milks, yogurt, ice cream, and reconstitutable powders, the protein quality of these products often being described in terms of protein efficiency ratio (PER) with appropriate amounts of vitamins and minerals (37).

The more improved processes of oilseed proteins include methods for making superior quality flours and grits, better extruded products, and high-quality protein concentrates and isolates (see Section II.A). Technically improved products have longer shelf life, higher product yields, and more efficient energy conservation (38). They also have higher PER ratings and a broad range of nitrogen solubility index. The texture of oilseed protein fractions is changed by mechanical and chemical means in specialized equipment and the processing conditions are closely controlled to ensure desired end product forms. Brian (39) has discussed the equipment, the nature of feed materials and details of processing conditions required to produce texturized proteins from soybean and other oilseeds.

5. Emulsifiers (Lecithin), Confections, Chocolates, and Other Specialty Fats and Tailor-made Fats

Food emulsifiers are primarily esters of fatty acids and polyol and/or water soluble organic acids. In surface-active agents, both polar and nonpolar parts are specially separated from each other in a balanced way. Soy lecithins are important emulsifiers used in foods, feeds, pharmaceuticals, and other industries. The major steps in the production of lecithin from soybean oil are as follows (40): (a) hydration of phosphatides, (b) separation of the sludge, (c) drying, and (d) cooling. Such lecithin has both water/oil and oil/water emulsifying properties. Products with improved emulsifying properties are obtained by modifications, involving mainly fractionation of alcohol, hydrolysis (enzymatic, acid, or alkali), acetylation, or hydroxylation. Lecithins of high chemical, physical, and bacteriological quality are produced by careful processing. Technically, lecithin can be obtained from egg yolk and various oilseeds such as flax, cottonseed, maize (corn) germ, sunflower seed, rapeseed, and soybean. Soybean lecithins are valued mainly because of their continuous availability and excellent emulsifying properties, color, and taste (41). Scocca (41) has discussed utilization of lecithin in industrial foods and cosmetics and their use in industrial applications, such as animal feeds, foods, chocolates, confections, hard candies, high sugar confection products, standard high salt-content margarines, and instant foods such as beverage powders, to improve their dispersion and in flour treatments to condition dough and increase water absorption.

Paulicka (42) reviewed the scope of certain specialty fats like hard butters and described the production technology with emphasis on raw materials and processing. The hard butters have been described in terms of their composition, thermal properties, and end uses in confectionery and imitation dairy products (42). Hard butters are produced from suitable refined oils that are modified by chemical and/or thermo-mechanical processes such as hydrogenation, interesterification, replacement of resterification, and fractionation.

Fractionation and winterization are basically separation processes of oils into two or more fractions with different melting points. In the winterization process, the oils are cooled and held at low temperature. The liquid and solid fractions are then separated by filteration. In the fractionation process, oil cooling and fractionation are performed in a more sophisticated way under controlled conditions. Both these processes have broad applications in edible oil technology, e.g., in the production of cocoa butter equivalents from cheaper vegetable oils such as palm oil, palm kernel oil, and shea fat; and hydrogenation and production of specialty fats from soybean and cottonseed oils (43). Cocoa butter, an ingredient of many candies and confectionery products, resembles mutton tallow in its fatty acid composition but differs greatly in physical properties. Whereas mutton tallow is a waxy solid at body temperature, cocoa butter is hard and brittle at ordinary temperatures and melts in the mouth with a pleasing and cooling sensation. The difference lies in the pattern in which the fatty acids are combined in the molecules of these two fats (26).

Several "tailor-made fats" are made from oils and fats for industrial uses, e.g., plastics, rubber-like products, high-grade linoleums, resins, synthetic waxes, detergents, emulsifiers, wetting-out agents, and other surface-active materials, shampoos, and quick-dissolving soaps.

6. Oilseed Cakes and Meals

Oilseed cake as discharged from a press has high temperature (90° to 160°C) and low moisture content (1% to 4%). It is passed through a cooler to lower the temperature quickly to a safe level, by spraying cold water on the cake conveyor ahead of the cooler, blasting cold air. Cooled and humidified cake may be ground directly into meal or stored and ground when required. Cake is ground in hammer mills or double revolving-disk attrition mills. Meals of almost all edible oilseeds are used as nutritious feed for poultry, dairy cattle, and other livestock, and those of non-edible oilseeds such as linseed, castor, tung, and tallow are mainly used as a manure and soil conditioner.

REFERENCES

1. Southgate, D.A.T., Meat, fish, eggs and novel proteins, *Human Nutrition and Dietetics*, 9th ed. (J.S. Garrow and W.P.T. James, eds.), Churchill Livingstone (Longman Groups), London, 1993, pp. 305–316.

2. D.H.S.S., Foods which simulate meat, Reports on Health and Social Subjects No.17, Dept. of Health and Social Security, H.M.S.O, London, 1980.

3. Desai, B.B., P.M. Kotecha, and D.K. Salunkhe, *Science and Technology of Groundnuts: Biology, Production, Processing and Utilization* (Chapter 16), Naya Prokash, Culcutta, 1998.

4. McWatters, K.H., and J.P. Cherry, Potential food uses of peanut seed proteins, *Peanut Science and Technology* (H.E. Pattee and C.T. Young, eds.), Am. Peanut Res. Edu. Soc. Yokum, Texas 1982, p. 689.

5. Ayres, J.L., and B.L. Davenport, Peanut protein: A versatile food ingredient, *J. Am. Oil Chem. Soc. 54*(A):109–111, 1977.

6. Natarajan, K.R., Peanut protein ingredients: Preparation, properties and foods uses, *Adv. Food Res. 26*:215–273 (1980).

7. Cater C.M., K.C. Rhee, R.D. Hagenmaier, and K.F. Mattil, Aqueous extraction—an alternative oilseed milling process, *J. Am. Oil Chem. Soc., 51*:137–141 (1974).

8. Arthur, J.C., Jr., Peanut protein: Isolation, composition and properties, *Adv. in Protein Chemistry* (M.L. Anson, K. Bailey, and J.T. Edsall, eds.), Academic Press, New York, 1953, pp 393–414.

9. Amantharaman, K., N. Subramanian, D.S. Bhatia, and V. Subramanian, Production of edible groundnut protein isolates, *Indian Oilseeds J. 3*: 85–89 (1959).

10. De, S.S., and J.A. Cornelius, Technology of production of edible flours and protein products from groundnut, FAO, UNO Agric. Serv. Bull.No. *10*:1 (1971).

11. Rhee, K.C., C.M. Cater, and K.F. Mattil, Effect of processing pH on the properties of peanut protein isolates and oil, *Cereal Chem. 50*:395–399 (1973).

12. Rhee, K.C., C.M. Cater, and K.F. Mattil, Aqueous process for pilot plant scale production of peanut protein concentrates, *J. Food Sci. 38*: 126–128 (1973).

13. Natraj, H.K., and N. Subramanian, Studies on groundnut protein concentrates prepared by alcohol and acid washing of the edible flour, *J. Food Sci. Technol. 11*: 54–57 (1974).

14. Rhee, K.C., K.R. Natarajan, C.M. Cater, and K.F. Mattil, Processing edible peanut protein concentrates and isolates to inactivate aflatoxins, *J. Am. Oil Chem. Soc. 54*:245A–249A (1973).

15. Rhee, K.C., C.M. Cater, and K.F. Mattil, Simultaneous recovery of protein and oil from raw peanuts in an aqueous system, *J. Food Sci. 37*:90–93 (1972).

16. Oke, O.L., and R.H. Smith, *Groundnut, Food Protein Sources* (N.W. Pirie, ed.), Cambridge Univ. Press, London, 1975, p. 105–116.

17. Cherry, J.P., L.C. Berardi, Z.M. Zarine, J.I., Wadsworth, and C.H. Vinnett, Cottonseed protein derivatives as nutritional and functional supplements in food formulations, *Nutritional Improvement of Food and Food Proteins* (M. Friedman, ed.), Plenum Pub.Co., New York, 1978, pp. 767–796.

18. Berardi, L.C., and J.P. Cherry, Preparation and composition of co-precipitated protein isolates from cottonseed, soybean, and peanut flours, *Cereal Chem. 56*:95–100 (1979).

19. Berardi, L.C., and J.P. Cherry, Functional properties of co-precipitated protein isolates from cottonseed, soybean and peanut flours, *Canadian Inst. Food Sci. Technol. J., 14*:283–288 (1981).

20. Pominski, J., W.O. Gorden, E.J. McCourtney, H.L.E. Vix, and E.A. Gastrock, Production of peanut protein, *Ind. Eng. Chem. 44*:925–928 (1952).

21. FAO, Production Yearbook, Food and Agriculture Organization, Rome, 1994s.

22. Clydesdale, F.M., and F.J. Francis, *Food Nutrition and Health*, AVI Pub.Co., Westport, 1984.

23. Pirie, N.W., *Leaf Protein: Its Agronomy, Preparation Quality and Use*, IBP Handbook No. 20, Blackwell Scientific Publications, Oxford, England, 1971.
24. Champagnat, A., *Protein from petroleum, Food, Readings from Sci. Am.*, W.H. Freeman & Co., San Francisco. 1973, p. 254.
25. Gray, W.D., *The Use of Fungi as Food and in Food Processing*, CRC Press, Cleveland, 1970.
26. Salunkhe, D.K., and B.B. Desai, *Postharvest Biotechnology of Oilseeds*, CRC Press, Boca Raton, 1986, p. 217.
27. Langstraat, A., Characteristics and composition of vegetable oil-bearing materials, *J. Am. Oil Chem. Soc.* *53*:430 (1976).
28. Sherwin, E.R., Antioxidants for vegetable oils, *J. Am. Oil Chem. Soc.* *53*:430 (1976).
29. Rewald, B., Phosphatides from oilseeds, *Biochem. J. 36*:822 (1942).
30. Crocker, W., and L.V. Barton, *Physiology of Seeds: An Introduction to the Experimental Study of Seed and Germination Problems*, Chronica Botanica, Waltham, Mass, 1957, p. 22.
31. Galloway, J.P., Cleaning, cracking, dehulling, decorticating and flaking of oil-bearing materials, *J. Am. Oil Chem. Soc. 53*:271 (1976).
32. Lesieur, B., Salad and cooking oils, *J. Am. Oil Chem. Soc. 53*:414 (1976).
33. Burkhalter, J.P., Crude oil handling and storage, *J. Am. Oil Chem. Soc. 53*:332 (1976).
34. Wright, L.M., Finished oil handling and storage in the United States, *J. Am. Oil Chem. Soc. 53*:408–409 (1976)
35. Johansson Gosta, M.R., Finished oil handling and storage in Europe, *J. Am. Oil Chem. Soc. 53*:410–415 (1976).
36. Bastiaens, F.G., Oilseed flour for human food, *J. Am. Oil Chem. Soc. 53*:316 (1976).
37. Achaya, K.T., Standards for protein-based foods in developing countries, *J. Am. Oil Chem Soc. 53*:316 (1976).
38. Becker, K.W., and E.A. Tiernan, New technology in oilseed proteins, *J. Am. Oil Chem. Soc. 53*:327 (1976).
39. Brian, R., Textured protein products, *J. Am. Oil Chem. Soc. 53*:325 (1976).
40. Van Nieuwenhuyzen, W., Lecithin production and properties, *J. Am. Oil Chem. Soc. 53*:425–427 9 (1976).
41. Scocca, P.M., Utilization of lecithin, *J. Am. Oil Chem. Soc. 53*:428 (1976).
42. Paulicka, F.R., Speciality fats, *J. Am. Oil Chem. Soc. 53*:421 (1976).
43. Kreulen, H.P., Fractionation and winterization of edible oils, *J. Am. Oil Chem. Soc. 53*:393 (1976).

13
Food Processing and Preservation

I. INTRODUCTION

Processing food for its preservation aims at arresting the biological deterioration of foodstuffs that is caused either by microorganisms contaminating the foods or by the endogenous enzymes present in the foods, which would bring about undesirable changes in appearance, odor, taste, texture, or nutritional quality. Foods gradually undergo deterioration or spoilage from the time they are harvested, slaughtered, or manufactured. Some foods such as fruits, vegetables, and fishes spoil rapidly; others, such as cereal grains can keep longer but for limited periods. The useful storage or marketable life of highly perishable foods such as leafy vegetables and fishes is less than a day or two at 21°C. The deteriorative changes (physiological, chemical, or biological) in such high-moisture foods are so rapid as to render them virtually useless for consumption in a matter of few hours (1–4).

The deterioration in foods may be microbial (bacteria, yeasts, and molds), enzymatic (enzymes in foods), other biological agents such as insects, parasites, and rodents and/or physical factors such as temperature (heat and cold), moisture, oxygen, light, and time. All these factors are not isolated in nature: at any one time, many forms of deterioration may set in depending on the type of food and environmental conditions. Manay and Shadaksharaswamy (5) have described the individual causes of food deterioration in detail.

II. FOOD SPOILAGE AND DETERIORATION

Food safety concerns both chemical and biological food spoilage as well as microbial spoilage. Clydesdale and Francis (6) preferred to call the former *deterioration* and the latter *spoilage*. Deterioration of food is commonly seen by the consumer but not always recognized. Deterioration or rancidity of fatty meats is caused by the chemical degradation of fat molecules, which form compounds that have certain odors and off-flavors. Milk deterioration is caused by microorganisms that break down the protein in the milk to smaller compounds that have very definite flavor and odor. However, such microorganisms are not harmful to the consumer and therefore this is not considered spoilage. Some other types of deterioration include wilting of leafy vegetables, toughening of beans and peas or sweet corn, and loss of texture in fruits such as berries and citrus fruits as the result of drying.

A. Microbial Spoilage

The term spoilage is often applied to microbiological hazards commonly encountered by the consumer. It has been estimated that as many as 20 million Americans suffer the effects of bacteria-contaminated food each year. Such contamination is primarily the result of unsanitary handling practices in restaurants, in catering establishments, and in the home.

Bacteria, yeast, and molds are the major types of microorganisms causing food spoilage. Around 50 different species of microbes have been found to cause food deterioration. Among them, bacteria are the major health problem. Yeast are not usually considered poisonous, but they do cause food decay. They are unicellular plants (fungi) widely distributed in nature and are commonly noticed in fruits, cereals and other foods containing sugar. They are also present in soil, in air, and on the skins and intestines of animals. They have been used for centuries for leavening of bread and fermentation of fruit juices. They are considered harmful to foods if they bring about undesired fermentation.

Molds are multicellular, filamentous fungi having a fuzzy or cottony appearance when they grow in foods. They are aerobes requiring oxygen for their growth and multiplication. Molds often thrive under conditions of acidity and osmotic pressures that are inhibitory to most bacteria. Molds are frequently found growing on the surfaces of jams and jellies. They require less free moisture for growth than yeasts and bacteria. The absence of bright light and presence of stagnant air favor their rapid growth and development. A few toxins, such as aflatoxins formed by certain fungi (*Aspergillus flavus*), in foods are dangerous and can cause a variety of health problems, including cancers.

Bacteria cause two types of food poisoning. In the first, *Salmonella* and *Shigella* bacteria that are present within the food can grow rapidly in the human intestinal tract, producing symptoms such as diarrhea and vomiting. In the second type, called food intoxication, bacteria first produce toxins in the food, which is consumed by a human to produce ill effects. In this case, it is not the bacteria themselves that cause food poisoning, but the toxins produced by the bacteria in the food. Some harmful toxin-producing bacteria are *Clostridium botulinum*, *C. perfringens*, *Staphylococcus aureus*, and some molds. Both food infection and food intoxication produce symptoms such as diarrhea, nausea, vomiting, convulsions, and so forth; *Clostridium botulinum* poisoning causes death in about 60% of all cases. Other types of food poisoning that cause dehydration and weakening may also result in debilitation and death, especially in young babies. Pathogenic organisms, *Listeria monocytogenes* and *Yersinia enterocolitica* have been reported to grow in milk at refrigerator temperature (6).

A common form of food intoxication caused by *Staphylococcus* bacteria can produce violent diarrhea and vomiting within 2 to 4 hours of ingestion of the poisoned food. Such contamination is often observed in cream pastries, tuna, canned chicken salads, and similar food mixtures. Such foods must be quickly refrigerated after handling, because these bacteria cannot grow and produce toxins at refrigerated temperatures. The toxins produced by *Staphylococcus* bacteria cannot be destroyed by heat. Mayonnaise and salad dressing, when added to salads or sandwiches, may retard the growth of harmful microorganisms because they contain acetic acid (vinegar), whose acidity inhibits bacterial growth.

Clostridium botulinum, an anerobic organism, cannot grow in the presence of oxygen. It is therefore normally found in canned foods and in sausage meats where oxygen is excluded. Like *C. perfringens*, it has a vegetative cell and a spore but unlike the perfringens, the spore has to vegetate within the foodstuff in the absence of oxygen and produce toxin prior to ingestion. Adequate processing, particularly heat processing, destroys both the vegetative cells and spores of *C. botulinum*.

Bacteria, yeast, and molds multiply best between 16° and 38°C, though some can grow even at 0°C and others at 100°C. They alter food constituents by hydrolyzing starch and other carbohydrates such as cellulose, pectin, and lignin; some can hydrolyze lipids producing rancidity; still others digest proteins, producing putridity and ammonia-like odors. They can decolorize foods and produce acids, gases, or toxins in the deteriorated foods.

B. Enzymatic Deterioration

Enzymes present in plant and animal foods continue to be present and are sometimes intensified after harvest and slaughter. During storage, these enzymes cause changes in color, texture, and flavor noted in the fresh produce. Some such changes may be desirable—e.g., continued ripening of tomatoes after harvest and natural tenderizing of meat on aging. However, if these changes are allowed to proceed too far, they can result in food deterioration. The enzymes responsible for deteriorative changes must be inactivated at the appropriate time to prevent food losses through deterioration.

C. Other Biological Agents

Insects, parasites, and rodents are other biotic factors causing food deterioration. Insects are especially destructive to cereal grains, pulses, fruits, and vegetables, causing heavy food losses. Insect eggs may persist in the foods even after processing, e.g. in flours. Apart from the loss due to the food eaten, insects cause greater damage because of bruises and cuts made in the foods, exposing them to microbial attack, resulting in further decay.

Parasitic nematodes can enter into pork when hogs eat uncooked food wastes. The live worms can infect humans if the pork is not thoroughly cooked. A parasitic worm, *Aniskis*, is found in fish and can infect human beings if it is eaten raw. A parasitic ameba, *Entamoeba histolytica*, contaminates foods causing amebic dysentry. Cooking, however, destroys most of these parasites.

Rodents cause substantial food losses in countries where they are not controlled. In addition to consuming large quantities of food, they also contaminate food by introducing disease-producing bacteria through their urine and droppings. Rats spread several human diseases such as typhus fever, plague, and typhoid.

D. Physical Factors

Heat and cold, though having an important role in food preservation, contribute significantly to food deterioration, if not regulated. The rates of all chemical reactions double for every 10°C rise in temperature. Excessive heat denatures food proteins, destroys most vitamins, breaks emulsions, and dehydrates food. Uncontrolled cold or chilling also can deteriorate food. Freezing and thawing of fruits and vegetables may alter their texture and structure. Skin rupture on fruits and vegetables makes them susceptible to microbial infection. Most tropical fruits and vegetables can be damaged permanently if held at refrigeration temperature (4°C). Such deterioration may include development of off flavors, surface biting, and various forms of decay.

Presence or absence of excessive moisture in foods may lead to food spoilage and deterioration. Moisture is essential for microbial growth and chemical reactions. Foods with high moisture content such as milk, fruits, leafy vegetables, fish, and meats deteriorate rapidly. Surface moisture changes due to variation in the relative humidity can cause lumping and caking, surface defects, crystallization and stickiness in foods. Condensation of moisture in foods can result in the multiplication of bacteria and molds. Fruits and vegetables can give off moisture through respiration and transpiration, even when packed in a moisture-free packages. Control of moisture thus is important for their preservation.

Air and oxygen bring about a number of oxidative changes in food components, resulting in destruction of food color, flavor, vitamins, and other food nutrients. Molds need oxygen for their growth. Foods are therefore protected by excluding oxygen by deaeration, vacuum packing or flushing containers with nitrogen or carbon dioxide, and by the use of oxygen-absorbing chemicals.

Light destroys riboflavin, vitamins A and C, and many food colors. Foods are required to be protected from light, using impervious packing or containers that screen specific wavelengths of light.

All the foregoing food-deteriorating factors are time-dependent—i.e., the longer the time, the greater the deterioration. Deterioration with time takes place with most foods, barring certain items, such as cheese, wine, and other fermented foods, which may even improve in their quality—up to a point—with time and aging.

III. FOOD PROCESSING SYSTEMS AND PROCESSED FOODS

Humans have been practicing food preservation through the ages, so as to store food supplies from the periods of plenty to make them available during seasons of little or no production. Food security and its year-round supply has become increasingly important in the existence of national governments.

Much of the food consumed by humans today undergoes some kind of food processing. According to Southgate and Johnson (7), many of the traditional methods of food processing, such as the milling of cereal grains to produce flours, the fermentation of cereals in the production of breads, and the enzyme and heat treatments used in the production of cheese, are so well established that they are regarded as "natural" by many food processing critics. The traditional techniques of food processing, such as drying, smoking, or preservation with salts, acetic acid (vinegar), or alcohol, have an ancient history and are therefore regarded as unexceptional. These traditional methods of food processing have come into use gradually and have played an important role in the improvement of nutritional value and acceptability of foodstuffs, in addition to providing a way of extending the availability of food supply beyond the periods of abundance and harvesting. The extension of food supplies into the periods when plant foods cannot be produced or animals maintained because of seasonal changes represents the most important contribution of food processing technology to human social evolution and the development of civilization, freeing human beings from the hunter-gatherer life of continuous search for food.

All modern methods of food processing and preservation have developed through centuries on the basis of traditional methods employed in the past. Industrial food processing began on a small scale in the 19th century and expanded tremendously in the following years. The processing industry, once established, was responsible for a number of technological advances in the food industry—e.g., development of heat processes for drying, pasteurization and canning of foods to control bacterial deterioration and spoilage of foods. This was followed by the development of refrigeration to control spoilage of meats and other perishables during their prolonged storage and transport. Deep-freezing was then developed for retaining quality of highly perishable foods such as vegetables and fish. In the highly developed countries such as the United State, the United Kingdom, and Japan, the majority of the food consumed has been processed in some way—and without the use of these processing methods, it would not be possible to maintain the population at its present size and nutritional status (7).

The basic principle of all preservation techniques, whether carried out in the home or commercially, is to restrict food spoilage caused either by biological or physical factors, to enable the food to be consumed safely at a later time. All preservation methods aim at inhibiting growth of organisms, the removal of organisms and/or their killing. These methods also arrest the biochemical degradation of tissues and transformation of cellular contents. This can be achieved by using heat, cold, drying, fermentation, radiation, and chemical preservatives. If not controlled carefully, these very techniques can bring about food deterioration. Therefore, the technique choosen should be such that harmful pathogenic microbes are killed or inhibited and biochemical attacks are lowered, and the food is still left unaltered.

Clydesdale and Francis (6) suggested the following possible ways of controlling the growth and development of microorganisms such as bacteria: (a) remove the food source, (b) change the temperature, (c) remove water, and (d) change the environment. Removal of the food source is not viable, for it would amount to taking away the food source for the human beings also.

A. Refrigerated and Frozen Foods

Most of the modern physical processing techniques aim at either changing the temperature or removal of water from food source. Temperature can be altered in a number of ways. Lowering of temperature (refrigeration) slows down the growth of bacteria and their multiplication, which causes food intoxication or food infection. Refrigeration effectively prevents deteriorations such as wilting of leafy vegetables, the rancidity of fats, and the souring of milk. A refrigerator maintained at 40°F (4.4°C) can about quadruple the keeping time of most foods.

Freezing is another effective way of preserving foods by changing the temperature. Freezing prevents the growth of microorganisms but will not kill them. The microbes do not get enough water for growth, because the available water is frozen. Also, at freezing temperatures microbes either cannot grow or do so very slowly. Though home freezing has become a common way of food preservation in the developed world, home-frozen foods are not as good quality as industrially frozen foods. The length of time the freezing process takes influences the product quality; i.e., the quicker the product is frozen, the higher will be its quality in terms of tissue damage and consequently its texture, color, flavor, and nutritive value. Industrial processes use techniques such as freezing by liquid nitrogen (–280°F, –137.8°C) and blast freezing, which uses a fan along with the freezer to create a wind effect. A low temperature coupled with a strong wind results in a wind-chill factor of about 60°F (16.5°C) or colder. Industrial blast freezers can attain the equivalent of very low temperatures and quick-freeze the food, which cannot be done in the home. The normal home freezer compartment therefore takes longer time to freeze food than industrial freezers.

It is necessary to blanch the food prior to its freezing, which involves subjecting the food to an elevated temperature (approx 190°F, 87.8°C) for a minute or so to destroy the enzymes present in fresh foods such as vegetables, thereby arresting the chemical reactions taking place in the frozen foods, which would give rise to off odors and off flavors.

Refrigeration has certain advantages over freezing. It takes less energy to cool a food to just above its freezing point than to freeze it. Refrigeration storage requires less insulation and refrigeration capacity. The refrigerated products do not normally suffer from texture and flavor losses caused by freezing. Also, the refrigerated foods do not have to be thawed before use—a process that may take as much as 48 hours with large frozen foods.

Most spoilage microbes grow above 10°C, some food poisoning organisms grow slowly up to 3.3°C, and cryophilic organisms grow slowly from –4.4° to –9.4°C, if the food is not frozen. These latter organisms, however, do not produce toxins or disease but can cause food deterioration. The organisms cannot grow below –9.4°C, though they are not totally destroyed at this temperature.

Chill-storage is an useful adjunct to other methods of food preservation. It requires controlled low temperature, which is achieved by taking the heat away from the storage area, using the principle of latent heat of vaporization. The commercial chill storage rooms are constructed taking into consideration the "refrigeration load," i.e., the quantity of heat that must be removed from the product and the storage area to alter the temperature from initial to selected final level and to maintain it for a specified time. The latter depends on the storage area and other factors that may generate heat within, or influence the heat removal from, the area. The specific heat of foods and rate of respiration of foods such as fruits and vegetables have an important bearing on the extent of refrigeration required.

Most foods can be deep frozen for 12 months or more without significant changes in their appearance, texture, color, and flavor. Such frozen foods have wide consumer acceptance.

Uncontrolled freezing of food, however, can result in the disruption of texture, breaking up of emulsion, denaturation of protein, and other undesirable physicochemical changes in foods. Because substances such as sugar, salts and soluble proteins dissolved in water lower the freezing point of water, these dissolved solids in a more concentrated solution (because of freezing of free water) require a still lower temperature to freeze it. Thus, different foods with varying levels of water and amount and nature of dissolved substances will have different freezing points and will require different times to reach a solid frozen state. Also, water present in the food does not freeze uniformly. The portion of food nearest to the container freezes first. As water continues to freeze, the concentration of dissolved solids increases, leaving the central core of highly concentrated liquid unfrozen, unless the temperature is sufficiently low to freeze the central core ultimately. Solid foods, such as pieces of meat held at −4°C may appear to be frozen solidly but may still contain about 3% of their water in an unfrozen condition. All the water in such foods does not get completely frozen even at −18°C. Such unfrozen water in frozen foods can cause their deterioration in terms of texture, color, flavor, and other quality parameters.

In slow freezing, water within and between cells of food tissues freezes and the ice crystals thus formed may cause physical rupture and separation of cells. However, if freezing is rapid, the minute crystals are formed only within the cells, minimizing the physical damage to the cells. Rapid freezing also minimizes concentration effects by decreasing the time of contact of solutes with food tissues during the transition from the unfrozen to the fully frozen state.

Like slow freezing, thawing also can have damaging effects on foods, repeated freezing and thawing being very detrimental to the quality of food. A fluctuation of even 3°C in freezing temperature above and below −18°C at which most foods are frozen and stored can damage foods. If thawing is slow, there is loss of quality due to concentration effects. Quick thawing helps to keep the microbial population in check. Use of microwave heating can bring about quick thawing.

Manay and Shadaksharaswamy (5) described three basic methods of freezing in commercial use: (a) freezing in air, (b) freezing by indirect contact with a refrigerant, and (c) freezing by direct contact with the freezing medium. Air freezing uses still air or an air-blast; in indirect contact freezing, food or food packages are placed on a surface cooled by a refrigerant. Immersion freezing or direct contact freezing, in which the food or food package is submerged in a cold liquid (or liquid is sprayed on the food), has several advantages. The intimate contact between the food and the refrigerant is especially important in freezing irregularly shaped food pieces. Also, immersion freezing minimizes the contact of food with air (oxygen) during freezing, thus decreasing oxidative deterioration of foods. The refrigerants used must be pure, nontoxic, and free from any taste, odor, color, or bleaching action. Low-freezing-point liquids cooled by indirect contact with another refrigerant or cryogenic liquids such as liquid nitrogen, liquid carbon dioxide, or freon are most commonly used. The low-freezing-point liquids employed are solutions of sugar, salt, or glycerol (a 23% NaCl or 62% sucrose solution can produce −21°C, and 67% glycerol-water solution can bring about −47°C). The cryogenic liquids are liquified gases of extremely low boiling point (liquid N_2, −196°C; liquid CO_2, −79°C; and freon 12, −30°C). The low boiling point of liquid nitrogen can bring about very quick freezing of large food materials maintaining their quality.

The packaging material used for freezing should be moisture-proof and impermeable to oxygen and flavor compounds, both during freezing and after thawing. It should also be resistant to chemical attack from the food constituents. The commonly used packaging materials include cans, metal foils, waxed papers, plastic-coated card-boards and plastic foils, cellophane, and parchment paper. Glass is generally not satisfactory for frozen foods.

B.   Baked and Canned Foods and Confectioneries

The other obvious way of utilizing temperature to control or kill microorganisms is heating. Cooking food destroys most of the harmful micobes; of course, cooking is also employed to make the food more palatable. Heat is the major method used in food processing and preservation by canning and in the preparation of baked foods and confectioneries. Home canning has become increasingly popular, but can be dangerous, if the guidelines for time and temperature applied to a given food in a given size container are not followed appropriately. The higher the temperature used, the shorter the heating time required. The modern food-processing industry is using higher temperatures and shorter times to process food by heating. The combination kills the bacteria effectively, without significantly destroying the essential nutrients.

The basic canning process consists of placing food in a suitable container, closing, heating, and cooling. In the developed world, large quantities of foods are canned and they form a significant part of the diet of the population. Most fruits and vegetables, a wide variety of meats, fish and their products, soups, and sausages are canned. Major steps in the canning process include cleaning, grading, and inspecting the raw commodity, blanching to inactivate enzymes, placing in the container with added brine or syrup and deaerating the product, heating in a retort at 1.05 kg/cm^2 pressure, using steam for metal cans or pressurized water for glass containers, partial cooling under pressure in the retort, followed by further cooling by water sprays or in a cooling tank, labeling, and racking or distribution.

In aseptic canning, food is pumped continuously through a plate-type or tubular heat exchanger that heats it very quickly to a high temperature, holding it at that temperature for the specified time and then cooling. Food is often sterilized at 150°C for 1 or 2 seconds (ultra-high temperature sterilization). The sterilized food is quickly cooled and placed in containers aseptically, and the lids are sealed in a sterile environment.

Low-acid foods (above pH 4.6) are usually pressure-canned ("*Flash 18*" process) by heating them above 100°C under pressure for sterility. The canning (sealing) process of these products is carried out in a chamber under a pressure of 1.05 to 1.40 kg/cm^2 to avoid violent boiling. Thus, low-acid foods are first presterilized by high temperature for a short time, and then the cans are transferred to a pressurized room and heated for specified time to obtain commercial-grade sterility, followed by sealing and cooling.

C.   Blanched and Pasteurized Foods

Blanching is often used in conjunction with vegetable processing to inactive degradative enzymes and to deaerate the product for further processing, rather than to kill the microorganisms. Unblanched products may give rise to off flavors and suffer from vitamin losses and color changes in frozen storage. Blanching is usually performed by dipping the products in boiling water for 2 to 3 minutes.

Pasteurization consists of heating food products either in containers or otherwise to a temperature below the boiling point of water for specified time. Pasteurization destroys most pathogenic organisms associated with food deterioration, thus extending a product's shelf life considerably, both by decreasing microbial population and inactivating some enzymes. The choice of temperature and time depends on the purpose of the process and the physicochemical composition of the food. Whereas milk, for example, is pasteurized at 62.8°C for 30 min, whole eggs are pasteurized at 64.4°C for 2 to 5 min to control dissemination of *Salmonella* sp. Sweetened condensed milk is given milder heat treatment because of the moderate heat resistance of yeasts, which are the only organisms that can grow in sweetened condensed milk. Beer, wines, fruit juices, and several other products are pasteurized to enhance their shelf life.

Pasteurized foods, being not sterile, contain vegetative organisms and spores that are capable of growing. Thus, many pasteurized foods must be stored under refrigeration. Pasteurized milk, for example, can remain in good condition only for a day or so at room temperature, but its life can be extended to about a week's time if stored in a refrigerator. High-temperature–short-time (HTST) methods (130°C and above for a few seconds to 6 min) may be used to obtain a germ-free stage.

D. Dried and Concentrated Foods

Food has been preserved by drying since the beginnings of human civilization. Nature also resorts to drying to preserve foods. Cereal and legume seeds in the field dry sufficiently on the stalk by exposure to the sun, without needing further drying for their preservation. Other foods, such as fruits, fish, meat, and vegetables, can be dried in the sun to increase their keeping quality. Natural drying is, however, feasible only under climatic conditions of high heat and low humidity.

Dried foods contain about 1% to 5% moisture and can keep at the ambient temperature for a year or longer. On reconstitution with water, most dried foods are very close to—or virtually indistinguishable from—their original quality.

Concentrated foods involve removal of part of their water (one-third to two-thirds) as in the preparation of syrups, evaporated/condensed milk, tomato paste, condensed soups, and sausages.

Microorganisms can grow on foods by using the water they contain. Such microbial spoilage of foods can be effectively stopped by drying foods to lower their moisture content at safe levels, e.g., dehydrated whole eggs, 10% to 11%, wheat flour, 13% to 15%; dehydrated fat-free meat 15%; dehydrated vegetables, 14% to 20%, and dehydrated fruits, 18% to 25%. Shelf life of dried foods is thus extended primarily by controlling the growth of microorganisms. Partial drying, as in concentrated foods, is less effective than total drying in this respect.

Drying and concentration, in addition to preserving food, help decrease the weight and bulk of food, thus resulting in great economy in storage, packaging, handling, and transport of food. Most convenience foods, such as instant foods, are prepared by drying.

The various factors influencing drying rates and the relationships between drying temperature and relative humidity, between evaporation and temperature, and time and temperature in food preservation have been described by Manay and Shadaksharaswamy (5). Thus, varying conditions such as temperature, humidity, air velocity and direction, thickness of food, and other factors influence drying of food.

Shrinkage of foods is the most obvious change brought about by drying, its type and magnitude depending upon the food and rate of drying. Quick high-temperature-dried foods absorb water, reconstitute quickly, and resemble the original fresh product more closely. With foods containing dissolved water and solutes in high concentration, drying may result in the shrinkage and sealing off of the surface pores and cracks, leading to trapping much of the remaining water with food, with the drying rate dropping off significantly. Such dried foods may contain voids, cracks, and pores of various sizes; shrinking and pore clogging by solutes is known as core hardening, which can be minimized by gradual drying with low surface temperature.

In addition to the physical changes, the chemical changes brought about by drying also can contribute to the quality of the dried foods and their reconstituted products in terms of color, flavor, texture, viscosity, nutritional value, and storage stability (8).

The common driers employed for liquid, solid, or mixture foods include air-convection driers, drum or roller driers, and vacuum driers. In air-convection drying, hot air supplies the heat for evaporation. The liquid food may be sprayed or poured into pans or on belts. Drum or roller driers are often used with liquid foods such as puree and mashes that are applied as thin films. Vacuum driers are used to lower the drying temperature. Various combinations of these drying methods are also used. Freeze-drying is used to dehydrate high-quality sensitive foods such as coffee, fruit juices, strawberries, and shrimps, which have delicate flavors, colors, and textures that cannot be preserved by other drying methods. In freeze-drying, water evaporates from ice without passing through the liquid state—i.e., water from ice directly becomes water vapor, at a temperature of 0°C or below and at a low pressure of 4.7 mm Hg or less. Frozen foods are dried in a vacuum chamber maintained at 0.1 to 2.0 mg Hg pressure and at a temperature below the melting point of ice. Under these conditions, water from frozen food evaporates at the maximum rate. Frozen food being rigid, the evaporation of water leaves voids behind, resulting in a porous, sponge-like, dried material. The vacuum in the dried food is then broken with inert nitrogen gas, the food being packed under nitrogen.

Foam (or puff)-dried products are made by dehydrating foods at atmospheric pressure. Liquid foods and purees are pre-foamed and then dried to obtain a product quality approaching that achieved through vacuum-drying. Foam exposes an enormous surface area for quick moisture escape, and drying of foams can take place rapidly even at atmospheric pressure at a reduced temperature, making the method more economic than vacuum drying. Whipping agents such as vegetable proteins, gums, and monoglycerides may be added prior to being whipped. Stable foams can be produced by casting them in thin layers into trays or belts followed by drying, employing various heating schemes (5).

Levels of water left in most concentrated foods are sufficient for microbial growth. Concentrated nonacid fruit juices and vegetable purees may undergo spoilage in time unless they are further processed. Concentrated sugar syrups, sauces, and jellies have relatively better shelf life than other products. Solutions containing 70% sugar or 18% to 25% salt prevent the growth of all microorganisms.

Common methods of concentration include those that use kettle evaporators, flash-evaporators, film-evaporators, vacuum evaporators, freeze-concentration and ultrafiltration, reverse concentration and ultrafiltration, and reverse osmosis. Open kettles and pans are heated by direct flame or steam. Higher temperatures and longer concentration times may damage most foods. Syrups are often concentrated by this method, as high heat is desirable to produce the color from caramealized sugar and develop typical flavor. Purees are usually concentrated by flash evaporation: superheated steam (150°C) is injected into the liquid food pumped into a vertical tubular steam-jacketed evaporator where boiling takes place. Use of film evaporators involves pumping food into a vertical cylinder that has a rotating element that spreads the food into a thin layer on the cylindrical wall. The latter is usually heated by steam. Water quickly evaporates from thin food layer and the concentrated food is simultaneously wiped from the cylinder wall.

Heat-sensitive liquid foods such as fruit juices are usually concentrated at low temperatures in vacuum evaporators. Several vacuumized vessels in series constitute multiple-effect evaporators. The first evaporator under vacuum is heated with steam and the water vapor boiled off from the food is sent to the next evaporator, maintained at a higher vacuum than the first. The water vapor acts as a heat source to evaporate food in the second evaporator. The water vapor from the second evaporator is then passed to a third one having a higher vacuum than the second, and so on. Grape and tomato juices are normally concentrated by this way.

Fruit juices may also be concentrated by freezing. When liquid food is frozen, all the water is not converted into ice simultaneously. Before the food freezes, the initially formed ice crystals are separated. A high percentage of water can be removed by repeating this process several times on the concentrated unfrozen food (9).

Ultrafiltration and reverse osmosis consist of pumping liquid foods at a high pressure against selective membranes that allow only water molecules to pass through, retaining organic macromolecules, sugar, salt, and so forth. In reverse osmosis, "tighter" membranes are used that do not allow passage of molecules. In reverse osmosis, under pressure, there is flow of water through membranes from a region of higher concentration to that of a lower concentration.

Most concentrated foods have a cooked flavor and darkened colors. Concentration may also bring about changes in the organoleptic and nutritional quality of foods. An increase in the levels of salts and minerals may result in the precipitation of proteins, which is often the cause of gel formation of evaporated milk after a few weeks or months of storage. Sugar may crystallize out as the concentration increases in foods containing sugar.

E. Fermented Foods

It is possible to preserve foods by changing the environment. Environmental factors can be manipulated as a means of controlling the quantity of microorganisms in a food material. Fermentation is a microbial process whereby microbes grow and produce an environment that is not suitable for the growth of other harmful microorganisms. This is how beer, hard liquor, and sauerkraut are made. Fermentation gives useful microorganisms an environment in which they can grow and multiply, excreting an acid that will inhibit the growth of harmful microbes. Acids produced naturally (e.g., malate from apples, citrate from oranges, and acetic acid from vinegar) can also prevent growth of undesired microorganisms. Acids may also be used as food additives to protect certain food products. *Clostridium botulinum* does not grow in acid foods having a pH of less than 4.5.

Natural fermentation also plays a vital role in preservation of foods—e.g. fruit juices left exposed to air under fermentation produces alcohol, and milk on standing turns acidic. Such changes have been traditionally used as a means of preserving perishable foods. The changes in the texture and taste of fermented foods are desirable. Some commonly used fermented foods are cheese, butter, alcoholic beverages, pickles, sauerkraut, vinegar, breads, *idli*, *dosa*, *khaman*, *dokla*, soy sauce, coffee, tea, and cocoa (10).

In fermentation, microbial enzymes break down carbohydrates under anerobic condition to organic acids. In common usage, the term *fermentation* refers to both the anaerobic and aerobic degradation of carbohydrates and carbohydrate-like materials to acids, e.g., conversion of lactose to lactic acid by *Steptococcus lactis* under anaerobic condition and conversion of ethanol to acetic acid by *Acetobactor aceti* under aerobic conditions.

During fermentation, a complex mixture of carbohydrates, proteins, and fats undergoes modifications simultaneously under the action of a variety of microorganisms and the enzymes thereof. Thus carbohydrates and like materials undergo fermentation, proteinaceous materials undergo proteolysis or "putrefactive" changes, and lipids undergo "lipolytic" breakdown. The nature and extent of these changes depend on the food, type of microorganisms, and conditions affecting their growth and metabolic pattern. The preservative effect of fermentation is brought about by the chemicals excreted by the microorganisms, principally the acids and alcohol that inhibit the growth of pathogenic microbes.

In addition to their preservative quality, fermented foods have better flavor and textural properties and higher nutritional value. Microorganisms, in addition to breaking down complex compounds, synthesize several vitamins and other growth factors, which are added to the fermented foods. The industrial production of certain vitamins is largely brought about by the fermentation process. Fermentation by certain molds breaks down the indigestible protective cellulosic and hemicellulosic coatings, thus enhancing the digestibility and nutritional value of the product.

Controlled fermentation is necessary to obtain a product of desirable quality. The factors influencing growth and metabolic activities of microorganisms during food fermentation include acidity (pH), level of alcohol, use of starters, and levels of oxygen and salts (5).

F. Irradiated Foods

Food irradiation involves the use of energy in the form of ionizing radiation to destroy insects and microorganisms without altering the food's composition and texture, as heating does. The decision of the Environmental Protection Agency (EPA) to suspend the use of ethylene dibromide (EDB) as a fumigant to control insects in stored grains, citrus fruits, and papaya has created the need for an alternative method, such as irradiation of foods, for their protection. The irradiation levels required in foods do not cause the food to become radioactive or dangerous in any other way. According to Clydesdale and Francis (6), 21 countries allow one or more of 31 foods to be irradiated. In the United States, irradiated foods available to the consumers include some spices and powdered vegetable seasonings approved by the FDA in July 1983. In February 1984, the FDA issued a proposal in the *Federal Register* to allowing low-dose irradiation to delay ripening of fresh fruits and vegetables and to kill insects that infest food. Poultry and shellfish also could be irradiated to increase their storage life, as well as pork to reduce the risk of trichinosis. Pigs fed garbage often become infected with *Trichinella spiralis*, a parasite. The latter can become lodged in human muscle, if it is not destroyed. This parasite can be controlled only by heating the entire piece of meat (ham, pork, etc.) until an internal center temperature of 137°F (58.3°C) is reached. Irradiation can be used more effectively to protect these foods.

This method has yet to gain general acceptance because the possible harmful effects of radiation on the human body have given rise to suspicion about the safety of the irradiated foods. Though much research work has been reported on the safety and wholesomeness of irradiated foods, more careful work is needed before allowing the use of irradiated food on a large scale.

Principal radiations used in food irradiation are gamma rays (less than 2A°) and electrons (beta-particles). Ultraviolet radiations are also used in preservation, but they have lower degree of penetration and are often employed to inactivate microorganisms of the food surface. Ionizing radiations are measured in terms of rads (and kilorad or megrad), a rad being 10 μJ of energy absorbed per gram of food material. The following doses of radiations are generally employed in food preservation: 10^4 to 10^7 rads (to kill microorganisms), 10^3 to 10^6 rads (to kill insects), and 10^3 to 10^4 rads (to inhibit sprouting of potatoes, onion, etc.). A dose of 10^2 to 10^3 rads may become lethal to human beings.

Ionizing radiations are used to sterilize foods in hermatically sealed packs, to reduce the load of spoilage flora on perishables, to eliminate pathogens in foods, to control infestation of stored grains as well as to prevent sprouting of potatoes, onions, and other foods.

Irradiation does not significantly affect the nutritional quality of foods, in comparison to heat processing. Because ionization can hydrolyse and modify proteins, starch, and cellulose, it can help improve the nutritive value of certain plant foods. Excessive doses, can alter however, the structure of organic biomolecules in foods, resulting in damage.

G. Smoked Foods

Smoking is one of the ancient methods of food preservation. It is another method of changing the environment that inhibits the growth of microorganisms. Smoking has traditionally been used to produce meat that is long-lasting, nutritious, and palatable. The smoke dries the surface of the meat, thereby preventing the growth of microorganisms to some extent. Certain compounds produced in the smoke specifically inhibit the growth of some organisms. Smoking, however, may produce certain carcinogenic compounds in the smoked foods.

H. Chemically Preserved Foods

A preservative is used to inhibit, retard, or arrest the growth of microorganisms or any deterioration of food due to microbes, or even to mask the evidence of such deterioration. Chemical preservatives interfere with cell membranes of microorganisms, their enzymes, or their genetic mechanisms. Commonly used preservatives include sugars, salts, acids, and some synthetic products.

The traditionally used sodium chloride (NaCl) stops the growth of microbes by interfering with the action of proteolytic enzymes. Salt also causes food dehydration by drawing out water from the tissue cells. It is normally used to control microbial population in foods such as butter, cheese, cabbage, olives, cucumbers, meats, fish, and bread. Brined foods have salt in the water phase. The preservative action of NaCl can be enhanced by controlling other factors such as pH, temperature, and partial pressure of oxygen.

Sugar brings about preservation through its osmotic effect. The high osmotic pressure of sugar creates an environment that is not favorable for the growth and reproduction of microbes. The preservative action of moderate-strength sugar solutions can be increased by using invertase to increase the concentration of glucose in relation to sucrose. Foods preserved by using sugars include syrups and confectionery products, fondant fillings in chocolates, honey, jams, jellies, marmalades, and conserves as well as fruits such as dates and currants.

Sulfur dioxide is used as a preservative to treat fruits and vegetables before and after dehydration, to extend shelf life of fresh fruits such as grapes, and to prevent growth of undesirable microorganisms during wine making and in the manufacture of fruit juices. Sulfur dioxide also effectively prevents the enzymatic browning reactions in dried fruits.

Sulfur dioxide may be used in its gaseous state (SO_2), the sodium or potassium bisulfites ($NaHSO_3$) or $KHSO_3$), sulfites (Na_2SO_3, K_2SO_3), and metabisulfite ($Na_2S_2O_5$, $K_2S_2O_5$). In aqueous solutions, sulfur dioxide and sulfite salts form sulfurous acid (H_2SO_3) and ions of bisulfite (HSO_3^-) and sulfite (SO_3^{2-}). At low pH (less than 4.5), the undissociated sulfurous acid predominates and inhibits the growth of yeasts and molds, whereas at high pH values, the HSO_3^- ions effectively inhibit bacteria but not yeasts. The use of sulfur dioxide leaves an unmistakable taste in the mouth and may cause breakdown of thiamin.

Nitrates and nitrites have been used as curing agents to preserve meats and to give them desirable color and flavor, as well as to prevent toxin formation through microorganisms. Nitrite ($NaNO_2$) when added to meat is converted to nitric oxide, which combines with myoglobin to form nitric oxide myoglobin (nitrosyl myoglobin), a heat-stable pigment. The curing also contributes flavor to the meat, inhibits the growth of *Clostridium* and *Streptococcus* bacteria, and lowers the temperature required to kill *C. botulinum*.

Cooking of nitrite-cured meats has been found to produce small amounts of N-nitrosamines which are potent carcinogenic compounds. Such nitrosation may also take place in foods during storage or processing. Evidence indicates that nitrosamines are formed under the strong acid condition in the human stomach when nitrite-cured meats are consumed. The reduction in the concentration of nitrate in the curing agents can help to alleviate this problem.

Reduction in the nitrate concentration can be achieved in the presence of another preservative that acts synergistically, because the diminished concentration of nitrite enhances the risk of food poisoning due to *C. botulinum*. According to Manay and Shadaksharaswamy (5), in the presence of isoascorbic acid, even very dilute concentrations of nitrite significantly decrease spoilage and toxin formation. Ascorbic acid and isoascorbic acid react with nitrite to produce nitric oxide, which accelerates the rate of formation of nitrosyl myoglobin and thus stabilization of color and flavor of the meat. Polyphosphates such as sodium triphosphate ($Na_5P_3O_{10}$) and sodium hexametaphosphate ($NaPO_3)_n$, where n = 10 to 15, are also used as meat-curing agents. These compounds act by enhancing water retention and increasing tenderness, juiciness, and flavor of the cured meats. They also improve the texture and act as antioxidants by chelating metal ions.

Straight-chain monocarboxylic acids and alpha-unsaturated fatty acid analogues such as sorbic acid (CH_3—CH=CH—CH=COOH) and its sodium and potassium salts have strong antimicrobial activity and inhibit molds and yeasts in foods such as cheese, bakery products, fruit juices, wines, and pickles. The molds are not able to metabolize the conjugated unsaturated structure of sorbate.

Acetic acid in the forms of sodium, potassium, and calcium acetates are used in a range of bakery products to prevent ropiness and growth of molds, but they do not interfere with yeasts. Acetate is also used in foods such as catsup, mayonnaise, and pickles for flavor and antimicrobial activity.

Propionic acid and its sodium and calcium salts also exert antimicrobial acitivity against molds and bacteria and are used in bakery products to prevent growth of *Bacillus mesentericus*, which produces ropiness in bread. The organisms are not able to metabolize the three-carbon unit of propionate.

Benzoic acid and its sodium salt are widely used in foods as antimicrobial agents against yeasts and bacteria; they are least active against molds. Benzoic acid has optimum activity in the pH range of 2.5 to 4.0 and is thus well suited for use in acid foods, such as fruit juices, carbonated beverages, pickles, and sauerkraut.

The alkyl (methyl, ethyl, propyl, and heptyl) esters of p-hydroxybenzoic acid (parabens) are used for their antimicrobial activity against molds and yeasts, but they are relatively ineffective against bacteria. They are active at pH 7.0 or higher and have little effect on flavor.

Cyclic ethers or epoxides such as ethylene oxide and propylene oxide can destroy all forms of microorganisms, including spores, and even viruses. They are often used in their gaseous forms for the intimacy of their contact with food. After adequate exposure, the residual epoxide is removed by flushing and evacuation. Their use is limited to dry foods such as nuts and spices. Spices often contain a high microbial load and cannot be sterilized by heat because of the instability of the flavor compounds to heat.

Antibiotics, produced naturally by a variety of microorganisms, have great chemotherapeutic value in controlling pathogenic disease-producing bacteria and molds. Antibiotics such as nisin, pimaracin, chlorotetracycline (aureomycin), and oxytetracycline (terramycin) have been used as food preservatives in some countries. Nicin is used to control the growth of spore-forming bacteria in dairy products such as cheese and condensed milk. Pimaracin is used to control the growth of fungi in cheese and sausages, and aureomycin and terramycin are used to control the growth of bacteria in fish and poultry.

Diethyl pyrocarbonate is used as an antimicrobial agent in fruit juices, wines, and carbonated beverages. It acts as a "cold sterilizing" agent for aqueous solutions, and after its action, it is readily hydrolyzed to ethanol and carbon dioxide. It is active in low concentration (120 to 300 ppm) and is an irritant in concentrated form. It may react with the ammonia generally present in plant and animal food tissues to form urethane (ethyl carbamate), a carcinogenic compound. Dimethyl pyrocarbonate, a lower member of this group of compounds, has a good potential to be used as a cold-sterilizing agent in foods.

IV. NUTRITIONAL VALUE OF THE PROCESSED FOODS

The nutritional value of "processed" food is sometimes compared with that of "natural" and "health" foods. In fact, many of the foods that are perceived as natural have been processed in some way, e.g., storage of fruits and vegetables in controlled atmosphere to extend their shelf life. Many of the specific claims about so-called health foods are also difficult to substantiate (7). Thus, the terms "natural" and "health" foods have no real scientific meaning. The techniques of animal and plant food production have developed simultaneously with those of food processing and preservation (11). Regulatory bodies such as the U.K. Ministry of Agriculture, Fisheries and Foods (MAFF), Food Advisory Committee also prefer to not use the term "natural" foods. The current legislation in the European Community (EC) and the United States positively discourages health claims by foods, especially when related to protection from, or treatment of, a specific disease because this is seen as making a medical or drug claim for a food, blurring the boundary between foods and medicines. The claims for most health foods rest on less substantial scientific evidence, some of which could almost be regarded as magical and sometimes even fraudulent (12) (see Chapter 23).

Food processing techniques such as canning, cooking, and irradiation do affect the concentrations of some nutrients in food, particularly the heat-labile vitamins. The genuine concerns about the techniques used in the processing of foods relate to the nature of the processes themselves, to the use of various kinds of additives. These issues relate basically to the safety of processed foods rather than to their nutritional value. Also, the concerns about the nutritional composition of processed foods relate primarily to their formulation in respect of the major components (7).

A. Effects of Processing On Food Losses

Losses of food occur throughout the food chain (1–4,9). Some of these losses are an inevitable consequence of converting the food from the field into an edible form; thus it may not be correct to consider such losses as "wastage." However, the food losses occurring during storage of food grains due to spoilage by rodents or insect pests or due to fungal and bacterial damage are, being avoidable, are considered wastage of valuable foods. These losses can be prevented or minimized at the cost of improved storage facilities and use of pesticides and antimicrobial agents.

Mechanical damage to fruits and vegetables during their harvesting is a common focus for the beginning of microbial damage. The availability of food in tropical developing countries is greatly influenced by the pre- and postharvest losses of foods, where temperature and humidity magnify the potential for biological damage.

Food processing results in various types of losses due to inefficient processing method and excessive peeling, trimming, or polishing and so forth. Carcasses are trimmed during butchering; cereal grains and pulses are cleaned and milled before use as food. Vegetables are trimmed to remove external leaves to prepare them for retail markets. Processes such as blanching of vegetables and cheese making can produce waste products that are not recoverable as food. However, some of the by-products of processing are used as animal feed—less since bran was recognized as a source of dietary fiber.

The preparation of foods for retail sale often produces significant food losses. Meats and fish are trimmed further, like vegetables, for the prepacked market. Such losses may also occur in the kitchen, followed by additional losses when all the edible material prepared is not consumed at the meal. In large-scale institutional catering, substantial wastage of edible material often occurs. Platt et al. (13) reported 25% to 35% wastage of the food served in hospital meals.

The household food waste collected from several hundred families during 1980 in the United Kingdom was analysed for energy and proximate constituents. The weekly waste amounted to 6.5% of the energy in summer and 5.4% in the winter (7). Southgate and Shirling (14) used a similar approach in a study of food consumption in a submarine, which showed substantial losses of edible or potentially edible food material.

Pets consume substantial quantities of food material. Conservative estimates show that 22 million dogs and 30 million cats in the United States of America eat food equivalent to 5% of the total human energy intake and 14% of the protein requirement, and 5 million dogs and 5 million cats in the United Kingdom eat about 3% of the energy and 2% of the protein required by the human population. Much of this food includes offal such as lungs, trachea, and carcass trimmings that are not fit for human consumption and hence cannot be regarded as waste. A substantial quantity of food prepared, such as scraps from plates and surplus food prepared for the family meal, however, is fed to pets in the developed world.

B. Effects of Processing on Nutritional Composition and Quality of Food

In addition to the quantitative losses, processing also has significant effects on the nutritive value and quality of the processed foods. Many changes in the proximate composition of the processed food are brought about by the heat and radiation energy applied to the foodstuff. Some of these changes may decrease the nutritional value of the food and others may produce potentially toxic compounds. However, processing by heat and radiation are important for the generation of flavor compounds and destruction of harmful microorganisms.

Heating or cooking food may denature protein, changing its tertiary structure. The protein may become insoluble and precipitate to form curd. Denaturation of protein, however, does not affect its nutritional value. A series of chemical changes (Maillard reactions) takes place when proteins are heated in the presence of carbohydrates, especially the reducing sugars. The reaction of the reducing sugar with the epsilon amino group of lysine reduces the biological value of the protein, by making lysine unavailable. Such effects are directly related to the severity of the heat used during processing, excessive heat treatment drastically decreasing the nutritional value of food. Mild heating produces browning (desirable in some processes) and only minor nutrient losses. According to Southgate and Johnson (7), upto 40% of the lysine may be damaged permanently when milk is roller-dried, whereas milder spray-drying of milk produces only about 10% losses. The baking and toasting of cereal products, associated with Maillard reactions, may also result in about 10% to 15% loss of lysine. The reactions between amino acids and other food components, however, are essential for the generation of flavor compounds and enhance consumer acceptance of the processed products.

Changes produced in fatty substances during processing arc mainly influenced by the fatty acid composition of the lipid, major changes involving the unsaturated fatty acids of the fat or oil. The double bonds present in the unsaturated fatty acids react with oxygen to produce highly reactive peroxides, superoxides, and other free radicals that may decompose to give a range of compounds; some of these contribute to the flavor of the fried foods and other are potentially toxic, carcinogenic compounds and cause darkening of the oil. Heat treatment of oils and fat may also result in the production of free fatty acids. These reactions, which occur slowly at normal frying temperatures, may be accelerated in the presence of metals such as iron and copper. Fats overheated for long periods darken, accumulating toxic compounds. Antioxidants may be used to minimize these changes.

Carbohydrates, in comparison with fats and proteins, are rather unreactive and heat processing or cooking has only minor effects on their nutritional properties. Reducing sugars take part in Maillard and browning reactions and contribute to the flavor of the processed products. In the absence of amino acids, sugar syrups react to form caramel, a mixture of condensation products of hexose (furfurals). Starch granules of unprocessed foods, when heated in an aqueous medium, absorb water and swell to produce a colloidal sol. These starch sols gel on cooling, the linear amylose molecules forming an insoluble precipitate that is very slowly hydrolyzed by alpha-amylase. The heating and cooling of starchy foods may thus decrease the digestibility of the food. Although heat processing of foods makes starch, as a whole, more digestible, the subsequent cooling makes a small proportion resistant to digestion. Heating brings about marked changes in the texture of foods, especially by its action on cell-wall polysaccharides and pectic substances.

Though heating per se has little effect on the minerological composition of foods, significant mineral losses can occur through leaching into the cooking medium. The heating effects on organic compounds may restrict bioavailability of minerals such as iron, zinc, and calcium. Heat-induced phytase enzyme may hydrolyse phytates in cereal foods to improve availability of minerals. The heat treatment may also inactivate the natural phytases present in the raw food, allowing the higher levels of phytate to be present in the processed food.

The most deleterious effects of food processing result from effects of heat treatment and cooking on the vitamin content of the food. The extent of losses depends on the nature of specific vitamin and the processing condition employed. The water-soluble vitamins, such as ascorbic acid, may be leached out in the cooking medium, and lost when the medium is discarded. Many vitamins are unstable and can be destroyed by heating in the presence of air; e.g., thiamin decomposes if heated in alkaline medium and vitamin C is easily oxidized by heating. The stability of some important vitamins under various conditions of processing, such as pH, acidity alkalinity, air, light, and heat, is shown in Table 1. The most heat-sensitive vitamins are vitamin C, thiamin, and riboflavin, though many other vitamins may be lost depending on the processing conditions employed.

Vitamin C is a powerful reducing agent and can be readily oxidized in the presence of air when food is heated. Oxidation proceeding beyond the stage of dehydroascorbic acid destroys all the vitamin C activity permanently, the processing being accelerated by the presence of oxidases in the food tissues, heat, alkalinity, traces of copper, and atmospheric oxygen. Vitamin retention can be increased by controlling these factors. The ascorbic acid oxidase released after the plant tissue is cut or macerated can be rapidly inactivated by placing fruits and vegetables in boiling water for a short time. Warm holding of cooked dishes can cause significant loss of vitamin C. Blanching of fruits and vegetables thus minimizes enzyme activity and vitamin losses; so does designing packages to exclude oxygen. The acidity of fruits is a major factor in the retention of ascorbic acid during the production of fruit juices. Special care is required to reduce the copper levels in the process water and production plant. Use of bicarbonate to retain the color of vegetables during cooking greatly destroys the ascorbic acid content. Also, the frying of potato crisps (chips) in shallow fat can may lead to significant losses of vitamin C.

When cereal foods such as rice are washed prior to cooking, the water-soluble thiamin is lost to some extent. As with vitamin C, alkaline conditions used during processing may lead to

Table 1   Stability of Vitamins Under Different Processing Conditions

Vitamin	pH7	Acid	Alkaline	Air	Light	Heat	Cooking losses[a] (%)
Retinol	S	U	S	U	U	U	0–40
Carotenes	S	U	S	U	U	U	0–30
Vitamin D	S	U	U	U	U	U	0–40
Vitamin E	S	S	S	U	U	U	0–55
Thiamin	U	S	U	U	S	U	0–80
Riboflavin	S	S	U	S	U	U	0–75
Niacin	S	S	S	S	S	S	0–75
Vitamin B_6	S	S	S	S	U	U	0–40
Vitamin B_{12}	S	S	S	U	U	S	0–10
Vitamin C	U	S	U	U	U	U	0–100

U = unstable, S = stable
[a]Losses depend on the duration of exposure to the conditions listed.
Source: Ref. 7.

significant loss of thiamin (10% to 20%). Thiamin is also destroyed by sulfur dioxide and sulfites used in foods.

Although riboflavin is comparatively stable during cooking, it is rather sensitive to light and decomposes by absorbing UV light. Milk left in sunlight or under fluorescent light can lose a significant quantity of riboflavin.

Folic acid is very susceptible to atmospheric oxidation when heated in neutral or alkaline conditions and is readily leached away in an aqueous medium. Substantial losses of folates can occur when dissolved oxygen is present in produce or a package is permeable to oxygen.

Vitamin B_6 (pyridoxal, pyridoxamine) is sensitive to oxidation during heat treatments, especially during canning when high temperatures are employed. Vitamin B_{12} (cyanocobalamin) although stable at normal cooking temperature, is lost by severe heat treatment as in HTST and UHT (ultra-heating) processes.

Both retinol and carotenes are stable at normal cooking temperatures, but high frying temperatures may lead to oxidative losses and isomerization of the carotenoids, losing their biological activity. Vitamin E (tocopherol) is slowly destroyed during frying and is decomposed by light (7).

Effects of processing methods other than heat treatment, such as deep-freezing, on nutrients are generally small. Some losses do occur during blanching, but deep-frozen foods are virtually equivalent to fresh products nutritionally, if not texturally. The vitamin losses taking place during extrusion cooking (HTST process) are comparable to those of conventional baking. The starch-like polysaccharides can undergo some depolymerization due to shear forces, and proteins are extensively modified physically, though with negligible nutritional changes.

The effects of irradiation on foods are similar to those of conventional thermal processes. The effects on biological value of proteins are very small at doses upto 10 KGy. Unsaturated fats may be oxidized, and bond scission can lead to unacceptable flavors, limiting the use of irradiation on fatty foods. Small depolymerization effects can occur in starchy foods. The labile vitamins are destroyed to a similar extent as that in normal thermal heating (7).

Table 2 Nutrient Retention in Solar-dried Mango and Papaya

Ripeness	Color	Texture	Treatment	2% Retention[a]	
				Vitamin C	Beta-carotene
Papaya					
Mature	Orange yellow	Firm	Citrate and sucrose	81.27	50.62
Ripe	Bright yellow orange	Soft, disintegrates on slicing	Citrate and sucrose	48.50	49.76
Mature	Orange yellow	Firm	Citrate and sucrose	90.63	50.74
Mature	Orange yellow	Firm	Sucrose only	84.30	40.93
Mango (Boribo)					
Mature	Golden yellow	Firm	Citrate and sucrose	57.22	81.15
Ripe	Orange yellow	Soft, spongy	Citrate and sucrose	38.61	85.40
Mature	Golden yellow	Firm	Steam blanched citric and sucrose	27.49	35.81

[a]On dry weight basis.
[b]Mature samples from different farms within the same area, and possibly from different cultivars.
Source: Ref. 8.

Gomez (8) reported the effects of drying on the nutritive value of foods. Carotene retention in the ambient temperature-dried treatments was lower than in the solar-dried treatments with continued losses in storage. Light-protected drying resulted in higher retention of carotene and vitamin C than light-exposed drying, and steam-blanching improved retention of these vitamins significantly. Papaya showed appreciably higher retention of vitamin C on drying than did mango, but the latter had significantly higher carotene retention. Steam blanching of mango prior to drying resulted in appreciable losses of both ascorbic acid and carotene (Table 2). Thus, it can be seen that significant changes do occur in the nutritional quality of food during processing.

REFERENCES

1. Salunkhe, D.K., and B.B. Desai, *Postharvest Biotechnology of Fruits*, Vol. I & II, CRC Press, Boca Raton, FL, 1984.
2. Salunkhe, D.K., and B.B. Desai, *Postharvest Biotechnology of Vegetables*, Vol. I & II, CRC Press, Boca Raton, FL, 1984.
3. Salunkhe, D.K., and B.B. Desai, *Postharvest Biotechnology of Oilseeds*, CRC Press, Boca Raton, FL, 1984.
4. Salunkhe, D.K., and B.B. Desai, *Postharvest Biotechnology of Sugar Crops*, CRC Press, Boca Raton, FL, 1988.
5. Manay, N.S., and M. Shadaksharaswamy, *Foods: Facts and Principles*, Wiley Eastern Ltd., New Delhi, 1987.
6. Clydesdale, F.M., and F.J. Francis, *Food Nutrition and Health*, AVI Publishing Co. Westport, 1985.
7. Southgate, D.A.T., and Johnson, I., Food processing, *Human Nutrition and Dietetics* (J.S. Garrow and W.P.T. James, eds.), 9th ed., Churchill Livingstone, London, 1993, p. 335.
8. Gomez, M.I. Effect of drying on the nutritive value of foods in Kenya, *Food Drying*, Proc. Workshop on 'Food Drying' held at Edmonton, Alberta, Ottawa, 6–9, July 1981, International Development Research Centre, Ottawa, Canada, 1982, p. 31.
9. Desai, B.B., and D.K. Salunkhe, Fruits and Vegetagles (Chapter 3) and Sugar Crops, (Chapter 4). *Foods of Plant Origin: Production, Technology and Human Nutrition* (D.K. Salunkhe and S.S. Deshpande, eds), Van Nostrand Reinhold, New York, 1991, p. 301 and p. 413.
10. Desai, B.B., and D.K. Salunkhe, Dhokla and Khaman (Chapter 10), *Legume-Based Fermented Foods* (N.R. Reddy, M.D. Pierson, and D.K. Salunkhe, eds.), CRC Press, Boca Raton, FL, 1986, p. 161.
11. Southgate, D.A.T., Natural and unnatural foods? *British Med. J. 288*: 881 (1984).
12. Bender, A.E., *Health or hoax*, Sphere Books, London, 1986.
13. Platt, B.S., T.P. Eddy, and P.L. Pellett, *Food in hospitals*, Oxford University Press, Oxford, 1963.
14. Southgate, D.A.T., and D. Shirling, The energy expenditure and food intake of the ship's company of a submarine, *Ergonomics 13*: 777 (1970).

14
Food Additives and Nutrification

I. INTRODUCTION

The use of food additives is one of the most debated subjects related to the food supply. It is also one of the issues least understood by the consumers and one of the most difficult to regulate, mainly because absolute food safety is not possible to demonstrate. Clydesdale and Francis (1) defined *food additive* as any minor ingredient added to a food to bring about some technical effect. In a broad sense, it may also include compounds unintentionally added during the production, distribution, and/or processing of food, barring those that may appear in foods accidentally. The term food additive, however, does not include compounds such as pesticides, color additives, new animal drugs, or substances used in accordance with a sanction or approval granted prior to effective date of the food additives amendment to the existing laws in 1958. According to the Federal Food, Drug and Cosmetic Act (U.S. Code, Section 321), legally a food additive is a substance, "the intended use of which results or may be reasonably be expected to result, directly or indirectly, in its becoming a component or otherwise affecting the characteristic of any food," with certain exceptions. Excluded from the requirements of this act are substances that are generally recognized by food experts to be safe under the conditions of their intended use. These substances are commonly referred to as GRAS (Generally Recognized As Safe) substances that have been used in foods over long periods without adverse effects and that are considered harmless by qualified scientists. Food additives have important uses in foods from a flavor, color, appearance, preservative, and economic point of view. They help to provide better food at lower price for more people and at minimum risk. The major categories of food additives include preservatives, colors, flavors, sweeteners, emulsifiers and stabilizers, antioxidants, flour improvers, and processing aids such as acids, acidity regulators, humactants, gelling agents, and antifoaming agents (2,3).

II. NEED FOR FOOD ADDITIVES

The use of food additives started at the beginning of human civilization, perhaps with the use of salt (sodium chloride) to preserve meat. The civilization of ancient Egypt used food colors; the Chinese burned of kerosine to ripen bananas, without knowing that the ripening agent present in combustion was ethylene. Many ancient civilizations have used flavorings and seasoning agents; as a result, spices and condiments were important items of commerce. The use and number of additives have increased with the improvements in preservation and processing technology. Over 3000 chemical compounds with more than 40 functions are used today in the food industry; they can be grouped into the following broad categories:

1. to provide protection against food spoilage and deterioration during storage, transport, distribution, or processing
2. to enhance the nutritional value of the product
3. to provide convenience foods such as "instant" or "ready-to-cook" foods, to industrialized societies
4. to increase consumer acceptability of foods, by improving their appearance, texture, color, flavor, and nutritive value.

Clydesdale and Francis (1) grouped additives into five broad categories:

1. flavors
2. colors
3. preservatives
4. texture agents
5. miscellaneous compounds

Spices and natural and synthetic flavors are used to complement, improve, and enhance the flavor of foods. Colors are used mainly to give food an appetizing appearance, because the way food looks has an effect on its palatability. Preservatives are used to prevent food spoilage, which is also achieved by food processing techniques such as heating, refrigeration, drying, freezing, fermentation, and curing. Some of these processes bring about only partial preservation, which is extended through additives. Food additives are thus primarily needed to prolong the food's keeping qualities, as an essential requirement of the modern urban society. Stabilizers and thickening agents are used to improve the texture of foods. Newer emulsifiers and stabilizers have given rise to most of the modern day convenience foods. Some of the additives used have numerous functions—e.g., addition of nutrients, such as vitamins and minerals; moisture retainers as well as acids, alkalies, buffers, and neutralizing agents used to improve the quality of baked goods, soft drinks and confectioneries.

III. FOOD ADDITIVES, GRAS SUBSTANCES, AND THEIR SAFETY

The permitted food preservatives (Table 1) are used to control the growth of harmful microorganisms in foods as well as to mask the evidence of microbial food deterioration. Food colors are used to improve the appearance and consumer acceptability of food. These materials include organic dyes and natural coloring pigments extracted from foods such as beetroots, anatto, and many other plant products. Caramels are important coloring materials used in large volume and are second only in importance to the yellow dye tartrazine, used in more than about 2000 foods (4). Some nutrients are used as food colors, providing unexpected sources of nutrient intake, unless nutritionists are aware of their use; e.g., E 101 is riboflavin, used in some sauces and mustard pickles, and B160(a) is beta-carotene. The red dye erythrosine E 127 has a high concentration of iodine.

Bixin, a red pigment, is derived from the seedcoat of *Bixa orellanta*, from which anatto dye is made by extracting yellow-to-red coloring material from the orange-red pulp of the seeds. Anatto is used in butter, cheese, margarine, and many other foods. A yellow pigment, carotene, derived from carrots is used in margarine. Safron is used both as a coloring and as a flavoring agent, and curcumin from turmeric is used to color meat products and salad dressings. Cochineal (or carnum) is a natural red color extracted from a female insect, *Coccus cacti*, and grape skin. The caramel and brown color obtained from burnt sugar are also used as food colors.

Flavors present in many fruits and vegetables are complex mixtures of aldehydes, esters of organic acids and alcohols, and a range of essential oils and terpenoids. Other savory flavors are

Table 1 List of Preservatives Permitted Under
U.K. Preservatives in Food Regulation, 1975

Benzoic acid
Methyl 4-hydroxy benzoate
Ethyl 4-hydroxybenzoate
Propyl 4-hydroxybenzoate
Biphenyl
Nisin
Sodium nitrate
Sodium nitrite
2-hydroxybiphenyl
Propionic acid
Sorbic acid
Sulfur dioxide
2-(thiazol-4-yl) benzimidazole
Hexamine

Source: Ref. 3.

derived from hydrolysates of cereals or proteins. A range of flavoring agents, both natural and synthetic (more than 2000 compounds), have been reviewed (5). Many synthetic substances are "nature identical"; i.e., they are found naturally in foods or are formed during cooking.

Flavor improvers such as monosodium glutamate (MSG) and other salts of glutamic acid, as well as some nucleotides, are also used as flavor enhancers. The latter are not flavors in themselves but they amplify the flavors of other substances synergistically. Most naturally occurring flavor substances, such as like spices, herbs, roots, essences, and essential oils, are used as flavor additives, but the flavors from such materials are not uniform in their chemical makeup.

Sucrose (from cane or beet) is the most widely used sweetening agent in foods, followed by glucose and high-fructose syrups (6), made by hydrolysing starch. In addition to providing sweetening, sugars are also sources of food energy. However, low-energy-content foods are also in demand from those who wish to regulate or reduce body weight and patients with *diabetes mellitus*, who must control their sugar intake. To meet these demands, a number of artificial sweeteners have been developed (7). Saccharin, which is about 400 times sweeter than sucrose, was widely used but its heat-unstability has limited its use in processed foods. Cyclamates (30 times sweeter than sucrose) are heat-stable but raise concerns about the possible carcinogenicity of their metabolites. The use of cyclamates has been banned in the United States, the United Kingdom, and some other countries.

Distinguished from "intense sweeteners" are a new category of "bulk sweeteners," such as the sugar alcohols (mono- or disaccharide alcohols), such as sorbitol or maltitol). Because these compounds are poorly absorbed from small intestine, they contribute to less metabolizable energy than the sugars. Aspartame (dipeptide of aspartic acid and phenylalanine), acesulfame K (potassium salt of acetyl sulfame), and thaumatin (natural extract from a tropical fruit) have been permitted to be used as food sweeteners (8).

Emulsions or foams improve the textural properties of processed foods, e.g. mono- and diglycerides and phospholipids such as lecithin, occurring naturally in many foods. Such improved textures are then stabilized by using stabilizers such as modified starches, pectins, and polysaccharide gums.

Antioxidants, such as BHA and BHT, are used to protect high-fat foods from oxidative rancidity. Ascorbic acid and its isomer erythorbic acid, and their salts, are also used as antioxidants in aqueous systems, e.g., to prevent darkening of fruit juices during processing, and to aid in retention of colors in processed meats.

Flour improvers are used during bread making to improve the elasticity of the dough, increase the volume of the loaf, improve the stability of the crumb, and slow the rate of redistribution of water in the bread during staling. Regulations in the developed countries allow the use only of ascorbic acid, which maintains a reducing environment during dough development in the Chorleywood bread process. Flour improvers may also bleach and mature the flour. Benzoyl peroxide is used as a bleaching agent in the flour. Materials used for bleaching and increasing chlorine gas are chlorine dioxide, nitrosylchloride, and nitrogen di- and tetraoxides. Other oxidizing agents used to improve dough quality are potassium bromate, potassium iodate, calcium iodate, and calcium peroxide (2).

Humectants are moisture-retaining agents used in foods to control viscosity, texture, bulking, moisture, and softness. They also help free-flowing of salts and other powders. They function by readily absorbing excess moisture and by coating particles to impart a degree of water repellency. Calcium silicate absorbs and remains free-flowing even after absorbing liquids in amounts two and half times its weight. Some anticaking agents can absorb oils and nonpolar organic liquids in addition to water. Calcium silicate is used to prevent caking in baking powders, salts, and other foods.

Several compounds are used as processing aids, e.g., organic acids such as citrate, tartarate, and malate to enhance food acidity, and the salts of these acids to buffer the acidity in foods. Many polysaccharide additives are used as thickening agents to alter or control the physical and textural properties of foods during heating, cooling, and storage.

Polyphosphates may be used in the processing of milk to prevent its gelation in the can, and in meat products to stabilize the water content and prevent water loss, thus leading to more succulent products.

In addition to yeast, other leavening agents may be used to produce light, fluffy baked products. In the presence of yeast, ammonium salts are added to dough to provide a ready source of nitrogen for their growth. Phosphate salts such as sodium and calcium phosphate are added to control pH. Chemical leavening agents such as baking powders help to generate carbon dioxide for leavening purposes, thus making the bakery products light and fluffy in texture.

In addition to the foregoing compounds, a number of other food additives are used in foods for different functions. Clarifying agents, such as bentonite and gelatin, and synthetic resins, such as polyamides and polyvinylpyrrolidone, are used to eliminate haziness, sediments, and oxidative deterioration products in fruit juices, beers, and wines. Enzymes may also be added to bring about desirable changes—e.g., rennin to produce milk curd and cheese, papain to tenderize meat, and pectinase to clarify beverages. Aluminium sulfate and calcium sulfate are used as firming agents to make the fruit and vegetable tissue crisp in the processed products. Liquid nitrogen and dichlorofluoromethane are used to chill foods; solvents such as ethanol, propylene glycol, and glycerine are used to dissolve suspended flavors, colors, and other ingredients. Insert gases are added to packets of instant foods to prevent oxidative deterioration.

The law does not really differentiate between "foods" and "food additives." Meat and potatoes, for example, may be considered as "additives" instead of "food" when served as stew, and more appropriately as GRAS substances. Preservatives such as sodium and calcium propionate are produced naturally in Swiss cheese. Citrate, a widely used food additive, is a natural constituent of citrus fruits. On the other hand, many so-called "natural" foods contain toxic substances, e.g., carcinogenic safrole present in sassafras roots, and acids used to flavor beverages. In 1960, the FDA banned use of safrole as a flavoring agent in root beer. Oxalates found in spinach and rhubard, goiter-inducing substances found in some vegetables, solanine (alkaloid) found in potatoes, a natural carcinogen, patulin, found in flour and orange juice, thiourea and related chemicals found in cabbage and turips, and tannin in tea and wine are all toxic substances in one way or another.

The alarm about additives may have directed people from some more serious concerns about food. Clydesdale and Francis (1) quote E.T. Larkin, who published an interesting article in an FDA consumer magazine (1983) regarding the safety of commonly used herbal teas. Larkin (9) pointed out that while many herbs such as peppermint, rose hip, orange, and others produce useful, delicious teas, as alternatives to traditional drinks containing caffeine—coffee and common tea (*Camellia sinensis*), it cannot be concluded that all herbal teas are safe, nor that it is safe to consume large amounts of any herbal tea over extended periods. Larkin pointed out the following cautions in weighing safety of this practice:

1. Some herbs contain the wrong kind of magic, and nature's most potent poisons are found among the herbs.
2. Enough is not known about the herbal teas to conclude that they are safe.
3. Doctoring oneself with herbs can be very dangerous.
4. Moderation in all things is advisable.
5. Not all persons are equal—genetic variation produces different reactions in different people.
6. Remember the cautionary proverb among the people gathering wild mushrooms: "There are old mushroom hunters, and there are bold mushroom hunters, but there are no old, bold mushroom hunters."

Thus, if one gathers one's own herbs to brew a cup of tea, one should be absolutely 100 percent certain that the herb picked is the one that was sought. Larkin (9) has listed herbs from some 28 plant sources that are not safe to be used in foods, beverages, or drugs.

The Delaney clause was added to the Pure Food and Drug Act as a result of an amendment offered by Congressman Delancy in 1958, which established a food additive regulation prohibiting the addition of any cancer-producing substance to human food. This admirable proposal, however, does not specify the amounts required for a substance to produce cancer. Many substances when added to the body in large enough quantities may cause cancer; e.g., one barbecued steak contains the same amount of benzopyrene (a potent carcinogen) as 600 cigarettes. Yet steak is generally not regarded as causing stomach cancer.

A. Testing for Regulated Food Additives

A substance proposed to be used as food additive must undergo strict testing designed to establish the safety of the intended use. A petition that is presented to the FDA should have the following information:

1. The identity of the additive, its chemical composition, how it is manufactured, specifications necessary to assure its reproducibleness, and any other means necessary to establish the composition of the additives.
2. Information on the intended use of the additive, including copies of the proposed labels.
3. Data establishing that the additive will accomplish the intended effect in the food and that the level sought for approval is not higher than that reasonably necessary to accomplish the intended effect.
4. An analytical method capable of measuring the amount of the additive present at the tolerance levels.

5. Data establishing that the intended use of the additive is safe. This requires experimental evidence, derived ordinarily from feeding studies using the proposed additive at various levels in the diets of two or more appropriate species of animals.

B. Safety of Food Additives and GRAS Substances

It is not possible to guarantee absolute safety of any product, as is the case in any area of life. Premarketing clearance requirements under the Food Additives Amendement to the Pure Food and Drug Act assure that the risk of the occurrence of unanticipated adverse effects is at an acceptably small level at least for food additives. Such assurances are possibly not available in the case of those GRAS substances that were exempted from the need for laboratory testing by the definition of the law. Eventually the FDA has reviewed the safety of each item on the GRAS list, and the evaluation has been recently completed.

It is reasonable that premarketing clearances for any substance should be established based on the scientific knowledge available at the time of establishment. Because the scientific knowledge is dynamic and expanding, the earlier decisions must be periodically reviewed to assure that the assessment of the safety of the substances added to foods is up to date.

A contract has been made with the Federation of American Societies of Experimental Biology to review the GRAS substances, by choosing a group of qualified scientists and designating the Select Comittee on GRAS substances (SCOGS). These scientists independently evaluated the GRAS compounds and published a series of reports known as SCOGS reports. Each GRAS compound reviewed was assigned into one of the five categories based on the conclusions reached about that compound as follows (1):

1. Category 1
   Conclusion: There is no evidence in the available information on [name of substance(s)] that demonstrates or suggests reasonable grounds to suspect a hazard to the public when it is (they are) used at levels that are now current or that might reasonably be expected in the future.
   Action Taken—Continue in GRAS status with no limitations other than good manufacturing practice.

2. Category 2
   Conclusion: There is no evidence in the available information on [name of substance(s)] that demonstrates or suggests reasonable grounds to suspect a hazard to the public when it is (they are) used at levels that are now current and in the manner now practiced. However, it is not possible to determine, without additional data, whether a significant increase in consumption would constitute a dietary hazard.
   Action Taken—Continue in GRAS status with limitations on amounts that can be added to food.

3. Category 3
   Conclusion: While no evidence in the available information on [name of substance(s)] that demonstrates a hazard to the public when it is (they are) used at levels that are now in current and in the manner now practiced is available, uncertainties exist requiring that additional studies should be conducted.
   Action Taken—Issue an interim food additive regulation requiring commitment within (specified number) days that necessary testing will be undertaken. GRAS status continues while tests are being completed and evaluated.

4. Category 4
   Conclusion: The evidence on [substance(s)] is insufficient to determine that the adverse effects reported are not deleterious to the public health when it is (they are) used at levels that are now current and in the manner now practiced.

Action Taken—Establish safer usage conditions as a food additive or remove ingredient(s) from food. Interested parties may subsequently submit a petition establishing conditions of safe use.

5.   Category 5
Conclusion: In view of the deficiency of relevant biological (and/or other) studies, the Select Committee has insufficient data upon which to base an evaluation of [substance(s)] when it is (they are) used as a food ingredient.
Action Taken—Insufficient data upon which to base on evaluation.

As a result of this evaluation of GRAS substances, 297 compounds were assigned to category 1, 69 to category 2, 21 to category 3, 5 to category 4, and 30 to category 5.

Most additives have been tested for their safety far more often than most naturally or traditionally processed foodstuffs, and it is possible that dozens of familiar foods would be banned if all foods were tested as much as additives are, and if Delaney Clause Standards dealing with possible carcinogenic effects of additives were applied to them. According to Clydesdale and Francis (1), per capita consumption of additives in the USA is only about 139 pounds per year compared to about 0.75 tons of food consumed. Thus, the threat posed by the use of the additive by itself may be relatively minor.

Boffey (10) quoted John Higinson, the founding director of the World Health's Organization International Agency for Research on Cancer, as stating that most cancers are caused by the environmental factors. However, "environment" does not simply mean "industrial pollution," but also lifestyle factors such as smoking, alcohol, exposure to the sun, and diet. Boffey (10) also discussed a study reported in June 1981 issue of the *Journal of the National Cancer Institute*. This study was conducted by two renowned British epidemiologists, Sir Richard Doll and Richard Peto of Oxford, who ranked the relative importance of the major factors as follows:

Factor	Percent of causes
Tobacco	25–40%
Diet (except food additives)	10–17%
Infection	1–10%
Sexual factors	1–13%
Occupation	2–8%
Alcohol	2–4%
Geography (sun, etc.)	2–4%
Environmental pollution	2–4%
Medicine (x-rays etc)	0–1%
Food additives	−5 (may prevent) 2%
Industrial products	1–2%

The above list indicates that a single number cannot be assigned to any cause, and it provides a rough measure of the relative contribution of each factor. It is interesting to note that food additives have been listed as preventive in some cases, which is consistent with the observation that two antioxidants, butylated hydroxytoluene (BHT) and butylated hydroxyanisole (BHA), prevented stomach cancer in mice. It has been suggested that addition of these compounds to breakfast cereals coincided with the decline in stomach cancer in the United States. Use of other antioxidants such as ascorbic acid and selenium has also shown beneficial effects.

Although such additives in foods are known to be safe at the levels normally used, their excessive use may lead to serious health problems. Solholz and Smith (11) quoted Durk Pearson and Sandy Shaw, as having stated in their book, *Life Extension*: *A Practical Scientific Approach*, that consumption of a mixture of water, vitamins, amino acids, prescription drugs (L-dopa) and other chemicals such as BHA retards aging and wards off illnesses from insomnia to cancer. Such recommendations, however, are potentially dangerous and their benefits remain unproven.

A committee on Diet, Nutrition and Cancer (1982) of the National Academy of Sciences, Nutritional Research Council, concluded that cancers of most major sites are influenced by dietary patterns, although data were not sufficient to quantitate the contribution of diet to the overall risk or to determine the percent reduction in risk that might be achieved by dietary modification. Some general recommendations made about diet and cancer are available (see Chapter 25).

There are many naturally occurring carcinogens in foods that are a normal part of our diet. According to Ames (12), plants in nature synthesize toxic substances in large quantities, apparently as a defense mechanism against bacteria, fungi, insects, and predators. The identification and chemical characterization of a range of these compounds have been completed during the past 100 years, and a large number of these natural toxicants have been shown to be carcinogenic. The scientific evidence available thus supports a recommendation for a wide variety of food with a somewhat decreased intake of calories as the safest diet. In this way, one can minimize the intake of any single carcinogen; humans do seem to have a natural resistance to small amounts of carcinogens that may be consumed inadvertently.

C. Amounts of Food Additives Consumed

The per capita consumption of food additives in the United States has been estimated to be about 140 pounds per year; the most widely used food additives are sweeteners, such as cane or beet sugar, corn sweeteners, glucose, fructose, and syrups, amounting to about 115 pounds per year (about 82%). The second most widely used food additive is common salt, about 15 pounds being consumed each year (about 1.7%), which may be decreasing due to current concerns about hypertension. Thus, barring sweeteners and salt, about 10 pounds of all other food additives are consumed by an individual in the United States per year. Of about 33 different additives used, 18 are used either as leavening agents or to adjust the food acidity. Of the 18 food additives, those used most often include yeast, sodium bicarbonate, citrate, black pepper, and mustard. The added vitamins and minerals are also included in the total. All these account to about 9 pounds and the remaining one pound is spread over the some 1800 other food additives used in different foods, i.e., about 0.5 mg per additive per year.

Mathews and Stewart (13) have described the reports prepared by committees of the National Academy of Sciences, giving the details of amounts and levels of specific food additives used in particular food products.

There is a basic dichotomy in the Food, Drug and Cosmetic Act in its treatment of imitation (synthetic) foods versus "natural" ones. This statutory provision has accorded favored treatment to "natural" foods and food ingredients. Despite these extremes, such a policy must still permit the manufacture and supply of food in an industrialized economy, often requiring a definition of natural as remarkable for its ingenuity as for its comprehensiveness. According to Section 402 of the U.S. law, a food shall be deemed to be adulterated, if it bears or contains any poisonous or deleterious substance that may render it injurious to health; but in case the substance is not an added substance (i.e., a "natural" one), such food shall not be considered adulterated under this clause, if the quantity of such substance in the food does not ordinarily render it injurious to health. An "added poisonous or deleterious substance," however, renders the food adulterated unless the additive is used within the other provisions of the Act, such as the Pesticide, the Food Additive, and the Color Additive Amendments. The regulations issued under these amendments extend, but do not clarify, the distinction between "added" and "not added" or between "natural" and "synthetic," e.g., the listing of synthetic and natural flavorings in CFR 121.1163 and 121.1164, where purification by distillation results in a "natural" product, whereas crystallization generally produces a "synthetic" one. The reason for this is that a higher degree of confidence is expressed in the safety of "natural" foods and ingredients than in wholly synthetic ones.

The toxicological approach of investigation of safety of compounds by animal feeding studies is an extremely useful tool and provides valuable insights into the degree and nature of hazards associated with food additives. But these methods also have their own strengths and limitations of both testing and experience.

Clydesdale and Francis (1) evaluated each food item in a reasonably attractive and elaborate dinner menu, not as treated under the law as natural food, but as it would be treated if manufactured from added ingredients. Among the toxic substances naturally present in certain foods are certain cholinesterase inhibitors of unknown structure that interfere with the transmission of nerve impulses (many potent pesticides are based on such activity). The cholinesterase inhibitors are present in measurable quantity in radishes, carrots, celery, and potatoes. In potatoes, the alkaloid solanine is often present with less than a tenfold safety factor between the normal level and levels causing human poisoning.

A number of foods contain glycosides that break down during cooking or digestion to yield hydrogen cyanide, e.g., almonds and lima beans. Lima beans, high in HCN, have been the cause of several serious poisoning outbreaks. Similarly, oxalates and oxalic acid occur in several foods such as spinach, cashews, almonds, cocoa, and tea.

Stimulents occur in a wide variety of foods. Nutmeg, for example, contains myristicin, and tea, coffee, cola, and cocoa contain caffeine. Tea also contains theophylline and cocoa, theobromine. Myristicin has been abused for its hallucinogenic property: nutmeg also contains small quantities of safrole, a carcinogenic compound. If nutmeg is used on spinach, coupled with consumption of untolerable limits of alcohol, it may lead to well-known hazards. High intakes of menthol have caused cardiac arrhythmia, and the glycerine in Cointreau is toxic at only small multiples of its normal use.

Goitrogenic substances promote goiter and are present in many common foods. The white turnip, for example, contains 1-5-vinyl-2-thiooxazolidone, and cauliflower contains a thiocyanate. However, it would take about 22 pounds per day of cauliflower to cause thyroid enlargement. Other foods such as peach, pear, strawberry, Brussels sprouts, spinach, and carrots have been demonstrated to produce goitrogenic activity in humans.

Pressor amines, serotonin and tyramine, raise the blood pressure and pose a danger to susceptible individuals, especially to those who are taking drugs like the tranquilizer Parnate.

Egg yolk has been reported to be carcinogenic in the diet of mice. The nitrates and nitrites present in foods are capable of causing methemoglobinemia in humans, and are transformed in the stomach to nitrosamines, which are potent carcinogens (also found in smoked meat products). Cured ham and bacon and certain vegetables such as spinach, especially when fertilized, contain substantial amounts of nitrites. Also, smoked foods almost invariably contain small amounts of polynuclear aromatic hydrocarbons; their role as dietary carcinogens in man has been confirmed by epidemiological surveys conducted in northern European countries where significant quantities of smoked foods are consumed, with unusually high prevalence of stomach cancers. Rolls present the ricket-promoting factor in yeast and the hazards of amino acid imbalance.

Food safety being a serious matter, all sources of relevant information should be used, which is also the basic concept of GRAS, where experience based on common use in food and scientific procedures are both used. Combined, these are still insufficient, and determination of food safety should always be open to new evidence. The crucial animal testing may also be irrelevant to human safety and human experience, with all its directness, still remains an enigma. The utility of both must be improved, which may be achieved partly by using animal species (in tests) that have shown to be suitable metabolic models for man. More detailed national dietary studies coupled with better reporting and analysis of individual health are needed, and use of mass human experience, not mass human experiments. Prior to the broad intentional use of a material in human food, information is necessary from animal and human studies to allow expert judgment to conclude with confidence that use of the material will not significantly increase the overall risk. It should be recognized that experience is the final determinant, no matter how encouraging the results from animal experiments are (1).

IV. NUTRIFICATION AND FORTIFICATION

Foods can be enriched through nutrification and fortification. Nutrients added in the form of vitamins, minerals, and other compounds such as essential amino acids and fatty acids can restore the values lost during processing and storage. Nutrification can also ensure higher nutritional value than what nature may have provided originally. When wheat is milled to produce white flour, the process often removes the brown-colored portion of the grain, rich in vitamins and minerals. Thus, to restore the nutritive value of the flour, thiamin, niacin, iron, and calcium are added to the flour. Similarly, vitamin C is added to canned citrus fruits to make up for the loss of the vitamin during processing.

The manufactured foods used as substitutes for natural ones often require addition of some nutrients to ensure that their nutritional value is at least equal to that of the natural product. Margarine, for example, is used as substitute for butter for economic reasons. Vitamins A and D thus need to be added to margarine to raise its nutritional value equal to that of the butter.

Certain foods may even be fortified by adding specific nutrients in excess of what nature provides. Milk, for instance, is a nutritious food, but is low in vitamin D content. The incidence of rickets in some countries has been eradicated by supplying milk fortified with vitamin D to the children. Other foods such as breakfast cereals, baby foods, and fruit juices can be fortified with vitamins and other essential nutrients to improve the nutritional value of the diet.

Some plant proteins are deficient in essential amino acids, e.g., most pulses are deficient in methionine and tryptophan and cereals are often deficient in lysine. Similarly, fatty foods may be fortified with an essential fatty acid, linoleic acid.

Iodine deficiency causes widespread endemic goiter, especially where seafoods are not available. Iodine in the form of potassium iodide (KI) is added to common salt (iodized salt) in controlled amounts to prevent goiter. Fluoride also may be added to drinking water to supply the mineral fluorine, required for normal tooth development in children

REFERENCES

1. Clydesdale, F.M., and F.J. Francis, *Food, Nutrition and Health*, AVI Publishing Co. Westport, Conn., 1985, p. 208.
2. Manay, N.S., and M. Shadaksharaswamy, *Foods: Facts and Principles*, Wiley Eastern Ltd, New Delhi, 1987, p. 451.
3. Southgate, D.A.T., and I. Johnson, Food Processing, *Human Nutrition and Dietetics*, 9th ed. (J.S. Garrow and W.P.T. James, eds.), Churchill Livingston, London, 1993, p. 335.
4. MAFF, Survey of color usage in food, Report of Steering Group on Food Surveillance, Ministry of Agriculture, Fisheries and Food, HMSO, London, 1987.
5. MAFF, Food Additives and Contaminants Committee review of the flavourings in food, Ministry of Agriculture, Fisheries and Food, HMSO, London, 1976.

6. Desai, B.B., and D.K. Salunkhe, Sugar Crops, *Foods of Plant Origin: Production, Technology and Human Nutrition* (D.K. Salunkhe and S.S. Deshpande, eds.), Van Nostrand Reinhold, New York, 413–489, 1991, p. 413.

7. Salunkhe, D.K., and B.B. Desai, *Postharvest Biotechnology of Sugar Crops*, CRC Press, Boca Raton, FL, 1988.

8. MAFF, Review of Food Advisory Committee on Use of Sweeteners in Foods, Ministry of Agriculture, Fisheries, and Food, HMSO, London, 1982.

9. Larkin, E.T., Herbs are often more toxic than magical, *FDA Consumer*, October, 5–10, 1983.

10. Boffey, P.M., Cancer experts lean toward steady vigilance but less alarm on environment, *The New York Times*, March 2, C-1-C-2, 1982.

11. Solholz, E., and J. Smith, How to live forever, *Newsweek*, March 26, 1984, p. 81.

12. Ames, B.N., Dietary carcinogens, *Science, 221*: 1256–1262 (1983).

13. Mathews, R.A., and M.R. Stewart, Report summarizes data from food additive surveys, *Food Technol. 38*: 3–58 (1984).

15

Food Labeling and Quality Assurance

I. INTRODUCTION

The human tendency to make a "fast buck" by trick or fraud has existed throughout the history of mankind. The need was therefore felt for consumer protection by safe-guarding the purchaser of foodstuffs from frauds due to the adulteration of food. Short weights of foods sold and addition of water to milk have been ancient practices of cheating the consumer, despite the existence of laws to prevent them. Old laws also existed in almost every country against the adulteration of costly spices such as pepper, which were mixed with local seeds, leaves, flour, or even sand, and against the sale of unsound meat and other foods.

During the Industrial Revolution (1750–1850), factory workers had to depend for their food on food manufacturers, some of whom practiced fraud and adulterated foods with chemicals that may have been poisonous. Toxicology and analytical methods to detect adulterants in foods were yet to be developed. In Britain, Dr. Wakeley, the owner and first editor of the *Lancet*, published in 1851 the names of about 3000 tradesmen who were found to practice food adulteration. *Lancet* had moral support from the public and the medical profession, and its efforts led to the passage by parliament of the "1860 Adulteration of Food and Drink Act", and when this proved ineffective, of the "1875 Sale of Food and Drugs Act", which eventually formed the basis for modern laws. Food science started developing rapidly since 1875 and newer knowledge of food chemistry and analysis enabled local governments to enforce food laws more effectively by appointing public analysts. Similar food laws were passed in other countries to check the fraudulent practices of food adulteration.

By the year 1900, food pathology was developed to identify most of the microorganisms involved in food poisoning, the cause of their spread, and the nature of diseases produced. Food hygiene became a branch of science, making it possible to control the spread of food poisoning by inspection of slaughterhouses, food warehouses, retail shops, and restaurant kitchens. Despite the understanding of the principles of control, their applications showed many lapses. New processes and methods of animal husbandry were responsible for giving rise to other food poisoning organisms (1). Pathogenic organisms posed the greatest danger to the health of people from foods, against which the consumer needed legal protection. The 20th century experienced new chemical hazards from foods, a large number of chemicals being used during the production, processing, and storage of foodstuffs, e.g. weedicides, pesticides, and antibiotics used in animal feeds to control disease and improve growth, some of which were carried into the foods. Several pesticides are used to control food losses during storage, transport, and distribution, due to senescence, ripening, or sprouting. The use of these highly active "agrochemicals" is closely controlled to regulate the levels of their residues in foods, in the form of prescription of intervals between the application of pesticides to crops and their entry into food distribution. Several countries today have effective surveillance program to sample market and imported foods for residue analysis. "Market basket" studies are undertaken in the United Kingdom and other countries to collect a typical day's samples of food intake for residue analysis (2).

At present, foods are supplied to the retailer and thence to the purchaser mostly in prepacked form, and the consumer must rely on the label for information on what the package provides. This information, therefore, must be accurate and not misleading, especially when the package contains a food prepared from several ingredients or consists of a whole meal. The choice of food by the consumer is influenced by many factors, including the advertising. Food legislation is thus primarily concerned with protecting the consumer by strictly regulating both food labeling and advertising (3).

Food legislation has grown with time to control the modern counterparts of the ancient fraudulent practices of tradesmen and food manufacturers. Most food manufactures and retailers are greatly concerned with the quality of their products, especially about the disclosure of an unsatisfactory or unsafe product in a competitive market, which may have disastrous effects on sales, not only of the product in question but subsequent other products from the same manufacturer. Modern legislation has arisen from a continuing dialogue between trade associations, consumer bodies, and enforcement authorities. The harmony in these dialogues leads to a common interest in making the food product safe and of high quality for all. The control of food quality is highly developed in the Western countries such as the United States of America, the United Kingdom, Germany, and others. The formation of the Economic Community in Europe has greatly influenced food legislation.

II. NUTRITIONAL LABELING FOR NUTRIENTS

The provision of accurate and informative labels on food containers is an essential part of consumer protection, especially when a food package contains many ingredients. According to Southgate (3), in the United Kingdom, most foods must have a list of all the ingredients on the label, in the decreasing order of their relative amounts. This requirement in some foods is waived, provided there are precise compositional food standards. Water, the common ingredient of most foods, is often not listed. Additives, being minor in amounts, usually appear toward the end of the list under their approved names or E numbers.

The law also requires that food labels should indicate an acceptable storage period, either in the shop as a "sell by" designation, or before consumption—a "best before" statement, usually including the appropriate conditions for storage.

In many countries, the claims on foods, especially the nutritional ones, are restricted. This protects the consumer from possible misleading claims regarding the benefits from the consumption of food. Such claims often escape prosecution under the law, unless a major food producer is involved. A misleading claim must be first brought to the attention of food authorities. Very often the time taken to make a legal case against the manufacturer is so long that it enables the manufacturer to withdraw the offending food.

In the United States of America, nutritional labeling was introduced during the period 1973–1975, and was intended to provide compositional information that would enable the consumer to judge the nutritional value of the food product. Thus, the consumer would be able to choose a dietary mixture to meet his or her nutrient requirements. The nutritional labeling was optional for many foods, unless a nutritional claim was made regarding the food product.

The legal regulations effectively prescribed the format for labeling and mode of its expression. The values of proximate components, energy (kcal), protein, fat, and carbohydrates were to be expressed in grams, and vitamins and minerals such as calcium as percentages of the RDAs (recommended daily allowances). The values chosen for these recommendations were the highest amounts required by an adult in the RADs prescribed by the National Research Council. The values were to be expressed per unit serving, to be given on the label.

The growth of knowledge about the possible relationship between the diet, nutrition, and the incidence of chronic diseases (see Part IV, Chapters 24 to 35) introduced a new dimension into nutritional labeling, enabling the consumer to choose foods to minimize the risks of diet-related chronic diseases. Nutritional labeling in the developed countries such as the United States thus has become a part of the public health strategy, in which the target is to reduce the long-term incidence of chronic diseases such as cancers and coronary heart disease, rather than just preventing bacterial food poisoning or long-term effects of food contaminants.

In the United States, the FDA is responsible for most food labeling, except for meat and poultry products, which are regulated by the USDA, and alcoholic beverages, which are controlled by the Bureau of Alcohol, Tobacco and Firearms. The Federal Trade Commission (FTC) regulates the advertising of food products and has authority to take action against unsubstantiated claims.

Food packaged and sold in U.S. supermarkets are often labeled with the product name, the name and address of the manufacturer, the amount of product in the package, and the ingredients, listed in descending order of their weight. Except for fresh fruits, vegetables, and meats, almost all other food products are labeled.

Foods such as catsup, ice cream, mustard, and mayonnaise are categorized as foods with a "standard of identity." These products must follow a certain recipe on file with the FDA, hence the manufacturer does not have to list ingredients, unless optional ingredients are included, such as extra spices or flavors. However, many manufacturers currently list the ingredients on labels of these foods, even though it is not required by law. This trend is caused by consumer demand. New labeling laws to be enacted are likely to eliminate this labeling exception.

Today, over 60 grams of foods under U.S. FDA control carry a nutrition label, of which about one-half are voluntary. Many foods, however, give no nutrient information, aside from their contents. A new law passed in 1990 requires most U.S. foods to be labeled.

The "nutrition label" lists the serving size of the product, servings per package, and kcalorie, protein, carbohydrate, fat and sodium amounts per serving. If the product contains more than 2% of the U.S. RDA for certain vitamins and minerals, these percentages must be listed. These nutrients include protein, vitamin A, vitamin C, thiamin, riboflavin, niacin, calcium, and iron. Additional information may be given on dietary fiber, the amount of sugars, and cholesterol.

Under the current law, manufacturers determine their own serving sizes, which may vary from one product to another. Thus, a product may be lower in kcalories than another similar one because the manufacturer simply listed a small serving size.

Proposed FDA labeling regulations are expected to bring changes: the new nutrition labels will, in general, have more information for the consumer, with a mandatory listing of saturated fat content, cholesterol content, total dietary fiber content, and total kcalories from fat in the food product.

The U.S. RDA will also be updated to more closely conform to the current RDA, with a name change to Reference Daily Intakes (RDIs). Serving sizes are expected to follow more uniform patterns. Daily Reference Values (DRVs) will also be set by the FDA for certain parts of the diet, not covered by the 1989 RDA, e.g., carbohydrate, fat, and dietary fiber. The DRVs will help the consumer to further evaluate food choices by comparing the food values of these substances to desirable (or maximum) nutrient intakes.

Some pitfalls accompany nutrition label reading. The meanings of certain healthy sounding terms are not always apparent, e.g. "no cholesterol," "low fat," "organic," and "sugar-free." It is difficult to know how trustworthy these claims are. Although technically true, many such claims may be irrelevant; others are misleading or paint only part of the picture.

The extent to which a food manufacturer can make health claims on a food product label has been debated. It is permissible to state that a food contains certain amounts of nutrients and a nutrition label can back up such a claim. The debate concerns whether a manufacturer can state that these nutrients will provide specific health benefits, e.g., dietary fiber in food helps to prevent certain types of cancer. Since the 1980s, the Kellogg Company has marketed its high fiber cereals as a possible preventive measure against certain forms of cancer. Many nutritionists think such claims lack scientific merit. Labeling regulations that are currently under development are expected to set standards for some more common claims such as "light" or "lite," "no cholesterol," and "high fiber." Currently, the FDA proposes to limit the use of health claims to six areas in which there is general scientific agreement of a relationship between a nutrient and a chronic disease, viz., fiber and cancer, fiber and heart disease, fat and cancer, fat and heart disease, sodium and hypertension, and calcium and osteoporosis.

Some groups oppose the use of any health messages on food labels, because these promote the "good food"/"bad food" comparison, ignoring the emphasis on total diet. It is important to focus one's total meal plan and nutrient intake because nutrients work together to maintain health, e.g. protein metabolism uses pyridoxine, iron metabolism uses ascorbic acid, and folate metabolism uses cobalamin (B_{12}). Again, health claims for specific foods or food supplements often ignore the significance of the entire diet. They may even turn out to be irresponsible because they do not warn of the dangers of excess intakes of the specific foods or supplements.

In the United Kingdom also, nutritional labeling was considered an essential part of implementation of nutritional guidelines to the people, such as those proposed in the NACNE discussion document (4). The report on health and social subjects, in regard to diet and cardiovascular disease (5), formally recommended the introduction of fat labeling of foods, to enable the consumer to reduce fat inake and select the degree of unsaturation of fats eaten to prevent cardiovascular disease. The government has accepted the recommendations and discussions have followed involving the food industry to examine how best the recommendations can be implemented. The MAFF, the department responsible for food labeling, has also produced guidelines for nutritional labeling. According to Southgate (3), currently the guidelines are voluntary and prescribe the format and mode of expression. The values of the nutrients must be expressed per 100 g of food and per portion if the package contains less than 100 g. Three levels of information are shown on the label; the first gives energy, protein, fat, and carbohydrate; the second includes dietary fiber and sodium; and the third lists sugar, vitamins, and minerals (only when the amounts present are greater than one-sixth of the recommended dietary intake (as is the position under current legislation regarding nutritional claims). The Food Advisory Committee (FAC) has currently proposed that nutritional labeling would become obligatory when a nutritional claim on a food product is made. The regulations also include obligatory fat labeling, giving the lists of percentages of saturated fatty acids as well as a more detailed breakdown of the fat used in the food.

The European Community Scientific Committee is also simultaneously developing the proposals for nutritional labeling, which are currently voluntary as long as specific nutritional claims have not been made. These proposals include labeling for the contents of energy, protein, fat, carbohydrates, total sugars, sodium, and dietary fiber in the minimum statement, with no breakdown of fat.

Pilot studies conducted on nutritional labeling in the United Kingdom have indicated that consumers find nutritional labeling difficult to use in the way its advocates desire to. Southgate (3) suggested that a more effective, parallel-running scheme on nutritional education of the general public is essential. Some food retailers have also supplemented the nutritional labeling with booklets containing more detailed information on nutrition to enable the consumer to choose an appropriate diet.

Nutritional labeling in the United States became effective on July 1, 1975; it required that the following specific information should be provided on the label (6):

1. The serving size and the number of servings per container
2. The calorie content to the nearest 10 calories per serving
3. The protein content to the nearest gram per serving, and also as a percentage of the RDA
4. The carbohydrate content to the nearest gram per serving
5. The fat content to the nearest gram per serving

The serving size is determined by aggreement between the manufacturer and the FDA authorities. The evaluation of the protein content posed a problem, in view of the difficulties in describing protein quality, the final compromise being an allowance of 45 grams (RDA) if its protein effeciency ratio (PER) is equal to or greater than that of casein, a high-quality milk protein. If the protein quality of the food is lower than that of the casein, the RDA of protein should be increased to 65 grams, and if PER of the protein is 20% or less of the PER of casein, no label declaration could be made. The PER is the simplest but not necessarily the best method of establishing protein quality. The overall solution to the problem of labeling of protein as a percentage of the RDA is a compromise of many complex considerations, and is probably one of the best available (6).

The type of fat and its quality have importance in relation to their effects on diseases of the circulatory system. Nutritional claims for fat must include the amounts of saturated and unsaturated fatty acids in grams per serving, and these two statements cannot be used if the food contains less than 10% fat or 2 grams per serving. If either fatty acids or cholesterol, or both are listed, the label must have the following disclaimer, viz., "Information on fat (and/or cholesterol, where appropriate) is provided for individuals who, on the advice of a physician, are modifying their total dietary intake of fat (and/or cholesterol, where appropriate)."

Although the listing of fat, protein, and carbohydrate in terms of grams per serving is easy to understand, the expression of the vitamin and mineral content on the label was difficult. After examining several methods, finally the U.S. RDA units proposed by the National Academy of Sciences—National Research Council (NAS-NRC), determined first in 1941 and revised eight times thereafter, were used. The U.S. RDA values of nutrients as revised in 1980 are shown in Table 1. These values represent the best nutritional information available on the daily intake of vitamins and minerals needed to maintain good health. The older Minimum Daily Requirements (MDR) units based on the minimum intake necessary to prevent deficiency diseases have been replaced by the NAS RDA units. Because individuals vary in their need for each nutrient, the NAS RDA requirement was set at two standard deviations above the average requirement, so as to include 97.5% of the population. The new U.S. RDAs (NAS/NRC) are given for a number of categories of people, based on age, sex, lactation, and pregnancy, and involve too many details to be declared on the label. Consequently the U.S. RDAs represent a selection, usually the highest of the NAS/NRC RDAs (Table 1). The estimated safe and adequate intake for some other nutrients has been established (Table 2). These estimates are based on a smaller database than the NAS/NRC values. Though the choice of US RDA for label declaration is sound and scientific, the consumer cannot easily determine the actual content of vitamins and minerals from the label. It is comparatively easy to calculate this information from the RDA values given in Table 1.

The FDA regulations require that the content of seven vitamins and minerals should be stated on the label—vitamin A, vitamin C, thiamin, riboflavin, and niacin, and the minerals iron and calcium. Nine other nutrients may be declared by the manufacturer, but this is not obligatory; these are vitamin D, vitamin E, folacin, vitamin B_6, vitamin B_{12} zinc, magnesium, phosphorus, and iodine. All the nutrients should be stated as percentage of the U.S. RDA contained in one serving. No other vitamin or mineral can be claimed on the label. The scientific community

Table 1 The U.S. RDA Values for Human Nutrition

Nutrient	Units
Vitamin A	100 µg RE[a]
Ascorbic acid	60 mg
Thiamin (B$_1$)	1.5 mg
Riboflavin (B$_2$)	1.7 mg
Niacin (B$_3$)	19 mg
Calcium	1.2 g
Iron	18 mg
Cholecalciferol (vitamin D)	10 µg
Tocopherol (vitamin E)	10 mg TE[b]
Pyridoxine (B$_6$)	2.2 mg
Folacin (folic acid)	0.4 mg
Cobalamin (B$_{12}$)	3 µg
Phosphorus	1.2 g
Iodine	150 µg
Magnesium	300 mg
Zinc	15 mg

[a]RE = Retinol equivalents.
[b]Tocopherol equivalents.
Source: Ref. 6.

Table 2 Estimated Safe and Adequate Daily Dietary Intakes for Adults of Additional Selected Vitamins and Minerals

Nutrient	Units
Vitamin A	70–140 µg
Biotin	100–200 µg
Pantothenic acid	4–7 mg
Copper	2–3 mg
Manganese	2.5–5.0 mg
Fluoride	1.5–4.0 mg
Chromium	50–200 µg
Selenium	50–200 µg
Molybdenum	15–500 µg
Sodium	1.1–3.3 g
Potassium	1.9–5.6 g
Chloride	1.7–5.1 g

Source: Ref. 6.

believes that other than the above 16, 17 more nutrients are necessary for humans. The sodium content in milligrams per serving must also be stated on the label.

III. DIETARY SUPPLEMENTS AND DRUGS

The original labeling laws regarding the classification of food products are very specific. Thus, foods with added nutrients, representing up to 50% of the US RDA are considered ordinary foods, whereas products with added nutrients that represent between 50% and 150% of the RDA are classified as "dietary supplements" and are so labeled. The regulations governing the sales of drugs and medicines are more stringent than those for food and it is not likely that the food manufacturers would choose to label their foods as drugs. However, several of the breakfast cereals contain 100% of the RDA of a number of nutrients and are labeled as "dietary supplements." The drug ruling makes an exception: if the nutrient occurs naturally in the food at levels above 150% of the RDA, then the product need not be labeled as a drug. The FDA has recently relaxed the ruling that food products with other 150% of the RDA be called "drugs"; instead, they can now be sold as dietary supplements.

Dietary supplements and health foods thus constitute a heterogeneous group of products that fall on the boundary between foods and drugs. In many cases, the advertising of such products includes the implications (which may be explicit) that the consumption of the product will confer health benefits on the consumer. Such claims may be either generalized ones or specifically related to a particular disease. Most food legislation in the United States of America, Europe, and other countries do not permit specific health claims for foods, mainly because they blur the distinction between foods and medicines (see Chapters 9 and 23).

IV. QUALITY ASSURANCE FOR CONSUMER PROTECTION

Nutrients have a specific function related to health, and consumer protection is concerned with the levels of their usage (recommended doses). In the case of nutrient supplements, an assumption is implicit that a consumer's diet is inadequate without the addition of the supplement. In certain cases, dietary supplements would clearly be of potential benefit, e.g., supplementing the diet of pregnant women with iron and folic acid; supplying iodized salt in areas where the soil source of iodine is poor; or supplementing vitamin A where the supply of fats and dairy foods is not adequate. In the developed Western world, specific nutrient deficiencies are rare, and the case for dietary supplements often rests on the concepts of optional intakes, rather than the need to prevent deficiencies. Consumer protection must therefore ensure that unwarranted claims for the benefits of dietary supplements are not made. It must also control the amounts available in products to prevent any possible hazards due to overdosing. The working Group of the Ministry of Agriculture, Fisheries and Food (7) has reviewed the supplements and recommended that the amounts of nutrients in such supplements should be limited to one-tenth of the undesirable dose levels for nutrients for which adverse effects of high doses were known (Table 3).

This report (MAFF, 1991) also considered health foods and concluded that many of the claims made for "health" foods were extremely difficult to substantiate. Many of these natural "health foods" contain biologically active substances, some of which are even toxic substances having undesirable effects at high doses. According to MAFF (7), these "health foods" should be regulated within the existing food legislation, without creating a special category for them. Deep concerns have been expressed on the continued sale of such products, emphasizing a need to increase awareness among consumers of the potential hazards of some products (3).

The Scientific Committee of the European Community has undertaken a consultation regarding the possible regulation of supplementary foods, health foods, and fortified foods. The legislation should include regulations to prevent false or undue claims for a food product, and to control the levels of nutrients, with reference to the nutritional requirements for health, as well as to stringently regulate the sale of food products containing potential toxic substances.

The nutritional labeling laws are voluntary with two exceptions. The label must state amounts of seven nutrients (five vitamins and two minerals) if a manufacturer adds nutrients or makes nutritional claims. However, if no nutrients are added and nutritional claims are not made, the product does not have to be labeled. The concept of voluntary labeling gives the manufacturer

Table 3 Recommended Levels of Nutrients in Foods

Nutrient	U.K. RNI	U.S. RDA	Undesirable dose Chronic (per day)	Acute
Vitamins				
Retinol	700 µg	800–1000 µg	6000 µg (3300 µg)[a]	
Vitamin D	10 µg	10 µg	50 µg	
Vitamin B_6	1.4 mg	1.4–2 mg	100 mg	
Vitamin C	40 mg	50–60 mg	6 g	
Niacin	17 mg	13–20 mg	500 mg[b]	
Minerals				
Iron	14.8 mg	10–15 mg	40 mg	20 mg/kg
Copper	1.2 mg	1.5–3 mg[c]	30 mg	
Zinc	7–9.5 mg	12–15 mg	20 mg	
Selenium	60–75 µg	40–70 mg	1 mg	
Sodium	1.6 g	X	8 g	
Cobalt	X	X	300 mg	
Chromium	>7–2.5 µg	50–200 µg	1 g	
Iodine	140 µg	150 µg	1 mg	
Fluorine	X	1.5–4 mg[c]	10 mg	
Molybdenum	50–400 µg	75–250 µg[c]	10 mg	

[a]During pregnancy.

[b]High doses of niacin have been associated with liver damage, sometimes severe. Most, but not all, of the formulations responsible for this association have been sustained-release products. It is not yet known whether the critical factor is the dose or the formulation or both.

[c]No RDA set, but an estimated safe and adequate daily dietary intake.

X = No recommended daily amount (RDA) set. Historically, previous UK committees felt either that not enough evidence was available to set RDAs for a number of nutrients, or that there was no public health need to do so. However, more evidence is now available about human needs, and in COMA's current review of RDAs, it is expected that the range of nutrients covered will be more extensive.

Source: Ref. 3.

the choice to label or not to label the product, which may soften the economic impact for complete, mandatory nutritional labeling that is desired. The pressure from competition in the marketplace is likely to persuade food manufacturers to comply with the new labeling laws whether or not nutrients are added to the foods.

Nutritional labeling laws will also have an indirect effect on the nutrient content and quality of the food products. Marketing departments in the future shall be hard pressed to promote a food product that has a label denoting that it contains less than 2% of U.S. RDA of the nutrients and will bring pressure on the producers to make their products appear better nutritionally.

The current legislation in the developed countries is sufficient to assure quality of the food products and to curb abuses in this area. Modest nutritional additions would be advantageous from a marketing point of view, the development likely to be encouraged by the marketing managers.

Purveyors of organic and health foods, who often make nutritional claims, however, may be hurt by the nutritional labeling laws. All those who sell food to the public must comply with the food laws and will have to label the nutrient content of their food products. Consumers today have an opportunity to compare the food quality in its nutritional and other terms, be it a health, natural, or commercial food. It is interesting to compare the nutritional quality of some of the non-fortified natural breakfast cereals with that of the fortified cereals.

Clydesdale and Francis (6) envisaged that the nutritional claims of some foods will be modified by the new laws, because all nutritional claims now must be substantiated by scientific nutritional data. Claims such as those mentioned below, for example, will not be allowed (6):

1. That the food, because of the presence or absence of certain dietary properties, is adequate or effective in the prevention, cure, mitigation, or treatment of any disease or symptoms
2. That a balanced diet of ordinary foods cannot supply adequate amounts of nutrients
3. That the lack of optimum nutritive quality of a food by reason of soil on which it was grown is responsible for an inadequacy or deficiency in the quality of the daily diet
4. That the storage, transportation, processing or cooking of a food is responsible for an inadequacy or deficiency in the quality of the daily diet
5. That the food has dietary properties when such properties are of no significant value or need in human nutrition

Elimination of such claims will help to prevent the spread of misinformation on human nutrition and enable consumers to obtain the benefits of legitimate nutrition claims.

It has been suggested that the amounts of nutrients on a label may be obtained from tables or nutritional data. At the time of adoption of nutritional labeling laws in the United States of America, in 1975, the existing nutritional tables were not adequate for this purpose. It is currently possible to make reasonable estimates of the nutrient content of a food product for nutritional labeling purposes from the mounting nutrient databanks. Some experts have objected to the inclusion of only seven mandatory nutrients of the thirty-three or so known to be required for optimum human nutrition. It is believed that if the seven mandatory nutrients are supplied adequately, it is very likely that all the remaining nutrients are also present in the food product. However, this is a rather tenuous assumption, especially when most of the seven nutrients in a food product have been added. A solution to this problem, therefore, would be continued surveillance of national nutrient intake to ensure that all population groups are not at risk from inadequate intake of one or more nutrients. If such problems do exist, they could be remedied by encouraging changes in food supply and consumption through nutritional education and by food legislation, if needed.

According to Clydesdale and Francis (6), the nutritional labeling laws are a very complex package of regulations, dealing with an exceedingly wide array of food products, and are open to many interpretations. The implementation of the nutritional labeling laws adds to the cost of food to the consumer. There is a large cost to the manufacturer for generating the initial data on nutrition, and a much smaller continuing cost entailed by making sure the data are current. A tremendous education campaign is necessary to enable consumers to take optimum advantage of the labeling laws. The cost of compliance and education will have to be balanced against the advantages derived by the consumers. The expenditure incurred on processed foods will also increase with increasing industrialization and urban societies.

National surveys have indicated that consumers pay little attention to the thiamin, riboflavin, and niacin content of the foods. Some people have even suggested that they should be dropped from the label. Major changes in the nutritional labeling laws are not expected, until sufficient time has elapsed to judge the successes or failures of the present law. In 1985, the sodium content of the food became mandatory for those using the nutritional labeling format. This change in law was in response to the public concern about sodium as related to high blood pressure.

The older concept of the four basic food groups (cereal products, meats, dairy products, and fruits and vegetables) of the balanced diet has become inadequate for nutritional guidance, with an increase in the number and types of nutritional disorders and diseases of the modern times.

Therefore more sophisticated yardsticks will have to be superimposed on top of the "basic four." The first step in this direction appears to be the declaration of the nutrient content on the food labels. If the educational goal is beyond the capacity of the common public, then the food fortification and nitrification program should progress to the point where it would be possible to maintain a balanced diet. Federal legislation in the developed countries is moving toward national nutritional-quality guidelines to encourage nitrification (8).

REFERENCES

1. Hobbs, B.C., and R.J. Gilbert, *Food Poisoning and Food Hygiene*, Edward Arnold, London, 1978.
2. MAFF. The British diet: finding the facts, Food Surveillance Paper No.23, Ministry of Agriculture, Fisheries and Food, HMSO, London, 1988.
3. Southgate, D.A.T. Consumer protection, In *Human Nutrition and Dietetics*, 9th ed. (J.S. Garrow and W.P.T. James, eds.), Churchill Livingstone, London, 1993, p. 368.
4. HEC, Proposals for nutritional guidelines for health education in Britain, National Advisory Committee on Nutrition Education (NACNE), Health Education Council, 1983.
5. DHSS, Diet and cardiovascular disease, Report on Health and Social subjects No. 28, Department of Health and Social Security, HMSO, London, 1984.
6. Clydesdale, F.M., and F.J. Francis, *Food Nutrition and Health*, AVI Publishing Co., Westport, Conn., 1985, p. 223.
7. MAFF, Dietary supplements and health foods, Report of the Working Group, Ministry of Agriculture, Fisheries and Food and Department of Health, HMSO London, 1991.
8. Deutsch, R.M., *Nutritional labeling: How it can work for you*? National Nutrition Consortium, Bethesda, Maryland, 1975.

16
Food Safety

I. INTRODUCTION

Food safety is primarily concerned with microbial food poisoning (see Chapter 13) and the presence of certain chemicals in food. The chemicals may either be present in foods as natural compounds or introduced to them through industrial accidents, food additives, pesticides, environmental pollutants, or even intentional fraud. All these sources require a different concept of food safety and a different approach to protect consumers from hazards (1).

Hundreds of compounds found naturally occurring in foods may have varying degrees of toxicity (2–7). There is meager information on the this subject in the form of quantitative data related to the magnitude of occurrence of the toxic substances and their effects on humans and animals.

Food additives found in food products are used to perform a variety of functions, such as antioxidants used to prevent rancidity of oils and fats, preservatives employed to check food spoilage from microorganisms, as well as colors, flavors, textural agents, and many others (see Chapter 14). Most of the chemicals added intentionally are generally regarded as necessary and safe.

Several chemicals such as fertilizers, pesticides weedicides, insecticides, fungicides, and bactericides, and growth hormones are used during the production of plant crops and animals as well to extend the postharvest life of the many food products. Many of these chemicals are essential for promoting growth of crops and health of animals and significant quantities of their residues may be found in the food products, e.g., DDT found in milk and milk products (2).

Industrial accidents are common in many technological societies. Clydesdale and Francis (1) cite an example of an unfortunate industrial accident involving food that occurred in May 1973. The Michigan Chemical Co. accidently shipped several 100-pound bags of Firemaster, a fire-retardant chemical, known as polybrominated biphenyls (PBBs) to a Farm Bureau Services feed mill, instead of a mineral nutrient preparation, magnesium oxide. The feed mill incorporated PBB into conventional feed mixes distributed widely in Michigan. The problem was noticed when the dairy cattle had decreased milk production and in October the animals showed obvious signs of sickness. PPB was identified as the cause only in April 1974. This was the worst single case of animal poisoning in the history of American agriculture: over 30,000 cattle, 1,500,000 chickens, 4,600,000 eggs, 4000 hogs, 750 tons of feeds, and thousands of pounds of cheese, ducks, and pheasants were condemned. The animals had PBB contents above the action levels set by the FDA, which refers to the amount of a compound in food—products having levels above the action level would be condemned by the FDA. This level is set by the FDA after considering all available information, including safety data. Tolerance levels, which are usually more permanent, are similar but require more formal procedures. Millions of animals had PBB levels below the FDA action level, and nothing could be done about it. Also, thousands of people were contaminated by PBBs, causing them mental anguish. Follow-up surveys for human problems caused by this contamination fortunately have not uncovered any deleterious effects (8).

The environmental pollutants often found in soil, air, and water can easily enter the food system, e.g., lead from gasoline, cadmium from industrial metal plating, and mercury in fish from the ocean. The polychlorinated biphenyls (PCBs) are a class of industrial chemicals that are very stable and virtually indestructible in the environment. They are widely used in electrical transformers, heat transfer systems, hydraulic fluids, plastics, adhesives, paints, varnishes, printing inks, fluorescent light starters, insulating tapes, sealants and many other industrial products. Their ubiquitous use and exceptional stability has led to a build-up in the environment. PCBs were found in milk samples collected from West Virginia in 1969 and were traced back to the use of transformer fluid added to a herbicide sprayed near cattle grazing areas (5–7).

The health problems related to PCBs were detected in the late 1930s as skin rashes, called chloracne, in industrial workers exposed to high levels of PCBs. PCBs are carcinogenic in animals, but evidence is insufficient to show that the low levels found in foods have any harmful effects on human beings. Social surveys have indicated that one-half of the U.S. population has detectable PCBs in their body tissues. The levels of PCBs in the environment are expected to decrease gradually in time to come, but at present they are everywhere. A judgment of safety, defined as an estimate of risk, is necessary for all such chemical compounds found in food products and the environment (3,4).

Chemicals added through intentional fraud can be controlled by passing and enforcing adequate food laws to punish unscrupulous operators endanging human health. The "cooking oil" incident that occurred in Spain in 1981 caused the deaths of 259 people and made over 20,000 seriously ill. An enterprising firm had imported denatured rapeseed oil intended for industrial use and reprocessed it for human use. After adding soy oil and pork fat, the mixture was sold at 25% discount as pure olive oil. The chemical contaminant that actually caused the deaths was not completely identified.

II. NATURAL TOXICANTS IN FOODS

Many substances present in foods may have adverse or toxic effects if the food is consumed in large quantities but the amounts normally present in foods are usually harmless. Walker (9) classified toxic substances present in foods into two major categories: toxins naturally present in foods, and chemicals used unintentionally or intentionally, as food additives (Table 1). Some common foods containing pharmacologically active agents known to have toxic effects on humans are given in Table 2. Toxicants naturally occurring in foods and food infections by pathogenic microorganisms have caused more human diseases leading to mortality than any categories of toxicants, though accidental chemical contamination and environmental pollution have been responsible for local disasters from time to time. The intentional additives used in food processing in the developed countries are considered safe by the food authorities (see Chapters 13 and 14). The standards of safety are rather strict, and those set for pure synthetic chemicals used in foods are even more strict than for the complex of substances present naturally in foods. According to Pyke (10), the tests for new foods and additives are so stringent that if the potato were put up as a new and unknown food now, it would not be accepted because of its solanine content.

A. Natural Food Toxins

Several natural toxicants and poisons present in foods have a great variety of acute and chronic pharmacologic effects on man (Table 2). Many of these toxins possibly evolved in plants as pro-

Table 1 Toxic Substances in Foods

Toxicants	Particulars
A. Natural toxicants	
1. Inherent	Usually present in the food and affects everyone if enough food is consumed, e.g., solanines in potatoes, and lathyrus toxin.
2. Toxin resulting from abnormal animal or plant conditions used for food	For example, neurotoxic mussel poisoning, honey from bees feeding on rhododendron or Azalea nectar
3. Abnormally sensitive consumer	Constitutional, e.g., celiac disease (wheat gluten), favism (broad beans), allergy to a particular food, or drug-induced, e.g., cheese reaction
4. Contamination from pathogenic bacteria	Acute illness, usually gastrointestinal, e.g., toxins produced by *Staphylococcus aureus* or *Clostridium botulinum*; food may not appear spoiled
5. Mycotoxins	Food moldy or spoiled, e.g., aflatoxin B_1 from *Aspergillus flavus* is a liver carcinogen
6. Mutagens and carcinogens	Produced by grilling, roasting, or frying meat and fish, e.g., free oxide radicals
B. Chemical contaminants	
1. Unintentional additives	
a. Chemical used in agriculture and animal husbandry	For example, fungicides, insecticides on fruits and grains, antibiotics or hormones given to animals
b. Environmental pollution	For example, organic mercury, cadmium, lead, aluminum, PCB and PBB, and radioactive fallouts affecting food chains
2. Intentional additives, preservatives, emulsifiers, colors flavors, and so on.	Many additives are naturally based and used in small amounts and are the most thoroughly tested and monitored of all chemicals used in food.

Source: Ref. 9.

tective mechanisms against other organisms feeding on them. Animals in turn have evolved elaborative biochemical reactions and cellular responses for disposing of toxins or at least partially neutralizing their poisonous effects.

1. Plant Food Toxins

Tares (vetches, pulses, and legumes) traditionally have been regarded as nutritionally unsatisfactory. One species of tare, *Lathyrus sativus*, also known as *khesari dhal* in India, is grown in several Asian and North African countries. Eaten in small quantities, lathyrus seeds are a valuable source of energy and protein. But if it is the main source of energy (providing more than 50%), a neurotoxin present in it, beta-N-oxalyl-amino-L-alanine (BOAA), causes a severe disease of the spinal cord, leading to crippling and permanent paralysis (11). White common vetch (*Vicia sativa*) contains BOAA (12) beta-N-oxalyl-L-alpha, beta-diaminopropionic acid has been isolated from the seeds of *Lathyrus sativus* (13). Both of these cause neurological lesions in primates; however, the relationship between intakes of these two toxins and the incidence and nature of neurological lesions in humans has not been established fully. Weaver (14) noted that when rats were fed certain vetches, especially the sweet pea, *Lathyrus odoratus*, a severe disturbance of collagenous structures developed, notably in skin and bones, known as osteolathyrism. Though not

Table 2 Possible Toxic Effects of Foods

Source	Active agent	Effects
Bananas and some other fruits	5-Hydroxytryptamine, adrenaline, noradrenaline	Effects on central and peripheral nervous system
Some cheeses	Tyramine	Raises blood pressure, enhanced by monoamine oxidase inhibitors
Almonds, cassava, and other plants	Cyanide	Interferes with tissue respiration
Quail	Due to consumption of hemlock	Hemlock poisoning
Mussels	Due to consumption of dinoflagellate, *Gonyaulax*	Tingling, numbness, muscle weakness, respiratory paralysis
Cycad nuts	Methylazoxymethanol (cycasin)	Liver damage, cancer
Some fish, meat, or cheese	Nitrosamines	Cancer
Mustard oil	Sanguinarine	Edema (epidemic dropsy)
Legumes	Hemagglutinins	Red cell and intestinal cell damage
Some beans	Vicine	
	Beta-aminopropionitrile	Hemolytic anaemia (favism) Interferes with collagen formation
	Beta-N-oxalyl-amino-L-alanine	Toxic effects on nervous system, lathyrism
Ackee fruit	Alpha-amino-beta-methylene cyclo-propane propionate	Hypoglycemia, vomiting sickness
Brassica seeds and other cruciferae	Glucosinolates, thiocyanates	Enlargement of thyroid gland (goiter)
Rhubarb	Oxalate	Oxaluria
Green potatoes	Solanine and other sapotoxins	Gastrointestinal upsets
Many fish	Various, often confined to certain organs or seasonal	Mainly toxic effects on nervous system
Many fungi	Various mycotoxins	Mainly toxic effects on nervous system

Source: Ref. 9.

a natural disease in man or animals, osteolathyrism can be produced experimentally in laboratory animals, and the neurotoxin responsible, beta-aminopropionitrile, is commonly used in the experimental study of collagen formation (9).

Many natural foods have been reported to contain carcinogenic substances that can produce tumors in experimental animals. Potent mutagens and carcinogens, such as aminoimidezo-aza-arenes, are produced by high-temperature cooking (grilling, roasting, frying) of meat and fish (15) (see Chapter 25).

Potatoes contain a potentially toxic alkaloid, solanine. Normal potatoes contain about 7 mg of solanine/100 g, which is concentrated in the skin, eyes, and sprouts. Potato poisoning is very rare, but McMillan and Thompson (16) reported an outbreak of suspected solanine poisoning in

London schoolboys; with symptoms including headache, vomiting, and diarrhea. Out of 78 boys affected, 17 boys were admitted to the hospital due to fever and circulatory collapse, and of these three were dangerously ill with neurological disturbances, stupor, and hallucinations. A sample of the potatoes that had been served at the school was found to contain 33 mg of solanine per 100 g. It has been suggested that solanine in potatoes eaten by mothers in early pregnancy may be responsible for spina bifida and other abnormalities of the central system, through there is no epidemiological or other evidence to support this hypothesis (9).

Seeds of cycad (*Cycas circinalis*) contain a toxin, cycasin, which has been shown to be a potent hepatotoxin and carcinogen in experimental animals. There was a high incidence of a type of motor neuron disease and parkinsonian dementia among the Chamorro people on the island of Guam and the neighboring Mariana Islands. These diseases were suspected to be due to the traditional high consumption of cycad seeds. Kurland (17) reported, however, that feeding adult animals with cycasin did not produce neurological damage, and the victims of the motor neuron disease could not be shown to have eaten more cycad seeds.

Several spices and flavouring agents contain volatile essential oils and hydrocarbons that stimulate glandular secretion and may have effects on the nervous system. Many of these substances when taken in large doses have toxic effects. Thousands of components of the essential oils of herbs and species are used as flavoring agents (food additives) in foods, but most of these components have not been tested toxicologically and pose difficulties in establishing a permitted list on a rational scientific basis (9).

Comfrey root and leaf, often used as a herbal tea, contain hepatotoxic and carcinogenic pyrollizidine alkaloids. Several other herbal teas may also contain toxic substances but have not been analyzed and tested (18).

Mustard oil was found to be responsible for endemic dropsy in Bengal and the Bihar parts of India (19,20). However, the toxin was not present in the oil from the mustard seeds themselves but in oil from the seeds of a poppy weed (*Argemone mexicana*) that commonly grows in the mustard crop. Seeds of poppy weed contain a toxic alkaloid, sanguinarine (21). The latter inhibits the oxidation of pyruvate, followed by cardiomyopathy, as in wet beriberi. Other vegetable oils may also become contaminated with argemone oil.

Jelliffe and Stuart (22) reported that ackee fruits (*Blighia sapida*) cause "vomiting sickness," a form of food poisoning in Jamaica. Williams (23), however, could not exclude a specific poison from ackee fruit. It was concluded that if such poison were indeed responsible, large amounts would have to be consumed, and the patients must be peculiarly susceptible to the poison, probably because of their undernourished state. Ackee fruit contains water-soluble alpha-amino-beta-methylene cyclopropyl-propionic acid, which causes accumulation of branched-chain fatty acids and acute hypoglycemia (hypoglycin) (24). This substance is thought to be responsible for the clinical features of vomiting sickness.

Rabbits and other experimental animals fed large amounts of raw leaves or seeds of Brassica species (cabbages, mustards, and rapes) develop goiter. This is due to the presence of glucosinolates and thiocyanates. Whereas glucosinolates act on the thyroid gland and prevent synthesis of thyroxine, thiocyanates reduce the iodine concentration in the thyroid gland. Brassicas such as cabbages eaten in normal amounts, however, have not been known to cause any harmful effects; rather, they are beneficial.

2. Animal Food Toxins

Several seawater fish from the Pacific Ocean and the Caribbean Sea have been reported to cause food poisoning, producing acute neuromuscular disorder with weakness and sensory changes. Most attacks are moderately severe; the symptoms may resolve in a few days, but itching may persist for several weeks and occasionally, widespread paralysis may be followed by coma and death.

A large number of species of fish are poisonous, some of which are always poisonous, others are poisonous at certain times of the year. The toxic substances from fish have not been identified and isolated. The toxins may be organo minerals entering into their feeding environment (25).

Hall and Strichartz (26) have reviewed the origin, structure, and molecular pharmacology of the marine toxins. Scombrotoxicosis arising from eating tuna, mackerel, and other related fish was thought to be due to histamine intoxication resulting from eating spoiled fish. Clifford and Walker (27) and Clifford et al. (28) have shown that outbreaks of scombrotoxicosis may be due to algal toxins relayed to the mackerel, possibly via shellfish and sand eels.

Saxitoxins are present in plankton, especially the dinoflagellate *Gonyaulax tamarensis*, ingested by bivalves such as mussels. The stable toxin remains in the tissues of shellfish that appear to be resistant to it and is not destroyed by cooking. Dinoflagellates occasionally multiply greatly, coloring the seas and such "red tides" cause heavy mortality of seabirds such as shags. Mussels, otherwise safe to eat, may then become toxic. A European Community directive insists on regular monitoring of paralytic shellfish poisoning (PSP) and a level of 80 μg/100 g in shellfish meat is the action level for increased sampling in an area, the results being made available daily. Okadaic acid, a potent carcinogen, is a diarrhetic shellfish toxin (PSP), produced by *Procentrum* and *Dinophysis* species of phytoplankton (9).

Outbreaks of acute paroxysmal myoglobinuria, accompanied by severe muscle pain, have occurred after eating eel or burbot fresh-water fishes. Fishermen and their families around Koeningsberg Haff in East Germany during World War I and II suffered from this malady and the condition became known as Haff disease. These fishes were found to contain a toxin that had entered the Haff with the industrial effluent from the nearby region. The toxin responsible has not been identified.

B. Antinutritional Factors

Dicoumarol, a compound related to vitamin K, was isolated from clover (29) and was found to cause a hemorrhagic disease in cattle feeding on spoiled sweet clover. The toxin produces hemorrhages by causing vitamin K deficiency in the tissues. Synthetic analogues of dicoumarol are used in clinical practice to decrease blood coagulation.

Compounds naturally present in foods can act as antinutritional (antivitamin) factors by preventing absorption of vitamins or destroying them in the gut. An outbreak of paralysis (chastek paralysis) was developed in silver foxes in the United States in 1936 on a farm belonging to Mr. Chastek. These foxes were fed on carp and the presence of thiaminase could be demonstrated in the flesh and viscera of the fish (30). An addition of thiamin can both prevent and cure the disease. Thiaminase enzyme is present in several fish species. Some plants (bracken) contain 3, 4-dihydroxy cinnamic acid, which also has thiaminase activity. However, thiamin deficiency due to the consumption of thiaminase has not been reported in humans.

Plants synthesize a multitude of chemicals that cause toxic reactions when consumed by man or animals (31–36). Pulses, for example, contain toxicants such as protease inhibitors, cyanogens, hemagglutinins, saponins, lathyrogens, and flavism agents. Cereals and potatoes may also contain protease inhibitors, and spinach and asparagus contain saponins. Goitrogens causing hypothyroidism and thioglucosides causing thyroid enlargement are present in brassicas such as cabbage and other related species (rapeseed and mustard). Most foods contain proteins that may act as allergens in sensitive individuals. The oxalic acid content of rhubarb, spinach, and beet may cause poisoning in certain individuals.

III. ADDED CHEMICAL TOXICANTS IN FOODS

Crops must be protected from weeds, insects, fungi, bacteria, and viruses, both during preharvest production and postharvest handling, storage, and transportation. Rodents, molds, and putrefying bacteria cause heavy postharvest losses of food crops. Also, animals need to be protected from external parasites, ticks, lice, maggots in the skin, and worms in the internal organs. A range of agricultural chemicals are used in crop and animal production to prevent or at least reduce these losses. In addition, chemical fertilizers and growth hormones are used to enhance the growth and development of crops and animals. These chemical agents, if not used properly, can enter the food chain and become toxic to consumers. The high yields of modern technical agriculture are mainly due to its dependence on the chemical industry.

A. Insecticides, Fungicides, and Herbicides

Manufacturers, distributors, and farm workers are often exposed to pesticides, resulting in several deaths every year. The cases of acute poisoning due to the residues of these pesticides left on a crop are comparatively rare. Karagaratnam et al. (37), however, reported an outbreak of organophosphate poisoning caused by eating barley contaminated with parathion, which is a powerful anticholinesterase agent. Prompt action contained the outbreak to 38 cases with nine deaths in Singapore. In Sri Lanka in 1981 young Tamil girls from tea estates suffered from toxic neuropathy by eating raw eggs and gingili oil. The oil had been stored in metal drums originally used for mineral oils. An insecticide, tri-cresyl phosphate, was detected in the oil sample. The girls had consumed 2.8 to 5.9 g of the poison during two weeks time, a dose sufficient to cause neuropathy (38). The clinical features of the poisoning included pain in the calves, weakness in the feet and hands, absent ankle jerks, and wrist drop, suggestive of polyneuropathy.

Organochlorine pesticides such as DDT have now been banned in most developed countries because of their widespread persistence in the food chain. Widespread use of DDT had adverse effects on hawks, eagles, and other birds living on the flesh of small animals. The eggs were not able to hatch due to the deficiency of estrogens, which are probably metabolized at increased rate by microsomal enzymes of the liver induced by DDT (9).

Many modern carbamate and organophosphorus pesticides are more toxic than organochlorines but are less persistent and thus cause fewer problems to consumers. Regulatory safety measures have led to the establishment of maximum residue levels (MRLs) of pesticides in foods (39). These issues have been reviewed recently (40).

Accidents often occur by eating seed grains treated with chemical fungicides, especially when previous crop harvests are small and instructions on seed are poor, e.g., alkyl-mercury poisoning that occurred in Iraq in 1972. Peters (41) reported that 3000 people in Turkey during the late 1950s suffered from porphyria with skin lesions precipitated by sunlight, after consumption of seeds treated with hexachlorobenzene.

B. Hormones and Antibiotics

Steroid sex hormones act as anabolic agents in beef cattle; their use is banned in the EEC but not in the United States (9). Bovine somatotropin (BST), for example, is used in the United States to improve milk production in dairy cattle. Scientific evidence is not sufficient that BST is harmful, though people find it difficult to accept. Comparable amounts of estrogens are naturally present in common foods such as soybeans and eggs. Moreover, the endogenous production of these hormones in humans and the amounts used in oral contraceptives are often much larger than used in anabolic agents. Therefore, the ban on the use of estrogens in the EEC does not appear to be logical. Hormonal feed additives are also not permitted in the EEC.

Several infectious diseases of farm animals are treated with antibiotics, which are also added to feeds to promote growth in pigs and poultry. In addition, antibiotics are used as food preservatives. Food contamination with antibiotics, however, has not shown to be directly harmful to man, though it has been suggested that indiscriminate use of antibiotics in animal husbandry may indirectly develop resistance to bacteria such as *Salmonella typhimurium* and *Escherichia coli*, often found infecting both humans and animals. Resistance to the action of antibiotics may be carried through the genetic material of the bacteria and transferred to other strains not previously exposed to the antibiotic. The Joint European Committee on Food Additives (JECFA) has discussed the problems of regulating veterinary drug residues in foods (42), the situation in the United Kingdom being monitored by MAFF (43). Martinez-Navaro (44) reported the illegal use of poisonous beta-agonist clenbuterol in beef production. According to Walker (9), strains of *Salmonella* resistant to antibiotics continue to be found in foodstuffs.

C. Industrial Pollutants and Radioactive Fallouts

Industrial poisons may contaminate foods and feeds in various ways through improper disposal of the waste products, accidents, and criminal adulteration.

Mercury and cadmium contaminations of food due to failure to dispose of industrial waste properly have been reported. According to a report by MAFF (45), lead from car exhausts has caused serious problem of increase in lead levels of food, compelling introduction of unleaded petrol and non-soldered can seams. A threshold value of lead for impairment of mental performance in infants and young children cannot be determined and deleterious effects are noted at very low exposure levels (46). Milk from several lead-affected herds was required to be withdrawn from the markets of the Netherlands and the United Kingdom (47,48). Skene et al. (49) reviewed the problems concerned with contamination of fish with PCBs from electrical insulation and plasticizers. Dioxins and tetrachlorodibenzofurans produced in incinerators and in the paper industry contaminate agricultural products, leading to tragic disasters (50,51).

A mysterious new disease caused by selling of rapeseed oil with adulterated aniline occurred in Spain in 1981, resulting in 13,000 people admitted to the hospital, with more than 100 deaths. Aniline is used to denature rapeseed oil for industrial purpose (52). The nature of the chemical poison causing the malady, however, remained unknown. The clinical features of the disease were diverse and unexplicable, ranging from fever, rashes, and myalgia to respiratory distress. Most of the deaths resulted from pneumonopathy. Also, intense muscular pain and numbness of the arms and legs were common symptoms. Walker (9) stressed that there is need for rapid enforcement of food safety laws, by providing adequate staff to the local authorities to promptly detect all breaches of food safety laws and regulations, together with the power to enforce them strictly.

Despite the Nuclear Test Ban signed in 1963 by the United States, the United Kingdom, and the Soviet Union, atomic explosions have occurred from time to time, liberating radioactive dust into the atmosphere. This dust has risen to the stratosphere, where it may drift over thousands of miles before sinking into the lower atmosphere and finally to the earth's surface. Radioactive fallouts contaminate cereal crops, fruits, and vegetables and also grasses and herbage eaten by cattle, whose milk and meat then contain radioactive poison. Foods of animal origin generally become more dangerous to humans than those of plant foods, owing to the concentration of radioactive material in milk and meat.

The major potentially dangerous radio-isotopes in the fallouts are iodine-131 (^{131}I), strontium-90 (^{90}Sr), and cesium-137 (^{137}Cs). ^{131}I has a half-life of only 8 days, thus most of it liberated into atmosphere becomes inactive in the upper strata, though unacceptable levels of ^{131}I have been reported in some milk samples. ^{90}Sr and ^{137}Cs have half-lives of 28 and 30 years, respectively, and are therefore potentially more dangerous. Like calcium, ^{90}Sr is concentrated in milk, and like potassium, cesium is concentrated in muscle (meats). ^{90}Sr is particularly dangerous because bones store it and bone marrow is rather susceptible to damage by radiation. Similarly the concentration of ^{90}Sr in milk is especially dangerous io infants and children (9). Hawthorn (53) described the effects of radioactive fallouts on food contamination in the United Kingdom. In recent times, the Chernobyl power plant accident caused a widespread food contamination with radionucleotides (54,55).

An International Reference Centre for Environmental Radioactivity was established at Le Vesignet, France, by the World Health Organization and the International Atomic Energy Agency (IAEA). This center enables national governments to collect information about all forms of radiation in the environment that are potentially dangerous to health and advises them on the control measures. Periodic reports are published on the levels of ^{90}Sr and ^{137}Cs in samples of milk from various countries. During emergency periods of radioactive fallouts, it is safe to eat foods that have been stored or packed in air-tight tins or jars or otherwise protected from atmospheric dust. An increase in dietary calcium is expected to decrease absorption of ^{90}Sr, because both calcium and strontium are metabolized by the same mechanism (9).

D. Chemical Food Preservatives and Additives

Extensive tests for toxicity and/or food safety must be carried out before deliberately adding any chemical to preserve food or to enhance its quality. Sulfiting agents and nitrates used as food additives often pose problems of food safety, some groups of people being more sensitive to these chemicals than other groups. Deaths have been reported among a group of severely afflicted, steroid-dependent asthmatics, following the use of sulfite-treated salads. The practice of using sulfites to prevent enzymatic browning in foods is not practiced in the United Kingdom (56,57). The nitrates added to foods are reduced to nitrites in the body, which can combine to form carcinogenic nitrosamines (implicated in stomach cancer). Walker (58) has reviewed occurrence of these compounds in foods and their safety aspects (see Chapters 14 and 15).

1. Cyclamate and Monosodium Glutamate Stories

According to the Soft Drinks Regulations (1964), a maximum amount of 1.35 g/liter of cyclamate was permitted in soft drinks as an artificial sweetener. This was based on the advice of the Food Additives and Contaminants Committee. The cyclamates were then permitted in the United States, based on extensive tests on animals and humans. However, in 1969, a study of cancer rates in the United States of America reported that high levels of cyclamate produced bladder cancer in 8 out of 240 rats. As a result of this study, cyclamate was immediately banned in the United States, and soon after in the United Kingdom. In the above study, a mixture of cyclamate and saccharine was used. Whereas saccharine has been shown to cause bladder tumors, cyclamate alone has not been shown to produce any cancer. Thus cyclamate was again reinstated to be used in soft drinks. Based on the metabolism of cyclamate to cyclohexylamine and the latter's "No Observed Adverse Effect Level" in Europe, an ADI value of 11 mg/kg body weight was allowed (59). However, the Committee on Toxicity in the United Kingdom has now set an ADI of 1.5 mg/kg body weight, based on a more conservative interpretation of the metabolic data on cyclohexylamine.

Kwok (60) reported a "Chinese-restaurant syndrome," with clinical features such as numbness of the back of the neck, gradually radiating to both arms and back, general weakness, and palpitation. The well-known syndrome is now presumed to be due to monosodium L-glutamate (MSG), which has been permitted to be used as flavoring agent in savory foods in the food industry. It has not been banned as a flavoring compound because the symptoms of its effects are transient, affecting only a minority of consumers, and lead to no permanent damage. Also, the symptoms are easily associated by the sufferer with excessive consumption of highly flavored foods, which can be avoided. The use of glutamate in infant foods has now been discontinued by most manufacturers (9).

The stories of cyclamate and monosodium glutamate present several messages to nutritionists. They show the uncertainty of contemporary knowledge, because newer information keeps on challenging the accepted opinions of the day. They also signify the value of a careful study of unusual and unexplicable symptoms appearing in humans or animals. These stories have well demonstrated the difficulty in making a decision regarding an acceptable risk, and the need to proceed slowly before making a judgment on any chemical. On the part of consumers, a comforting fact is that human beings have not usually suffered in any serious way as a consequence of taking a permitted food additive, barring an occasional individual allergic to one of such compounds. This, however, does not mean that the present standards of toxicity testing and food safety should be relaxed. On the countrary, there is a need to make present tests more precise and to continue to devise better tests in time to come.

IV. PATHOGENS IN FOODS

The dangers from pathogenic agents in food are much greater than those of naturally occurring toxicants or man-made chemicals added to foods or present as contaminants. A larger number of pathogenic organisms, such as fungi, bacteria, protozoa, viruses, and helminth worms, may gain access to foods and enter the body of humans and animals to cause a well-defined disease. Southgate (61) has given a detailed account of the pathogenic agents present in food.

A. Fungal Toxins

Certain species of mushrooms and fungi, such as *Amanita phalloides* (Britain) and *Amanita serna* (America) are poisonous, each containing two types of toxins. Phallotoxins are heptapeptides that act quickly and cause vomiting, diarrhea, and abdominal pain. Amatoxins are octapeptides and act after their absorption by hepatocytes and renal tubular cells. Oliguria leading to renal failure may occur only after the gastrointestinal symptoms have subsided. Kidney damage can be fatal if hemodialysis is not available. Short et al. (31) reported an incidence of mushroom poisoning in the north of Scotland, wherein three young people on holiday had gathered and eaten mushrooms with orange gills (*Cortinarius speciosissimus*). Gastrointestinal symptoms of varying severity followed: one person showed evidence of slight renal damage but recovered later on; the other two also survived, thanks to hemodialysis and subsequent renal transplantation.

Epidemics of the disease known as St. Anthony's fire in France in the 18th century caused intolerable burning pain in the limbs, which became black, shrivelled, and dropped off. Convulsions, palsies, and disordered movements in some patients indicated that the central nervous system as well as the peripheral vascular system were affected. The disease was associated with eating rye infected by a fungus, *Claviceps purpura*. King (32) reported five cases of gangrenous ergotism associated with eating wild oats infected with *Claviceps* species in Ethiopia. In India, the pearl millet (bajra), *Pennisetum typhoides*, infected with *Claviceps fusiformis* produces alkaloids of the clavine group, which are different from the ergot alkaloids (33). The clinical features of the poisoning include severe nausea and vomiting, accompanied by giddiness and drowsiness, but recovery is rather rapid.

Allcroft et al. (34) reported an outbreak of widespread fatal disease of young turkeys in England during 1960. The birds were fed with a ration containing imported peanut meal. The disease was characterized by acute enteritis and hepatitis. The toxic factor, aflatoxin, was produced by a fungus, *Aspergillus flavus*, in peanuts that were harvested, stored, and processed under high humid conditions. Aflatoxins can contaminate several human foods, especially nuts and grains produced and stored in warm, moist climates. Aflatoxins damage the liver and lead to carcinoma in many animals. Aflatoxin B_1 is the most potent known natural hepatocarcinogen, at least in susceptible species such as rats and ducklings. A dose of 0.05 mg/kg can be toxic to primates. Krishnamachari et al. (35) reported a widespread epidemic caused by eating maize contaminated with aflatoxin in Gujarat and Rajastan (India) during 1974. An acute illness had clinical features such as jaundice, ascites, portal hypertension, and a high mortality. The patients had probably consumed 2 to 6 mg of aflatoxin daily for one month. Ueno (36) has reviewed toxicology of mycotoxins in animal husbandary.

Other mycotoxins include sterigmatocystin from *Aspergillus versicolor* on maize, which is carcinogenic to animals but is much less potent than the aflatoxins, and patulin from *Penicillium expansum*, found in rotten apples, which is also carcinogenic. Also, the trichothecenes produced by *Fusarium* species on moldy cereals cause a human disease known as alimentary toxic aleukia in Russia, and ochratoxin from *Aspergillus ochraceus* on moldy barley has been reported to cause a kidney disease in swines in Denmark. Recently, fumonosins have been added to the long list of mycotoxins that are more likely to contaminate foods grown and processed without the use of fungicides, preservatives, and chemical additives.

B. Bacterial Poisoning

Serological typing has identified and distinguished over 1600 types of salmonella, which are the most common food poisoning organisms (62). These organisms infect most species of vertebrates and are especially widespread in poultry and other intensively reared animals. *Salmonella typhimurium* and *S. enteriditis* are the strains most commonly associated with human infections. They are often confined to the intestines, where they cause an acute gastroenteritis with diarrhea and vomiting, but they may also enter the bloodstream and invade tissues, causing enteric fever such as typhoid. Mites and rats infected with *S. typhimurium* commonly excrete the organism in their feces and urine, thus infecting the foods. *S. enteriditis* can be spread from the intestines of infected poultry during processing of the carcasses and through the eggs from the oviducts of infected birds (61). Several pathogenic bacteria and viruses excreted in human feces and urine may become the cause of fecal-oral infections, including dysentary and acute gastroenteritis.

Bacterial food poisoning, such as acute gastroenteritis, is often short and self-limiting. The number of fatal cases is small and deaths usually occur among young children with weakened immunological defences. Diarrhea with severe dehydration and loss of electrolytes is the major cause of infant mortality in the developing world.

Food provides an ideal culture medium for the growth of pathogenic organisms, including bacteria. In addition to the supply of nutrients from the food, other factors influencing their growth and development are temperature, pH, water activity, and atmosphere. Cooking temperatures often kill most of the pathogenic organisms, certainly the vegetative cells, if not the spores; the latter are killed by higher canning temperatures. Low temperatures slow the rate of growth, and refrigerated storage helps to control food poisoning.

Many pathogens do not grow in acid media and their growth can be synergestically inhibited by combining pH and use of preservatives such as sodium chloride and nitrates, as in cured meats (63). Low O_2 atmospheres encourage the growth of obligate anerobic pathogens, whereas the growth of other species is inhibited by high CO_2 concentrations in the atmosphere. Controlled atmosphere (C.A.) storage is now being used to preserve most perishable foods.

Low water activity being inhibitory to the growth of microorganisms, use of salt and sugar can preserve most foods osmotically. The most common food poisoning organisms include *Staphylococcus aureus*, *Bacillus cereus*, *Clostridium botulinum*, *Clostridium perfringens*, *Sal-*

monella sp., *Campylobacter jejuni*, *E. coli*, *Yersinia enterocolitica*, *Vibrio parahemolyticus*, and *Listeria monocytogenes*. The characteristics of some of these species, along with sources of their infection, period of incubation, site of toxin production, and control measures are given in Table 3.

C. Other Microbial Toxins

1. Viral Infections

Many viruses infect human beings through the intestinal tract and have been isolated from feces. Blacklow and Cukor (64) established that Norwalk and rotaviruses as major causes of gastroenteritis. Unlike bacteria, viruses cannot multiply in foods, but they may be transferred to feeds through dirty utensils and food handlers, infecting the intestinal tract after consumption of such food.

2. Other Disease Agents

Helminth parasites are transmitted to humans through consumption of raw or under-cooked pork and beef or raw salads that have been washed or irrigated with contaminated water. Pig and beef tapeworms, *Taenia solium* and *T. saginata*, form cysts in muscle tissue. When consumed by humans, the adult worms develop in the gut; the segments of these worms and ova are shed with feces. The ova may also develop into larvae, invading muscle and other tissues, where they form cysts (cysticercosis), a condition leading to neurological disorders. Consumption of undercooked pork containing larvae of *Trichinella spiralis* may lead to a febrile illness (61). Similarly, consumption of raw or undercooked fish containing the tapeworm *Diphyllobothrium lactum* causes a megaloblastic anemia, because the adult worm (15 m in length) competes with the host for dietary vitamin B_{12} (65).

A bovine spongiform encephalopathy (BSE), detected in 1985, has been implicated in human disease. It is believed to be transmitted between several animal species and is caused by a strain of a scrapie-like agent. Feeding of cattle with protein supplements prepared from the ren-

Table 3 Characteristics of Bacterial Food Poisoning

Organism	Source of infection	Incubation period (hr)	Size of toxin production	Control measures
Staphylococcus aureus	Skin and mucous membranes of carriers	2–6	Food	Storage of food below 5°C
Bacillus cereus	Airborne spores	1–16	Food (rapid), intestine (slow onset)	Refrigeration to control growth
Clostridium perfringens	Soil, raw meat	18–20	Food	Heating to 80°C to inactivate heat-labile spores
Clostridium botulinum	Soil, fish	12–96	Food (heat-labile)	Storage at low-temperatures, pH less than 4.6, low water activity, curing salts
Salmonella sp.	Excreta, intestinal contents	3–36	Intestine	Thawing and cooking of food thoroughly
Listeria monocytogenes	Soil, widely distributed	Days to weeks	Intestine	Freezing low-acid foods

dered offal derived from scrapie-infected sheep carcasses may establish the disease in the animals. There is, however, no evidence as yet of its transmission to humans.

V. FOOD ALLERGIES AND INTOLERANCES

An "allergy" to foods, food additives, beverages, and even water may cause a wide range of distressing physical and psychological problems and chronic, disabling diseases (66). The precise diagnosis of either allergy or food intolerance, however, relies on clinical methodology. Advances in understanding the immunological and pharmacological mechanisms of food intolerance have helped to distinguish allergies from psychologically based reactions to foods. AAAI and NIAID (67) and Metcalf et al. (68) have given a detailed account of allergic phenomena, classifying about 400 diseases associated with foods.

According to Ferguson (66), food allergy is a form of food intolerance in which there is both reproducible food intolerance and evidence of an abnormal immunological reaction to food. Food aversions are based on psychological food reactions and comprise both psychological avoidance and psychological intolerance, which is an unpleasant bodily reaction caused by emotions associated with the food, rather than the food itself; it does not occur when the food is given in an unrecognizable form.

It is very difficult to elucidate the exact relationship between dietary constituents and the clinical phenomena observed in an individual patient or a specific disease. It has become an established practice to use the objectively monitored effects of exclusion diets and provocation tests, as diagnostic criteria. The objective measures include serial recordings of forced expiratory volume or of nasal airflow, mapping of the extent and severity of skin rashes, daily aphthous ulcer counts, measurements of fecal characteristics, intestinal permeability tests, morphometry of mucosal biopsies and so forth.

The patient's perceptions and the doctor's diagnosis of food intolerance in elimination diet and challenge protocols are not always correct. In patients with clear and convincing histories of adverse reactions, less than 50% are confirmed as intolerant on objective testing. Moreover, double-blind protocols reveal a high rate of symptomatic responses to placebo in some adult groups, which is rare in children (66).

Food aversion, intolerance, and allergy symptoms are often very difficult to distinguish from one another. Despite the presence of objective changes, food intolerance can be diagnosed only if the symptoms disappear with an elimination diet and if a controlled challenge then leads to a recurrence of symptoms.

Food intolerance in children includes a wide range of conditions, such as eczema, wheeze, urticaria, alterations in moods, angio-edema, epilepsy, failure to thrive, diarrhea, vomiting, and gastrointestinal blood loss. Milk-induced colitis can be distinguished from ulcerative colitis by clinical and pathological features. Cow's milk protein intolerance is well documented by small intestinal damage with malabsorption, which can also occur with soy, chicken, rice, fish, and egg intolerance.

The classic allergic symptoms in adults are urticaria, asthma, or anaphylaxis. The urticaria in response to food additives can develop from prostaglandin release, rather than from an allergy mechanism. Food sensitivity is related to migraine in a complex way and has a pharmacological rather than an allergic basis. It is produced by a direct effect of a chemical on the walls of blood vessels. Similarly, arthritis appears to be associated with food allergy, though there is little evidence to establish this relation scientifically. Irritability and depression may accompany certain manifestations of food intolerance, which remain to be established fully. Some other food-provoked symptoms are of gastrointestinal origin, e.g., nausea, bloating, abdominal pain, constipation, and diarrhea, produced by so-named irritable bowel syndrome.

Psychological attitudes to food vary very greatly, dieting, overeating, and food fads being very common. Vague symptoms ranging from irritable bowel syndrome to serious allergic disease such as atopic eczema or progressive chronic diseases such as multiple sclerosis, rheumatoid arthritis, and schizophrenia may appear, leading patients to embark on a radical elimination diet without proper medical or dietary advice. In the absence of dramatic cure, patients try to identify substances in foods or in the environment that may be possibly responsible for their symptoms or disease, turning to costly and highly unorthodox investigations and treatments such as homeopathy, iridology, medical herbalism, and acupuncture as alternative medicines. However, food intolerance is not widespread and unrecognized, posing a danger to society (66).

A. Lactose Intolerance

Lactose is a milk sugar containing glucose and galactose. Mammalian enzyme, lactase (beta-1, 4 galactosidase) present in the brush border hydrolyzes lactose to glucose and galactose. In the absence of lactase, consumption of milk in certain groups of people may produce diarrhea, abdominal pain, and distension because of nonabsorption of lactose, resulting in an osmotic effect in the small intestine and accumulation of large amounts of fluid and sugar in the large intestine. In the latter part of bowel, sugar is rapidly fermented, producing gas, ensuing osmotic diarrhea in the presence of enough lactose (66,70). Though some human populations retain the ability of digesting lactose after weaning, lactase activity declines rapidly in all species of animals, including humans. Populations with their ancestors in the Aryan races of the Middle East and North India drink milk traditionally. Thus a majority of northern Europeans and white people of North America, Australia, and New Zealand retain their ability to digest lactose after weaning, except for about 5% to 15% alactasic individuals (71,72). According to Cummings (73), in most parts of the world, including Asia, Africa, South America, and the Mediterranean, milk drinking (with the exception of fermented milk) is uncommon because of very low lactase activity in these populations.

Lactose intolerance resulting from lactase deficiency in humans may be either genetic, either inborn (rare) or declining after weaning (usual), or acquired. The latter may result from gastrointestinal diseases affecting mucosa, including protein-energy malnutrition, celiac disease, tropical sprue, small-bowel resection, Crohn's disease, acute gastroenteritis, chronic alcoholism, immunodeficiency syndrome, and cow's milk protein intolerance (73).

Lactose intolerance can be diagnosed with certainty only by jejunal biopsy and assay of disaccharidase (lactase) activity. Also a rise in blood glucose of less than 20 mg/100 ml after a standard dose of 50 g of lactose to adult humans or an increase in breath hydrogen over fasting levels (more than 20 ppm) indirectly indicate lactose intolerance. Lactose intolerance is often associated with lactose malabsorption and delivery of unabsorbed carbohydrate into the colon. It may occasionally be caused by the osmotic effects of a carbohydrate load in the upper small intestine even in a lactose absorber; e.g., after peptic ulcer surgery, rapid stomach emptying presents a concentrated load to the upper gut, shifting of fluid from the bloodstream into the gut, followed by an accelerated passage down the intestine.

A low-lactose diet in the form of reduced intake of milk and its products helps to manage the malady. Most cheeses are low in lactose, though certain soft types may contain a small amount of lactose through added milk. Naturally made yoghurt or *dahi* is virtually lactose-free, but milk or milk solids may be added to many yoghurts, giving them the lactose levels of fresh milk (5 g/100 ml). Symptoms that are attributed to lactose intolerance, secondary to gastrointestinal disease, are often due to intolerance of other components of food. According to Bayless et al. (69)

and Haverberg et al. (74), most people with low lactase activity can tolerate reasonable amounts of lactose in their diet (10–15 g/day), provided it is taken in small amounts at a time.

Deficiencies may also occur for other disaccharides, besides lactase, e.g. sucrase, isomaltase, and trehalase as well as certain isolated monosaccharide transport defects for glucose and galactose. These conditions are very rare and often manifest during early childhood.

The adverse reactions and the clinical effects (nausea, bloating, abdominal pain, and diarrhea) of lactose ingestion during the diagnostic tests are related to dose, and there is a wide variation among individuals in dose-response phenomenon. The conventional lactose load of 50 g used in tolerance tests produces symptoms in 70% to 80% of malabsorbers, whereas 10 to 15 g of lactose (equivalent to half a pint of milk) will produce abdominal symptoms in only 30% to 60% of people. When an oral dose of lactose causes the foregoing symptoms and the ingestion of a similar dose of another carbohydrate does not produce these effects, lactose malabsorption is likely to be present. However, about 10% of healthy individuals will always develop symptoms such as dizziness, nausea, and palpitation after eating 50 g of any carbohydrate. Hence, it is necessary to be cautious while interpreting these clinical effects. Also, for reasons not well understood, lactose presented in a food is less likely to induce symptoms than an identical load of pure lactose taken in solution. The fat content of the food or drink consumed may slow the entrance of lactose into the small intestine, thus altering the rate of gastric emptying of lactose (66).

A number of inherited disorders of carbohydrate metabolism such as galactosemia and fructose intolerance also occur.

REFERENCES

1. Clydesdale, F.M., and F.J. Francis, *Food, Nutrition and Health*, AVI Publishing Co., Westport, Conn., 1985, p. 239.
2. Anonymous, *Toxicants Occurring Naturally in Foods*, Report of Committee on Food Protection, National Academy of Sciences, Washington, D.C., 1973.
3. Anonymous, *Regulation of Potential Carcinogens in the Food Supply*: The Delany Clause. Report No. 89, Council for Agricultural Science and Technology, Ames, Iowa, 1981.
4. Anonymous, *The Risk/Benefit Concept as Applied to Food*. A Scientific Status Summary by the Institute of Food Technologists, Chicago, Illinois, 1981.
5. Havender, W.R., *Of Mice and Men*, Report by the American Council of Science and Health, New York, 1984.
6. Lawrence, N.N., *Of Acceptable Risk: Science and Determination of Safety*, William Kaufman Inc, Los Altos, California, 1976.
7. Sterrett, F.S., and B.L. Rosenberg, *Science and Public Policy* 11, Academy of Sciences, New York, 1982.
8. Brilliant, L.B., K. Wilcox, G.V. Amburg, E. Eyster, J. Isbister, and A.W. Bloomer, et al., Breast-milk monitoring to measure Michigan's contamination with polybrominated biphenyls, *Lancet 2*: 643 (1978).
9. Walker, R., Food toxicity, *Human Nutrition and Dietetics*, 9th ed. (J.S. Garrow and W.P.T. James, eds.), Churchill Livingstone, London, 1983, p. 354.
10. Pyke, M., *Food and Society*, Murray, London, 1971, p. 102.
11. Sleeman, W.H., Rambles and reflexions of an Indian Official, (New ed., 1893), (V.A. Smith, ed.), Westminster Press, London, 1844.
12. Ressler, C., Isolation and identification from common vetch of the neurotoxin beta-cyano-1-alanine, a possible factor in neurolathyrism, *J. Biol. Chem. 237*: 733 (1962).
13. Adiga, P.R., S.L.N. Rao, and P.S. Sarma, Some structural features and neurotoxic action of a compound for *L. sativus* seeds, *Curr. Sci. 32*: 153 (1963).
14. Weaver, A.L., Lathyrism: A review, *Arthritis and Rheumatism 10*: 470 (1967).

15. Sugimura, T., Mutagens, carcinogens and tumour promoters in our daily food, *Cancer 49*: 1970 (1982).

16. McMillan, M., and J.C. Thompson, An outbreak of suspected solanine poisoning in school boys, *Quaterly J. Med. 227*. 243 (1979).

17. Kurland, L.T., An appraisal of the neurotoxicity of cycad and the etiology of amyotrophic lateral sclerosis in Guam, *Federal Proceedings 31*: 1540 (1972).

18. WHO, Environmental Health Criteria No. 80, Pyrollizidine alkaloids, World Health Organization, Geneva, 1989.

19. Lal, R.B., and S.C. Roy, Investigations into the epidemiology of epidemic dropsy, *Indian J. Med. Res. 25*: 163 (1937).

20. Lal, R.B., S.P. Mukherji, A.C. Das Gupta, and S.R. Chatterji, Quantitative aspects of the problem of toxicity of mustard oil, *Indian J. Med. Res. 28*: 163 (1940).

21. Sarkar, S.N., Isolation from argemone oil of disanguinarine and sanguinarine: toxicity of sanguinarine, *Nature 162*: 265 (1948).

22. Jelliffe, D.B., and K.L. Saturat, Acute toxic hypoglycaemia in the vomiting sickness of Jamaica, *British Med. J. 1*: 75 (1954).

23. Williams, C.D., Report on vomiting sickness in Jamaica, Government Printer, Jamica, 1954.

24. Holt, C. Von, J. Chang, M. Von Holt, and H. Bohm, Metabolism and metabolic effects of hypoglycin, *Biochem. Biophys. Acta 90*: 611 (1964).

25. Jardin, C., Organo-minerals and ciguatera, *FAO Nutrition Newsletter 10*: 14 (1972).

26. Hall, S., and G. Strichartz (eds.), Marine toxins: origin, structure and molecular pharmacology, *Am. Chem. Soc. Symp. Series No. 418*, American Chemical Society, Washington, 1990.

27. Clifford, M.N., and R. Walker, The aetiology of Scombrotoxicosis, *Inter. J. Food Sci. Technol. 27*: 721 (1992).

28. Clifford, M.N., R. Walker, and P. Ijomah, Do saxitoxin-like substances have a role in scombrotoxicosis? *Food Additives and Contaminants* (in Press), cited by Walker (Ref. 9).

29. Link, K.P., The anticoagulant 3, 3′-methylene bis- [4-bis (4-hydroxycourmanin)], *Federal Proceedings 4*: 176 (1945).

30. Green, R.G., W.E. Carlson, and C.A. Evans, The inactivation of vitamin B_1 in diets containing whole fish, *J. Nutr. 23*: 165 (1942).

31. Short, A.I.K., R. Watling, M.K. Macdonald, and J.S. Robson, Poisoning by *Cortinarius speciosissimus*, *Lancet 2*: 942 (1980).

32. King, B., Outbreak of ergotism in Wollo, Ethiopia, *Lancet 1*: 1411 (1979).

33. Krishnamachari, K.A.V.R., and R.V. Bhat, Poisoning by ergoty bajra (Pearl millet) in man, *Indian J. Med. Res. 64*: 1624 (1976).

34. Allcroft, A., R.B.A. Carnaghan, K. Sargeant, and J. O'Kelly, A toxic factor in Brazilian groundnuts, *Veterinary Record 73*: 428 (1961).

35. Krishnamachari, K.A.V.R., R.V. Bhat, V. Nagaragan, and T.B.G. Tilak, Hepatitis due to aflatoxicosis: an outbreak in Western India, *Lancet 1*: 1061 (1975).

36. Ueno, Y. The toxicology of mycotoxins, *CRC Crit. Rev. in Toxicology. 14*: 99 (1985).

37. Karagaratnam, K., W.K. Bron, and T.K. Hoh, Parathion poisoning from contaminated barley, *Lancet 1*: 538 (1960).

38. Senanayake, N., and J. Jeyaranam, Toxic polyneuropathy due to gingili oil contaminated with tri-cresyl phosphate affecting adolescent girls in Sri Lanka, *Lancet 1*: 88 (1981).

39. WHO, IPCS Environmental Healthy Criteria No. 104, Principles for the toxicological assessment of pesticide residues in food, World Health Organization, Geneva, 1990.

40. M.A.F.F./H.S.E., *Annual report of the Working Party on Pesticide Residues: 1991*. Supplement to the Pesticides Register, Ministry of Agriculture, Fisheries and Food/Health and Safety Executive 1992, HMSO, London, 1992.

41. Peters, H.A., Hexachlorobenzene poisoning in Turkey, *Federal Proceedings 35*: 2400 (1976).

42. WHO, Evaluation of certain veterinary drug residues in food, 38th report of the Joint FAO/WHO Expert Committee on Food Additives, Technical Report Series No. 815, World Health Organization, Geneva, 1991.

43. MAFF, Veterinary residues in animal products, 1986–1990, 33rd report of the Steering Group on Chemical Aspects of Food Surveillance, Food Surveillance Paper No. 33, Ministry of Agriculture, Fisheries and Food, HMSO, London, 1992.

44. Martinez-Navarro, J.F., Food poisoning related to the consumption of illicit beta-agonist in the liver, *Lancet 336*: 1311 (1990).

45. MAFF, Lead in food: progress report: The 27th report of the Steering Group on Food Surveillance, the Working Party on Inorganic Contaminants in Food, 3rd supplementary report on lead, Ministry of Agriculture, Fisheries and Food, HMSO, London, 1989.

46. WHO, IPCS Environmental Health Criteria No. 85, Lead—environmental aspects, World Health Organization, Geneva, 1989b.

47. Baars, A.J., H. Van Beek, and I.J.R. Visser, Lead intoxication in cattle: a case report, *Food Additives and Contaminants 9*: 357 (1992).

48. Crews, H.M., M.J. Baxter, and T. Bigwood, Lead in feed incident multi-element analysis of cattle feed and tissues by inductively coupled plasma-mass spectrometry and co-operative quality assurance scheme for lead analysis of milk, *Food Additives and Contaminants 9*: 365 (1992).

49. Skene, S.A., I.C. Dewhurst, and M. Greenberg, Polychlorinated dibenzo-p-dioxins and polychlorinated dibenzofurans: The risks to human health. A review, *Human Toxicol. 8*: 173 (1989).

50. WHO, IPCS Environmental Health Criteria No. 88, Polychlorinated dibenzo-p-dioxins and dibenzofurans, World Health Organization, Geneva, 1989c.

51. WHO, IPCS Environmental Health Criteria No. 140, Polychlorinated biphenyls and terphenyls, World Health Organization, Geneva, 1992.

52. WHO, Toxic oil syndrome: current knowledge and future perspectives. Regional Publication series No. 42, World Health Organization, Copenhagen, 1992.

53. Hawthorn, J., The occurrence of radio strontium in foodstuffs, *Proceedings of the National Society 18*: 44 (1959).

54. Fry, F.A., and A. Britcher, Doses from Chernobyl radiocaesium, *Lancet 2*: 160 (1987).

55. Mondon, K.J., and B. Walters, Measurement of radiocaesium, radio-strontium and plutonium in whole diets following deposition of radioactivity in the UK originating from the Chernobyl power plant accident, *Food Additives and Contaminants 7*: 837 (1990).

56. FASEB, The re-examination of the GRAS status of sulphiting agents. Report by Life Science Research Office of FASEB, prepared for the Center for Food Safety and Applied Nutrition, Federation of American Societies of Experimental Biology, US FDA, Washington, DC, 1985.

57. Walker, R., Toxicological aspects of food preservatives, *Nutritional and Toxicological Aspects of Food Processing*. (R. Walker and E. Quattrycci, eds.) Taylor and Francis, London, 1988, p. 25.

58. Walker, R., Nitrates, nitrites and N-nitroso compounds: a review of the occurrence in food and diet and the toxicological implications. *Food Additives and Contaminants 7*: 717 (1990).

59. WHO, Evaluation of certain food additives and contaminants, 26th report of the Joint FAO/WHO Expert Committee on Food Additives, Technical Report Series No. 683, World Health Organization, Geneva, 1982, p. 27.

60. Kwok, R.H.M., Chinese-restaurant syndrome, *New England J. Med. 278*: 796 (1968).

61. Southgate, D.A.T., Pathogenic agents in food, *Human Nutrition and Dietetics*, 9th ed. (J.S. Garrow and W.P.T. James, eds.), Churchill Livingstone, London, 1993, p. 349.

62. Moss, M.A., Microbial food poisoning, *Essays in Agriculture and Food Microbiology*. (J.R. Norris and G.L. Petripher, eds.), John Wiley, Chichester, 1987.

63. Egan, A.F., and T.A. Roberts, Microbiology of meats and meat products. *Essays in Agriculture and Food Microbiology* (J.R. Norris and G.L. Petripher, eds.), John Wiley, Chichester, 1987, p. 167.

64. Blacklow, N.R., and G. Cukor, Viral gastroenteritis, *New England J. Med. 304*: 397 (1981).

65. Passmore, R., and J.S. Robson (eds.), *A Companion to Medical Studies*, Blackwell Scientific Publications, Oxford, Vol. 3, 1974, p. 36.

66. Ferguson A., Nutrition and the immune system, *Human Nutrition and Dietetics*, 9th ed. (J.S. Garrow and W.P.T. James, eds.), Churchill Livingstone, London, 1993, p. 685.

67. AAAI and NIAID, Adverse reactions to foods, NIH Publication No. 84–2442, July 1984, American Academy of Allergy and Immunology and National Institute of Allergy and Infectious Diseases, 1984.

68. Metcalf, D., R. Simon, and H.A. Sampson (eds.), *Adverse Reactions to Foods and Food Additives*, Blockwell, Cambridge, Mass., 1992.

69. Bayless, T.M., B. Rothfield, C. Massa, et al., Lactose and milk intolerance: Clinical implications, *New England J. Med. 292*: 1156 (1975).

70. Tandon, R.K., Y.K. Joshi, D.S. Singh, et al., Lactose intolerance in North and South Indians, *Am. J. Clin. Nutr. 34*: 943 (1981).

71. Cook, G.C., Primary and secondary hypolactase (lactase deficiency), *Tropical Gastroenterology*, Oxford University Press, Oxford, 1980, p. 325.

72. Neale, G., The diagnosis, incidence and significance of disaccharidase deficiency in adults, *Proc. Royal Soc. Med. 61*: 1099 (1968).

73. Cummings, J.H. Nutritional management of diseases of the stomach and bowel, *Human Nutrition and Dietetics*, 9th ed., (J.S. Garrow and W.P.T. James, eds.), Churchill Livingstone, London, 1993, p. 480.

74. Havenberg, L., P.H. Kwon, and N.S. Scrimshaw, Comparative tolerance of adolescents of differing ethnic backgrounds to lactose-containing and lactose-free dairy drinks. I. Initial experience with a double-blind procedure, *Am. J. Clin. Nutr. 33*: 17 (1980).

17
Food Transportation, Storage, and Marketing

I. INTRODUCTION

Food is required to be transported from the place of its production to the place where it is processed and from the processing plants to warehouses where it may be temporarily stored and again from these places to the consumer through various marketing channels. The transport of raw food, such as fruits, vegetables, and other perishables to the place of processing as well as the transfer of the clean, processed food to the consumer is not a simple and speedy operation; its transit involves a variety of modes of transportation, such as carts, trucks, railroads, and ships. The food may have to travel long distances by a variety of means and it can be subjected to jolting and rough handling during transportation. Its journey may be interrupted by periods of storage prior to sale. The safe handling, transportation, storage, and distribution of food throughout its journey is a basic requirement of food production and technology.

II. FOOD TRANSPORTATION

A. Modes of Transport

Trucks, railroads, and ships constitute the major modes of food transportation all over the world. The primary users of these facilities are middlemen and food merchants, who assemble, process, store, and ship the food from large-scale food producers to other middlemen, who sell it to the retailers. A substantial quantity of food is transported on a global basis.

All modes of transport are used for hauling different food items. In most countries, transportation of food by railroads predominates, representing primarily the long-haul movement of food, whereas the short-haul movement of food from the farm to the country assembly point and retailers is mostly accomplished by trucks. The long-haul movement of food may also involve use of boats and airplanes. The food shipped by air is a high-value food such as fruits and vegetables for which the buyer is willing to pay the high cost of this premium service.

Privately owned and leased trucks are gnerally used to transport short-haul food shipments. These trucks are either owned or leased by food producers and wholesale buyers who haul foods from the farm to the country assembly point for reshipment, as well as by the retailers who distribute food to the consumers.

According to Holman and Snitzler (1), two types of leased carriers engage in food transportation in the United States: exempt carriers and regulated carriers. The distinction is based on the Motor Carrier Act of 1935, which provides exemptions for vehicles hauling nonmanufactured food commodities such as fresh fruits and vegetables, poultry, eggs, livestocks, and food grains. Exempt carriers haul only exempt commodities and are subject to rules of the Interstate Commerce Commission (ICC) as to safety and hours of service of drivers. The regulated carriers are authorized by the ICC to transport other than exempt commodities. They may haul exempt commodities but then are not subject to regulation by the ICC. Food items such as seeds serve to balance out return trips for many regulated motor carriers. Both types of motor carriers haul seeds from the production centers or warehouses of seed wholesalers to their retailers (2).

Rail transportation can save money, although sometimes it is cheaper to use trucks for either inbound or outbound trips. Convenience of loading and unloading of foods is another advantage of rail transportation. The shipper or receiver of foods has 48 hours free of charge for loading or unloading the car after it has been placed at his disposal, and any time beyond the 48 hours is chargeable as per the published demurrage rates. Also, the rail carriers can handle large shipments on long hauls at cheaper rates.

Trucks often deliver food items from the warehouse of a wholesaler to customers in less time than it would take to move them by rail. Speed of transportation is important, particularly for perishable food products and during emergency conditions such as floods and droughts.

A large portion of the food-marketing business may not require fast delivery service. However, in order to reduce storage risks and to ensure more orderly distribution, shipments of foods to the retailers are done using both rail and truck transportation. Trucks provide pickup and delivery service, which is particularly important to customers who are not near railroads. Both railcars and trucks can be partially loaded at one place, completing the loading somewhere else. They may also be stopped for unloading at more than one place. Stopping in transit to load or unload some of the food allows buyers to obtain the benefit of lower carload rates usually available on heavier shipments.

B. Food Losses During Transport

Both the shippers and carriers are responsible for taking protective care and measures to ensure that food lots arrive at their destination in satisfactory condition. The shippers are responsible for food being properly loaded and protected from ordinary transportation hazards, and carriers must deliver the food items to the destination in the same condition in which it was received.

A major cause of loss and damage to shipments such as food grains is torn sacks or bags (normally associated with railway shipment), causing losses of both the food grain and its container. Protruding nails and bolts and loose or splintered boards are common causes of torn bags during transport. Water may cause the containers to split apart, damaging the food quality. Leaky roofs, loose-fitting doors, and worn tarpaulins may lead to such damage, which occurs more frequently in truck shipments.

Industrial chemicals and oil residues not removed from the railcar or truck before loading may cause the food bags to disintegrate. The container may soak up some of the residues or take up an odor from them. Freezing injuries to certain foods such as potatoes may occur during transportation. Portable heaters may need to be placed in the truck or car for shipments of such foods in winter, taking care that they do not overheat. Food grain lot that is moved in bulk into the wholesaler's plant for further processing may suffer damage and loss during transit because of loose doors, loose or broken floorboards, or cracks in the floor.

C. Precautions and Protective Measures for Quality Preservation

The shipper must critically inspect the carrier's equipment to ensure that it is fit to haul the food material in cool and dry conditions, which are especially important in the transport of perishable food products such as fruits, vegetables, poultry, and eggs as well as for other foods. Such inspections should reveal the presence of loose or broken wallboards or floorboards, protruding nails or bolts, broken pieces of wire strapping, chemical or oil residues, or other material that might damage the food quality or its container. The shipper should ask the carrier to replace the equipment if it is found unsatisfactory.

Before loading, cars or trucks should be swept carefully and the floor, sidewalls, and ends lined with heavy paper. Special precautions need to be taken for bags or cartons of foods stacked near the doorway of a railcar, which may be strapped with heavy paper strips, reinforced at regular intervals with steel strapping, and nailed to the doorposts through prepunched holes in the strappings. For bulk shipments of foods, one-piece wooden doors or heavy duty water-repellent paperboard, reinforced with steel strapping, are placed inside the regular car doors for additional protection.

The heaviest bags should be placed on the bottom to prevent other bags from splitting open from the overhead weight. The bags should be stacked tightly together in an interlocking pattern to reduce chances of shifting the load during transit. While unloading the shipment, bags must not be dragged over the car floor and the bottom and outside layer of bags must be removed with care to avoid any possible damage. Care should be taken to remove all nails and bolts before loading, but some may work out in transit.

Food materials should be handled with great care during loading and unloading. Modern automated equipment is available for safe handling of most kinds of foods, e.g., bucket elevators to move the food grains vertically in bulk and self-cleaning vertical elevators for handling the bulk; pneumatic conveyors to carry materials through a pipe in a high-velocity stream of air; high-pressure fluidized conveyors to avoid physical damage to foods during handling; belt-conveyors to move food grains in bags or in bulk in a horizontal or inclined condition; flat-belt conveyors for bagged or packaged foods; and troughed-belt conveyors to move the food grain in bulk. Portable belt conveyors with platform elevators are used in warehouses for piling bagged food grains, removing them from the piles, and moving bagged grain into and out of the warehouse (2).

The industrial forklift is used with pallets to handle bagged or packaged food material in large warehouses having suitable floors and column arrangements. Unit loads (group of bags or packages) can be picked up and stacked by this method, enabling the transport of loads of 150 million tons or more. Forklift trucks with a capacity of 1500 to 2000 kg are suited to handle bagged food grains in many warehouses. Smooth, level floors and runways speed the movement of such trucks. Pallets form a natural base for transporting unit loads. The wooden pallet (1.2 × 1.2 m) is used widely because of its low cost, light weight, and fair durability. More costly metal skids of various types and sizes are also available. A pusher-bar installed on the front end of a forklift is used to push the food load off a pallet onto the floor of a rail car or truck. If pallets accompany rail and truck shipments, the charges for their return shipment can be sizable. Therefore, expendable, one-trip paper pallets are often used to save the cost of the return freight.

III. IDEAL FOOD STORAGE ENVIRONMENT

A. Storage of Food Grains

The principal biological agents of food deterioration during their storage are fungi and insects, whose development is influenced by the moisture content of the food material and temperature of the storage facility. Important fungi and insect pests associated with some stored food legumes (pulses and oilseeds) and cereal grains are given in Tables 1 and 2, respectively. Beetles, such as the granary weevil, bore into the food grain and lay their eggs internally; the larvae then feed on the endosperm and the embryo. In some foods, the eggs are laid on the surface and the larvae bore into the grain (3).

The limiting relative humidity (RH) for the growth of fungi is about 65% to 70%, corresponding to the equilibrium moisture content of 14% to 15% in starchy food grains and 8% to 9%

Table 1   Important Fungi Associated with Some Stored Food Legumes

Legume crop	Fungal species
Cowpea	*Aspergillus niger, Rhizoctonia bataticola, Cladosporium herbarum, A. flavus, Absidia* sp. *Rhizopus* sp.
Pea	*Aspergillus* sp.
Peanut	*A. flavus, A. parasiticus*
Phaseolus sp.	*A. glaucus, A. restricus, Penicillium* sp.
Soybean	*A. flavus, A. glaucus, A. restricus, A. ochreus, A. niger, A. fumigatus, A. repens*

Source: Ref. 3

Table 2   Important Insect Pests of Some Stored Food Grains

Order and pest	Common name
Order Coleoptera	
Sitophilus granarius	Granary weevil
S. oryzae	Rice weevil
S. zeamais	Corn (maize) weevil
Tribolium castaneum	Red flour beetle
T. confusum	Confused flour beetle
Ginathocerus cornutus	Broad-horned flour beetle
Trogoderma granarium	Khapra beetle
Steobium paniceum	Drugstore beetle
Oryzaephilus surinamensis	Saw-toothed grain beetle
Achanthosclelides obtectus	Common bean weevil
Callosobruchus sp.	Cowpea weevil
Bruchus pisorum	Pea weevil
Bruchus rufimanus	Bean weevil
Order Lepidoptera	
Ephestia kaehniella	Mediterranean flour moth
Cadra cautella	Almond moth
Plodia interpunctella	Indian meal moth
Nemupogon granellus	Grain moth

Source: Ref. 3.

in oilseeds (Table 3). Both the moisture content of the food grain and humidity within the grain air spaces determine the growth of insects (4). Insects generally do not develop at grain moisture contents equivalent to 40% RH, i.e., about 10% to 11% in starchy grains and 5% to 7% in oilseeds, but there is a considerable variation between different species of food crops (Table 3). Even if fungi and insects do not develop because of an unfavorable storage environment (too dry and too cold), food grains will still deteriorate with age and lose quality. Deterioration in quality due to aging alone becomes significant only in long-term storage of food materials but it does not seriously affect short-term (season-to-season) or reserve storage of most kinds of foods.

In addition to the moisture content of the food material and its storage temperature, availability of oxygen plays an important part, because of its role in respiration of food material. Oxygen may become limiting in hermetically sealed storage.

Table 3 Typical Moisture Content (%) of Food Grains in Equilibrium with a Range of Relative Humidities (RH)

Crop	Percent moisture at				
	30% RH	40% RH	50% RH	60% RH	70% RH
Wheat, rye	9	10	12	13	15
Barley, oats	8	10	11	12	14
Corn (maize)	9	11	12	13	14
Sorghum	9	10	11	12	14
Rice	8	9	11	12	13
Ryegrass	9	10	11	12	14
Lucerne	8	9	10	12	14
Phaseolus	7	10	12	14	16
Pea	8	10	12	13	15
Beet, onion	7	8	10	11	13
Soybean	7	7	8	10	12
Cotton	6	7	8	9	10
Brassica	5	6	7	8	9
Peanut	4	5	6	7	9

Source: Ref. 4.

Barring extreme conditions, the effects of food grain moisture and temperature can be summarized in terms of Harrington's values (5), namely, "the storage life of food grains (seeds) is halved for each 1% increase in moisture content and for every 5°C in storage temperature." These rules operate with grain moisture contents ranging from 5% to 14% and temperatures from 0° to 50°C and are independent of one another. Above 14% moisture, molds can grow on food grains, and heating can occur above 18% moisture. Insect activity is greatest between 21° and 27°C, and therefore food grains should be stored below 20°C whenever possible (6).

The ideal storage environment to preserve the high quality of food grains can be expressed simply as "dry and cool," but the material and mechanical resources required to provide this ideal storage environment vary enormously according to the prevailing climate. Duration of storage is another important variant that must be taken into account. Most food grains required to be stored do not require elaborate storage conditions, but seed stocks to be stored as planting material for more than a year will need more stringent storage conditions. A rule of thumb would be that the temperature (in °F) added to the RH should not exceed 100 (4).

In the dry hot tropics and subtropics, insects are the principal cause of deterioration of food grains. Because temperature control of large warehouses is costly and difficult, the most effective preventive measure is to dry food grains to a moisture content in equilibrium with 50% RH or even 35% in some cases (Table 3), which is not very difficult. Fumigants or contact insecticides may also be used for carryover stocks.

Of all regions, the humid tropics present the most difficult situation. It is possible to store most food grains between harvest and their resowing without air conditioning, if the temperature and RH remain below 30°C and 70%, respectively. Natural drying of food grains to a moisture content low enough for storage is possible only if the grain is exposed to the sun. Sun-drying is limited to small quantities of food grains; also it is slow and erratic. To guard against both fungi and insects under the prevailing temperatures, the grains must be dried to a moisture content in equilibrium with 40% to 50% RH, or less than 40% for carryover stocks (Table 3). The high ambient humidity will tend to increase the moisture content of the stored grain; when the humidity is not too high, cool air can be circulated to lower the temperature. The refrigeration and dehumidification necessary for long-term storage in the humid tropics are prohibitively expensive for large quantities of food grains. On a medium scale, insulated rooms filled with a capacity of about 100 tons of grains in bags have been successfully operated at 22°C and 50% RH. Because dehumidification creates heat, the refrigeration unit used should be powerful enough to counteract it (3).

Alternatively, food grains can be stored in sealed, air-tight plastic containers in the wet tropics using a high-quality polyethylene film. For this kind of storage, however, the grain must be drier than for open storage, with a moisture content in equilibrium with 30% to 40% RH or even lower for long-term storage. A slight rise in the humidity during storage (due to grain respiration) is not enough to permit mold development. Desai et al. (2) have described various methods and structures of grain (seed) storage, including conditioned storage, cryogenic storage, hermetic storage, and containerized grain storage.

Apart from grain moisture content and storage temperature, other factors influencing the grain quality during storage include initial grain quality, damage caused by rough handling, and the extent of cleaning. Grains damaged during harvesting and processing and containing a high proportion of rubbish matter—broken pieces of straw or leaf—will not store well. Grain storability is also influenced by the kind of grain and its variety, some kinds being more naturally short lived (e.g. onion, soybean, peanut) than others. However, the amount of moisture content in the food grain is the single most important factor influencing the grain quality during storage. Over the most commonly encountered grain moisture ranges, cereal grains stored at temperatures not exceeding 90°F (32.2°C) will have a storage life as shown in Table 4. (5).

Since the life span of food grains revolves around moisture content, grains should be dried to their safe moisture content to avoid losses due to mold growth (12–14%, moisture) and heating (18–20% moisture). The safe moisture content depends on kind and variety of the grain, the length of storage period desired, and the type of storage structure and packaging material employed. The use of fungicides and insecticides to protect food grains from pathogenic organisms during storage involves an element of toxicity to both the grain (e.g., seed germinability) and the consumer. Thomson (4) stated the following general rules to be observed in the management of stored seed grains:

1. The seed stocks should be kept under continuous observation, especially looking for hot spots.
2. Seeds should be fumigated between outgoing and incoming stocks.
3. Floors should be swept thoroughly and all rubbish material burned.
4. Ventilation should be encouraged within and between stocks.
5. Seed should not be piled against a wall.

Table 4   Moisture Content and Storage Life of Cereal Grains[a] at Temperatures Not Exceeding 90°F (32.2°C)

Grain moisture (%)	Storage life
11–13	6 months
10–12	1 year
9–11	2 years
8–10	4 years

[a]Grains of high germination and vigor.
Source: Ref. 5.

6. The storage house should be repaired and kept in good condition.
7. Seed showing the best storage potential should be selected for carryover stock.
8. Seed stored in bulk require frequent turnings to prevent deterioration due to heating.

B. Storage of Fruits and Vegetables

Metabolism of freshly harvested foods such as fruits and vegetables continues until an overripe stage is reached, when the produce is almost unmarketable. Although these metabolic processes cannot be stopped, they can be retarded by one or more of the following measures, both during their transportation and storage.

1   Reduction in temperature (cold storage)
2. Controlled atmospheric (CA) storage
3. Modified atmospheric (MA) storage
4. Reduced pressure (hypobaric or subatmospheric storage)

Lower holding temperatures retard the rate of respiration of food material during their storage and transport. The temperature must be maintained above the freezing point and for most tropical fruits should be at least 10°C to avoid chilling injury. The RH should preferably be 85% to 90%. Hartoungh (7) recommended temperature and RH as well as probable period of storage for a variety of fruit crops (Table 5). Storage requirements vary considerably depending on crop and stage of fruit ripeness. According to Wills et al. (8), the storage life (in weeks) of some fruits should be as follows: at 5° to 9°C—orange, 6 to 12; mandarin, 4 to 6; ripe pineapple, 4 to 5; avocado, 3 to 5; mango, 2 to 3; passionfruit, 3 to 5; and at 10°C—grapefruit, 6 to 12; lemon 12 to 20; banana, 1 to 2, and green pineapple, 4 to 5.

Table 5 Recommended Holding Conditions for Various Fruits

Fruit	Temperature (°C)	Relative humidity (%)	Period[a]
Orange	1–7	85–90	1–6 mo
Mandarin	4–7	85–90	3–12 wk
Grapefruit	10–15	85–90	3–13 wk
Lemon			
Green	11–14	85–90	1–4 mo
Yellow	0–10	85–90	3–6 wk
Lime	8–10	85–90	3–8 wk
Banana			
Green	11–14	90–95	10–20 d
Ripe	13–16	85–90	5–10 d
Pineapple			
Green	10	90	2–4 wk
Ripe	5–10	85–90	2–6 wk
Avocado	5–13	85–90	2–4 wk
Brazil nuts	0	70	8–12 mo
Cashew	0–1	85–90	4–5 wk
Guava	7–10	85–90	3–4 wk
Mango	7–10	85–90	4–7 wk
Papaya	4–10	85–90	2–5 wk
Passionfruit	5–7	80–85	4–5 wk

[a]d = days, wk = weeks, mo = months
Source: Ref. 7.

Low-temperature storage decreases ethylene production and lowers the rate of response of the fruit to the applied ethylene. Storage at high RH may predispose the produce to microbial infection, causing decays and rots. A compromise is generally effected by providing adequate air movement via ventilation and using moderately high RH for the freshness of the stored product. Lutz and Hardenburg (9) determined the optimum storage temperature and RH for several tropical fruits. Fidler and Coursey (10) reviewed the effects of low-temperature injury in different tropical and subtropical fruits. Banana and grapefruit often suffer chilling injury at low temperature storage, resulting in decays as pathogens enter the weakened tissue. Chilling injury of grapefruit can be reduced by holding fruits at high RH (more than 90%) and hypobaric storage (11), by thiabendazole and benomyl treatments (12), and by applying benomyl several months before harvest (13). Grierson (14) noted that the green citrus fruits were most susceptible to chilling injury, the yellow ones somewhat less so, and the orange fruits most resistant.

The general compatibility of temperature and humidity requirements for fresh produce must be observed carefully during transport and storage. Lipton and Harvey (15) classified fruit compatibility along with the recommended temperatures and relative humidities during transport for each group of fruits (Table 6). The following four types of compatibility must be taken into consideration while storing or transporting mixed loads.

1. *Temperature compatibility*: Differences in temperatures needed for various products in a load; e.g., strawberries must be kept near 0°C and hence should not be shipped with summer squash, cucumbers, or tomatoes, all of which are sensitive to chilling injury below about 12.5°C.
2. *Ethylene production and sensitivity compatibility*: Commodities that produce large amounts of ethylene, e.g., apples, pears, avocados and certain musk-melons, should not be shipped with commodities that are very sensitive to ethylene, e.g., broccoli, carrots, lettuce, kiwi fruit, and most ornamentals and flowers. The incidence of russet spotting on lettuce (caused by exposure to ethylene) is about three times greater in mixed loads than in straight loads in truck shipments.
3. *Product odor compatibility*: Some food products produce odors (e.g., onions and garlic) that can be absorbed by other products, causing the latter to have an objectionable odor and decreased consumer acceptability.

Table 6 Grouping of Compatible Fruits for Transport in Mixed Loads

Group 1 (1.0–1.1°C 90–95% RH)	Group 2 (12.8–18.3°C, 85–90% RH)	Group 3 (2.2–5.0°C, 90–95% RH)
Apple	Avocado	Cranberry
Apricot	Banana	Lemon
Berries (except cranberry)	Grapefruit	Litchi
Cherries	Guava	Orange
Fig	Lime	Tangerine
Peach	Mango	
Pear	Olive	
Persimmon	Papaya	
Plum	Pineapple	
Pomegranate		
Quince		

Source: Ref. 15.

4. *Moisture compatibility*: Some food products benefit from package-ice or a high RH in the ambient atmosphere, e.g., leafy vegetables, sweet corn and berries, while other commodities benefit from intermediate humidity levels, e.g., garlic and dry onions. Humidity control is especially important during long transit periods (16,17).

As an adjunct to low-temperature storage or a substitute for refrigeration, the addition or removal of gases resulting in an atmosphere different from that of normal air—as in controlled atmosphere (CA), modified atmosphere (MA), or subatmospheric (hypobaric or low-pressure) storage—has been widely employed to extend the shelf life of fruits, vegetables and other perishable foods. These methods aim at reducing respiration and other metabolic reactions by increasing the CO_2 and decreasing the O_2 concentrations. They also lower the rate of natural ethylene production (as in fruits such as banana), as well as the fruits sensitivity to ethylene. Controlled atmospheres with high CO_2 inhibit breakdown of pectic substances and retain fruit texture, firmness, and flavor for a long period (18). Not all fruits, however, respond favorably to atmospheric regulation, and some are little affected by CA or MA storage. The use of these techniques is advantageous where the produce is harvested over a relatively short period and where increasing the shelf life of high-value foods can improve their marketability. CA storage, being expensive, is advocated only when there is a distinct financial gain from its use (16–20). Hypobaric storage is a form of atmospheric control in which the food produce is stored in a partial vacuum. The vacuum chamber is vented continuously with water-saturated air to maintain desirable O_2 levels and minimize water loss. Reductions in the partial pressure of oxygen as well as in ethylene levels delays fruit ripening, extending shelf life (16,17,21–23).

Like fruits, vegetables also must be stored to ensure their continual supply through seasons when fresh produce is not available. Market prices reflect the availability of the produce and the cost of transportation. Vegetable storage may range from short-term (one day, in the case of lettuce and other leafy vegetables) to long-term storage (e.g., onions may be stored throughout the entire winter and spring). Only clean and healthy produce should be stored for prolonged periods, keeping the food material free from diseases and insect pests. Disease infections can occur long before the food crop enters the store; e.g., neck rot (*Botrytis allii*) of onion, contracted in the field, may cause serious storage losses (18).

Grading, sorting, and appropriate packing of foods is essential before its long-term storage. Grading or sorting may be limited to removal of splits, punctures, deformed fruits, and incipient rots. Effective packaging is necessary to assemble the produce in convenient units for handling and transport and protect it during the subsequent storage and marketing operations. Precooling and commodity treatments, such as waxing of fruits, disinfection (fumigation) or the use of fungicides and growth regulators are employed to prolong the shelf life of fresh fruits.

Considerable developments are taking place in the area of packaging and containerization of foods, newer techniques and packaging materials being added every year. The use of laminates and plastics has increased in recent years. There are many types of flexible material used singly or in combination. Fruits to be cold-stored are wrapped in flexible film, and a mixture of gases is then inserted to delay postharvest biochemical changes (gas flushing). Salunkhe and Desai (17) have reviewed these developments in food packaging technology, discussing such aspects of packaging materials as mechanical strength for adequate protection of food; their inherent toxicity; handling and marketing requirements in terms of weight, size, and shape related to packaging; and standardization for mechanical handling. Rapid cooling of the food material in its package, permeability of plastic films to respiratory gases, and cost of the package in relation to the value of the food material are the most important factors (24,25).

Salunkhe and Desai (26) have described various prestorage treatments such as precooling, hydrocooling, vacuum cooling, curing, and treatment with ethylene to prolong the storage life of vegetables. Leafy vegetables are difficult to cool with water or air refrigeration but they can be field-packed and then cooled rapidly and uniformly by vacuum cooling, i.e., by reducing the atmospheric pressure in hermetically sealed chambers until the reduced vaporizing point of water cools the produce. The speed and uniformity of cooling are the obvious advantages of this system. Other vegetables adapted to vacuum cooling are globe artichoke, asparagus, broccoli, brussels sprout, cabbage, celery, sweet corn, and peas (27).

Nagy and Wardowski (28) have reviewed the effects of various storage methods on the nutritional composition of fruit crops. Grierson and Wardowski (29) studied the length of holding after harvest and the usual cause of the end of storage life of several fruits and vegetables. Overmaturity and the resulting decay during prolonged storage lead, in turn, to a virtually complete loss of nutrients in fruits. Most storage studies with fruits have reported changes in keeping quality, decay, and weight loss, and in the case of citrus, changes in sugar and acid content.

IV. FOOD MARKETING AND DISTRIBUTION

The basis of food marketing is that food must be stored, transported, processed, and delivered in the form, at the time, and to the places that consumers desire to purchase it. These functions are performed more and more by specialists and less and less by food growers and farmers. Their competition for the consumers' money encourages efficiency. The price of the food product is decided by the wholesalers and retailers. Although marketing begins at the farm gate, many things happen afterward: assembling the fresh produce, transportation, preparation, storage shifting and sharing risks, changes in ownership, pricing and exchange, wholesaling, and retailing. Seeking the consumers' favor, expressed through their purchases, is a major activity of marketing. Producers, handlers, wholesalers, retailers, and processors have come to appreciate more and more the importance of knowing what consumers want to buy.

Agricultural food crops follow many paths from the producer to the consumer, as shown in the generalized food-marketing scheme (Fig. 1). According to Copeland and McDonald (30), marketing of food grains may be simple or complex, involving several contributive functions. The simplest marketing cycle is completed when the producer sells the food material to his or her neighbour. Marketing of most food, however, calls for a more sophisticated chain of events when the food enters the marketing channel, similar to that illustrated in Fig. 1.

A. Marketing Requirements and Research

Most of the agriculturally produced food is a perishable commodity of high value and is expensive to produce, store, and transport food, its production must be geared to realistic marketing and distribution targets. While assessing marketing requirements, one must answer the following questions (31):

1. How much, where, and when is the food needed?
2. What standards of quality are required?
3. At what price can it be sold?

Only after getting answers to these questions, can one plan both the scale and the timing of food production to meet the expected market demand.

Based on crop statistics, cropping area and local food demand, it is easy to compute the total food requirement for a particular crop in a specific country. In addition to the total food requirement of a state or country, it is also necessary to know what proportion of food can be exported to other countries. Such estimates require market research.

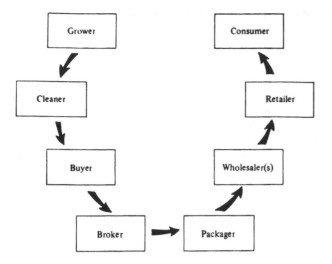

Figure 1 A generalized food-marketing scheme. (From Ref. 30.)

Food production also needs to be planned to make fresh food materials such as fruits and vegetables available continuously, for both local and outside markets.

B. Quality Control and Food Standards

Both the consumer's needs and the difficulty and cost involved must be taken into consideration when deciding on the standards of food quality required. The quality standards should have a real practical value for the food producer. Whereas too high standards will increase the cost of food production, too low standards will not serve a useful purpose to the consumer. The desire to make claims for a high-quality standard as an aid to sales usually conflicts with the realistic situation in relation to its actual needs, often necessitating a compromise between the two.

The price of food should include all direct and indirect costs of its production plus a reasonable profit, with a regard to what the consumer will pay. The consumer must be able to perceive some benefit at the price of food being asked.

The postwar farming revolution throughout Europe and North America resulted in a substantial increase in food production, bringing down prices. This was brought about through proliferation in agricultural research institutes and boosting government subsidies to farmers, linked to the development of free national agricultural advisory services. Marketing boards and farming cooperatives were established. Tax advantages and price support schemes to producers ensured maximum food production, e.g., milk, butter, cheese, cream, meat, poultry as well as food grains. Food mountains of unsold food had to be stored before being disposed. The United States and EEC began to compete on the world market, selling butter, cereals, beef, and other foods below world prices to the former Soviet Union and Eastern Europe. By maintaining high food prices for Western farmers and selling cheaply abroad, farmers in most developing countries were at a disadvantage because they had little incentive to produce food crops for export. In the 1990s, the Europeans attempted to adjust their subsidy policies, while arguing with the United States, Australia, and other countries about their need to maintain the viability of the farming community. According to James (32), this is part of the adjustment of the European Community's Agriculture Policy (CAP) to the General Agreement on Tariffs and Trade (GATT) as part of longstanding international trading agreement.

The social and economic pressures on the urban communities of the developing countries have brought about dietary changes, such as an increase in the intakes of fat, sugar, and salt. With the postwar emphasis on improving food production for a balanced diet, it was also important to ensure that the foods were safe in terms of their toxicological and compositional content, requiring development of complex regulatory procedures (see Chapters 13 through 16). On an international basis, FAO and WHO established a standing committee, known as Codex Alimentarius, composed mostly of industrial food technologists and toxicologists, to agree with the internationally binding regulations on analytical methods, food labeling issues, and toxicological problems.

The emphasis on regulatory aspects of food safety, combined with consumer choice, has led the food industry and the governments to agree on a common basis of food labeling (Chapter 15), including standard displays of the absolute amounts of nutrients per 100 g of food product. These labels were made meaningful for consumers, justifying fortification policies and health claims, by agreeing to present the weights and units of each nutrient in terms of the national or internationally accepted and scientifically determined values for the requirements of each nutrient. These values are traditionally set as the recommended dietary allowances (RDA).

Compositional standards were originally introduced as a form of consumer protection, so that food products could be guaranteed to have a minimum content of meat, fat, or fruit (Chapter 15). The need to guarantee the quality of food stemmed from concern about having enough protein, energy, or other nutrients such as vitamins and minerals in a food and to prevent the adulteration of good-quality products. Regulations had to be introduced specifying standards for production of traditional food products, such as cheeses. Regulations were then made to protect special foods or drinks from being copied through the patent laws.

C. The Food Industry, Food Retailing, and Supermarkets

With postwar national priorities for cheap food production, the food industries in North America and Northern Europe blossomed spectacularly. Luxury food items, such as confectionery, cakes, biscuits, butter, cream, cheese, meat, and other more unusual foods, became more readily available at a price most people could afford.

In most Western countries, World War II brought women to play a major role in national economic activity. This new-found freedom, amplified by the widespread introduction of reliable forms of contraception, brought women into jobs before, during, and after their childbearing years. The demand for simplification of food preparation and cooking, thus opened up a major opportunity for the sale of kitchen gadgets, refrigerators, and a variety of labor-saving devices. Foods that could be bought in bulk, preserved for longer periods of time, and then easily and quickly cooked were in great demand. As the purchasing power of the consumer increased, seasonal foods became available throughout the year, as air, rail, and road transport were revolutionized to move foods in chilled or frozen form across continents and half-way round the world. Food manufacturers offered traditional foods in newly packaged forms: in tins, plastic containers, vacuum packs, and ready-cooked varieties of dishes. The challenge for a food manufacturer was to establish a market niche and develop specific brands of foods to retain consumer loyalty. Food was no longer a matter of survival and health, but a pleasure, with major social connotations.

With market pressures increasing, more than 70% of all the foods consumed in Northern Europe and the United States was processed, preserved, and/or packaged in some way. Consumers had to pay higher prices for the "value-added" food products, in return for their preservation or modification into some "appetizing" food produced in a form that is more convenient in purchasing, preservation, or serving terms (convenience foods). Thus, consumption of potatoes in the form of chips and crisps has increased, rather than in their fresh state. Also, consumption of sugar products, such as soft drinks, ice creams, and confectionery, has increased.

The food industry has developed products that are rich in sugar, salt, and fat. New processing techniques have improved the flavor of products with added sugars, fats, salt, and species. Poorer sections of the community thus had access to readily available, attractively packaged, cheap foods.

Major national and international food companies began to control networks of wholesale and retail outlets, which resulted in an intense competition, leading to a major source of advertising revenue for television and radio companies, through marketing of these new foods and drinks.

Most Western countries have seen profound changes in food production, processing, and distribution. The traditional selling of the produce to local distributors or to individual village shops has been converted into a highly organized purchasing and retailing business, as is seen in the United States. With improvement in the standard of living, most people have a car and find it convenient to shop once a week or even once a month, instead of daily. The efficiency of supermarkets means cheaper food, often of a high quality and in a far greater variety than could be bought at a small local shop. During the 1970s and 1980s the distribution and selling of foods was revolutionized, with supermarkets accounting for about three-quarters or more of all food sales in the United Kingdom and the United States. Supermarket buyers have accelerated the fall in food prices and forced even more efficient ways of providing foods. Supermarkets have now begun to realize that they can sell more profitably by concentrating on the quality of their products. The West thus seems to be changing from a cheap food policy based on older concerns to food being chosen by consumers as a social and enjoyable feature of life, to which are now added new concerns for human health. According to James (32), eatings for health is once more on the national agenda of the Western countries, for almost the first time since World War II.

REFERENCES

1. Holman, L.E., and J.R. Snitzer, Transporting, handling and storing seeds, *Seeds: The Yearbook of Agriculture*, U.S. Department of Agriculture, Washington, D.C. 1961, p. 338.
2. Desai, B.B., P.M. Kotecha, and D.K. Salunkhe, *Seeds Handbook: Biology, Production, Processing and Storage*, Marcel Dekker, New York, 1997, p. 532.
3. Deshpande, U.S., and S.S. Deshpande, Legumes, *Foods of Plant Origin: Production, Technology and Human Nutrition* (D.K. Salunkhe and S.S. Deshpande, eds.), Van Nostrand Reinhold, New York, 1991, p. 137.
4. Thomson, J.R., *An Introduction to Seed Technology*, Leonard Hill, London, 1979.
5. Harrington, J.F., and J.E. Douglas, *Seed Storage and Packaging: Applications for India*, National Seeds Corporation, New Delhi, 1970.
6. Kelly, A.F., *Seed Production of Agricultural Crops*. Longman Scientific and Technical, New York, 1988.
7. Hartoungh, J.C.C., Bewaring van vruchten en gronten in de tropen, Lecture notes, Wageningen, 1978 (unpublished).
8. Wills, R.B.H., T.H. Lee, D. Graham, W.B. McGlasson, and E.G. Hall, Postharvest: *An Introduction to the Physiology and Handling of Fruits and Vegetables*, Granada, London, 1981.
9. Lutz, J.M., and R.E. Hardenburg, The commercial storage of fruits, vegetables and florist and nursery stocks, *Agriculture* Handbook No. 66 US GPO, Washington, D.C. 1968.
10. Fidler, J.C., and D.G. Coursey, Low temperature injury in tropical fruit, Proc Conf. on Tropical and Subtropical Fruits, 15–19 Sept. 1969, Tropical Products Institute, London, 1969.
11. Burg, S.P., and E.A. Burg, Fruit storage at subatmospheric pressure, *Science 153*:314 (1966).
12. Schiffman-Nadel, M., E. Chalutz, J. Waks, and M. Dagan, Reduction of chilling injury in grapefruit by thiobendazole and benomyl during longterm storage, *J. Am. Soc. Hortic. Sci. 100*: 270 (1975).

13. Wardowski, W.F., L.G. Albrigo, W.P. Grierson, C.R. Barmore, and T.A. Wheaton, Chilling injury and decay of grapefruit as affected by thiabendazole, benomyl and CO_2, *Hort Science 10*: 381 (1975).

14. Grierson, W.P., Preservation of citrus fruits, *Refrig. Serv. Eng. Soc. Sect. 7*: 1 (1976).

15. Lipton, W.J., and J.M. Harvey, Compatibility of fruits and vegetables during transport of mixed load, *Agri. Res. Sta. Bull.* No. 1, USDA, Washington, DC, 1972.

16. Salunkhe, D.K., and B.B. Desai, *Postharvest Biotechnology of Fruits*, Vols. 1 & 2, CRC Press, Boca Raton, FL, 1984a.

17. Salunkhe, D.K., and B.B. Desai, *Postharvest Biotechnology of Vegetables*, Vols. 1 & 2, CRC Press, Boca Raton, FL, 1984.

18. Desai, B.B., and D.K. Salunkhe, Fruits and Vegetables, *Foods of Plant Origin: Production, Technology and Human* Nutrition (D.K. Salunkhe and S.S. Deshpande, eds.), Van Nostrand Reinhold, New York, 1991, p. 301.

19. Do, J.Y., and D.K. Salunkhe, Controlled atmosphere storage. I. Biochemical considerations, *Postharvest Physiology, Handling and Utilization of Tropical and Subtropical Fruits and Vegetables* (E.B. Pantastico, ed.), AVI Publishing Co., Westport, 1975, p. 175.

20. Ulrich, R., Controlled atmosphere II. Physiological and practical consideration, *Postharvest Physiology, Handling and Utilization of Tropical and Subtropical Fruits and Vegetables* (E.B. Pantastico, ed.), AVI Publishing Co. Westport, 1975, p. 186.

21. Salunkhe, D.K., and M.T. Wu, Effect of subatmospheric pressure storage on ripening behaviour and some chemical changes in certain deciduous fruits, *J. Am. Hortic. Sci. 98*: 113 (1973).

22. Salunkhe, D.K., and M.T. Wu, Subatmospheric storage of fruits and vegetables, *Postharvest Biology and Handling of Fruits and Vegetables* (N.F. Haard and D.K. Salunkhe, eds.), AVI Publishing Co., Westport, 1975, p. 153.

23. Burg, S.P., Hypobaric storage and transportation of fresh fruits and vegetables, *Postharvest Biology and Handling of Fruits and Vegetables* (N.F. Haard and D.K. Salunkhe, eds.), AVI Publishing Co., Westport, 1975, p. 172.

24. Hardenburg, R.E., Principles of packaging I. General considerations, *Postharvest Physiology, Handling and Utilization of Tropical Fruits and Vegetables* (E.B. Pantastico, ed.), AVI Publishing Co., Westport, 1975, p. 283.

25. Hall, C.W., R.E. Hardenburg, and E.B. Pantastico, Principles of Packaging. II: Consumer packaging with plastics, *Postharvest Physiology, Handling and Utilization of Tropical and Subtropical Fruits and Vegetables* (E.B. Pantastico, ed.), AVI Publishing Co., Westport, 1975, p. 303.

26. Salunkhe, D.K., and B.B. Desai, Effects of agricultural practices, handling, processing and storage on vegetables, *Nutritional Evaluation of Food Processing*, 3rd ed. (E. Karmas and R.S. Harris, eds.), AVI/Van Nostrand Reinhold, New York, 1988, p. 23.

27. Ryall, A.L., and W.J. Lipton, *Handling, Transportation and Storage of Fruits and Vegetables*, Vol. 1, 2nd ed., AVI Publishing Co., Westport, 1979.

28. Nagy, S., and F. Wardowski, Effects of agricultural practices, handling, processing and storage on fruits, *Nutritional Evaluation of Food Processing*, 3rd ed. (E. Karmas and R.S. Harris, eds.), AVI/Van Nostrand Reinhold, New York, 1988, p. 73.

29. Grierson, W., and W.F. Wardowski, Relative humidity effects on postharvest life of fruits and vegetables, *Hort Science 13*: 570 (1978).

30. Copeland, L.O., and M.B. McDonald, *Principles of Seed Science and Technology*, 3rd ed., Chapman & Hall, New York, 1995.

31. Kelly, A.F., *Seed Production of Agricultural Crops*, Longman Scientific and Technical, New York, 1988.

32. James, W.P.T., Historical perspective, *Human Nutrition and Dietetics*, 9th ed., (J.S. Garrow and W.P.T. James, eds.), Churchill Livingstone, Edinburgh, London, 1993, p. 1.

18
Adequacy of Diet

I. INTRODUCTION

Adequacy of diet for fitness and health is like chasing a moving target because the appetite does not have a solely scientific basis. This is so partly because eating is a social act. It is often said that "all animals feed but humans alone eat." Humans also like and dislike individual foods for other than sociological reasons. Fallon and Rozin (1) categorized food rejection into the following four types, each with its own profile of psychological characteristics.

1. *Distaste*, a sensory rejection with no objection to the presence of such food in the body or in untastable amounts of other food
2. *Disgust*, based on what the substance *is* with an objection to having it in the body or in other foods
3. *Danger*, based on anticipated harmful consequences of eating the food
4. *Inappropriate*, the substances which are not considered to be food.

Image is another important aspect in food choice (2) Hertzler et al. (3) stated the following examples of some image foods: supercultural foods or prestige foods (snobbish, exotic, gourmet); body image food (beautiful, athletic); reward foods (good behavior, success); status food (rich, elite); magic foods (cure-all, quick weight loss), and foods for sickness. In addition to these critical effectors of food choice, Clydesdale (4) pointed out that "purchase appeal" also must be considered within the framework of such factors as nutrition, cost, safety, availability, convenience, and quality. It is thus obvious that the consumer is faced with many questions when making food choices—adequacy of diet probably being given only a minor importance. These questions, along with a barrage of alternative advice offered by government, academics, industry, consumer groups, self-appointed nutritionists, exercise gurus, neighbors, and myriad other sources, often result in confusion and frustration.

Choosing a healthy and adequate diet requires checking the composition of one's diet to compare it with the nutritional needs of the body. A healthy diet is a varied diet and perhaps the healthiest way to eat is to consume a wide variety of foods, restricted to the caloric needs of the body. The basic four group plan may help one to choose an adequate diet: two servings from the meat group (meat, fish, poultry, eggs, nuts, and beans); two from the milk group; four from the vegetable-fruit group (including one good source of vitamin C per day and one of vitamin A every other day); and four servings from bread-cereal group. More recently, a fifth group including fats, sweets, and alcohol, has been added (2). Simple as it may look, this system may be misused if foods are chosen unwisely.

II. DIET DURING PREGNANCY AND LACTATION

A continuum of adjustments in maternal body composition, metabolism, and the functions of different physiological systems form the basis of successful pregnancy and lactation (5). A diet meeting the maternal nutritional needs is required for these adjustments to safeguard maternal well-being with the birth of a healthy, thriving infant. Garza (5) listed several factors that influence both maternal and infant outcomes (Table 1).

Nutritional needs during pregnancy and lactation are presented for distinct physiological states, pregnancy normally being divided into quarters of 10 weeks or trimesters of about 13 weeks' duration, though duration of lactation is highly variable. The infants are, in general, expected to be predominantly breast-fed for the first 4 to 6 months and may be partially breast-fed, for periods up to 2 or 3 years', infants thus have varying nutritional needs during these periods.

According to FAO/WHO/UNU (6), the estimations of nutrient needs during pregnancy and lactation are based on the principle that they should conform with long-term health and in terms of energy should allow for the maintenance of "economically necessary and socially desirable physical activity". The goal of promoting the well-being of not one individual but two (mother and fetus, or infant) often complicates the estimate. The nutritional well-being of the fetus and the exclusively breast-fed infant depends totally on the mother. For some nutrients, the infant's nutritional status is maintained solely at the expense of the mother; for some nutrients, mother and offspring compete more evenly; and for others, the infant may suffer more severe consequences of deficiency than the mother.

The nutritional needs are often estimated by factorial approaches, balance methods, and dietary surveys of presumably well-nourished populations. The factorial approaches are commonly used to estimate nutrient needs during pregnancy and lactation, by adding the extra nutrient needs imposed by pregnancy and lactation to the baseline estimates for nonpregnant, nonlactating women. Thus, to estimate energy needs during lactation, the sum of energy secreted into milk and the energy required to synthesize all the milk components must be calculated. The difference between the energy cost of milk production and secretion and the energy represented by the weight lost during lactation is added to the baseline energy needs of nonpregnant, nonlactating women (5).

Table 1 Factors Influencing Maternal and Infant Outcomes

Demographic/socio-economic/lifestyle characteristics	Medical history	Previous reproductive history	Complications	
			Intrapartum	Postpartum
Maternal age	Chronic diseases,	Spontaneous abortion	Premature rupture	Mastitis
Unwanted pregnancy	such as diabetes,	Premature delivery	of aminiotic sac	Nipple erosion
Education	hypertension,	Uterine anomalies	membranes	Breast engorgement
Income	anatomical	Unsuccessful attempt	Amnionitis	
Illicit drug addiction	abnormalities of	to breast-feed	Vaginal bleeding	
Alcohol consumption	the mammary			
Smoking	gland			

Source: Ref. 5.

A. Physiological Changes During Pregnancy and Lactation

The amount of weight gained and change in body's composition primarily determine the extra energy and nutrient needs during pregnancy, the amount of weight gained significantly influencing the pregnancy outcomes. Mother's pregnancy weight also influences the gestational weight gain associated with a desirable pregnancy outcome, i.e., a full-term infant weighing 3 to 4 kg. A greater gain is required in women with a low prepregnancy body mass index (BMI) to achieve a desirable birth weight (7).

Various sociodemographic characteristics significantly influence the gestational weight gain. The individual factors influencing weight gain include maternal age, genetics, and ethnicity; socioeconomic factors are diet, smoking, physical activity, and prepregnancy weight-for-height.

The rate of weight gain varies considerably during the course of pregnancy. About 5% of the total is normally gained in the first quarter, the remainder being gained fairly evenly during the rest of the period. The distribution of weight gain among maternal and fetal tissues indicates that of the total weight increased, about 62% is water, with increased blood volume accounting for about 10% and extracellular fluid for 13%, the fat and protein contributing about 30% and 8%, respectively (8). The gain in body water is larger than that occurring during normal weight gain. Thus, measurements of body composition relying on assumption of a constant proportion of water in lean tissue are difficult to evaluate. Gains in maternal body fat are also neither constant during pregnancy, nor are distributed uniformly (9). The adipose tissue accumulates most rapidly in midpregnancy, the most marked increase in body fat occurring in abdominal, subscapular, and upper thigh areas. The fetus accounts for about 25% of the total weight gained, but for only about 10% of the fat; placental tissues together gain about 60% of the protein (8).

The changes in body composition during lactation are not well known. However, the expansion of extracellular and blood volumes during pregnancy are not reversed immediately after delivery, though there is a modest increase in plasma volume during lactation both in humans and animals. The adipose tissue gained during early part of pregnancy meets the needs of fetal growth in the last quarter of gestation and the enhanced energy demands of lactation. Breast-feeding is, therefore, regarded as potentially beneficial in preventing the progressive weight gain and obesity associated with multiple pregnancies. However, the food intake also usually increases during lactation, and the difference between total expenditure and energy intake is not great enough to ensure the loss of all the fat gained during pregnancy. Heinig et al. (10) observed that women in western societies who breast-fed their infants exclusively during the first 4 to 6 months lost 0.6 to 0.8 kg/month, the rate of weight loss slowing in later stages. The energy content of the weight lost during lactation varies among individuals (11,12); more than 90% of loss is only fat, the subscapular and suprailiac fat depots being the most labile.

B. Energy Requirements

It is estimated that the average energy cost of pregnancy is about 293 MJ for women who have a pregnancy weight of about 60 kg (13); about 60% of this energy is required for the development of the fetus and maternal tissues, and the remaining 40% is due to a higher BMR and the extra cost of moving a heavier body. Both the maternal weight gain and increases in BMR, however, vary greatly among women living in diverse environments (Table 2). The data reported in Table 2 show about fourfold difference in the energy content of maternal adipose tissue gained during pregnancy, and an eightfold difference in BMRs. The energy content of the fetal and maternal tissues approached the expected 167 MJ only for women in Scotland.

The basal metabolism is expected to increase its activities during pregnancy, because of the enhanced metabolic activity of maternal and fetal tissues and the extract work done by the mater-

Table 2 Energy Requirements of Pregnancy as Estimated in Five Countries

	Energy cost and additional intake during pregnancy (MJ)				
Factors	Scotland	Netherlands	Gambia	Thailand	Philippines
Energy cost					
Fetus	34	34.5	30	30	29
Placenta	3	3.1	2	2.5	2.5
Subtotals	37	37.6	32	32.5	31.5
Maternal tissues	12	12.3	10	10.5	10
Maternal fat	106	59.9	28	64.5	60
Subtotals	118	72.2	38	75	70
Basal metabolism	126	144.2	8	100.5	79.5
Total energy cost	281	254	78	208	181

Source: Ref. 14.

nal cardiovascular, renal, respiratory, and other systems. Nevertheless, metabolic efficiency during pregnancy may change at low planes of energy status, as seen in the women of Gambia (Table 2) (14).

The postprandial thermogenesis is usually reduced in well-fed pregnant and lactating women, which appears to be another metabolic adaptation occurring during pregnancy. The energy saving on this account may not exceed more than 2% to 5% of the total food eaten (15).

With the potential for metabolic adaptation and changes in physical activity, the known costs of accumulating the extra tissues during pregnancy may not match with a need to increase food intake by an equivalent amount. The direct measurements of food intake in pregnancy therefore often show only a small increase in late pregnancy (16). Despite these observations, it would be unwise to assume that pregnancy does not require an increase in intake. Food supplements often benefit maternal weight gain and infant birth weight in the most undernourished women. It is thus not surprising that committees differ in their assessment of the extra energy needs of pregnancy. Whereas FAO/WHO/UNO (6) recommended the highest increment of 1.3 MJ, 300 kcal/day throughout the pregnancy, the UK panel recommended only 0.84 MJ (300 kcal) daily for the last trimester. Fasting is not advisable during pregnancy, because there is a more rapid fall in circulating glucose, insulin, and gluconeogenic amino acids than in nonpregnant fasting women (17). Fasting accelerates production of ketone bodies, which may be transferred to the fetus, leading to possible fetal metabolic derangements and even brain damage.

Lactation requires much more energy than pregnancy, with about one month's lactation being equivalent to the full cost of pregnancy, not counting the maternal fat storage. The energy content of the milk produced is the major determinant of the extra energy needed during lactation. Milk production in well-nourished women is about 600 to 750 ml/day for the first 4 to 6 months of full lactation. The gross energy content of milk is approximately 2.8 kJ/ml or 2.1 MJ/day. Considering the 80% to 90% efficiency range of milk production (18), the energy cost to synthesize 750 ml milk would be 0.1 to 0.5 MJ/day, depending upon efficiency.

The BMR falls to normal levels after delivery in well-nourished women, but the low BMR in some women (Gambia) can persist into lactation if the usual diet is maintained (19). The estimates of cost of milk synthesis and secretion vary (15,20), thus the estimates of the full energy costs of lactation do not allow for changes in BMR or PPT. In the first 6 months of full lactation, the energy costs vary from 2.2 MJ (525 kcal/day) to 2.6 MJ (625 kcal/day). Assuming that 146 MJ (35000 kcal) are stored in adipose tissue during pregnancy and are mobilized during lactation for 6 months, energy costs would be offset by about 0.84 MJ (200 kcal/day). Therefore, an additional dietary energy of about 1.4 to 1.8 MJ (325–425 kcal/day) above prepregnant levels would be necessary during lactation.

Successful lactation with a gradual weight reduction is possible, at a rate of 2 kg/month, without affecting volume or composition (21), though more rapid weight loss is not advisable. It is difficult to establish relationship between total energy intake and milk production due to variation in the body size, BMR, physical activity, and the demands of infants in women; poorly nourished women generally produce less milk (22). Under normal dietary conditions, the total intake of dietary protein, carbohydrate, or fat do not seem to have any detectable impact on either milk quantity or quality, although the fatty acid composition of diet does affect the composition of milk fat. Undernourished women produce more milk when supplemented during either pregnancy or lactation. The most severe effects on milk production are observed when poor intakes during pregnancy are followed by poor intakes during lactation (5).

C. Protein Requirements

Extra protein during pregnancy is gained at a variable rate, with a marked increase seen during the second trimester, slowing down in the last. A total of about 925 g of protein can be accumulated during pregnancy. From these assessments of protein storage, it is possible to estimate protein requirements and dietary allowances during pregnancy (Table 3). The average rate of nitrogen accumulation is first estimated, and this value is then increased by 30% to cover the +2 SD limits of the variability in protein accumulation expected in healthy women. Their variable needs are estimated from the ±15% CV in birthweight, this allowance further being adjusted based on a 70% conversion efficiency of dietary protein to body protein.

People with a ready access to food normally consume more protein than the RDAs/RNIs, but the protein supplements given to mothers in developing countries did not increase the amounts stored (23,24).

The protein losses of lactation are also calculated by the factorial method based on milk volumes of 750 ml/day for the first 6 months and 600 ml/day thereafter. Assuming 1.1 g/dl mean protein concentration, with a 30% variability in milk production and an efficiency of 70% (0.70) conversion, the RDIs are estimated at 15 g protein/day for first 6 months of full lactation and 12 g/day thereafter (25).

D. Fat Requirements

Essential fatty acids are thought to play a role in pregnancy; they are transferred by placenta to sustain fetal cell division and brain growth. Olsen et al. (26) assessed the role of *n*-3 fatty acids in

Table 3 Safe Levels of Additional Protein During Pregnancy

Trimester	N gain (g/d)[a] Average	N gain (g/d)[a] (+ 30%)	Efficiency[b] (0.70)	Additional protein required (g/day)[c]
First	0.104	0.14	0.20	1.2
Second	0.525	0.68	0.98	6.1
Third	0.922	1.20	1.71	10.7

[a]Estimated tissue *N* gained in a pregnancy producing a 3.3 kg infant, cv of birth weight 15%.
[b]Assuming 70% efficiency of conversion of dietary to tissue protein.
[c]In terms of absorbed protein.
Source: Ref. 6

altering the time of delivery and in promoting fetal growth. The long chain *n*-3 fatty acids are particularly needed for neuronal structures and the fetal requirements are high in the later stages of pregnancy (27), the premature infant thus being vulnerable (see Chapter 30).

E. Requirements of Vitamins and Minerals

The blood or plasma levels of vitamins and minerals often used to assess nutrient status of the body are difficult to employ in pregnancy and lactation because the normal expansion of blood volume during pregnancy dilutes circulating nutrient concentrations. Also, there is a highly efficient transport of some nutrients from the placenta to the fetus, which may have higher concentrations of these nutrients than in the maternal circulation. The activities of coenzyme (vitamin)-dependent enzymes are frequently higher in pregnant than in nonpregnant women (5).

1. Fat-soluble Vitamins

The U.S. RDAs for the fat-soluble vitamins during pregnancy include substantial increases above the nonpregnant levels for vitamin D (100%) and vitamin E (25%), but no increases for vitamin A and K (Table 4). The allowances recommended during lactation are the same or slightly higher than in pregnancy (25).

Vitamin D deficiency during pregnancy may cause maternal osteomalacia, reduced birthweight, and neonatal hypocalcemia and tetany. The maternal effects of vitamin D deficiency during lactation remain to be elucidated completely. The risk factors for vitamin D deficiency include low sun exposure, dark skin, and living in a northern climate. Vitamin D toxicity can cause hypercalcemia in women. The placental transfer of vitamin D to the infant is especially important because of the low vitamin D levels of human milk. Vitamin D concentrations (0.3–0.9 µg/l) vary

Table 4 Recommended Dietary Allowances of Vitamins During Pregnancy and Lactation

Vitamins	Pregnancy	Lactation 1st 6 months	Lactation 2nd 6 months
Fat-soluble			
A (µg RE)[a]	800 (0%)[e]	1300 (62%)	1200 (50%)
D (µg)[b]	10 (100%)	10 (100%)	10 (100%)
E (mg alpha-TE)[c]	10 (25%)	12 (50%)	11 (38%)
K (µg)	65 (0%)	65 (0%)	65 (0%)
Water-soluble			
C (mg)	70 (17%)	95 (58%)	90 (50%)
Thiamin (mg)	1.5 (36%)	1.6 (45%)	1.6 (45%)
Riboflavin (mg)	1.6 (23%)	1.8 (38%)	1.7 (31%)
Niacin (mg NE)[d]	17 (13%)	20 (33%)	20 (33%)
B_6 (mg)	2.2 (38%)	2.1 (31%)	2.1 (31%)
Folate (µg)	400 (122%)	280 (45%)	260 (44%)
B_{12} (µg)	2.2 (10%)	2.6 (30%)	2.6 (30%)

[a]Retinol equivalents, 1 RE = 1 µg retinol or 6 µg beta-carotene.
[b]As cholecalciferol, 10 µg cholecalciferol = 400 IU vitamin D.
[c]Alpha-tocopherol equivalents, 1 mg alpha-tocopherol = 1-alpha-TE.
[d]Niacin equivalent, 1 NE = 1 mg niacin or 60 mg of dietary tryptophan.
[e]Percentage increase above levels for nonpregnant, nonlactating women.
Source: Ref. 25.

substantially, partly because of differences in maternal vitamin D status, which in turn depend on vitamin D intake and exposure of body to sun. Exclusively breast-fed infants are often at risk of vitamin D deficiency if maternal vitamin D intake is limited and sun exposure of mother and infant is low. According to Specker et al. (28), a fully clothed infant without a hat requires about 2 hours of sun exposure per week to maintain normal serum 25-OH vitamin D levels.

The intakes of retinol and its precursors usually meet baseline needs and extra needs of pregnancy (25) in the Western countries. However, in the developing countries and in populations with restricted access to vitamin A–containing foods, vitamin A intakes may be inadequate. Vitamin A deficiency during pregnancy is related to intrauterine growth retardation and premature birth (29). Subclinical vitamin A deficiency in children is probably associated with increased childhood mortality (see Chapter 7), suggesting the preventive role of vitamin A supplementation during pregnancy. Careless supplementation may, however, induce teratogenicity, which is of special concern among malnourished women who may be exposed to increased risk of vitamin A toxicity (30).

Requirements of vitamin A during lactation are determined from estimates of milk output of vitamin A, which is about 500 µg/day. Under the conditions of marginal vitamin A adequacy, milk vitamin A levels respond to maternal supplementation. Breast-feeding appears to protect infants against vitamin A deficiency following weaning (31), because of the infants' ability to store the vitamin.

Maternal consequences of vitamin E deficiency during pregnancy or lactation have not been described in humans. However, US RDAs have recommended increased allowances for vitamin E during pregnancy (25), expecting that higher vitamin E levels are required to promote fetal growth. As with other nutrients, most vitamin E transfer from mother to fetus probably takes place during the last quarter of pregnancy, hence premature infants are likely to be born with inadequate stores. Hemolytic anemia in the premature infant has often been found to respond to vitamin E administration. Inadequate vitamin E status in premature infants has also been found to be associated with bronchopulmonary dysphasia, retinopathy and intraventricular hemorrhage, though the causative role for vitamin E deficiency in these disorders remains to be demonstrated conclusively.

Maternal needs for vitamin E during lactation are based on the expected amount of milk produced and its tocopherol content (25).

A vitamin K-deficient neonate may develop a fetal hemorrhagic disease with intracranial hemorrhage (5). The babies are born with inadequate stores of vitamin K (see Chapter 7), and vitamin K injection for the infant at birth have been recommended (13,32). Administration of vitamin K to pregnant women at term does not appear to influence the clotting factors, II, IX, and X in their infants, though giving vitamin K to women who deliver prematurely offers some short-term protection to the infant (33).

Vitamin K output in milk is about 1.5 µg/day, mostly in the form of phylloquinone, though its concentration in milk varies greatly. Maternal vitamin K supplements increase its milk concentrations markedly, but a seemingly adequate vitamin K status of the mother does not appear to ensure adequate vitamin K intakes for the exclusively breastfed neonate, which is at increased risk of vitamin K deficiency if vitamin K is not supplied from external source, especially in the first month of life. There is a need to study the relative significance of placental transfer of vitamin K, its intake from milk, the limited ability of the neonate's intestinal microbes to synthesize vitamin K and its ability to absorb vitamin K (5,21).

2. *Water-soluble Vitamins*

Both the U.S. and U.K. committees have recommended special allowances for water-soluble vitamins during pregnancy and lactation, which are about 10% to 100% higher than those for non-pregnant women and sometimes increase further to meet the needs during lactation (Table 4).

The allowances for folate (folacin) are set considerably higher in pregnancy than in lactation, which reflects the key role of folacin in cell division and development. Folate deficiency during pregnancy results in megaloblastic anemia and is associated with high rates of spontaneous absorption, toxemia, intrauterine growth retardation, premature delivery, fetal malformation, and antepartum hemorrhage. The U.S. RDAs for folate have been set at 400 μg/day in excess of the average amount consumed by nonpregnant women (25); the U.K. RDIs are much lower, at 200 to 300 μg/day.

Adequate folate intake may be needed to avoid neural tube defects; therefore, an adequate folate status must be ensured before pregnancy, because by the time a woman realizes that she is pregnant, the critical stage when the fetal neural tube closes by further cell division may be passed. This has created new medical and public interest in prepregnancy nutritional counseling and the widespread use and abuse of preconceptual vitamin supplementation. A double-blind controlled trial of 4 mg of folate daily in European women who had already had a child with a neural tube defect showed a highly significant reduction in the chances of having a second abnormal child (34). However, the results of this trial cannot be extrapolated to all women, although Smithells et al. (35) have claimed that women on poor diets were particularly liable to have a child with neural tube defects. This uncontrolled trial with 0.36 mg of folate/day appeared to be protective. The U.S. Department of Health now recommends consumption of at least 0.4 mg (but less than 1 mg) of folate/day to reduce the risk of neural tube defects (36). The U.K. (Department of Health, 1992) report recommends that all young women should consume 0.4 mg folate daily to ensure adequate folate stores, whether they have a planned or unplanned pregnancy, and 4 mg folate/day should be taken to prevent recurrence of neural tube defects.

About 40 μg/day of folate is expected to be lost through milk during lactation. Considering about 50% efficiency of absorption of folate from food and a CV of 12.5% in milk production, milk content and absorption efficiency (25), 60 μg of folate/day has been recommended in the United Kingdom whereas U.S. RDAs are a substantial 260 μg/day (25).

Because folate concentrations of milk are not correlated with the mothers' plasma folate concentrations and the milk folate does not increase with maternal folate supplementation, folate concentrations in milk appear to be regulated. However, folate stores accumulated during fetal life are influenced by the maternal folate status and the stores transferred to the infant in utero probably play an important role in maintaining folate status in infancy (21).

Pregnancy and lactation in vegetarians can decrease vitamin B_{12} levels, though omnivorous women do not seem to be affected because of their substantial hepatic stores of cobalamin. About 0.4 μg/day of vitamin B_{12} is lost in milk during lactation in well-nourished women, but it may not drop to one-tenth of that level in depleted women. Thus, urinary concentrations of methylmalonate (an index of B_{12} deficiency, see Chapter 6) are higher in ovo-lacto-vegetarian mothers and their breast-fed infants compared with those in omnivorous women and their infants (37). Infants are more vulnerable to B_{12} deficiency than the mothers, infantile deficiency occurring before any clinical manifestation of maternal deficiency. The infant uses up fetal stores by about 6 months of age (5).

Thiamin requirements (erythrocyte transketolase activation assay, see Chapter 6) are increased throughout pregnancy. Severe cardial decompensation in pregnant women may lead to congestive heart failure in the newborn babies because of marked thiamin deficiency. Thiamin supplementation programs in women at risk for vitamin B deficiency have shown reductions in stillbirths, maternal and perinatal mortality, and toxemia, though the causative role of B_1 in these disorders remains to be proved conclusively.

About 160 μg/day of thiamin outputs in milk during lactation are taken as a basis for thiamin intakes during lactation. Also, there is an additional increment of thiamin required for the extra energy during lactation, because thiamin needs are directly related to energy requirements of the body. Maternal intakes influence milk thiamin concentrations, which may decrease substantially in women eating high-carbohydrate diets with low B_1 levels, leading to the development of beriberi in exclusively breast-fed infants.

Because of the higher rate of conversion of tryptophan to niacin induced by estrogens, niacin needs during pregnancy may not be increased significantly (25). The increased conversion efficiency is thought to partly compensate for the additional needs of fetal growth and maternal metabolism, so that niacin allowance for pregnancy is increased by about 13% (Table 4).

Based on the about 2.3 mg/day output of niacin in human milk, U.S. RDAs for niacin have been increased to 4 mg/day during lactation.

Riboflavin deficiency develops during pregnancy, as indicated by fall in the urinary excretion of riboflavin, and rise in erythrocyte glutathione reductase activation coefficeints, which respond to riboflavin supplementation (7).

Riboflavin intakes during lactation are based on estimates of riboflavin outputs in milk (about 260 µg/day) and an overall efficiency of 70% in the dietary utilization of riboflavin from milk products (25). The mothers' riboflavin intakes significantly influence milk riboflavin levels.

The role of pyridoxal and pyridoxamine phosphate coenzymes in the transamination and other aspects of protein metabolism probably increases the requirements of vitamin B_6 during pregnancy and lactation (25). Inadequate maternal status of vitamin B_6 has been associated with toxemia, low birthweight, and a poor general condition of newborns of deficient mothers (7). Mature human milks vary in their vitamin B_6 concentrations substantially and depend on maternal dietary intake. The vitamin B_6 output in milk is about 70 mg/day. Kirksey and Roepke (38) postulated that reductions in milk B_6 levels can become sufficiently severe to cause abnormalities in central nervous system functions of neonates.

Plasma ascorbic acid levels fall during pregnancy, probably because of the normal expansion of blood volume and fetal vitamin C concentrations by special placental transfer mechanisms (25). Considering this transfer and the presumably higher metabolic demands of pregnancy for vitamin C, the U.S. RDAs are set at 10 mg/day above those required by nonpregnant women. The U.K. RNIs recommend similar allowance during the last trimester of pregnancy. The vitamin C requirements of lactation are much higher (30 mg/day) based on milk outputs of about 2 mg/day and 25% variation in milk output. This increment and an allowance for about 85% absorption efficiency for vitamin C raises the figure to 35 mg/day during lactation in the United States though COMA report (13) restricts the value to 30 mg/day in the United Kingdom. It should be noted that the ascorbic acid output in milk is highly variable and responsive to maternal intake levels (5).

3. Minerals

The general metabolic roles of minerals, viz., structural components (Ca, P), cofactors for metalloenzymes (Zn, Se), and constituents of vital organic molecules such as vitamins and hormones (Co, Fe, I) are unaltered by pregnancy and lactation. However, it is necessary to take into account the enhanced mineral needs in pregnancy and lactation because of their transfer to fetus and milk losses (Table 5). Certain adaptive measures have been recognized that alter the rates of mineral absorption and utilization during pregnancy and lactation.

The total body calcium content of a 55-kg woman, with 25% body fat, is about 0.9 to 1.0 kg, considering the Ca content of about 23 g/kg fat-free mass in adults. Most of the neonate's calcium content (about 30 g) is deposited during the last trimester of pregnancy. The maternal calcium store therefore declines to meet this high fetal demand, despite the increased efficiency of calcium absorption (39). The loss of maternal calcium indicates that the calcium balance in late pregnancy is not sufficiently positive to account for the calcium transferred to the fetus, despite the enhanced calcium absorption in early pregnancy to boost maternal stores. The fetal accumulation of calcium amounts to only about 2.5% of the maternal stores (5).

Table 5 Recommended Dietary Allowances of Minerals

Minerals	Pregnancy	Lactation	
		1st 6 months	2nd 6 months
Calcium (mg)	1200 (50%)[a]	1200 (50%)	1200 (50%)
Phosphorus (mg)	1200 (50%)	1200 (50%)	1200 (50%)
Magnesium (mg)	320 (14%)	355 (27%)	340 (21%)
Iron (mg)	30 (100%)	15 (0%)	15 (0%)
Zinc (mg)	15 (25%)	19 (58%)	16 (33%)
Iodine (μg)	175 (17%)	200 (33%)	200 (33%)
Selenium (μg)	65 (18%)	75 (36%)	75 (36%)

[a]Percentage increase above levels for nonpregnant, nonlactating women.
Source: Ref. 25.

Approximately 40 g (210 mg/day) calcium are lost during 6 months of lactation. Considering the significant potential calcium losses that occur during pregnancy and lactation, allowances for calcium have been increased by 400 mg/day.

About 800 to 900 mg of iron is needed during pregnancy, of which around 500 mg is required for increases in maternal erythrocyte volume and hematopoietic tissues and 300 to 400 mg for the development of placenta and fetus. Delivery bleeding iron loss amounts to about 250 mg; thus, the net loss of iron to the mother after parturition totals about 500 to 650 mg.

The healthy infant body iron concentration is about 50% higher than that of the normal adult. These significant iron reserves and the high bioavailability (around 50%) of iron in human milk are sufficient to maintain iron status within normal limits in exclusively breast-fed infants for about 6 months. The daily output of iron in milk is around 0.2 mg/day which is much less than the average menstrual losses of iron of 0.7 mg/day. Unlike most other nutrients, iron demands of pregnancy are greater than those of lactation (5).

Women in lower social-economic groups, teenagers, and multiparous women are at greater risk for iron deficiency, both in the economically developing and developed countries. Iron-deficient women risk greater complications during pregnancy from the blood loss accompanying parturition, maternal iron deficiency (Hb less than 10 mg/dl) being associated with enhanced rates of prematurity, low birthweight, and perinatal mortality (7,21,25).

III. INFANT NUTRITION AND WEANING

Human nutrition achieves its highest significance during infancy, when the tissue and organ synthesis rates are highest and maturation processes continue rapidly. These changes demand a balanced but relatively high intake of specific nutrients and energy—when the infant's tolerance to "food" is relatively limited by the immaturity of the gastrointestinal tract, liver, and kidneys. Also, unlike adults, young infants cannot consume solid foods and do not tolerate foods that contain large amounts of fiber, toxins, and salts. Thus, they rely, for at least the first few months, on milk for all their nutritional needs. Therefore, it is important that both the composition and supply of this sole food, milk, is as near optimal as possible (40). The estimated energy and selected nutrient needs for the normal development of infants are given in Table 6 (41,42).

Table 6 Estimated Needs of Energy and Selected Nutrients in Normal Infants

Nutrient	Age (months)	
	0–6	6–12
Based on normal infant's intake		
Energy (MJ/kg)	0.42	0.38
Protein (g/kg)	1.46	1.16
RDAs for Fat-soluble vitamins		
Vit A (μg RE)[a]	375	375
Vit E (μg alpha-TE)[a]	3	4
Vit K (μg)	5	10
Vit D (μg)	7.5	10
RDAs for water-soluble vitamins		
Vit C (mg)	30	35
Thiamin (mg)	0.3	0.4
Riboflavin (mg)	0.4	0.5
Niacin (mg NE)[a]	5	6
Pyridoxine (mg)	0.3	0.6
Folic acid (μg)	25	35
Vit B_{12} (μg)	0.3	0.5
RDAs for major and trace elements		
Calcium (mg)	400	600
Phosphorus (mg)	300	500
Magnesium (mg)	40	60
Iron (mg)	6	10
Zinc (mg)	5	5
Iodine (μg)	40	50
Selenium (μg)	10	15

[a]1RE = 1 μg retinol or 6 μg beta-carotene.
1 alpha TE = 10 g d-alpha tocopherol.
1 NE = 1 mg niacin or 60 mg dietary tryptophan.
Source: Refs. 40, 41, and 42.

A. Breast-feeding

A normal human neonate, put on its mother's chest, spontaneously learns to suckle within the first hour of its life (43). This behavior, which is common to all mammals, enables the offspring to obtain the initial milk called colostrum through the action of suckling. Colostrum is necessary for the survival of neonates in most mammalian species, though not in humans. Nevertheless, both early suckling and intake of early maternal milk are vital in infants' psychological and physical development.

The suckling of breast-feeding allows mutual somatosensory stimulation and responsiveness between mother and child (44). An increase in postpartum sensitivity of the mother's sensitive buccal mucosa aid in the mutual stimulation by contact which leads to hormonal responses. Whereas the infant's gastrin and cholesystokinin levels rise and somatostatin levels fall, the mother's prolactin and oxytocin levels rise. These effects stimulate milk production in the mother by starting a let-down reflux that brings milk to the point of delivery, milk ejection, and local skin vasodilatation, providing warmth for the infant in contact and often a pleasing, calming sensation. The endocrine changes in the infant help to stimulate growth and development of the gastrointestinal tract, enhance nutrient absorption, and induce satiety and sleepiness. Breast-feeding ensures rapid "bonding" between mother and infant. The infant learns to trust early, such a relationship fostering normal psychological development. Breast-feeding also suppresses the mother's reproductive system, thereby delaying further conception as the result of the increased postpartum circulating levels of prolactin, which fall with time as fertility improves.

1. Human Milk

Human milk provides sufficient energy and essential nutrients for the growth and development of the child at least for the critical first 4 months. In addition, it contains antimicrobial substances and hormones, enzymes, growth factors, binding proteins, and other ill-defined functional substances. However, human milk does not appear to provide sufficient vitamin K and fluoride for optimum health (45). Also, human milk does not supply enough iron after 4 months and it may not provide sufficient vitamin D. The various constituents of human milk as compared to those of cow's milk and a typical cow's milk whey-based formula are shown in Table 7 (46). The composition of maternal milk varies widely among individuals, with the time of day, and with the length of time postpartum.

Milk produced during the first 4 to 5 days (colostrum) contains relatively large amounts of protein, especially the secretory immunoglobulin A (Secr IgA), along with albumin, serum immunoglobulins, and lysozyme (45). It also contains a higher proportion of cholesterol than mature milk and several trace elements such as zinc and selenium (47), but relatively less fat.

Human milk fat has 98% triglycerols and contributes 50% to 60% of the total milk energy. It has substantial amounts of unsaturated fatty acids, with the predominance of oleic and linoleic acids. The fat occurs as globules enclosed in membranes, which protect it from lipolysis and oxidation. The membranes also contain phospholipids, cholesterol, proteins and trace elements. Human milk fat is hydrolysed mainly to beta-monoglycerides, which are more easily absorbed than alpha-monoglycerides, the products of fat hydrolysis in cow's milk (40). The fat content of "mature" milk (after 10–15 days) is variable; its concentration increases during a feed and often in the morning. Maternal diet also influences the content of fat-soluble vitamins in milk.

Mature milk proteins are composed of whey proteins and caseins in the ratio of 60:40. About one-third of whey proteins is alpha-lactalbumin, which along with caseins constitutes the predominant source of essential amino acids. Other important whey proteins are lactoferrin and Secr IgA, which have nonnutritional functions. Human milk contains Secr IgA antibodies to microbes in the G.I. and respiratory tracts of both mother and infant (48). These antibodies bind bacterial antigens, preventing them from attaching to the intestinal mucosal cell membrane; they also neutralize toxins and viruses. Secr IgA is thought to play a role in the prevention of allergic food sensitization in infants. Food sensitivity mainfestations such as diarrhea, vomiting, eczema, and asthma are markedly reduced in breast-fed infants, especially when their mothers exclude potent allergens such as cow's milk and eggs from their diets (see Chapter 23). Lactoferrin binds iron, thus withholding it from bacteria so that their intestinal growth is inhibited. Whey proteins present in small amounts bind corticosteroids, thyroxine, and vitamins such as folate, vitamin D, and vitamin B_{12}. Many proteins are enzymes—e.g., lysozyme (which is bacteriostatic) and lipases, alpha-amylase, antiproteases, and lactoperoxidase. Caseins are linked together with calcium and phosphate to form small micelles, resulting in a soft, flocculent coagulum in the infant's G.I. tract that aids casein digestion.

About one-fourth of total nitrogen in human milk is in nonprotein form (49), largely present as N-acetyl glucosamine and urea, whose functions are not known. Other nonprotein nitrogenous compounds include amino acids, (e.g., taurine, required for formation of bile salt), peptides (epidermal growth factor), somatomedins, insulin, thyroxine (thyroid-stimulating hormone), and thyrotropin-releasing hormone, carnitine, creatinine, and creatine (40).

Table 7 Approximate Composition of Mature Human Milk, Cow's Milk and a Cow's Milk Whey-based Infant Formula for Selected Constituents[a]

Constituents	Human milk	Cow's milk	Typical formula[b]
Energy[c](MJ/1)	3.1	2.9	2.8
Total protein (g/l)	8.9	31.4	15.0
Total whey (g/l)	6.4	5.8	9.0
Alpha-lactalbumin (g/l)	2–3	1.1	9.0
Beta-lactalbumin (g/l)	0	3.6	0
Lactoferrin (g/l)	1–3	Trace	0
Secr IgA[d](g/l)	0.5–1.0	0.03	0
Lysozyme (g/l)	0.05–0.25	Trace	0
Total casein (g/l)	2–3	27.3	6.0
Non-protein nitrogen, % total N	18–30	5	–
Total fat (g/l)	42	38	36
Cholesterol (mg/l)	160	110	–
Essential fatty acids (g/100 g fatty acids)			
18:2 linoleic	7.2	1.6	–
18:3 linolenic	0.8	0.4	–
20:4 arachidonic	0.3	0.1	–
Carbohydrate			
Lactose (g/l)	60–70	47	72
Oligosaccharides (g/l)	12–13	1	0
Fat-soluble vitamins			
Vit A (μg/l)	600	350	605
Vit E (μg/l)	3500	1400	7400
Vit D (μg/l)	0.1	0.8	10
Vit K (μg/l)	2.1	35	40
Water-soluble vitamins			
Vit C (mg/l)	38	18	60
Thiamin (μg/l)	160	430	400
Riboflavin (μg/l)	300	1700	500
Niacin (μg/l)	2300	950	4000
Pantothenic acid (μg/l)	2600	3600	4000
Biotin (μg/l)	7.6	40	11.3
Folic acid (μg/l)	52	55	100
Vit B_{12} (μg/l)	0.1	4.5	1.5
Major and trace elements			
Sodium (mg/l)	150	450	180
Calcium (mg/l)	350	1200	590
Phosphorus (mg/l)	150	940	350
Magnesium (mg/l)	28	120	60
Iron (mg/l)	0.8	0.6	8
Zinc (mg/l)	3	3	4
Iodine (μg/l)	70	80	40
Selenium (μg/l)	14	30	–

[a]Ref. 45.
[b]Cow's milk whey-based formula (Aptamil, Milupa).
[c]*Source*: Ref. 46.
[d]Secr IgA = Secretory immunoglobin A.

Lactose is the predominant carbohydrate of human milk and unlike other constituents varies little in concentration. Lactose provides about 38% of the total energy in human milk. Intestinal microflora convert unabsorbed lactose to lactate, which decreases the pH, thus increasing the solubility and absorption of calcium.

The calcium and phosphorus in human milk are associated with the casein fraction, whereas the other elements are associated primarily with the whey fraction. Some essential trace elements are also associated with the fat globules. About 28% of zinc and 40% of copper are found bound partly to serum albumin in milk, and 30% to 40% of iron is bound to lactoferrin, which also binds manganese and perhaps zinc (47). Selenium is present largely as selenomethionine and selenocysteine. Fluoride in human milk is present in very low concentration, so that fluoride supplements are recommended for infants solely breast-fed after 6 months of age (50).

According to Hambraeus (47), the vitamin content of human milk is related closely to the maternal vitamin status. The levels of water-soluble vitamins are generally adequate, though thiamin deficiency (beriberi) was reported in a S.E. Asian breast-fed infant (51). Whereas vitamin E levels tend to be high, vitamin A levels are moderate but variable; vitamin D deficiency (rickets) has been reported to occur in breast-fed infants of Middle Eastern ancestry residing in the United Kingdom: lack of exposure to sunlight, rather than dietary deficiency, appears to be the main reason (52). Though rickets is rather uncommon in Caucasian infants, vitamin D supplements have been recommended for breastfed infants (32). Human milk appears to be deficient in vitamin K, as evidenced by occurrence of hemorrhagic disease in breast-fed newborns, not in bottle-fed infants (53). This disease is entirely preventable by supplying vitamin K immediately after birth, either through intramuscular injection or the oral route, which is safer and effective (40).

Water, cells, and "contaminants" are some other components of human milk. The water intake of an entirely breast-fed infant is quite adequate, even in hot tropical climates. The functions of different types of cells appear to be antimicrobial in the infant's G.I. tract. The majority are macrophages and polymorphonuclear leukocytes, with small numbers of lymphocytes (50% are T-lymphocytes), whose numbers fall dramatically during the first month of lactation. The epithelial cells present in colostrum, however, increase in numbers in mature milk. The major role of macrophages is probably phagocytosis and killing of microorganisms. The lymphocytes are thought to have a role in the production of interferons, a glycoprotein group rendering cells less susceptible to viral infection.

Many varied types of contaminants are present in human milk, some of which are actively secreted while others are passively diffused into the milk. They include hormones, drugs, pesticides, other pollutants, and viruses. Both oral contraceptives (47) and smoking reduce milk volumes. Acidic drugs pass readily into milk, the concentration of lipid-soluble drugs depending on the milk fat content. Breastfeeding is not advised when the mother is receiving phenobarbitone, thiouracil, or cytotoxic drugs. Alcohol and many other drugs also appear in significant amounts in human milk. Many lipid-soluble pollutants pose risk to infants if they are accumulated in the mother's adipose tissue and are released during lactation. Although there is little clinical evidence of the toxic effects of pollutants in breast-fed infants, there is evidence of transmission of a variety of viruses, including the human immunodeficiency virus (HIV) (54); therefore infected mothers in the United Kingdom are advised not to breast-feed their offspring (55). According to Lederman (56), for certain poorer communities of Africa, the risk of HIV infection from breast-feeding is much less than the risks of other infections and undernutrition associated with bottle-feeding.

2. Cow's Milk and Formula Milks

Cow's milk made naturally for calves is different from human milk in many respects (Table 7) and unless modified, it is not appropriate for young infants. It is associated with a renal solute load that is about threefold larger than that of human milk due to its higher concentrations of protein and inorganic ions. Skim milk, which is popular in adult diets, is also not very appropriate for infant nutrition. However, a good substitute for human milk can be produced by manipulating the casein/whey ratio and adding certain essential nutrients, such as linoleic acid, iron, zinc, copper, and vitamins, with subsequent dilution.

The major problem of formula milks is feeding by bottle, which loses the advantages of suckling to both infant and mother. Bottles become contaminated by pathogenic organisms especially under poor hygienic conditions where the ambient temperature is high. Also, bottle feeds are more expensive than the extra cost of feeding the mother to permit normal lactation and maintain health. The composition of formula milks remains suboptimal in several circumstances. Infants may become quickly intolerant to milk, without basic cause; and by the time the etiology is established, secondary effects of intolerance are manifested. The sensitivity of the infant's G.I. tract to bovine protein, mainly beta-lactoglobulin, appears to play a part in milk intolerance. Some infants are born with genetic primary or secondary disaccharidase deficiency, for whom specialized formulas are now available, e.g., with the protein hydrolysed to reduce its antigenicity, with different carbohydrates and fat, or with extra trace elements and vitamins needed for health. Although formula milks allow the mother freedom to work outside the home and increase possible cares for the child, they will probably never match the remarkable properties of maternal milk; at least for the first 4 months, after which the non-nutritional advantages of human milk become less important; many infants gain weight faster if supplemented with formula milk (40).

3. Other Milks

Like cow's milk, goat's and sheep's milks also have higher renal solute loads and lack certain minerals and vitamins, especially folate (57). Soy milk–based formulas have been developed for infants being reared as vegans (vegetarians who eat no animal foods) and for those intolerant of cow's milk–based formula. Soy "milk" differs greatly from both human and cow's milk—e.g., it lacks methionine and carnitine; thus soy-based formulas are now supplemented with both (58). Also, soy milk contains phytates that bind mineral nutrients such as calcium, zinc, and iron, thus reducing their availability (59), which may occur even at low phytate concentrations. Most soy milk formulas still contain phytates, because they are difficult to remove completely. Like cow's milk, soy milk protein is also antigenic (60) and may contain high concentrations of aluminum (61).

According to Golden (40), the newer cow's milk formulas containing hydrolysed protein are normally better tolerated and should be recommended rather than soy milk formula in cases of sensitivity. However, much milk intolerance is due to secondary lactase deficiency, following gastro intestinal infection. In such cases, soy formulas can be recommended, because they usually contain sucrose, glucose, or polysaccharides instead of lactose (see Chapter 16).

B. Weaning

Weaning is the infant's gradual transition from a single-food (milk) diet to a mixed diet containing a variety of foods. Whereas in countries like the UK, weaning occurs earlier and earlier, in very traditional societies it may occur late. In some poor urbanized communities of the tropical countries, the weaning period is a particular time of risk for the infant's nutrition (62).

The range of time over which weaning occurs successfully varies considerably, within limits. Too-early weaning is harmful to the young infant's G.I. tract, liver, and kidneys, and too-late weaning is also harmful if milk is not sufficient to permit normal growth, development, and metabolism; e.g., when human milk provides little iron and copper, young breast-fed infants normally use their hemoglobin and hepatic stores of these elements, leading to their depletion and low serum ferritin levels, as the iron stores are used up by 6 months or so. Wharton (63) found that serum ferritin in infants fed unmodified cow's milk was low by 4 months. Most infant formulas are currently therefore supplemented with iron, copper, and vitamins A, D, and K.

Based on the current limited knowledge of nutritional requirements, breast-fed infants should be weaned earlier than formula-fed infants (40). It is still not known what precisely governs nutrient availability from human milk. It is generally agreed that weaning in infants should begin between 4 and 6 months of age, because all types of milks are good sources of energy and essential nutrients and can very well supplement infant nutrition of the weaning child. Maternal milk may also continue to confer some protection against infection. Though the levels of Secr IgA and lactoferrin fall during the first 6 months of lactation, lysozyme levels rise and remain high up to 2 years postpartum. Prolonged breast-feeding, for at least up to a year, should therefore be encouraged, especially in poor households of developing countries, where nutrition and hygiene are often compromised (40).

Weaning foods aim to be more energy-dense than milk, with well balanced essential nutrients, especially with improved levels of those nutrients that are found short in milk (iron, copper, vitamins A, D, and K). The staple food of the region, a cereal or root crop, may be given during weaning. Cereal-based (except wheat) weaning foods, precooked with milk or soya to improve nutritional quality and supplemented with specific micronutrients, are manufactured commercially under available guidelines (64). Initially weaning foods are served as a fluid gruel given once a day, followed by thicker gruels given more often. Germinated cereal grains can be used in the preparation to reduce cereal viscosity without altering its energy density (62). New foods may be introduced in small quantities at intervals of several days. Slow feeding, taking care to avoid choking, is important. Milk-based custards, cooked cereals, and root crops, eggs, and bananas are some of the early weaning foods. High-fiber foods, highly acidic fruits and vegetables, and highly seasonal foods should be avoided. Solid foods should be crushed or later, cut into small pieces, until the eruption of the infant's deciduous teeth (30–36 months), by which time weaning is almost complete.

Some long-term effects of infant nutrition have recently been reported (65,66) to show statistically significant correlation between birthweight and weight at 1 year as well as between cardiovascular disease and impaired glucose tolerance. These data imply that growth, and therefore, pre- and postnatal nutrition, may affect morbidity and mortality many decades later. The composition of the infant's diet affects his or her lipid metabolism: breast-fed infants have higher circulating total LDL (low-density liporotein) and VLDL (very low-density lipoprotein) cholesterol than those fed commercial formulas. Barclay et al. (67) suggested that this pattern in breastfed infants may decrease their serum cholesterol in adulthood, and thereby the risk of ischemic heart disease, by chronically suppressing hepatic HMG CoA reductase activity, required for cholesterol synthesis (68).

Glinsmann et al. (68) have pointed out that many diet strategies designed to promote adult health and nutrition in the 1995 edition of Dietary Guidelines for Americans (69) are inappropriate for infants and children under the age of two. The guidelines, developed in 1994 by Gerber Products Company (68), seek to distinguish the unique dietary needs of this vulnerable population group. Infants and young children are not simply small versions of adults and they have special needs with respect to nutrient requirements and the acquisition of healthy feeding patterns. Advantages of breast-feeding and the importance of developing preferences for "natural" or "traditional" foods are increasingly being recognized.

Widespread misconceptions prevail among parents regarding healthy infant feeding practices. The most common error, probably, is to follow the *Dietary Guidelines for Americans* when choosing foods for children under 2 years of age. Many parents encourage their older infants to consume high-fiber diets and introduce low-fat milks during the second year of life. These choices can lead to nutrition imbalances or adequacies. Alternatively, some parents may try to maximize weight gain and performance on growth charts. The long-term impact of such practice on children's ability to moderate food intake and prevent excess body weight gain is not known.

The Dietary Guidelines for Infants first developed in 1989 by Gerber Products Company were updated in 1994 to integrate recent scientific work in infant nutrition with a new component—infant development. The updated version provides a better understanding of how the developmental factors that affect infant nutrition evolve during the first 2 years of life, highlighting the significance of the mealtime environment and communication to a healthy parent-child feeding partnership (68).

During the first months of life, infants have a very large energy requirement, 3 to 4 times that of adults, on a body weight basis (70). Young infants have immature digestive and excretory systems, not equipped to handle a wide variety of foods. Their basic need is for energy-dense foods that are readily digestible and metabolizable, with appropriate micronutrients to maintain normal physiological functions and growth. Human milk or infant formulas are ideal foods in the first months of life, as they contain high-quality protein and readily digestible sugars and fats, with a appropriate mix of vitamins, minerals, and certain non-nutritive factors (in human milk).

All mammalian milk fats contain two saturated fatty acids on the second position of glycerolmyristic and palmitic acids, which enhance serum cholesterol levels. This would seem to indicate that while milk fat may be undesirable for some adults with hypercholesterolemic atherosclerosis problems, it could have some important functions in early childhood development. Milk fat may be important to maintain a large enough circulating pool of LDL cholesterol to support growth (71), and also to maintain circulatory cholesterol levels to support adequate synthesis of bile acids required for emulsification of high-fat infant diet. The role of long-chain fatty acids such as docosahexanoic acid and arachidonic acid of milk fat in the development of visual acuity and cognitive function (72,73) and the possible role of lactoferrin in immune function and as a growth factor for intestinal mucosal cells (74) are being elucidated. In the light of these studies, infant formula compositions are likely to be modified to incorporate new research data.

According to Glinsmann et al. (68), in addition to nutrition benefits, human milk confers several functional advantages on the breast-feeding infant. Breast-feeding helps newborn infants to make the abrupt transition from intrauterine to oral feeding and the shift from glucose to lipid as an energy source. The breast-fed infant is exposed to dietary variety, as the flavor of some foods are transferred from the mother's diet to the infant through her milk. Such exposure may facilitate the transition to a varied diet, because the familiar flavors may help an infant more readily accept complementary foods. As the normally developing infant moves through the transitional and modified-adult periods of infant feeding, there is an increasing need to provide developmentally appropriate and nutritious foods in positive mealtime experiences, so that the infant achieves normal growth and development, learns to accept and enjoy a wider variety of nutritious foods, and starts the smooth transition from dependent to independent feeding. Glinsmann et al. (68) have provided the following guidelines for feeding infants:

1. Build to a variety of foods.
2. Pay attention to your baby's appetite to avoid overfeeding or underfeeding.
3. Since babies need fat, restricted fat-diets and low-fat milks are not appropriate for infants and children under the age of 2 years.
4. Introduce fruits, vegetables, and grains but don't overdo high-fiber foods.
5. Babies need sugars in moderation.
6. Babies need sodium in moderation.
7. Choose foods with iron, zinc, and calcium.

The parents of young children eating supplemental foods need to view nutrition in terms of total diet—not necessarily one food or food group, or one meal, or one day. Older infants and young children who eat a variety of foods over the course of several days are most likely to receive adequate nutrition. Glinsmann et al. (68) concluded that pediatric care providers should be urged to counsel parents about the risks of over interpreting the adult guidelines, to ensure that nutritional needs of the younger population are met adequately. The Dietary Guidelines for Infants can thus serve a useful guide to parents as they choose foods for their infants and young children, develop positive mealtime communication, and help youngsters to develop healthy and active lifestyles.

IV.   DIET DURING CHILDHOOD, YOUTH AND OLD AGE

Childhood, youth, and old age are the periods during the life cycle of humans when physiological needs for nutrients are as important as the psychological aspects of food for the maintenance of good health. The following discussion on diet and nutrition during childhood, adolescence, youth, and old age is mainly based on Dwyer (75).

A.   Childhood Nutrition

Supplements to breast-feeding become necessary by the age of 4 to 6 months for the infant's further developmental growth (76). Gradual weaning of the infant from breast-feeding or bottle-feeding begins with the transition to family diets and stepwise introduction of solid foods having appropriate texture, consistency, and non-allergic properties. This helps the infant learn to chew, to eat solid foods, and to use fingers and spoons, and other eating skills. Weaning helps to provide the needed energy and other nutrients. As the infant gains experience in eating, foods that must be chewed, chopped foods, and small pieces of foods can be introduced. Normal children of the same age will vary in weight and height because of the variation in their genetic potential for growth.

Overfeeding and underfeeding of the child can be avoided if parents are sensitive enough to the child's ways of expressing hunger. Poor appetites may be associated with growth, teething, growing independence, attempting to change too many aspects of the child's diet at once, and illness. The infant and child should not be unduly forced to finish every bit of food on the plate, nor should the child be constantly fed when he expresses discontent for any reason.

By 18 months of age, most normal infants successfully complete the transition to family fare, and after about 2 years of age, moderation is in order with respect to several dietary components that should not be restricted. Prior to 2 years of age, children should not be placed on modified diets without medical supervision.

The growth rates of preschool children, who are nutritionally vulnerable, are slower than they were in infancy, with corresponding reduction in their nutrient needs. Toddlers and preschool children require a physical and social environment that supports their physical growth as well as their emotional, intellectual, and motor skill development (75).

Parents must ensure that the child's levels of physical activity and rest each day are sufficient to foster and maintain a good appetite and normal growth. Children should be provided nutritious food in the home as well as in infant care centers, nursery schools, and preschools. The child should be taught to choose and eat nutritious food by emphasizing nutrition in family meal and snack planning, and by stocking food supplies to match. Preschool child feeding outside the home should be an adjunct to and not a substitute for home efforts. Home food intakes should be supplemented with healthy food that is provided in a timely, safe, sanitary manner in the child care setting outside the home. Meals served in preschool programs should be adequate in their proportions of protein, vitamins, and minerals in line with energy supplied.

1. Refusal to Eat

Good child nutrition can be promoted by avoiding counterproductive behavior while feeding children. The expressions of real physiological need on the child's part must be distinguished from other emotional and physical needs, often expressed in terms of food refusal. The child's normal striving for greater independence may be expressed through temporary refusals to eat, dawdling, and use of food and eating to attempt to exert control over the parent or others who feed. Such food-related struggles should be handled calmly, without becoming emotionally involved in the issues to avoid the development of long-term feeding problems in children. It should be recognized that child appetites wax and wane from day to day and that some food waste is inevitable. Undue concerns about the ill-effects of short-term (meal to meal or a few days) fluctuations in child's food intakes, and counterproductive measures such as forcing, coaxing, nagging, and above all physical punishment or emotional isolation to remedy food refusal must be avoided. Excessive use of food for rewarding, pacifying, or punishing the young child may set a stage for emotional battles that may result in immediate or long-term feeding problems. These should be recognized and dealt with before they become well established. Refusal of specific foods during temporary periods of negativity on the child's part are best coped with by ignoring them and waiting for a better time to introduce the food again. Poor appetite may be due to many causes, and steps should be taken to eliminate those that are remediable, which may include small size for age, or small appetite compared to other children in the family, poor appetite due to illness or recovery from illness, and wide variations in day-to-day physical activity. Severe feeding problems associated with persistent negativism and multiple food dislikes on the child's part should be resolved by seeking advice from a nutritionist, psychologist, or pediatrician. Undetected health problems or increased health risks may be involved in bizarre food choices for longer periods of time and need a physician's help. Special care needs to be taken to teach children to avoid ingestion of harmful or poisonous substances.

Because vitamin or mineral supplements in otherwise healthy children do not produce any biochemical or functional improvements, they are recommended only for high-risk schoolchildren, such as those from very poor families, those with poor appetites and eating habits, and those who are ill (77).

Dietary excesses are more common than insufficient dietary intakes in children. Intakes of total fat, saturated fat, sodium, and cholesterol are often in excess, leading to obesity in the children, especially those of the affluent societies. Action to prevent obesity and to intervene by non-pharmacological means to decrease the diet-related risk of hyperlipidemia and hypertension in high-risk children has been recommended by health authorities, though countroversy exists regarding the intake of fat and sodium-modified diets for schoolchildren in general (78–81).

2. Snacking

Snacking by children is inevitable and there is no evidence to show that snacking is unhealthy as long as snack choices are appropriate and carry their share of vitamins, minerals, and calories, and are without excessive amounts of saturated fat, sodium, and cholesterol. Children, however, need help in making wise snack choices. The principles of moderation and balanced nutrient intake are often violated by the notion that foods at meals should be healthy and nutritious, but that snack foods need not be so; for many children snacking is very common and regular meals are frequently missed. Healthy snacks include fruit, vegetables, bread, and low-fat milk products. Snack foods high in calories, and sticky, sugary, and starchy ingredients should be deemphasized. Sweet foods, in addition to their high calories and low contributions of other nutrients, increase the risk of dental caries and should be restricted to once or twice a week at family meals. Also, children should be urged to rinse out their mouths with water and to brush their teeth after eating sticky, sugary snacks to minimize the risk of dental caries.

Moderation on the part of parents and other adults in the use of food rewards, especially sweets, is important. Expressing affection and rewarding good behavior on the part of the child by verbal praise and non-food treats are preferable to constant rewards with candies or sweets (75).

3. Meal Planning

Breakfast in the morning provides children a good portion of total intakes of ascorbic acid and other nutrients that are often at lower than recommended levels in their diets. Parents can help children to be good consumers by resisting the pressures of advertisements on commercial programs, and not buying foods they do not wish their children to eat. Parents need to alter their family food buying practices to avoid sweet-starchy-sugary foods that are low in protective nutrients and to include food items that are healthy and nutritious. Children need to be taught to understand what is undesirable in some food items, and why they should consume specific foods.

4. Obesity and Malnutrition in Children

Obesity in schoolchildren is common and reflects the interactions of genetic predisposition and permissive environments (82). Despite continuing emphasis on prevention and treatment, the prevalence of child and adolescent obesity appears to be increasing (83), especially among some minority groups, such as blacks (84). This may be partly because of increasingly sedentary lifestyles, which for many children include excessive television viewing and other sedentary activities (85). The root cause of child obesity is rarely endocrine; low energy outputs relative to needs are involved more frequently than high energy intakes.

Obesity adversely affects child development, even in the school years. It stimulates and reinforces patterns of physical inactivity, intensifies family tensions, and contributes to the development of a negative and distorted body image and a sense of self-worthlessness. Obese children are also at higher risk of obesity in later life, and obesity continued in adulthood has very negative effects on social mobility and physical and mental health (see Chapter 26).

Even if obesity cannot be eliminated, efforts should be made to reduce its severity and progression. In addition to the medical aspects involved, it is necessary to address psychological factors, to foster more tolerance of diversity in bodily appearance, to emphasize prevention by manipulation of the food environment, and to educate both parents and children about food and physical activity. Non-food-oriented forms of emotional release must be sought, and distorted communications between children and parents should be rectified (86).

Fat loss, and not necessarily weight loss, should be the goal in preventing and treating obesity in children. The child is permitted to grow up into fatness by very modest alterations in energy inputs and increased emphasis on physical activity. Drastic weight reduction diets, below 1000 calories, are unwarranted except in medical emergencies, as linear growth and lean body mass may be retarded (see Chapter 26). Social and physical environments are needed to promote moderation in eating and vigorous physical activity, which are conducive to maintaining normal body fitness and cardiovascular fitness. Healthy family behaviors, such as regular and vigorous physical activity several times a week, should be encouraged.

B. Adolescent Nutrition

The second period of most rapid growth after infancy in the human life cycle is marked by the pubertal growth spurt that heralds adolescence. An individual child's growth rates can be followed with the help of growth charts for height and height velocity (87), which are also useful in problem cases to judge whether a child's growth is normal or otherwise.

1. Nutritional Requirements

Adolescent nutritional needs are unique from the biological, psychological, and social points of view. Although their biological nutritional requirements are similar in the types of nutrients needed, adolescents require larger amounts of protective nutrients such as protein, vitamins and minerals per unit of energy consumed than prepubertal children or adults. Energy needs are only slightly increased, but the needs for other nutrients imposed by growth and sexual maturation are much increased over younger individuals, approaching those of adults by late adolescent stage. Thus, adolescents require diets that are high in nutritional quality, the growth spurt itself requiring both energy and nutrients as structural materials.

Changes in physiological function after sexual maturity also alter nutrient needs, e.g., the requirement of iron after the menarche, which increases iron needs because of menstrual blood losses. Diseases present in some adolescents may also alter nutrient needs because of changes they induce in absorption, nutrient metabolism, or excretion.

Nutrient needs correlate rather poorly with chronological age during adolescence, but are more closely linked to biological or maturational age as determined from bone age or sexual maturity ratings. However, due to difficulty in determining biological age, RDAs are given currently by sex on a chronological age basis (see Chapter 22). The margins of safety in these recommendations are sufficiently large to be satisfactory for most purposes and to allow for individual variation in needs. However, special attention may be needed to be given in the application of RDAs for very early or very late maturers. Quantitatively, adolescent nutrient needs differ by sex and change with growth during adolescence. Females reach their full height about 2 years before males and adult men are on an average 15 cm taller and more than 15 kg heavier than women. Tanner (88) noted that for a brief period during puberty, girls are often larger than boys.

Adolescents who live in poverty or have other social or health disadvantages are more likely to be malnourished than their affluent counterparts, but prevalence and severity of such problems is less. Those at high risk include ethnic or racial minorities, especially if they are also poor and have chronic illnesses (75).

Much progress has been made to improve adolescent nutrition and health on the global scale. Undernutrition due to lack of money or environmental access to food is also rare. Inadequate food intakes may occasionally occur due to intentional dieting of various types or due to the effects of pathophysiological and social problems. Inappropriate food choices due to lack of access, lack of knowledge, habit, or cultural and other influences are, however, common, as are the adolescent food habits leading to overnutrition and imbalances due to excessive intakes of total and saturated fat, cholesterol, sodium, and energy during mid to late childhood and early adolescence stages.

Adolescent problems associated with dietary inadequacy include emaciation due to anorexia nervosa among affluent youth and obesity among the poor. Co-morbidities that combine both under- and overnutrition, such as iron deficiency anemia and obesity, may exist in a single person. Healthy dietary habits during adolescence can be maintained by meeting needs for energy and protective nutrients such as proteins, vitamins, and minerals and identifying and altering eating habits that are not conducive to good nutrition, e.g., excessive intake of high-calorie low nutrient- dense foods, high-fat foods, highly irregular and unplanned eating, and alcohol abuse. Many adolescents need professional help in maintaining their weight at appropriate levels for their growth status, and in altering weight either downwards or upwards.

To reduce fatness in adolescents, physical activity is to be encouraged to prevent obesity and to lose weight in the already obese. Vigorous aerobic physical activity for at least 20 minutes at 60% or more of maximal aerobic capacity is important among obese adolescents, because their problems with fatness are often linked with low energy outputs rather than elevated intakes. Moderation in dietary habits instead of drastic dieting programs are advisable. Reductions in caloric intakes by 50 to 100 calories are in order, with increased outputs, until linear growth has ceased. However, decreasing fatness by dietary means during puberty must not stunt growth, and unless obesity is very pronounced, dietary treatment is often best delayed until physical maturity has been reached.

The goal of dietary treatment is not weight loss, but fat loss and the growth of lean tissue. Modest caloric reduction and a vigorous physical activity program that expends energy favors development of muscles and bones. Obese adolescents also need help in recognizing and avoiding ineffective reducing diets and the perils of fasting and self-induced vomiting to achieve weight control. Very lean adolescents need help in assessing their weight status and reaching more healthy weights (75).

Adolescent pregnancy and lactation further increase the need for many nutrients. Pregnant adolescents may need special help in meeting their needs while increasing both the quality of their diets and satisfying their food preferences.

Nutritional well-being is only a part of the development of a healthy body; other important aspects include aerobic fitness, muscle strength, flexibility, and adequate fat stores. Some immediate benefits of physical fitness include fun, new ways to combat boredom, exercise, stress or tension relief, and a positive mental attitude; the long-term benefits are better physical appearance, increased self-confidence, better tolerance of physical exertion, and better control of body weight. Some common fears and problems that pose as barriers to physical activity include lack of time, fear of soreness or overheating, and among girls, concerns that exercise will make them unfeminine and cause ravenous appetites that in turn will lead to excessive weight gain.

The easiest way to improve fitness during adolescence is to increase the daily physical activities and exercise training. All activities involving moving the body, such as walking, lifting objects, climbing stairs, and the like can lead to considerable energy outputs, because the total time spent in these activities is considerably more than that spent in vigorous exercise, even though outputs per minute are lower than for more vigorous exercise. Life-long aerobic exercise patterns tend to foster cardiovascular fitness, e.g., walking, bicycling, jogging, soccer, and tennis. Adolescents themselves could choose the type of physical activity and exercise that suits them well and is best to meet their needs.

The importance of good nutrition in childhood and adolescence in determining later health is being realized increasingly; it is thought to decrease the risk factors of coronary artery disease associated with dietary fat and cholesterol intakes in early life; also recognized is the importance of achieving high peak bone mass on later risk of osteoporosis (75) (see Chapter 27).

C. Diet During Old Age

Quantitative needs for most nutrients, notably energy, decrease as the human organism ages, though the qualitative needs for all essential nutrients remain the same. Because the energy intakes during old age are lower than in adulthood, there is a rise in the nutrient density needs. Foods that are high in nutrient density but low in fat (energy) and that provide protein, vitamins, and minerals are helpful for elderly people—e.g., lean meat, fish, eggs, low fat milk, and fruits and vegetables.

Diet-related diseases and disorders (see Chapters 24 through 34) afflict many people during aging; some elderly persons require therapeutic diets (89) and many others have difficulties in undertaking the purchase, preparation, and cooking of food (90). Also, eating difficulties in old age may necessitate alterations in food constituents, in the physical form of food, or in the manner of feeding.

Nutritional goals among persons over 65 years of age are improved quality of life and the promotion of continued autonomy. Good nutritional status is essential for a high quality of life, because food contributes to the quality of life through psychological, social, and physical mechanisms (91,92).

It is assumed that in terms of functional capacity, physical conditions, and social, economic, and lifestyle situations, the elderly population is more heterogeneous than any other age group. Also, the research base for making nutritional recommendations for older people is still evolving (75), needing updates of specific recommendations periodically. There is a need to find ways not only to moderate the aging process, but also to decrease the consequences of the diseases of old age. The impairments, disabilities, and handicaps arising from diseases associated with old age have impacts on the activities of daily living, including eating.

1. Nutritional Needs of Old Age

The U.S. RDAs (1989) have recommended intakes for most nutrients, including for energy, for individuals 55 years and older, which are not divided separately for lack of data (93). Suter and Russell (94) have shown how requirements for vitamins and minerals change with aging: in general they decrease with age as the result of reduction in physical activity and decreases in resting energy expenditure. The lean body mass, the metabolically active tissue of the body, declines by about 3 kg per decade after age 50, though it is likely that these declines in lean body mass are not totally inevitable but instead reflect the more sedentary lifestyle of older people; and to a lesser extent they may also signal the presence of one disease or another (95–97). Cellular metabolic rates also decline significantly with aging, but these are much smaller than decreases in physical activity.

Based on the current knowledge of nutrition, it is assumed that energy allowances should decrease by about 6% between 51 and 75 years of age, and by another 6% after 76 years, about two-thirds of the decrease being due to decreased physical activity, and one-third to decreases in the resting metabolism (98). The currents RDA of about 80 mg/day of high quality protein for aging adults appears to be reasonable, though some researchers have indicated that older adults may require more protein than younger adults (99). The nutrients involved in energy metabolism (thiamin, riboflavin, niacin) are required in lower quantities in old age than in adulthood, whereas calcium requirements may be even higher in estrogen-deprived postmenopausal women (100). Vitamin D supplements (10 mg/day) for institutionalized or housebound old people can be improved especially during the winter months; also beneficial is increasing their exposure to sunlight wherever possible. The Committee on Diet and Health stresses the avoidance of excess and imbalances and achieving sufficiency for adults of all ages (101).

The increasing evidence indicates that the marked decrease in physical activity observed in elderly people today is not desirable, and they should have a reasonable, individually tailored physical activity and exercise program, after consulting a physican.

2. Old Age, Body Weights, and Intake of Macronutrients

Whereas men tend to become overweight between 35 and 64 years of age, women continue to rise in weight throughout their lives at least up to 65 years. There is a slight lifetime loss in stature, probably about 3 cm in men and 5 cm in women (102). Russell and McGandy (103) observed that the weight-for-height reference standards based on desirable weight for lowest mortality derived for people 25 to 59 years of age may not be useful for elderly people. Normative standards, which include data on people up to age 75, also have disadvantages, because such data simply report the weights and heights of the elderly and are based on what is rather than on the actuarial standard of lowest mortality, or some other index showing that at these weights function is improved. The data summarized from several studies indicated that minimal mortality did not occur in the leanest segments of the population, as was commonly believed, but in individuals who were somewhat plumper (104–106). Data from the longitudinal aging study also showed that mild or moderate overweight among the elderly was not a potent risk factor, even after correcting for smoking (107).

The optimal weights from the standpoint of morbidity and improved functional status appear to be in the range of the adjusted values presented by Frisancho (108). It is known that height decreases with age, and when it is not possible to obtain weights for height because height cannot be measured, segmental measurements, such as lengths from ankle to knee, can be made, and these are related to overall height. Tables are available for making these conversions.

Recommendations for macronutrients such as carbohydrate are at least 100 g per day, to avoid ketosis. The dietary guidelines for Americans suggest that intakes of complex carbohydrates and fiber should increase; fiber intakes of 25 to 30 g/day from natural sources are necessary for normal laxation with recourse to medication. Avoidance of between-meal foods that are high in fermentable carbohydrates (sugary-starchy mixtures), and the importance of good oral hygiene have been stressed to prevent tooth root caries. Maintenance of ideal weight and modest reduction in sugar in the diet are suggested for diabetic individuals (especially type II, non-insulin-dependent). Also, among most diabetics, increased calories from carbohydrates and decreased proportion of calories from fats have been suggested, because all types of diabetics are at high risk for atherosclerosis.

The type and amount of dietary fat and cholesterol are risk factors for elevated serum cholesterol, at least among middle-aged persons, and probably also among older individuals, especially because most of the age-related rise in serum cholesterol is in LDL (low-density lipoprotein) cholesterol, the levels of which can be modified by dietary alterations. Along with the emphasis on moderation with respect to fat and cholesterol consumption, it is also vital for elderly people to follow other health recommendations regarding smoking and antihypertensive medications, the two health behaviors that are likely to have great and well-documented impacts on arteriosclerotic and cardiovascular diseases, among the elderly.

The water content of the body decreases with age, with a reduction in the urine-concentrating capacity, so that more water is required to excrete smaller quantities of wastes from the body. It is therefore important that fluid needs are liberally met by the elderly. Also, moderation in the use of alcohol among the aged is warranted, because the barbiturates taken by some may interact adversely with alcohol. Because of the lower body water of the aging individual, the same amount of alcohol leads to far greater blood alcohol levels in older than in younger individuals. Drug-drug and drug-nutrient interactions should be discovered and measures should be taken to avoid or minimize them. It is also necessary to ensure that the home and other living environments of elderly people are safe, to avoid any possible accidents (75).

V. DIETS FOR SPORTSMEN AND ATHLETES

The notion that certain constituents of the diet can confer exceptional virtues or abilities, and a primitive but understandable belief that "you are what you eat," has raised the interest of sportsmen and athletes in nutritional rituals for centuries. This is illustrated by the Zulus, who reputedly increased their valor by eating the hearts of their prisoners, as the ancient gladiators and Olympic competitors increased their strength by eating bull's testicles (the first use of anabolic steroids).

Success and failure in modern sports can be separated by millimeters or 100ths of a second. These fractional differences in the performance leading to fame and fortune from anonymity have been ascribed to a champion's diet, especially if it contains anything exotic. Lesse Viren, Finnish Olympic champion at 5000 and 10,000 m in both 1972 and 1976, claimed that his success was based on a diet that included reindeer milk, though sceptics believed that it was due to blood doping—the infusion of extra blood a few days before competition (109).

Computerized assessment of energy expenditure during football has been employed to produce precisely calculated diets for individual players. This method has an accuracy of about 20% in calculating energy expenditure, and since there is only about 20% accuracy in following a feeding formula, the average athlete would be around 10 to 20 times more accurate in the long term by relying on body mechanisms and appetite instead of the computerized assessment.

Hard and strenuous training is part of modern athletics, developed in the 1960s and 1970s. It was believed that he or she who trained hardest and longest triumphed, which resulted in training schedules for athletes consisting of several hours a day of severe exertion; the training loads distributed into two or more sessions per day, each lasting as long as 2 hours. Because exercise must be taken more than 1 to 2 hours after meals, fitting in the meals between the training sessions can be a major problem, resulting in skipping of meals. For an amateur, self-supporting athlete, arranging the training and adequate meals can be very difficult and expensive.

Severe exertion of training burns up a large amount of carbohydrate, depleting muscle glycogen stores. Running or jogging a mile expends about 100 kcal, and runners running 20 miles or more a day may exceed 2000 kcal energy. Saris et al. (110) estimated that cyclists in the Tour de France expended more than about 6000 kcal/day, a caloric intake that is rather difficult to achieve by conventional means.

A.   Metabolic Requirements During Exercises

1.   Aerobics

Aerobic exercise involves a sustained level of exertion, usually of large muscle groups (e.g., walking, jogging, swimming, or cycling) that can be maintained for several minutes without excessive breathlessness. The exertion is performed with the aerobic metabolism of glycogen and fat, without accumulation of lactate from anerobic glycolysis.

With a steadily increasing exercise load on ergometer, e.g. bicycle or treadmill with increasing speed/gradient, the oxygen uptake gradually increases to a maximum, in this case 4 liters/min. The oxygen uptake thereafter plateaus as does the heart rate: 50% and 75% of maximum oxygen uptake are marked. The blood lactate remains steady during the early, totally aerobic phase of the exercise, but begins to increase at point, and rapidly thereafter. This is the anerobic threshold (or lactate threshold). No units are given for this idealized representation. The lactate threshold in this case is at about 65% of VO_2 max and can be increased with aerobic training. Close to VO_2 max, glycogen is the sole muscle fuel, but at lower levels fat contributes up to 50% of the energy (109). Thus, aerobic exercise can be performed only until a certain point, then there is a sudden increase in the respiration, which becomes more labored and is associated with a large increase in the level of perceived exertion. At this point glycogen is metabolized anaerobically as well as aerobically, with the accumulation of lactate in the muscles and in the blood (anerobic threshold). Incremental exercise after this point is often of limited duration, and the O_2 consumption rate plateaus at a high level of perceived exertion, with a heart rate close to its maximum, and any further exertion will render the subject severely short of breath. The blood activity becomes more marked, with the normal pH of around 7.35 dropping to 7.0 or even lower on severe exertion. The low pH causes breakdown of carbonic acid, with the release of CO_2 and an increasingly high respiratory quotient with more CO_2 being expired than O_2 being taken up. Exertion above the level of O_2 consumption plateaus, becomes increasingly anaerobic, and is eventually limited by fatigue in the muscle caused by an excess of protons generated by anerobic glycosis. Further severe exertion after this point is usually not possible until the lactic acid in the muscles and blood is metabolized aerobically in the liver (109).

2. Anerobic Exercise

Anerobic exercise is that which takes place above the anerobic threshold in which the predominant source of energy is anaerobic glycolysis of glycogen. This is often short lasting because it is limited by accumulation of lactate in the muscle and blood, e.g., sprint or a series of push-ups.

The above picture of aerobic and anaerobic exercise is based on whole-body measurements. Even below the anerobic threshold, some individual muscle fibers will be functioning anaerobically and the lactate will be metabolized by other fibers or by the liver, without rising the blood lactate level. Above the anerobic threshold, there will still be many muscle fibers working aerobically, depending on the fiber types, the intensity of the exercise, the degree of 'training' of the muscle, and its perfusion.

Maximum oxygen uptake (VO_2 max) is the level of exertion at which O_2 uptake plateaus, expressed in liters/min or ml of O_2/kg body weight/min for comparisons between people of different build—e.g., an 80 kg man with VO_2 max of 4 liter/min may have a value of 50 ml/kg body wt/min. These values range between 20 and 90 ml/kg/min, with the highest values being found in exceptional athletes having very little body fat. The maximum O_2 uptake is related to the lean body mass; the lowest values of VO_2 max, expressed in ml O_2/kg/min are found in obese people. VO_2 max indicates the potential for aerobic exercise and can be increased with training by up to 20% in the previously unathletic subject.

Exercise at maximum O_2 uptake levels cannot be sustained for long; the stimulus for this appears to be partly anaerobic and this level of exertion can be maintained for about 7 min in the well-trained athlete. Thus, the anerobic threshould is a better measure of what can be sustained for long periods, often expressed as a percentage of VO_2 max. This value varies greatly with the degree of training, e.g., an elite marathon runner may run for more than 2 hr at 80% to 90% of VO_2 max. whereas the untrained person may have difficulty in maintaining a value of 60%.

Anaerobic exercise and exercise close to the VO_2 max is almost entirely catered for by glycogen metabolism, whereas the fuel for aerobic exercise at levels below 60% of VO_2 max is about 50% fat. Aerobic training increases the percentage of fat used.

Levels of exertion can be expressed in various ways, in addition to relating them to VO_2 max: The O_2 demand in ml/kg body wt is a commonly used method, and is expressed in terms of multiples of the resting O_2 uptake, which is 200 to 250 ml/min for the average man or 3.5 ml/kg/min for a 70 kg man. Severe exertion in an elite endurance athlete would be 20 times this value (20 metabolic equivalents, METS), giving totals of 70 ml/kg/min or 5 liter/min, the average level of O_2 uptake required to run 11 to 12 miles/hr (17.5 km/hr) on a flat surface. This level of exertion generates about a kilowatt of heat (109); moderate exercise costs about 10 METS or consumes 2.5 liters O_2/min, a level that can be sustained by a moderately fit person.

B. Requirements of Energy

Energy required for both immediate and prolonged exertion is supplied from the muscle stores that are replaced late from outside stores. The type of exercise and extent of exertion determines the utilization energy source, such as ATP, creatine phosphate, muscle glycogen used anaerobically and aerobically and the body fat; e.g. sudden exertion is catered for by ATP, a very short burst of exercise by creatine phosphate, and longer periods of exercise by anaerobic and then aerobic utilization of glycogen, and an increasing utilization of body fat as the exercise becomes less intense and more prolonged (111).

The relatively smaller stores of energy in the form of ATP and creatine phosphate and the inhibition of further anerobic degradation of glycogen due to acidosis exert a protective effect on the muscle to prevent its overheating and possible enzyme denaturation. The division between aerobic and anerobic energy sources is seen in events involving maximum exertion lasting about 2 min (800 m running), where around 50% of the energy comes for each aerobic and anerobic degradation of muscle glycogen.

According to Holloszy and Coyle (112), fat metabolism on its own can only maintain exercise at about 50% of VO_2 max. and this type of exercise with depleted muscle glycogen is extremely arduous. Fat cannot be oxidized at rates comparable to glycogen degradation, though fat releases more than twice the energy of glycogen for each gram oxidized. Also fat is stored in the cell as pure fat, whereas glycogen is stored with about three times its weight of water. Data in Table 8 show the running time and distance that can be supported by the energy stores of an average human subject (113).

The much larger energy stores in the form of fat are of limited value in most sports because they do not allow a sufficiently high energy output and may have an adverse effect on the power/weight ratio. In addition to providing insulation against cold, such as in swimming, fat is used as a fuel source during all endurance events. It is probably used in conjunction with other fuel supplies such as carbohydrates.

One of the most important dietary essentials is adequate fluid replacement during exercise. The athlete is advised to drink sufficient fluid to maintain a pale, straw-colored urine, and plenty of it, and to drink copiously if the volume of urine decreases and becomes darker. A 70 kg man has a total body water of 50 liters, of which about 36 liters is intracellular, 10.5 liters intestinal, and only about 3.5 liters in the blood plasma. Because water moves between these compartments, severe dehydration from sweat loss may deplete water from plasma and intestinal compartments as well as from the cells. Total rehydration after severe dehydration is rather gradual and often takes more than 24 hours.

C. Requirements of Water

Thirst reflecting plasma volume, stomach contents, and mouth breathing is a poor indicator of fluid requirement, and is even worse when there is intracellular water and salt loss and contraction of the plasma volume. If this occurs, water is perhaps not the best fluid for replacement for rapid correction of dehydration (114). Water in large volumes renders the blood plasma hypotonic, promoting a brisk diuresis; an electrolyte solution does not. The latter also allows greater fluid retention and replacement of intracellular water loss. Beer, the common athlete's beverage, can potentiate dehydration, because it gives an illusion of satisfying thirst but may produce a bigger volume of diuresis than the volume consumed.

Loss of water in the form of sweat during prolonged exertion can be as high as 1 to 2 liters/hour, the loss of about 8% body water (4 liters) or even more being common during

Table 8 Energy Stores as Fat and Glycogen in an Average Man

Source	KJ	Running time (min)	Miles
Adipose triglycerols	337500	4018	550–630
Liver glycogen	1660	20	3–4
Muscle glycogen	5880	71	10–14
Blood glucose	48	Less than 1	0

Source: Ref. 113.

marathons lasting 2 to 4 hours. Fluid replacement being difficult while running, the dehydration produced can have profound physiological effects, not least in limiting sweat production, which is the principal means of controlling body temperature during exertion. Exercise is thermodynamically very inefficient, because it generates twice as much heat energy as the mechanical energy used. Nadal et al. (115) noted that sustained production of around 1 KW of heat energy is stored to produce a temporary rise in body temperature; the rest has to be dissipated to the environment, principally by evaporating sweat. If this heat is not dissipated, it could raise body temperature by 1°C/5 min, which would theoretically be lethal after 30 to 40 min. In practice, it produces heat collapse or heat stroke in athletes who stop sweating.

A 70 kg man running 10 miles (16 km) in 1 hr produces a heat of 1000 kcal (4000 kJ), which must be dissipated to maintain normal body temperature. Evaporation of 1 liter of sweat loses about 600 kcal (2500 kJ) of heat, and considering lower sweating efficiency, the runner would be required to sweat at least 1.7 liters or more to retain thermal equilibrium of the body. During severe exertion, practical experience shows that on an average runners can consume about 500 ml fluid/hr without producing discomfort and nausea (116). Drinking on the run causes much air swallowing, and both gastric emptying and intestinal absorption are rate limited and influenced by several factors (117).

With exertion rising over 70% VO_2 max., sweating becomes profuse; the highest recorded sweat rates of 5 liters/hr are found on exposure of body to hot environment at rest where the skin blood flow is at maximum and not competing with circulation to active muscle. Athletes may train for as much as 20 hr/week with sweat rates of 1 to 2 liter/hr, which may lead to chronic dehydration.

Fluid losses are best made good as soon as they occur, with water or fruit cordials of various types, supplemented perhaps by beer after competition. Beer, however, promotes diuresis by inhibiting antidiuretic hormone and thus prevents complete rehydration. Several newly introduced sports drinks claim to put back fluid faster than water and replace electrolytes lost in sweat, as well as to supplement carbohydrate intake to delay fatigue by putting back lost energy fast (109).

D. Requirements of Sodium and Other Electrolytes

Isotonic drinks containing small quantities of sodium and other electrolytes (Cl^-, K^+) and glucose, taken during endurance events, such as marathon runs, are absorbed better than water and may have benefits over plain water in preventing, correcting, or delaying dehydration. Chronic salt depletion in athletes is very unlikely but may occur in some non-endurance athletes who are not heat acclimatized on sudden exposure to heat conditions. They may be advised to put extra salt on their food or in their drinks without making it a lifetime habit. The use of slow-release salt tablets (slow sodium) in sports appears to be extravagent and unnecessary. Excess of potassium and other electrolytes lost during exercise can be readily met by dietary intakes and through fruit juices (109).

E. Requirements of Carbohydrates

Muscle glycogen stores limit sustained exercise at between 60% and 80% of VO_2 max, after 1 to 3 hrs of continuous exercise (118), the exercise becoming more strenuous as the muscle glycogen levels fall and fat becomes the main fuel source. The exercise then becomes slower (50% of VO_2 max), requiring higher O_2 cost, with fat as the fuel instead of carbohydrate, as more O_2 is used per unit of ATP produced. This may be followed by a risk of hypoglycemia when the muscle carbohydrate level is severely depleted (119). Liver glycogen is broken down to maintain blood sugar level, some of which may be taken up by muscle with a fall in blood glucose. Exercise at

60% to 80% VO_2 max in trained athletes can be maintained for longer times, if the muscle glycogen is at a high level before exercise begins. Endurance athletes often have higher-than-normal muscle glycogen levels and are on high carbohydrate diets after resting for a few days. This increase in muscle glycogen is known as "carbo loading." A week before the marathon event, the athletes severely deplete their muscle glycogen stores with long runs followed by repeated fast strides. During the next 3 days, they train moderately hard while eating a low carbohydrate diet, predominantly composed of protein and fat to further deplete muscle glycogen. For the last 4 days, they train only lightly but eat a very high carbohydrate diet. The muscles deprived of glycogen would be supercompensated with much higher than normal glycogen stores (120,121). This regimen, however, does not suit all runners; some find that training on a low-carbohydrate diet is very uncomfortable, and they start the race stiff and heavy. Brewer et al. (122) suggested that endurance runners can have high muscle glycogen by tapering off their training for the few days before the race and eating a very high carbohydrate diet. Thus, a well-trained endurance athlete can load his muscle with about 2 kg of glycogen bound with water, which is released as the glycogen is metabolized and acts as an additional source of water.

Foster et al. (123) postulated that a high-carbohydrate meal or snack taken an hour before exercise carries the risk of producing a dramatic insulin response, increased glycogen utilization, and premature fatigue, leading to hypoglycemia. This does not occur if a carbohydrate drink is taken just before the commencement of exercise. The circulating catecholamines during vigorous exercise suppress the insulin response and prevent the negative effect of carbohydrate feeding (124). It has also been shown that these drinks, or indeed solid carbohydrate, may prolong exercise endurance or improve performance if taken repeatedly during an endurance event, although studies by Coyle et al. (125) showed no muscle glycogen is used by the exercising muscle. Saris et al. (110) similarly demonstrated that the average requirements, about 6000 kcal/day energy of Tour de France cyclists, could be met by continuous feeding with high carbohydrate drinks, which accounted for 50% of their caloric intake on race days. Simulation of the race in a calorimeter indicated that without the maltodextrin drink, cyclists could not maintain their energy balance and catabolized muscle protein (126). Cyclists who could not maintain the required energy intake in the Tour de France dropped out from fatigue, and only those who matched their caloric intake to the energy expended day by day (presumably by conserving and replacing muscle glycogen) did well.

The progressive depletion of muscle glycogen and fatigue encountered during high-intensity training, both aerobic and anerobic, can take up to 48 hrs to replace glycogen, and rest days may be essential to do this. Glycogen is taken into muscle most avidly within 2 hr of exercise (127) and may be better supplied through repeated carbohydrate meals than in one or two large ones. A high carbohydrate diet (60%–70%) may be necessary for rapid replacement and maintenance of high glycogen in muscle (109).

F. Requirements of Protein

Maintenance of extraordinary physical bulk and powerful muscle would require consumption of a high protein diet, such as steak, eggs, milk, and so on. However, in certain sports events, power to weight ratio may be more important than mere physical bulk, wherein a high carbohydrate intake could benefit the athlete. This controversy has been complicated by the wide use of anabolic steroids by sportsmen in strength events, and an abnormally high protein intake may have been found essential to obtain the dramatic anabolic effects of steroids, causing spurts of power and energy for short times.

It is apparent that negative nitrogen balance may occur with inadequate carbohydrate intake during a heavy training load, which can be readily remedied by consuming increased carbohydrate diet as well as by an increase in protein. According to Lemon (128), endurance athletes require a higher than normal protein intake, about twice the usual RDA, which is also true of the strength athletes, provided both these groups have adequate carbohydrate intake. The strength athletes may require more than 200% of the RDA to maintain nitrogen balance when they are on a muscle-building/weight-reduction regimen. An accelerated rate of protein turnover rather than the formation of new muscle tissue during the training appears to be the reason for the extra protein requirement. The accelerated rate of protein turnover in athletes during training also demonstrated increased protein catabolism.

According to FAO/WHO/UNU committee estimates from the results of the best nitrogen balance studies, the average need of adults for high-quality proteins is 0.6 g/kg body weight/day. The FAO/WHO's "safe" intake limit was set at 0.75 g of high-quality protein/kg/day. The RDA for adults in the United States of America is 0.8 g/kg/day. Men and women do not differ in their protein requirements per unit of body weight, but women, because they generally weigh less, need less total protein than men. No extra allowance for protein is recommended for physically active people.

The recommended intakes of protein for different age groups are sufficient to meet protein needs if there is adequate consumption of all other essential nutrients and energy. These amounts of protein are less than most people desire, which is evident from the average U.S. intake of nearly 100 g/day. The committee that established the recommended intakes of nutrients (RNI) for the United Kingdom proposed a guideline for protein of not less than 10% of calories. Recommendations of 10% to 15% of kcalories as protein on the basis of evidence that diets rich in protein are ordinarily highly nutritious are not likely to pose a risk to human health. As caloric expenditure declines during aging, the appropriate guideline for the elderly should probably be toward the upper end of the range, but as kidney function also tends to decline with increasing age, it should not exceed 15% of total calories.

G. Requirements of Iron

Risser et al. (129) noted that about 30% of women cross-country runners were iron deficient, which they attributed to probable use of 'junk food' or food fads. Some iron loss may occur in sweat and slightly increased gastrointestinal blood loss in runners, especially when they take aspirin or other nonsteroidal anti-inflammetory drugs for an injury or stiffness. The occasional hematuria from bladder trauma and hemoglobinuria is often well compensated by the increased total dietary intake associated with high-calorie diets of athletes. Iron supplements are thus not normally considered necessary and may cause gastrointestinal disturbances or even hemosiderosis. Brotherhood et al. (130) studying hematological paramters in a group of 40 male distance runners and 12 control subjects observed no significant differences between those on iron or iron and folate supplements, and those on a normal diet.

Iron deficiency may be suspected in endurance athletes having a slightly lower than average hemoglobin (athletes' anemia; a hemoglobin less than 14 g% in men and less than 12 g% in women). This is often a training-induced physiological condition caused by an increase in plasma volume (10%–30%), which is greater than the training-induced increase in red cell mass. However, despite a slightly reduced hemoglobin, the total red cell mass is often normal or greater than normal in these athletes. Athletes' anemia, thought to be associated with low serum ferritin, has not been found to be correlated with poor performance, and does not respond to iron supplementation. Thus, hemoglobin and ferritin levels can be misleading. Iron therapy for one month may be justified only when the mean cell hemoglobin level is less than 25 μg or the ferritin is more than 5 μg lower than the laboratory limit (131,132); if iron deficiency is really present, the hemoglobin level should rise by 1 g. Women athletes may, however, have genuine iron deficiency, either from menstrual losses, dietary fads, or both.

H. Requirements for Amino Acids, Vitamins and Trace Elements

Amino acids may be used as a source of fuel by active muscle (133). It has been suggested that the overtraining syndrome of endurance athletes with its attendant immune deficiency may be prevented by glutamine supplements (134). Several studies have failed to show any advantages of super supplementation with trace elements and antioxidants such as vitamin C and E when the diet is adequate in these nutrients. Despite the lack of positive evidence, many athletes dose themselves every day with cocktails of amino acids, vitamins, trace elements, royal jelly, ginseng, and so on, whose promoters seem to be producing the required "scientific evidence" of their benefits. Some sports doctors have given vitamin B_{12} (cyanocobalamin) injections as placebos to athletes to boost their performance, to suggest that something is missing in the normal diet. The athletes are often found to overindulge in dietary supplementation of nutrients after dehydration and inadequate carbohydrate intake.

The International Congress on Sports Nutrition held in 1990 has suggested the following guidelines for sportsmen and athletes (109):

1. A diet adequate, in terms of quantity and quality, during and after training and competition will produce maximum performance. Carbohydrates probably contribute about 60% to 70% of the total energy intake, protein about 12%, and the remainder fat in the optimum diet for most sports.
2. Total energy intake must be raised to meet the enhanced energy expenditure during training. The maintenance of energy balance can be assessed by monitoring body weight, body composition, and food intake. Body weight should be reduced gradually, if necessary and not immediately after competition.
3. High-intensity and long-duration athletic events, such as multiple sprint and endurance sports, require a good supply of carbohydrate for better performance. High carbohydrate diets (greater than two-thirds of total energy) and maximum glycogen stores are responsible for improved performance in such activity and are also needed to sustain high-intensity training on a daily basis. The requirement for sugars and starches, in both solid and liquid forms, varies depending on the duration and nature of the physical activity in the sport.
4. Increased fluid intake may be necessary to avoid dehydration and improve performance during prolonged exercise, especially when sweat loss is high in hot climates. Normal food intakes after exercise can replace electrolytes and salts when sweat losses are relatively small in short-duration exercises.
5. The protein requirements for individuals involved in physical training programs are relatively higher than in inactive people. Most athletes, however, consume sufficient proteins as a consequence of their increased energy intake.
6. Fat consumption should be restricted to 30% of the total energy intake; body is able to mobilize its large energy store which must be maintained between the periods of exercise by ingesting sufficient energy.
7. Vitamin supplements are not needed for athletes eating an adequate diet, both in respect of its quantity and quality. The iron and calcium status of the body should be maintained at desired levels, especially in those individuals who may be at risk.

REFERENCES

1. Fallon, A.E., and P. Rozin, The psychological bases of food rejection by humans, *Ecol. Food Nutr.* *13*: 15 (1983).

2. Clydesdale, F.M., and F.J. Francis, *Food Nutrition and Health*, AVI Publishing Co., Westport, 1985.
3. Hertzler, A.A., N. Wenkam, and B. Standall, Classifying cultural food habits and meanings, *J. Am. Med. Assoc. 80*: 421 (1983).
4. Clydesdale, F.M., Nutritional realities—where does technology fit? *J. Am. Diet. Assoc. 74*: 17 (1979).
5. Garza, C., Pregnancy and lactation, *Human Nutrition and Dietetics*, 9th ed. (J.S. Garrow and W.P.T. James, eds.), Churchill Livingstone, Edinburgh, London, 1993, p. 376.
6. FAO/WHO/UNU, Expert Consultation, Energy and Protein Requirements, Technical Report Series 724, World Health Organization, Geneva, 1985.
7. Anonymous, Nutrition during pregnancy, Subcommittee on 'Nutritional Status and Weight Gain During Pregnancy' and Subcommittee on 'Dietary Intake and Nutrient Supplements During Pregnancy,' Institute of Medicine, National Academy Press, Washington, DC, 1990.
8. Hytteen, F.E., and G. Chamberlain, *Clinical Physiology in Obstetrics*, Blackwell Scientific, Oxford, 1980, p. 193.
9. Taggart, N.R., R.M. Holiday, and W.Z. Billewicz, Changes in skinfold during pregnancy, *British J. Nutr. 21*: 439 (1967).
10. Heinig, M.J., L.A. Nommsen, and K.G. Dewey, Lactation and postpartum weight loss, *FASEB J. 4*: 362A (1990).
11. Butte, N.F., C. Garza, and J.E. Stuff, Effect of maternal diet and body composition on lactational performance, *Am. J. Clin. Nutr. 39*: 296 (1984).
12. Brewer, M.M., M.R. Bates, and L.P. Vannoy, Postpartum changes in maternal weight and body fat depots in lactating vs. nonlactating women, *Am. J. Clin. Nutr. 49*: 259 (1989).
13. COMA, Reference values for food energy and nutrients for the United Kingdom, Committee on Medical Aspects of Food Policy, HMSO, London, 1991.
14. Durnin, J.V.G.A., Energy requirements of pregnancy, An integrated study in 5 countries: background and methodology, Nestle Foundation Annual Report, Nestle Foundation, Lausanne, 1986.
15. Illingworth, P.J., R.T. Jung, and P.W. Howie, et al., Diminution in energy expenditure during lactation, *British Med. J. 292*: 437 (1986).
16. Mertz, W., J.C. Tsui, and J.T. Judd, What are people really eating? The relationship between energy intake derived from estimated diet records and intake determined to maintain body weight, *Am. J. Clin. Nutr. 54*: 291 (1991).
17. Tyson, J.E., K. Austin, J. Fairnholt, Endocrine metabolic response to acute starvation in human gestation, *Am. J. Obstet. Gynecol. 125*: 1073 (1976).
18. Frigerio, C., Y. Schutz, and A. Prentice, Is human lactation a particularly efficient process? *European J. Clin. Nutr. 45*: 459 (1991).
19. Frigerio, C., Y. Schutz, R. Whitehead, and R. Jequier, Lactation and infant feeding, *Am. J. Clin. Nutr. 54*: 526 (1991).
20. Whitehead, R.G., M. Lawrence, and A.M. Prentice, Maternal nutrition and breast feeding, *Human Nutr. Appl. Nutr. 40*A (Suppl.): 1 (1986).
21. SNDL, Nutrition during lactation, Subcommittee on Nutrition During Lactation, Institute of Medicine, National Academy Press, Washington, DC, 1991.
22. Brown, R.H., N.A. Akhtor, A.D. Robertson, and M.G. Ahmed, Lactation capacity of marginally malnourished mothers: relationships between maternal nutritional status and quantity and proximate composition of milk, *Pediatrics 78*: 909 (1986).
23. Lechtig, A., J.P. Habicht, and H. Delgado, Effect of food supplementation during pregnancy on birthweight, *Pediatrics 56*: 508 (1975).
24. Delgado, H.L., V.E. Valverde, R. Martorell, and R.E. Klein, Relationship of maternal and infant nutrition to infant growth, *Early Human Development 6*: 273 (1982).
25. NRC, *Recommended Dietary Allowances*, 10th cd., National Research Council, National Academy Press, Washington, DC, 1989.
26. Olsen, S.F., J.D. Sorenson, and N.J. Sacher, Randomised controlled trial of effect of fish-oil supplementation on pregnancy duration, *Lancet 339*: 1003 (1992).
27. Nettleton, J.A., Are *n*-3 fatty acids essential nutrients for fetal and infant development? *J. Am. Dietet. Assoc. 93*: 58 (1993).

28. Specker, B.L., B. Valanis, and V. Hertzberg, Sunshine exposure and serum 25-hydroxy vitamin D concentrations in exclusively breastfed infants, *J. Pediatrics 107*: 372 (1985).

29. Shah, R.S., and R. Rajalakshmi, Vitamin A status of the newborn in relation to gestational care, body weight and maternal nutritional status, *Am. J. Clin. Nutr. 40*: 794 (1984).

30. Malheiros, L.R., F.J. Paumgarten, T.R. Riul, and V.A. DeSilva. Protein-energy malnutrition increases teratogenicity of hypervitaminosis A in rats, *Brazilian J. Med. Biol. Res. 21*: 659 (1988).

31. Sommer, A., *Nutritional Blindness: Xerophthalmia and Keraltomalacia*, Oxford University Press, New York, 1982.

32. Anonymous, *Pediatric Nutrition Handbook*, 2nd ed, Committee on Nutrition, American Academy of Pediatrics, Elk Grove Village, IL, 1985.

33. Pomerance, J.J., T.G. Teal, and J.F. Gogolock, Maternally administered antenatal vitamin K: effect on neonatal prothrombin activity, partial thromboplastin time, and intraventricular hemorrhage, *Obstet. Gynecol. 70*: 295 (1987).

34. MRC, Vitamin study group 1991, Prevention of neural tube defects: results of the Medical Research Council Vitamin Study, *Lancet 338*: 131 (1991).

35. Smithells, R.W., S. Sheppard, and C.J. Schorah, Vitamin deficiencies and neural tube defects, *Arch. Dis. Childhood 51*: 944 (1976).

36. Rosenberg, I.H., Folic acid and neural tube defects time for action, *N. Engl. J. Med. 327*: 1875 (1992).

37. Specker, B.L., D. Miller, and E.J. Normal, Increased urinary methylmelonic acid exeretion in breast-fed infants of vegetarian mothers and identification of an acceptable dietary source of vitamin B_{12}, *Am. J. Clin. Nutr. 47*: 89 (1988).

38. Kirksey, A., and J.L.B. Roepke, Vitamin B_6 nutrition of mothers of three breastfed neonates with central nervous system disorders, *Fed. Proc. FASEB, 40*: 864 (1981).

39. Purdie, D.W., Bone mineral metabolism and reproduction. *Contemp. Rev. Obstet. Gynecol. 1*: 214 (1989).

40. Golden, B.E., Infant nutrition, *Human Nutrition and Dietetics*, 9th ed. (J.S. Garrow and W.P.T. James, eds.), Churchill Livingstone, Edinburgh, London. 1993, p. 387.

41. FNB, Recommended dietary allowances, Revised 1989, Food and Nutrition Board, National Academy of Sciences, National Academy Press, Washington, DC, 1989.

42. Fomon, S.J., Requirements and recommended dietary intakes of proteins during infancy, *Pediatric Res. 30*: 391 (1991).

43. Widstrom, A.M., A.B. Ransjo-Arvidson, K. Christensson, A-S. Marthiesen, J. Wingberg, and K. Uvnas-Moberg, Gastric suction in healthy newborn infants. Effects on circulation and developing feeding behaviour, *Acta Paedic. Scandinavica 76*: 566 (1987).

44. Uvnas-Moberg, K., and J. Winberg, Role for sensory stimulation in energy economy of mother and infant with particular regard to the gastrointestinal endocrine system, *Textbook of Gastroenterology and Nutrition in Infancy*, 2nd ed. (E. Lebenthal, ed.), Raven Press, New York, 1989, p. 53.

45. Williams, A.F., Lactation and infant feeding, *Textbook of Paediatric Nutrition*, 3rd ed. (D.S. McLaren, D. Burman, N.R. Belton, and A.F. Williams, eds.), Churchill Livingstone, Edinburgh, London, 1991, p. 21.

46. George, D.E., and B.A. Defrancesca, Human milk in comparison to cow milk, *Textbook of Gastroenterology and Nutrition in Infancy*, 2nd ed. (E. Lebenthal, ed.), Raven Press, New York, 1989, p. 239.

47. Hambraeus, L., Human milk: Nutritional aspects, *Clinical Nutrition of the Young Child* (O. Brunser, F.R. Carrazza, M. Gracey, et al., eds.), Raven Press, New York, 1991, p. 289.

48. Hanson, L.A., B. Carlsson, and F. Jalil, Antiviral and antibacterial factors in human milk, *Biology of Human Milk* (L.A. Hanson, ed.), Nestle Nutrition Workshop Series, Vol. 15, 1988, p. 141.

49. Carlsson, S.E., Human milk non-protein nitrogen: Occurrence and possible functions, *Advances in Pediatrics*, Vol. 32 (L.A. Barness, ed.), Year Book Medical, Chicago, 1985, p. 43.

50. Anonymous, Fluoride supplementation: revised dosage schedule, American Association of Pediatrics, *Pediatrics 63*: 150 (1979).

51. Rascoff, H., Beriberi heart in a 4-month-old infant, *J. Am. Med. Assoc. 120*: 1292 (1942).

52. Bachrach, S., J. Fisher, and J.S. Parks, An outbreak of vitamin D deficiency rickets in a susceptible population, *Pediatrics 64*: 871 (1979).

53. Motohara, M., M. Matsukura, and J. Matsuda, Severe vitamin K deficiency in breastfed infants, *J. Pediatrics 105*: 943 (1984).

54. Oxtoby, M.J., Human immunodeficiency virus and other viruses in human milk: placing the issues in broader perspective, *Pediatr. Inf. Dis. J. 7*: 825 (1988).

55. DHSS, Present-day practice in infant feeding: third report, Report on Health and Social Subjects No. 32, HMSO, London, 1988.

56. Lederman, S.A., Estimating infant mortality from human immunodeficiency virus and other causes in breast-feeding and bottle-feeding populations, *Pediatrics 89*: 290 (1992).

57. Taitz, L.S., and B.L. Armitage, Goat's milk for infants and children, *Br. Med. J. 288*: 428 (1984).

58. Fomon, S.J., E.E. Ziegler, and L.J. Filer, Methionine fortification of a soy formula fed to infants, *Am. J. Clin. Nutr. 32*: 2460 (1979).

59. Lonnerdal, B., Dietary factors affecting trace element bioavailability from human milk, cow's milk and infant formulas, *Progr. Nutr. Food Sci. 9*: 35 (1985).

60. Estham, E.J., T. Lichauco, M.I., Grade, and W.A. Walker, Antigenicity of infant formulas: role of immature intestine on protein permeability, *J. Pediatr. 93*: 561 (1978).

61. Bishop, N., M. McGraw, and N. Ward, Aluminium in infant formulas, *Lancet 1*: 490 (1989).

62. Rowland, M.G.M., The weanling's dilemma: are we making progress? *Acta Paediatrica Scandinavica 322* (Suppl.): 33 (1986).

63. Wharton, B.A., Weaning and early children, *Textbook of Paediatric Nutrition*, 3rd ed. (D.S. McLaren D. Burman, N.R. Belton, and A.F. Williams, eds.), Churchill Livingstone, Edinburgh, London, 1991, p. 47.

64. Anonymous, Guidelines on infant nutrition II. Recommendations for the composition of follow-up formula and Beikost, ESPGAN Committee on Nutrition, *Acta Paediatrica Scandinavica 287* (Suppl.): 1 (1981).

65. Barker, D.J.P., P.D. Winter, and C. Osmond, Weight in infancy and death from ischaemic heart disease, *Lancet 2*: 577 (1989).

66. Hales, C.N., D.J.P. Barker, and P.M.S. Clark, Fetal and infant growth and impaired glucose tolerance at age 64-years, *Br. Med. J. 303*: 1019 (1991).

67. Barclay, S., A. Ralph, and W.P.T. James, Childhood diet and adult disease, *Textbook of Paediatric Nutrition*, 3rd ed., (D.S. McLaren, D. Burman, N.R. Belton, and A.F. Williams, eds.), Churchill Livingstone, Edinburgh, London, 1991, p. 531.

68. Glinsmann, W.H., S.J. Bartholmey, and F. Coletta, Dietary guidelines for infants: a timely reminder, *Nutr. Rev. 54* (Suppl. 1): 50 (1996).

69. Anonymous, Dietary Guidelines Advisory Committe, Report of the Dietary Guidelines Advisory Committee on the dietary guidelines for Americans, 1995, to the Secretary of Agriculture and the Secretary of Health and Human Services, Washington, DC, 1995.

70. NRC, Energy, *Recommended Dietary Allowances*, 10th ed, National Academy Press, National Research Council, Washington, DC, 24, 1989.

71. Hayes, K.C., Dietary impact on biliary lipids and gallstones, *Annu. Rev. Nutr. 12*: 299 (1992).

72. Anonymous, Report of the 103rd Ross Conference on Pediatric Research, *Lipids, Learning, and the Brain*: *Fats in Infant Formulas* (J. Dobbing, ed.), Ross Laboratories, OH, 1993.

73. Carlson, S.E., S.H. Workman, J.M. Peeples, and W.M. Wilson, Long-chain fatty acids and early visual and cognitive development of preterm infants, *Eur. J. Clin. Nutr. 48* (Suppl. 2): 27 (1994).

74. Lonnerdal, B., and S. Iyer, Lactoferrin: molecular structure and biological function, *Annu. Rev. Nutr. 15*: 93 (1995).

75. Dwyer, J.T., Childhood, young and old age, *Human Nutrition and Dietetics*, 3rd ed. (J.S. Garrow and W.P.T. James, eds.) Churchill Livingstone, Edinburgh, London, 1993, p. 394.

76. AAP/CN, The feeding of supplemental foods to infants, American Academy of Pediatrics, Committee on Nutrition, *Pediatrics 65*: 1178 (1980).

77. AAP/CN, Toward a prudent diet for children, American Academy of Pediatrics, Committee on Nutrition, *Pediatrics 66*: 1015 (1980).

78. AAP/CN, Toward a prudent diet for children, American Academy of Pediatrics, Committee on Nutrition, *Pediatrics 71*: 78 (1983).

79. AAP/CN, *Pediatric Nutrition Handbook*, 2nd ed., American Academy of Pediatrics, Committee on Nutrition, Elk Grove Village, IL, 1985.

80. AAP/CN, Prudent life style for children: Dietary fat and cholesterol, American Academy of Pediatrics, Committee on Nutrition, *Pediatrics 78*: 521 (1986).

81. NCEP, Report of the Expert Panel on 'Blood Cholesterol Levels in Children and Adolescents,' National Cholesterol Education Program, U.S. Department of Health and Human Services, Public Health Services, National Institutes of Health, 1991.

82. Rosenbaum M., and R.L. Liebel, Obesity in children, *Pediatrics Rev. 11*: 53 (1989).

83. Shear, C.L., D.S. Freedman, G.L. Burke, D.W. Harsha, L.S. Webber, and G.S. Berenson, Secular trends of obesity in early life: the Bogalusa Heart Study, *Am. J. Public Health 78*: 75 (1988).

84. Harlan, W.R., J.R. Landes, K.M. Flegal, C.S. Davis, and M.E. Miller, Secular trends in body mass in the US, 1960–1980, *Am. J. Epidemiol. 128*: 1065 (1988).

85. Tucker, L.A., The relationship of television viewing to physical fitness and obesity, *Adolescence 21*: 797 (1986).

86. Peck, E.B., and H.D. Ulrich (eds.), Adhoc Interdisciplinary Committee on 'Children and Weight: a Changing Perspective,' Nutrition Communications Associates, Berkeley, CA, 1988.

87. Tanner, J.M., and P.S.W. Davies, Clinical longitudinal standards for height and weight velocity for North American children, *J. Pediatrics 107*: 317 (1985).

88. Tanner, J.M., *Growth at Adolescence*, 2nd ed., Blackwell Scientific Publications, Oxford, 1962.

89. Gaffney, J.T., and G.R. Singer, Diet needs of patients referred to home health, *J. Am. Diet. Assoc. 85*: 198 (1985).

90. Posner, B.M., and M.M. Krachenfels, Nutrition services in the continuum of health care, *Clinics Geriatric Med. 3*: 261 (1987).

91. Anonymous, Surgeon Generals Report on 'Nutrition and Health, U.S. Dept. of Health and Human Services, US Govt. Printing Office, Washington, DC, 595 (1988).

92. Anonymous, Surgeon Generals Report on 'Nutrition and Health', U.S. Dept. of Health and Human Service, US Govt. Printing Office, Washington, DC, 1988, p. 593.

93. Anonymous, Surgeon General's Workshop on 'Aging,' Surgeon General's Workshop: Health Promotion and Aging, US Depth of Health and Human Services, Washington, DC, 1988.

94. Suter, P., and R.M. Russell, Vitamin requirements of the elderly, *Am. J. Clin. Nutr. 45*: 501 (1987).

95. Perizkova, J., Age-dependent changes in dietary intakes related to work output, physical fitness and body composition, *Am. J. Clin. Nutr. 49*: 962 (1989).

96. Powell, K.E., C.J. Caspersen, J.P. Koplan, and E.S. Ford, Physical activity and chronic disease, *Am. J. Clin. Nutr. 49*: 999, (1989).

97. Ravussin, E., and C. Bogardus, Relationship of genetics, age and physical fitness to daily energy expenditure and fuel utilization, *Am. J. Clin. Nutr. 49*: 968 (1989).

98. McGandy, R.B., C.H. Barrows, A. Spanias, A. Meredith, J.L. Stone, and A.H. Norris, Nutrient intake and energy expenditure in men of different ages, *J. Gerontology. 21*: 581 (1966).

99. Young, V.R., Protein and amino acid metabolism with reference to aging and the elderly, *Progress in Clinical and Biological Research.* (D.M. Prinsley and H.H. Sandstead, eds.), Vol. 326: *Nutrition and Aging*, Alan R. Liss, New York, 1990, p. 279.

100. Recker, R.R., and R.P. Heaney, Calcium nutrition and its relationship to bone health, *Human Nutrition: A Comprehensive Treatise* (H.N. Munro and D.E. Danford, eds.), Vol. 6, *Nutrition, Aging and the Elderly*, Plenum Press, New York, 1989, p. 245.

101. CDH, Diet and health—implications for reducing chronic disease risk, Committee on 'Diet and Health,' National Research Council, National Academy Press, Berkeley, CA, 1989.

102. McDowell, A., A. Engel, J.T. Massey, and K. Mauer, Plan and operation of the second national health and nutrition examination survey, 1976–1980, Vital and health statistics series 1, No. 15, DHHS Publication No. (PHS) 81-1317, US Dept. of Health and Human Services, Washington, DC, 1981.

103. Russell, R.M., and R.D. McGandy, Reference weights: practical considerations, *Am. J. Med. 76*: 767 (1984).

104. Andres, R., Effect of obesity on total mortality, *Int. J. Obesity 4*: 381 (1980).

105. Andres, R., Aging, diabetes, and obesity: standards of normality, *M Sinai J. Med. 48*: 489 (1981).

106. Andres, R., D. Elahi, J.D. Tobin, D.C. Muller, and L. Brant, Impact of age on weight goals, *Ann. Intern. Med. 103*: 1030 (1985).

107. Andres, R., Influence of obesity on longevity in the aged, *Aging, Cancer and Cell Membranes* (C. Borck, C.M. Frengolio, and D.W. King, eds.), Thieme-Stratton, New York, 1980.

108. Frisancho, A.B., New standards of weight and body composition by frame size and height for assessment of nutritional status of adults and the elderly, *Am. J. Clin. Nutr. 40*: 808 (1984).

109. Tunstall Pedoe, D.S., Exercise, sport and athletics, *Human Nutrition and Dietetics*, 9th ed. (J.S. Garrow and W.P.T. James, eds), Churchill Livingstone, Edinburgh, London, 1993, p. 409.

110. Saris, V.H.M., M.A. van Erp-Baart, and F. Bronus, Study on food intake and energy expenditure during extreme sustained exercise: The Tour de France, *Int. J. Sports Med. 10*: 526 (1989).

111. Krogh, A., and J. Lindhard, Relative value of fat and carbohydrate as a source of muscular energy, *Biochem. J. 14*: 290 (1920).

112. Holloszy, J.O., and E.F. Coyle, Adaptations of skeletal muscle to endurance exercise and their metabolic consequences, *J. Appl. Physiol. 56*: 831 (1984).

113. Newsholme, E., and T. Leech, *The Runner: Energy and Endurance Fitness*, Walter L. Meagher, New Jersey and Oxford, 1983.

114. Nose, H., G.W. Mack, S. Xiangong, and E.R. Nadel, Role of osmolality and plasma volume during rehydration in humans, *J. Appl. Physiol. 65*: 325 (1988).

115. Nadel, E.R., B. Wenger, and M.F. Roberts, Physiological defences against hyperthermia of exercise, *Ann. NY Acad. Sci. 31*: 98 (1977).

116. Maughan, R.J., Thermoregulation in marathon competition at low ambient temperature, *Int. J. Sports Med. 6*: 15 (1985).

117. Rehrer, N.J., Aspects of dehydration and rehydration during exercise, *Advances in Nutrition and Top Sport*, Medical Sports Sciences, Vol. 32 (F. Bronus, ed.) Basel, Karger, 1991, p. 128.

118. Bergstrom, J., and E. Hultman, The effect of exercise on muscle glycogen and electrolytes in normals, *Scand, J. Clin. Invest. 18*: 16 (1966).

119. Coyle, E.F., J.M. Magberg, and B.F. Hurley, Carbohydrate feeding during prolonged strenuous exercise can delay fatigue, *J. Appl. Physiol. 55*: 230 (1983).

120. Bargstrom, J., L. Hermansen, E. Hultman, and B. Saltin, Diet, muscle glycogen and physical performance, *Acta Physiol. Scandinavica 71*: 140 (1967).

121. Astrand, P.O., Diet and athletic performance, *Fed. Proc. 26*: 1772 (1967).

122. Brewer, J., C. Williams, and A. Patton, The influence of high carbohydrate diets on endurance running performance, *Eur. J. Appl. Physiol. 57*: 698 (1988).

123. Foster, C., D.L. Costill, and W.J. Fink, Effects of pre-exercise feeding on endurance performance, *Med. Sci. Sports Exercise 11*: 1 (1979).

124. Galbo, H., *Hormonal and Metabolic Adaptations to Exercise*, George Thieme Verlag, New York, 1983.

125. Coyle, E.F., A.R. Coggan, M.K. Hemnert, and J.L. Ivy, Muscle glycogen utilization during prolonged strenuous exercise when fed carbohydrate, *J. Appl. Physiol. 61*: 165 (1986).

126. Bronus, F., W.H.M. Saris, J. Stroecken, et al., Eating, drinking and cycling: A controlled Tour de France–simulated study. 11. Effects of diet mainpulation, *Int. J. Sports Med. 10* (Suppl.): 41 (1989).

127. Ivy, J.L., A.L. Katz, C.L. Cutler, et al., Muscle glycogen synthesis after exercise: effect of time of carbohydrate ingestion, *J. Appl. Physiol. 65*: 1480 (1980).

128. Lemon, P.W.R., Does exercise alter dietary protein requirements, *Advances in Nutrition and Top Sports*, Medical Sports Sciences Vol. 32 (F. Brouns, ed.), Karger, Basel, 1991, p. 15.

129. Risser, W.L., E.J. Lee, and H.B.W. Poindexter, Iron deficiency in female athletes: its prevalence and impact on performance, *Med. Sci. Sports Exercise 20*: 116, (1988).

130. Brotherhood, J., B. Brozovic, and L.G.C. Pugh, Haematological status of middle and long distance runners, *Clin. Sci. Molecular Med. 48*: 139 (1975).

131. Magnusson, B., L. Hallberg, and L. Roossando, Iron metabolism and "sports anaemia"—a haematological comparison of elite humans and control subjects, *Acad. Med. Scandinavica 216*: 157 (1984).

132. Watts, E., Athlete's anaemia, *British J. Sports Med. 23*: 81 (1989).

133. Brooks, G.A., Amino acid and protein metabolism during exercise and recovery, *Med. Sci. Sports Exercise 19*: 5150 (1987).

134. Newsholme, E.A., M. Parry-Billings, N. McAndrew, and R. Budgett, A biochemical mechanism to explain characteristics of over training, *Advances in Nutrition and Top Sports*, Medical Sports Sciences, Vol. 32 (F. Brouns, ed.), Karger, Basel, 1991, p. 79.

19

Digestion, Absorption, Metabolism, and Excretion

I. INTRODUCTION

Nutrition is one of the most obvious and important components of the wellness approach to good health. Food provides nutrients that supply energy, construction materials, blueprints, and machinery to maintain the body and to make it run. As a remarkably designed machine, the body continually rebuilds itself, every cell in the body being in a dynamic and ever-changing flux; e.g., the cells making up the lining of small intestine are lost by extrusion into the intestine at a rate of 20 to 50 million cells per minute. The food that we eat supplies all the necessary chemicals to replace these cells at the same rate. The old saying that "we are what we eat" implies that all the essential chemicals and materials of the human body are provided by the food consumed.

The highest single component of the human body is water, made of hydrogen and oxygen. These two basic elements, along with nitrogen and carbon in different combinations, also form fat, carbohydrates, and proteins of the body. Considering the total body makeup, approximately 98% of its weight comes from compounds formed from C, H, O, and N, the remaining 2% made up of many other diverse elements, some of which are known to be essential and others we are not so sure about, but which are found in the body (Sn, Si, Ni, and V). All these elements combine to form the various compounds that make up the human body (see Chapter 1), including water, carbohydrates, protein, fats (lipids), vitamins, and minerals (see Chapters 2 to 7).

The gastrointestinal (G.I.) digestive tract is a hollow tube, extending through the body from the mouth, where the food is ingested, to the anus, where the waste products are excreted. As the food travels down this G.I. tract, it is cut, ground, (mouth), mixed with various digestive juices (mouth, stomach, and small intestine), absorbed (stomach, small intestine) and assimilated in the form of chemicals that are required to maintain the body. The food ingredients that are not digested and absorbed are excreted. During digestion the food is broken down into smaller and smaller compounds, until they can be absorbed by the intestinal wall for their further utilization by the body.

II. CARBOHYDRATES

A. Digestion and Absorption

The digestion of carbohydrates begins in the mouth, where chewing disintegrates the food and mixes it with saliva containing alpha-amylase (ptyalin); the resulting bolus is swallowed easily. Starch digestion begins in the bolus (in the mouth) but lasts a relatively shorter time because the amylase is inactivated by the gastric acid when the bolus is broken in the stomach. Much of the starch gets digested in the small intestine by the action of pancreatic anylase, which hydrolyses starch to short-chain dextrins and maltose. Glucosidases present in the brush border of the intestinal epithelium further hydrolyse the dextrin to maltose and specific disaccharidases—maltase, sucrase, and lactase—and convert them to monosaccharides. Glucose, fructose, and galactose are transported across the epithelial cells and enter the portal vein. Free concentration of monosaccharides in the intestine or at the mucosal surface is often high enough for passive or facilitated absorption, but the active transport against a concentration gradient, requiring energy, becomes necessary as their concentrations fall. The active transport involves expenditure of ATP and presence of Na^+, as in the absorption of glucose from the renal tubules. Glucose and galactose are absorbed faster than fructose (1).

The blood glucose level, after a meal, may rise to a maximum within about 30 min, returning slowly to the fasting level after 90 to 180 min; this varies with the nature of the meal and indicates the rate at which starchy foods are digested in the small intestine. The glycemic index can be used as a physiological measure to estimate the relative rates of glucose absorption from different foods (2). The subjects are asked to ingest a portion of the test food containing 50 g carbohydrate, and peripheral blood glucose levels are measured every 30 min for 3 h. The area under the resultant glucose curve is then compared with the area under the curve obtained by feeding the subject 50 g of standard carbohydrate, usually glucose or white bread. The values of glycemic index obtained for different foods range from less than 50 for legumes to more than 100 for mashed potato. Such values may be useful in planning diabetic diets to keep the blood glucose as low as possible. However, a diet that is mixed with several types of foods affects the rate of carbohydrate absorption. Wahlqvist (3) noted that glucose, dextrins, and soluble starch are all absorbed at equal rates, indicating that luminal digestion of these soluble glycans per se is not a limiting factor in glucose absorption.

B. Effects of Cooking and Food Preparation on Carbohydrate Absorption

The rate and extent of starch digestion in the small intestine depend on the physical form of food, crystallinity of starch granules and its retrogradation after cooking. Thus, the proportion of dietary starch that enters the colon is significantly influenced by the way the food is processed and prepared in the factory and/or at home.

Pancreatic amylase cannot hydrolyze the starch granule discretely present in the whole grains or seeds, but crushing, chopping, and milling enhance the accessibility of the starch, the rate of starch digestion depending on the final particle size (4,5). The density of the product, which decreases enzyme access, retards starch hydrolysis in foods like pasta (6). Physical accessibility of the starch to amylase may decrease starch hydrolysis significantly so that the undigested starch particles may enter the large intestine, and starch contained within discrete structures such as seed grains may even be excreted in the feces totally undigested.

In vitro digestibility of starch varies widely among foods, the digestibility of starch from a single source being affected by different processing methods (Table 1). Raw white wheat flour, consisting mainly of ungelatinized starch granules with an A-type crystalline structure, is digested more slowly, about 48% of the starch measuring as slowly digestible starch (SDS). Baking the flour into shortbread, which involves cooking in the presence of very little water, results in limited disruption of granular structure, giving a product that is digested slowly. However, baking the flour into bread, a process that requires a long cooking time in the presence of a moderate amount of water, causes extensive gelatinization of the starch granules, resulting in a rapidly digestible product. Only a small amount of retrograded amylose (RS_3) is produced during baking. Spaghetti made of wheat flour is also digested more slowly, like shortbread, despite being cooked by moist heat, because the dense structure of the pasta impedes its enzymatic hydrolysis,

Table 1 In Vitro Digestibility of Starch in Some Foods

Source	% RDS	% SDS	% RS$_1$	% RS$_2$	% RS$_3$
White flour	49	48	—	3	T
Shortbread	56	43	—	—	1
White bread	94	4	—	—	2
White spaghetti	52	43	3	—	3
Banana biscuits	39	23	—	38	T
Potato biscuits	47	27	—	25	1
Haricot beans	18	42	18	9	12
Pearl barley	41	41	9	—	2

RDS = Rapidly digestible starch
SDS = Slowly digestible starch
RS = Resistant starch
T = Trace
Source: Ref. 1.

as demonstrated by the 3% of starch measuring as RS$_1$ (physically inaccessible), in the cases of haricot beans and pearl barley (Table 1). Biscuits made with a 1:1 mixture of wheat flour and either banana or potato flour contain substantial amounts of RS$_2$, because no water is used in the formulation and thus starch granules retain their crystalline structure, leading to a product containing about one-third of its starch that resists digestion (7,8).

According to Englyst and Kingman (1), the digestibility of starch within the small intestine depends on starch crystallinity and the physical form of the starchy food itself as well as on a number of other variable factors such as the extent of chewing, the transit time of the food in the small intestine, the concentration of the amylase, the amount of starch, and the presence of other food components hindering enzymatic hydrolysis. Thus, it is rather difficult to predict accurately the digestion of starchy food in an individual human sugject.

Soundarapandian et al. (9) reported the effect of different feeds on midgut gland digestive enzymes in juveniles of fresh water prawn (*Macrobrachium malcolmsonii*). Different feeds had significant effect on protease activity in the midgut, although they did not affect amylase activity. Dietary protease significantly altered growth but not amylase. Among five feeds (three types of live foods, viz., adult Artemia, earthworm, and oyster, and two types of artificial feeds), adult Artemia was found to be the best food for *M. malcolmsonii*.

C. Fate of Undigested Carbohydrate

A range of potentially fermentable substrates enters cecum, mainly the nonstarch polysaccharides (NSP) and starch along with a significant amount of protein that escapes digestion in the small intestine (Table 2) (10). Studies with ileostomy subjects (people who have their large intestine removed for medical reasons) have indicated that dietary NSPs are almost completely recovered in the ileostomy effluent, though for many foods starch rather than NSP reaches the colon. Cummings and Englyst (11) showed that the quantity of starch escaping digestion and available for fermentation in the colon may range from 2% in oats to 89% in bananas.

Endogenous carbohydrates from mucin and glycoproteins that line the gut also contribute to the extent of 3 to 5 g of fermentable substrate per day, with normal intestine epithelial turnover in adults on a Western diet. Other potential substrates for colonic fermentation include fructose, sorbitol, and other poorly absorbed monosaccharides; lactose in lactase-deficient individuals; raffinose; stachyose; verbascose; and fructans such as inulin as well as some synthetic carbohydrates

Table 2   Principal Substrates Available for Fermentation in the Human Colon[a]

Substrate	Amount (g/day)
Carbohydrates	
Resistant starch	8–40
Non-starch polysaccharides	8–18
Unabsorbed sugars, sugar alcohols	2–10
Oligosaccharides	2–6
Chitin and amino sugars	1–2
Nitrogenous substrates	
Dietary protein	3–9
Pancreatic enzymes and secretions	4–6
Urea and nitrate	0.5
Other substrates	
Mucin	2–3

[a]The amounts estimated are based on subjects consuming a Western diet.
Source: Ref. 10.

such as polydextrose, palatinite, and neosugar. All these compounds together may provide about 5 g of carbohydrate a day in a typical U.K. diet and are considered normal, except in some disease states (1).

In the large intestine, these carbohydrates are degraded by colon microflora, which ferment them to short-chain fatty acids (SCFA), with evolution of gases such as CO_2, H_2, and CH_4. The type and nature (solubility) of the substrate influences the extent of fermentation. The soluble carbohydrates such as pectin are degraded completely, other insoluble polymers in lignified materials, such as present in wheat bran, are attacked to a much smaller extent. During colonic fermentation, initially large polymers are broken down to constituent monomers, predominantly glucose, galactose, arabinose, xylose, and uronic acids. Sugars are glycolytically converted to pyruvate, following different routes, depending on microbial species present and nature of the substrate. The main SCFAs produced during fermentation are acetate, propionate, and butyrate as well as isobutyrate, valerate, isovalerate, lactate, and succinate present in small amounts, contributing to low pH (5.6–6.6) in the large intestine. The SCFA production efficiency and the molar ratios of acetate, propionate and butyrate generated from carbohydrate vary according to the substrate being utilized; e.g., while fermentation of starch will produce SCFA with a large proportion of butyrate (29%), pectins when fermented will produce only about 2% of butyrate.

Acetate and propionate produced in the colon are rapidly absorbed and transported through the portal vein to the liver. Butyrate is actively metabolized to ketone bodies (acetoacetate and beta-hydroxybutyrate), carbon dioxide, and water. Kim et al. (12) demonstrated that buyrate rather than glucose or glucosamine used by the colonic epithelium had beneficial effects (antitumor action) in vitro. Most of the SCFAs are metabolized by the liver to form acetate that is released to be used as fuel by the peripheral tissues (13,14).

The fermentation gases include hydrogen, carbon dioxide, and in some individuals methane (CH_4) produced from CO_2 and H_2; the latter diminishes the total volume of the gas accumulating in the colon (one volume of CH_4 is produced from four volumes of H_2). Also, sulfate-reducing bacteria in some individuals may incorporate hydrogen to hydrogen sulfide (H_2S), especially after a high intake of dietary sulfate (15).

Gases may be excreted from the rectum when their production exceeds the absorptive capacity of the colon; however, most of these gases are absorbed by the body and excreted through the lungs. Anderson et al. (16) employed measurement of the hydrogen expired in breath as an index of carbohydrate fermentation. This may be used in a clinical setting to detect pancreatic inefficiency, though it may not be useful for reproducible assessment of the quantity of carbohydrate entering the colon (17). Blaxter (18) showed that the energy obtained from the fermentation of carbohydrates of SCFA and their utilization by the body tissues represents to the extent of about 60% to 70% the energy potentially available, had the carbohydrates been completely hydrolyzed and absorbed from the small intestine. Thus, most of undigested carbohydrate material, referred to earlier as "unavailable," is utilized by the body to produce energy (18).

The principal carbohydrate escaping digestion in small intestine is NSP (dietary fiber) and starch. The concept of resistant starch introduced recently has not helped to investigate the consequences of starch reaching the colon.

D. Dietary Fiber

Trowell (19) observing that all the common non-infective diseases of the large bowel, known as "diseases of civilization", a group of 17, including constipation, appendicitis, diverticular disease, hemorrhoids, colorectal cancer, coronary heart disease, and gallstones, were rarely noted in sub-Saharan blacks, postulated that the protective factor might be the soft and bulky nature of their stools, which passed easily and frequently owing to their high-fiber diet. It has now been shown that lack of dietary fiber is a major factor involved in several gastrointestinal diseases. A highly refined diet results in hard, dry stools that pass sluggishly through the large intestine and require a large increase in luminal pressure for their evacuation. A diet that is rich in refined carbohydrates and fats is often associated with the development of diabetes, coronary heart disease, and obesity in the affluent societies, though it is not generally accepted that fiber deficiency is the cause of these conditions. The quantity and type of dietary fiber are important in determining the extent of increase in fecal weight, decrease in intestinal transit time, and improvement in glucose and lipid metabolism.

Cummings et al. (20) showed that individuals consuming a typical U.K. diet excreted on an average 106 g of stool per day, with wide individual variation in the weight of stool and the frequency of bowel movement. Both dietary fiber and starch have effects on stool weight, though there is a poor correlation between fecal weight and total dietary fiber intake per se, because this effect mainly depends on the type of fiber consumed.

Two factors are involved in the fecal bulking effect of dietary fiber. Soluble fiber is readily fermented and leads to increased fecal weight through proliferation of the bacterial population, but insoluble fiber, especially if lignified as in wheat bran, partially survives the fermentation process and acts directly as a bulking and water-holding agent. More insoluble cereal fibers generally increase fecal weight and also have an important laxative action. Also, the stool weight is closely associated with transit time, and fecal weights below 150 g per day are associated with increasing transit time. Constipation commonly occurs when the fecal output falls below 100 g/day. Epidemiological studies have indicated that low stool weights and extended transit time are associated with increased risk from diverticular disease and bowel cancer. Cummings et al. (20) suggested that bowel diseases in the United Kingdom could be reduced by increasing the mean fecal output to 132 g/day, which would require consumption of a mean 17.9 NSP/day.

The intestinal transit time (the time taken for a meal to pass from the mouth to the anus) may be measured by administering a marker such as carmine red by mouth and knowing the time taken for this to appear in the feces. The whole-gut transit time is conveniently divided into two phases: mouth to cecum transit and colonic transit. The latter takes approximately ten times as long as mouth-to-cecum transit.

The mouth-to-cecum transit is influenced by gastric emptying and small-intestinal transit, both of which may be altered by consuming viscous polysaccharides such as guar gum, gum tragacanth, and oat bran; the viscosity of these fibers prolongs gastric emptying, resulting in greater satiety and a delay in the delivery of nutrients to the small intestine (21). Viscous dietary fibers also delay the absorption of low-molecular weight nutrients like sugars within the small intestine, especially in its distal region, where the viscosity is increased by the absorption of water from the gut contents.

The colonic transit is influenced less by the viscosity of polysaccharides, which is rapidly reduced as the fermentation advances. Insoluble dietary fibers such as wheat bran decrease colonic transit time and produce larger and softer stools. It is not known whether increase in fecal bulk stimulates colonic peristalsis or whether dietary fiber has any direct effect on colonic motor activity. However, it is likely that a number of different factors, such as the retention of fluid in the fiber matrix, the presence of poorly absorbed SCFA (lactate), a low pH that inhibits salt and water absorption, an increase in bacterial cell mass and distension due to gas production, all possibly contribute to reduce the intestinal transit time.

Epidemiological studies have also indicated that the consumption of dietary fiber is inversely related to the incidence of diseases such as coronary heart disease and gallstones that are associated with steroid metabolism, especially the level of cholesterol in the serum. Physiologically, also, it has been shown that addition of certain plant fibers to the diet significantly reduces the serum cholesterol concentration, the soluble NSP fractions (pectins, gums, etc) being most effective in this respect. Mostly, the low-density lipoprotein (LDL) fraction is reduced and is accompanied by decreases in the cholesterol content of the liver, aorta, and other tissues. This effect is explained in terms of bile acid metabolism. Bile salts and neutral steroids are synthesized from liver cholesterol, secreted in the bile, and again returned to the liver via resorption in the small intestine (the enterohepatic cycle). Dietary fiber is thought to interrupt this cycle by absorbing bile acids and preventing their reabsorption, thus necessitating their replacement from the cholesterol pool (1). Several NSP fractions from fruit and vegetables have been reported to bind bile acids in vitro and several fiber fractions have been shown to increase the daily fecal output of bile acids in vivo. The bile acids binding is probably not the sole factor involved. Chen and Anderson (22) postulated that hepatic cholesterol synthesis may be altered by SCFAs derived from the colonic fermentation of soluble fibers. Propionate was shown to inhibit hydroxylmethylglutaryl CoA reductase, the rate-limiting enzyme of cholesterol synthesis, which may result in lower serum cholesterol levels (see Chapter 24).

III. PROTEINS

A. Digestion and Absorption

The ingested proteins are denatured by the acid in the stomach and they are further hydrolyzed by a variety of proteolytic enzymes in the stomach and intestine, including trypsin, chymotrypsin, elastin, and carboxypeptidase. The resulting mixture of free amino acids and small peptides is absorbed by the gut cells through a series of carrier systems. The free amino acids may be transported through a bloodstream or metabolized within the gut.

For a number of reasons, protein digestion and absorption remain incomplete. Some proteins, owing to their physicochemical structure, are resistant to proteolytic hydrolysis. The free amino acids and peptides may not be absorbed totally, especially when gut function is impaired or when certain antinutritional factors such as lectins or trypsin inhibitor proteins are present in the diet. The unabsorbed amino acids, peptides, and protein pass into the colon and are metabolized by colon bacteria. These amino acids, however, are not available to the body and are eliminated in the feces as bacterial proteins. The absorbed amino acids are transported to the liver through the portal vein, where a portion of the amino acids pool is used, and the remainder is sent to various tissue cells of the body through the circulation for their further utilization (23–25).

B. Utilization of Amino Acids

Protein synthesis is a continuing process that takes place in almost all types of cells in the body. During the steady-state condition, protein synthesis is balanced by an equal amount of protein degradation. Bond and Butler (26) and Mortimore et al. (27) have described the mechanism and regulation of protein degradation in the liver. The proess by which all proteins are continuously broken down to amino acids and resynthesized again is termed protein turnover (see Chapter 5). In the adult human body, more than about 250 g of protein are synthezied and degraded daily, which compares with a dietary intake of only 70 g of protein. The magnitude of protein turnover is highest in the infants and decreases with age, and is much less in elderly people than in young adults on a body weight basis (Table 3) (28,29). The relationship between protein turnover and age is similar to that between protein requirement and basal metabolic rate (BMR) and age. Certain tissues of the body have more active protein turnover than others; e.g., the liver and intestine, despite their rather small contribution to the total body's protein content, contribute to about 50% of the whole body protein turnover. The skeletal muscle, which constitutes approximately 50% of the body's protein mass, on the contrary, contributes only about 25% of body protein turnover. The active protein turnover appears to be a sensitive means of regulating the amount of each separate enzyme or structural protein. Other proteins may be secreted from the cell after their synthesis and may be subsequently degraded at a distant site from their synthesis; e.g., serum albumin is synthesized in the liver, antibodies are synthesized in the betalymphocytes, digestive proteases and other enzymes in the pancreas, and peptide hormones in the endocrine glands.

C. Amino Acid Metabolism

Around 10 to 15 g of nitrogen is excreted daily in the urine of a healthy adult human, mostly in the form of urea, with smaller proportion of ammonia, uric acid, creatinine, and some free amino acids (Table 4) (30). These are the end products of the body's nitrogen metabolism, arising from the oxidation of amino acids (urea and ammonia). Reversible transamination uses the keto acids of glucose metabolism to receive amino nitrogen. Taking part in this reaction, most amino acids are concentrated into alanine (from pyruvate), aspartate (from oxaloacetate), and glutamate (from

Table 3 Whole-body Protein Synthesis in Humans at Different Ages

Growth phase	Protein synthesis		
	g/kg/day	g/g protein requirement	g/kcal BMR
Newborns (premature)	17.4	5.4	0.15
Infants (1 year)	6.9	4.1	0.13
Young adults	3.0	5.2	0.11
Elderly	1.9	4.5	0.11

Source: Ref. 28, as modified by Ref. 29.

Table 4 Approximate Distribution of
Nitrogen in Urinary Constituents in Human
Subjects Eating a Normal Balanced Diet

Compound	g nitrogen/24 h
Urea	12.90
Ammonia	0.70
Amino acids	0.70
Creatinine	0.65
Uric acid	0.30
Hippuric acid	0.05
Total	15.30

Source: Ref. 30.

alpha-keto-glutarate). Most amino acids can thus be synthesized in the liver, but the metabolism of three branched-chain amino acids, viz., leucine, isoleucine, and valine, is brought about mainly by peripheral transamination, especially in the skeletal muscle tissue, by transferring their amino nitrogen mainly to alanine and glutamine, which are then passed into circulation. These are very important carriers of nitrogen from the periphery to the intestine and liver. In the small intestine, glutamine is metabolized to ammonia, alanine, and citrulline, which are transported to the liver.

A number of amino acids can be deaminated to form ammonia and keto acids, either directly (histidine), by dehydration (serine, threonine), through the purine nucleotide cycle (aspartate), or by oxidative deamination (glutamate). Glutamate in turn can be formed specifically through deamination of arginine and lysine. Thus nitrogen from any amino acids can be converted into two precursors of urea, viz., ammonia and aspartate.

Urea is synthesized in the liver by the Krebs-Henseleit cycle through hydrolysis of arginine by enzyme arginase to urea and another amino acid, ornithine (not found in protein). The arginine is then resynthesized from ammonia and asparate. The urea thus formed is transported from the liver to the kidney to be excreted in the urine.

In the purine nucleotide cycle, purine nitrogen is converted to ammonium ions, mainly in the skeletal muscle and transported into blood as glutamine, some of which is metabolized in the kidneys to form ammonia ions and glutamate. This glutamate is used to synthesize glucose in the kidney (gluconeogenesis). The generation of ammonia ions of glutamine has an important role in acid-base homeostasis, ammonia ions excreted in this process serving as the main vehicle for the excretion of excess protons (H^+) formed during acidosis (23).

Keto acid analogues are formed after deamination of most amino acids, many of which can enter into TCA cycle for their oxidation (Fig. 1); e.g., alpha-ketoglutarate derived from glutamate and pyruvate from alanine are intermediates of the TCA cycle through which glucose is oxidized completely to CO_2 and water. All amino acids can be specifically degradated to form the intermediates of this oxidative pathway. Thus, proteins can serve as a source of body's energy supply, especially in non-growing adults, who may use about 10% to 15% of their dietary protein for the production of energy. Protein oxidation may rise considerably in highly traumatized or septic individuals (see Chapter 33), whereas proteins contribution to energy during chronic starvation or in protein-restricted diets is limited (23).

The deaminated keto acid skeletons of most amino acids after entering into TCA cycle or the glycolysis pathway can be utilized to synthesize either glucose or fat, depending on their points of entry into the general metabolism (Fig. 1). If amino acids enter in the form of acetyl CoA, then only fat or ketone bodies can be formed (if not for energy production). Other amino

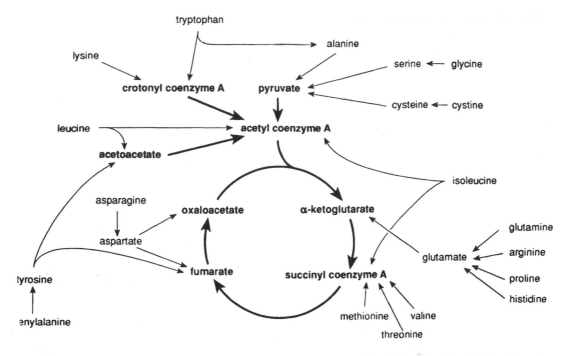

Figure 1 Metabolism of the carbon skeletons of the amino acid chains (light arrows) and their points of entry into the general pathways of glucose and fat metabolism (bold arrows). (From Ref. 23.)

acids may enter metabolism in such a way that their carbon skeletons are used to form glucose. Thus, amino acids may be nutritionally categorized into ketogenic (ketones) or glucogenic (glucose). Many amino acids, however, can give rise to both the products.

The predominant precursors of glucose during gluconeogenesis are alanine, glutamate, and aspartate. A significant proportion of glucose synthesized by this route represents recapture and recycling of amino acids derived from the amination of 3-carbon units of glucose metabolism in the liver. This is referred to as the glucose-alanine cycle (a direct parallel of the Cori cycle) and the glucose-glutamine cycle. Because the nitrogen donors may be either glucogenic or ketogenic amino acids, these cycles serve as a mechanism to transport nitrogen from the peripheral tissue to the liver for glucose production. The transport of glutamine from the periphery to the G.I. tract is also important for the synthesis of arginine and proline and is critical in preventing the buildup of excessive ammonia in the circulation.

In addition to their predominant utilization in the synthesis of numerous body proteins, amino acids are also required to synthesize a range of non-proteinous nitrogenous compounds of vital importance in the physiological function of human body (Table 5). Some of these pathways have the potential to exert a substantial impact on the utilization of certain amino acids, such as glycine (Table 5), which is involved in several synthetic pathways; e.g., it is required in substantial quantities to synthesize creatine (muscle function), heme (oxygen transport and oxidative phosphorylation), and glutathione (protective reactions) (23). In the absence of a dietary source of creatine, an adult human requires at least 1.2 g of glycine daily to sustain adequate rates of creatine and heme synthesis. According to Jackson (31), a supply of glycine is needed in the diet of milk-fed premature infants for optimal growth and thus glycine may then be termed as condi-

Table 5 Non-Protein Pathways of Amino Acid Utilization

End product	Precursor amino acids
Serotonin	Tryptophan
Nicotinic acid	Tryptophan
Catecholamines	Tyrosine
Thyroid hormones	Tyrosine
Melanin	Tyrosine
Carnitine	Lysine
Taurine	Cysteine
Glutathione	Glutamate, cysteine, glycine
Nucleic acid bases	Glutamine, aspartate, glycine
Heme	Glycine
Creatine	Glycine, arginine, methionine
Bile acids	Glycine, taurine
"Methyl group metabolism"	Methionine, glycine, serine

Source: Ref. 23.

tionally essential. Similarly, the lysine supply in the diet may become quantitatively significant because it is needed for the synthesis of creatine, involved in intracellular fatty acid transport. However, these may be nutritionally important considerations only in individuals consuming very low amounts of proteins of plant origin (32).

D. Body Reserves of Amino Acids and Proteins

A 70 kg man has about 11 kg total protein that is distributed among the various body tissues as shown in Table 6. Nearly one-half of the protein is present as skeletal muscle, the remainder largely in the skin and blood; the visceral tissues such as liver and kidney contain relatively small amounts of protein (1% of the total). A newborn infant has comparatively less muscle but more protein in the brain and visceral tissues than the adult human (Table 6) (33).

Table 6 Body Content of Proteins in Adults and Newborn Babies and Approximate Distribution of Protein Among the Tissues

Protein content	Newborn	Adult
Whole body (kg)		
Body weight	3.5	70
Total protein	0.41	11
Tissue protein (% total)		
Muscle	29	43
Skin	21	15
Blood	19	16
Liver	5	1.8
Brain	6	1.5
Kidney	1	0.3

Source: Ref. 33.

The myosin, actin, collagen, and hemoglobin of the human body together contain over 50% of body protein, one-half of which is present only as collagen. This proportion may rise considerably in an individual suffering from malnutrition when there is a substantial loss of non-collagen proteins, collagen itself being retained by the body (34).

Munro and Allison (35) described the concept of "labile protein reserve" to indicate re-equilibrium of body protein to make up for the temporary gain or loss of protein over the first few days of a variety of nutritional and pathological conditions. The liver and visceral tissues in animals appear to serve as labile stores of body protein to be used in an emergency (as much as 40% of protein may be lost during severe starvation). The labile protein reserve in the human being is about 3% of total protein (300–400 g). The body adapts to a wide range of variation in dietary intake as well as to pathological conditions such as starvation, injury, infection, cancer, and diabetes. However, if these conditions go unchecked for more than few days, serious depletion of body protein mass may become life threatening.

A very small proportion of the body's total mass of amino acids is present as free amino acids, which have an important function in the nutritional and metabolic control of the body's proteins (23). The content of free and protein-bound amino acids in rat muscle was found to vary considerably, with no relationship between their concentrations in the free pool and body proteins (36).

In the human body, free phenylalanine constitutes less than 0.2% of the total body pool, corresponding to only about 1.5 hours worth of protein synthesis or one-quarter of the day's intake of protein. Although free glutamate and alanine make up a much larger proportion of their respective body pools, they cannot be considered as reserves for more than a very short time. Human muscle has a very large free pool of glutamine (10–15 g N), which becomes depleted to about 50% after trauma, thus contributing to a significant total loss of body's nitrogen.

The concentration of most amino acids is higher in the intracellular pool of tissue than the plasma compartment. The concentration of large neutral amino acids such as leucine and phenylalanine is 1–2 times higher in muscle than in plasma, whereas that of glutamine, glutamate, and glycine may be as high as 10 to 50-fold more concentrated in the muscle. Both dietary changes and pathological conditions can significantly alter the concentrations of individual free amino acids in the plasma and tissue pools (36,37).

E. Amino Acid and Protein Requirements

The FAO/WHO/UNU Expert Consultation has modified the policy on the essential amino acid requirements of adults (38), on which tables of requirements are set out. The method used in calculating the protein requirements in children is shown in Table 7. Protein requirements are based on the total intake and nitrogen content of breast milk fed directly or by bottle during the first 4 to 6 months. About 20% of the total nitrogen in breast milk is in the form of non–amino acid nitrogen such as urea. Because babies grow well on this milk, provided it is supplied in the required quantity, it is assumed that all the milk nitrogen is utilized by the body as though all the nitrogen was protein. From 6 to 12 months, the breast-fed child is still growing rapidly but is now relying on other supplementary food sources. To obtain these requirement values, short-term nitrogen balance studies using milk or egg protein are carried out. Additional studies are done on children up to 1 to 5 years of age using soya milk or mixed protein sources, along with nitrogen-balance measurements conducted with milk. Different nitrogen intakes are chosen, allowances are made for skin losses, and a slope of nitrogen retention in relation to intake is computed to obtain maintenance requirements. Adjustments are made for the digestibility of different proteins. Mixed feeding leads to additional fecal nitrogen loss, compared to those of a milk diet, hence the true maintenance needs of absorbed amino acids are less than the protein intake. After the estimation

Table 7 Calculating the Safe Level of Milk Protein and Other Dietary Proteins for Children

	Age (Years)			
	0–2	2–3	5–6	9–10
Maintenance needs (mg N/kg/day)	120	118	115	111
Growth needs (mg N/kg/day)	80	28	17	17
Estimated average requirement (mg N/kg/day)	200	146	132	128
CV (%)	16	12	12	12
Add 2 SD	264	181	164	155
Ref. nutrient intake (RNI) (g protein/kg/day)	1.65	1.13	1.02	0.99
Type of diet	Wheat and Vegetable	Rice, 70%; Fish, 30%	Beans & corn, 95% vegetable, 5%	Mixed, animal, 45%
Digestibility (%)[b]	66	73	59	80
RNI with allowance for digestibility (g protein/kg/day)[c]	2.5	1.5	1.7	1.2
Amino acid score (%)[d]	76	81	89	100
RNI with allowance for both digestibility and protein quality (g protein/kg/day)	3.3	1.9	1.9	1.2

[a]CV% = Coefficient of variation, which combines a CV for maintenance of 12.5% and for growth of 35%.
[b]Digestibility (D%) = $100 \times (I-F)/I$, I = N intake, F = fecal N on the diet.
[c]The diets and corresponding digestibility values are taken from individual studies cited in the report to illustrate the varying values. Adults in general have about 85% digestibility of N on unrefined diets and 95% on refined diets.
[d]Amino acid scores take into account the limiting amino acids of the mixed diet.
Source: Ref. 38.

of protein requirements for growth and maintenance in children, the true needs for dietary proteins are to be increased to make allowance for incomplete digestiblity or additional endogenous nitrogen excreted from the intestine in response to the specific diet. Thus, to obtain RDAs or RNI values, allowances must be made for the individual variability in requirements which are about 12.5% CV in healthy children.

The variation in the weight gained by children during growth needs to be considered while assessing the protein requirements. If energy intakes are high and both quality and quantity of protein are inadequate, children, especially when recovering from malnutrition, can put on weight as fat, with only modest increases in body protein. Thus, during the rapid growth period, children must be provided with enough protein to maintain an adequate growth rate. Also, children in the developing countries are often ill with respiratory or gastrointestinal infections that arrest growth, impair absorption, and reduce body weight. Additional protein (and energy) may therefore be needed for catch-up growth. Allowing for the variation in the maintenance requirements of individual children (CV, 15%) and for the greater natural variation in growth rate (CV, 35%) the RNIs that have taken into account these factors are likely to meet the needs of many children for catch-up growth. The higher the rate of growth, the greater will be the need for both total protein and for protein with a high nutritional quality (Table 7) (38).

The nutritional quality of a protein in terms of its amino acid composition has traditionally been assessed by comparing it with milk or egg protein, which have an amino acid composition similar to that found in total body protein. Animal studies have established the significance of having the correct complement of amino acids for growth, emphasizing the importance of animal proteins in the human diet. A vegetarian diet based completely on cereals would be most limiting in the essential amino acids, such as lysine, methionine plus cysteine, threonine, and tryptophan. A mixed diet with beans or a mixture of different cereals and pulses will balance and compensate for the amino acid deficiencies. An inclusion of a small amount of animal protein in the diet will most likely supply all the essential amino acids required by human beings. The lysine score of a food like wheat, 0.73, means that 37% (1–0.73/0.73) more wheat would theoretically be needed to make up the deficiency. Alternatively, an addition of an animal protein will improve the score and enhance the child's ability to grow.

Digestibility of food varies with age and tends to be lower in children than in adults (Table 7). The digestibility values shown in Table 7 only refer to the output of fecal nitrogen in excess of that observed on a milk diet, because the maintenance requirements in these cases were calculated assuming some fecal nitrogen loss. In adults protein requirements are calculated by providing no allowance for growth, although there is a need to add high-quality protein for dietary estimates of people gaining weight during recovery from illness.

IV. LIPIDS

A. Digestion and Absorption of Fats

Triacylglycerols, which form the bulk of the fats in the human diet, are broken down to partial glycerides, fatty acids, and glycerol by the pancreatic lipase in the small intestine, before their absorption by the small intestine. In most adult humans, more than 90% of about 100 g of fat consumed daily is digested and absorbed, though higher quantities of fat (up to 250 g/day or more) can be digested and absorbed during shortages of energy (39).

The newborn baby adapts to the fat content of breast milk, with a low fat digestion efficiency because the pancreatic and biliary secretions are yet to be developed fully (40). According to Hamosh (41), neonatal fat digestion is aided by the lipase enzyme secreted from the lingual serous glands and carried into the stomach, where it is hydrolysed without the need of bile salts (at pH of about 4.5–5.5). The lipase activity is probably stimulated by the sucking action and the presence of fat in the mouth. The hydrolysis products include 2-monoacylglycerols, diacylglycerols, and nonesterified fatty acids. The lipase in human breast milk may also contribute to fat digestion in newborns (42). During the later stages of life, fat digestion also begins in the stomach, the churning action helping to form a coarse fat emulsion. Though the latter is not hydrolyzed, it enters the small intestine and is modified after mixing with bile and pancreatic juice (43). The biliary secretion increases with an increase in the amount of dietary fat (44), and contains bile acids that are synthesized in the liver from cholesterol. 7-Hydroxycholesterol and cholic acid (primary bile acids) are excreted in the bile as conjugates of taurine or glycine. The polar groups and the shape of the molecules of these bile acids make them effective detergents to solubilize the fats present in the small intestine (39).

Fat is digested predominantly in the duodenum and catalyzed by the pancreatic lipase, the fat is hydrolyzed to 2-monoacylglycerols and non-esterified fatty acids. Phospholipids are broken down to lysophosphoglycerides and a fatty acid released from position 2 of the phosphoglycerides by pancreatic phospholipase. Cholesterol esters present in dietary fat are hydrolysed by a pancreatic cholesterol esterase before they can be absorbed. Mixed micelles containing large molecular aggregates of monoacylglycerols, fatty acids longer than C12, bile salts, and phospholipids form as the digestion proceeds, with a decrease in the volume of oil phase. The mixed micelles are then able to draw into the hydrophobic core the less water-soluble molecules such as cholesterol, the carotenoids, tocopherols, and some undigested triacylglycerols.

Most lipid absorption takes place in the jejunum (middle) part of small intestine, where the hydrolyzed products pass into the enterocyte membrane by passive diffusion (43), the diffusion gradient being maintained by the presence of a fatty acid binding protein that binds fatty acids entering the cell, as well as by the rapid re-esterification of fatty acids to monoacylglycerols (Fig. 2). Cholesterols are re-esterified by the action of acyl-CoA:cholesterol acyltransferase or by the reversal of cholesterol esterase before being absorbed. The triacylglycerols and cholesterol esters resynthesized in the enterocytes are esterified with fatty acids having more than 12 carbon atoms

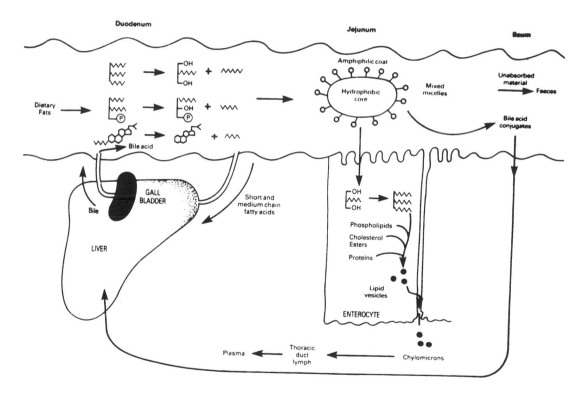

Figure 2 Digestion and absorption of lipids in the small intestine. The enzyme pancreatic lipase hydrolyzes ester bonds in positions 1 and 3 of triacylglycerols, releasing 2 moles of fatty acids per mole of triacylglycerol and 1 mole of 2-monoacylglycerol. Bile salts aid in the emulsification of the fat droplets, and CO-lipase anchors the enzyme to the surface of the fat droplets. The phospholipids are split by a pancreatic phospholipase A_2, releasing the fatty acid in position 2 and leaving a lysophospholipid. A cholesterol ester hydrolase splits the fatty acid from cholesterol esters. Liposis products are then stabilized in mixed micelles comprising surface-active components (see text). Short-chain fatty acids are absorbed as free acids into the portal blood, and monoacyl-glycerols and long-chain fatty acids from mixed micelles are transported across the brush borders and re-esterified in the enterocytes. Re-formed triacylglycerols are stabilized with phospholipids and apo-proteins and exported into plasma as chylomicrons. (From Ref. 39.)

in their chain (Fig. 2). The short ($C_4 = C_6$) and medium ($C_8 = C_{10}$) chain fatty acids can be directly absorbed into the portal blood and transported to the liver, where they can be rapidly oxidized for energy (Fig. 2); they thus do not contribute to plasma lipids and are not deposited in adipose tissue to any significant extent (39).

Defects either in digestion or absorption of lipids may lead to their failure to assimilate by the body (45). Incomplete lipolysis can result in maldigestion, which may be caused by pancreatic inefficiency (pancreatitis), a pancreatic tumor, or diseases of malnutrition such as kwashiorkor, leading to pancreatic failure to secrete enough lipase. Alternatively there may be enough lipase but a defect in the production of bile because of biliary disease, with obstruction of the bile duct, or chronic liver disease. One of the most common causes is bile-salt deficiency arising from surgical resection of the ileum, the site of active transport of bile salts. The deficiency of bile salts leads to the failure of micellar solubilization of lipolysis products. Gastric disorders also may affect fat digestive efficiency of the body.

Despite normal functioning of the digestion process, malabsorption may occur as the result of defects in the absorptive surfaces of the small intestine, e.g., bacterial invasion or sensitization of the gut to dietary components such as gluten, as in coeliac disease. Malabsorption syndrome, often referred to as sprue, is characterized by dramatic changes in the morphology of the intestinal mucosa, such as flattened and irregular epithelium and atrophy of the villi decreasing the total absorbing surface. Sprue results in a massively increased excretion of fat in the feces (steatorrhea), arising from unabsorbed dietary material and from the proliferating bacterial population in the gut. Because of poor fat absorption, sprue patients are at increased risk of deficiencies of energy, fat-soluble vitamins, and essential fatty acids. Fat malassimilation can be clinically managed by replacing normal dietary fats by medium-chain triacylglycerols (MCT) (45). A refined coconut oil containing mainly C_8 and C_{10} saturated fatty acids that are more efficiently digested and absorbed directly into the portal blood is often used.

B. Metabolism of Lipoproteins and Fatty Acids

The triacylglycerols produced in the enterocyte acquire a stabilizing coat of phospholipids and apolipoproteins (apo A and apo B) during active fat absorption. These large spherical particles (75–600 nm in diameter), known as chylomicrons, are secreted into lymphatic vessels (Fig. 2) and are passed to the jugular vein, via the thoracic duct. In the bloodstream they acquire apolipoproteins C and E (33).

The chylomicrons pass through the lungs and the ventricles of the heart with little modification, and then rapidly enter the capillaries of the skeletal muscles, heart, mammary glands, and adipose tissues, where they are acted upon by an enzyme, lipoprotein lipase (LPL), which hydrolytically breaks triacylglycerols into fatty acids. The latter are then transported to the cells of the target tissue. After a meal, an elevated insulin concentration directs most of the chylomicron breakdown to adipose tissue by activating the adipose tissue LPL. The hormonal balance during a fast activates muscle LPL, whereas during lactation, the LPL of mammary glands is elevated under the stimulation of prolactin, to ensure the supply of substrates for the synthesis of milk fat. Approximately one-half of the chylomicron triacylglycerols are hydrolysed in 2 to 3 minutes, but the particles are not completely degraded. The remnants, which contain relatively less triacylglycerol and more cholesterol, are poor substrates for the LPL and are taken up by the liver, where the cholesterol is utilized for membranes or new lipoproteins, or converted into bile acids (Fig. 3) (39).

The endogenous fatty acid and triacylglycerol biosynthesis is suppressed when the diet contains an appreciable amount of fat, although the process of lipid turnover occurs continuously in

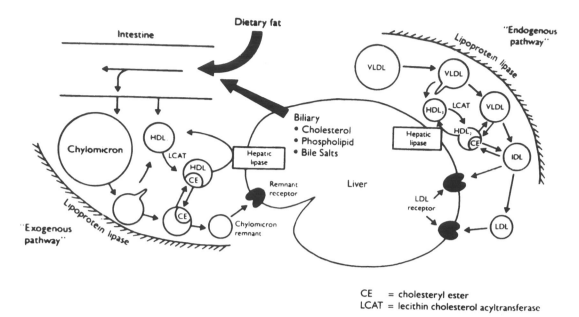

CE   = cholesteryl ester
LCAT = lecithin cholesterol acyltransferase

Figure 3 The metabolism of lipoproteins. The exogenous pathway is concerned with the transport and metabolism of dietary fat. The fats are packaged as chylomicrons which circulate and are removed from plasma by lipoprotein lipase, mainly in the adipose tissue. The chylomicron remnants (remain to be digested by enzyme) are transported to the liver. Parts of chylomicrons also go into making HDL which, in conjunction of the enzyme LCAT, remove excess cholesterol from membranes and other lipoprotein particles, converting them into cholesteryl esters. This process involves interconversion of two forms of HDL (HDL$_2$ and HDL$_3$) and cholesteryl esters are taken to the liver for further processing. The endogenous pathway involves the transport and metabolism of fats made in the body itself. The products are VLDL, which are metabolized similarly to the chylomicrons. Their remnants are called intermediate-density lipoproteins (IDL) and are further metabolized to LDL, which is carried by specific LDL-receptors. (From Ref. 39.)

all tissues (46,47). Sjostrom (48) noted that fatty acid synthesis in human adipose tissue (measured in isolated adipocytes and subcellular fractions) may increase up to 11-fold when subjects change from a high-fat to a high-carbohydrate diet. Liver is the predominant organ for lipid biosynthesis and the newly formed fat is exported as very low-density lipoproteins (VLDL), which are similar to chylomicrons but are less dense and contain relatively more phospholipids, cholesterol, and proteins.

High rates of the medium-chain fatty acids, caprylic (octanoic) and capric (decanoic) occur in mammary glands during lactation, especially when the amount of fat in the diet is very low (49). The proportion of these fatty acids is highest after the main meal and falls within a few hours (50).

The chylomicrons and VLDL are the molecular aggregates of lipids and proteins, called lipoproteins (51); they function in the transport of lipids from the plasma to tissues, where they are needed as sources of energy components of membranes or precursors of biologically active metabolites.

There are several apolipoprotein peptides, identified by a series of letters A to E, more subclasses being discovered as research continues. Apolipoprotein C is now divided into apo C-I, II, and III. Many of these peptides are involved in receptor recognition, and some in the functioning of enzymes of lipoprotein metabolism; e.g., apo C-II is required for the activation of LPL and apo A-1 for an enzyme involved in cholesterol esterification (46). An individual's apolipoprotein profile is determined genetically and any variation in it may result in specific metabolic disorders (39).

The chylomicrons are the major carriers of fat from the diet and VLDLs are involved in the transport of endogenously synthesized lipids. The VLDL remnants are known as intermediate-density lipoproteins (IDL), the further degradation yielding particles called low-density lipoproteins (LDL), which are major carriers of cholesterol in human beings. A person with a plasma cholesterol of 5 mmol/l may carry about 70% of this on LDL. These particles are 18 to 22 nm in diameter and contain 20% protein and 80% lipid. The lipid portion is about 50% cholesterol, 80% of which is cholesterol ester, mainly in the form of 18:2, 18:1, and 16:0. LDLs deliver cholesterol to tissues for the vital functions of membrane synthesis and repair. Cholesterol may be discharged by passive endocytosis or by a specific receptor-mediated uptake process (52). Endogenous cholesterol biosynthesis is regulated by the amount available from the diet. Familial hypercholesterolemia is an inherited disorder characterized by high circulating concentrations of LDL, resulting from the absence of the LDL receptor (52).

The high-density lipoproteins (HDL) carry cholesterol from the peripheral cells to the liver, where it is degraded or repackaged (reverse cholesterol transport). A low plasma concentration of HDLs may be indicative of increased risk of cardiovascular heart disease (CHD), and it has been postulated that HDLs may have a protective role in this regard. However, it remains to be established that procedures leading to an elevation of HDL do indeed reduce the risk of CHD. Protein (predominantly apoA-I and II, with some C, D, and E peptides) constitutes about 50% of HDL mass, with about 22% phospholipid, 20% cholesterol ester, and 8% triacylglycerol. A key step in reverse cholesterol transport is catalyzed by the enzyme lecithin cholesterol acyltransferase (LCAT). A fatty acid is transferred from phosphatidylcholine to cholesterol to form a cholesterol ester. In human plasma, LCAT is associated with HDL and the phospholipid substrate is also present in HDL, which has been transferred from chylomicron remnants or IDL (during degradation of chylomicrons or VLDL). The cholesterol substrate is obtained from the surfaces of plasma lipoporteins or plasma membranes of cells. LCAT consumes cholesterol and promotes its net transport from cells into plasma. The cholesterol ester molecules transferred to lipoproteins containing apo B or apo E are taken up by the liver, thus completing the 'reverse cholesterol transport' process (Fig. 3) (39).

The influx of digestion products from lipids and carbohydrates after the consumption of a meal influences the amounts and proportions of lipoproteins in the plasma, especially the chylomicrons and VLDLs. The intakes of fats and carbohydrates may influence the levels of lipoproteins in the following ways (39):

1. Increasing the dietary intake of cholesterol increases plasma cholesterol by only a small extent (about 0.5 mmol/1 or 2 mg/dl) for every 100 mg of cholesterol consumed daily, mainly in the form of LDL fraction.
2. Substitution of saturated fatty acids by monounsaturated or *n*-6 polyunsaturated fatty acids decreases the concentration of LDL cholesterol. HDL cholesterol is not reduced unless linoleic acid provides more than about 12% of dietary energy.
3. The addition of long-chain *n*-3 PUFA (mainly 20:5 and 22:6) to diets decreases the concentration of VLDLs, but not LDL or HDL.

4. The replacement of dietary saturated fatty acids with carbohydrates decreases the concentrations of LDL and HDL and in some people may increase concentrations of VLDL.

5. The replacement of dietary *n*-6 PUFA with carbohydrates increases LDL-cholesterol concentrations, with little change in HDL, and in some people may increase concentrations of VLDL.

These changes probably occur by reducing the rate at which the apo B receptors in the liver remove LDL. This is in turn brought about by some saturated fatty acids (especially 12:0 and 14:0), and reversal of this effect by some unsaturated fatty acids. Alternatively, different types of fatty acids and carbohydrates may influence rates of biosynthesis of LDL from VLDL (53).

The fatty acids are enzymatically synthesized and esterified into triacylglycerols, phospholipids, and other lipids in most of the body tissues (46,54). It is known that a low-fat diet enhances rates of fatty acid synthesis, especially in the liver, to provide the body's needs of structural and storage fat, the main products being palmitate and oleate. However, when the needs of storage and structural fats are satisfied from dietary intake alone, as in Western peoples, the enzymes of fatty acid synthesis may be switched off. Diet may regulate the body's fatty acid biosynthesis by altering the synthesis or activities of biosynthetic enzymes through the availability of cofactors, such as pantothenic acid or biotin or even by influencing the concentrations of circulating hormones which either induce or suppress the synthesis of the enzymes of lipid metabolism, e.g., insulin suppresses glucose synthesis in the liver, induces glycogen and fatty acid synthesis, stimulates uptake of glucose into adipose tissue, and inhibits the breakdown of fat in that tissue.

A high degree of unsaturation is required to achieve the desired physical properties of lipid in cells that is brought about by the enzymatic introduction of double bonds, through desaturases present in almost all tissues; e.g., palmitic and stearic acids, arising either from the diet or biosynthesis in the tissues, are desaturated to palmitoleic (*cis*-9-hexadecenoic) and oleic (*cis*-9-octadecenoic) acids, respectively. Similarly, polyunsaturated fatty acids may be produced by enzymatic introduction of further double bonds, giving rise to several families of PUFA, depending on the structure of the precursor fatty acid. The most important families are the n-3, n-6, and n-9 series.

In the course of evolution, human beings have lost the ability to synthesize enzymes that catalyze the introduction of double bonds between carbon 12 and 13 and between 15 and 16 as present in linoleic and alpha-linolenic acids, formed in plants. Because these fatty acids are essential for human life, they have become dietary essential fatty acids.

Because the same desaturases are involved in the metabolism of various PUFA families, it has been shown that substrates on different pathways compete with each other for desaturases, thus influencing the proportions of the end products formed. The affinity of the 6-desaturase for its substrate is highest for 18:3, followed by 18:2 and 18:1. The pathway beginning with linoleic acid (the *n*-6 series) normally predominates, arachidonic acid being the major end product. If the diet has a very small amount of linoleic acid, compared with oleic acid, the *n*-9 pathway will begin to predominate, giving rise to an excessive production of 5, 8, 11-20:3. This explains why the ratio of 20:3 (*n*-9) to 20:4 (*n*-6) is an indicator of essential fatty acid (EFA) deficiency. Other acids, such as the isomeric fatty acids formed during hydrogenation, can also compete with linoleic acid, and diets with excessive amounts of these isomers, and limiting amounts of linoleic acid, could also give rise to EFA deficiency, as defined by these biochemical criteria. Although this occurs rarely for most individuals, some people who eat diets predominating in hardened fats are likely to be exposed to EFA deficiency (39).

A diet containing a larger proportion of fish oils rich in *n*-3 fatty acids will tip the balance of PUFA metabolism in favor of the *n*-3 family, stimulating the production of eicosanoids derived from these precursors. These eicosanoids have been shown to reduce the ability of platelets to aggregate, possibly explaining why the Eskimos, whose diets are rich in *n*-3 fatty acids, have very low incidences of thrombosis, despite their extremely high total fat intakes. However, it cannot be assumed that the indiscriminate use of these highly unsaturated fatty acids is entirely without risk.

The conversion of PUFA into eicosanoids is an example of enzymatically controlled oxidation, whereas uncontrolled oxidation of PUFA can be brought about by free radical chain reaction in the presence of oxygen and a catalyst such as iron. The human body is protected against such uncontrolled peroxidation by two main mechanisms (39):

1. The organization of lipids in membrane bilayers in juxtaposition with lipid-soluble antioxidants such as vitamin E, and
2. The presence of enzyme systems such as superoxide dismutase (SOD) that destroy initiating radicals.

Growing evidence indicates that diets deficient in natural antioxidants such as vitamins E and C, and environmental factors producing free radicals (e.g. smoking), can cause oxidative stress, which if uncontrolled by an individual's capacity to scavenge free radicals may lead to degenerative changes over a period of time (55).

C. White and Brown Adipose Tissues

There are two types of adipose tissues in the human body with different functions. White adipose tissue functions as storage of fat, whereas brown adipose tissue has evolved to provide heat to maintain body temperature. White adipose tissue provides a reserve of fuel for energy. It consists mainly of mesenchymal connective tissue cells, called adipocytes (56). These cells store fat as a single droplet, pushing the nucleus and cytoplasm to the periphery. Adipocytes have enormous capacity to expand when more fat needs to be stored. These cells have a capillary network and receive nerves from the autonomic nervous system, whose fibers terminate in close relation to both cells and blood vessels.

Adipose tissues have significant amounts of non-fat cellular material; e.g., healthy man carrying 10 kg of adipose tissue (about 15% of body weight, of which 85% is fat) has 1.5 kg of fat-free adipose tissue, containing about 200 g protein. A healthy woman has more fat (about 25%) in relation to her body weight than a man. Amounts of adipose tissue can vary widely, from about 1 kg in very emaciated persons to as high as 100 kg or more in very obese people. Health problems are often associated with excessive adipose tissue mass (see Chapter 26).

In humans, approximately two-thirds of adipose tissue is located under the skin (subcutaneous) and one-third internally (visceral). In addition to storage fuel, visceral fat provides a protective cushion for the delicate internal organs; the external fat acts as an insulator as well as providing a cushioning effect. Men tend to deposit more adipose tissue around the abdomen, which is accentuated with age; women tend to deposit more fat in the upper and lower body, over the hips and thighs. Abdominal adipose tissue appears to be closely associated with health problems such as raised blood pressure, diabetes, and an increased risk of cardiovascular disease (57).

According to Hausman (56), white adipose tissue begins to develop in fetal life and a newborn baby weighing 3.5 kg has about 560 g adipose tissue; mainly synthesized from glucose. Fat cells possess all the enzymes needed to make lipids de novo, which are suppressed by high fat intakes in later stages of life. Adipose tissue undergoes continuous lipid turnover, even when the total mass of body fat remains more or less constant. Hirsch et al. (58) observed that half of the linoleic acid in adult adipose tissue is replaced within 350 to 750 days. The insulin-regulated LDL activity governs the rate of entry of fatty acids from circulating lipids into the fat cell, whereas a hormone-sensitive triacylglycerol lipase activity controls the lipolysis of the stored fat, prior to the export of fatty acids into the blood for their further metabolism by beta-oxidation (46,47) in muscle, liver, and other tissues.

Diet influences the composition of adipose tissue. Widdowson et al. (59) demonstrated that the concentration of linoleic acid in Dutch babies fed a formula milk containing a vegetable oil rich in linoleic acid was very high (50% of total fatty acids) compared with British babies fed cow's milk (2%–4% of total fatty acids). There was even a slight difference at birth, suggesting that the Dutch mothers' diets also contained more linoleic acid than their British counterparts.

Linoleic acid of adipose tissue makes an ideal marker for the type of dietary fat consumed. Small pieces of fat tissue taken by needle biopsy are analyzed by gas-liquid chromatography, which is a more reliable measure of habitual fatty acid intake than dietary surveys (60,61). The relationship between dietary intake and adipose tissue composition, however, does not hold true for all fatty acids, e.g., the adipose tissue concentrations of alpha-linolenic and arachidonic acids tend to be lower than predicted from their amounts in the diet. Wood et al. (62) noted a lower content of linolenic acid in the adipose tissue of men living in Edinburgh (where incidence of CHD is relatively high) compared to those in Stockholm (where it is lower), and in healthy Scottish men, compared with patients prone to CHD (see Chapter 24).

1. Thermogenic Brown Adipose Tissue

In most mammals, including humans, newborns have a special type of adipose tissue called brown fat, in which substrates are oxidized not to produce ATP, but to generate heat to keep the newborn warm. This specialized adipose tissue, located at the back of the neck of human infants, is brown in color because of the presence of large numbers of mitochondria and thus large amounts of cytochromes, whose heme groups strongly absorb visible light. The brown fat mitochondria oxidize fuels (especially fatty acids) through normal electron transport chains. The brown fat mitochondria have a unique protein in their inner membrane, called thermogenin or uncoupling protein (UCP), present as an integral membrane protein, which provides a path for protons to return to the matrix without passing through the F_0, F_1, complex. This short-circuiting of protons causes dissipation of energy as heat, rather than conservation by ATP formation.

Mammals can react to cold by muscular activity, typically by shivering, which produces heat. Heat is also produced in the body through certain thermodynamically inefficient chemical reactions, referred to as futile cycles. At birth, heat production by shivering in response to cold is ineffective, and the activation of brown adipose tissue is the chief mechanism for controlling body temperature in a cold environment (63). Some animal species use activation of brown adipose tissue as a means of disposing of excess dietary energy to control body weight, but its significance in human beings remains to be established.

REFERENCES

1. Englyst, H.N., and S.M. Kingman, Carbohydrates, *Human Nutrition and Dietetics*, 9th ed. (J.S. Garrow and W.P.T. James, eds), Churchill Livingstone, Edinburgh, London, 1993, p. 38.
2. Jenkins, D.J.A., D.M. Thomas, T.M.S. Wolever, R.H. Taylor, et al. Glycaemic index of foods: a physiological basis for carbohydrate exchange, *Am. J. Clin. Nutr. 34*: 362 (1981).
3. Wahlqvist, M.L., E.G. Wilmshurst, C.R. Murton, and E.N. Richardson, The effect of chain length on glucose absorption and the related metabolic response, *Am. J. Clin. Nutr. 31*: 1998 (1978).
4. Crapo, P.A., and R.R. Henry, Postprandial metabolic responses to the influence of food form, *Am. J. Clin. Nutr. 48*: 560 (1988).

5. Heaton, K.W., S.N. Marcus, P.M. Emmett, and C.H. Bilton, Partical size of wheat, maize and oat test meals: effect on plasma glucose and insulin responses and on the rate of starch digestion in vitro *Am. J. Clin. Nutr. 47*: 675 (1988).

6. Hermansen, K., O. Rasmussen, J. Arnfred, E. Winther and O. Schnitz, Differential glycaemic effect of potato, rice and spaghetti in Type 1 (insulin-dependent) diabetic patients at constant insulinaemia, *Diabetalogia 29*: 358 (1986).

7. Englyst, H.N., and J.H. Cummings, Digestion of the polysaccharides of some cereal foods in the human small intestine, *Am. J. Clin. Nutr. 42*: 778 (1985).

8. Englyst, H.N., and J.H. Cummings, Digestion of the carbohydrates of banana (*Musa paradisiaca sapientum*) in the human small intestine, *Am. J. Clin. Nutr. 44*: 42 (1986).

9. Soundarapandian, P., T. Kannupandi, and M.J. Samuel, Effect of feeds on digestive enzymes of juveniles of *Macrobrachium malcolmsonii* (H. Milne Edwards), *Indian J. Exp. Biol. 36*: 720 (1998).

10. Macfarlane, G.T., and J.H. Cummings, The colonic flora, fermentation and large bowel digestive function, *The Large Intestine: Physiology, Pathophysiology and Diseases* (S.E. Philips, J.H. Pemberton, J.H. Shorter, eds.) Raven Press, New York, 1990.

11. Cummings, J.H., and H.N. Englyst, Fermentation in the human large intestine and the available substances, *Am. J. Clin. Nutr. 45*: 1243 (1987).

12. Kim, Y.S., D. Tsao, A. Morita, and A. Bella, Effect of sodium butyrate on three human colorectal adenocarcinoma cell lines in culture, *Colonic Carcinogenesis* (R.A. Malt and R.C.N. Williamson, eds), Falk Symp. 31, MTP Press, Lancaster, 1982, p. 317.

13. Pomare, E.W., W.J. Branch, and J.H. Cummings, Carbohydrate fermentation in the human colon and its relation to acetate concentration in venous blood, *J. Clin. Invest. 75*: 1448 (1985).

14. Skutches, G.L., C.P. Holroyde, R.N. Myers, P. Paul, and G.A. Reichard, Plasma acetate turnover and oxidation, *J. Clin. Invest. 64*: 708 (1979).

15. Christl, S.U., G.R. Gibson, and J.H. Cummings, The role of dietary sulphate in the regulation of methanogenesis in the human large intestine, *Gut*, 32:1 (1992)

16. Anderson, I.H., A.S. Levine, and M.D. Levitt, Incomplete absorption of carbohydrate in all-purpose wheat floor, *N. Engl. J Med. 304*: 891 (1981).

17. Cummings, J.H., and H.N. Englyst, Measurement of starch fermentation in the human large intestine, *Can. J. Physiol. Pharmacol. 69*: 121 (1991).

18. Blaxter, K.L., *The Energy Metabolism of Ruminants*. Hutchinson, London, 1962.

19. Trowell, H., *Non-Infective Disease in Africa*, Edward Arnold, London, 1960, p. 217.

20. Cummings, J.H., S.A. Bingham, K.W. Heaton, and M.A. Eastwood, Fecal weight, colon cancer risk and dietary intake of non-starch polysaccharides (dietary fibre), *Gastroenterology 103*: 1783 (1992).

21. Holt, S., R.C. Heading, D.C. Carter, L.F. Prescott, and P. Hothill, Effect of gel fibre on gastric emptying and absorption of glucose and paracetamol, *Lancet 2*: 636 (1979).

22. Chen, W.L., and J.W. Anderson, Propionate may mediate the hypocholesterolemic effect of plant fibers in cholesterol fed rats, *Proc. Soc. Exp. Biol. Med. 175*: 215 (1984).

23. Garlick, P.J., and Reeds, P.J., Proteins, *Human Nutrition and Dietetics*, 9th ed. (J.S. Garrow and W.P.T. James, eds.), Churchill Livingstone, Edinburgh, London, 1993, p. 56.

24. Alpers, D.H., Digestion and absorption of carbohydates and proteins, *Physiology of Gastrointestinal Tract*, 2nd ed., Vol. 2, (L.R. Johnson, ed.), Raven Press, New York, 1987, p. 1469.

25. Hopfer, U., Membrane transport mechanisms for hexoses and amino acids in the small intestine, *Physiology of the Gastrointestinal Tract*, 2nd ed., Vol. 2 (L.R. Johnson, ed.), Raven Press, New York, 1987, p. 1499.

26. Bond, J.S., and P.E. Butler, Intracellular proteases, *Ann. R. Biochemistry 56*: 333 (1987).

27. Mortimore, G.E., A.R. Poso, B.R. Lardeux, Mechanism and regulation of protein degradation in liver, *Diabetes/Metabolism Rev. 5*: 49 (1989).

28. Young, V.R., W.P. Steffee, P.B. Pencharz, J.C. Winterer, and N.S. Scrimshaw, Total human body protein synthesis in relation to protein requirements at various ages, *Nature 253*: 192 (1975).

29. Waterlow, J.C., P.J. Garlick and D.J. Millward, *Protein Turnover in Mammalian Tissues and in the Whole Body*, North Holland, Amsterdam, 1978.

30. Diem, K., *Documenta Geigy Scientific Tables*, 6th ed., Geigy UK, Macclesfield, 1962, p. 528.

31. Jackson, A.A., Optimizing amino acid and protein supply and utilization in the newborn, *Proc. Nutrition Soc. 48*: 293 (1989).

32. Reeds, P.J., Amino acid needs and protein scoring patterns, *Proc. Nutrition Soc. 49*: 489 (1990).

33. Lentner, C., Units of measurement, body fluids, composition of the body, nutrition, *Geigy Scientific Tables*, 8th ed. Vol. 1, Ciba-Geigy, Basle, 1981.

34. James, W.P.T., Research in malnutrition and its application to parenteral feeding, *Advances in Parenteral Nutrition* (I.D.A. Johnston, ed.), Proc. Int. Symp. Bermuda, 1977, p. 521.

35. Munro, H.L., and J.B. Allison, *Mammalian Protein Metabolism*, Vol. I, Academic Press, New York, 1964.

36. Waterlow, J.C., P.J. Garlick, and D.J. Millward, Protein turnover in mammalian tissues and in the whole body, North Holland, Amsterdam, 1978 (Quoted by Garlick and Reeds, Ref. 23).

37. Furst, P., Regulation of intracellular metabolism of amino acids, *Nutrition in Cancer, Trauma and Sepsis* (F. Bozzetto and R. Dionigi, eds.), Proc. Sixth ESPEN Congr., Karger, Basle, 1985, p. 21.

38. FAO/WHO/UNU, Energy and protein requirements, Report of a joint expert consultation, WHO Technical Report Series No. 724, World Health Organization, Geneva, 1985.

39. Gurr, M., Fats, *Human Nutrition and Dietetics* (J.S. Garrow and W.P.T. James, eds.), Churchill Livingstone, Edinburgh, London, 1993, p. 77.

40. Hamosh, M., The role of lingual lipase in neonatal fat digestion, *Development of Mammalian Absorptive Processes*, CIBA Foundation Symp. No. 70, Excerpta Medica, Amsterdam, 1979, p. 92.

41. Hamosh, M., Fat digestion in the newborn: role of lingual lipase and preduodenal digestion, *Pediatric Res. 13*: 615 (1979).

42. Fredrikzon, B., O. Hernell, L. Blackberg, and T. Olivecrona, Bile salt-stimulated lipase in human milk: evidence of activity in vivo and of a role in the digestion of milk retinol esters, *Pediatric Res., 12*: 1048 (1978).

43. Carey, M.C., D.M. Small, and C.M. Bliss, Lipid digestion and absorption, *Ann. Rev. Physiol. 45*: 651 (1983).

44. Hill, M.J., Colon cancer: a disease of fibre depletion or of dietary excess? *Digestion 11*: 289 (1974).

45. Sickinger, K., Clinical aspects and theory of fat malassimilation with particular reference to the use of medium-chain triglycerides, *The Role of Fats in Human Nutrition* (A.J. Vergroescn, ed.), Academic Press, London, 1975, p. 116.

46. Gurr, M.I., and J.L. Harwood, *Lipid Biochemistry: An Introduction*, Chapman and Hall, London, 1991.

47. Vance, D.E., and J.E. Vance (eds.), *Biochemistry of Lipids and Membranes*, Benjamin Cummings Publishing Co., Menlo Park, California, 1985.

48. Sjostrom, J., Carbohydrate-stimulated fatty acid synthesis de novo in human adipose tissue of different cellular types, *Acta Medica Scandinavia 194*: 387 (1973).

49. Read, W.W.C., P.G. Lutz, and A. Tashjian, Human milk lipids. II. The influence of dietary carbohydrates and fat on the fatty acids of mature milk. A study in four ethnic groups, *Am. J. Clin. Nutr. 17*: 180 (1965).

50. Read, W.W.C., P.G. Lutz, and A. Tashjian, Human milk lipids. III. Short-term effects of dietary carbohydrates and fat, *Am. J. Clin. Nutr. 17*: 184 (1965).

51. Segrest, J.P., and J.J. Albsers, The lipoproteins: Vol. 128, Preparation, structure and molecular biology; Vol. 129, Characterization cell biology and metabolism, *Methods Enzymol.* Academic Press, New York, 1986.

52. Brown, M.S., P.T. Kovanen, and J.L. Goldstein, Regulation of plasma cholesterol by lipoprotein receptors, *Science: 212*: 628 (1981).

53. Grundy, S.M., and M.A. Denke, Dietary influences on serum lipids and lipoproteins, *J. Lipid Res. 31*: 1149 (1990).

54. Vance, D.E., and J.E. Vance (Eds.), *Biochemistry of Lipids and Membranes*, Benjamin Cummings Publishing Co., Menlo Park, California, 1985.

55. Gey, K.F., On the antioxidant hypothesis with regard to arteriosclerosis, *Bibliotheca Nutritia Deita 37*: 53 (1986).

56. Hausman, G.J., The comparative anatomy of adipose tissue, *New Perspectives in Adipose Tissue: Structure, Function and Development* (A. Cryer and R.L.R. Van, eds.), Butterworths, London, 1985, p. 1.

57. Stern, M.P., and S.M. Haffner, Body fat distribution and hyperinsulinaemia as risk factors for diabetes and cardiovascular disease, *Arteriosclerosis 6*: 123 (1986).

58. Hirsch, J., J.W. Farquar, E.H. Andrews, M.L. Peterson, and W. Stoffel, Studies of adipose tissue in man: a microtechnique for sampling and analysis, *Am. J. Clin. Nutr. 8*: 499 (1960).

59. Widdowson, E.M., M.J. Dauncy, D.M.T. Gairdner, J.H.P. Jonxis and M. Pelikan-Filipkova, Body fat of British and Dutch infants, *B. Med. J. 1*: 653 (1975).

60. Katan, M.B., W.A. Van Staveren, P. Deurenberg, et al., Linoleic and *trans*-unsaturated fatty acid content of adipose tissue biopsies as objective indicators of the dietary habits of individuals, *Progr. Lipid Res. 25*: 193 (1986).

61. Berry, E.M., J. Hirsch, J. Most, D.J. McNamara, and J. Thornton, The relationship of dietary fat to plasma lipid levels by factor analysis of adipose tissue fatty acid composition in a free-living population of middle-aged American men, *Am. J. Clin. Nutr. 44*: 220 (1986).

62. Wood, D.A., R.A. Riemersma, S. Butler, Linoleic acid and eicosapentaenoic acid in adipose tissue and platelets and risk of coronary heart disease, *Lancet 1*: 177 (1987).

63. Hull, D., and M.J. Hardman, Brown adipose tissue in newborn mammals, *Brown Adipose Tissue* (O. Lindberg, ed.), Elsevier, New York, 1970, p. 97.

20
Hormonal Regulation of Food Intake

I. INTRODUCTION

A number of hormones of endocrine systems, such as insulin, glucagon, and others that are involved directly or indirectly in the regulation of glucose, as sensed by the hypothalamus, are thought to be involved in the regulation of food intake.

II. ENDOCRINE SYSTEMS

The word *hormone* is derived from the Greek verb *"horman,"* meaning "to stir up or excite." Hormones are chemical messengers (peptides, amines, or steroids) that are secreted by certain body tissues to the blood, and serve to regulate the activity of other tissues. Hormones act in a hierarchy of functions. Nerve impulses first stimulate the hypothalamus to send specific hormones to the pituitary gland, either stimulating or inhibiting the release of tropic hormones. The anteriar pitutary hormones in turn stimulate other endocrine glands (thyroid, adrenals, pancreas) to secrete their own characteristic hormones, which in turn stimulate specific target tissues to bring about the metabolic coordination among separate organs, tissues, and cells of the body.

The concept of hormones was recognized in the nineteenth century, "internal secretions" into the bloodstream being distinguished from "external secretions" such as sweat and tears. Ernest Henry Starling introduced the term hormone in 1905 in his lecture on "The chemical correlation of the functions of the body." In addition to regulating different aspects of metabolism, hormones also control cell and tissue growth, heart rate, blood pressure, kidney function, motility of the gastrointestinal tract, secretion of digestive enzymes and other hormones, lactation, and functioning of the reproductive systems (1).

A. Endocrine Hormones

Hormones are chemically diverse and biologically potent molecules; they can be classified into three distinct groups based on their chemical nature:

1. Peptide hormones
2. Amine hormones
3. Steroid hormones

A fourth group of extracellular signals, the eicosanoids, has been recognized; they are hormonelike in their actions but act locally (Table 1). The peptide hormones, which have 3 to more than 200 amino acid residues, include all the hormones of the hypothalamus and pituitary and pancreatic hormones such as insulin, glucagon, and somatostatin. The amine hormones are low-

Table 1 Classification of Hormones and Hormonelike Substances, Their Secreting Organs/Cells, and Function/Activity

Hormones	Secreting organ/tissue/cells	Function or activity
1. Peptide hormones		
Thyrotropin-releasing hormone (TRH)	Hypothalamus	Stimulates thyrotropin release from anterior pituitary
Corticotropin (ACTH)	Anterior pituitary	Stimulates synthesis of adrenocortical steroids in adrenal cortex
Vasopressin (antidiuretic hormone, ADH)	Posterior pituitary	Increases blood pressure, promotes water reabsorption by kidney
Insulin	Pancreas	Stimulates glucose uptake and utilization
Glucagon	Pancreas	Stimulates glucose production by liver
2. Amine hormones		
Epinephrine (adrenaline)	Adrenal medulla	Controls responses to stress, increases heart rate
Thyroxine (thyroid hormone)	Thyroid	Stimulates metabolism in many tissues
3. Steroid hormones		
Cortisol	Adrenal cortex	Limits glucose utilization, increases blood glucose
Aldosterone	Adrenal cortex	Regulates sodium retention and blood pressure
Beta-estradiol	Ovary	Regulates activity in female reproductive tissues
Testosterone	Testis	Regulates activity in male reproductive tissues
Progesterone	Corpus luteum (in ovary)	Regulates activity in female reproductive organs during menstrual cycle and pregnancy
4. Eicosanoids (hormonelike compounds)		
Prostaglandins	Most tissues	Trigger smooth muscle contraction, fever, and inflammation
Leukotrienes	Leukocytes (WBC)	Cause bronchial constriction, involved in hypersensitivity reactions
Thromboxanes	Platelets and other tissues	Regulate blood clotting, vasoconstriction, and platelet aggregation

Source: Ref. 1.

molecular-weight compounds derived from the amino acid tyrosine, and include water-soluble epinephrine and norepinephrine of the adrenal medulla, and the less water-soluble thyroid hormones. The steroid hormones are fat-soluble substances and include the adrenal cortical hormones, hormone forms of vitamin D $[1, 25\text{-}(OH)_2D_3]$, and the androgens and estrogens (the male and female sex hormones). They move through the bloodstream bound to specific carrier proteins. The eicosanoids are derivatives of the 20-carbon PUFA, arachidonic acid. All types of eicosanoids (prostaglandins, leukotrienes, and thromboxanes) are unstable and insoluble in water and do not move far from the tissues producing them—they act primarily on cells very near their point of release (2).

Hormones normally occur in very low concentrations in the blood, ranging from micromolar (10^{-6} M) to picomolar (10^{-12} M) levels, in contrast to much higher concentrations of blood glucose (4×10^{-3} M). Hormones are therefore difficult to identify, isolate, and measure accurately and need extremely sensitive techniques such as radio-immunoassays and enzyme-linked immunosorbent assay (ELISA). Hormones exist in blood for very short periods of times, often only for minutes, and are inactivated enzymatically as soon as their functions are completed. Some hormones, such as epinephrine, yield immediate (within seconds) physiological or biochemical responses, whereas others, such as thyroid hormones and estrogens, promote maximal responses in their target tissues only after hours or even days. These different responses correspond to their difference in mode of action. The fast-acting hormones generally lead to a change in the activity of one or more preexisting enzyme(s) in the cell, through allosteric mechanisms or covalent modification of the enzyme(s), whereas the slow-acting hormones often alter gene expression, resulting in the synthesis of more or fewer copies of the regulated protein(s). All hormones act through specific receptors present in hormone-sensitive target cells to which hormones bind with high specificity and affinity (3).

Water-soluble peptide and amine hormones do not penetrate cell membranes readily, their receptors being located on the outer surface of the target cells; the lipid-soluble steroid and thyroid hormones readily pass through the plasma membrane of their target cells and their receptors are specific proteins located in the nucleus. Upon the binding of hormone to a plasma membrane receptor, the receptor protein undergoes a conformational change, analogous to that produced in an allosteric enzyme by effector binding. In its altered form, the receptor either produces or causes production of an intracellular messenger molecule, often referred to as "second messenger," e.g., adenosine 3′, 5′-cyclic monophosphate (cAMP). The second messenger conveys the signal from the hormone receptor to some enzyme or molecular system in the cell, which then responds. The second messenger either regulates a specific enzymatic reaction or changes the rate at which a specific gene or set of genes is translated into proteins. In the case of steroid and thyroid hormones, the hormone-receptor complex itself carries the message and alters the expression of specific genes (1).

B. Endocrine Glands

The major endocrine glands of the human body are the hypothalamus, pituitary, thyroid, adrenals, pancreas, kidneys, and testis (males) and ovaries (females). The word endocrine comes from the Greek *endon*, meaning "within," and *krinein*, "to release," indicating that secretions of such glands are internal, i.e., they release into the blood. In contrast, the exocrine glands secrete their products (tears, sweat, digestive enzymes) "outward," through ducts that lead to the body surface or intestinal lumen.

The hypothalamus is a specialized portion of the brain and a coordination center of the endocrine system, receiving and integrating messages from the central nervous system. In response to these messages, the hypothalamus produces a number of regulatory hormones that pass to the anterior pituitary gland, located below the hypothalamus. Whereas some hypothalamic hormones (releasing factors) stimulate the anterior pituitary to secrete a given hormone, others are inhibitory in their action. The stimulated anterior pituitary secretes hormones that are carried in the blood to the next rank of endocrine glands, viz., the adrenal cortex, the thyroid gland, the ovary and testis, and the endocrine pancreatic cells, which in turn are stimulated to secrete their specific hormones to be carried by the blood to hormone receptors on or in the cells of the target tissues.

The posterior pituitary contains the axonal endings of many neurons that originate in the hypothalamus. Two short peptide hormones, oxytocin and vasopressin, are synthesized in these neurons from longer precursor peptides. The hypothalamus thus functions at the top of the hierarchy of many hormone-producing tissues. It receives neural input from diverse regions of the brain and feedback signals from hormones circulating in the blood. These signals are integrated in the hypothalamus, which responds by releasing appropriate hormones to the pituitary. The anterior pituitary responds by producing six tropic hormones (tropins) (from the Greek *tropos*, meaning "turn"), relatively long polypeptides that activate the next rank of endocrine glands; viz., ACTH stimulates the adrenal cortex, thyrotropin stimulates the thyroid gland, follicle-stimulating hormone (FSH) and luteinizing hormone (LH) act on the gonads, and growth hormone, somatotropin, stimulates the liver to produce several growth factors.

Thyroid hormones are released when the hypothalamus secretes thyrotropin-releasing hormone, which stimulates the thyroid gland to secrete 1-thyroxin (T_4) and 1-triiodothyronine (T_3), which in turn stimulate energy-yielding metabolism, especially in liver and muscle. These hormones bind to a specific intracellular receptor protein. The hormone-receptor complex then activates certain genes encoding energy-related enzymes, increasing their synthesis and thereby the basal metabolic rate.

The basal metabolic rate (BMR) is a measure of the rate of oxygen consumption by an individual at complete rest, 12 hours after a meal. Hyperthyroid individuals (i.e., those who oversecrete thyroid hormones) have an elevated BMR and are likely to have higher food intake than hypothyroid people with lowered BMR (4).

The major steroid hormones are the adrenocortical hormones, the sex hormones (androgens and estrogens), and vitamin D–derived hormones. These are fat-soluble hormones and readily pass through plasma membrances into the cytosol of target cells where they combine with specific intracellular receptor proteins, which in turn act in the nucleus to effect some gene expressions. Whereas most steroid hormone receptors are localized in the nucleus, others may move from the cytosol to the nucleus after binding to the hormone. Steroid hormones are produced by cells in the outer portion (cortex) of the adrenal glands, located on top of the kidney. Under stress conditions, the hypothalamus secretes corticotropin-releasing hormone, which stimulates the anterior pituitary to release corticotropin into the blood, which in turn signals the adrenal cortex to produce its characteristic corticosteriod hormones, including cortisol, corticosterone and aldosterone. The adrenal cortex produces over 50 different types of corticosteroid hormones, which can be classified into two general groups: glucocorticoids and mineral corticoids. While the glucocorticoids primarily influence carbohydrate metabolism, the mineral corticoids regulate the concentrations of electrolytes (Na^+, K^+, Cl^-) in the blood.

The testes and ovaries secrete the androgens (testosterone) and the estrogens (estradiol, progesterone), respectively. These influence sexual development and sexual behavior and are involved in a range of other reproductive and non-reproductive functions. Steroid hormones produced from vitamin D by enzymes in the liver and kidney [1, 25(OH)$_2$D$_3$] control the uptake and metabolism of Ca^{2+} and phosphate ions, including the formation and mobilization of calcium phosphate in bone.

Water-soluble amine hormones, epinephrine, norepinephrine, dopa and dopamine are all derived from catechol (catecholamines). Epinephrine (adrenaline) and norepinephrine (noraderenaline) are closely related hormones, made and secreted by the inner portion (medulla) of the adrenal glands in response to signals from the central nervous system. The normal blood epienphrine level of about 10^{-10}M may lead to its increase in concentration, 1000-fold within seconds or minutes, after the sensory stimuli alarm the animal and galvanize it for action. The brain and other neural tissues also make the catecholamines that function as neurotransmitters.

The exocrine cells of the pancreas produce digestive enzymes for secretion into intestine (amylase, protease, and lipase) and endocrine cells produce and secrete peptide hormones that regulate fuel metabolism throughout the body. The clusters of specialized pancreatic cells called the islets of Langerhans produce the peptide hormones, insulin, glucagon, and somatostatin, each islet cell type producing a single hormone: alpha cells produce glucagon; beta cells, insulin; and delta cells, somatostatin.

Insulin is a small protein with two polypeptide chains, A and B, joined by two disulfide bonds. It is synthesized as an inactive single chain precursor, preproinsulin, with an amino-terminal "signal sequence" that directs its passage into secretory vesicles. Proinsulin is produced by proteolytic removal of the "signal sequence" and formation of three disulfide bonds. Proinsulin thus made is stored in secretory granules of beta cells. After the triggering of insulin secretion by elevated blood glucose, proinsulin is converted into active insulin by specific peptidases that cleave two peptide bonds to form the mature insulin molecule.

Glucagon is a single polypeptide chain of 29 amino acids, and like insulin is derived from larger precursors (preproglucagon and proglucagon) by precise proteolytic cleavages. Somatostatin is also a polypeptide hormone and functions by inhibiting the secretion of both insulin and glucagon by the pancreas. In addition to the delta cells of the pancreas, somatostatin is also produced and secreted by the hypothalamus and certain intestinal cells (1).

III. HORMONAL REGULATION OF BLOOD GLUCOSE

The blood glucose level is maintained constant, near 4.5 mM, by minute-to-minute adjustments brought about by the combined actions of insulin, glucagon, and epinephrine on metabolic processes in many body tissues, but especially those of liver, muscle, and adipose tissue. Insulin signals these tissues that the blood glucose concentration is higher than normal; as a result, the excess glucose is taken up from the blood into cells and converted into storage compounds, glycogen and triacylglycerols. Conversely, when glucagon carries the message that blood glucose is too low, the tissues respond by producing glucose through glycogen breakdown and gluconeogenesis, and by oxidizing fats to reduce the use of glucose. Epinephrine is released into the blood to prepare the muscle, lungs and heart for a burst of physical activity. Thus, insulin, glucagon, and epinephrine primarily determine the metabolic activities of muscle, liver, and adipose tissue (5).

During stressful situations requiring increased physical activity—fighting and fleeting, in the extreme case—neuronal signals from the brain trigger the release of epinephrine and norepinephrine from the adrenal medulla. Both these hormones increase the rate and strength of the heartbeat; raise the blood pressure, thereby increasing the flow of oxygen and fuel to the tissues; and dilate the respiratory passages to facilitate O_2 uptake. Epinephrine primarily acts on carbohydrate metabolism in the muscle, liver, and adipose tissue, by activating glycogen phosphorylase and inhibiting glycogen synthesis (through cAMP-dependent phosphorylation of enzymes), thus stimulating the conversion of liver glycogen into blood glucose, the fuel for anaerobic muscular work.

Glycogen synthase and glycogen phsophorylase are reciprocally regulated through the action of hormones. The breakdown of glycogen is regulated by both covalent and allosteric modulation of glycogen phosphorylase. Phosphorylase a (the active form), which contains essential phosphorylated serine residue, is dephosphorylated enzymatically (phosphorylase a phosphatase) to yield phosphorylase b (relatively inactive form), which can be stimulated by its allosteric modulator, AMP. Phosphorylase b can be converted back into its active phosphorylase a form by the enzyme phosphorylase b kinase, by phosphorylating the essential serine residues (6).

Like glycogen phosphorylase, glycogen synthase also occurs in phosphorylated and dephosphorylated forms and is regulated in a reciprocal manner, but opposite to that of glycogen phosphorylase. Glycogen synthase a (the active dephosphorylated form) can be converted to a less active form, glycogen synthase b, by phosphorylating at two serine hydroxyl groups enzymatically, by a protein kinase. The conversion of the less active glycogen synthase b back into the active form in turn is promoted by phosphoprotein phosphatase enzyme, by removing the phosphate groups from the serine residues. Both glycogen phosphorylase and glycogen synthase enzymes are thus reciprocally regulated through phosphorylation and dephosphorylation cycle, i.e., when one is stimulated, the other is automatically inhibited, the two enzymes never being active simultaneously. The balance between glycogen synthesis and its breakdown in liver is ultimately controlled by the hormones glucagon and insulin, by regulating the level of cAMP in their target tissues. These hormones also regulate the concentration of fructose-2, 6-diphosphate, and thereby the balance between gluconeogenesis and glycolysis. Epinephrine has effects similar to those of glucagon, but its target is primarily muscle, whereas glucagon's primary action is on liver (7).

Epinephrine stimulation of anerobic breakdown of glycogen in the skeletal muscle produces lactate by fermentation (glycolytic ATP formation). This is accomplished by raising the concentration of fructose-2, 6-bisphosphate, a potent allosteric activator of the key enzyme phospho fructokinase-1. Epinephrine also stimulates fat mobilization in adipose tissue, activating the triacylglycerol lipase (through cAMP-dependent phosphorylation). Finally, epinephrine stimulates the secretion of glucagon and inhibits the secretion of insulin, to reinforce its effect on the mobilization and storage of body fuels.

The blood glucose level falls to below 4.5 mM several hours after the intake of dietary carbohydrate, even in the absence of significant physical activity or stress. This is due to the continued oxidation of glucose by the brain and other body tissues. The lowered blood glucose level triggers secretion of glucagon hormone, simultaneously decreasing the release of insulin. Glucagon increases blood glucose in the following two ways: (a) Like epinephrine, glucagon stimulates the net breakdown of liver glycogen by activating glycogen phosphorylase and inactivating glycogen synthase (through phosphorylation of the regulated enzymes, triggered by cAMP) (8). However, unlike epinephrine, glucagon inhibits glucose breakdown by glycolysis in the liver and stimulates glucose synthesis by gluconeogenesis; both of these effects result from lowering the level of fructose-2, 6-bisphosphate, an allosteric inhibitor of the gluconeogenic enzyme, fructose-1, 6-bisphosphatase and an activator of phosphofructokinase-1. The fructose-2, 6-bisphosphate level is ultimately controlled by a cAMP-dependent protein phosphorylation reaction. Glucagon also inhibits the glycolytic enzyme pyruvate kinase by promoting its cAMP-dependent phosphorylation, thus blocking the conversion of phosphoenol pyruvate to pyruvate, and preventing pyruvate oxidation via tricarboxylic acid (TCA) cycle. The resulting accumulation of phosphoenolpyruvate then favors formation of glucose by gluconeogenesis. Thus, glucagon restores blood glucose to its normal level by enabling the liver to export glucose by stimulating glycogen breakdown and preventing glucose utilization in the liver, as well as by promoting gluconeogenesis (8).

Although its primary target is the liver, glucagon, like epinephrine, also influences adipose tissue by activating triacylglycerol lipase through cAMP-dependent phosphorylation. The free fatty acids released in this process are exported to the liver and other tissues to be used as fuel, thus sparing glucose for the brain. The net effect of glucagon is to mobilize fatty acids from adipose tissue to be used instead of glucose as fuel for tissues other than the brain, all the effects of glucagon being mediated through cAMP-dependent protein phosphorylation (8,9).

A. Fuel Metabolism During Starvation

There are three types of fuel reserves in a normal adult human being.

1. Glycogen stored in the liver and in muscle in relatively small quantities.
2. Larger quantities of triacylglycerols in the adipose tissue.
3. Tissue proteins that can be degraded if necessary to provide fuel for energy.

Significant changes take place in fuel metabolism during starvation. After an overnight fast, almost all of the liver glycogen and most of the muscle glycogen are depleted, and within about 24 hours, the blood glucose level begins to fall, insulin secretion slows down, and glucagon secretion is stimulated. These hormonal signals cause the mobilization of triacylglycerols in the adipose tissue, which then constitute the primary fuels for muscle and liver. The liver begins to degrade certain proteins (those most expendable in an individual not ingesting food). The amino acids resulting from the protein degradation are oxidized in the liver for energy and the nitrogen is excreted by the kidney in the form of urea. The carbon skeletons of glucogenic amino acids in the liver are converted into keto acids such as pyruvate and other intermediates of TCA cycle (alpha-keto-glutarate, oxaloacetate). These intermediates as well as the glycerol derived from the hydrolysis of triacylglycerols in adipose tissue, provide the starting materials for gluconeogenesis in the liver to produce glucose required for the brain.

Eventually the use of TCA cycle intermediates for gluconeogenesis depletes oxaloacetate, thus preventing the entry of acetyl-CoA into the citric acid cycle. The acetyl-CoA produced by fatty acid oxidation begins to accumulate, favoring the formation of ketone bodies like acetoacetyl-CoA in the liver. If the fasting continues, the level of ketone bodies in the blood rises as these fuels are exported from the liver to heart and skeletal muscle and the brain, which use them for energy instead of glucose.

Normal adult human beings store triacylglycerols in adipose tissue to provide enough fuel to maintain basal metabolic rate for about three months, and very obese adults may store fuel to endure a fast of more than an year or so. However, prolonged fasting can be extremely dangerous, as it leads to severe overproduction of ketone bodies (ketosis) and eventually death. After the depletion of fat reserves, the degradation of essential proteins begins, leading to loss of heart and liver function, and death.

Conversely when glucose enters the bloodstream from the intestine, after a normal carbohydrate-rich food intake, the resulting increase in blood glucose will stimulate secretion of insulin and decrease secretion of glucagon. Insulin in turn stimulates glucose uptake by the muscle tissue, converting glucose to glucose-6-phosphate. Insulin also activates glycogen synthase and inactivates glycogen phosphorylase to channel much of the glucose-6-phosphate into glycogen. The blood glucose level then falls to the normal level, as a consequence of accelerated uptake of glucose from the blood. The decreased blood glucose slows down the rate of insulin release from the pancreas. This closely regulated feedback relationship between the rate of insulin secretion and blood glucose concentration maintains the blood glucose level constant around 4.5 mM in an healthy individual, despite large fluctuations in the dietary intake of glucose (10).

Insulin also stimulates the storage of excessive fuel consumed in the diet as fat, by activating both the oxidation of glucose-6-phosphate to pyruvate via glycolysis, and that of pyruvate to acetyl-CoA. The acetyl-CoA not oxidized further for energy production is used for fatty acid synthesis in the liver; these fatty acids are exported as the triacylglycerols of plasma lipoproteins (VLDLs) to the adipose tissue. Insulin stimulates synthesis of triacylglycerol in the adipocytes, using fatty acids released from the VLDL triacylglycerols. These fatty acids are ultimately derived from the excess glucose obtained from the excessive intake of food above the body's needs. Thus, insulin favors the conversion of excessive blood glucose from the diet into two storage forms: glycogen in the liver and muscle, and triacylglycerols in the adipose tissue (1,11,12).

IV. REGULATION OF FOOD INTAKE

All animals, including humans, must eat to live, and there are mechanisms that direct them to take food through hunger, appetite, and satiety. According to Manay and Shadaksharaswamy (13), in almost every case some sort of control is exerted over the amount and kind of food consumed by the animal. Hungry animals respond by locating and ingesting food to satisfy the hunger and stop eating when hunger is satieted.

A. Hunger, Appetite, and Satiety

A holistic theory of the mechanism(s) controlling normal eating behavior provides the basis for a computer model that is an integrated quantitative basis for a central and peripheral physiology of appetite. It also provides a cognitive psychological framework for the cultural anthropology of eating habits. The theoretical concepts included were backed by evidence from laboratory and field. All the postulated mechanisms were observed independently of the operation of the system as a whole; e.g., the limited control of body weight that can be actually observed could be achieved without set points in the computer-modeled theory. The behavior processes that integrate sensory and visceral signals and form a basis for cognitive aspects of appetite and satiety, were explicitly analyzed by laboratory experiments with adult and infant rats, lean and obese monkeys, and adult human subjects.

Appetite and associated phenomena of hunger, satiety, palatability, craving, liking, and distaste can be specified and measured as aspects of the overall behavioral performance. The cognitive postulate that eating is a set of learned reactions to configurations of sensory, somatic, and social cues has provided the basis for fundamental methodological progress in the analysis of the influences on an individual's appetite: this takes the form of linear causal analysis of influences from sensory characteristics of the diet and their integration with the perceived bodily effects or socioeconomic attributes of eating specific menus and foods.

Hunger is often considered as an unpleasant sensation that compels a person to seek and eat food. It is a physiological condition associated with the contraction of the stomach muscle, which may be controlled through the action of hormone-like substances, such as prostaglandins and others. Such contractions are forceful and occur for a period and then subside as the stomach passes into a resting stage. Hunger conditions that subside without eating will reappear later with greater intensity. In addition to stomach contractions resulting in tenseness, rumbling, and a feeling of emptiness, a hungry person may experience certain general sensations, such as weakness, irritability, occasional headache, or even nausea (13).

In contrast to hunger, appetite in many people can be a pleasant sensation that causes a person to desire and anticipate food; it can be experienced for a certain kind of food. Appetite also has physiological components controlled hormonally, but it is basically a psychological state. It is less easily localized than hunger, and is often felt in the mouth or palate. It depends more on the odor or flavor and the pleasant memory of food. Appetite is a clearly distinct sensation from hunger: a person may express a desire for some particular food at the end of dinner when he is comfortably replete.

Satiety is the sensation accompanying the satisfaction of the desire for food after eating it. It is not just the opposite of hunger and has far fewer sensations. Whereas hunger builds up slowly, satiety occurs more rapidly. The absence of desire for food, even when it is needed by the body, is an abnormal or diseased condition, often called anorexia.

Syndromes of eating disorders known as *anorexia nervosa* and *bulimia* (nervosa) are certainly pychopathological in nature. The mechanisms that establish normal appetite for food explain the eating disorder when coupled with socially induced distortions of feelings about body shape. Such syndromes can result from a process of cultural inveiglement of the sufferer into extreme operation of normal learning of appetite and normal physiological adaptations to starvation or vomiting. Thus, the causes of such disorders do not necessarily involve anything organic or dysfunctional in the hypothalamus, the limbic system, the gastrointestinal tract, or any other part of the brain or body involved in the physiology of appetite, emotions, or endocrine control.

Any biologically normal person may become susceptible to eating disorders with abnormal attitudes to foods and to the body.

The term *compulsive overeating* (CO) has been used in many ways, some of which make it synonymous with bulimia nervosa, whereas others simply suggest regularly eating large portions of food. It has also been viewed as eating to avoid feeling and dealing with emotional pain and is performed without regard to biological need for nutrients and done in a repeated, ritualized fashion to induce a sense of well-being, numbness, or freedom from anxiety. The behavior pattern may result in continuously eating food throughout a defined period of time (grazing) or cycles of bingeing interpersed with normal eating. Compulsive overeating is different from anorexia nervosa, and particularly bulimia nervosa, because it does not necessarily involve a persistent concern with body shape, weight, or thinness. CO behavior is seen in people who have not learned to appropriately express and deal with their feelings. They often come from alcoholic families or have been victims of sexual abuse.

It has been hypothesized that eating is controlled by learned responses to the physiological consequences and social contexts of food intake. The physiological and cultural bases for eating disorders are concerned with people's physiological, psychological, and social capacities. In addition, the "slimming culture," an individual's weight control, and the physiology of fat deposition are an interlinked causal network, operating within energy balance across the skin. Treatment of eating disorders should include dietary advice, behavior modification, and cognitive restructuring, to restore normal eating.

According to Hollmann and Struder (14), eating disorders are associated with a wide range of biochemical changes. Corticotropin-releasing hormone (CRH), released from the hypothalamus, attenuates appetite produced by norepinephrine. While the latter hormone enhances appetite through two post-synaptic receptors, most studies support an inhibitory role of serotonin on food intake, which is mediated through mechanisms in the hypothalamic area (15). CRH is also most probably involved in this because 5-HT is an excitatory transmitter for hypothalamic production and release of this neuropeptide. Benzodiazepines, which enhance food intake, suppress limbic-hypothalamic pituitary-adrenocortical activity, possibly by activating the GABA-mediated inhibition of CRH-release (16). On the contrary, inverse benzodiazepine-receptor ligands not only oppose the behavioral complex of benzodiazepines but also their neuroendocrine effects, as they increase cortisol, probably through elevated CRH. CRH apparently induces anorexia by suppressing hunger. Brown et al. (17), for example, noted that CRH is able to maintain blood glucose level by enhancing sympathetic outflow in several brain areas. Accordingly, CRH concentration was found to be elevated in major brain areas of starving rats (18). It is thus difficult to recognize hypercortisolism in anorexia as a phenomenon solely secondary to food abstinence. A primary role of enhanced CRH release, resulting in anorectic behavior—and concomitantly in neuroendocrine alteration—must also be considered (14).

Experimental weight loss in human subjects has resulted in exaggerated limbic-hypothalamic pituitary-adrenocortical activity and subsequent suppression of the gonadal axis (19). Elevated CRH resulting from stress or physical exercise, starvation, or a primary disturbance of CRH regulation also suppresses gonadal activity, impairing reproductive function (20).

According to Kurzer (21), despite the paucity of data about the relationship between food and mood in women, food intake appears to increase premenstrually, although the causes of food cravings or the usefulness of foods or nutrients to improve mood are not known. The possibility that food intake has a strong influence on mood is intriguing, but the supporting data are weak. There is some evidence that a high-carbohydrate, low-protein meal will improve mood in women who experience premenstrual syndrome (PMS), but there are few data to show that this same effect will occur in healthy women or in women with psychological disorders such as depression. Many foods, such as chocolates, contain bioactive compounds, but few studies show that consumption of these foods actually improves mood. The claims that women with PMS or depression consume carbohydrate (or chocolate) to self-medicate are based on interesting speculation, but have little scientific support. Women most likely crave these foods for their sensory properties (they taste good) and positive emotional associations, rather than for the nutrients or bioactive compounds they contain. The psychological basis for food cravings and cause-effect associations between food and mood remain to be elucidated (21).

B. Regulation of Food Intake

Hypothalamus of the brain has been identified as the site that basically evokes the sensation of hunger and satiety in animals. In the central portion of the hypothalamus (the ventromedial hypothalamus), the destruction of a small area causes animals to eat voraciously and become obese because of the destruction of the satiety center. Again, the destruction of a small center at the side of the hypothalamus (the lateral hypothalamus) results in the opposite effect: i.e., animals stop eating due to the destruction of the hunger center and become anorexic. Thus, stimulation of the satiety center causes animals to stop eating and stimulation of the feeding center causes them to eat.

The satiety and the hunger centers of the hypothalamus are connected by nerve fibers. After stimulation, the satiety center sends signals to the feeding center to inhibit feeding activity—i.e., the feeding (or hunger) center controls the feeding behavior and the satiety center regulates it.

Numerous physiological factors stimulate the satiety center to regulate the feeding center. Manay and Shadaksharaswamy (13) described the following sensory, metabolic, and hormonal influences that control food intake in humans and animals:

1. Sensory Influences

Stomach contraction results in hunger for food, but this is not the only feature of food intake regulation, as hunger contractions may continue even when the main nerve to the stomach is severed. There are stretch and chemoreceptors in the gastrointestinal system that record the distensions of the stomach and the presence of food after a meal; this information is relayed to the brain, resulting in short-term regulation of food intake.

Several other stimuli inolved in the gastrointestinal system appear to contribute to the eating sensation. Sensory stimuli coming from the taste, smell (flavor), textural appearance, and color of food are relayed to the cortex of the brain and are then transmitted to the satiety center in the hypothalamus, which in turn sends signals either to stop or continue to eat. Certain psychological factors associated with food may also influence this center.

2. Metabolic Factors

Glucose receptors in the satiety center are involved in glucose utilization by the body (see Section III above). Blood sugar level increases after food consumption and the rate of glucose utilization by the body tissues also increases. The glucose receptors are then stimulated, which cause the satiety center to send signals to stop eating. Some hours after eating, the blood glucose level falls, resulting in its low utilization rate, which causes the satiety center to stop sending signals to the hunger (feeding) center. This mechanism of metabolic regulation of food intake is known as glucostatic regulation.

Long-term food intake is regulated by the amount of fat stored in the adipose tissues (lipostatic regulation). The precise information on the fat stores is thought to be relayed from the adipose tissues to the nervous control center. When the fat stores are full, signals are given to stop eating and vice versa, until the satiety center is activated again.

The plasma concentration of amino acid patterns produced by the diet also appear to have an effect on the amount of food intake by an individual. Many brain neurotransmitters are influenced by the supply of amino acids, such as tyrosine; thus it has been suggested that feeding behavior in animals could also be regulated through amino acids (aminostatic regulation).

3. Hormonal Factors

Several hormones, such as insulin, glucagon, and epinephrine, are directly or indirectly involved in the regulation of glucose utilization by the body, as sensed by the hypothalamus glucose receptors, and are also involved in the regulation of food intake (see Section III above). A number of peptide hormones, of which cholecystokinin (CCK) is the most important, are able to inhibit food intake; other peptides (e.g., opioids) stimulate food intake. Injection of neuropeptide Y into the paraventricular nucleus (PVN) induces an increased preference for carbohydrate, whereas injection of galanine induces an increased preference for fat. Several neurotransmitters in the central nervous system (CNS) must be present for optimal functioning of normal food intake, the most important being noradrenaline, dopamine, and serotonin. Changes in serotonin metabolism were found in several disorders of feeding behavior, e.g., anorexia nervosa, bulimia, and obesity. Increased serotonergic neurotransmission is known to inhibit food intake. Evidence available indicates that the intake of major nutrients such as carbohydrates, fat, and protein is regulated separately, and these food preferences depend on the daily rhythm of food intake. Animal experiments have shown that rats prefer to eat carbohydrate during day-time and the beginning of the dark phase; later in the dark phase, protein and fat are also consumed.

It is known that nutritional inadequancy in a relative or absolute way lowers the activity of hypothalamic gonadotropin releasing-hormone (GRH) neurons that are extremely sensitive to the ambient metabolic milieu. Consequently, the pulsatile release of luteinizing hormone (LH) and follicle-stimulating hormone (FSH) by the pituitary decreases, preventing adequate ovarian follicular maturation, and estrogen and progesterone synthesis. Thus, the reproductive capacity of an animal may be aborted during times of undernutrition. The loss of normal reproductive development and established menstrual cyclicity with undernutrition is reversible with weight gain, better nutrition, or recovery from anorexia nervosa. The transient and reversible nature of the menstrual dysfunction associated with undernutrition is indirect evidence for the sensitivity of the reproductive axis to the nutritional environment. It has been suggested that these alterations in fertility and reproductive capacity associated with undernutrition are simply nature's way of birth control in times of scarcity.

Polyamines have been known to act as secondary messengers, thereby mediating the action of all known hormones and growth factors. Thus, polyamines fulfill an indispensable role in human metabolism. Bardocz (22) reviewed the role of polyamines in food and their consequences for food quality and human health. According to Bardocz (22), polyamines (putrescine, supermidine, and spermine) fulfill an array of roles in human cellular metabolism and in the synthesis of protein, RNA, and DNA. Only a proportion of polyamines are synthesized *in situ* according to needs. However, as is the case for semiessential amino acids, food is an important source of the polyamines required to support cell renewal and growth. Although the bioavailability and the mechanism(s) of the uptake of polyamines in the gastrointestinal tract remain to be established fully, it is evident that at least some proportion of the polyamines in the diet can be absorbed and utilized by the body.

REFERENCES

1. Lehninger, A.L., D.L. Nelson, and M.M. Cox, *Principles of Biochemistry*, 2nd ed., CBS Publishers and Distributors, New Delhi, 1993, p. 736.

2. Wilson, J.D., and D.W. Foster (eds.), *Williams Textbook of Endocrinology*, 8th ed., W.B. Saunders Company, Philadelphia, 1992.

3. Crapo, L. *Hormones: The Messengers of Life*, W.H. Freeman and Company, New York, 1985.

4. Harris, R.A., and D.W. Crabb, Metabolic interrelationships, *Textbook of Biochemistry with Clinical Correlations*, 3rd ed., (T.M. Devlin, ed.) John Wiley and Sons, Inc. New York, 1992, p. 576.

5. Pilkis, S.J., and T.H. Claus, Hepatic gluconeogenesis/glycolysis: regulation and structure/function relationships of substrate cycle enzymes, *Annu. Rev. Nutr. 11*: 465 (1991).

6. Roach, P.J., Control of glycogen synthase by hierarchal protein phosphorylation, *FASEB* J. *4*: 2961 (1990).

7. Kennelly, P.J., and E.G. Krebs, Consensus sequences as substrate specificity determinants for protein kinases and protein phosphatases, *J. Biol. Chem. 266*: 15555 (1981).

8. Krebs, E.G., Role of the cyclic AMP-dependent protein kinase in signal transduction, *J. Am. Med. Assoc. 262*: 1815 (1989).

9. Taylor, S.S., J.A. Buechler, and W. Yonemoto, cAMP-dependent protein kinase: framework for a diverse family of regulatory enzymes, *Annu. Rev. Biochem. 59*: 971 (1990).

10. Sutherland, E.W., Studies on the mechanisms of hormone action, *Science 177*: 401 (1972).

11. Hue, L. Gluconeogenesis and its regulation, *Diabetes Metab. Rev. 3*: 111 (1987).

12. Pilkis, S.J., M.R. El-Maghrabi, and T.H. Claus, Hormonal regulation of hepatic gluconeogenesis and glycolysis, *Annu. Rev. Biochem. 57*: 755 (1988).

13. Manay, N.S., and M. Shadaksharaswamy, *Foods: Facts and Principles*, Wiley Eastern Ltd., New Delhi, 1987.

14. Hollmann, W., and H.K. Struder, Exercise, physical activity, nutrition and the brain, *Nutr. Rev. 54* (Suppl.): 371 (1996).

15. Blundell, J.E., Serotonin and appetite, *Neuropharmacolosy 23*: 1537 (1984).

16. Cooper, S.J., and L.B. Estall, Behavioral pharmacology of food, water, and salt intake in relation to drug actions at benzodiazepine receptors, *Neurosci. Biobehav. Rev. 9*: 5 (1985).

17. Brown, B.S., T. Payne, C. Kim, et al., Chronic response of rat brain norepinephrine and serotonin levels to endurance training, *J. Appl. Physiol. 46*: 19 (1979).

18. Suemaru, S., K. Hashimoto, T. Hattori, et al., Starvation induced changes in rat brain corticotropin releasing factor (CRF) and pituitary-adrenocortical response, *Life Sci. 39*: 1161 (1986).

19. Fichter, M.M., K.M. Pirke, and F. Holsboer, Weight loss causes neuroendocrine disturbances: experimental study in healthy starving subjects, *Psychiatry Res. 17*: 61 (1986).

20. Holsboer, F., Psychiatric implications of altered limbic-hypothalamic-pituitary-adrenocortical activity, *Eur. Arch. Psychiatr. Neurol. Sci. 238*: 302 (1989).

21. Kurzer, M.S., Women, food and mood, *Nutr. Rev. 55*: 268 (1997).

22. Bardocz, S., Polyamines in food and their consequences for food quality and human health, *Trends Food Sci. Technol. 6*: 341 (1995).

21
Nutrient Evaluation and Analysis Methodology

I. INTRODUCTION

Use of computers in nutrition and dietetics has increased during the past couple of decades, several Nutrient Data Bank Directory and nutrient analysis systems having been listed in the United States and Sweden (1,2). The first Annual National Nutrient Data Bank Conference was held in the United States of America in 1976. A Nordic project group (NORFOODS) was created in 1982 for the coordination of food composition tables and of nutrient data banks, immediately followed by an international (INFOODS) and European (EUROFOODS) colllaboration groups. The activities of INFOODS (International Network of Food Data Systems) began with a planning conference (Food and Nutr. Bull., Vol. 2, 1983), aiming to improve the amount, quantity, and availability of food composition data (3). INFOODS, therefore, has set up a secretariat and established international working committees on different topics of common interest, e.g. users' needs information systems, and data quality and terminology. In addition, several regional committees working independently and together with INFOODS have been established, as are NORFOODS and EUROFOODS (2,4). Both INFOODS and the regional committees are composing food tables and nutrient database systems for user needs (5).

II. FOOD COMPOSITION DATA

Food composition data are needed for various purposes, by individuals as well as by the local, national, and international organizations who require such data for calculating food supplies. Epidemiologists use food composition data to trace the relationship between diet and disease. Also, national government agencies need nutritional information on foods and diets for planning agricultural policies, and for evaluating national food supplies as well as for assessing the nutritional status of the population, through different social surveys. Such surveys—e.g., National Health and Nutrition Examination Surveys (NHNES) and the Nationwide Food Consumption Survey (NFCS) in the United States—have provided objective data on which a government can base decisions regarding nutrition-related public policies. The food industry requires data on nutrition and dietetics to optimize recipes by replacing a specific component with another that has improved nutrient content, for nutrition labeling, and for creating new food products.

Local hospitals and other institutions need to plan their menus and special diets systematically, which includes purchasing, production, preparation, menu, and fiscal controls (6), for which food composition data are required. These data are also used in research projects of several disciplines, such as nutrition and dietetics, medicine, odontology, food science and technology, economics, home science, psychology, sociology, ethnology, and cultural anthropology.

At the individual level, diet counseling and consumer guidance require use of food composition data. A person can check the intake of special nutrients on a computer with a special nutrient analysis program (5).

III.   NUTRIENT DATABASE SYSTEMS

According to Bergstrom (5), a nutrient analysis system or a nutrient database system has the following three parts:

1.   A computer (hardware)
2.   Program(s) (software)
3.   A nutrient data bank.

Computers used in nutrition and dietetics are often categorized into three types, based on their size and capability: maxi (or main) computers, mini-computers, and micro-computers. The boundary lines between the sizes of computers, especially between mini and micro are diffusing quickly with the fast developments in computer technology, thus necessitating careful examination of all new information (7,8).

The unbiased reports and information from colleagues working with analysis systems help to select appropriate software. An entire issue of the *Journal of Nutrition Education* (No. 2, 1984) was devoted the use of computers in nutrition education; software programs with short descriptions were listed on 40 pages of this issue. The *Journal of Dietetic Software* also deals with this subject. The Consumer Nutrition Center of the U.S. Department of Agriculture has one of the best-known nutrient data banks in the world, called "The National Nutrient Data Bank" (NOB). It is a computer-based management system analyzing nutrient values in food and is designed for storage, summary and retrieval of food composition data. These data are from published scientific literature or are unpublished data from government and university laboratories, industry laboratories, and contract research.

The following three databases are employed for data evaluation and food identification coding before they are entered into the system for processing (5):

1.   Individual analysis
2.   Average values of like items
3.   Representative values.

The third database was used to revise the USDA Agriculture Handbook No. 8 (USDA 1976–1984), and different data bases are available for purchase (9–11). These databases, together with other nutrient data sources are found in the U.S. systems. However, countries with limited resources cannot use the same procedures to create food composition tables and nutrient databases as the USDA. Often the country's own comprehensive or abbreviated food composition tables are the principal nutrient data sources in the different systems, aided by nutrient data from national laboratories and information from the food industry and literature. Many databases have a recipe file and programs for calculating nutrients in various food dishes (5).

Developing computerized nutrient analysis system is expensive, laborious, and time-consuming and it requires accuracy and knowledge of nutrition, chemistry, biochemistry, physiology, medicine, food science and technology, cooking, mathematics, statistics, and computer technology. Thus, developing such a system requires teamwork involving experts from various disciplines.

Careful planning involves definition of the purpose of the system to select foods, nutrients, and programs. The nutrient analysis systems can be divided into three major types (5):

1. Comprehensive, for nearly all purposes
2. Abbreviated, for use in schools, slimming courses, etc.
3. Specialized, for research in a special field.

The comprehensive systems need information on raw foods, the products purchased in the particular country, and recipes or analyses for dishes generally consumed by the people. In the abbreviated system, only selected core foods and recipes for the most common dishes are included; in a specialized system, the foods included in the comprehensive base are supplemented with special foods.

The comprehensive nutrient analysis system may include as many nutrients as possible, although many may eventually be missing, and these gaps must be flagged. The nutrients included in the national nutrition recommendations are generally enough for an abbreviated base, using only approximations. However, for a specialized system, foods must be analyzed for special nutrients (12).

The comprehensive nutrient analysis systems include input and output programs for recalls, records, dietary histories, food frequencies, menu planning, meal patterns, consumption analyses, nutrition calculations, dietary analyses of different kinds, energy content of protein, fat, carbohydrates, and alcohol, national and special nutrition recommendations, P:S ratios, and statistical parameters. The abbreviations may include only a simple input program of food items and outputs for nutrition calculation, energy percentages, percentages of nutrition recommendations, and perhaps P:S ratios, whereas specialized system programs depend on particular topics.

Thus, while designing a nutrient analysis system, it is necessary to choose a flexible database management system and programs for easy and continuous revisions. A system should be well documented with manuals, flow charts, and so forth (5).

IV. NUTRITIONAL EVALUATION

All users of nutrient analysis systems aim to work with reliable nutrient data. Analyses of nutrients in foods are costly and for some specific nutrients extremely expensive, so nutrient data for the compilation of food composition tables are often borrowed from others, for which it is necessary to know the corresponding name of the food in a particular foreign language. Use of scientific/botanical names can be of some help in this respect and INFOODS and some other committees are currently working on thesauri of food names. In addition, information on the food standards, food additives (vitamins and minerals), the analysis methods employed, and the number of analyses carried out is also required. According to Schaefer (13), analysis of food composites has several advantages. It enables fairly precise estimations of the nutrients actually consumed, in which cooking losses have already been accounted for. It also takes into account variations of nutrient content of different foods, and provides means of estimating other nutrients that cannot be calculated from usual food composition tables, e.g., pantothenic acid, cobalamin (B_{12}), pyridoxine, fluorine, iodine, and total sodium chloride. Pearson (14) has described various biochemical methods that are used for the assessment of nutritional status and concluded that biochemical data are no better than the methods that produce them.

Food products with or without brand names and cooked dishes without the mention of ingredients are rather difficult to identify correctly with only a name. It is therefore necessary to provide lists of principal ingredients, preferably in grams, and recipes as well. The natural variations in the composition of plant foods, due to soil and climatic conditions, fertilizers, harvest times, storage and processing, also need to be accounted for. Similarly in animal foods, the breed, sex, addition of vitamins and minerals to the feeds, and seasonal variations in food composition (e.g., fish, milk) are important.

According to Southgate (15), significant variations in the nutrient content of foods result from different processing and preparation methods; especially fortification, enrichment, and foreign food standards result in great variability. An accurate description of food analyses is thus very necessary.

Methods for analyzing food nutrients are being developed in the United States and elsewhere. The state of methodology for some common nutrients is conflicting, and it is missing for some unusual nutrients. The state of knowledge of nutrition composition for different food groups has been surveyed. Stewart (16) has suggested the use of quality indices and confidence codes for foods in the compilation of food composition data.

Bergstrom (5) has compared nutrient contents in some selected foods, deriving the food values from published German, Danish, British, and American food composition tables and the Swedish and Finnish (Helsinki University) nutrient database systems (17–23). The values in these tables are assumed to include the nutrient databases of the concerned country. However, the values might not be current, because computerized systems can be easily updated, but they can very well be used for purpose of comparison. Bergstrong (5) offered the following general comments on these nutrition composition tables of various countries:

1. Dairy products in different countries are often regulated by different food standards (e.g., fat content). Low-fat milk products are also commonly fortified with vitamins. If a product is missing in a database, it is replaced by a similar food product (e.g., quark for cottage cheese). When beef meat was compared with pork, it was found that the thiamin content was higher in pork, but the iron content was higher in beef than in the pork.

2. In the calculation of food supplies, the edible portion values are important and waste must be described carefully. The energy values of foods depend on different methods of calculation. Calculation of vitamin D in fish indicated that the low and high retinol contents in American (and Swedish) tuna and shrimp are probably due to the use of old methods of analyses.

3. For fats and oils, different kinds of standards may be used for various products. Margarine is often supplemented with vitamins A and D, and some oils also might be enriched with these vitamins. Fatty acids in margarine depend on the use of oils and fats, which vary from one country to other.

4. Cereal food products are also very often enriched with vitamins and minerals such as thiamin, riboflavin, niacin, pyridoxine and iron. Information on such enrichment practices must be known before borrowing a value from another country.

5. Variation in the edible portion of core vegetables, such as cabbage, carrots, and potatoes, is important, as is the high protein quality in peas and potatoes.

6. Fruits are usually consumed for their vitamin C content. Processing of fruit products such as orange juice will seriously lower the vitamin C level. Vitamin C content in some fruits varies with variety (e.g., apples). Also, apples with skin have higher vitamin C content than the peeled ones.

7. Nuts are important contributors of protein and fat to the diet in some parts of the world. They are very rich in fat (more than 50%) and potassium and have interesting fatty acid composition.

8. Although confectionary and sweets (sugary products) constitute predominantly "empty calories," some nutrients other than carbohydrates (usually fat) are found.

9. About 10 cups (1 dl) of coffee daily for a woman will provide 50% of the RDA of niacin in England, but only about 20% in the United States of America. Also, coffee seems to provide more energy than tea.

Today, computers are increasingly being used to produce food composition tables. Although three decimal figures of food values appear to be appropriate in computer calculations, the output may perhaps be rounded off, because too many figures give a wrong impression of accuracy. The calculation of recipes is an important source of error in the nutrition evaluation studies. According to Bergstrom (5), different food yields, lack of food yields, "guesstimated" yields, and different factors used for the calculation of nutrient losses and gains make recipe-calculated food values very uncertain. It is ideal to analyze all food dishes, which is often not possible for economic reasons, and calculations are used instead. The following three methods are used at the USDA to calculate the nutrient content of a cooked dish (24):

1. Apply a retention factor to each raw ingredient for each nutrient to be determined.
2. Use nutrient data for cooked ingredients together with information about yield of cooked ingredients from raw materials.
3. Use retention factors for each nutrient for the whole dish.

The comparison of different nutrient analysis systems reveals that discrepancies can be related to the nutrient database, calculating procedures, computer programs, as well as to the user. These discrepancies are mainly due to different sources of data in the bases, particularly those entering as additional data to a standard data set. The data must be reliable, valid, and current; all missing, uncertain, or estimated values should be marked. In research, there should be enough food items in the base to avoid substitutions of foods to similar items. Also, sufficient choices of household measures and serving choices must be provided to reduce possible errors in such measurements.

Recipes' calculations have not been standardized; different food yields and loss and gain factors are used at present. Accuracy of computer programs must be checked before being used in standard procedures. The food items are often entered with codes, and an input of a wrong code or wrong weight of a food item can lead to unpredictable results. A nutritionist or dietitian has to be familiar with food values to detect such errors. Hoover (25) and Dwyer and West Suitor (26) have compared several studies of nutrient analysis systems, and methods are now available for appraisal of nutrient database system capabilities (5,27). Efforts are being made to improve the quality, quantity, and accessibility of food composition data by various international and national network systems of food composition data (INFOODS, EUROFOODS, ASIA FOODS, NORFOODS, LATIN FOODS, MEDIFOODS, and NOA FOODS).

In response to U.S. dietary guidelines and health goals, the food industry has introduced a variety of innovative food products designed to help the American public lower its fat intake. Gershoff (28) reviewed the physical characteristics and safety considerations of these products as well as their association with chronic disease prevention. The availability of a wide array of low-fat foods, some using fat substitutes, has the potential for expending the ways in which Americans, with the assistance of health care providers, can control their weight. Although they may be misused by some, their potential value to those with weight, lipid, and associated chronic disease problems should not be discounted (28).

It has been envisaged that the increasing availability of low-fat foods may soon make it easier for people to conveniently follow diets consistent with national dietary goals. It should be relatively simple to determine whether these diets on the chronic diseases of aging would be more time consuming and expensive to assess.

With the exception of the olestra studies, other-studies have rarely used foods made with fat substitutes; instead they have provided low-fat food replacements, such as skim milk or reduced the consumption of high-fat foods like butter or margarine. It has been suggested that when fat substitutes are used, there are likely to be net decreases in fat intake and net increases in carbohydrate and protein intakes, as indicated by several studies. Also, for people who are primarily interested in maintaining body weight or altering serum lipids, a large decrease in caloric intake would not be as desirable as for obese dieters. In all the reported studies, the feeding of low-fat diets has been accompanied by an immediate decrease in caloric intake, followed by caloric adaptation, which is far from complete in a number of studies.

In a crossover study of 10 obese men and women, over a 20-day low-fat diet period, Glueck et al. (29) replaced 40 g fat with 40 g of olestra for every 1200 kcal in their meals, resulting in a 30% reduction in meal time caloric intake. Total daily caloric intake dropped 23% during the low-fat study period. Lissner et al. (30) fed 24 healthy, non-smoking, 22 to 41 year-old women three diets *ad libitum* for 2 weeks. The diets contained either 15% to 20%, 30% to 35% or 40% to 45% calories from fat, and were similar except for their fat content (fat substitutes were not used). Changes in body weight were consistent with the variations in caloric intake. The individuals on the low-fat diet lost weight and those on the high-fat diet gained weight. Caloric compensation on the low-fat diet occurred but was less than 37% complete. It was concluded that unrestricted consumption of low-fat diets may be an effective approach to weight control. In the long-term study, Kendall et al. (31) obtained similar results. Although intakes on the low-fat diet increased over the experimental period, caloric compensation was only 35% at the end of 11 weeks. In contrast to these findings, other studies have shown that there is full replacement of calories when low-fat diets are fed to subjects who are able to regulate food intake fairly well (28). The results of four studies showed that fat consumption was reduced, but energy consumption was not significantly changed.

Studying the effects of low-fat diets on 29 healthy boys and girls, 2 to 5 years of age, Birch et al. (32) concluded that use of a fat substitute at 10% of energy from dietary fat did not significantly reduce 24-hour energy intake. Levitsky (33) pointed out the difficulties in accurately measuring food intake on low-fat diets in laboratories and suggested that the differences seen in energy adaptations to low-fat diets may have to do with behavioral differences in the subjects studied; e.g., lean young men may display better caloric compensation than females.

While one may argue about the extent of caloric compensation, it appears that when low-fat foods are fed, fat is not replaced. Sheppard et al. (34), supporting this hypothesis, concluded that weight loss in 200 to 300 women over a 2-year period was more strongly associated with change in percent energy from fat, rather than with change in total energy intake.

Barring olestra, there are few published reports that relate the feeding of low-fat diets using fat substitutes to serum lipid levels. Crouse and Grundy (35) also reported that olestra lowered both total and LDL cholesterol at all levels of cholesterol feeding. It was suggested that olestra might reduce the absorption of cholesterol. Jandacek et al. (36) noted that olestra feeding at a level of about 14 g/day decreased cholesterol absorption by 17%.

In controlled feeding studies, it is possible to produce acceptable American-style diets that are low in fat and will help people control their weights and serum lipids. These diets make use of both naturally low-fat foods and foods in which fat is replaced by nutritive and non-nutritive fat substitutes. The use of such diets, which are consistent with national dietary goals, has the potential of reducing many obesity-related diseases in people. Although nutrition professionals are optimistic about this, most are waiting to see what the new foods will look like and how they are presented to the public. There is a large number of low-fat and fat-free salad dressings currently available on the market, but if people do not eat fresh salads, the effect of the dressings on health, if any, will be very limited. According to the NIH (37), 33% to 40% of adult women and 20% to 24% of men are currently trying to lose weight, with an additional 28% of each group trying to maintain weight. It is estimated that the economic costs of illness associated with overweight in the United States of America was approximately 39 billion dollars in 1986 (38). It was noted that the prevalence of overweight in America has increased by 8% between surveys done in 1976–1980 and again in 1988 and 1991, alarmingly. One-third of Americans over 20 years of age were estimated to be overweight, with overweight representing 124% of the desirable weight for men and 120% for women. The desirable weight is defined as the midpoint of the range of weights for a medium frame from the 1993 Metropolitan Height and Weight tables, after appropriate adjustments for clothes (28).

Awareness of adverse effects of excessive dietary fat intake is virtually universal. Consequently, health-conscious individuals are modifying their dietary habits and eating less fat (39,40). Consumer acceptance of any product depends on taste—the most important sensory attribute. Although consumers want foods with minimal to no fat calories, they also want the foods to taste good. Because several foods formulated with fat replacers do not compare favorably with the flavor of full-fat counterparts, it is difficult for some people to maintain a reduced-fat dietary regimen. Food manufacturers continue to search for the elusive 'ideal fat replacer' that tastes and functions like conventional fat without the potential adverse health impact. Akoh (39) has briefly reviewed key characteristics and functions of fat replacers that are commercially available and a few that are under development. Akoh (39) concluded that at present there is not a single ideal fat replacer that can recreate all the functional and sensory attributes of fat. As a result, a systems approach using several ingredients individually or in combination is frequently used to achieve the characteristic of fat (41). Further development in fat replacement is needed, particularly with respect to the effect of water on food formulations containing fat replacers. Much emphasis is being placed on heat-stable fat substitutes to maintain the taste and texture of fried foods. A desirable further outcome will include successful development of fat replacers that do not interfere with nutrient or drug utilization and that are safe, inexpensive, noncaloric, and suitable for frying as well as cooking. Genetic engineering is expected to play a role in future fat replacement. There is no "magic bullet" to achieving dietary goals. A prudent approach would be combining proper nutrition and dietary variety with a healthy lifestyle, regular exercise, and a reduction of total dietary fat, aided by choosing foods formulated with fat replacers (39).

According to Akoh (42), fat substitutes contain the fatty acids found in conventional fats and oils, with all the physical and organoleptic properties of fats, but provide few or no calories in the diet. Some fat substitutes are modified triacyl glycerols with reduced digestion and absorption, others are digestible and non-digestible carbohydrate fatty acid esters and polyesters, respectively. Sucrose polyester (Olestra®), a sucrose molecule esterified with six to eight fatty acids, is the best studied of the lipid-based fat substitutes containing a carbohydrate backbone. After approval by the FDA, the sucrose polyester has found application in almost all fat-containing foods. Specialty fats or fat substitutes targeted to people with special needs are being developed. Among these are the medium-chain triacylglycerols and structured lipids (glycerol backbone) or "neutraceuticals" with reduced absorption and medical applications. Enzyme biotechnology is another tool available to lipid chemists to selectively modify, esterify, transform, trans-esterify, and inter-esterify fats and oils or synthesize new lipids such as structured lipids of food, nutritional, and medical importance. These designer fats may be the trend in the future for producing lipids that do not occur normally in nature. Akoh (42) has reviewed different types of lipid-based fat substitutes with respect to their synthesis, analysis, metabolism, potential application/uses, and the future of fat substitutes. Some potential applications/uses of nondigestible fat substitutes include replacing saturated fat in the diet, providing few to zero calories, reducing total fat intake in the diet, reducing total cholesterol (cholesterol dissolves in the sucrose polyester), reducing serum and plasma triacylglycerol levels, reducing LDL ("bad") cholesterol, maintaining ideal body weight or promoting weight loss and helping obese persons to lose weight, maintaining HDL ("good") cholesterol (sucrose polyester has little or no effect on HDL cholesterol), reduc-

Table 1   Some Potential Uses of Sucrose Fatty Acid Esters

Products	Functions
Bread	Increase loaf volume
Noodles	Prevent sticking of mixed dough
Cake	Increase cake volume, shorten whipping time
Cracker, cookies	Stabilize emulsion, prevent stickiness
Ice cream	Improve overrun by preventing excessive cohesion of fat during freezing due to stable emulsion
Whipping cream	Prevent water separation
Margarine and water-in-oil emulsion	Emulsification, prevent spattering
Shortening	Stabilize emulsion, increase water-holding capacity
Emulsion, oil-in-water	Stabilize emulsions at a wide HLB value
Processed meat	Increase water-holding capacity of sausages, prevent separation of bolognas
Fruits	Coating to maintain freshness and extend shelf life
Drugs	Stabilize fat-soluble vitamins, as lubricants, binder, and filler
Cosmetics	Softness to skin, smoothness
Detergents	Cleaning baby bottles, vegetables, and fruits
Antimicrobials	Prevent growth of microorganisms

Source: From Ref. (42).

ing CHD risk factors, and other applications such as frying, cooking, baking, salad dressing, sour cream, margarine, butter, cheese, formed meat, and so forth. Some potential uses of sucrose fatty acid esters are given in Table 1. The effects of fat substitutes on the immune system, tolerance levels/dosage, essential fatty acid availability, degradation in the soil, smoke and fire point, more physical properties, applications, stability and analysis in food matrices, and so forth, need further research. Fat substitutes are likely to offer new strategies for reducing fat content in the diet. Although there are no recommendations as yet, Akoh (42) suggested that partial replacement rather than total replacement of dietary fats and consumption in moderation should be the method of choice when approved for use in foods.

V.   NUTRIENT ANALYSIS METHODOLOGY

The methods of analyses of nutrients in foods must be precise, accurate, simple, and rapid in order to accommodate an analytical load involving large numbers of samples and replicates and to provide data suitable for accurate modeling as well as for routine quality-control applications in the food industry, for nutritional data gathering, or for regulatory purposes. Potential nutritional effects of food processing (see Chapter 13) may include enhancement or impairment of protein digestibility and amino acid bioavailability, alterations in the chemical form and bioavailability of certain minerals, reduction in the biological activity or availability of certain vitamins, and changes in compounds that affect the biological activity of some nutrients.

Gregory (43,44) described the methodology for vitamin analyses of foods. While many of the vitamins can be quantitified in fairly pure form employing direct spectrophotometric, fluorometric, or electrochemical methods, more specific procedures are required for the analyses of foods and other biological materials. Chemical methods that are suitable for food analysis ordinarily employ spectrophotometric techniques for quantitation, after the formation of specific chromophores or fluorophores, or high efficiency isolation methods such as high-performance liquid chromatography (HPLC). In addition to these methods, certain vitamins have been assayed traditionally by microbiological methods based on the specific nutritional requirements of different microorganisms. Other biologically specific assay methods for certain vitamins involve quantitation of binding to specific binding proteins (ligand binding assays), and those based on coenzymatic activity of certain vitamins having coenzyme functions (enzymatic assays), e.g., folacin, riboflavin, pantothenic acid, and pyridoxine and vitamin B_6 compounds. Animal bioassays provide a great deal of otherwise unobtainable information concerning nutritional quality of foods despite considerable length, expense, relatively low precision, and other problems associated with these methods (43).

A. Automated Vitamin Assay Methods

Several automated high-precision, rapid techniques have now been developed using either absorption and fluorescence spectrophotometric methods or high-performance liquid-chormatographic systems.

1. Spectrophotometric Methods

Traditionally several vitamins, such as ascorbic acid, niacin, thiamin, and riboflavin have been assayed by using absorption and fluorescence spectrophotometry. The chemical reactions involved in the formation of absorbing or fluorescing species in these methods impart greater sensitivity and specificity than by direct spectrophotometric examination of a food extract. Though cumbersome for large-scale multiple analyses, these procedures can be used reliably, with minimum expense (45). The documented accuracy and comparative simplicity of these methods are well suited for automation, resulting in a variety of continuous-flow type methods, widely used to determine various vitamins (46–54). Roy (55) reviewed application of automated methods to the determination of water-soluble vitamins. The automated methods have greatly enhanced the research on the nutritional effects of food processing. Continuous-flow techniques have been found to improve analysis rate, reduce technician time requirements, and improve the precision of analysis (46,47,49,56). The segmented-flow technique of continuous-flow analysis is based on the use of air bubbles to provide segmentation between adjacent portions of the mixed sample-reagent stream to minimize carryover and enhance mixing (57,58).

An alternative method for automated analysis is flow-injection analysis, which is a continuous-flow method based on narrow-bore flow manifolds and valve injection of small sample volumes to provide controlled dispersion in the absence of air segmentation (59–63). Flow injection systems yield fast sampling rates (60 to 200/hr) with baseline resolution between samples, require little stabilization time, often consume less reagent and are more versatile than segmented flow systems (59,62,63). The flow-injection techniques have been extensively used in organic and inorganic analysis as well as in enzyme assays, but their application to vitamin analysis has been limited to some preliminary reports on ascorbic acid and thiamin (62,64–66).

2. High-Performance Liquid Chromatography

Analytical chromatographic vitamin assay techniques are based mainly on high-performance liquid chromatography (HPLC). Most vitamins are poorly suited for gas chromatography, whereas HPLC provides a wide range of applications in separation and detection techniques, and also offers the potential for limited multivitamin analysis of a single food sample extract (43). Methods have been developed for the simultaneous determination of thiamin and niacin in pasta and cereals (67); niacin, riboflavin, and thiamin in rice products (68); pyridoxine, thiamin, and riboflavin in fortified cereals (69), vitamins A and E in fortified cereal products (70); and vitamins A, D, and E in animal feeds and premixes (71). The further developments of HPLC methods for multivitamin determination are limited, however, by the complexity of resolving and quantifying all biologically active forms of several vitamins, the need for multiple detectors to maximize detection sensitivity and specificity, and development of suitable techniques for sample extract purification depending on the chemical nature of the analytes (43).

Foltz et al. (72) and Yeransian et al. (73) have reviewed the application of HPLC techniques for the determination of water-soluble and fat-soluble vitamins. Several authors have reported vitamins A, D, and E and other metabolites in foods and biological materials using HPLC methods (70,74,75). These methods have also been used to determine vitamin K in milk and formula products (76); ascorbic acid (77,78), thiamin and riboflavin (79), and niacin (68). Gregory and Kirk (80) have reviewed and reported vitamin B_6 compounds using semiautomated continuous-flow and chromatographic methods. Postcolumn derivatization technique, using the principles of flow-injection analysis, have been employed in the HPLC determination of folic acid to enhance the sensitivity and specificity of analysis (81).

3. Ligand-binding Methods

Many water-soluble vitamins can be analyzed by the simple, rapid, and highly-sensitive ligand binding assays (43), based mainly on the interaction of the vitamin with either a naturally occurring binding protein or an antibody formed against a protein-analyte conjugate. The vitamin present is quantified on the basis of competition for the binding protein between the vitamin in a food extract (or standard solution) and a known quantity of a radiolabeled derivative. An innovative concept of ligand binding assays was developed to determine biotin based on a biotinyl-lysozyme conjugate and the inhibition of lysozyme activity by its complexing with avidin (82). The degree of avidin binding to free biotin in standards or sample extracts forms the basis of quantification, which influences the lysozyme conjugate activity. This technique may be applied to other vitamins for which specific binding proteins exist (e.g., riboflavin, thiamin, folacin, and vitamin B_{12}), thus eliminating the need for radiochemicals in ligand-binding assays. Viceps-Madore et al. (83) prepared monoclonal antibodies that could be used to quantify all the biologically active vitamin B_6 compounds using an enzyme-linked immunosorbent assay (ELISA) technique. According to Gregory (43), such techniques show a great promise for many water-soluble vitamins. Further research on ligand-binding methods in this regard may evolve suitable alternatives to microbiological assays.

4. Enzymatic Methods

Enzymatic assays based on the coenzymatic activity of certain vitamins, such as folacin, vitamin B_6, riboflavin, pantothenic acid, and pyridoxine compounds, have been employed in the analysis of foods. However, the use of this technique in the determination of total vitamin activity would be limited by the need to convert other vitamins to a coenzymatically active form. The sensitivity of enzymatic assay is inversely proportional to the Michaelis constant (Km) for each coenzyme. According to Haarasilta (84), an enzymatic assay for the determination of biotin, using pyruvate carboxylase, is an attractive alternative to other methods available.

REFERENCES

1. Hoover, L.W., *Nutrient Data Bank Directory*, 4th ed., Presented at the Ninth Annual National Nutrient Data Bank Conf., 1984.

2. Bergstrom, L., Review of food composition tables and nutrient data banks in Europe: Sweden. Activities of NORFOODS. The Nordic project on food composition tables and nutrient data banks, *Ann. Nutr. Metab. 29* (Supl.1):11 (1985).

3. Rand, W.M., The need for an international food system, Paper presented at ASIAFOODS Conf. Sept, 1984.

4. West, C.E., (ed.) Towards compatability of nutrient data banks in Europe, *Ann. Nutr. Metab. 29* (Suppl. 1):1 (1985).

5. Bergstrom, L., Nutrient data banks for nutrient evaluation in foods, *Nutritional Evaluation of Food Processing*, 3rd ed. (E. Karmas and R.S. Harris, eds.), Van Nostrand Reinhold Co., New York, 1988, p. 745.

6. Moore, A.N., and B.H. Tuthill (eds.), *Computer-Assisted Food Management Systems*, Univ. of Missouri, Columbia, 1971 (3rd printing, 1982).

7. Williams, C.S., and L.W. Burnet, Future applications of the micro-computer in dietetics, *Hum. Nutr. 38A* (8):99 (1984).

8. McMurray, P., and L.W. Hoover, The educational uses of computers: Hardware, software and strategies, *J. Nutr. Educ. 16*(2): 39 (1984).

9. Butrum, R.R., and S.E. Gebhardt, Nutrient data bank: Computer-based management of nutrient values in foods, *J. Am. Oil Chem. 53*: 727A (1977).

10. Rizek, R.L., B.p. Perloff, and L.P. Postai, USDA's nutrient data bank, *Food Technol* (Austr.) *33*: 112 (1981).

11. Hepburn, F.N., The USDA national nutrient data bank, *Am. J. Clin. Nutr. 35*: 1297 (1982).

12. Bruce, A., and L. Bergstrom, User requirements for data bases and applications in nutrient research, *Food Nutr. Bull. 5*: 24 (1983).

13. Schaefer, A.E., Assessment of nutritional status: Biochemical methods, *Nutrition: A Comprehensive Treatise*, Vol. III, *Nutritional Status: Assessment and Application* (G.H. Beaton and E.W. McHenry, eds.), Academic Press, New York, 1966, p. 217.

14. Pearson, W.N., Assessment of nutritional status: Biochemical methods, *Nutrition: A Comprehensive Treatise*, Vol. III, *Nutritional Status: Assessment and Application* (G.H. Beaton and E.W. McHenry, eds.), Academic Press, New York, 1966, p. 265.

15. Southgate, D.A.T., *Guide Lines for the Preparations of Food Composition*, Karger, Basel, 1974.

16. Stewart, K.K., The state of food composition data: An overview with some suggestions, *Food Nutr. Bull. 5*: 54 (1983).

17. Greenfield, H., and D.A.T. Southgate, *Guidelines to the Production, Management and Use of Food Composition Data Systems*, 4th ed., 1985 (MS).

18. Souci, S.W., W. Fachmann, and H. Kraut, *Food Composition and Nutrition Tables*, 1981/82, Wissenschaftliche Verlagsgesellschaft, Stuttgart, 1981.

19. Moller, A., Levenedsmiddltabeller, Danish National Food Agency, Soborg, 1983.

20. Paul, A.A., and D.A.T. Southgate, *McCance and Widdowson's The Composition of Foods*, HMSO, London, 1978.

21. USDA, *Agriculture Handbook No. 8*, Vol. 1–12, United States Government Printing Office, Washington, DC, U.S. Dept. of Agriculture, 1976–1984.

22. Kost, Swedish National Food Administration, Nutrient Database, 1981.

23. Food System, Department of Nutrition, University of Helsinki, Nutrient data base, 1981.

24. Marsh, A., Problems associated with recipe analysis, Paper presented at the Ninth Annual National Nutrient Data Bank Conference, 1984.

25. Hoover, L.W., Computerized nutrient data bases. 1. Comparison of nutrient analysis systems, *J. Am. Diet. Assoc. 82*: 501 (1983).

26. Dwyer, J., and C. West Suitor, Caveat emptor: Assessing needs, evaluating computer options *J. Am. Diet. Assoc. 84*: 302 (1984).

27. Hoover, L.W., and B.P. Perloff, Computerized nutrient data bases. 2. Development of model for appraisal of nutrient data base system capabilities, *J. Am. Diet. Assoc. 82*: 506 (1983).

28. Gershoff, S.N., Nutrition evaluation of dietary fat substitutes, *Nutr. Rev. 53*: 305 (1995).

29. Glueck, C.J., M.M. Hastings, and C. Allen, Sucrose polyester and convert caloric dilution, *Am. J. Clin. Nutr. 35*: 1352 (1982).

30. Lissner, L., D.A. Levitsky, B.J. Strupp, H.J. Kalkwarf, and D.A. Roe, Dietary fat and the regulation of energy intake in human subjects, *Am. J. Clin. Nutr. 46*: 886 (1987).

31. Kendall, A., D.A. Levitsky, B.J. Strupp, and L. Lissner, Weight loss on a low fat diet: consequence of the imprecision of the control of food intake in humans, *Am. J. Clin. Nutr. 53*: 1124 (1991).

32. Birch, L.L., S.L. Johnson, M.B. Jones, and J.C. Peters, Effects of a nonenergy fat substitute on children's energy and macronutrient intake, *Am. J. Clin. Nutr. 58*: 326 (1993).

33. Levitsky, D.A., Imprecise control of food intake on low-fat diets, *Nutrition in the 90s*, Vol. 2. (F.N. Kotsonis and M.A. Mackey, eds.), Marcel Dekker, New York, 1994, p. 45.

34. Sheppard, L., A.R. Kristal, and L.H. Kushi, Weight loss in women participating in a randomized trial of low-fat diets, *Am. J. Clin. Nutr. 54*: 821 (1991).

35. Crouse, J.R., and S.M. Grundy, Effects of sucrose polyester on cholesterol metabolism in men, *Metabolism 28*: 994 (1979).

36. Jandacek, R.J., M.M. Ramirez, and J.R. Crouse, Effects of partial replacement of dietary fat by olestra on dietary cholesterol absorption in man, *Metabolism 39*: 848 (1990).

37. N.I.H., Methods for voluntary weight loss and control, National Institute of Health technology assessment conference statement, March 30-April, 1, 1992, Office of Medical Applications of Research, Bethesda, MD, 1992.

38. Kuczmarski, R.J., K.M. Flegal, S.M. Campbell, and C.L. Johnson, Increasing prevalence of overweight among US adults, The National Health and Nutrition Surveys, 1960 to 1991, *JAMA 272*: 205 (1994).

39. Akoh, C.C., Fat replacers, *Food Technol. 52*: 47 (1998).

40. Miller, G.D., and S.M. Groziak, Impact of fat substitutes on fat intake, *Lipids 31* (S): 293 (1996).

41. CCC, *Fat Reducation in Foods*, Calorie Control Council, Atlanta, Ga, 1996, p. 111.

42. Akoh, C.C., Lipid-based fat substances, *Crit. Rev. Food Sci. Nutr. 35*: 404 (1995).

43. Gregory, J.F., (III), Methodology for nutrient analysis, *Nutritional Evaluation of Food Processing*, 3rd ed. (E. Karmas and R.S. Harris, eds.), Van Nostrand Reinhold Co., New York, 1988, p. 719.

44. Gregory, J.F. (III), Methods of vitamin assay for nutritional evaluation of food processing, *Food Technol. 37*: 75 (1983).

45. Thornberg, W., Devil's advocate—the AOAC manual methods, *J. Assoc. Offic. Anal. Chem., 60*: 1255 (1977).

46. Kirk, J.R., Automated method for the analysis of thiamin in milk, with application to other selected foods, *J. Assoc. Offic. Anal. Chem. 57*: 1081 (1974).

47. Kirk, J.R., Automated method for the analysis of riboflavin in milk, with application to other selected foods, *J. Assoc. Offic. Anal. Chem. 57*: 1085 (1974b).

48. Kirk, J.R., and N. Ting, Fluorometric assay for total vitamin C using continuous flow analysis, *J. Food Sci. 40*: 463 (1975).

49. Egberg, D.C., and R.H. Potter, Improved automated determination of riboflavin in food products, *J. Agric. Food Chem. 23*: 815 (1975).

50. Roy, R.B., A. Conetta, and J. Salpeter, Automated fluorometric method for the determination of total vitamin C in food products, *J. Assoc. Offic. Anal. Chem., 50*: 1244 (1976).

51. Egberg, D.C., R.H. Potter, and J.C. Heroff, Semiautomated method for the fluorometric determination of total vitamin C in food products, *J. Assoc. Offic. Anal. Chem. 60*: 126 (1977).

52. Jocobson, B.S., Hydroxylamine hydrochoride in automated and manual methods for riboflavin determination, *J. Assoc. Offic. Anal. Chem. 60*: 147 (1977).

53. Pelletier, O., and R. Madere, Automated determination of thiamin and riboflavin in various foods, *J. Assoc. Offic. Anal. Chem., 60*: 140 (1977).

54. Behrens, W.A., and R. Madere, Improved automated method for determining vitamin C in plasma and tissues, *Anal. Biochem. 92*: 510 (1979).

55. Roy, R.R., Application of the Technicon Auto Analyser II to the analysis of water-soluble vitamins in foods, *Topics in Automatic Chemical Analysis*, Vol.1 (J.K. Foreman and P.B. Stockwell, eds.), Ellis Horwood Ltd., Chichester, UK, 1979.

56. Snyder, L.R., and S.J. Vander Wal, Precision of assays based on liquid chromatography with prior solvent extraction of the sample, *Anal. Chem. 53*: 877 (1981).

57. Snyder, L.R., J. Levine, R. Stoy, and A Conetta, Automated chemical analysis: update on continuous-flow approach, *Anal. Chem. 48*: 942A (1978).

58. Snyder, L.R., Continuous-flow analysis: Present and future, *Anal. Chim. Acta. 144*: 3 (1980).

59. Ruzicka, J., and E.H. Hansen, Flow injection analysis. 1. A new concept of fast continuous flow analysis, *Anal. Chim. Acta 78*: 145 (1975).

60. Stewart, K.K., G.R. Beecher, and P.E. Hare, Rapid analysis of discrete samples: The use of non-segmented continuous flow, *Anal. Biochem. 70*: 167 (1976).

61. Betteridge, D., Flow injection analysis, *Anal. Chem. 50*: 832 A (1978).

62. Ruzicka, J., and E.H. Hansen, Flow injection analysis. 10. Theory, techniques and trends, *Anal. Chem. Acta. 99*: 37 (1978).

63. Ranger, C.B., Flow-injection analysis: Principles, techniques, applications, design. *Anal. Chem. 53*: 20A (1981).

64. Karlberg, B., and S. Thelander, Determination of readily oxidized compounds by flow injection analysis and redox potential detection, *Analyst 103*: 1154 (1978).

65. Karlberg, B., and S. Thelander, Extraction based on the flow-injection principle. 3. Fluorometric determination of vitamin B_1 by the thiochrome method, *Anal. Chim. Acta. 114*: 129 (1980).

66. Strohl, A.N., and D.J. Curran, Flow injection analysis with reticulated vitreous carbon flow-through electrodes. *Anal. Chem. 51*: 1045 (1979).

67. Kamman, J.F., T.P. Labuza, and J.J. Warthesen, Thiamin and riboflavin analysis by high performance liquid chromatography, *J. Food Sci. 45*: 1497 (1980).

68. Toma, R.B., and M.M. Tabekhia, High performance liquid chromatographic analysis of B-vitamins in rice and rice products, *J. Food Sci. 44*: 263 (1979).

69. Wehling, R.L., and D.L. Wetzel, Simultaneous determination of pyridoxine, riboflavin, and thiamin in fortified cereal products by high performance liquid chromatography, *J. Agric. Food Chem. 32*: 1326 (1984).

70. Widicus, W.A., and J.R. Kirk, High-pressure liquid chromatographic determination of vitamin A and E in cereal products, *J. Assoc. Offic. Anal. Chem. 62*: 637 (1979).

71. Cohen, H., and M. Lapointe, Methods for the extraction and cleanup of animal feed for the determination of liposoluble vitamins D, A and E by high-pressure liquid chromatography, *J. Agric. Food Chem. 26*: 1210 (1978).

72. Foltz, A.K., J.A. Yeransian, and K.G. Sloman, *Food Anal. Chem. 55*: 164 R (1983).

73. Yeransian, J.A., K.G. Sloman, and A.K. Foltz, *Food Anal. Chem., 57*: 278 R (1985).

74. McMurray, C.H., and W.J. Blanchflower, Application of a high performance liquid chromatographic fluorescence method for the rapid determination of alpha-tocopherol in the plasma of cattle and pigs and its comparison with direct fluorescence and high-performance liquid chromatography—ultraviolet detection methods, *J. Chromatography 178*: 525 (1979).

75. Howell, S.K., and Y.M. Wang, Quantitation of physiological alpha-tocopherol, metabolites and related compounds by reversed-phase high-performance liquid chromatography, *J. Chromatography 227*: 174 (1982).

76. Haroon, Y., M.J. Shearer, S. Rahim, W.G. Gunn, G. McEnergy, and P. Barkhan, The content of phylloquinone (vitamin K) in human milk, cow's milk and infant formula foods determined by high-performance liquid chromatography. *J. Nutrition 112*: 1105 (1982).

77. Vanderslice, J.T., and D.J. Higgs, High-performance liquid chromatography analysis with fluorometric detection of vitamin C in food samples, *J. Chromatogr. Sci. 22*: 485 (1984).

78. Kacem, B., M.R. Marshall, R.F. Matthews, and J.F. Gregory, Simultaneous analysis of ascorbic acid and dehydroascorbic acid by high-performance liquid chromatography with post-column derivatization and UV absorbance, *J. Agric. Food Chem. 34*: 271 (1986).

79. Fellman, J.K., W.E. Artz, P.D. Tassinari, C.L. Cole, and J. Augustin, Simultaneous determination of thiamin and riboflavin in selected foods by high-performance liquid chromatography, *J. Food Sci. 47*: 2048 (1982).

80. Gregory, J.F., and J.R. Kirk, Determination of vitamin B_6 compounds by semiautomated continuous-flow and chromatographic methods, *Methods in Vitamin B_6 Nutrition* (J.E. Leklem and R.D. Reynolds, eds.), Plenum Press, New York, 1981, p. 149.

81. Day, B.P., and J.F. Gregory, Determination of folacin derivatives in selected foods by high-performance liquid chromatography, *J. Agric. Food Chem. 29*: 374 (1981).

82. Gebauer, C.R., and G.A. Rechnitz, Ion selective electrode estimation of avidin and biotin using a lysozyme label, *Anal. Biochem. 103*: 280 (1980).

83. Viceps-Madore, D., J.A. Cidlowski, J.M. Kittler, and J.W. Thanassi, Preparation, characterization and use of monoclonal antibodies to vitamin B_6, *J. Biol. Chem. 258*: 2689 (1983).

84. Haarasilta, S., Enzymatic determination of biotin, *Anal. Biochem. 87*: 306 (1978).

22
Dietary Allowances and Goals

I. INTRODUCTION

The dietary intake of individuals or a group of population can be assessed by various methods, each having its own advantages and limitations. It is therefore important that published work giving the results of dietary assessment gives an adequate description of the technique used. Ralph (1,2) has described the methods employed for dietary assessment and the dietary reference values used in different countries.

II. DIETARY ASSESSMENT METHODS

Dietary assessment is a broad term used to indicate any method used to evaluate the dietary intake of the human subject. The past intakes are often assessed either by interviews or using a questionnaire, whereas the current intakes can be known by records at the time of eating or by direct analysis.

A. Interviews/Questionnaire

Whereas the term dietary questionnaire has no precise meaning or adequate description, it may include one or other of the following techniques (1):

1. Diet Recall

In this technique, the respondent is asked to recall the actual food and drink consumed on specific days, often in the immediate past 24 hours (24-hr recall), but sometimes for longer periods.

2. Diet History

In this technique, the respondent is questioned about the "typical" or "usual" food intake in a 1 to 2 hour interview, with an objective of constructing a typical week's eating pattern. Each meal and inter-meal period in turn, or each day of the week in turn, is discussed in detail. A fully structured interview may be employed, although open-ended questions are often asked. The diet history may be preceded by a 24-hour recall and/or supplemented with a checklist of foods usually consumed during the period.

3. Food Frequency (and Amount) Questionnaire (FFQ)

This technique presents the respondent with a list of foods, and he or she is asked how often each food item is consumed per day/week/month etc. Food lists that serve as important sources of particular nutrient may be chosen, though these will not be able to assess the total diet. The FFQ may be self-completed or done through interviews. This technique may include an assessment of the quantities of food consumed on each eating occasion or day.

4. Study-Specific Dietary Questionnaire

This technique covers all dietary assessments, using a set of predetermined questions (questionnaire) not conforming to any of the above-mentioned techniques. The method is defined by the questionnaire itself, which may be either self-completed or conducted by interview.

B.   Record Methods

Diet record is a broad term used to refer to all record techniques. A record of actual food and drink consumed by the subject on specific days, after the first contact by the investigator, is maintained for about a week's duration or so; the number of days recorded, however, may be fewer or more.

1. Food Frequency (or Menu) Record

The term menu record is used preferably to avoid confusion with FFQ (1). This is obtained by quantifying the portions of food items, which may be subsequently analysed in terms of frequency of food consumption. Alternatively, an investigator may assign "average" weights to food portions consumed. It is not possible to assess the actual quantity or weight of individual portion of the food consumed, because the quantity consumed is not indicated.

2. Estimated Record

This method aims to estimate the actual quantity of food consumed by keeping a record of the portions consumed using the usual household measures, such as cups, tablespoons, and so forth, with or without aid of diagrams or photographs.

3. Weighed Record (Weighed Inventory Technique)

A record of weights of food portions served and the plate wastes is maintained in this technique. These records are rarely fully weighed; estimated portions are often for foods eaten away from home.

4. Precise Weighed Record

In this technique, a respondent keeps a precisely weighed record of all ingredients used in the food preparation, and also of inedible waste, total cooked weight of meal items, cooked weight of individual portions of food, and plate waste.

5. Cardiff Photographic Record

The respondent photographs food on the plate before its consumption. Portions are then quantified by comparing these photographs with the reference photographs of portions of known weight, projected alongside the survey photographs (3).

6. Semi-Quantitative Method

This method is used to measure the family food intake (4), wherein the total quantity of food served to a family is weighed and quantities served to individuals are given in household measures like spoons and cups. This term has been mistakenly used by some authors for a weighed diet record wherein it is acknowledged that not all food in fact is weighed (1).

C. Direct Analysis Methods

1. Duplicate Diets

In this method, respondents keep a weighed record and also weigh out and put aside a duplicate portion of each food item consumed, for later direct analysis in the laboratory by the investigator.

2. Aliquot Sampling

In this technique, the respondents keep a weighed record of the food portions, and subsequently a combined sample of raw foods, equivalent to the mean daily amounts of foods eaten, is made by the investigator for laboratory analysis.

In certain situations, the foods used need to be described in detail because of the relevance of the method of food preparation or cooking employed or even the variety used. Ralph (1) has provided a checklist of information that should be given while writing a report or publishing work on dietary assessment (Table 1).

It is desirable to include the questionnaire as an appendix, even if it is much reduced in its size or condensed. The questionnaire describes the method and shows the questions asked and the foods and frequencies chosen. Information provided in the form "available from the authors" is unsatisfactory, because it does not permit immediate evaluation of the study, which may be even unobtainable in later years. At the least, a copy of the questionnaire should be made available for review purposes.

Ralph (1) has defined the terms relating to the quantification of food portions as follows:

1. *Qualitative (unquantified) assessment*: An assessment is made only in terms of foods eaten, often by counting the frequency of consumption.
2. *Quantitative assessment*: An assessment quantifies the portions of diet consumed to calculate the nutrient (s) intake.
   a. *Average portions*: The "average" portion weights derived from previous studies, experience, or publications are assigned (5). Terms such as small, medium, or large may be used to indicate portion size in relation to the average.
   b. *Household measures*: The food portions are described in terms of household measures, e.g., cups, spoons, and so forth, assigning standard weights to the descriptions.
3. *Photographic measures*: Respondents are shown photographs of portions of known weight and asked to relate their own portion to the pictures. (This should not be confused with the Cardiff Photographic Record.)
4. *Food models/replicas*: Respondents are shown three-dimentional models of foods and asked to relate their own portions to the models, which may be realistic replica foods, or a variety of neutral shapes and sizes.
5. *Weighed*: The human subjects weigh and keep a record of each food item consumed.

D. Use of Computers in Dietary Assessments

Computers are being used successfully in the methods of dietary assessments described above. Computer-conducted assessments differ from person-conducted assessments only in the mechanics used, i.e., the computer may substitute for the paper and pencil of a self-completion questionnaire or at most it may substitute for the interviewer in a diet history by fully structured interview.

Table 1   Checklist of Information Required for Dietary Surveys

A. Sample Characteristics	
Sample (and control) recruitment	How subjects were recruited
	Sampling framework
	Number contacted and recruited, and of completed study
	Reasons for non-completion
	Use of incentives
Sample (and control) characteristics	Age, sex, height, weight, social class
	Other demographic/clinical information
	Representativeness of the sample
	Geographic coverage
Other relevant information	Timing in relation to diseases
	Timing in relation to interventions
	Timing in relation to season
B. Method of Dietary Assessment	
1. Information Required for all Methods	
Method of dietary assessment	See definition above
Validity of the method	Rationale for choice of method
	Pre-testing of techniques on similar populations
	Validation of method with any other dietary method or external markers of intake
	Assessment of repeatability
Methods used for quantifying portions	See definitions above
	Specify:
	Sources of "average" portions
	Details of aids used to quantify portions
	Scales used for weighing
	Methods to quantify unweighed foods in a weighed record
Food composition detabase used	Specify database used
	Dealing of foods not in the database
	Any supplementary analytical work
Interviewers or field workers	Qualifications (dietitians/nutritionists)
	Training given to unqualified field workers
	Same workers have collected data and coded it for analysis?
Data collection procedures	Details of data collection (where/how), home/clinic/by interview—face-to-face or telephone/self-completed—by post or by computer
	Number of interviews/subject
	Duration of interviews
Checking procedures	Frequency of record checking with respondents, when checked
	Any checks for coding errors
	Any checks on the consistency of field workers
2. Information Required Specific to Different Methods	
a. Recall method	How many and which days recalled?
	Were all days of week included?
	If not, were results weighed?
b. Diet history	Attempted time scale (current/recent distant past/past/season/whole year)
	Open-ended questions or fully structured interview
	Structure of interview (a 24-hr recall?)
	Any cross-checks for types or frequency of foods consumed?

Table 1 Continued

c. Food frequency (and amount) questionnaires	Interviewer-administered or self-completed Rationale for choice of foods? Pre-testing of technique in a similar population? Foods covered and options for frequency.
d. Study-specific questionnaire	Interviewer-administered or self-completed? Rational for the questionnaire form Pre-testing for technique in similar populations? Inclusion of questionnaire as appendix
e. All record methods	Days of study (how many and which) Inclusion of all days of week? Quantification of home used food? Instructions and equipment given to respondent for quantification

Source: Ref. 1.

Computerized interviews may, however, be combined with nutrient analysis of food to provide "instant" information on nutrient intake. The assumptions necessary to code foods and quantify their portions are built into the computerized program. The computer also can substitute for the investigator in performing the post-interview coding tasks.

E. How are Dietary Assessment Data Compared and Used?

Cameron and Van Stavern (6) have described the methodology of food consumption studies in detail, giving the coding of foods and the conversion to nutrients, using different analyses of food tables and databases (see Chapter 21). Bingham (7,8) also provided further reviews and recommendations on methods of collecting dietary intake data and their analyses, giving an emphasis on the importance of the validity and precision of the techniques used, giving the possible sources of errors (Table 2).

The analyses of coefficient of variation (CV) within individuals, between individuals, and between the methods indicated that some of these errors are random, and there is scope to

Table 2 Source of Errors in Dietary Surveys

Source of error	Records with weights	Records with estimated weights	Daily recalls	Dietary history and questionnaires
Food tables	+	+	+	+
Coding errors	+	+	+	+
Wrong weights of food	−	+	+	+
Reporting error	−	−	+	+
Variation with time	+	+	+	−
Wrong frequency of consumption	−	−	−	+
Change in diet	±	±	−	−
Response bias	±	±	±	±
Sampling bias	+	+	+	+

+ = Error known to be present, − = Error not present
± = Error may be present
Source: Ref. 8.

improve precision by increasing the number of observations on each individual or the number of individuals in a group. A systematic bias, due either to different methods of dietary assessment or from consistent over- or underreporting by the subjects, can constitute a more serious potential source of error in the use of dietary assessment data. Independent methods for validating dietary assessments, such as the 24-hour urine nitrogen output or the double-labeled water technique (see Chapter 8), therefore, should be included in any study of a free-living individual. The accuracy of dietary assementa data can be increased by reducing both the random and bias errors.

Dietary intake data may be used along with health data in policy making. Per capita food consumptions estimated from national food balance sheets, or even from national institutions or households, do not indicate individual variation. The World Health Organization has provided a critical assessment of the use of different sources of data and their limitations (9).

III. DIETARY REFERENCE VALUES

Dietary reference values (DRVs), previously known as recommended daily amounts (or allowances) (RDAs), refer to the range of intakes based on an assessment of the distribution of requirements for each nutrient. The DRVs apply to groups of healthy people and are not appropriate for those with physiological diseases or metabolic abnormalities. Also, the DRV for one nutrient presupposes that requirements for energy and all other nutrients are met.

A. Terminology Used

Various terminology has been used in different countries, such as the United Kingdom, the United States, and Europe and by the World Health Organization.

1. United Kingdom

The Department of Health, revised the DRVs in 1991. For most nutrients, the values have been expressed as:

LRNI	Lower Reference Nutrient Intake, 2 SD below EAR
EAR	Estimated Average Requirement, which assumes normal distribution of variability
RNI	Reference Nutrient Intake, 2 SD above EAR; where only one value is given in summary tables, this value (RNI) is chosen.
Safe intakes	For some essential nutrients, sufficient data on human requirements are not available to set any DRVs. A safe intake for such nutrients was judged to be a level or range of intakes above which there is no risk of deficiency and below which there is risk of undesirable effects.
Individual minimum	
Individual maximum	Used for specifying carbohydrates (fiber) and fat needs
Population averages	

2. United States of America (National Research Council, 1989)

The National Research Council and Food and Nutrition Board of the National Academy of Sciences, revised their Recommended Daily Allowances (RDAs) in 1989. These are designed for the maintenance of good nutrition in healthy people (10).

RDA	This is the average daily intake over time; it provides for individual variations among most normal persons living in the United States under the usual environmental stresses.
Safe intakes	Estimated safe intakes and adequate daily dietary intakes are given for some vitamins and minerals for which there is less information on which to base RDAs, recommending ranges of intakes, because the toxic levels for many trace elements may not be much greater than the safe intakes (e.g., for copper); these safe levels should not be habitually exceeded.

3. Europe (European Community)

European DRVs were revised in 1992 (11,12) but the values given in DRV tables were provided prior to final publication of the report (2) and those for carbohydrate, fat, and non-starch polysaccharide population goals were obtained from James (13).

LTI	Lowest Threshould Intake
ARI	Average Requirement Intake
PRI	Population Reference Intake: Mean requirement + 2 SD. This is the value chosen for most of the DRV tables.
Acceptable range	Range of safe values given where insufficient information is available to be more specific.

4. World Health Organization (WHO)

The FAO/WHO have revised requirements for groups of nutrients from time to time (14,15) and FAO/WHO/UNU (16), with the addition of trace elements in 1992 (17).

a. Population Requirement Safe Ranges (1992)

Basal	Lower limit of safe ranges of population mean intakes
Normative	Population mean intake sufficient to meet normative requirements. This value is used in most DRV tables.
Maximum	Upper limit of safe ranges of population mean intakes

b. Recommended Intakes (1974).
Average requirement augmented by a factor that takes into account inter-individual variability. The amounts are considered sufficient for the maintenance of health in nearly all people.

B. Units of Dietary Reference Values

These vary for different nutrients:

1. Energy (kcal/day, KJ/day or MJ/day)

All energy values are based on the Schofield equations (16) and hence should be similar for each source. Variation may occur because the equations are based on weight and activity within broad age bands. The mean weight and activity level used for each age band is not the same in each source (see Chapter 8).

2. Carbohydrate and Fat

These are expressed as a percentage of total energy intake, including 5% alcohol, or as a percentage of food energy, excluding alcohol.

3. Protein (g/day or g/kg/day)

Protein requirements are all based on the FAO/WHO/UNU (16) Report, and like energy should be similar from various sources, the only difference being the average weight chosen for each age group.

4. Iron and Zinc

Requirements for Fe and Zn depend on their bioavailability in the diet, which may be low, moderate, or high (see Chapter 7). In the DRV tables, levels were chosen for medium availability from WHO values. The U.K. and U.S. values assume that Western diets have high availability of iron and zinc.

5. Most Nutrients (g/day, mg/day or μg/day)

Some nutrient interactions:

Niacin	:mg/1000 kcal or mg/MJ
Vitamin B_6	:μg/g protein
Vitamin E	:mg/g polyunsaturated fatty acids

C. Age Bands

Various national and international sources of data have used slightly different age bands in some instances, which have been adjusted to correspond as nearly as possible with the most frequently used age bands, where necessary (2).

D. World Nutrient Guides

Canada has its own version of RDAs, called Recommended Nutrient Intakes (RNIs) set by the Department of National Health and Welfare, as does the United Kingdom and other countries. The World Health Organization, together with FAO/WHO of the United Nations, publishes a counterpart to the RDAs to apply worldwide. All these nutrient recommendations are set by separate groups of scientists; and they do not always agree, so the recommended nutrient levels may differ from one country to another, although they are usually close. If they are not close, a good explanation for the difference often exists; e.g., different populations worldwide consume different amounts of protein, which can lead to varying vitamin and mineral needs. Philosophies on the role of dietary allowances vary in different countries, altering the amounts set.

The RDAs represent the nutrient needs of groups, not individuals, and they are established for specific age and gender categories. The individual's personal nutritional requirements are not known. The best general rule is that the further one strays from the RDAs for one's age and gender, the greater is the chance for experiencing a nutritional deficiency.

The Food and Nutrition Board of NRC, USA, revises the RDAs every 4 to 6 years to add new scientific information. In 1980, *Estimated Safe and Adequate Daily Dietary Intakes* (ESADDI) were listed for several nutrients that previously had no RDA, e.g. copper, biotin, and chromium. The data were not sufficient to set an RDA for these nutrients, but enough data existed to suggest a range for a reasonable intake for groups. In 1989, the tenth edition of RDAs included a category called *minimum requirements* for sodium, potassium, and chloride, rather than ESAD-DIs as in the ninth edition. Some nutrients—such as carbohydrates, fats, boron, and nickel—are still not covered by specific numerical amounts and have no set number. Meeting all nutrients stated by the Food and Nutrition Board through diet, not with supplements, should account for these other nutrients.

One practical application of the U.S. RDAs is recommended daily allowances (D stands for daily). The U.S. RDA, set in 1974 by the FDA, is used on nutrition labels on foods, which replaced minimum daily requirements (MDR). The U.S. RDA for adults basically represents a combination from the 1968 publication of the RDAs and uses the highest RDA values within specific age groups; e.g., in 1968 the RDAs for iron for adult men and for adult women and adolescents were 10 and 18 mg/day, respectively. The U.S. RDA for adults used the higher value of iron, 18 mg/day. The U.S. RDAs have included a category referred to as "children over 4 years of age through adults." Also, the highest adult and adolescent RDA for calcium in 1968 was 1200 mg/day, which is now 1000 mg/day. Four age versions of the U.S. RDAs exist: (1) children over 4 years and adults, (b) infants less than 1 year, (c) toddlers 1 to 4 years, and (d) pregnant and lactating women. Most nutrition labels that list the US RDA use the adult version, infant formulas use the infant U.S. RDA, junior baby foods use the toddler U.S. RDA, and vitamin supplements designed for pregnant women use the U.S. RDA for pregnant and lactating women.

For economic reasons, the U.S. RDAs have not been updated since 1968, but new food labeling laws are expected to lead to changes. The new name for U.S. RDA will be *Reference Daily Intakes* (RDIs); the values are based on the 1989 RDAs and represent an average value of the RDA for the nutrient over the age range to which the RDI is applied to. In addition, daily reference values (DRVs) will also be set by the FDA for certain parts of a diet having no true 1989 RDA (carbohydrate, fat, sodium, potassium, and dietary fiber). The DRVs are expected to help people to further evaluate food choices, by comparing food values of these substances to desirable (or maximum) intakes.

IV. NUTRITION EDUCATION AND DIETARY GOALS

The United States is considered to have one of the most varied, abundant, safest, and appealing food supply systems in the world, associated with a very nutritious food supply and a national awareness of the importance of nutrition (18). The health care cost in the United States has increased substantially, from 5% of gross national product (GNP) to 10% in 1982. Even allowing for inflation, the rate of increase in health care was far outstripping increases in the GNP. This situation obviously could not continue indefinitely and has formed the political background behind the recent emphasis on dietary goals (19,20). The prospect of lowering the costs of national health care by improvements in the diet can be most appealing to any country, for the simple reason that healthy people need less medical care.

A. Nutritional Education

The "dietary goals" are another way of encouraging consumer awareness of good nutrition. In the mid 1950s (1954), food was divided into 13 groups and consumers were encouraged to partake of each group to obtain a varied diet. The groups were then reduced to nine, then to seven and later to four. In 1982, five groups were recognized, which are called the "Basic Five" or sometimes the "four plus one."

1. Milk and milk products
2. Fruits and vegetables
3. Meat, poultry, fish, and eggs
4. Bread, flour, and cereals
5. Fats and sweets

The last group was added recently to conform to the reality of what people were actually eating. This placed the USDA in the peculiar position of appearing to recommend the consumption of fats, candies, soft drinks, and so on, whereas the actual recommendations are to reduce the consumption of fats and sweets. This dilemma was solved by promoting the fifth group only as a source of needed energy.

The "Basic Five" concept is a simple and effective way to promote nutritional knowledge in schools, colleges, and consumer groups. It has served very well in the past few decades, when staple foods were more recognizable. With the development in food science and technology, highly processed and even some ethnic foods have arrived in the market that are difficult to classify into basic groups; e.g., a taco has a vegetable portion (Group 2), a meat portion (Group 3), and a shell (Group 4). The "Basic Five" may be an effective teaching tool, but something more than that is needed. The nutritional labeling program (see Chapter 15) lists the nutrients, but again we eat food, not nutrients. Therefore, both approaches are needed. Nutritional labeling is only a part of the solution to the problem of consumer ignorance of nutrients in foods. For a meaningful labeling program, serving size, the nutritional makeup in terms of the percentage of the RDA for each nutrient as well as calories, proteins, carbohydrates, fats, and a system of freshness dating (date before which food must be consumed) must be included on each label. Since 1973, the U.S. Food and Drug Administration has required complete nutritional labeling if a nutrient is added to a food or a nutrient claim is made by a manufacturer. A 1990 law made the formerly voluntary full nutritional labeling necessary for all products, including meats, fruits, and vegetables and has set standards for common terms such as "low fat." Nutritionists, physicians, and dietitians are faced with the problems of acquainting people with nutritious foods available to them, supplying them with the knowledge to make good nutritional decisions, and educating them to the dangers of poor food habits. Introducing people to wholesome food is not enough; they must also come to enjoy and actually prefer nutritious food to derive its benefits in the long run.

The national governments' efforts to increase food supply, improve the nutrient content of food, and implement programs that enable consumers to judge nutrient control will succeed only when food scientists are able to judge what is an optimum diet and convey this information to consumers. In spite of understanding the problem well and the unparalled political and economic motivation, this has remained a controversial area and much remains to be done.

The goal of an optimum diet is almost the same now as it was at the dawn of civilization. People still want a diet that will enable them to live well and enjoy the good life. Frivolous claims are made in the popular press about diets curing cancer, diabetes, arthritis, heart disease, stroke, and intestinal problems, or even diets that would make one smarter, able to talk better, run faster, look better, enjoy sex, and almost anything one wishes. Some of the claims for medical benefits are serious and worth considering but most others are frauds. This is another important area where people need to be educated by the professionals.

B. Dietary Goals

The possible relationship between diet and various diseases (see Chapters 24 through 34) has also been studied professionally, as seen in a number of official reports, such as "Dietary Goals for the

United States," published in 1977 by the Select Committee on Nutrition and Human Needs, headed by Senator George McGoven (19). A number of eminent scientists were asked to give their views on "Diet, Nutrition and Health" to the Senate Committee. This 83-page report included fascinating data on historical food consumption in the United States and made a number of recommendations for optimum health, including reducing fat content of the diet from 42% to 30% of calories and increasing carbohydrates from 46% (22% sugars) to 58%, of which only 10% should be in the form of refined and processed sugars. This report created a real controversy, with ardent supporters on both sides. The Committee was disbanded in 1977, and responsibility for nutritional concerns was assigned to two government departments, the Department of Agriculture (USDA) and the Department of Health and Human Services (USDHHS), which together published another report entitled, "Nutrition and Your Health: Dietary Guidelines for Americans" (21). It was similar to the previous report but was less controversial. Its recommendations included the following advice:

1. Eat a variety of foods daily
2. Maintain ideal weight
3. Avoid too much fat, saturated fat, and cholesterol
4. Eat foods with adequate starch and fiber
5. Avoid too much sugar
6. Avoid too much sodium
7. If you drink alcohol, do so in moderation.

Another report (20) published in the same year by the U.S. Surgeon General's office, entitled "Healthy People," supported the low-fat, high-carbohydrate theme of the earlier report. In 1979, the National Cancer Institute, previously uncommitted on dietary policy, in a "Statement on Diet, Nutrition and Cancer" also supported the low-fat recommendations of the earlier reports (22).

In 1980, the National Academy of Sciences published a report entitled, "Toward Healthful Diets," which received the most public attention. It included the following recommendations (23):

1. Select a nutritionally adequate diet from the foods available, by consuming each day appropriate servings of dairy products, meats or legumes, vegetables and fruits, and cereals and breads.
2. Select as wide a variety of foods in each of the major food groups as is practicable in order to ensure a high probability of consuming adequate quantities of essential nutrients.
3. Adjust dietary energy intake and energy expenditure so as to maintain appropriate weight for height; if overweight, achieve appropriate weight reduction by decreasing total food and fat intake and by increasing physical activity.
4. If the requirement for energy is low (e.g., reducing diet), reduce consumption of foods such as alcohol, sugars, fats, and oils, which provide calories but few other essential nutrients.
5. Use salt in moderation; adequate but safe intakes are considered to range between 3 and 8 g of sodium chloride daily.

These recommendations are very general, probably because the committee members felt that there was no sufficient scientific evidence to link diet with diseases to warrant sweeping changes in the diet.

Another report published by the National Academy of Sciences in 1982, entitled "Diet, Nutrition and Cancer," was probably based on sufficient evidence to warrant the following conclusions of this report (24):

1. *Eat less fat*: Fat consumption should be decreased to 25% of the total energy. However, the committee found insufficient evidence to recommend changes in the type of fat ingested (e.g., saturated vs. polyunsaturated).
2. *Consume adequate amounts of vitamins A and C, and selenium*: Vitamin supplements are discouraged because excessive vitamin A and selenium are toxic. The best sources of these nutrients are fruits, vegetables, and whole grains.
3. *Eat less cured meat products and smoked products*: Such products are often of concern because of the possible formation of nitrosamines and complex cyclic hydrocarbons.
4. *Drink alcohol only in moderation*: Smokers, especially, were advised to restrict alcohol consumption.

Thus, the NRC recommendations are very similar to the USDA nutritional guidelines and to those of the McGoven Report.

In 1984, the American Cancer Society produced the following recommendations:

1. Avoid obesity.
2. Cut down on total fat intake.
3. Eat more high-fiber foods such as fruits, vegetables, and whole-grain cereals.
4. Include foods rich in vitamins A and C (fruits and vegetables) in the daily diet.
5. Include cruciferous vegetables such as cabbage, broccoli, brussels sprouts, kohlrabi, and cauliflower in the diet.
6. Be moderate in consumption of alcoholic beverages.
7. Be moderate in consumption of salt-cured, smoked, and nitrite-cured foods.

The common element in all these reports is a reduction in fat, an increase in fiber, and an increase in complex carbohydrates. It was understandable that the recommendation of decrease in the fat content of diet in the forms of beef, pork, eggs, chicken, and dairy products could not have been taken very kindly by the industries producing these products, but it seemed strange even to some consumers, who had been taught for generations that meat, eggs, and dairy products were highly desirable, now to be told that they were not so good after all.

The changes in eating habits needed to achieve the USDA Dietary Guidelines for Americans are given in Table 3. Betty Peterkin of USDA calculated the diets that would meet the Senate Dietary Goals, as follows:

a. 2.5 to 3 cups of cereal
b. 13 slices of bread or other equivalent baking products.
c. 2.5 cups of vegetables or fruit
d. 1.5 egg

Table 3   Means to Achieve the USDA Dietary Goals

Increase	Decrease
Fruits	Sugar
Vegetables	Red meat
Whole grains	Whole milk
Poultry	Total fat
Fish	Butterfat
Nonfat milk	Eggs
Polyunsaturated fat	Salt

Source: Ref. 18.

    e.   5 oz lean meat, poultry, or fish

    f.   1½ cups skim milk

The above diet is not exactly primed to whet the appetite. According to Clydesdale and Francis (18), it is likely that the dietary goals that were set perhaps went too far too fast and the public was not ready to accept such radical changes. A number of consumers moving toward the goals, even to a small degree, will be a welcome idea.

C. The Food Pyramid

To reflect the recent research findings on nutrition, in 1992, the USDA and Department of Health and Human Services changed the daily diet recommendations from the "Basic Five" concept or the earlier "four food groups" to a food pyramid, with foods that should be eaten more often at the base and those used less frequently at the top. The emphasis is on consuming less of the meat and meat substitutes, dairy products, and oils and fats, and more of the breads, cereals (complex carbohydrates), and fruits and vegetables. When properly followed, the food pyramid teaches the use of a wide variety of food items, moderation in total food intake, especially in the industrially developed societies of the Western countries, and proportionality among the food groups to ensure adequate nutrient intake.

D. Dietary Nutritional Goals

"Nutrition recommendations" suggest that it is advisable to consume 30% of the dietary energy as fat and 55% of energy as carbohydrate, from a variety of sources. While much emphasis has been placed on reducing fat intake, less work has been done on changing carbohydrate intake, with the results that little change in intake of this nutrient has been seen over the past 2 to 3 decades. According to Stephen (25), new evidence indicates that there may be direct advantages for health of increasing carbohydrate consumption, rather than just as a substitute energy source when fat intake is reduced. Research since 1980 has indicated that not all starch consumed is digested and absorbed in the small intestine, but that 8% to 10% may reach the colon, where it is fermented by the intestinal microflora. Fermentation of starch results in a higher proportion of the short chain fatty acid, butyric acid, than fermentation of dietary fiber. This may be of importance because butyrate is a preferred energy source for the colonic mucosal cells and has been shown to have anticancer properties *in vitro*. Benefits for health of starch consumption are emerging with new research and therefore the public must be informed and encouraged to consume a high-starch diet (25).

The fourth edition of *Nutrition and Your Health: Dietary Guidelines for Americans (1995)* recommended that consumers choose a diet with "most of the calories from grain products, vegetables, fruits, low-fat milk products, lean meats, fish, poultry and dry beans" and with "fewer calories from fats and sweets" (26). The importance of exercise has also been stressed, stating that "nearly all Americans' lifestyle is unhealthful." It is noted that most dietary calories should come from grain products, vegetables, and fruits, because they provide vitamins, minerals, complex carbohydrates (starch and dietary fiber) and other substances that are important for good health. They are also low in fat, depending on how they are prepared and what is added to them at the table.

Some dietary fat is needed for good health. Although an increasing number of consumers now eat less fat, saturated fat, and cholesterol-rich foods, there are still many people who continue to eat high-fat diets. Thus, guidelines recommend that not more than 30% of calories in the diet should come from fat, with a maximum of 10% from saturated fat, emphasizing continued importance of choosing a diet with less total fat, saturated fat, and cholesterol. Partially hydrogenated vegetable oils, such as those used in many margarines and shortenings, contain a particular form of unsaturated fat known as *trans* fatty acids that may raise blood cholesterol levels, although not as much as saturated fat does. One can keep the daily cholesterol intake at 300 mg level or lower by eating more grain products, vegetables, and fruits and by limiting intake of high-cholesterol foods. The following general recommendations have been made in the latest edition of Dietary Guidelines:

1. Eat a variety of foods.
2. Choose most foods from the grain group (6–11 servings daily), vegetable group (3–5 servings), and fruit group (2–4 servings). Eat moderate amounts of foods from the milk group (2–3 servings daily) and the meat and beans group (2–3 servings).
3. Choose different foods within each food group. Choosing a variety of foods within and across food groups improves dietary patterns because foods within the same group have different combinations of nutrients and other beneficial substances.
4. Choose sparingly foods that provide few nutrients and are high in fat and sugars.
5. Choose a diet moderate in salt and sodium.
6. Balance the food you eat with physical activity. Try to do 30 minutes or more of moderate physical activity on most—preferably all—days of the week, maintaining or improving the weight.

Limiting fat intake may help to prevent excess weight gain in children, but fat should not be restricted for children younger than two years of age. Changes to children's diets should be phased in gradually, so that by age 5, no more than 30% of calories are from fat. If one drinks alcoholic beverages, moderation in drinking has been advised—no more than one drink a day for women and two drinks a day for men (26).

A report of a Joint Expert Consultation (27) on "Fats and Oils in Human Nutrition" has provided minimum desirable intakes of fats and oils for adults, infants, and young children, giving upper limits of fat/oil intakes. The report has also given recommendations for saturated and unsaturated fatty acids and cholesterol, isomeric fatty acids, and substances associated with fats and oils, viz., antioxidants and carotenoids, and essential fatty acids (EFA).

For most adults, dietary fat should supply at least 15% of their energy intake. Women of reproductive age should consume at least 20% of their energy from fat. Infants should be fed breast milk if at all possible. The fatty acid composition of infant formulas should correspond to the amount and proportion of fatty acids contained in breast milk. During weaning and at least until 2 years of age, a child's diet should contain 30% to 40% of energy from fat, providing similar levels of EFAs as are found in breast milk.

Active individuals who are in energy balance may consume up to 35% of their total energy intake from dietary fat, if their intakes of EFAs and other nutrients are adequate and the level of saturated fatty acids does not exceed 10% of the energy consumed. Sedentary individuals should not consume more than 30% of their energy from fat, particularly if it is high in saturated fatty acids, derived primarily from animal sources.

Intakes of saturated fatty acids should provide no more than 10% of energy. Desirable intakes of linoleic acid should provide between 4% and 10% of energy. Intakes in the upper end of this range are recommended when intakes of saturated fatty acids and cholesterol are relatively high. A reasonable restriction of dietary cholesterol, to less than 300 mg/day, has been advised.

Consumers should substitute liquid oils and soft fats for hard fats to reduce both saturated fatty acids and *trans* isomers of unsaturated fatty acids (USFA). Food manufacturers should reduce the levels of *trans* isomers of fatty acids arising from hydrogenation. Governments should monitor the levels of isomeric fatty acids in the food supply; and should limit the claims concerning saturated fatty acid content of foods that contain appreciable amounts of *trans* fatty acids, and should not allow foods that are high in *trans* fatty acids to be labeled as being low in saturated fatty acids.

In countries where vitamin A deficiency is a public health problem, the use of red palm oil, wherever readily or potentially available, should be encouraged. If the oil is refined, processing techniques that preserve the carotenoid and tocopherol content of red palm oil should be utilized. Tocopherol oils in edible oils need to be adequate to stabilize the unsaturated fatty acids present. Therefore, foods high in polyunsaturates should contain at least 0.6 mg tocopherol equivalents per gram of PUFA. Higher levels may be necessary for fats that are rich in fatty acids containing more than two double bonds.

The ratio of linoleic to alpha-linolenic acid in the diet should be between 5:1 and 10:1. Individuals with a ratio in excess of 10:1 should be encouraged to consume more *n*-3–rich foods such as green leafy vegetables, legumes, fish, and other seafoods. Particular attention must be paid to promote adequate maternal intakes of EFAs throughout pregnancy and lactation, to meet the requirements of fetal and infant development.

Salalkar et al. (28) recently showed that green leafy vegetables and sprouted pulses and peanuts have significantly improved nutritional composition (Tables 4, 5, and 6) and these foods

Table 4 Composition of Some Leafy Vegetables[a]

Constituent	Broccoli (sprouting)	Brussels sprout	Cabbage	Cauliflower	Lettuce	Spinach
Water (g)	85.7	84.3	92.0	88.4	94.7	89.7
Energy (kcal)	35	43	24	34	16	25
Protein (g)	3.9	3.5	1.6	3.6	1.0	2.8
Fat (g)	1.1	1.4	0.4	0.9	0.6	0.8
Sugars (g)	2.4	3.4	3.6	2.6	1.7	1.5
Calcium (mg)	204	26	38	21	21	171
Iron (mg)	1.9	0.8	0.4	0.7	0.6	2.1
Vitamin C (mg)	—	115	48	43	6	26
Thiamin (mg)	0.04	0.15	0.11	0.17	0.12	—
Riboflavin (mg)	0.12	0.06	0.03	0.05	0.02	0.09
Niacin (mg)	0.1	0.2	0.7	—	0.6	1.2
Folates (μg)	—	137	40	15	—	150

[a]Per 100 g edible portion.
Source: Ref. 32.

Table 5 Improvement in Major Nutritional Constituents of Pulse, *Vigna radiata* (mungbean) During Sprouting

Sprouting time (days)	Protein (mg/g)	Carbohydrate (mg/g)	Free amino acids (mg/g)
Unsprouted	2.5	14.13	0.98
First	5.5	26.25	1.81
Second	6.9	33.00	2.79
Third	9.25	37.40	4.20
Fourth	12.7	46.12	5.30

Source: Ref. 28.

Table 6 Improvement in Major Nutritional Constituents of Peanut, *Arachis hypogaea* (L.), During Sprouting

Sprouting time (days)	Protein (% increase)	Carbohydrate (% increase)	Lipids (% decrease)
Unsprouted	100	100	100
First	229	187	58
Second	315	247	50
Third	410	199	38
Fourth	562	79	27

Source: Ref. 28.

Table 7 Recommended Diets for Women (Recommended by the ICMR)

Nutrients	For women doing moderate work (g/day)	For pregnant women (g/day)
Cereals	350	400
Pulses	55–70	55–70
Green leafy vegetables	125	150
Other vegetables	75	75
Roots and tubers	75	75
Fruits	30	30
Milk	100–200	200–325
Fats and oils	35–40	35–40
Sugar and Jaggery	30	40

Source: Indian Council of Medical Research as modified by Ref. 28.

Table 8 Recommended Daily Intake of Nutrients for Pregnant Women

Nutrients	Quantity
Energy (kcal)	2500
Protein (g)	38–45
Vitamin A (μg)	750
Vitamin D (μg)	10
Vitamin B_{12} (μg)	3.0
Folic acid (μg)	400
Thiamin (mg)	1.0
Riboflavin (mg)	1.5
Niacin (mg)	16.3
Ascorbic acid (mg)	30
Iron (mg)	14–30
Calcium (mg)	1.0 1.2

Source: Ref. 28.

provide most appropriate amounts of minerals, vitamins, proteins, free amino acids, and carbohydrates. The recommended diets and daily intake of nutrients by pregnant women are given in Tables 7 and 8, respectively (28).

In addition, the WHO/FAO (27) have passed the following recommendations regarding dietary information and program needs:

1. Standard methods and reference materials should be used in the analyses of the fatty acid content of foods and in the preparation of nutrient data bases.
2. Adequate composition data on fats should be made widely available and accessible, with each food item identified by unambiguous descriptive factors.
3. The standard Atwater factor of 9.0 kcal/g of fat (37.7 kJ) should be used for calculating the energy value of fat in all nutrition surveys and food composition tables.

Table 9 Summary of Examples of Recommended Nutrients Based on Energy Expressed as Daily Rates

Age	Sex	Energy (kcal)	Thiamin (mg)	Riboflavin (mg)	Niacin (NE[b])	n-3 PUFA[a] (g)	n-6 PUFA (g)
Months							
0–4	Both	600	0.3	0.3	4	0.5	3
5–12	Both	900	0.4	0.5	7	0.5	3
Years							
1	Both	1100	0.5	0.6	8	0.6	4
2–3	Both	1300	0.6	0.7	9	0.7	4
4–6	Both	1800	0.7	0.9	13	1.0	6
7–9	M	2200	0.9	1.1	16	1.2	7
	F	1900	0.8	1.0	14	1.0	6
10–12	M	2500	1.0	1.3	18	1.4	8
	F	2200	0.9	1.1	16	1.1	7
13–15	M	2800	1.1	1.4	20	1.4	9
	F	2200	0.9	1.1	16	1.2	7
16–18	M	3200	1.3	1.6	23	1.8	11
	F	2100	0.8	1.1	15	1.2	7
19–24	M	3000	1.2	1.5	22	1.6	10
	F	2100	0.8	1.1	15	1.2	7
25–49	M	2700	1.1	1.4	19	1.5	9
	F	2000	0.8	1.0	14	1.1	7
50–75	M	2300	0.9	1.3	16	1.3	8
	F	1800	0.8[c]	1.0[c]	14[c]	1.1[c]	7[c]
75+	M	2000	0.8	1.0	14	1.0	7
	F[d]	1700	0.8[c]	1.0[c]	14[c]	1.1[c]	7[c]
Pregnancy (additional)							
1st Trimester		100	0.1	0.1	0.1	0.05	0.3
2nd Trimester		300	0.1	0.3	0.2	0.16	0.9
3rd Trimester		300	0.1	0.3	0.2	0.16	0.9
Lactation (additional)		450	0.2	0.4	0.3	0.25	1.5

[a]PUFA, polyunsaturated fatty acids.
[b]Niacin equivalents.
[c]Level below which intake should not fall.
[d]Assumes moderate physical activity.
Source: Ref. 29.

Table 10 Summary Examples of Recommended Nutrient Intake Based on Age and Body Weight Expressed as Daily Rates

Age	Sex	Weight (kg)	Protein (g)	Vit. A (RE[a])	Vit. D (μg)	Vit. E (mg)	Vit. C (mg)	Folate (μg)	Vit. B$_{12}$ (μg)	Calcium (mg)	Phosphorus (mg)	Magnesium (mg)	Iron (mg)	Iodine (μg)	Zinc (mg)
Months															
0–4	Both	6.0	12[b]	400	10	3	20	50	0.3	250[c]	150	20	0.3[d]	30	2[d]
5–12	Both	9.0	12	400	10	3	20	50	0.3	400	200	32	7	40	3
Years															
1	Both	11	19	400	10	3	20	65	0.3	500	300	40	6	55	4
2–3	Both	14	22	400	5	4	20	80	0.4	550	350	50	6	65	4
4–6	Both	18	26	500	5	5	25	90	0.5	600	400	65	8	85	5
7–9	M	25	30	700	2.5	7	25	125	0.8	700	500	100	8	110	7
	F	25	30	700	2.5	6	25	125	0.8	700	500	100	8	95	7
10–12	M	34	38	800	2.5	8	25	170	1.0	900	700	130	8	125	9
	F	36	40	800	5	7	25	180	1.0	1100	800	135	8	110	9
13–15	M	50	50	900	5	9	30	150	1.5	1100	900	185	10	160	12
	F	48	42	800	5	7	30	145	1.5	1000	850	180	13	160	9
16–18	M	62	55	1000	5	10	40[a]	185	1.9	900	1000	230	10	160	12
	F	53	43	800	2.5	7	30[a]	160	1.9	700	850	200	12	160	9
25–49	M	74	61	1000	2.5	9	40[a]	220	2.0	800	1000	250	9	160	12
	F	59	44	800	2.5	6	30[a]	175	2.0	700	850	200	13	160	9
50–74	M	73	60	1000	5	7	40[a]	220	2.0	800	1000	250	9	160	12
	F	63	47	800	5	6	30[a]	190	2.0	800	850	210	8	160	9
75+	M	69	57	1000	5	6	40[a]	205	2.0	800	1000	230	9	160	12
	F	64	47	805	5	5	30[a]	190	20	800	850	210	8	160	9
Pregnancy (additional)															
1st trimester			5	100	2.5	2	0	300	1.0	500	200	15	0	25	6
2nd trimester			20	100	2.5	2	10	300	1.0	500	200	45	5	25	6
3rd trimester			24	100	2.5	2	10	300	1.0	500	200	45	10	25	6
Lactation (additional)			20	400	2.5	3	25	100	0.5	500	200	6.5	0	50	6

[a]Retinol equivalents.
[b]Protein is assumed to be from breast milk and must be adjusted for infant formula.
[c]Infant formula with high phosphorus should contain 375 mg calcium.
[d]Breast milk is assumed to be the source of the mineral.
[d]Smokers should increase vitamin C by 50%.
Source: Ref. 29.

Table 11 Intermediate or Ultimate European Nutrient Goals[a]

	Intermediate nutrient goals[b]		Ultimate nutrient goals
	General population	High cardiovascular risk group	
Body weight	BMI[c] 20–25	BMI 20–25	BMI 20–25
Total fat (% energy)	35	30	20–30
Saturated fat (% energy)	15	10	10
P:S ratio	0.5	Increase upto 1.0	Increase upto 1.0
Cholesterol (mg/4.18 MJ)	—	100	100
Sugar (% energy)	10	10	10
Complex carbohydrates[d] (% energy)	40	45	Increase (45–55)
Dietary fiber[e] (g/day)	30	30	30
Nutrient density	Increase	Increase	Increase
Salt (g/day)	7–8	5	5
Protein (% energy)	No change	No change	No change (12–13)
Alcohol	Limit	Limit	Limit
Water fluoride (mg/liter)	0.7–1.2	0.7–1.2	0.7–1.2
Iodine prophylaxis	+	+	+

[a]The goals are based mainly on what is considered to be an ideal nutritional pattern for the prevention of cardiovascular diseases.

[b]The intermediate targets are particularly applicable to northern European countries where the average nutrient intakes are far removed from those considered ideal. Those at high risk for cardiovascular disease are advised to have a diet more closely conforming to the ultimate goal.

[c]The body mass index (BMI) values are not necessarily appropriate for the developing world, where the average BMI may be 18.

[d]The figures are implications of the other recommendations.

[e]The values are based on analytical methods that measure non-starch polysaccharides and enzyme-resistant starch produced by food processing or culinary methods. All values given as % of energy refer to alcohol-free total energy intakes.
Source: Ref. 30.

4. Periodic surveys of the weight status (body mass index) of adults are desirable in all countries to help identify trends and populations affected by or at greater risk of undernutrition and diet-related noncommunicable diseases and to monitor the impact of interventions.

The summary of the recommended nutrient intakes by the Scientific Review Committee of the Ministry of National Health and Welfare, Canada, is given in Tables 9 and 10 (29).

James (30) presented a summary of the proposals for a European Nutrition Policy, (Table 11). The intermediate goals shown in these proposals are suitable for northern countries. Each country is advised to assess its current pattern of consumption and choose the intermediate or ultimate (ideal) WHO goals; countries that already have a low-fat diet should ensure that they do not follow the British pattern of agriculture and food production, which is particularly true of Easter European countries where central planning in theory means that much can be done on a central government policy-making basis. In Italy, Greece, Spain, and Portugal, current dietary changes, which seem to be moving away from the traditional Mediterranean diet, are seen as disadvantageous and need to be discouraged.

According to James (30), it is not easy to generate a new food and nutrition policy, because it promptly becomes a major social issue, immediately highlighting for each country how these changes can be made. In North America there seems to be a greater flexibility due to the power and effectiveness of consumer organizations. In Europe, however, there are fewer consumer organizations and culturally there is a tradition in which central government plays a more dominant role. Governmental policy making in the economic, agricultural, and health fields can be used very effectively to promote public awareness of health and dietary changes, as was done by Britain during World War II. The European governments should reassess a complex range of their long-standing policies. Major economic issues concerning agricultural policy are likely to provide the stimulus for governmental change. Without these pressures, most of the developments in health benefits from agriculture and the food industry are likely to come from consumer-led changes in demand (30).

Lloyd and Cronier (31) concluded that agriculture must be prepared to accept the consequences on any segment of the industry that may be negatively affected by sound dietary guidelines. It must also insist on scientific substantiation for all dietary guidelines. The agriculture and food industries together must accept the responsibility of maintaining a nutritious food supply, because the nutritional status of a population depends on the quality of the food products made available to it. The health professions and agriculture can become productive partners in ensuring optimal nutritional health for the human population.

REFERENCES

1. Ralph, A., Appendix 1. Methods for dietary assessment, *Human Nutrition and Dietetics*, 9th ed., (J.S. Garrow and W.P.T. James, eds.), Churchill Livingstone, Edinburgh, London, 1993a, p. 777.
2. Ralph, A., Appendix 2. Dietary reference values, *Human Nutrition and Dietetics*, 9th ed. (J.S. Garrow and W.P.T. James, eds.), Churchill Livingstone, Edinburgh, London, 1993b, p. 782.
3. Elwood, P.C., and G. Bird, A photographic method of diet evaluation, *Human Nutrition: Appl. Nutr. 37A*: 473 (1983).
4. Nelson, M., and P.A. Nettleton, Dietary survey methods. 1. A semi-weighed technique for measuring dietary intake within families, *J. Human Nutr. 34*: 325 (1980).
5. Crawley, H., *Food Portion Sizes*, Minstry of Agriculture, Fisheries and Food, HMSO, London, 1988.
6. Cameron, M.E., and W.A. Van Staveren, *Manual on Methodology for Food Consumption, Studies*, Oxford University Press, Oxford, 1988.
7. Bingham, S.A., The dietary assessment of individuals, methods, accuracy, new techniques and recommendations, *Nutrition Abstr. Rev.* (Ser. A) *57*: 705 (1987).
8. Bingham, S.A., Limitations of the various methods for collecting dietary intake data, *Ann. Nutr. Metabol.*, *35*:117 (1991).
9. WHO, Food and health data. Their use in nutrition policymaking, WHO Regional Publications, European Series No.34, World Health Organization, Copenhagen, 1991.
10. NRC, Commission on Life Sciences, 1989, *Recommended Dietary Allowances*, 10th ed., National Research Council, Food and Nutrition Board, National Academy Press, Washington, DC, 1989.
11. Anonymous, Report on Health and Social Subjects, 41. Dietary reference values for food energy and nutrients for the United Kingdom, Committee on Medical Aspects of Food Policy, Department of Health, HMSO, London, 1991.
12. EEC, Reference nutrient intakes for the European Community, EEC Scientific Committee for Food EC, Brussels, 1992.
13. James, W.P.T., Healthy nutrition preventing nutrition-related diseases in Europe, WHO Regional Publications, European Series No. 24, WHO, Copenhagen, 1988.
14. WHO, *Handbook on Human Nutritional Requirements*, Monograph Series No.61, World Health Organization, Geneva, 1974.

15. WHO, Diet, Nutrition and the Prevention of Chronic Diseases, Technical Report Series No.797, World Health Organization, Geneva, 1990.
16. FAO/WHO/UNU, Energy and protein requirements, Report of a Joint FAO/WHO/UNO Expert Consultation, Technical Report Series No. 724, WHO, Geneva, 1985.
17. WHO, Trace Elements in Human Nutrition, World Health Organization, Geneva, 1992.
18. Clydesdale, F.M., and F.J. Francis, *Food Nutrition and Health*, AVI Publishing Co., Westport, Conn. 1985, p. 231.
19. Anonymous, Dietary Goals for the United States, Select Committee on Nutrition and Human Needs, 2nd ed., U.S. Govt. Printing Office, Washington, DC, 1977.
20. Anonymous, Healthy People; The Surgeon General's Report on Health Promotion and Disease Prevention, DHEV (PHS) Publ. No.79-55071, Department of Health, Education and Welfare, Washington, DC, 1979a.
21. Anonymous, Nutrition and Your Health, Dietary Guidelines for Americans, U.S. Department of Agriculture and Health and Human Services, U.S. Govt. Printing Office, Washington, DC, 1979b.
22. Upton, A.C. Statement on Diet, Nutrition and Cancer, National Cancer Institute, Hearing of the Senate Committee on Nutrition, Washington, DC, 1979.
23. Anonymous, Toward Healthful Diets, Food and Nutrition Board, National Research Council, National Academy of Sciences, Washington, DC, 1980.
24. CDNC, Committee on Diet, Nutrition and Cancer, Assembly of Life Sciences, National Research Council, National Academy of Sciences, Washington, DC. 1982.
25. Stephen, A.M., Increasing complex carbohydrate in the diet: Are the benefits due to starch, fibre or decreased fat intake? *Food Res. Intl. 27*: 69 (1994).
26. Anonymous, New dietary guidelines show slight changes, *INFORM 7*: 282, (1996).
27. WHO/FAO, Fats and oils in human nutrition: Report of a Joint Expert Consultation (WHO/FAO), 1994, *Nutr. Rev. 53*: 202 (1995).
28. Salalkar, B.K., B.B. Desai, R.M. Naik, A.A. Kale, and M. Dikshit, Dietary guidelines for women's health during pregnancy, Paper presented at the Int. Conf. on '*Women and Child Health, Empowerment, Right and Development*', Rural Medical College, Loni, Maharashtra, India, Nov. 14–16, 1998, p. 114 (Abstract).
29. Anonymous, Summary of Recommended Nutrient Intakes, The Report of the Scientific Review Committee, 1990, The Ministry of National Health and Welfare, Canada, 1990.
30. James, W.P.T., Dietary guidelines and the development of a European policy, *Diet, Nutrition and Health* (K.K. Carroll, ed.), McGill-Queen's Univ. Press, London, 1989, p. 3.
31. Lloyd, L.E., and C. Cronier, Dietary guidelines: Implications for agriculture, *Diet Nutrition and Health* (K.K. Carroll, ed.), McGill-Queen's Univ. Press, London, 1989, p. 268.
32. Southgate, D.A.T., Vegetables, fruits, fungi and their products, *Human Nutrition and Dietetics* (J.S. Garrow and W.P.T. James, eds.), Churchill Livingstone, Edinburgh, London, 1993, p. 289.

23
Diet Therapy and Clinical Nutrition

I. INTRODUCTION

The role of diet in disease prevention and treatment is being recognized increasingly, although traditionally food products have been developed for taste, appearance, value, and convenience to the consumer. This has motivated the food industry and companies involved in formulating health foods into new areas of research, such as health risk, risk benefit analysis, evaluation of efficacy and toxicity, and health regulations (1). Regulations governing the nutrient content of food and health protection within legislation have often been viewed as barriers to product development and economic growth (2). According to Rowland (3), food regulations have generally been viewed negatively by many consumers, suggesting that government legislation is detrimental to the pursuit of appropriate food choices for health. The health agencies, on the other hand, insist that newly developed food products should have the well-determined active component(s) in the natural product evaluated for effectiveness in human trials. Such quality-control measures are essential for both consumers and product developers (1).

The fitness movement, through "high-teach" measures and technology, and the use of drugs in sports have affected people of all ages. Fortunately enough, "aging" has become a better accepted phenomenon and the long search for perpetual youth seems to have peaked. A healthy image and the notion of being responsible for one's own health is rather refreshing. However, food and diet are being either blamed or credited for nearly everything, which seems to be forcing unwise decisions on naive and gullible consumers. Although what one eats does affect how one feels and thus constitutes an integral part of health, food and diet are not likely to provide cure-alls for every health problem. An appropriate and prudent diet will allow people to live up to their genetic potential, helping them maintain healthy bodies, but the alleged dietary cure-alls and magic foods are not backed by scientific experimentation, thus their merits and demerits are difficult to prove.

II. ROAD TO FITNESS AND HEALTH

A. Exercise

Use of appropriate exercises and a prudent diet have often been credited with providing good health. However, it is difficult to find in the scientific literature a definitive study on the effects of exercise on health. Forbes (4) investigated the effects of exercise such as jogging, weight lifting, exercise machines, and so forth on the total amount of lean body mass in athletes and concluded that exercise and/or training did not result in a significant augmentation in lean body mass for the majority of the subjects. It was further pointed out that although athletes tend to possess a larger lean body mass than sedentary individuals, this is not proof that training accounts for the difference, because the athlete may have possessed a larger lean body mass from an early age. Training certainly decreases the weight of an individual due to the calories expended, but it is doubtful whether one can increase lean body mass over one's genetic predisposition (5).

The benefits of weight control through exercise however, are very obvious. Aerobic exercise, such as walking, swimming, jogging, and so forth, done on a routine basis (4 to 5 times a week) tends to maintain the basal metabolic rate (BMR), even while one loses weight. The BMR is a measure of the calories required to sustain life in the resting state. If BMR is maintained instead of decreased during weight loss, the amount of food does not have to be decreased continually. Women, because of their smaller size, after a certain weight loss, reach a plateau where they virtually cannot lose any more weight on a nutritious diet. In such cases, exercise becomes essential to maintain health and lose weight.

Aerobic exercise generally improves the oxygen capacity of the body and lowers the resting pulse rate. Exercise is also thought to decrease calcium loss from bone, thereby decreasing the risk of osteoporosis and bone fractures. And exercise seems to be a factor in controlling blood pressure and in maintaining HDL (the right kind of cholesterol) in the blood. However, the evidence equating exercise with increased life span is contradictory (5). Exercise is not a panacea for all health problems and it will not ensure protection against disease. In moderation, exercise does not seem to hurt anyone, and evidence indicates that it will help, provided it is not overdone.

B.   A Prudent Diet

A vegetarian diet is often correlated with health. Strictly speaking vegetarianism means a diet completely devoid of all animal products and by-products such as meat, milk, egg, cheese, poultry, fish, and yogurt. Such a diet may be dangerous: groups such as the "vegans" in Britain, who maintain such a diet, have a long history of poor health because this type of diet may be deficient in certain nutrients such as vitamin B, iron, and zinc, among others. However, most people are ovo-vegetarians (ovo=eggs), lacto-vegetarians (lacto=milk), ovo-lacto-vegetarians, fish-ovo-lacto-vegetarians, or poultry-fish-ovo-lacto-vegetarians. The addition of food groups to the vegetarian diet is likely to reduce the risk of nutrient deficiency. A shift in diet to plant foods is often recommended, but not the elimination of meat from the diet. An inclusion of 3 to 5 ounces of lean meat, fish, or poultry per day contributes to a balanced diet.

"Organic" and "natural" foods have not been defined suitably by the Federal Trade Commission, but they almost always cost more. However, fresh foods available in season, are not necessarily organic natural foods. Chemophobia (a fear of chemicals) has developed in some industrially developed countries like the United States with some basis in fact. Problems certainly exist with pollution due to the misuse and abuse of agricultural chemicals such as fertilizers, pesticides, and growth regulators, leading to the widespread belief that all processed food is bad, that any food that is manipulated by man is bad, and that the addition of any chemical to a food is harmful. Foods are in fact simply chemicals; the human body contains the same chemicals found in foods, such as sugars, starches, and other polysaccharides, fatty acids, oils and fats, amino acids, and proteins. Therefore, the addition of chemicals to foods, as long as such chemicals are safe, is at times necessary to enhance sensory and nutritional qualities of food. Unfortunately, a minority of the scientific community has sometimes proclaimed, on the basis of very poor evidence, that certain foods are bad for one's health and consumers should not eat them.

According to Feingold (6), food colorants and many other food additives may be responsible for hyperactivity in children. Despite meager scientific evidence, this idea was accepted immediately by many. Scientific studies conducted by the National Institute of Mental Health, however, failed to show a significantly high correlation between food intake and hyperkinesis (7).

At a 1982 conference on food and behavior at the Massachusetts Institute of Technology, it was reported that although folk wisdom maintains that refined sugars and carbohydrates cause children to be hyperactive, scientific studies show that the more likely effect of the consumption of sugars is to make people sleepy because of their role in the formation of serotonin, a neurotransmitter in the brain that induces sleep (8,9).

Frank Konishi of Southern Illionis University described how much of certain foods must be consumed to obtain the recommended daily allowances of selected nutrients (Table 1). The data indicated that none of these foods is a good source of the nutrients mentioned, although some people believe them to be. There is no single source, natural or otherwise, that can provide all the key nutrients needed by the human body.

Controversy exists surrounding the role of diet in either preventing or curing various human disorders, such as diabetes, obesity, diseases of blood, heart, and circulation, diseases of kidney and liver, of teeth and bones, and of the nervous system, among many others (see Chapters 24 through 34). Our recommendations for the 80% of the population without an inherited trait for high blood lipids are that the exclusion of any one food group from the diet is not only unnecessary but in fact may be harmful. However, some of the general recommendations include lowering total calories, decreasing consumption of meat to about 3 to 5 ounces of lean meat per day, eating dairy products in moderation, increasing consumption of grains, fruits, and vegetables, and using unsaturated fats and oils in foods and for cooking because meats and dairy products provide saturated fats.

Most diseases, including heart disease, have a multifactorial etiology and are influenced by several factors, such as genetics, weight, alcohol, and stress; food and diet can be a part of a program to decrease risk but can hardly ensure freedom from disease.

Unfortunately, in the realm of diet, we have few cause-and-effect relationships between food and disease. Therefore diseases such as cancers, whose exact causes are not known, cannot be entirely prevented by changing diet. However, the committee on Diet, Nutrition and Cancer (1982), has summarized in its report the evidence relating dietary patterns with incidence of cancers (see Chapter 25). The committee has further stated that there was insufficient evidence to reach conclusions on the effects of dietary fiber, cholesterol, vitamin E, chlorinated water, sugar, eggs, caffeine, coffee, or tea (10). The committee has not examined the effects of "nutritional therapy" or smoking with regards to cancer.

Thus, choosing a prudent and healthy diet is not very difficult. According to Clydesdale and Francies (5), a healthy diet is a varied diet. Checking the composition of one's diet is also not a

Table 1 Quantities of Foods That Must Be Eaten to Obtain the RDAs of Selected Nutrients

Nutrient	Food
Protein	30 slices of bread, 82 "protein pills," or 40 servings of gelatin dessert
Vitamin A	22 pounds of sunflower seeds
Vitamin B	60 raw eggs
Vitamin C	10 apples
Niacin	36 glasses of beer
Riboflavin	230 tablespoons of honey and vinegar
Thiamin	25 tablespoons of blackstrap molasses
Calcium	68 raw oysters
Iron	45 doughnuts
Iodine	6.5 quarts of seawater

Source: Ref. 5.

difficult task, and everyone should match diet to his or her nutritional needs. Clydesdale and Francies (5) have proposed general concepts for those who wish a simple method of changing their diet. The healthiest way to eat is to consume a wide variety of foods but to cut down on the total caloric intake. Therefore, in order to keep calories down or at least at the same level, one must cut down on fats or fat-rich protein foods and increase consumption of complex carbohydrate foods, such as grains, potatoes, fruits, and vegetables. The diet of the most people living in the industrially developed countries is generally slightly deficient in fiber. The ingestion of more unrefined carbohydrates in the form of whole grains, fruits, and vegetables will provide the necessary fiber, along with the required calories. Most people are also deficient in iron, vitamin A, vitamin C, and certain vitamins of the B group, even in the United States. Nutritional labeling can be used to the consumer's advantage by keying in on foods that are high in these nutrients.

The "Basic Four" food group plan can also help one to choose an adequate diet. It recommends two servings from the meat group (meat, fish, poultry, eggs, nuts, and beans), two from the milk group, four from the vegetable-fruit group, and four from the bread-cereal group. Recently a fifth group, containing fats, sweets, and alcohol, was added. This is a reasonably simple system for building a foundation for good nutrition, provided the foods are chosen wisely and the system is not misused.

Utilizing the newfound knowledge, common sense, and the Basic Four food group, Clydesdale (9) put forth the following recommendations for a healthier way of living:

1. Reduce calories to lose and then maintain a weight consistent with age, sex, body size, and shape.
2. Increase exercise up to to a moderate level.
3. Within the confines of the maintenance-calories level, choose a variety of foods, increasing consumption of grains, fruits, and vegetables, with an appropriate nutrient/calorie ratio to meet the RDA.
4. Stop smoking.
5. Reduce alcohol consumption to no more than 100 calories a day; if this is not possible, quit drinking alcohol.

Good nutrition is essential to ensure soundness of body and health. Some types of malnutrition can be alleviated by an increase in dietary fats to supply energy, essential fatty acids, and vitamin A. Conversely, many persons in the more effluent societies suffer from obesity and vascular diseases, which may be treated by decreasing the intake of dietary fats while ensuring an adequate intake of essential fatty acids (EFA). The balance between the essential and non-essential nutrients in the diet is important. Some of the signs of EFA deficiency may occur when an otherwise adequate intake is swamped by an excess of non-essential fat. Such an imbalance may affect metabolism by altering the properties of biological membranes and cellular function or by modifying the production pattern of prostaglandins. These changes in turn may affect the fine-tuning of the immune or the endocrine systems. Subtle modifications of this kind may lead, in susceptible individuals, to pathological changes that form the basis for diseases. Dietary fats and the balance between them may thus be involved both in the etiology of disease or in its nutritional management.

Similarly, ketonuria can be easily produced by nutritional imbalance aggravated by exposure to cold or hard work. Transient albuminuria can be produced by an unbalanced diet or vigorous exercise. Microscopic hematuria and cylindruria could also be produced by starvation or unbalanced diets, especially those consisting of pure carbohydrates. It has been shown that many alterations can be provoked in renal function by nutritional imbalance, caloric deficit, dehydration, physical work, and temperature extremes.

Diet therapy has been employed in the primary lipid transport disorders. Often dietary manipulations alone will allow normalization of plasma lipid levels. If use of drugs proves necessary, diet should be continued because the effects of diet and drugs are often additive and more effective than either alone. The success of dietary management of diseases depends on the rapport of the physician, dietitian, and patient. The doctor should explain the significance of the nutrient(s). The dietitian should understand the patient's disease and dietary needs and counsel him or her on its practical aspects. Frequent return visits, teaching aids, and family dietary counseling are all of benefit. The patient should be encouraged to call or write for additional information. The patient's motivation and understanding of the diet are essential in the dietary management of diseases.

C. Dietary Cure-Alls, Food Fads, and Fallacies

Most people commonly search for dietary cure-alls for disorders other than heart disease and cancer; e.g., some people take vitamin C to cure the common cold, despite recent findings that vitamin C neither cures nor prevents the onset of the common cold. There are some indications that the length of time one has a cold may perhaps be lessened due to the intake of vitamin C. Similarly, there is a completely unfounded belief that vitamin E increases sexual potency. Vitamin E also has been claimed to reduce heart disease and atherosclerosis, without much scientific backing.

Food fads and fallacies often lead people to take extraordinarily large doses of vitamins or other nutrients in order to prevent or cure certain organic disorders that by and large are not curable by the ingestion of food. Howsoever illogical these food fads may seem, they are followed by many people, mainly because it is easy to ingest food in an attempt to cure a disease. However, this type of cure-all can be extremely dangerous. Certain diseases, such as malignant tumors, are recessive—i.e., the pain or other effects may disappear for a short time, only to return again after some time. If a person with such a disease (whose symptoms may disapperar for short periods of time) eats a certain food when the symptoms go away naturally again, the belief that the food has curative powers may be reinforced. When the pain becomes intolerable after a year or so, a person may then go to a physician only to find that he has a cancer that could have been cured had he seen the doctor a year ago. Thus, use of food as a cure-all may sometimes lead to irreparable damage to health.

III. MANAGEMENT OF CLINICAL MALNUTRITION

Malnutrition is a broad generic term encompassing various clinical manifestations resulting from a lack of nutrients in general (undernutrition) or their imbalance (malnutrition). Clinical malnutrition may result from a variety of factors, including an inability to eat, malabsorption, loss of endogenous nutrients, prolonged administration of hypocaloric solutions, or inadequate use of defined nutritional mixtures (11). The imbalance between intake and requirements of nutrients leads to wasting of muscle, negative nitrogen balance, and multisystem dysfunction, ultimately promoting disease conditions such as infection, poor wound healing, and increased mortality (12,13).

About 50% of hospitalized patients appear to suffer from malnutrition, even in countries with a high standard of living, and malnutrition-related disorders have in recent years increased hospital costs to such an extent that nutritional support is thought to be cost-saving strategy (14). Nutritional support has especially become important because improvements in the treatment of disorders such as sepsis, cardiorespiratory failure, and electrolyte abnormalities have allowed patients to survive to a point where malnutrition becomes a limiting factor in their progress. Nutritional deficiency particularly occurs in patients with prolonged inability to eat (e.g., in those who have undergone surgery and radio-chemotherapy and those with gastrointestinal diseases compromising absorption of an oral diet) (15,16).

A.   Effects of Fasting/Starvation

Starvation leads to metabolic changes that are designed to decrease energy needs and loss of lean body mass. Starvation results in the reduction of insulin levels, insulin promotes the mobilization of adipose tissue fat as free fatty acids (FFA), which in turn provide energy. Hepatic glucose production continues through glycogenolysis and gluconeogenesis. Muscle proteins are catabolized to alanine, glutamine, and other amino acids, despite enhanced output of FFA in early fasting. Deaminated ketoacids (carbon-skeletons) of alanine and glutamine are utilized to produce glucose in the liver and kidney, nitrogen being excreted as urea and ammonia. Thus, muscle breakdown provides substrates for gluconeogenesis and other metabolic activities of the liver, kidneys, and intestine at the cost of a negative nitrogen balance. The latter averages around 10 g/day during the first 4 days of complete fasting, and falls to about 3 g/day when starvation extends beyond one week. Along with reduction in nitrogen loss, the metabolic rate also falls to about 30%, which decreases energy needs. Complete starvation, such as in hunger strikes, may lead to death in 40 to 60 days (17), and survival during fasting depends on conserving body proteins and supplying energy to vital body organs. These opposing needs are met during starvation by decreasing energy expenditure up to one-third and by reducing gluconeogenesis, because ketoacids needed for gluconeogenesis are now increasingly used as a brain fuel instead of glucose (see Chapter 20).

The metabolic effects of energy and protein deficits may be aggravated in patients with gastrointestinal disorders by an insufficient uptake and enhanced loss of micronutrients from the G.I. tract (fistula, drainage, and diarrhea). Wolman et al. (18) noted that zinc losses can lead to catabolic effects, and retention of nitrogen in tissues depends on the availability of zinc and several other micronutrients such as potassium, phosphorus, and magnesium (19).

Clinical malnutrition often tends to be polymorphic because it results from a variety of situations, involving combined macro- and micronutrient deficiencies.

1.   Protein Metabolism

When protein intake is reduced, the loss of nitrogen initially continues at the previous rate, and then exceeds the current intake. The discrepancy between intake and output is greatest in persons who have previously eaten a high-protein diet and is least in those already depleted or living on a low-protein diet. After a few days, however, the nitrogen excretion progressively falls, plateauing at about 2 mg/cal of metabolic rate (20). The latter is mediated partly by increasing availability of fat energy to meet the body's requirements and in part by changing the "labile nitrogen stores" of about 30 to 50 g of nitrogen (20).

In healthy humans, total body potassium (TBK) and total body nitrogen (TBN) exist in a constant proportion (21–24), and in malnourished persons the ratio of TBK/TBN increases significantly in males but is not changed in females, as compared with control subjects. Thus, the loss of different body components may change with malnutrition and may be disproportionate in males, but not in females (22,23).

Isotopic studies by Long et al. (25) of surgical patients with sepsis indicated that the observed negative nitrogen balance may be due to increased protein synthesis, with an even greater increase in protein breakdown. It has also been shown that in trauma, hormones (glucagon, glucocorticoids, and catecholamines) that oppose the action of insulin are elevated and cause increased nitrogen loss (see Chapter 33).

2. *Energy Metabolism*

The fall in the BMR due to malnutrition is proportional to the loss of lean body mass (26), although the lean body tissue in malnourished subjects has been shown to be relatively hypermetabolic (27). Spontaneously decreased physical activity is associated with altered profile of certain hormones such as catecholamines, thyroid metabolites, insulin, glucagon, glucocorticoids, and growth hormone. The respiratory quotient (the ratio of CO_2 excreted to O_2 consumed) changes significantly with the type of diet, i.e., with a mixed carbohydrate fat diet, the ratio varies between 0.85 and 0.90, reaching 1.0 if carbohydrate is the sole source of energy and decreasing to 0.70 when fat is the main source of energy. Malnourished patients have respiratory quotients of around 0.70, suggesting that the major source of their energy is fat.

The fatty acids must undergo beta-oxidation in the mitochondria to provide energy. However, fatty acids require the carrier, carnitine, to enter into mitochondria. Carnitine is present in most natural foods (meat, vegetables), but is not present in the artificial diets used for nutritional support. Patients with malnutrition and other diseases kept on total parenteral nutrition (TPN) may develop carnitine deficiency (28,29). It has been found that 1-carnitine supplementation (20 mg/kg/day) may be beneficial to some patients on TPN (11).

Starvation coupled with stress and sepsis mobilizes the energy stored in adipose tissue, but in addition, increased breakdown of muscle protein greatly enhances loss of muscle mass. Thus, malnourished patients who are also stressed run a high degree of risk for profound muscle wasting.

3. *Vitamins and Minerals*

Vitamins, trace elements, and essential fatty acids form three major groups of micronutrients. Whereas the vitamins and trace elements are essential cofactors (coenzymes) of enzymes and are vital for normal cellular activity, essential fatty acids are needed for prostaglandin synthesis. Rudman et al. (19) demonstrated that in patients receiving parenteral nutrition, nitrogen could be retained only when TPN was supplemented with K and P. Thus, positive nitrogen balance depends not only on providing calories, but also on the major intracellular electrolytes. Freeman (30) also showed that in the absence of adequate amounts of magnesium, nitrogen retention is decreased.

Among the essential trace elements (iron, copper, chromium, selenium, iodine, cobalt and zinc), zinc is an essential constituent of a number of tissues, including muscles. Zinc is lost in proportion to the nitrogen in urine during the catabolic phase of injury. Golden and Golden (31) demonstrated that there was a rapid fall in the plasma zinc levels when malnourished patients were re-fed with a zinc-free diet. In contrast, starved individuals had normal zinc levels prior to refeeding. These authors further showed that in the absence of zinc supplementation, even when high-energy formulas were fed to children with protein-calorie malnutrition, there was very little change in the body weight. Zinc supplementation, keeping all other parameters of energy and protein constant, thus appears to be associated with an increase in body weight and resumption of growth in children. Wolman et al. (18) also noted that a positive zinc balance in patients fed TPN resulted in a better nitrogen balance. During TPN, the attainment of a positive zinc balance was found to be associated with a higher insulin concentration in the plasma and reduced glucose levels. Zinc thus improves carbohydrate utilization during artificial nutritional support (11,18).

B. Nutrient Needs of Malnourished Subjects

Whereas animal refeeding is often associated with a rapid weight gain and restoration of lean and fat masses, adult human subjects who are not growing may respond differently. Both oral and enteral feeding rapidly improves muscle function and enhances intracellular potassium, with a modest gain in body nitrogen later on. Chan (32) noted that a 2-day infusion of glucose, potassium, and insulin restored muscle function in malnourished patients who were to undergo surgery. In contrast, patients receiving home parenteral nutrition, over a longer period of time, gained body nitrogen and weight, and restored both lean and fat masses. Thus, nutrient requirements must be defined in terms of the goals of feeding and its duration. Also, the excessive feeding of severely malnourished or injured patients may be associated with other complications. A modest balanced nutrient intake is therefore advised for hospital patients receiving short-term feeding, and progressive feeding with increased calories and proteins may be used over the longer term to rehabilitate patients recovering from illness.

1. Protein Requirements

In the mid 1960s, it was shown that protein and energy interact to maintain nitrogen balance, and when protein is limiting an excess of energy does not improve nitrogen retention (33). Similarly, giving protein without significant energy was also not effective in maintaining nitrogen balance. These studies were conducted in normal subjects who were replete in body protein, indicating that both nitrogen and energy are required to maintain normal body nitrogen.

The human body cell mass is fixed in relation to the person's genetic stature. Thus, in a normal human subject, there is little potential for long-term nitrogen gain through diet alone. Long-term nitrogen retention in normal subjects, however, can occur by increasing muscle mass with exercise and/or by supporting structure with nitrogen, which occurs with deposition of adipose tissue.

In the malnourished subject, the results are somewhat different. Greenberg et al (34) found that preoperative patients receiving 1 g protein/kg/day had one-half the negative nitrogen balance of those receiving only 5% dextrose providing 550 kcal/24 hr, without protein. Examination of the substrate-hormone profiles revealed that the patients receiving 5% dextrose had high levels of lactate, pyruvate, and insulin, whereas the groups receiving fat or no additional non-protein energy substrate had high levels of FFA and ketones with lower levels of insulin. Despite the different hormone profiles, the nitrogen balance was determined not by the substrate-hormone profile but the presence or the absence of nitrogen. Thus, the primary effect of nitrogen was nitrogen-sparing irrespective of the substrate-hormone profile. These results were confirmed in a crossover design wherein these patients received either 1 or 2 g protein/kg/day, and it was found that providing higher amounts of amino acid (AA) resulted in a net positive balance in contrast to the negative balance with lower intake (35). Thus, in postoperative malnourished patients, it was possible to maintain nitrogen balance or even induce a slightly positive nitrogen balance without providing added nonprotein calories. This finding is in complete contrast to that obtained in replete subjects. Hill et al. (36) also similarly showed that giving AA without calories maintained total body nitrogen, in sharp contrast to unfed controls who lost their body nitrogen during the same period. It has been shown that the nitrogen required for balance in stable adults is only 0.8 g/kg/day (37), although nitrogen retention increased with increasing intake and the gain was linear over a range of 0.25 to 2 g/kg/day. An AA load of 1.0 to 1.5 g/kg/day of a balanced AA mixture appears to be ideal (11).

There are eight essential amino acids (AA), among 20 to 21 AA found in the protein of human tissue. Two nonessential AA, arginine and histidine, may become essential under certain circumstances, such as in childhood or in patients with renal failure. Three branched-chain AA (BCAA) (leucine, isoleucine, valine) have distinct biochemical properties. Rose (38) noted that AA mixtures have to be given in certain proportions and in specified minimal amounts. The AA mixtures with correct proportions have since then been referred to as "balanced." Thus, the quantity of protein required to maintain nitrogen balance depends on the quality of protein given, as determined by its AA profile. If an AA mixture is deficient in an essential AA or if there is an imbalance in the essential AA, nitrogen balance cannot be achieved in patients receiving parenteral nutrition (39). Even the AA solutions containing only the essential AA are not as well utilized as the balanced AA mixtures of both essential and non-essential AA (37). Leucine and its transaminated analogue, alpha-keto-isocaproic acid, appear to enhance protein synthesis and inhibit proteolysis (40,41).

Attempts have been made to optimize AA solutions for patients in acute renal failure in order to minimize azotemia and avoid dialysis. A mixture containing only essential AA was found to improve survival in patients with acute renal failure as compared with the control patients receiving glucose, without reducing the need for dialysis (42,43). Feinstein (44), however, observed no difference between a balanced AA mixture and that containing only essential AA.

In patients with hepatic failure, a perturbed plasma AA profile and disturbances of water and electroyte balance are observed. In chronic hepatic encephalopathy, low levels of BCAA appear to be associated with elevated aromatic AA and tryptophan levels, which has led to the use of BCAA-enriched mixtures in such patients. Use of BCAA, however, has not consistently shown clinical improvement over the standard acid solutions (11,45).

2. Energy Requirements

The basal energy expenditure (BEE) of a fasting person depends on weight, height, age, and sex. Harris Benedict (46) employed the following equation to predict BEE:

Men (kcal/24h) = $66 + (13.7 \times W) + (5 \times H) - 6.8 \times A$

Women (kcal/24h) = $655 + (9.6 \times W) + 1.9 \times H) - 4.7 \times A$

where W = weight in kg, H = height in cm, and A = age in years (see Chapter 8 for more recent WHO equations).

The resting energy expenditure (REE) of a bedridden patient can be approximated by adding the specific dynamic activity of food (diet-induced thermogenesis) to the BEE. Kinney (47) suggested that the REE can be approximated by increasing the BEE by 10%. Malnutrition may decrease BEE by about 35% and physical activity, injury, and sepsis (especially burns) are thought to increase energy expenditure by about 30%, 60%, and 100%, respectively. This concept of hypermetabolism has now been disproved (48–50). According to Pichard and Jeejeebhoy (11), an increase of even 60% in the BEE (about 20–25 kcal/kg/day) works out to be a requirement of only 40 kcal/kg/day or 2800 kcal/day for a 70 kg person. Thus, there is no evidence for feeding 4000 to 6000 kcal to critically sick patients, as was recommended earlier.

Indirect calorimeters are currently used to customize nutritional support to the patients' needs. Using the Harris-Benedict equation and increasing it at most by 30% has been found to meet the needs of most patients, barring research studies where precise measurements are required. Energy requirements calculated on the body weight basis, though less accurate, will be adequate for most clinical situations, except in cases of obesity or cachexia. Basal energy requirements are thought to be about 20 kcal/kg/day and ambulatory or stressed patients require about 25 to 30 kcal/kg/day, which may be increased to a maximum of 35 kcal/kg/day (11).

Malnourished patients receiving either glucose-based or lipid-based TPN have shown equivalent nitrogen retention (50,51). Using a balanced glucose-lipid TPN can prevent the complications associated with the administration of substantial amounts of glucose—e.g., hepatic steatosis, CO_2 retention, essential fatty acid deficiency, hypo- or hyperglycemia, and the need to add insulin to the TPN regimen.

3. Vitamins and Minerals

Vitamins, trace elements, and essential fatty acids are required for the proper utilization of protein, carbohydrate, fat, and electrolytes. The actions and deficiencies of some vitamins given with enteral and parenteral nutrition are given in Table 2. Precise vitamin requirements during nutritional support in malnourished patients are not known. Although water-soluble vitamins may be given liberally without apparent toxicity, fat-soluble vitamins, especially A and D, can become toxic in higher quantities. Shike et al. (52) showed that prolonged parenteral administration of vitamin D enhanced metabolic bone disease, which was associated with hypercalcemic pancreatitis. Home TPN patients are therefore not given vitamin D and are instead exposed to sunlight. Patients with gastrointestinal disorders resulting in specific malabsorption or a loss of vitamins for a prolonged period of time are given special prescriptions for vitamins only after a clinical examination made to detect vitamin deficiencies. Table 3 shows general recommendations for parenteral and enteral intakes of vitamins.

Table 2 Roles and Clinical Deficiency Symptoms of Selected Vitamins

Vitamin	Roles	Symptoms
B_1 (thiamin)	Coenzyme involved in the removal of CO_2 (alpha-keto acids and glucose metabolism)	Beriberi, hypoglycemia, blood acidosis
B_2 (riboflavin)	Constituent of flavin nucleotide coenzymes involved in energy metabolism	Photophobia, glossitis, cheilosis, skin pruritus
B_6 (pyridoxine)	Coenzyme involved in amino acid metabolism	Dermatitis, intertrigo, seborrhea, irritability, somnolence, neuropathy
B_{12} (cyanocobalamin)	Nucleic acid and amino acid metabolism	Megaloblastic anemia, glossitis, diarrhea, neuromyelopathy
C (ascorbic acid)	Maintenance of intercellular matrix of cartilage, bone and dentine; collagen synthesis, antioxidant	Scurvy
Biotin	Coenzyme related to fat synthesis, amino acid metabolism and glycogen formation	Fatigue, depression dermatitis, and myalgia
Choline	Constituent of phospholipids, precursor of neurotransmitter acetylcholine	Not reported
Niacin	Constituent of NAD and NADP coenzymes involved in oxidation-reduction reactions	Pellagra
Pantothenic acid	Component of coenzyme A involved in energy metabolism	Asthenia, paresthesia, mental disorders, epigastric discomfort
A	Constituent of retinal pigment, maintenance of epithelium, Infection defense	Xerophthalmia, night blindness, infection
D	Calcium absorption and depletion in bone	Osteomalacia, rickets
E (and selenium)	Antioxidant preventing cell membrane lesions	Myalgia, cardiomyopathy
K	Blood clotting	Blood dyscrasia

Source: Ref. 11.

Table 3 Standard Vitamin Recommendations in
Parenteral and Enteral Nutrition

Vitamin	Recommended dose
Water-Soluble	
B₁ (thiamin)	5 mg/day
B₂ (riboflavin)	5 mg/day
Pantothenic acid	15 mg/day
Niacin	5 mg/day
B₆ [pyridoxine]	50 mg/day
Folic acid	0.6 mg/day
C [ascorbic acid]	300 mg/day
B₁₂ [cyanocobalamin]	12 µg/day
Fat-Soluble	
A	Home TPN: 2500 IU/day
D	Home TPN: none added
	Hospital TPN: 400 IU/day
E	50 IU/day[a]
K	10 mh/week

[a]Fat emulsions contain vitamin E in different amounts [i.e., 35 IU in
1 liter of Nutralipid[R].]
Source: Ref. 11.

Malnutrition is often associated with major changes in electrolyte balance. The importance of fluid and electrolytes for promoting tissue perfusion and ionic equilibrium has been recognized. Malnutrition leads to loss of the intracellular magnesium, potassium, and phosphorus ions, along with a gain of sodium and water. A positive balance of sodium and water may be seen during refeeding with carbohydrate (53): this process, referred to as "refeeding edema," usually disappears with improvement in the mineral status. Refeeding of malnourished patients, especially elderly subjects and those with cardiopulmonary disease or renal insufficiency, must be undertaken very carefully because of the risk of pulmonary edema. The standard electrolyte recommendations for parenteral and enteral nutrition are as follows (11):

Sodium	100–120 mmol/day
Potassium	80–120 mmol/day
Calcium	8–10 mmol/day
Phosphorus	14–16 mmol/day
Magnesium	12–15 mmol/day

These recommendations have to be altered to meet special needs such as in cardiac, renal, or hepatic dysfunction.

Iron and zinc deficiencies are very common and may develop more rapidly than for other elements such as copper, chromium, selenium, iodine, and cobalt (as vitamin B₁₂). Clinical situations with increased requirements are common (e.g., iron in chronic bleeding, zinc in diarrhea, gastrointestinal fistula, surgical drainage, and hypermetabolism) and the normal requirements are higher than for other trace elements. The general recommendations for parenteral intakes of trace elements are given in Table 4.

Table 4 Standard Trace Element Recommendations in Parenteral and Enteral Nutrition

Element	Recommended dose
Iron	
Men	1 mg/day
Women	Premenopausal: 2 mg/day
	Postmenopausal: 1 mg/day
Zinc	2.2 mg/day + 12.2 mg/1 small bowel fluid loss + 17.1 mg/1 stool loss
Copper	300 μg/day
	None with severe liver disease
Chromium	20 g/day
Selenium	120 g/day
Iodine	120 g/day
Molybdenum	20 g/day
Manganese	700 g/day
	None with severe liver disease

Source: Ref. 11.

The main essential fatty acid is linoleic acid, which is a precursor of arachidonic acid, needed for prostaglandin synthesis. Patients given fat-free TPN have been shown to develop biochemical evidence of essential fatty acid deficiency within 2 weeks (54), without any change in linoleic acid stores (12% of total fatty acids). Suppressed lipolysis resulting from the high insulin level secondary to the glucose infusion rapidly develops linoleic acid deficiency (55), clinical deficiency of which can be avoided by giving 2% to 4% of total calories as linoleic acid.

According to Pichard and Jeejeebhoy (11), the rational use of nutritional support depends on the identification of malnutrition or its potential, definition of the risks involved, and demonstration of the reversal of such risks by nutritional support. The history of the patient's food intake, the present nutritional state, and the patient's ability to metabolize nutrients are important considerations. Clinical nutrition may consist of a range of approaches that need to be integrated, proceeding from a normal oral diet to parenteral nutrition and vice versa. Normal or modified oral diet may be used whenever possible, monitoring the nutrient intake and tolerance. Enteral feeding should be started if oral intake is consistently poor, and TPN should be given if there is intolerance to enteral feeding or if the gut is not functional.

C. Assessment of Malnutrition

Early malnutrition and its nutritional status are difficult to define clinically, especially with a view to initiate nutritional support before complications begin. Earlier methods to assess the nutritional status depend on objective anthropometric measurements (age, sex, weight, height, skin-fold thickness, arm muscle circumference) and laboratory tests such as body composition (creatinine-height index, 3-methylhistidine excretion, total body nitrogen and potassium, total body water); hepatic secretory proteins levels (albumin, prealbumin, transferrin, retinol-binding protein, thyroxine-binding protein); immunological tests (delayed cutaneous hypersensitivity); combination of above (as in the prognostic nutritional index), and physiological methods (muscle function, dynamometry). Most of these techniques, however, lack specificity in relation to their ability to predict a clinically significant adverse effect, which may lead to an erroneous conclusion, because all these measurements provide information about the body's composition, rather than outcome (clinically significant event).

Table 5   Methodology for Subjective Global Assessment (SGA)

History
  Weight change
    Overall loss in past 6 months in Kg and in % loss change in past 2 weeks in kg
  Dietary intake change
    Duration in weeks, gradation from nerve to starvation.
  Gastrointestinal symptoms that have persisted for more than 2 weeks
    none
    nausea
    vomiting
    diarrhea
    anorexia.
  Functional capacity
    Optimal
    duration and dysfunction
    type (working, ambulatory, bedridden)
  Disease and its relation to nutritional requirements, primary diagnosis, metabolic
  demand (none to high stress)

Physical examination
  Loss of subcutaneous fat
  Muscle wasting
  Ankle edema
  Sacral edema
  Ascites

SGA rating
  Well nourished
  Mildly malnourished
  Severely malnourished

Source: Ref. 11.

A more practical method of assessing the risks of malnutrition is to evaluate the patient at the bedside—subjective global assessment (SGA). The SGA methodology is described in Table 5. This technique has been found to be reproducible and can predict adverse clinical events (56). The subjective global assessment is a composite evaluation of the ability to eat, disease stress, functional impairment, and clinical wasting. The SGA can be conducted anywhere, because it requires only the clinical judgment of the examiner. Good clinical judgment is the best available method to assess nutritional status in the normal hospital setting.

D.   Needs for Enteral and Parenteral Nutrition

When a patient is not able to meet his or her nutritional requirements by eating a normal diet, he or she is a candidate for enteral nutrition (EN). The clinician and the nutritionist should together set a target for the patient's nutrients. After a short trial period, if nutrient intake is found insufficient, nutritional support should be provided. In the following situations, oral intake is often insufficient, even in the presence of a usable G.I. tract, necessitating use of nasogastric or nasointestinal tube feeding:

1.   Severe systemic illness
2.   Neurologic impairment preventing oral feeding

3. Increased requirements with relative anorexia (e.g., burn cases)
4. Chronic obstructive lung disease with severe dyspnea or pharyngeal surgery.

Enteral feeding often may be necessary in diseases of the esophagus, stomach, and pancreas; short bowel with more than 60 cm of small intestine available; inflammatory bowel disease; chronic partial bowel obstruction; and postoperative reduced bowel motility. The success of enteral feeding depends on delivering diets carefully with the aid of a pump to avoid a surge of nutrient, consequent bowel distension, and interruption of feeding (57). Some patients will show intolerance and complications, and when EN fails or cannot be used then TPN must be used.

Total parenteral nutrition (TPN) is an expensive nutritional support. Though controversial because of conflicting conclusions regarding the patient's outcome (58), it has positively influenced rehabilitation and morbidity after surgery (59,60). Thus, TPN is essential in cases of prolonged bowel obstruction and for patients with extended intestinal resection. TPN is often needed in patients with acute pancreatitis and those with high output fistula, where enteral feeding will not be tolerated and may even aggravate the clinical problem.

Pragmatic use of TPN has been suggested for the following clinical conditions, where TPN may be started to save time and EN instituted if possible (11):

1. Starving patients intolerant to EN—TPN is indicated in patients in the intensive care unit (ICU) who are intolerant to enteral feeding, especially those who have starved for a week or more and those who at the outset are malnourished.
2. Gastrointestinal symptoms compromising oral feeding—Severe illness is often due to gastrointestinal motility disorders, when enteral feeding becomes impossible because of nausea, vomiting, diarrhea, or bloating. Patients undergoing chemo- or radiotherapy may also be constantly nauseated and unable to eat. In severe G.I. disorders, symptoms worsen with oral feeding, e.g., pain related to acute pancreatitis may increase as the result of oral feeding. In patients with high small-bowel fistula, the output will increase and fistula will open if oral feeding is undertaken, and TPN is thought to promote fistula closure.
3. Cancer—In case of cancer producing malnutrition by obstructing the bowel, TPN may be beneficial, as in the case of starving patients who cannot be fed enterally and those with gastrointestinal symptoms that preclude oral feeding.
4. Renal and hepatic disorders—The parenteral route should be used when the G.I. tract is nonfunctional and nutrient intake needs to be modified because of the metabolic abnormalities of liver and renal diseases. Patients on chronic hemodialysis are prone to infection and if they are put on TPN (as after major surgery), special care needs to be taken to avoid catheter-related infection.
5. Patients with immunodeficiency or immunosuppression—Severely ill patients and those receiving chemo- or radiotherapy are mostly allergic to EN. TPN is routinely administered when enteral feeding is not possible. In immunosuppressed patients undergoing major surgery for organ transplantation, if TPN is needed for less than a week, the associated risk of infection should be weighed against the beneficial effects of nutrition.

Pichard and Jeejeebhoy (11) have described various techniques of administering enteral and parenteral nutrition and the complications involved therein.

IV. MANAGEMENT OF PROTEIN-ENERGY MALNUTRITION

Malnutrition is a clinical condition that includes several overlapping syndromes, such as growth failure in children and muscle wasting in adults. These may result, primarily or secondarily, from an inadequate supply, relative to the body's needs, of energy and/or essential nutrients. Primary malnutrition is associated with poverty and is common in the developing world. It was also evident in Europe until the late 19th century, but now it is rare except in the east, where war and political reorganization have caused large-scale deprivation (61).

Various terms have been used to describe the scientific basis of malnutrition and great controversy exists regarding use of these terms, which describe apparently different syndromes with different views as to their etiology. Williams (62) first introduced the term 'kwashiorkor' to describe the disease of Ghanaian children deposed from the breast by the birth of the next one, with the often total syndrome characterized by initial growth failure and irritability, followed by skin lesions, edema, and fatty liver. Despite criticism, the term kwashiorkor remains one of the most useful to describe the syndrome because it does not imply any cause.

Most children with malnutrition, however, do not show the classic features of kwashiorkor; they are simply underweight, usually short for their age, and sometimes thin. Jelliffe (63) proposed the term "protein-calorie malnutrition" to include all the syndromes relating to inadequate feeding. This term has now largely been replaced by protein-energy malnutrition (PEM) or simply malnutrition.

A. Assessing Nutritional Status

There is a need to deveop simple, reliable methods to assess nutritional status, especially in children and to classify the results according to severity. Childhood malnutrition is often characterized by growth failure, resulting in lower weight than ideal for the child's age, so measurement of weight and assessment of age are particularly important. These are generally easy and accurate to define, except in communities where the child's age is not known accurately. In these cases, the number of teeth erupted is a better indicator of age than height, head circumference or developmental milestones. PEM classifications based on weight and age are still the backbone of nutritional assessment methods for both population and individual assessments. Height or length in children too young to stand, and edema, are more difficult to measure accurately, but help to discriminate individual cases among the syndromes, which require different management.

Golden (61) put forward the following definitions that can be used for classification: Weight-for-age (%) = 100 × child's wt/reference wt of a child of the same age, Height-for-age (%) = 100 × child's ht/reference ht of a child of the same age, Weight-for-height (%) = 100 × child's wt/reference wt of a child of the same ht.

The term 'reference' value must be carefully chosen because few scientists agree on what can be considered as ideal weight or height. The values of the National Center for Health Statistics (NCHS) collected from U.S. children between birth and 18 years are considered as reference vaues.

Gomez et al. (64) classified population based on weight-for-age as follows:

% Reference	(NCHS) Nutritional class
90–109	Normal
75–89	Grade I or mild malnutrition
60–74	Grade II or moderate malnutrition
Less than 60	Grade III or severe malnutrition

Estimating the proportions of children with grade II and grade III malnutrition has remained a widely used and efficient method of comparing different populations. However, the cut-off point of 90% for 'normal' is thought to be too high, because many well-nourished children are below this limit,and yet fall within the range of the NCHS reference values. Edema that contributes to weight is ignored in this classification.

The Welcome Classification (65) uses both weight-for-age and the clinical qualitative assessment of the presence or absence of edema as follows:

% Reference	Nutritional class
No edema	Edematous
60–79	Undernourished kwashiorkor
Less than 60	Marasmus, marasmus kwashiorkor

Edema is the most consistent clinical feature of the kwashiorkor syndrome (62) which was frequently fatal. In the above classification, kwashiorkor is used strictly to include only children with pitting edema, whereas marasmus applies only to children with less than 60% weight-for-age.

Waterlow (66) classified population on the basis of both height-for-age and weight-for-height, excluding edema, as follows:

% Reference	Nutritional class
Ht-for-age	Stunting
90–94	Mild
85–89	Moderate
Less than 85	Severe
Wt-for-ht	Wasting
80–89	Mild
70–79	Moderate
Less than 70	Severe

The height-for-age estimates show how short or "stunted" a child is compared with the reference height for his age, whereas weight-for-height estimates show how thin or 'wasted' he is, relative to a reference child of the same height. For the latter calculation, it is assumed that a stunted child (e.g., 2 years old) of the same height as a younger, reference child (e.g., 5 months old) should have the same weight as the reference child (of 5 months), which is not quite true, especially when older children are compared with young infants (because of different shapes). However, the Waterlow classification is still used in nutritional management. Wasted children given short-term vigorous treatment recover within weeks, whereas stunted children require prolonged support over months or years to recover their expected height. According to Golden (61), it is advisable to use both the Welcome and the Waterlow classifications to choose the best available form of treatment for the individual malnourished child.

Some other indices of PEM include measurement of mid-upper arm circumference (MUAC) in relation to height, MUAC/head circumference (HC), triceps skinfold (TF) and mid-upper arm muscle circumference (MUAC-πTF). These are all less 'sensitive' indicators of PEM. Somatic quotient (SQ), which is the mean of weight, height, MUAC, and HC, each expressed as percentage reference value for age, also has been used but has proved to be too complex and limited even for individual assessment.

Body mass index (BMI), i.e., weight/height^2 in metric units has been employed to assess adult nutritional status (67). The term chronic energy deficiency (CED) is based on BMI with different degrees of CED. With a decreased body weight, the risks of illness increase in both men and women. The ill-health associated with underweight adults may potentially handicap the next generation. Adult nutrition has generally been neglected by nutritionists, because children, pregnant women, nursing mothers, and the elderly are often most at risk, but new data suggest adults as a major new area of nutritional concern (61).

B. Prevalence of Primary Malnutrition

The nutritional status for the most-free-living groups of children with primary malnutrition may be regarded as a continuous variable and may be described as the "iceberg phenomenon." The majority of children in a community may have a mild malnutrition, but far fewer have moderate malnutrition, and only a very few, the "tip of the iceberg," have severe malnutrition. These facts have been reported repeatedly (68,69).

Assessments of children in Asia, Africa, the Americas, and the Caribbean (70,71) has shown prevalence levels of malnourished children under 5 years and general trends over the past 25 years. The greatest problem of malnutrition is in south and southeast Asia, followed by Africa (Table 6), where the prevalence of underweight children is 2 to 3 times higher than elsewhere (72).

The worldwide economic recession in the 1980s, which caused rapidly increasing food prices; massive national debts in the developing world; and "natural disasters," such as droughts in Africa, have all increased the prevalence of malnourished children in Africa, Asia, and American regions after 1980. With each drought, harvest failure, earthquake, financial setback, and measles epidemic, the prevalence of malnutrition has increased within a few months and this could persist for several years. According to the WHO (71) report, the nutritional status of young children is probably the most sensitive indicator of sudden changes in food security and health status, acting as an early signal of distress, ill-health, famine and eventually, death.

The likely prevalence of malnourished children in 17 regions within Africa, Asia, and the Americas has been forecast up to 2005 (72) based on a statistical model of each country. This model includes previous prevalence rates of PEM, population densities, average per capita dietary energy supplies, infant mortality rates, and various variables for particular countries. Based on this model, Kelly (72) has predicted that the total numbers of malnourished children below 5

Table 6 Estimated Number and Prevalence of Malnourished Children, Younger Than 5 Years of Age in Selected Regions During 1990

Region	Number (millions)	Prevalence (%)
North America	0.3	2
South America	4.3	12
Caribbean	0.5	21
Africa	23.6	23
South Asia	91.0	69
East Asia	47.4	35

[a]Less than –2 SD NCHS reference weight-for-age.
Source: Ref. 72.

years will not change, but their prevalence will continue to fall slowly from 54% in 1975 to 49% in 1990 to 46% in 2005. This world average is very high because of the dominant effect of South Asia, including India and Bangladesh (Table 6).

The above studies, however, have not distinguished edematous malnutrition (kwashiorkor and marasmic kwashiorkor) from growth failure (undernutrition and marasmus). In the developing world, these conditions coexist in poor communities, often in the same family, and even in the same child at different stages of growth. Children with edematous malnutrition often lose their edema to become marasmic children, and those at high risk of developing edema are ones who are already malnourished.

Kwashiorkor and marasmus vary widely in different communities and with time. Gopalan (73) estimated that in India in the 1960s there was about 80% prevalence of growth failure, but only a 1.0% to 1.5% point prevalence of frank kwashiorkor and 2% to 3% of marasmic kwashiorkor. McLaren (74) noted that kwashiorkor was especially common in Tanzania but rare in the Labanon, where marasmus was common. Kwashiorkor tends to dominate in wet rather than drier regions of Africa, and it also tends to occur during the wet season of the year, rural rather than urban communities especially being affected.

Growth failure in malnourished children is characterized by suboptimal rates of gain in skeletal and soft tissues, conveniently estimated as a slowing of linear growth, or stunting. A normal child's height velocity is maximum in the first 6 months (about 3 cm/month), lesser in the second 6 months (abour 1.5 cm/month) and less than 1 cm/month thereafter. The growth failure is particularly obvious in infancy, at the time when weaning occurs, often with a fall in the nutrient intake.

The analysis by Golden (75) indicates that protein rather than energy intake is the predominant determinant of growth in height. Thus, selectively supplementing stunted children with milk protein can stimulate a spurt in height, whereas supplementation with energy (e.g., margarine) may lead to increase in weight but little or no spurt in height. Malcolm (76) in Papua New Guinea also found that protein-containing foods were particularly useful in allowing children to grow rapidly, which is in line with the proposal of Millward and Rivers (77) that the 'anabolic' drive depends on sufficient protein to stimulate the complex interactions of growth hormones (insulin and other growth factors) to allow a spurt in the growth of long bones.

Increasing evidence shows that stunting induced by environmental factors (including diet), is linked to increased risks of infections, illness, and even death (78). Also, slower mental development may be noticed in stunted children (79). These authors have further shown that both mental development and growth in height can be improved by food supplementation alone. The skills and capacity for physical work in PEM children are adversely affected and these effects are likely to persist into adulthood, leading to poorer development of societies. Thus, emergency measures to cope with malnourished children having a low weight for height must be matched by renewed efforts to promote children's growth.

Children with severe malnutrition, below 60% weight-for-age, are often also wasted, as are those with weight-for-height below 80%. Whereas the stunting measures the cumulative history of stress episodes, wasting signals a deteriorating condition at the time of measurement (80). According to Golden (61), poverty, which is the common denominator of primary malnutrition in childhood, is usually associated with illiteracy, inadequate sanitation, poor personal hygiene, insufficient access to medical services, poor earning capacity, poor agricultural practices, overpopulation, and inefficient and inappropriate use of resources both at a national and family level.

With the beginning of supplementary feeding, the growth rates of poor infants tend to fall, with frequent infections. With recurrence of infections, immune function also fails, increasing the duration of each infection. This leads to progressive deficits in the child's weight and deterioration in health (81).

C. Clinical Features of Malnutrition

Children at particular risk of malnutrition are characterized by the following:

Home: Very poor
Mother: Adolescent, multiparous
Guardian: Not a parent, low intelligence or knowledge; active or passive deprivation.
Child: less than 3 years old; birth weight less than 2.5 kg; congenital abnormality.

The main topics to be addressed in the history of the malnourished child include (61):

1. Present illness
2. Mother's pregnancy; birth, birthweight, parinatal events
3. Family history: parents' heights, causes of sibling illness/death
4. Socioeconomic history
5. Medical history: frequency of hospital visits, infections
6. Developmental milestones: regression
7. Past body weights with dates
8. Dietary history, before and since present illness
9. Appetite: vomiting, stools before and since present illness
10. Swelling, before and since present illness

In the developing countries, many children are born at home, hence brain damage and other congenital problems tend to go undiagnosed until the child presents with secondary malnutrition. A child's appetite is one of the best guides to early prognosis, a recent decrease in appetite being the main evidence of infection.

Golden (61) listed the following major features of malnutrition in children:

1. *Weight deficit*—stunting, general and local (buttocks, upper arm) wasting
2. *Mood abnormality*—misery, irritability
3. *Reduced activity*—milestone delay or regression
4. *Edema*—feet and lower legs; later periorbital hands'
5. *Jowls hepatomegaly*—variable, often firm with sharp lower edge
6. *Abdominal distension*—gaseous (ascites very rare)
7. *Skin lesions*—Hyper- and hypopigmentation and keratinization, "flaky paint"/"crazy pavement", delayed wound healing, pallor; purpura, jaundice.
8. *Mouth lesions*—Smooth tongue, stomatitis, angular, general.
9. *Eye lesions*—sunken, conjunctival pallor, scleral jaundice, signs of vitamin A deficiency.
10. *Hair changes*—Easily plucked out, thin, fragile, straight, depigmented, "forest sign," "flag sign," persistent lanugo, long eyelashes.
11. *Bone changes*—signs of rickets, especially "rosary" and "bossing."

After examining the child's nutritional status by anthropometric means (Welcome and Waterlow classification), other clinical features may be present that help to differentiate between primary and secondary malnutrition characteristics of particular deficiencies. Children with edematous malnutrition have much higher fat in their liver (up to 50% on wet basis) than the marasmic children.

There is often a depression of digestion and absorption of protein, fat, and carbohydrate in malnourished children, owing to low outputs of gastric acid and intestinal and pancreatic enzymes. Bile salt deconjugation occurs with small-bowel overgrowth with presence of mucosal atrophy. Overt gastrointestinal infection is very common. Exocrine pancreatic deficiency and small-bowel overgrowth may cause mild fat malabsorption, limiting the supply of fat-soluble vitamins A, D, E, and K. The output of all disaccharidases is decreased, lactase being the most severely affected and apparently, the slowest to return to normal with rehabilitation.

The endocrine system is often grossly atrophic, but fairly well preserved. There are marked changes in hormonal balance (reduced insulin, glucagon and thyroxine), which reflect the body's adaptation to an inadequate dietary intake. However, plasma thyroid-stimulating hormone, growth hormone, cortisol, and aldosterone levels are usually raised, especially in edematous malnutrition.

Glucose intolerance is a consistent feature of malnutrition, caused by low insulin production and high peripheral insulin resistance, high plasma cortisol and growth hormone levels, and probably due to chromium and potassium deficiencies. Mild to moderate anemia is common in malnourished children (70–100 g Hb levels/l).

Malnutrition and infection are synergistic, since as malnutrition increases, the susceptibility to invasion by pathogens also increases. Profound anorexia, hypothermia, hypoglycemia and neutropenia infections are common in very ill children (61).

D. Management of Protein-Energy Malnutrition

Wasted children can be managed at home successfully. Recovery in stunted children with catch-up to reference height-for-age values is uncommon, even with medical care. It requires the concerted efforts of the family, the community, and the support of the welfare and medical services over several years.

Ideally, each child needs to be examined to exclude the possibility of underlying disease. When any disease is present, the child's treatment and prognosis may be different, which must be explained to the mother to gain her trust and cooperation. Primary malnutrition is also usually associated with frequent intercurrent infections, which must be treated as early and effectively as possible. Acute respiratory viral infections especially take longer periods to resolve, leading to greater weight losses and risk of bacterial infections such as pneumonia.

Management of acute gastroenteritis should begin early, with frequent closely supervised feeds of oral rehydration solution (ORS) (20 volumes) to water (1 volume). With some care, ORS can be made at home as shown in Table 7. However, international agencies such as WHO and charity groups have made sachets of ORS powder that can be readily reconstituted with boiled, cooled water. The combination of sugar and salt allows glucose-linked sodium absorption to occur, while the enterotoxin-induced intestinal secretion continues. Feeds should be encouraged, not withheld, to avoid further weight loss.

Table 7   Oral Rehydration Solution

Composition (mmol/L)	WHO[a]/UNICEF	BNF[b]	Home (approx.)
Na^+	90	35	85
Cl^-	80	37	85
K^+	20	20	0
HCO_3	30	18	0
Glucose	110	200	117 (sucrose)
Method of preparation	Dissolve sachets of powder in water		1 level teaspoon salt and 8 level teaspoons sugar are dissolved in 1 liter water

[a]World Health Organization, *A Manual of the Treatment of Acute Diarrhea* (1984).
[b]BNF compound: NaCl and oral glucose powder.
Source: Ref. 61.

The management of the malnourished child at home requires improvement in the child's micro- and macro-environment and hygiene, diet, and feeding practice. Energy intakes should be increased by substituting high-energy, low-cost foods for relatively expensive items and by using food supplements.

Children with kwashiorkor, marasmus, and severe wasting will need hospital management for quicker recovery. Golden (61) divided hospital management in three stages. In stage I, the child's acute problems are diagnosed and treated vigorously, employing antibiotic therapy, maintenance feeds, and supplements. In stage 2, "high-quality" feeds are given *ad libitum* in increasing amounts to permit rapid catch-up to about the 50th centile weight-for-height. In stage 3, the child is weaned to home feeds.

Stage 1 should begin as soon as possible after the child's admission to the hospital. After the clinical history and examination, investigation of blood for hemoglobin, serum electrolyte, urea, and creatinine, microbiological tests for ova and cysts, urine examination for sugar and protein, and chest x-ray will help to treat the child subsequently for any particular infectious diseases. Severely malnourished children are often infected with gram-positive and gram-negative organisms.

Efforts must be made to feed the malnourished child sufficient energy (maintenance energy) and protein to prevent further tissue catabolism, taking care not to overfeed at this stage. About 400 KJ and 2.0 g protein/kg/day are usually advised, with a protein/energy (P/E) ratio of about 5 g/MJ. The P/E ratio of most commercially available feeds is higher than this. By substituting vegetable oil and sugar for some of the water added to infant formula powder one can devise a feed with an appropriate P/E ratio, which is not hyperosmolar or deficient in water. Such feed is given at the rate of 100 g/kg/child/day, as frequent small feeds. Extra water or 4.3% dextrose/0.18 normal saline may be given if the child is dehydrated or having excess fluid loss. Feed may be offered in smaller volumes more frequently, or even at half strength in cases of refusal or persistent vomiting, and then increased in volume or strengths as appropriate at daily intervals. If this fails, a finc, soft nasogastric or nosojejunal tube can be inserted gently to commence feeding continuously. Intravenous 'feeding' should be avoided, as a small mistake in rate or composition may be fatal. With enteral feeding, the intestinal mucosa acts as a barrier buffer against such mistakes. Intravenous fluids however, may be necessary when a child is severely dehydrated and will not tolerate any enteral fluid. The extremely ill child, unable to take feeds, may benefit from a small (10 ml/kg) intravenous infusion of fresh, cross-matched whole blood, although there is a high risk of circulatory overload and cardiac failure in this.

According to Goden (61), when a marasmic child retains "maintenance energy," he begins to maintain weight, and when an edematous child retains this intake, he generally tends to lose weight as he loses edema. With an improvement in mood and appetite, most of the children begin to crave more feed, usually within a week of being on maintenance energy.

Malnourished children often experience intracellular deficiency of K^+ and Mg^{2+}, which may be supplemented orally, if possible. The ongoing diarrhea increases their requirements. Low plasma Zn^{2+} levels are occasionally evident in the form of severe skin lesions (zinc status is rather difficult to quantify in malnutrition), which heal quickly when zinc is supplied. Copper supplements should be given, even in the absence of overt copper deficiency, and iodine may be given in endemic goiter regions. Large amounts of Na^+, as in 0.5 or 1 N saline solutions, should be avoided, as most severely malnourished children have an excess of body Na to eliminate. Iron should not be given until children reach stage 2, and all malnourished children should be given oral or nasogastric vitamin supplements containing vitamins A, C, D, E, B_1, B_2, B_6, niacin, and folic acid.

Some of the common problems encountered during stage 1 include persistent anorexia, persistent edema, hypothermia, hypoglycemia, persistent vomiting, persistent diarrhea, congestive cardiac failure, breathlessness, paralytic ileus, purpura, and jaundice. Septicemia is almost invariably fatal without the correct antibiotic given in adequate dosage.

Stage 2 management can begin after a few days, by increasing daily the amounts of feed followed by *ad libitum* feeding within week's time, with eight 3-hourly feeds/day and later six 4-hourly feeds. The K, Mg, vitamin, and trace element supplements should continue, with oral iron, about 4 mg/kg/day, as ferrous sulfate. Feed volumes are increased gradually, once the edema is lost, as the weight gains begin to rise. After the child reaches the 50th centile of weight-for-height, the feed intake decreases to less than 500 kJ/kg/day, when weaning to an *ad libitum* mixed diet would be appropriate. This adjustment takes a few days before the child returns to steady weight gain, after which he is ready for home.

Such hospital treatment and care are unusual in practice because of overloads; often children are sent home early to allow for others to be treated. The benefits of stage 2 recovery are considerable, provided the guardians are also helped to improve their child care, with knowledge of appropriate diets. Breast-feeding, family planning, and preventive measures (e.g., immunization) all need to be integrated into the hospital management scheme for the greater advantages (61).

V.   DIET, NUTRITION, AND THE IMMUNE SYSTEM

Intuitively, it is realized that persons that are well fed and well cared for are often healthier than those who are not well fed or cared for. Nutritionists have long been concerned with minimum nutrient requirements for maximal growth rate and maintenance, but researchers have not begun to look at the nutritional intakes that provide optimal health. The increasingly sophisticated methods of immunology have allowed investigators to define indicators of resistance to disease such as cell-mediated immunity, lymphocyte functions, and macrophage functions. The combination of these immunological tools with the classical methods of nutrition research is expected to bring out how dietary constituents influence each of these cellular immune systems, and to understand how these systems may influence resistance to various diseases (82).

While relating nutrition to either infection or the immune system, two important areas, viz., public health [the prevention and treatment of human diseases and metabolic disorders] and livestock and poultry production must be considered. The production of meat, poultry, and animal materials continues to become a more intensive operation in the world's agriculture, and the number of such high-density systems or "confinement operations" will continue to rise. Newer and more severe problems of disease control are appearing with the expansion of these operations. Nutritionists have to develop diets not only to provide the basic nutrient requirements but to optimize the health of humans and animals through diet and nutrition to reduce the impact of infection and other physiological stresses.

The information contained in Chapters 24 to 34 in this volume is devoted to diet, nutrition, and human health; these chapters discuss how human diet and nutrition influence various clinical disorders and diseases, including heart and circulation disorders; cancers; obesity and diabetes; diseases of the bones, teeth, skin and hair; diseases of the kidney and liver; and the disorders of the nervous system.

Keusch (83) reviewed effects of protein energy malnutrition on immune responses in the human host. These studies document major impairment of the T-cell and complement systems in severe PEM, and less profound, but probably significant, effects on B cells and immunoglobulins, particularly secretory IgA (SIgA). While mild-to-moderate malnutrition also alters the T-cell system, predisposing the individual to infection, the evidence available is not enough to suggest that complement is similarly affected. Evidence, however, indicates that a host with mild-to-moderate malnutrition is still able to respond to stress with an acute phase serum protein response and to boost serum levels of complement and complement activity. Such a functionally significant distinction may serve to separate the more from the less severely ill individuals. Many factors alter immune response, including vitamins, calories, and trace elements, and few clinical studies have investigated these parameters. Therefore, it is not certain how much of the problem in malnutrition is due to protein, to energy intake, to iron, to other micronutrients, trace elements, and vitamins alone or in combination with protein and energy deficiencies.

Vitamin A is known to subserve a number of important physiological functions that contribute to effective host defense. Moderately large doses have an immunostimulatory effect and can reverse the suppression produced by pharmacological agents, such as cortisone. Vitamin A acts as an adjuvant and influences both cell membranes and intracellular composition and function. This applies to both lymphocytes and monocytes. Vitamin A deficiency is thus associated with an increased incidence of infection and disease, which may be brought about through epithelial changes and reduced cell-mediated and mucosal immunity. Recent research work suggests that moderately large but nontoxic doses of vitamin A or its derivatives have a protective effect for certain tumors or that such therapy may reduce tumor size or change the morphological type and differentiation of the malignant cell (84). Vitamin A thus appears to have a wide-ranging immunological and antitumor effects. However, the relevance of scientific data for human diseases still remains uncertain until more research work is carried out with human subjects.

According to Watson (85), some dietary changes, such as deficiency of protein, zinc, or fat, act as stresses in mammalian systems, resulting in an elevation in serum corticosteroids. These stresses often result in suppression of cellular immune function. An excess of dietary vitamin E was found to decrease serum corticosteroid levels, showing an apparent stress-reducing action, as monitored by either serum corticosteroid levels or the normalcy of immune functions. Thus, diet can be either stress-promoting or stress-reducing with accompanying changes in immune functions and defenses.

Infectious diseases deplete host nutrient stores in various ways and, reciprocally, nutritional factors influence host susceptibility to infection. Nutritional factors influence immune functions and other host defensive measures. Beisel (86) envisioned a complex interrelationship between nutritional factors and immune functions, because acute or chronic infections also initiate changes in defense system functions as well as in the nutritional status of the host. Infection and immune functions are also closely linked and have reciprocal interrelationships. Thus, possible effects of infection cannot be ignored when nutritional status is being evaluated for its role in influencing immunological functions.

According to Beisel (86), generalized infectious illnesses cause predictable biochemical, metabolic, and hormonal responses. In combinations with fever and anorexia, these responses lead to hypermetabolic losses of cellular constituents and deplete body nutrient stores. Concomitantly, infectious processes stimulate defensive measures that include both organism-specific immunological responses and an activation of generalized nonspecific defenses. A concomitant suppression of some immune system functions may also occur. The possible presence and impact of an infectious process should therefore be considered whenever nutrition–immune system interrelationships are studied in animals. In clinical situations, nutritional depletion and weakened host defenses must be recognized as expected sequels of acute infectious diseases; conversely, the presence or development of an infectious process must be anticipated in patients with malnutrition, both before and during nutritional rehabilitation.

The immune system performs many important functions, including the control of pathogenic infections and inflammatory responses and the prevention of the growth of cancer cells. According to Kelley (87), two major branches of the immune system include (a) the innate immune response (IR), which is present at all times in normal individuals and is fully functional before infectious agents enter the body, and (b) the adaptive immune response, which is activated only after a pathogen has evaded the innate response and has entered the body. While the innate IR does not distinguish between microbes of different species and its response time does not change with repeated exposures, the adaptive IR is specific to the attacking microbes, and the response time is reduced during repeated exposures. Examples of innate immunity include mechanical barriers such as the skin and the epithelial linings of lungs and gut, secreted products such as saliva and tears, and the immune cells, including macrophages, neutrophils, and the natural killer (NK) cells. Adaptive immunity has two major classes: humoral immunity mediated by B lymphocytes and cell-mediated immunity that is mediated by T lymphocytes and activated macrophages (87).

In vitro studies conducted with the cells of the immune system demonstrated that essential fatty acids (EFA) are required for the growth and maintenance of these cells and that free fatty acids are produced and secreted during the activation of immune cells. Fatty acid concentrations up to 10 µg/ml stimulated several functions of immune cells in vitro, whereas concentrations higher than 10 g/ml were inhibitory, PUFA being more inhibitory, than saturated fatty acids (SFA) at a given high concentration. Also, both n-6 and n-3 PUFAs were equally inhibitory. Animal studies have shown that both deficiency and excess of EFA inhibit IR.

Human epidemiological studies have also indicated that there exist possible links between fat intake and certain types of cancer, and the severity of autoimmune disorders. Thus, enough evidence suggests that dietary fat may modulate IR. Several human studies have shown the effects of total fat and its composition on human IR. Reduction in total fat intake was found to enhance IR (88) and increase the number and activity of NK cells (89,90). The inhibitory effect of n-6 PUFA was possibly overcome by the stimulatory effect of reduced fat intake, and n-6 PUFA may inhibit IR in a high-fat or low-antioxidant nutrient diet. An increase in linoleic acid (LA), accompanied with an increase in total fat (from 22% to 28% of energy), inhibited NK cell activity in healthy men. Rasmussen et al. (90) noted that the plasma and adipose tissue levels of n-6 PUFA presumably reflect dietary intake, significant negative correlation being found between NK cell activity and the plasma levels of total PUFA, n-6 PUFA, and LA. Thus, the effect of n-6 PUFA on IR may be modified by the intake of total fat, antioxidant nutrients, duration of feeding, and a number of other factors.

LA is rapidly oxidized with only a limited conversion to arachidonic acid (AA), a precursor for a variety of eicosanoids, including prostaglandin E_2 (PG E_2) and leukotriene B_4 (LTB$_4$), which have a profound effect on the cells of the immune system. Kelley et al. (91) examined the effect of dietary AA on IR and several other health parameters of young men. The healthy men were fed a basal diet containing 30% energy from fat (10:10:10, saturated/monounsaturated/polyunsaturated) and 200 mg/day for 15 days, after which the diet of 6 men was supplemented with 1.5 g additional AA from ARASCO oil (Martek Bioscience Corp., Columbia, MD) for 50 days, the other four remaining on the basal diet. The diets of two groups were crossed over for the next 50 days. AA supplementation did not have any adverse effect on a number of indexes of IR tested. However, it significantly increased the number of circulating neutrophils and also the second response to influenza vaccine. The feeding of the low-fat, nutritionally balanced diet was found to enhance several indices of IR. Moderate levels of AA fed as natural triglycerides do not appear to have any adverse effects on human IR, even if AA is a precursor for the inflammatory eicosanoids.

The n-3 PUFA have been found to be beneficial in the management of some human autoimmune diseases and to reduce the incidence of certain types of cancer in animal models. Studies examining the effect of n-3 PUFA on human IR have been conducted with the 18 C (vegetable source) n-3 PUFA, alpha-linolenic acid (ALA), marine oils containing 20 and 22 C n-3 PUFA, eicosapentenoic acid (EPA), and docosahexenoic acid (DHA). Most of these human studies indicate inhibition of human IR by n-3 PUFA.

Fish oils have been found to inhibit several aspects of neutrophil, monocyte, and lymphocyte functions in several human studies (92–94). Fish oil intake of 18 g/day, in addition to the fat content of the basal diet, inhibited neutrophil and monocyte functions within 6 weeks, although it failed to inhibit T-cell functions. Kelley et al. (95) also noted that high fish intake [EPA + DHA = 1.23 g/day or 0.54 energy %] for 6 months significantly inhibited several indexes of IR, although low intake of fish (EPA + DHA) = 0.27 g/day or 0.13% energy) for the same period did not inhibit any of these indices. The lymphocyte proliferation and DTH were actually enhanced by the low fish diet. The total fat, the ratios between n-6 and n-3 PUFA, the age, and the antioxidant nutritional status are important factors determining the impact of n-3 PUFA on human IR (87).

The immuno-inhibitory effects of n-3 PUFA along with their beneficial effects for cardiovascular health have promoted a number of studies in the management of autoimmune and inflammatory diseases. Kremer et al. (96) reported that the diets of rheumatoid arthritis patients, when supplemented with fish oils, led to a reduction in swollen and tender joints, morning stiffness, and pain index. Fish oil supplementation has also been reported to decrease symptoms of lupus, psoriasis, cystic fibrosis, ulcerative colitis, and inflammatory bowel disease and to decrease early restenosis after angioplasty as well as to improve renal functions in patients maintained on cyclosporin after kidney or liver transplant.

Although the results from clinical trials with fish oils seem encouraging, any benefit from their intake must outweigh the risk associated with overall suppression of IR. Fish oils being rich in cholesterol, the risk of increased cholesterol intake should also be considered. The risk/benefit ratios may vary in different individuals and for the same individual under different sets of conditions. Kelley (87) proposed several mechanisms of action, including serum lipoproteins, escosanoid type and concentration, oxidative stress, and membrane fluidity. Any single dietary intervention may involve more than one of these mechanisms. In addition to these mechanisms, it is also possible that some fatty acids may have direct effects on the cells of the immune system (87).

According to Hanson et al. (97), early diet influences development of the immune system. New experimental data suggest that the mother's immune response to fetal antigens determines the growth of the trophoblasts and placenta by production of certain cytokines. The size of the placenta may determine the size of the fetus. Maternal undernutrition may increase the risk and endanger the immune system, causing intrauterine growth retardation (IUGR) by production of the untoward cytokines, IFN-gamma and TNF-alpha. IUGR in the form of "small for gestational age" (SGA) can cause severe and long-lasting disturbances of the infant's immune system.

Breast-feeding has numerous immediate, long-term, and probably lasting effects on the B cells as well as T cells of the offspring. Vitamin A deficiency of the mother and the infant will cause a severe secondary immunodeficiency that may have consequences either immediately or presumably later on in life. In early life, it is determined whether immune responsiveness or tolerance will develop toward food proteins. However, little is known about this important area, although new research data are producing interesting results (97).

REFERENCES

1. Stephen, A.M., Regulatory aspects of functional foods, *Functional Foods: Biochemical and Processing Aspects* (G. Mazza, ed), Technomic Publishing Co. Lancaster, 1998, p. 403.

2. I.F.F.L., Neutraceutical/Functioning Foods. An exploratory survey of Canada's Potential, International Food Focus Limited, Agriculture and Agri-Food, Ottawa, 1995.

3. Rowland, D.W., Foods or quasi-drugs?, *Healthy Naturally 28*: 14 (1997).

4. Forbes, G.B., Some influences on lean body mass: exercise, androgens, pregnancy and food, *Diet and Exercise: Synergism in Health Maintenance* (P.L. White and T. Mondeike, eds.), American Medical Association, Chicago, Illinois, 1982.

5. Clydesdale, F.M., and F.J. Francis, *Food, Nutrition and Health*. AVI Publishing Co., Westport, 1985.

6. Feingold, B., *Why Your Child is Hyperactive?* Random House, New York, 1975.

7. Kolata, G., Food affects human behavior, *Science 218*: 1209 (1982).

8. Clydesdale, F.M., Culture, fitness and health, *Food Technol. 38*: 108 (1984a).

9. Clydesdale, F.M., View of a view point: nutritional considerations, *J. Learning Disabil. 17*: 450 (1984b).

10. Anomymous, Assembly of Life Sciences, Committee on *Diet, Nutrition and Cancer*, National Research Council, National Academy of Sciences, Washington, D.C., 1982.

11. Pichard, C., and K.N. Jeejeebhoy, Nutritional management of clinical undernutrition, *Human Nutrition and Dietetics*, 9th ed. (J.S. Garrow and W.P.T. James, eds.), Churchill Livingstone, Edinburgh, London, 1993, p. 421.

12. Mullen J.L., G.P. Buzby, D.C. Matthews, B.F. Smale, and E.F. Rosato, Reduction of postoperative morbidity and mortality by combined preoperative and postoperative nutritional support, *Ann. Surgery 92*: 604 (1980).

13. Rombeau, J., L.R. Barot, C.E. Williamson, and J.L. Mullen, Reduction of postoperative morbidity and mortality by combined preoperative total parenteral nutrition and surgical outcome in patients with inflammatory bowel disease, *Am. J. Surgery 143*: 139 (1982).

14. Lennard-Jones, J.E., A positive approach to nutrition as treatment, Report of a working party on enteral and parenteral nutrition, King's Fund Centre, London, 1992.

15. Willicuts, H.D., Nutritional assessment of 1000 surgical patients in an affluent suburban community hospital, *J. Paren. Ent. Nutr. 1*: 25 (1977). (Abstr.)

16. Brennan, M.F., Metabolic response to surgery in the cancer patient, *Cancer 43*: 2053 (1979).

17. Lowe, A.H.G., Prolonged starvation, *Extremes of Nutrition*, First British Society of Gastroenterology, Glaxo International Teaching Days, 1982.

18. Wolman, S.L., G.H. Anderson, E.B. Marliss, and K.N. Jeejeebhoy, Zinc in total parenteral nutrition: Requirements and metabolic effects, *Gastroenterology 76*: 458 (1979).

19. Rudman, D., W.J. Millikan, T.J. Richardson, T.J. Bixler, W.J. Stackhouse, and W.C. McGarrity, Elemental balances during intravenous hyperalimentation, *J. Clin. Investigation 55*: 94 (1975).

20. Munro, H.N., *Mammalian Protein Metabolism* (H.N. Munro and J.B. Allison, eds.), Academic Press, New York, 1964, p. 381.

21. Moore, F.D., K.H. Olsen, J.D. Mc.Murray, H.V. Parkar, M.R. Ball, and C.M. Boyden, *The Body Cell Mass and its Supporting Environment: Body Composition in Health and Disease*, W.B. Saunders, Philadephia, 1968.

22. Lukaski, H.C., J. Mendez, E.R. Buskirk, and S.H. Cohn. A comparison of methods of assessment and body composition including neutron activation analysis for total body nitrogen, *Metabolism 30*: 777 (1981).

23. MacNeill, K.G., J.E. Harrison, J.R. Mernagh, S. Stewart, and K.N. Jeejeebhoy, Changes in body protein, body potassium, and lean body mass during total parenteral nutrition, *J. Parent. Ent. Nutr. 6*: 106 (1982).

24. Russell, D.Mc. R., P.J. Prendergast, P.E. Darby, et al., A comparison between muscle function and body composition in anorexia nervosa: the effects of refeeding, *Am. J. Nutr. 37*: 229 (1983).

25. Long, C.L., B. Jeevanandam, B.M. Kim, and J.M. Kimney, Whole body protein synthesis and catabolism in septic man, *Am. J. Nutr. 30*: 1340 (1977).

26. Kinney, J.M., Assessment of energy metabolism in health and disease, Report 1st Ross Conf. Med. Research, 1978, p. 42.

27. Rosa, A.M., and H.M. Shizgal, The Harris, Benedict equation reevaluated: resting energy requirements and the body cell mass, *Am. J. Clin. Nutr. 40*: 168 (1984).

28. Pichard, C., M. Roulet, C. Rossle, R. Chiolero, E. Jequier, and P. Furst, Effects of 1-carnitine supplemented total parenteral nutrition on lipid and energy metabolism in post operative stress, *J. Paren. Ent. Nutr. 12*: 55 (1988).

29. Pichard, C.M. Roulet, Y. Schutz, C. Rossle, P. Furst, and E. Jequier, Clinical relevance of 1-carnitine supplemented total parenteral nutrition in postoperative trauma. Metabolic effect of continuous or acute carnitine administration with special reference to fat oxidation and nitrogen utilization. *Am. J. Clin. Nutr. 49*: 283 (1989).

30. Freeman, J.B., Magnesium requirements are increased during total parenteral nutrition, *Surgery Forum 288*: 61 (1977).

31. Golden, M.H.N., and B.E. Golden, Trace elements: Potential importance in human nutrition with particular reference to zinc and vanadium, *British Med. Bull. 37*: 31 (1981).

32. Chan, S.T.F., Muscle power after glucose-potassium loading in undernourished patients, *Br. Med. J. 293*: 1055 (1986).

33. Calloway, D.H., and H. Spector, Nitrogen balance as related to calorie and protein intake in active young men, *Am. J. Clin. Nutr. 2*: 405 (1954).

34. Greenberg, G.R., E.B. Marliss, G.H. Anderson, et al., Protein sparing therapy in postoperative patients. Effects of added hypocaloric glucose and lipid, *N. Engl. J. Med. 294*: 1411 (1976).

35. Greenberg G.R., and K.N. Jeejeebhoy, Intravenous protein sparing therapy in patients with gastrointestinal disease. *J. Paren. Ent. Nutr. 3*: 427 (1979).

36. Hill, G.L., R.F.G.J. King, R.C. Smith, et al., Multi-element analysis of the living body by neuro-analysis. Application to critically ill patients receiving intravenous nutrition, *Br. J. Surg. 66*: 868 (1979).

37. Anderson, G.H., D.C. Patel, and K.N. Jeejeebhoy, Design and evaluation by nitrogen balance and blood aminograms of an amino acid mixture for total parenteral nutrition of adults with gastrointestinal disease, *J. Clin. Invest. 53*: 904 (1974).

38. Rose, W.C., Amino acid requirements of man. *Federal Proc. 8*: 546 (1949).

39. Petel, D., G.H. Anderson, and K.N. Jeejeebhoy, Amino acid adequacy of parenteral casein hydrolysate and oral cottage cheese in patients with gastrointestinal disease as measured by nitrogen balance and blood aminogram, *Gastroenterology 65*: 427 (1973).

40. Sherwin, R.S. Effect of starvation on the turnover and metabolic response to leucine, *J. Clin. Invest. 62*: 1471 (1978).

41. Li, J, and L. Jefferson, Influence of amino acid availability on protein turnover in perfused skeletal muscle, *Biochim. Biophys. Acta 544*: 351 (1978).

42. Saba, T.M., B.C. Dillon, and M.E. Lanser, Fibronectin and phagocytic host defense: relationship to nutritional support, *J. Paren. Ent. Nutr. 7*: 62 (1983).

43. Walser, M., Therapeutic aspects of branched-chain amino acids, *Clin. Sci. 66*: 1 (1984).

44. Feinstein, E.I., M.J. Blumentanz, and M. Healer, Clinical and metabolic responses to parenteral nutrition in acute renal failure. Controlled double blind trial, *Medicine 60*: 124 (1981).

45. Wahren, J., J. Densis, and P. Desurmont, Is intravenous administration of BCAA effective in treatment of hepatic encephalopathy? A multicenter study, *Hepatolgy 3*: 475 (1981).

46. Harris, J.A., and F.G. Benedict, Standard basal metabolism constants for physiologists and clinicians, *A Biometric Study of Basal Metabolism in Man*, Carnegie Institute of Washington, J.B. Lippincott, Philadelphia, 1919, p. 233.

47. Kinney J.M., Indirect calorimetry in malnutrition: nutritional assessment or therapeutic reference, *J. Paren. Ent. Nutr. 11*: 90 (1987).

48. Askanazi, J., Y.A. Carpentier, D.H. Elwyn, et al., Influence of total parenteral nutrition on fuel utilization in injury and sepsis, *Ann. Surgery 191*: 40 (1980).

49. Roulet, M., A.S. Detsky, E.B. Marliss, et al., A controlled trial of the effect of parenteral nutritional support on patients with respiratory failure and sepsis, *Clin. Nutr. 2*: 97 (1983).

50. Baker, J.P., A.S. Detsky, S. Stewart, et al., Randomised trial of total parenteral nutrition in critical ill patients: Metabolic effects of varying glucose lipid ratios as the energy source, *Gastroenterology 87*: 53 (1984).

51. Nordenstrom, J., J. Askanazi, D.H. Elwyn, et al., Nitrogen balance during total parenteral nutrition: glucose vs. fat. *Ann. Surgery 197*: 27 (1983).

52. Shike, M., W.C. Sturtridge, C.S. Jam, et al., A possible role of vitamin D in the genesis of parenteral nutrition-induced metabolic bone disease, *Ann. Intern. Med. 95*: 560 (1981).

53. Mac Fie J., R.C. Smith, and G.L. Hill, Glucose or fat as non-protein energy source. A controlled clinical trial in gastroenterological patients requiring intravenous nutrition, *Gastroenterology 81*: 285 (1981).

54. Goodgame J.T., S.F. Lowry, and M.F. Brennan, Essential fatty acid deficiency in total parenteral nutrition: time course of development and suggestions for therapy, *Surgery 84*: 271 (1978).

55. Wene, J.D., W.E. Connor, and L. Den Besten, The development of essential fatty acid deficiency in healthy men fed fat free diets intravenously and orally, *J. Clin. Invest. 56*: 127 (1975).

56. Baker, J.P., A.S. Detsky, D.E. Wessen, et al., Nutritional assessment: A comparison of clinical judgement and objective measurements, *N. Engl. J. Med. 306*: 969 (1982).

57. Pichard, C., and M. Roulet, Constant rate enteral nutrition in bucco-pharyangeal cancer care, *Otolaryngology 9*: 209 (1984).

58. Koretz. R.L. What supports nutritional support? *Dig. Dis. Sci. 29*: 577 (1984).

59. Young, G.A., J.P. Collins, and G.L. Hill, Plasma proteins in patients receiving intravenous amino acids or intravenous hyperalimentation after major surgery, *Am. J. Clin. Nutr. 32*: 1192 (1979).

60. Bastow, M.D., J. Rawlings, and S.P. Allison, Benefits of supplementary tube feeding after fractures of the neck of femur, *Br. Med. J. 287*: 1589 (1983).

61. Golden, B.E., Protein-energy malnutrition. *Human Nutrition and Dietetics*, 9th ed. (J.S. Garrow and W.P.T. James, eds.), Churchill Livisngstone, Edinburgh, London, 1993, p. 440.

62. Williams, C.D., Kwashiorkor, *Lancet 2*: 1151 (1935).

63. Jelliffe, D.B., Protein-calorie malnutrition in tropical preschool children. *J. Pediatrics 54*: 227 (1959).

64. Gomez, F., R. Ramos-Falvan, S. Frenk, et al., Mortality in second and third degree malnutrition, *J. Trop. Pediatrics 2*: 77 (1956).

65. Anonymous, Classification of infantile malnutrition, *Lancet 2*: 302 (1970).

66. Waterlow, J.C., Note on the assessment and classification of protein energy malnutrition in children, *Lancet 2*: 87 (1973).

67. Ferro—Luzzi, A., S. Sette, M. Franklin, and W. P.T. James, A simplified approach to assessing adult chronic energy deficiency, *Eur. J. Clin. Nutr. 46*: 173 (1992).

68. Bengoa, J.M., The problem of malnutrition, *WHO Chronicle 28*: 3 (1974).

69. Ashworth, A., and D. Piou, Nutritional status in Jamaica (1968–74), *West Indian Med. J. 25*: 23 (1976).

70. WHO, Administrative Committee on Coordination—Subcommittee on Nutrition (ACC/SCN), First Report on the World Nutrition Situation, World Health Organization of United Nations, Geneva, 1987.

71. WHO, ACC/SCN, Update on Nutrition Situation. Recent trends in 33 countries, World Health Organization of United Nations, Geneva, 1989.

72. Kelly, A.W., Technical Working Paper for United Nations Administrative Committee on Coordination—Subcommittee on Nutrition (ACC/SCN), 1991.

73. Gopalan, C., Protein versus calories in the treatment of protein calories malnutrition: Metabolic and population studies in India, *Protein Calories Malnutrition* (R.E. Olsen, ed.) Academic Press, New York, 1975, p. 329.

74. McLaren, D.S., The great protein fiasco, *Lancet 2*: 93 (1974).

75. Golden, M., The consequences of protein deficiency in man and its relationship to the features of kwashiorkor, *Nutritional Adaptation in Man* (K. Blaxter and J.C. Waterlow, eds.), John Libbey, London, 1985, p. 169.

76. Malcolm, L.A., Growth retardation in a New Guinea boarding school children and its response to supplementary feeding, *British J. Nutr. 24*: 297 (1970).

77. Millword, D., and J.P.W. Rivers, The need for indispensible amino acids: the concept of the anabolic drive, *Diabetes Metab. Rev. 5*: 191 (1989).

78. Waterlow, J.C., A. Ashworth, and M. Griffiths, Faltering in infant growth in less-developed Countries, *Lancet 2*: 1176 (1980).

79. Grantham-McGreger, S.M., C.A. Powell, S.P. Walker, and J.H. Himes, Nutritional supplementation, psychosocial stimulation and mental development of stunted children: the Jamaican study, *Lancet 338*: 1 (1991).

80. Martorell, R., Child growth retardation: a discussion of its causes and its relationship to health, *Nutritional Adaptation in Man* (K. Blaxter and J.C. Waterlow, eds.). John Libbey, London, 1985, p. 13.

81. Mata, L.J., R.A. Kromal, J.J. Urrutia, and B. Garcid, Effect of infection on food intake: perspective as viewed from the village, *Am. J. Clin. Nutr. 30*: 1215 (1977).

82. Philips, M., and A. Bactz (eds), *Diet and Resistance to Disease, Advances in Experimental Medicine and Biology*, Vol. 135, Plenum Press, New York, 1981.

83. Keusch G.T., Host defence mechanism in protein energy malnutrition, *Diet and Resistance to Disease* (M. Philips and A. Baetz., eds), *Advances in Experimental Medicine and Biology*, Vol. 135. Plenum Press, New York, 1981, p. 183.

84. Vyas, D., and R.K. Chandra, Vitamin A and immunocompetence, *Nutrition, Disease Resistance, and Immune Function* (R.R. Watson, ed.), Marcel Dekker, New York, 1984, p. 325.

85. Watson, R.R. Stress caused by dietary changes: Corticosteroid production, a partial explanation for immunosuppression in the malnourished, *Nutrition, Disease Resistance and Immune Function* (R.R. Watson, ed.), Marcel Dekker, New York, 1984, p. 273.

86. Beisel, W.R., Nutrition, infection, specific immune responses and non specific host defenses: A complex interaction, *Nutrition, Disease Resistance and Immune Function* (R.R. Watson, ed.), Marcel Dekker, New York, 1984, p. 3.

87. Kelley D.S., Dietary fat and human immune response, *INFORM 7*: 857 (1996).

88. Kelley, D.S., R.M. Doughterty, L.B. Branch, P.C. Taylor, and J.M. Iacon, Concentration of dietary n-6 polyunsaturated fatty acids and human immune status, *Clin. Immunl. Immunopath. 62*: 240 (1992).

89. Barone, J., J.R. Hebert, and M.M. Reddy. Dietary fat and natural killer cell activity, *Am. J. Clin. Nutr. 50*: 861 (1989).

90. Rasmussen, L.B., B. Kiens, B.K. Pedrson, and E.A. Richter, Effects of diet and plasma fatty acid composition on immune status in elderly men, *Am. J. Clin. Nutr. 59*: 572 (1994).

91. Kelley, D.S., P.C. Taylor, G.J. Nelson, P.C. Schmidt, and B.E. Mackery, Effects of dietary arachidonic acid on human response *FASEB J. 10*: A 557 (1996).

92. Endres, S.S., N. Meydani, R. Ghorbani, R. Schindler, and C.A. Dinarello, Dietary supplementation with n-3 fatty acids suppresses interleukin-2 production and mononuclear cell proliferation *J. Leukocyte Biol. 54*: 599 (1993).

93. Krammer, T.R., N. Schoene, L.W. Douglass, J.W. Judd, J.T. Ballard-Barbash, R. Taylor, P.R. Bhagawan, and P.P. Nair, Increased vitamin E intake restores fish oil induced suppressed blastogenesis of mutogen-stimulated T lymphocytes, *Am. J. Clin. Nutr. 54*: 896 (1991).

94. Meydani, S.N., S. Endres, M.M. Woods, B.R. Goldin, C. Soo, A. Morrill-Labrode, C.A. Dinarello, and S.L. Gorbach, Oral n-3 fatty acid supplementation suppresses cytokine production and lymphocyte proliferation: comparison between young and old women, *J. Nutr. 121*: 547 (1991).

95. Kelley, D.S., G.J. Nelson, L.B. Branch, P.C. Taylor, Y.M. Rivera, and P.C. Schmidt, Salmon diet and human immune status, *Eur. J. Clin. Nutr. 46*: 4039 (1992).

96. Kremer, J.M., D.A. Lawrence, G.F. Petillo, L.L. Litts, P.M. Mullay, R.I. Rynes, R.P. Stocker, N. Pirhami, N.S. Greenstein, B.R. Fuchs, A. Mathur, D.R. Robinson, R.I. Sperling, and J. Bigaouette, Effect of high-dose fish oil on rheumatoid arthritis after stopping nonsteroidal anti-inflammatory drugs, *Arthritis Rheumat 38*: 1107 (1995).

97. Hanson, L.A., M. Hahn-Zoric, U. Wiedermann, S. Lundin, A. Dahlman-Hoglund, R. Saalman, V. Erling, U. Dahlgren, and E. Telemo, Early dietary influence on later immunocompetence, *Nutr. Rev. 54*(Suppl. 2): 23 (1996).

24
Diet, Cholesterol, and Heart Disease

I. INTRODUCTION

Diseases of the heart and circulation disorders account for a significant proportion of total morbidity and adult deaths throughout the world and especially in the industrially advanced countries. Rheumatic heart disease appears to be common in the developing countries but in most affluent societies, new cases of this disease are relatively low. Coronary heart disease (CHD), however has reached epidemic proportions in the developed nations. Mann (1) described these diseases of heart and circulation and the role of food and nutrition in their etiology and management.

II. CAUSES OF HEART AND CIRCULATION DISORDERS

An atheromatous plaque that occludes one or more coronary arteries to a varying degree is the basic pathological lesion underlying CHD; the superimposition of a thrombus or clot on the plaque often leads to occlusion of an artery. The pathogenesis of the atherosclerotic plaque and arterial thrombus involves a variety of cells and lipids, including lipoproteins, cholesterol, triacylglycerols, platelets, monocytes, endothelial cells, fibroblasts and smooth-muscle cells. Food and nutrition may influence the development of CHD by modifying one or more of these factors. Two major clinical features of CHD are *angina pectoris* characterized by pain and discomfort in the chest from exertion or stress, caused by a reduction or temporary blockage of blood flow through the coronary artery to the myocardium. The pain often passes with rest and seldom lasts for more than 15 minutes. The second major feature is coronary thrombosis (myocardial infarction) due to prolonged total occlusion of the artery, which causes infarction or death of some of the heart muscle and is associated with prolonged and often excruciating central chest pain (2).

A. Effects of Environment and Behavior

Population studies have indicated that CHD is the most common single cause of death in most industrially developed countries; e.g., about 27% of all deaths in England and Wales are reported to be the result of CHD. Approximately 60% of all fatal myocardial infarctions lead to deaths within the first hour of the attack, without giving the sufficient time for treatment to influence the prognosis (1).

Marked international/regional differences have been noticed in the rate of occurrence of CHD. In one population study of men aged 40 to 59, initially free of CHD, the annual incidence (occurrence of new cases) ranged from 15 per 100,000 in Japan to 198 per 100,000 in Finland (3). Even among the industrialized countries, mortality rates vary considerably (Table 1). Some of the variation observed between countries, however, may arise from differences in diagnostic practice

Table 1 Age-standardized Mortality form Coronary Heart Disease in 1985 in Selected Countries, Based on the Population of Europe (Rates per 100,000, Aged 30–69 Years).

Country	Males	Females	Country
N Ireland	406	142	Scotland
Scotland	398	130	N. Ireland
Finland	390	125	U.S.S.R
U.S.S.R.	349	105	Hungary
Czechoslavakia	346	104	Ireland
Ireland	339	101	Czechoslavakia
Hungary	326	94	New Zealand
England and Wales	318	94	England and Wales
New Zealand	296	80	USA
Norway	266	79	Finland
Australia	247	76	Australia
Sweden	243	56	Sweden
USA	235	55	Norway
Canada	230	54	Poland
FRG	204	52	FRG
Switzerland	140	33	Italy
Italy	136	30	Switzerland
Spain	104	24	Spain
France	94	20	France
Japan	38	13	Japan

Source: Ref. 1.

and coding of death certificates. Numerous studies using comparable methods have shown that real differences do exist in the frequency of CHD. In Europe, France, Italy, and Spain appear to have significantly lower incidences of CHD than Finland, Scotland, and Northern Ireland, which have about fourfold higher rates of death due to CHD (4). These variations between countries may be chiefly the effects of environmental and behavioral differences among the people of different countries. People who have migrated from a low-risk country, such as Japan, to a high-risk country, such as the United States, tend to have the rate of CHD approaching that of the host country, although there are some reports showing just the reverse—e.g., Finns living in Sweden have apreciably lower rates of CHD than those in their country of origin. Stamler (5) noted that in the United Kingdom, where CHD rates are much higher in Scotland and Northern Ireland than in England, CHD risk depended on the country of residence at the time of death rather than the country of birth.

Major charges in the CHD rates of many countries have taken place during recent times. Male populations in many European countries, Australia and New Zealand showed an increase in CHD rates during the period 1952–1967, with continued increase in eastern Europe during 1970–1985, whereas in nearly all western European countries, North America, and Oceania (Australia and New Zealand), CHD rates declined appreciably during 1970–1985. In most countries, except for those of eastern Europe, the CHD rates in women have been declining, especially in countries where preventive efforts are being made, indicating that CHD is preventable if its causes can be noticed in time and modified (3–6).

Accumulated evidence thus far has clearly shown that patients with high plasma total and LDL cholesterol levels are at higher risk of developing CHD, and that the risk of CHD is decreased following the lowering of serum LDL cholesterol. In response to these findings, the National Cholesterol Education Program (NCEP) has published specific guidelines for lowering serum LDL cholesterol concentrations. The NCEP has suggested screening individuals by measuring plasma cholesterol levels and recommending decreased intake of saturated fat. However, having a high blood cholesterol level (hypercholesterolemia) is only one of several metabolic abnormalities that increase the risk of heart disease. It is now known that significant risk exists in populations and individuals without elevated serum LDL cholesterol concentrations. Studies of Asian Indians dwelling in London have demonstrated that these populations have a death rate from CHD approximately 50% higher than the British national average, which is already one of the higher rates in the world—this despite the fact that the plasma total cholesterol levels of Asian Indians were actually lower. In addition, Indians in northwest London were found to have lower dietary intake of saturated fat and a higher intake of polyunsaturated fat than the British average. The high rates of heart disease in Asian Indians now have been attributed to their higher blood insulin levels (hyperinsulinemia), higher blood triglyceride levels (hypertriglyceridemia), and lower blood HDL cholesterol levels than the British nationals. All these metabolic abnormalities have been identified as risk factors for CHD, and. their presence in Asian Indians is strongly related to the high prevalence of heart disease in this ethnic group (1).

These same risk factors also apply to individuals of European descent; e.g., data from Framingham, Mass., have shown that if the total cholesterol level is low (less than 200 mg/100 ml), and the HDL cholesterol level is also low (less than 40 mg/100 ml), then the risk of heart attack within the next 4 years is as great as if the total cholesterol level were more than 260 mg/100 ml. These high-risk individuals with low IIDL cholesterol would be missed by screening and treatment programs that focus only on total and LDL cholesterol levels (6).

Data from recent prospective studies have also confirmed that hypertriglyceridemia is a primary risk factor for heart disease in women. The results of the Paris prospective study have indicated that triglyceride levels can be a significant, independent predictor of death from CHD in subjects with total cholesterol levels lower than 220 mg/100 ml, as well as in subjects with impaired glucose tolerance or diabetes. Gerald M. Reaven of Palo Alto, California, a nationally recognized expert in both diabetes and heart disease, has suggested that a cluster of risk factors tends to occur in individuals, and the underlying defect may be resistance to insulin-stimulated glucose uptake. The hyperinsulinemic individual with either normal or impaired glucose tolerance, in general, tends to have high triglyceride levels and blood pressure, and lower HDL cholesterol levels. This cluster of risk factors has been referred to as "Syndrome X," to emphasize the existence of an entity that may have an important role in the etiology of CHD. Dr. Reaven has further suggested that a substantial proportion of risk is not just linked to high LDL cholesterol levels but is also related to a series of associated abnormalities of carbohydrate and lipoprotein metabolism and blood pressure regulation (1).

Knowledge of an individual's "cholesterol count" will not necessarily serve to identify all subjects at increased risk for development of heart disease; heart attacks may occur in individuals with cholesterol levels under 200 mg/100 ml—a value that would not be considered to be high by NCEP guidelines in an otherwise healthy individual. Also, the public health measures to reduce the risk through dietary changes, aimed at lowering serum LDL cholesterol levels, need to be reconsidered for people whose metabolic abnormalities require another intervention—e.g., the advised "prudent diet," which replaces saturated fat by carbohydrate, will lead to a fall in the LDL cholesterol level but will tend to increase serum glucose, insulin, and triglyceride concentrations and cause a fall in HDL cholesterol concentration. The advocacy of this "prudent diet" in individuals who already are insulin resistant and glucose intolerant, and have high triglyceride and insulin and low HDL cholesterol levels, can be questioned. In this situation, replacing saturated fat with monounsaturated and polyunsaturated fat would seem more useful dietary advice (1).

Thus, increases in serum total and LDL cholesterol levels are important in the etiology of CHD, but increasing evidence indicates that a cluster of associated changes in carbohydrate and lipoprotein metabolism and blood pressure control are equally important. The hither-to-followed narrow approach of focusing on hypercholesterolemia at the expense of other metabolic processes in efforts to reduce morbidity and mortality from CHD will no longer be appropriate for all people at risk (1).

Antioxidants, which function chiefly by protecting us and our food supply from the ravages of oxygen, are now being considered as agents in the prevention of CHD, cancer, and other diseases, usually chronic types. Dietary supplementation of beta-carotene may help to resist the development of CHD. This may be described as use of nutrients as drugs (nutraceuticals). "Antioxidants and CHD" is an exciting new area of research that shows much promise. Much evidence available supports the idea that lipid oxidation products are damaging to coronary arteries and that antioxidants can help to prevent such damage, which is the forerunner to atherosclerosis and CHD. It now appears that LDL must first undergo oxidation before plaque accumulations can occur. Because LDL is the primary carrier of fatsoluble vitamins, it seems logical that antioxidant vitamin supplementation can fortify LDL with antioxidant power to resist autoxidation. Enough epidemiological evidence supports the hypothesis that elevated dietary and serum levels of antioxidants are associated with decreased CHD risk (3–6).

Platelets, the blood-clotting agents, create blood clots that trigger heart attacks by blocking arteries with plaques. Antioxidants such as vitamin E may reduce the tendency of platelets to form clots.

The risks of antioxidant supplementation are virtually nonexistent, provided some knowledge and common sense is applied. People taking extremely high levels of antioxidants may be occasionally at risk for various disagreeable effects. For example, administration of high levels of vitamin E can exacerbate blood coagulation defects in vitamin K–deficient individuals, including those who are given a vitamin K antagonist as medication to decrease chances for clots and ongoing risk of CHD. Also, high amounts of vitamin C may pose a risk for those who tend to overstore iron (hemochromatosis). Vitamin C can inhibit copper absorption. Conditions suggesting the use of supplemental antioxidants are smoking, living in a smoggy environment, and a familial risk of CHD and/or cancer. However, more scientic data would be required to establish the positive effects of antioxidants in the prevention of various diseases (1–2).

B. Effects of Dietary Factors

Data relating dietary factors directly to CHD are sparse, although much indirect evidence shows a close relationship between CHD rates and food intake or diet. Early attempts to investigate dietary determinants of CHD rates, based on national food consumption data, the balance sheets of the Food and Agriculture Organization, or more reliable household food surveys conducted in the United Kingdom, showed positive association of CHD with saturated fat, sucrose, animal protein, and coffee and negative correlations with flour (and other complex carbohydrates) and vegetables. Recent studies conducted in the United States, the United Kingdom, Australia, New Zealand, and Iceland (6–10) have shown a downward trend of CHD rates in relation to dietary changes. Associations between falling CHD rates in relation to changes in foods and nutrients in these countries are apparent. However, in view of the strong correlations (positive and negative) among different dietary constituents, it is difficult to be sure which dietary factor is mainly involved or indeed whether dietary change is simply occurring in parallel with some other more important environmental factor, e.g., increasing physical activity and reduction in cigarette smoking.

Keys and associates noted strongest correlations between CHD death rates and the percentage of energy derived from saturated fat, after measuring food consumption by people in 16 defined cohorts in seven countries (3,10). Weaker inverse associations were noticed between percentages of energy derived from mono- and polyunsaturated fat and CHD; and total fat was not significantly correlated with CHD death rate. Among other risk factors for CHD investigated in this study, only cholesterol and blood pressure appeared to explain the geographical variation, suggesting that it is mainly the nutrition-related factors that determine the presence of high CHD rates. Evidence obtained in this study indicated that the degree of risk conferred by factors not specifically related to nutrition is strongly influenced by the nutrition-related factors, as illustrated by the powerful relationship between cigarette smoking and CHD in the United States and Europe.

Meager data are available to show a relationship between the dietary intake of individuals within a country and subsequent CHD risk. In one such study with a 7-day weighed dietary record, employing male bank staff, bus drivers, and bus conductors in London, it was found that those with a high intake of dietary fiber from cereals had a lower rate of CHD subsequently than the rest of the group. A high-energy intake, apparently reflecting higher physical activity and to a lesser extent, a high ratio of polyunsaturated to saturated fatty acids in the diet, were also features of men who subsequently remained free of CHD (11).

Shekelle et al. (12) noted an inverse correlation between CHD mortality and consumption of polyunsaturated fatty acids and a positive association between CHD mortality and dietary cholesterol and with the Keys score among the employees of the Western Electric Company in Chicago. However, no association was found between CHD and saturated fat intake considered in isolation.

An appreciable reduction of CHD risk in vegetarians (Seventh Day Adventists and people shopping in health food stores) was noted, taking into account possible confounding factors such as cigarette smoking. However, it was not possible to determine which aspects of the vegetarian diet might be protective, or indeed whether the protective effect could be explained by some associated but unstudied factor (13,14).

Miettinen et al. (15) and Riemersma et al. (16) reported that low levels of long chain polyunsaturated fatty acids of both n-3 and the n-6 series in the blood and adipose tissue are associated with an increased risk of subsequent CHD. The composition of the tissue lipid reflects the type of fat eaten. According to Mann (1), such studies provide reinforcement for the importance of the nature of dietary fat in etiology of CHD, although dietary fat alone cannot be the only epidemiological determinant.

The potential important protective effects of antioxidants and certain trace elements obtained through fruits and vegetables in reducing CHD rates have been stressed (17). It is difficult to establish, even with most sophisticated epidemiological studies, the relationship between foods nutrients and CHD (1).

III. NUTRITIONAL DETERMINANTS OF CARDIOVASCULAR RISK FACTORS

Studies on pathological processes underlying CHD and identification of individuals at risk have revealed that there is no single cause of the disease. Detailed examination of the role of diet in the etiology of CHD may lead to better understanding of the characteristics that put individuals at particular risk of developing CHD. The term *risk factor* has been used loosely to describe features of lifestyle and behavior as well as physicochemical attributes predicting the possibility of developing CHD. Potential risk factors can be identified by comparing people who have developed CHD with healthy control subjects (case-control studies) and can be confirmed through cohort studies in which these factors are measured in a large group of apparently healthy people who are followed prospectively, relating the presence, absence, or degree of each factor to the risk of

Table 2 Risk Factors for Coronary Heart Disease

Irreversible factors
Masculine gender
Increasing age
Genetic traits, including monogenic and polygenic disorders of lipid metabolism
Body build
Potentially reversible factors
Cigarette smoking
Hyperlipidemia: increased levels of cholesterol and triglyceride
Low levels of high-density lipoprotein (HDL)
Obesity
Hypertension
Physical inactivity
Hyperglycemia and diabetes
Increased thrombosis: increased hemostatic factors and enhanced platelet aggregation
Psychological factors
Low socioeconomic class
Stressful situations
Coronary-prone behavior patterns: type A behavior
Geographic factors
Climate and season: cold weather
Soft drinking water

Source: Ref. 1.

developing CHD. A list of some of the most important risk factors is given in Table 2. Weatherall et al. (2) have reviewed the irreversible psychological and geographic factors and Mann (1) reviewed the potentially reversible dietary factors, on which the following discussion is primarily based.

A. Hyperlipidemia

Hyperlipidemia is a term used to describe raised levels of blood lipids, found in lipoproteins in the form of cholesterol and triacylglycerol, placing individuals at higher risk of CHD in two ways: (a) a relatively small proportion of people inherit a disorder of lipid metabolism, with an exceptionally high CHD risk, and (b) a large number of people (about one-half the adult population in high-risk countries) have a slight to moderately high risk because of their higher-than-normal blood lipids levels. The latter probably results from an interaction between polygenic and environmental (largely dietary) factors (1).

The blood cholesterol level among peoples of different countries, regions, and races varies widely; the mean serum cholesterol from New Guinea to east Finland ranges from 2.6 to 7.0 mmol/1 (100–270 mg/100 ml) among people of the same age and sex group (18). No other blood constituent varies so much between different people as cholesterol, thus it appears to be the most important determinant of the geographic variation in the distribution of the risk factor for CHD. Keys (3), in the seven-country study, showed that median cholesterol values were highly correlated with CHD death ($r = 0.8$), accounting for 64% of the variance in the CHD death rates among the cohorts. Even among individuals within a population group, the association between blood cholesterol level and CHD death rate is equally strong, as shown in over 20 prospective studies in different countries. The total plasma cholesterol was shown to be related to the rate of development of CHD, the association being 'dose' related, occurring in both sexes, and being independent of all other measured risk factors. Martin et al. (19) showed that the risk of CHD varied over about fivefold in relation to the plasma cholesterol levels found in an average American population. However, there is no discernible critical value, because the risk tends to increase throughout the range, although the absolute risk associated with any given cholesterol level may vary in people living in different regions of the world.

The association of total cholesterol with CHD mortality appears to derive predominantly from the low-density lipoprotein (LDL) fraction, with which it is highly correlated. Macrophages appear to take up the oxidized form of LDL and deposit it in the atheromatic plaque. It has been suggested that inhibition of LDL oxidation through dietary intakes of antioxidants, vitamins C and E, and carotenoids may protect LDL cholesterol against oxidation and help to slow the progression of the atherosclerotic lesions (17,20). Mann (1) has cautioned about the possible confusion in research and clinical practice arising from measurement of cholesterol immediately after a myocardial infarction, because levels tend to fall and readings may be falsely low for up to 3 months after this event.

The mean cholesterol levels in adult men and women tend to be similar, with slightly higher total and LDL cholesterol levels in men, up to age 50, after which these levels in women rise higher than in men. Hormonal factors have been implicated but there is no convincing explanation for these sex differences, nor it is clear to what extent they account for the differences in CHD rates in men and women (21).

1. Effects of Diet on Cholesterol Levels

Dietary factors determine total body cholesterol level via an effect on LDL. Also overweight and obesity are strikingly correlated to both total and LDL cholesterol; there is a gradual increase in cholesterol with increasing body mass index. In the seven-country study, Keys (3) noted that mean concentrations of cholesterol of each group were highly correlated with percentage of energy derived from saturated fatty acids, and even more strikingly related to the intake of polyunsaturated fatty acids. Careful feeding studies conducted in the 1950s and 1960s have confirmed that plasma cholesterol was raised by saturated fatty acids (SFA) and lowered by polyunsaturated fatty acids (PUFA). Various formulas were developed to calculate the change in cholesterol indicated to be the result of changing the proportions of SFA and PUFA in the diet. Keys et al. (22) suggested that SFAs raise plasma cholesterol twice as much as PUFAs lower it, as follows:

Plasma cholesterol (mmol/l) = 0.035 (2 S – P)

where S and P represent the changes in percentages of dietary energy derived from SFAs and PUFAs, respectively.

In practice, however the formula provides only a rough prediction of the changes that occur, partly because of the genetic variations in response among individuals.

Early studies conducted in 1960s and 1970s indicated that palmitate (C16:0), myristate (C14: 0), and laurate (C12:0) raised plasma cholesterol more than fats with either shorter or longer chain fatty acids. Bonanome and Grundy (23) reestablished that stearate (C18: 0) consumption is associated with lower levels of total and LDL cholesterol than palmitate (C16:0), and indeed the cholesterol-lowering effect of stearate was similar to that seen with oleate.

According to Mann (1), the effects of unsaturated fatty acids on total and LDL cholesterol are rather more complex than suggested by early research work. Experiments with monounsaturated fatty acids (MUFA) have mainly involved oleic acid (C18:1), which appeared to lower cholesterol about the same extent as the n-6 PUFAs from plant sources, especially linoleic acid (C18:2). The n-3 PUFAs predominating in marine oils (eicosapentenoic acid [C 20: 5] and docosahexenoic acid [C 22:6]) had variable effects on the LDL cholesterol of healthy individuals; large quantities decrease LDL as a result of a reduction in very low-density lipoprotein (VLDL).

Most unsaturated fatty acids have double bonds in the *cis* form, but a small proportion of the fatty acids in animal foods such as meat and dairy products exist in *trans* form. Occasionally *cis*-unsaturated fatty acids shift to the *trans* form during processing, making the oil more solid, with a higher melting point. *Trans* fatty acids appear mostly as MUFAs, and the *trans* isomers of oleic acid (the main *trans* fatty acids of manufactured food such as margarine) appear to raise LDL cholesterol to the same extent as the saturated fatty acids (24).

The ratio of polyunsaturated to saturated fatty acids (P/S) has been widely employed to demonstrate the cholesterol-lowering potential of the diet; low P/S ratios of about 0.2 are often associated with high cholesterol levels and a high risk of CHD. Higher P/S ratios of around 0.8 are found in persons living in Mediterranean countries and are associated with more favorable cholesterol levels and decreased CHD risk. However, P/S ratio may be an unacceptable oversimplication of the problem (1). Ulbricht and Southgate (25) suggested that P/S ratio should be replaced by an index of atherogenicity (IA), which involves an inversion of the P/S ratio, so that IA would be highest for the most atherogenic dietary components. The lower-chain-length saturated fatty acids and strearic acid are omitted from S, and P includes MUFAs, so that their proposed ratio becomes (25).

$$IA = \frac{aS^1 + bS^{11} + cS^{111}}{dp + eM + fM^1}$$

Where S^1 = C12:0, S^{11} = C14: 0 and S^{111} = C 16:0; P = sum of *n*-6 and *n*-3 PUFAs, M = oleic acid (C18:1) and M^1 = sum of other MUFA, a-f are empirical constants, with b set at 4 because C14:0 appears to have the most powerful effects in elevating LDL, and a,c,d,e and f set at unity in the absence of firm evidence to assign other values.

The indices of atherogenicity for some foods and diets are shown in Table 3. These indices, however, do not take into account the effects of *trans* MUFAs, nor the fact that *n*-3 and *n*-6 fatty acids do not have comparable effects on LDL. Moreover a detailed breakdown of fat composition of foods is often not available in the food composition tables used in many countries.

The effects of different dietary fatty acids on cholesterol levels (Table 4) indicate that both total and plasma LDL cholesterol levels fall when the dietary energy provided through fats is reduced. It is not known whether this effect is entirely owing to a reduction in the saturated fatty acid intake: controversy exists regarding the significance of dietary cholesterol as a determinant of plasma cholesterol in view of contrasting effects of extreme cholesterol intakes (e.g., 800 mg and 100 mg/day) on the plasma cholesterol levels, in the context of a diet relatively high in saturated fatty acids. Keys formula has been thus modified to include changes in dietary cholesterol as follows:

$$\Delta \text{Cholesterol in mmol/1} = 0.035 (2 \Delta S - \Delta P) + 0.08\Delta \sqrt{chol/MJ}$$

where chol/MJ is the cholesterol intake in mg/MJ.

Some individuals are thought to be hyperresponders to dietary cholesterol, i.e., they show exaggerated increase in plasma cholesterol when dietary cholesterol is increased in contrast to the hyporesponders, who show little or no response. Very high intake of dietary cholesterol down-regulate LDL receptors that are necessary for LDL to be internalized and broken down in cells, implying that dietary cholesterol does have an important influence on blood levels. However, the majority of these experiments have involved extreme doses of dietary cholesterol, instead of comparing within the usual range of intakes, when increased intake may be readily balanced by inhibited endogenous production. Data are not sufficient to show that dose-response gradient occurs over the usual range of intake found in the affluent societies (200–500 mg cholesterol/day). Recent research has shown that when saturated fatty acid intake is decreased, the effects of dietary cholesterol on plasma cholesterol are minimal and there is little evidence for the hyperresponse

Table 3 Indices of Atherogenicity (IA) and Thrombogenicity (IT) for Some Foods and Diets

Food/Diet	Index of atherogenicity (IA)	Index of thrombogenicity (IT)
Coconut oil	13.63	6.18
Milk, butter, cheese	2.03	2.07
Palm oil	0.88	1.74
Lamb:		
Roast breast, lean and fat	1.00	1.58
Chop, lean only	1.00	1.33
Beef:		
Topside roast, lean	0.72	1.06
Raw, minced	0.72	1.27
Grilled sausages	0.74	1.39
Pork:		
Roast leg, lean	0.60	1.37
Grilled sausages	0.58	1.35
Fried streaky bacon, lean and fat	0.69	1.66
Hard margarine (vegetable oils only)	0.56	1.26
Stewed ox liver	0.41	0.82
Chicken, roast meat and skin	0.50	0.95
PUFA margarine	0.35	0.53
Olive oil	0.14	0.32
Sunflower oil	0.07	0.28
Raw mackerel	0.28	0.16
Eskimo diet	0.39	0.28
Danish diet	1.29	1.51
British diet	0.93	1.21

Source: Ref. 1.

phenomenon. Average intakes of around 300 mg cholesterol/day thus are not expected to influence total and plasma LDL cholesterol in any significant manner (26–28).

Carbohydrates per se have little direct effect on total and LDL cholesterol levels, although increasing carbohydrates in the diet causes a reduction of saturated fatty acids, which in turn are associated with a decrease in this lipoprotein fraction. Soluble dietary fiber in the form of nonstarch polysaccharide (NSP) is though to reduce total and LDL cholesterol. NSP derived from *guar* gum, oat bran, and dried beans has been used in experiments (29), although there is no evidence to show that these foods have any special merits over other foods high in soluble fiber, such as barley and rye products, lentils, chickpeas, and high-pectin fruits. Also, the results of these studies have not been entirely consistent; some show no effects of dietary soluble fiber. Perhaps very high intakes of soluble fiber are required to produce an effect on LDL cholesterol, and soluble fiber exerts its effects only when the fat consumption of the diet has also been changed. Also soluble fiber may exert its effects by enhancing satiety and reducing the intake of saturated fatty acids and other high-energy nutrients (30). Thus, at least under certain specific circumstances, soluble fiber does have an effect on total and LDL cholesterol, but its effect appears to be almost certainly less than that of dietary fat. Leadbetter et al. (31) showed that at least in normal subjects, the effects of fiber and fat modification are additive. Judd and Truswell (32) proposed that soluble fiber may act like the lipid-lowering drug cholestyramine and promote sterol excretion and

Table 4 Dietary Determinants of Plasma Lipids

1. Unfavorable or possibly unfavorable effects	
Saturated fatty acids (SFA) (especially C12:0, C14:0, C16:0)	↑↑↑LDL cholesterol
trans monounsaturated fatty acids (MUFA)	↑↑↑LDL, HDL cholesterol
Dietary cholesterol	↑LDL cholesterol when fed in large amounts with high SFA intake
Fiber-depleted complex carbohydrates[a]	↑VLDL and triglyceride, HDL if carbohydrate makes up 60% or more total energy
Sucrose[a]	↑VLDL and triglyceride if taken in large amounts (more than 140 g/day) and with high SFA
2. Beneficial effects	
cis monounsaturated fatty acids (MUFA) (C18:1)	↓↓LDL cholesterol
Soluble dietary fiber	↓LDL cholesterol
3. Beneficial as well as possibly unfavorable effects	
n-6 polyunsaturated fatty acids (C18:2)	↓↓LDL cholesterol, HDL if taken in large amounts
n-3 polyunsaturated fatty acids (C20:5, C22:6)	↓↓VLDL cholesterol
	↑LDL especially in hyperlipidemia

[a]Effects probably transient.
↓↓↓ or ↑↑↑ appecialbe change, ↓↓ or ↑↑ modest change, ↓ or ↑ some change.
Source: Ref. 1.

LDL-receptor-mediated removal. Insoluble fiber has not been reported to influence lipid metabolism appreciably.

The effects of dietary protein on lipids and lipoproteins have not been well established. Descovich et al. (33) noted that complete replacement of mixed animal proteins by a soybean protein preparation decreased plasma cholesterol substantially in normal and hypercholesterolemic subjects. Van Raaij et al. (34) however, reported smaller effects of proteins on LDL cholesterol.

Despite the influence of dietary manipulations on total and LDL cholesterol and correlations between dietary variables and cholesterol in cross-cultural comparisons, it has not been possible to establish a relationship between reported intake of macronutrients and dietary fiber and plasma cholesterol level within a population. This has been often attributed to the lack of appropriate methods for assessing dietary intake in the population studies. Also, within the relatively narrow range of dietary intakes observed in affluent societies, polygenic determinants of lipid metabolism override the differences due to dietary factors. Thorogood et al. (35) found that vegetarians and vegans, as groups, had lower total and LDL cholesterol than non-vegetarians. These authors, in a subsequent study of vegetarians, vegans, fish-eaters who do not eat meat, and carnivores in Britain, observed an association between total and LDL cholesterol and intakes of saturated fatty acids and cholesterol as well as an inverse relationship between these lipids and PUFA and dietary fiber, over a wide range of intake within a single population.

Sindhurani and Rajamohan (36) reported the hypolipidemic effect of hemicellulose component of coconut fiber. The neutral detergent fiber (NDF) isolated from coconut kernel was digested with cellulase and hemicellulase and the residual fiber rich in hemicellulose, (without cellulose) and cellulose (without hemicellulose) was fed to rats and compared with a fiber-free group. The results indicated that hemicellulose-rich fiber showed decreased concentration of total cholesterol LDL + VLDL cholesterol and increased HDL cholesterol, whereas cellulose-rich fiber had no significant effect. The activity of HMG (hydroxymethyl glutaryl) coenzyme A increased, along with an increase in incorporation of labeled acetate into free cholesterol. Rats fed hemicellulose-rich coconut fiber had lower concentration of triglycerides and phospholipids and lower release of lipoproteins into circulation. The concentration of hepatic bile acids also increased, along with an increased excretion of fecal sterols and bile acids. The results of this study indicated that the hemicellulose component of coconut fiber was responsible for the observed hypolipidemic effects. Somochowiec and Czerny (37) treated 25 atherosclerotic patients with allicin (metabolite of *Allium sativum*) in combination with essential phospholipids (EPL). The hypolipidemic effects of allicin were increased with EPL. A direct-lipid lowering action and a carrier function of these phospholipids for allicin have been discussed (37).

Dwivedi (38) listed plants showing cardioprotective, antiplatelet, hypolipidemic, hypotensive, and hypoglycemic activities. Cardiovascular activity of the following plants has been discussed: *Allium sativum, Cicer arietinum, Commiphora mukul, Coleus forskohlii, Curcuma longa, Emblica officinalis, Inula racemosa, Ocimum sanctum, Pterocarpus marsupium, Terminalia arjuna,* and *Trigonella foenum-graecum.*

Muriana et al. (39) noted that *trans*-bilayer movement of erythrocyte membrane cholesterol is impaired in patients with essential hypertension. This inherited disorder also involves environmental factors. Dietary fats play a role in the prevention and/or treatment of this abnormality. Muriana et al. (39) tested this hypothesis by using a diet (with 30% energy from fat) rich in olive (*Olea europaea*) oil or in high-oleic sunflower (*Helianthus annuus*) oil as natural sources of monounsaturated fatty acids (MUFAs). The influence of these oils on the movement of cholesterol into the lipid bilayer of the erythrocyte membrane was determined after a 4-week period. It was observed that olive oil was helpful in normalizing the impaired transbilayer movement of membrane cholesterol in erythrocytes of eight normocholesterolemic and eight hypercholesterolemic hypertensive patients. However, the effects could not be attributed exclusively to the content of MUFAs in the diet, as high oleic sunflower oil did not induce favorable changes.

Reuter et al. (40) reviewed the therapeutic effects and applications of garlic and its preparations on several human diseases, including cardiac and circulatory disorders. Of all the effects of garlic reported over the years, perhaps the most interesting are those on the heart and circulatory system. According to Reuter et al. (40), by appropriate application, garlic may protect the blood vessels from the deleterious effects of free radicals, increase capillary flow, and lower elevated blood pressure levels, meaning that development of arteriosclerosis can be prevented or an already existing condition favorably influenced. The cardiovascular effects of garlic were essentially rediscovered in the late 1960s, although garlic is an old constituent of folk medicine for treating cardiovascular problems in Asian and European countries. The antiatherosclerotic effects of garlic are based on the reduction of thrombocyte adhesiveness and aggregation. The effective constituents of garlic have been reported to significantly decrease the tendency of the platelets to aggregate and to form thrombi. In addition, fibrinolysis is enhanced, resulting in more rapid dissolution of coagulated blood, plaques, and clots. The decrease of lipoprotein circulating in the blood (LDL form) and of cholesterol occurs through increased formation of antiatherogenic HDL lipoprotein at the expense of LDL (41,42). The effects of garlic on free radicals must be considered in connection with the decreased levels of blood lipids and decreased deposition of cholesterol into the vessel walls (43,44). Blood fluidity can be maintained by eating fresh garlic or by corresponding doses of pharmaceutically manufactured garlic products (40).

Several recent studies have shown that a correlation exists between the concentration of blood lipids and the narrowing of coronary vessels. A significant correlation between serum cholesterol and the risk of heart disease in both men and women also has been demonstrated (45). A major 25-year follow-up study in the United States, Europe, and Japan has recently shown that increased serum total cholesterol levels are directly associated with enhanced CHD in all cultures (46). In several studies and reports dealing predominantly with garlic and onion preparations, it has been documented that this disease process can be stopped or even reversed by lowering the cholesterol level (47–51). The most important risk factors for developing arteriosclerosis with its secondary effects, such as myocardial infarction, stroke, and occlusive arterial disease, are hyperlipidemia and hypercholesterolemia in addition to obesity, high blood pressure, diabetes, and nicotine and alcohol abuse (40).

B. Hypertriglyceridemia (Hypertriacyglycerolemia)

Patients with myocardial infarctions tend to have higher levels of triacylglycerols and VLDLs than controls. Prospective studies have shown this to be a CHD risk factor. However, it is not known whether it is independent of other factors known to be associated with both raised levels of triacylglycerol and cardiovascular risk, e.g., obesity, hyperglycemia, hypercholesterolemia, and hypertension. Castelli (52) postulated that raised levels of triacylglycerol are linked with increased CHD risk only in the presence of decreased HDL cholesterol to a level less than 1 mmol/l. West et al. (53) noted that raised levels of triacylglycerol are especially important in determining cardiovascular risk in diabetic people. Triacylglycerol levels showed less cross-cultural variation than cholesterol levels with similar trends for age and sex, although men at all ages had higher levels of triacylglycerol than women. Increased physical activity was found to be associated with a reduction in triacylglycerol levels.

Obesity and alcoholism are the most important dietary factors influencing triacylglycerol levels. Alcohol-associated hypertriacylglycerolemia is often associated with very high alcohol intakes, but some susceptible individuals may develop appreciably raised levels of triacylglycerol even with modest intakes. Patients with lipid metabolic disorders are most likely to develop hypertriacylglycerolemia due to an excessive intake of alcohol. Banaona and Lieber (54) hypothesized that alcohol may result in hypertriacylglycerolemia by providing an increased energy intake and possibly by stimulating hepatic synthesis of triacylglycerol. The latter mechanism is also thought to increase fasting triacylglycerol levels when either starch or sugar is added to an experimental diet, when an appreciable proportion of the usual fat intake is isoenergetically replaced by fiber-depleted carbohydrate, or when sucrose or fructose are given in substantial quantities to replace energy previously provided by complex carbohydrates. This effect is seen only when substantial quantities of sucrose (140 g or more) are consumed, and when a relatively high proportion of dietary fat is derived from saturated fatty acids. Evidence indicates that such adaptation may occur and that the effect of these manipulations of dietary carbohydrate do not persist longer than 6 weeks (55). Eicosapentenoic and docosahexenoic acids can appreciably reduce triacylglycerol levels (56).

Several genetically determined well-defined disorders of lipid metabolism are characterized by raised levels of cholesterol and/or triacylglycerol that are distinguished from the polygenic form of hyperlipidemia. Lewis (57) has described the characteristics of most of these important inherited disorders. Familial hypercholesterolemia is characterized by marked elevation of total and LDL cholesterol resulting from a reduction in LDL receptors on the cell surfaces, an autosomal dominant trait, with cholesterol-filled xanthomas in exterior tendons (on hands) and a very high risk of premature CHD. About 85% of untreated males with this disorder will have myocardial infarctions before the age of 60 years. Familial combined hyperlipidemia is characterized by enhanced LDL and VLDL levels, resulting from their increased production. This condition is also associated with a great risk of cardiovascular disease. Despite drug treatment, dietary modification remains extremely important in the management of these disorders. Evidence indicates that even in these clearly inherited disorders, environmental factors, including dietary factors, influence the pretreatment lipid levels. It is found that the levels of total and LDL cholesterol in people with heterozygous familial hypercholesterolemia in China, for example, are lower than in people with the same condition in affluent Western countries. This difference has been attributed to dietary factors, among others (58).

Table 5 Levels of High-Density Lipoprotein (HDL) Cholesterol and Subsequent Incidence of Coronary Heart Disease (CHD)

HDL cholesterol		
Mg/dl	mmol/l.	CHD rate/1000 population
All levels		77
Less than 25	less than 0.65	177
25–44	0.65–1.38	103
45–64	1.40–1.64	54
65–74	1.64–1.90	25

Source: Ref. 59.

C. High-Density Lipoproteins (HDL)

Women have been found to have higher HDL levels than men and a lower risk of CHD (1). Data reported in Table 5 indicate that people with high levels of HDL had an appreciably lower rate of CHD. Gorden et al. (59) produced similar evidence to show a gradient effect. It has been further shown that an increment of 0.026 mmol/l (1 mg/100 ml) is associated with a 2% to 3% reduction in CHD (60). Physical activity and cigarette smoking appear to influence HDL levels favorably and unfavorably, respectively, although age does not have any marked effect on HDL levels.

Dietary factors also do not have a profound influence on HDL levels. However, regular fish eaters (who do not also eat meat) are reported to have significantly higher HDL levels than vegetarians, vegans, and regular meat eaters (35). Grundy (61) found that increasing carbohydrate up to about 60% of total energy from the more usual levels in the affluent societies (around 45%) was associated with a small but significant decrease in HDL in short-term studies. The HDL-lowering effect of high-carbohydrate diets may be prevented or decreased if the carbohydrate is high in soluble fiber (62). Very high intakes of polyunsaturated fatty acids with a P/S ratio of more than 1.0 have been found to decrease HDL levels (63). This effect is seen more with diets high in *trans* MUFAs than *cis* ones (64).

Effects of dietary factors on the subfractions of HDL have not been investigated fully. According to Mann (1), HDL_2 is the subfraction that is inversely related to CHD, and dietary modifications are thought to alter mainly the HDL_3 fraction, which is probably not related to CHD risk factor. The reported positive association between moderate levels of alcohol intake and HDL (65) also need further confirmation.

D. Apoproteins and Lipoprotein (a)

Protein components of the plasma lipoproteins, known as apoproteins, maintain the structural integrity of lipoproteins and are involved in receptor recognition and enzyme regulation (1). Apoproteins are classed A, B, C, D, and E, with subclasses. Apoprotein B (Apo B), constituting around 90% of LDL protein, is also a major protein of chylomicrons and VLDL and is believed to have a vital function in the metabolism of these lipoproteins (LDL, IDL, and VLDL). Also, ApoB levels appear to be predictive of subsequent CHD, an effect found to be independent of total cholesterol levels. Dietary factors that influence LDL also have an effect on ApoB levels and the latter are thought to explain some of the genetic variations in LDL response to changes in dietary fat. ApoA, the major protein of HDL, which determines its production and metabolism, is very strongly correlated with HDL cholesterol measured on a stable diet and explains the variation in HDL response to changes in dietary fat (from high to low fat diet). The interactive effects between diet and apoproteins need further investigation (66).

Lipoprotein(a) [Lp(a)], which is assembled from LDL and apolipoprotein (a), may vary in its concentration from near zero to more than 1000 mg/l in the plasma. Rosengren et al. (67) have put forward convincing evidence to show a strong independent association between Lp(a) and CHD. However, the plasma levels of Lp(a) are determined more by genetics, and diet modifications have not been known to decrease serum Lp(a) concentrations (68)

IV. THROMBOGENETIC FACTORS

The clinical features of CHD cannot be described in terms of atheroma alone, and thrombogenetic factors have not been given enough attention. Arterial thrombosis certainly involves platelets, but their function has not been assessed in large-scale epidemiological studies, partly due to the lack of international standardization and the time required for the measurement of platelet function. Thus, small-scale epidemiological studies and clinical and basic nutritional studies have provided some evidence to support relationship between diet, platelets, and heart disease.

Low death rates from CHD in Eskimos living in Greenland, despite the fact that they consumed a diet high in cholesterol and total fat, have renewed the interest of the researchers. The fat in the diet of the Greenland Eskimos is derived almost exclusively from the fish and other marine foods, which contain large quantities of the n-3 fatty acids, eicosapentenoate (EPA, C 20:5) and docosahexenoate (DHA, C 22:6). Substantial evidence suggests that the low CHD incidence in Eskimos at least partly is attributable to their high intake of n-3 fatty acids (69,70).

The effects of fatty acids on thrombogenesis are complex. According to Mann (1), there are three series of prostanoids and thromboxanes that have profound and different effects on platelet function and vascular tone. Each series of prostanoids is derived from a different fatty acid as follows: (a) the first series from dihomogammalinoleic acid (DHLA), (b) the second from arachidontic acid (AA), and (c) the third from eicosapentenoic acid (EPA). Most diets contain little DHLA and AA, but significant quantities of these fatty acids, especially AA, are produced in the body from linoleic acid. When a vessel wall is injured, platelets are stimulated to release AA from their membrane phospholipids and AA is immediately converted to thromboxane A_2 (TxA_2), a potent proaggregatory and vasoconstrictive compound. Simultaneously, the endothelial cells of the arterial wall metabolize significant quantities of AA to prostacyclin (PGI$_2$), a compound exerting strong antiaggregatory and vasodilatory activity. A proper balance between TxA_2 and PGI$_2$ production is thought to be essential for normal arterial health, and an overproduction of TxA_2 is associated with an enhanced risk of thrombogenesis (71). The fatty acids of the n-3 series, EPA and DHA particularly, have a powerful antithrombogenic effect (56), and they act by inhibiting conversion of AA to TxA_2 and by facilitating the production of prostacyclin PGI$_2$, a protein inhibitor of aggregation (72,73). These effects are noticed with purified forms of fish oil fed in capsules or diets containing appreciable quantities of only fish. The fatty acids of n-6 series also decrease platelet aggregation by providing series 1 prostanoids and by increasing the fluidity of platelet membranes (74).

Along with the antithrombogenic effects of PUFAs in humans, the thrombogenic effects of the saturated fatty acids also have been investigated in laboratory animals. The consistent findings in this regard indicate that all the longer-chain saturated fatty acids (C14:0, C16:0, and C18:0) accelerate the process of thrombosis probably, by inhibiting the antiaggregatory prostacyclin (75). Stearic acid (C18:C), which has no apparent adverse effects on LDL, also has thrombogenic properties.

The P/S ratios used earlier as an indicator of thrombogenicity and atherogenicity are now regarded as an oversimplification to the extent of being misleading (1); e.g., sunflower oil, according to its P/S ratio, should be more antithrombotic than fish oil. Ulbricht and Southgate (25) also developed an index of thrombogenicity (IT), which appears to be more complex than their index of atherogenicity:

$$IT = \frac{mS^{iv}}{nM + oM^1 + p\,(n\text{-}6) + q\,(n\text{-}3) + \dfrac{n\text{-}3}{n\text{-}6}}$$

where S^{iv} = sum of C14:0, C16:0 and C18:0, n-6 = n-6 PUFA; n-3 = n-3 PUFA, M and M^1 are defined for IA, and m, n, o, p, and q are unknown empirical constants; m has arbitrarily been set at unity, n, o, and p are asigned the value of 0.5, because MUFA and n-6 PUFA are less antithrombogenic than n-3 PUFA, and has a value 3.

The denominator was devised to give fish (high in MUFA as well as n-3 PUFA) the lowest IT, and to take into account the effects of various fatty acids. The IT values of various foods and diets more or less show a similar trend as the IA values (Table 3). There are several difficulties in the routine use of IT values, warranting further research: (a) insufficient evidence to set accurate values for the constants, (b) non-accounting of possible different effects of *trans* MUFA, and (c) non-availability of detailed fatty acid composition of many foods.

Dietary factors appear to influence thrombogenesis via their effect on the blood coagulation system. The hemostasis in this system is secured by promoting production of thrombin in response to an injury, which then converts soluble fibrinogen to insoluble fibrin. A number of factors involved in coagulation, including factor VIIc and fibrinogen, are important predictors of CHD, suggesting that an inappropriately high level of coagulability may predispose an individual to accelerated thrombogenesis (76). These authors reported the determinants of the coagulation factors and characteristics associated with high and low levels of factor VIIc and fibrinogen (Table 6) (77).

Obesity and cigarette smoking appear to induce high levels of fibrinogen, and dietary factors are associated with the production of factor VII. Miller et al. (78) noted that increasing dietary fat can elevate levels of factor VII within 24 hours, suggesting that raised levels of blood cholesterol, which are strongly correlated with factor VII, are possibly not responsible for the elevation

Table 6 Characteristics Associated with Higher or Lower Than Usual Levels of Factor VIIc Activity and Fibrinogen

Factor VIIc	Fibrinogen
High levels	
Increasing age	Increasing age
Obesity	Obesity
Oral contraceptive use	Oral contraceptive use
Menopause	Menopause
Diabetes	Diabetes
High-fat diet	Smoking
	Low employment grade
Low levels	
Black ethnic group	Moderate alcohol intake
Vegetarians	

Source: Ref. 77.

of this coagulation factor, because the hypercholesterolemic effects of saturated fatty acids are not expected to manifest so rapidly. Thus, raised levels of both factor VII and blood cholesterol may be a parallel consequence of a higher intake of saturated fatty acids. Meade and North (79) recorded lower levels of a range of clotting factors, including factor VII, in groups of population eating a low-fat, high P/S ratio, and high-fiber diet. Also, the individuals changing to such a diet showed reduction in these factors. Thus, the total fat intake appears to be the predominant determinant of blood coagulation (1).

Reddy (80) has reviewed newer recombinant thrombolytic drugs such as pro-urokinase, saruplase, alteplase, K_1K_2Pu, and staphylokinase, which have shown promise in animal models of arterial and venous thrombosis and also in pilot-scale clinical studies in patients with myocardial infarction. More trials are needed to determine whether these agents show improved efficiency and fibrin specificity, with minimal bleeding tendencies. The currently used thrombolytic agents in arterial thrombosis leading to cardiovascular diseases such as myocardial infarction, stroke, and pulmonary thromboembolism include plasmogen activators to restore blood flow. The fibrinolytic system consists of an inactive proenzyme, plasminogen, which is converted by plasminogen activators to the enzyme plasmin, which degrades fibrin (80).

V. CHD, DIABETES, AND HYPERTENSION

Diabetic people with impaired glucose tolerance have been shown to have increased risk of CHD. In addition to strong genetic influences, dietary factors also have been found to play a role in the etiology of non-insulin-dependent (type 2) diabetes. Higher obesity with a body mass index of more than 30 is associated with a considerable increase in the risk of diabetes, although lesser degrees of obesity also have been found to confer some risk. However, the obesity-mediated risk is greatest in people with truncal obesity, but there is less evidence to indicate the role of specific dietary factors. Type 2 diabetes appears to be very uncommon in populations eating a high-fiber, high-carbohydrate, and low-fat diet, although there is no evidence to show that any of these dietary factors have protective effects, and that fiber depletion or a high intake of fat or sucrose in themselves are predisposing to produce diabetes. However, these factors may influence the risk of diabetes indirectly by encouraging increased energy intake (1) (see Chapter 26).

Obesity and an excessive intake of alcohol are strikingly related to blood pressure, and both weight reduction and alcohol restriction have been reported to lower blood pressure levels (81). The roles of other dietary factors, such as excessive sodium, saturated fat, coffee, and meat and low potassium and calcium, have not been well established. There is a striking relationship between systolic and diastolic blood pressures and CHD (1).

On the basis of critical reviews of 27 published studies, Gliberman (82) concluded that although there exists a relation between salt intake and blood pressure, it is not known whether salt, or cultural changes, or both are responsible for the increase in blood pressure. The Intersalt—a study involving 24-hour urinary sodium excretion, which collected data on over 10,000 people aged 20 to 59 years in 32 countries—indicated that an overall association between sodium and median blood pressure or prevalence of hypertension was less striking and statistically not significant, except for four centers with very low sodium intakes (83). These findings showed that a 100 mmol/day reduction in dietary sodium might reduce systolic blood pressure by 3.5 mm Hg and diastolic pressure by 1.5 mm Hg. The reasons for the underestimation of the relationship between dietary sodium and blood pressure are unreliability of assessing dietary intake or even a single measurement of urinary sodium, a narrow range of intakes among populations, and genetic variability (84).

Law et al. (84) analyzed data from published reports of blood pressures and sodium intakes for 24 different communities in the world and suggested that the Intersalt study may have appreciably underestimated the association of blood pressure with sodium intake, and that the association increases with age and initial blood pressure; e.g., at age 60–69 years, the estimated systolic blood pressure reduction in response to a 100 mmol/24-hr reduction in sodium intake was on average 100 mm Hg, but varied from 6 mm Hg for those on the 5th blood pressure centile to 15 mm Hg for those on the 95th centile. From the results of the intervention trials involving sodium restriction, aggregating the results of 68 crossover trials and 10 randomized controlled trials of dietary salt reduction, Law et al. (84) concluded that a reduction in salt intake by a whole Western population would decrease the incidence of stroke by 26% and of CHD by 15%. A reduction in the amount of salt added to processed foods would lower blood pressure by twice as much and could prevent as many as 70,000 deaths per year in Britain.

In the Intersalt study, urinary potassium excretion, an assured indicator of intake, was negatively correlated with blood pressure, as was the urinary Na^+/K^+ ratio (83). Despite the conflicting conclusions of the trials, pooled analysis indicated that potassium supplementation decreases blood pressure in normotensive and hypertensive subjects by an average of 5.9 and 3.4 mm Hg, respectively (85).

Vegetarians are known to have lower blood pressure than meat eaters. A series of carefully controlled studies from Perth, Western Australia, have shown that significant reductions in both systolic and diastolic pressures occurred when subjects were switched from a typical Western diet to a vegetarian diet (86). In addition to excluding meat and fish, vegetarian diets have less saturated fat and cholesterol, more dietary fiber and complex carbohydrates, and various differences with regard to micronutrients when compared with a usual diet. It is not known, however, which specific aspects of the vegetarian diet are particularly relevant in the reduction of blood pressure.

Thus, the importance of avoiding (and reducing when necessary) obesity and excessive alcohol intake has now been well established in the prevention and management of hypertension and related disorders. Salt restriction is much more important than was previously recognized (84), and even moderate salt restriction by the population at large could confer substantial public health benefits, and for patients with diagnosed hypertension, an appropriate reduction of dietary sodium should be regarded as the most important aspect of therapy. An increase in potassium may also confer significant benefit, but should be obtained through a diet rich in fruit and vegetables rather than by increasing high-potassium salt substitutes (87).

Considerable epidemiological evidence suggests that dietary changes certainly decrease CHD risk, although the most direct evidence for the benefits of dietary change should come from clinical trials that include a sufficient number of human subjects. Most recent studies have adopted a multifactorial approach in which various dietary changes are made to achieve maximum cholesterol lowering. Such changes are also likely to influence risk factors other than cholesterol. Attempts are also made to modify risk factors that are not related to the diet, e.g., cigarette smoking. The clinical trials conducted to lower cholesterol have been reviewed (1,88).

The Los Angeles Veterans Administration study, the first of the major intervention studies, with 846 male volunteers (55–89 years), showed that during 8 years of follow-up the beneficial effect of the cholesterol-lowering diet was most evident in those with high cholesterol levels at the onset of the study. An increase in noncardiovascular mortality in the experimental group indicated for the first time a possibility that cholesterol lowering might be harmful in some respects, despite the reduction in CHD (89).

In the Oslo trial (90,91), men at high CHD risk (due to smoking or higher cholesterol levels of 7.5–9.8 mmol/l) were divided in to two groups, one receiving intensive dietary education and advice to stop smoking, and the other serving as a control group. A significant reduction in total coronary events was observed with a 13% fall in cholesterol and 65% reduction in tobacco consumption, reflecting a marked improvement in total mortality. About 60% of the CHD reduction could be attributed to serum cholesterol change and 25% to smoking reduction. There were no significant differences between the two groups with regard to noncardiac causes of death. The total and saturated fat of the experimental diet was markedly reduced without any appreciable increase in *n*-6 PUFA, but fiber-rich carbohydrate was increased, which might account for the different results obtained with regard to noncardiovascular diseases.

The diet and reinfarction trial (DART) by Burr et al. (92) examined the effects of diets high in *n*-3 PUFA, by randomizing 2,033 men who had survived myocardial infarction to receive, or not to receive, advice on each of three dietary factors: a reduction in fat intake and an increase in the P/S ratio; an increase in fatty fish intake; and an increase in cereal fiber within a short follow-up period of 2 years. The group advised to eat fatty fish had a 29% reduction in all causes of mortality compared with other groups. The other two diets were not associated with significant reduction in mortality, but fat modification achieved a 3% to 4% reduction in serum cholesterol. It is possible that diets aimed to reduce atherogenicity are likely to take longer to show beneficial effects than those aimed to reduce thrombogenicity.

The lifestyle heart trial (93) was an attempt to study the effects of lifestyle change on coronary atherosclerosis, rather than morbidity and mortality. Subjects who were randomized to a strict low-fat vegetarian diet and advised to stop smoking and increase physical activity, and given stress-management training, showed a striking trend toward regression of coronary narrowing, compared to the control group. However, these diets were extremely low in fat (6.8% of dietary energy), and hence not appropriate for dietary recommendations.

Two large multifactorial trials (Multiple Risk Factor Intervention Trial Research Group 1982) (94) and WHO collaborative trial (95) showed no difference between treated and control groups, which may be attributed to negligible difference in cholesterol reduction achieved through intervention in these studies. Also, the two countries participating in the WHO study that did achieve risk factor reduction (Italy and Belgium) showed reduction in all causes of mortality as well as CHD. Peto et al. (96) pointed out that in all these studies, especially the smaller ones, the results are subject to a considerable margin of error.

Several studies have shown an increase in some non cardiac causes of mortality; as a result, total mortality was not decreased significantly (97). A possibility that cholesterol lowering diets, especially those high in PUFA, might increase the risk of cancer was first indicated by the Los Angeles study. PUFA are liable to peroxidation and diets very high in these fatty acids may paradoxically actually initiate cancer or CHD. There is no evidence to confirm this hypothesis and a meta-analysis of several primary prevention trials also found no convincing evidence of increased cancer risk (98). Nevertheless, there are no populations that consume high amounts of *n*-6 PUFA, such as were used in some clinical trials. Also, owing to an increased risk of gallstones in people taking a diet high in PUFA (P/S ratio of 1.5 or more), such high intakes would not be recommended. According to Lewis et al., (99), there is no evidence for a usual association between low cholesterol levels and noncardiac mortality. Although most authorities consider that the diets currently recommended for reducing CHD risk (8–9% cholesterol reduction) are not associated with any appreciable risk of noncardiac mortality, these diets should be reserved for those with particularly high cholesterol levels, who are likely to benefit most from cholesterol reduction, and not for the general population (1,97).

VI. NUTRITIONAL STRATEGIES AND RECOMMENDATIONS

It has widely been accepted that the high CHD rates prevailing in most countries call for nutritional strategies to decrease the frequency and extent of CHD risk factors. The nutritional approach primarily aims at decreasing both atherogenic and thrombogenic risk factors by reducing obesity, lowering total and LDL cholesterol and triacylglycerol levels, increasing HDL cholesterol level, lowering blood pressure, and reducing platelet aggregation. Despite the fact that the dietary changes required to modify risk factors are more complex, it is possible to recommend a range of dietary principles to facilitate one or more of these changes. Lewis et al. (99) put forth two main approaches to achieve theses results: a population strategy and an individual strategy.

A. Population Strategy

A "high risk" preventive strategy aimed solely at people with greatest CHD risk (cholesterol levels more than 7 mmol/l) will have little impact on the epidemic proportions CHD has reached in many countries. For an overall impact, it is necessary to shift the entire distribution of cholesterol and other risk factors to a range where overall risk is low. The main disadvantage of this approach is that while many individuals are being asked to make changes that are likely to produce relatively small reduction in their personal CHD risk, those at much greater risk are unaware that they require more radical lifestyle changes or preventive medical care, including drug therapy (99).

The desirable levels of cholesterol that are likely to be associated with the lowest achievable levels of lipoprotein-mediated risk of CHD have been much debated. While a multidisciplinary workshop in 1979 suggested that the mean serum cholesterol of an adult population should not exceed 4.7 mmol/l, the WHO Expert Committee in 1982 recommended that mean levels of total cholesterol in adults should be below 5.2 mmol/l (200 mg/100 ml) (100). The justification for the latter was that populations with high CHD rates have higher cholesterol levels; CHD is relatively infrequent in countries with lower mean levels; and that within single populations, subgroups with the lowest levels have the lowest CHD risk. A National Institutes of Health Consensus Development Conference has regarded this level as an attainable goal for individuals and populations, and suggested a lower level of 4.7 mmol/l as an appropriate target for younger adults (1).

Earlier recommendations concentrated almost exclusively on the need for reduction in blood cholesterol, emphasizing lowering of total dietary fat and dietary cholesterol. However current recommendations acknowledge the importance of thrombogenesis and other cardiovascular risk factors and that lipoprotein-mediated risk and its determinants involve more than a simple consideration of blood cholesterol. Recently published dietary reference values for fat and carbohydrate in the United Kingdom (Table 7) (101) emphasize that total fat should be calculated from the sum of fatty acid intakes and glycerol, though restriction of total fat is important for obese people. The reduction in saturated fatty acids to 10% of total dietary energy is much greater than earlier recommendations, and is more in line with North American and WHO recommendations, which acknowledge the particular importance of SFA in both atherogenesis and thrombogenesis. Although stearic acid is not associated with an elevation of LDL, as is the case with SFA of shorter chain length, it is impractical to distinguish between different saturated fatty acids, because stearic acid may be thrombogenic, if not atherogenic. It has also been advised that *cis* MUFA should continue to provide on average 12% of dietary energy. British recommendations do not suggest an increase in MUFA, but some increase would seem acceptable in the light of current knowledge, which has been incorporated into recent recommendations in New Zealand (102). It is suggested that *cis* PUFA should continue to provide an average of 6% of total energy, derived from a mixture of *n-6* and *n-3* PUFA. Dietary energy of PUFA should not exceed 10% of total energy, a slightly higher average intake (up to 8%) being recommended in some countries. *Trans* fatty acid intake should not exceed the current estimated average of 5 g/day or 2% of dietary energy. The total fatty acid intake should thus average 30%, and total fat (including glycerol) 33% of total dietary energy, including alcohol, or 35% of energy derived from food. Little emphasis has been given to dietary cholesterol, although populations' mean intake should be below 300 mg/day (1).

Dietary reference values given for carbohydrates and nonstarch polysaccharides (Table 7) are not specifically aimed at reducing cardiovascular risk. Whereas an increase in nonstarch poly-

Table 7 Dietary Reference Values for Fat and Carbohydrate for Adults as a Percentage of Daily Total Energy Intake (Percentage of Food Energy)

	Individual minimum	Population average	Individual maximum
Fat		10(11)	
Saturated fatty acids			
Cis polyunsaturated fatty acids	*n*-3: 0.2	6(6.5)	10
	n-6: 1.0		
Cis monounsaturated fatty acids		12(13)	
Trans fatty acids		2(2)	
Total fatty acids		30(32.5)	
Total fat		33(35)	
Carbohydrate			
Non-milk extrinsic sugars	0	10(11)	
Intrinsic and milk sugars and starch		37(39)	
Total carbohydrate		47(50)	
Non-starch polysaccharide (g/day)	12	18	24

The average percentage contribution to total energy does not total 100% because figures for protein and alcohol are excluded. Protein intakes average 15% of total energy, which is above the RNI. Since many individuals derive some energy from alcohol, it is assumed to average 5%, approximating current intakes. However, the panel allowed some groups not to drink alcohol, and thus for some purposes nutrient intakes as a proportion of food energy (without alcohol) might be useful. Therefore, average figures are given as percentages both of total energy and in parenthesis of food energy.
Source: Department of Health, 1991.

saccharide is recommended, there is no specific advice to increase soluble forms of carbohydrates. A high intake of fruit and vegetables, as given in all dietary guidelines, should provide an adequate intake of antioxidants. A reduction of dairy products and red meats is an important means of decreasing intakes of SFA, with suitable alternatives like skimmed or semi-skimmed milk, reduced-fat cheese, and predominantly unsaturated margarines, especially those high in oleic acid. Moderate amounts (up to 180 g/day) of lean meat with less SFA and more MUFA and PUFA may be incorporated into dietary advice aimed at achieving optimal lipoprotein profiles (103). Similarly, eating fish, especially oily fish, several times a week may confer additional benefit.

Full compliance with the above dietary recommendations would be expected to reduce cholesterol levels by at least 16%, reducing the mean adult population's cholesterol levels in countries such as the United Kingdom from the present levels of around 5.9 to 5.0 mmol/l or even less. Farquhar et al. (104) and Tuomilehto et al. (105) evaluated the effects of intervention programs in the United State of America and Finland, respectively. In both countries, the most impressive results were seen from the reduction of cigarette smoking. The reductions in cholesterol (around 3%) and blood pressure were much lower than expected, indicating that dietary advice, for some reason, was not complied with fully; possible explanations for disappointing results include inappropriate information and educational programs, lack of availability of appropriate foods, and unsatisfactory food labeling (1).

Based on cholesterol levels of people in Britain, the data presented in Table 8 show that with full compliance with the WHO or British recommendations, only about 5% of the population, as compared with 25% at present, would remain at appreciable risk of CHD due to hypercholesterolemia (cholesterol more than 6.5 mmol/l) and 15% of the population would be at some risk as compared with just under 50% at present. However, with a more realistic expectation of an 8%

Table 8 Percentage of Population in the United Kingdom Aged 25–59 Years with Cholesterol Levels Exceeding 6.5 and 5.2 mmol/l, and Percentage Predicted to Exceed These Limits After Adoption of Dietary Recommendations

	Serum cholesterol level (mmol/*l*)	
	>6.5	>5.2
Prevalence study 1984–1985 (Mann et al., 1988)	25%	47%
Mean cholesterol reduction 16.5% (WHO, 1982) (British Dietary Reference Values, Dept. of Health, 1991)	4.5%	15%
Mean cholesterol reduction 8% (Optimistic estimate of what might be achieved in practice)	13%	31%

Source: Ref. 1.

reduction in serum cholesterol (half of what would be predicted from full compliance with recommendations), about 13% of the population would remain at considerable risk. In countries with a higher mean level than in Britain, this figure would be much greater. Mann (1) concluded that highly energetic attempts should be made to achieve population changes, which may include educational measures aimed at the population as well as legislative measures to facilitate change, e.g., higher taxes on cigarettes and widespread availability of appropriate, relatively low-cost foods. The greater the reduction in mean cholesterol, the fewer the number that will remain at high risk. The risk-reducing strategy in such individuals would be an essential complement to the population strategy until high-risk populations make major lifestyle changes. Also, various population strategies need to be evaluated with regard to the risk reduction achieved, because programs suitable for one community may not be necessarily appropriate to others.

B.   Dietary Guidelines for High-Risk Individuals

Principles of dietary advice for individuals are primarily based on reductions of lipid levels in high-risk populations, with more strict targets. An average 15% reduction in cholesterol levels and up to 25% reduction in cholesterol and 20% to 40% in triglyceride levels have been frequently reported in individuals receiving advice from dietitians in lipid clinics. All individuals having cholesterol levels higher than 6.5 mmol/l and/or triacylglycerol greater than 3 mmol/l should receive such individual advice from professional nutritionists or dietitians. Some basic principles of diet for high-risk people are given in Table 9. Individuals will also require advice regarding recipes and methods of food preparation, especially where cooking habits differ appreciably from those recommended. Widely differing diets used for various forms of hyperlipidemia in the past have proved to be unnecessary in view of the current simple approach (Table 9). The recent report of the Joint Expert consultation (106) on "fats and oils in human nutrition" has provided minimum desirable intakes of fats and oils for adults, infants, and younger children, giving upper limits of fat oil intakes. Recommendations are also given in this report for saturated and unsaturated fatty acids and cholesterol, isomeric fatty acids as well as for substances associated with fats and oils, *viz.*, antioxidants and carotenoids and essential fatty acids (see Chapter 22, for details).

The relative risk of cardiovascular disease associated with recognized risk factors appear to decrease with aging and there have been few clinical trials showing benefits of risk reduction in elderly people. Although aging limits advantages to dietary changes, there is no clear cutoff point

Table 9 Principles of Diet Modification for Individuals with Hyperlipidemia

	Initial advice for hypercholesterolemia and endogenous hypertriglyceridemia	Advice for resistant hypercholesterolemia	Advice for chylomicronemia syndrome
Total fatty acids (% total energy)	<30	About 25	15[a]
Saturated fatty acids and *trans* unsaturated fatty acids	<10 (range 6–10)	6–8	
Polyunsaturated fatty acids	About 8 (range 6–10)	6–8	
Monounsaturated fatty acids	up to 18 (range 10–18)	10–15	
Dietary cholesterol (mg/day)	<300	<200	<200
Dietary fiber (g/day)[b]	35	45	35
Protein (% total energy)	12	12	20

[a]This usually involves reducing total fat to below 25 g/day. Medium-chain triglycerides that are not transported in chylomicrons may be added if liver function is normal. Supplementary fat-soluble vitamins may be required.
[b]Special emphasis given to soluble dietary fiber
Source: Ref 1.

for age, and thus older people are also likely to benefit from relatively simple advice that is compatible with the nutritional recommendations for high-risk people.

Fad diets, such as those based on advice to increase oat bran and niacin, may be without scientific justification and are often based on half-truths. Oat bran may be rich in soluble forms of NSPs, which have some cholesterol-lowering properties, and nicotinic acid (niacin) can also lower LDL and VLDL levels; however, such diets may have small overall beneficial effect, unless attention is paid to other more important determinants of cardiovascular risk factors, because pharmacological doses of nicotinitic acid are required to produce an effect on lipoproteins. Similarly *n-3* PUFAs (omega-3 fatty acids) sold as concentrates in capsules are often advertised as a useful means of lowering cholesterol. Although these preparations have a profound effect on thrombogenesis and VLDL, and may indeed reduce the risk of CHD, they do not have consistent effects on LDL and total cholesterol, except in pharmacological doses. Also, the safety of such preparations in large amounts has not been established. Although it appeals to recommend an increased intake of fish, it is not appropriate to advise large amount of *n-3* fatty acids in concentrated form, until their requirements and safety have been well established.

Merolli (107) has reviewed the health benefits of medium-chain lipids. Many medical nutritional products for critically ill hospital patients and for outpatients with chronic disease contain medium-chain triglycerides (MCT) as part of the fat blend. Medium-chain lipids are used as components of liquid diet formulas for patients with diverse medical conditions, such as AIDS and cystic fibrosis, for certain postoperative cancer patients, and for patients with multiple trauma, burn injury, respiratory distress, hepatic or renal disease, and conditions requiring fluid restriction, such as congestive heart failure. For the critically ill, hypermetabolic due to trauma and/or sepsis, MCTs provide a quick and concentrated source of energy that is rapidly absorbed and easily digested (108). MCTs also improve the absorption of other fats as well. When medium-chain fatty acids (MCFAs) are part of a structured lipid of optimal configuration, with MCFA at sn-1 and -3 only, the triglyceride, molecule hydrolyses more rapidly, as does absorption of essential fatty acids (109,110).

Use of MCT for outpatients includes products for nutritional supplementation of persons with cystic fibrosis or AIDS/HIV. The MCTs in these products improve nitrogen balance, provide energy, and help to prevent weight loss. Flavored shake mixes such as scandishake (Scandipharm, Birmingham, Alabama) and energy bars such as NuBar (NCT Medical Foods, Irwindale, California) are on the market. MCT oil can also be used in cooking and baking for a whole foods diet for persons with chromic fat malabsorption (107).

MCFAs have been found to be synergistic with fish oil to develop immune system function (111). MCT products have been designed specifically for patients with suppressed immune systems. MCFAs are not eicosanoid precursors and thus do not aid in the overproduction of inflammatory eicosanoids such as prostaglandin E_2, which in turn promotes secondary infection in burn and trauma patients.

MCFA have long been considered to be cholesterolemically neutral (112). MCTs have been used for decades at moderate to high dietary levels for various conditions, including cardiac failure, without causing concern over levels of total cholesterol. Experimental evidence available indicated that MCFA may be weakly cholesterolemic, but considerably less so than palmitic acid (113), the major saturated fatty acid in typical U.S. diets. Thus, substituting MCFA for palmitate in processed foods could yield a more healthful product.

Effects of MCT on serum lipids and lipoproteins have not been established. The effects of MCT per se are thought to vary from those of MCFA in a structured lipid or MCFA oil (107). Thus, each new medium-chain lipid will need to be evaluated on its own merits. Kritchevsky (114) clearly demonstrated that site of placement of saturated fatty acids on the triglyceride molecule has profound impacts on both cholesterol levels and atherogenicity of a lipid. An MCFA oil produced in canola may have comparatively less effect on cholesterol levels than MCT, because saturated fatty acids are excluded by the canola plant from sn-2 (115). MCTs also have been known to elevate serum triglycerides (as do carbohydrates), which may be a risk factor for heart disease in middle-aged women (116), although Lanza Jacoby et al. (117) have reported that structured lipid composed of MCFA and fish oil fatty acids did not raise triglyceride levels relative to soybean oil. Merolli (107) envisaged that during the next decade, research strategies will explore insertion of a series of unsaturated fatty acids to provide specific nutritional benefits, e.g., fatty acids targeted for the adult population may include *n-3* fatty acids (EPA and DHA) and *n-6* gamma-linolenic acid. For infant formulas, specific fatty acid targets may include polyunsaturates, arachidonic acid DHA, as well as palmitate.

According to Rickard and Thompson (118), flaxseed is the richest known plant source of *n-3* fatty acid, alpha-linolenic acid, as well as of lignan precursors and soluble fiber. These components, in addition to the oil, appear to contribute to the beneficial effects observed for flaxseed in chronic diseases. Flaxseed feeding has been shown to antagonize the action of platelet activating factor (PAF), thereby reducing the ability of platelets to aggregate (119). Thus, lignans in flaxseed may have beneficial effects in the prevention and/or treatment of cardiovascular disease (118). The benefits seen for both the mucilage and lignan components of flaxseed suggest that these components may be excellent candidates for preventive and therapeutic uses in a number of other chronic diseases such as cancer and gastrointestinal disorders (as a soothing balm for inflammation and as a laxative) and diabetes.

Clinton (120) reviewed the chemistry, biology, and implications of lycopene for human health and disease. A diet rich in carotenoid-containing foods is known to be associated with a number of health benefits. Lycopene, which provides the familiar red color to tomato products, is one of the major carotenoids in the diets of Western populations. Interest in lycopene is growing rapidly following the recent publication of epidemiologic studies implicating lycopene in the prevention of cardiovascular disease and cancers of the prostate or gastrointestinal tract. Lycopene has unique structural and chemical features that may contribute to its specific biological properties. Clinton (120) has reviewed the data concerning lycopene bioavailability, tissue distribution, metabolism, excretion, and biological actions in animal experiments and human studies. The knowledge in these areas and the associations between lycopene consumption and human health has been summarized. The strategies to decrease the progression of atherosclerosis in cardiovascular disease include hypertension and diabetes and treatment of hyperlipidemias. In addition to these, many dietary factors are also important, and much emphasis is being placed on caroteniods and antioxidant nutrients, such as vitamins C and E. Accumulating evidence favors the hypothesis that oxidatively modified macromolecules, particularly those derived from lipoproteins deposited in the vessel wall, may be critical factors that initially activate the cellular and cytokine networks involved in lesion formation and progression (121,122). It is possible that carotenoids such as lycopene may be involved in the pathogenesis of cardiovascular disease, although this hypothesis remains to be fully established. Frei (123) proposed that carotenoids in conjunction with vitamins E and C may protect lipoproteins and vascular cells from oxidative damage. Epidemiologic evidence supports the hypothesis that foods rich in carotenoids and antioxidant vitamins are associated with decreased risk of atherosclerotic vascular disease (124).

Kohlmeier et al. (125) conducted a multicenter study of men with myocardial infarction and matched controls in 10 European countries. Adipose tissue needle aspiration biopsies of each participant were analyzed for carotenoid profiles and tocopherols. After adjusting for age, body mass, socioeconomic status, smoking hypertension, and family history, the lycopene concentration remained independently protective, with an odds ratio (OR) of 0.52 for the 10th versus the 90th percentiles. Interestingly, the protective effect of lycopene was attenuated in persons who smoked and in those with lower concentrations of adipose tissue PUFAs. However, the earlier finding by Street et al. (126) examining serum carotenoids, rather than adipose tissue concentrations and risk of myocardial infarction in a case-control study, did not support the results of Kohlmeier et al (125).

Fuhrman et al. (127) recently investigated the ability of lycopene to modulate cholesterol metabolism in cell culture and a very small clinical trial. The incubation of human macrophage cell lines with lycopene was found to inhibit cholesterol synthesis and augment production of macrophage LDL receptors. Dietary supplementation of 60 mg lycopene/day in six males for 3 months was found to be associated with a 14% reduction in plasma LDL cholesterol levels. Fuhrman et al. (127) proposed that lycopene may be a modest hypocholesterolemic agent, secondary to the inhibition of macrophage 3-hydroxy-3-methly-glutarly-coenzyme A (HMGCoA reductase), the rate-limiting enzymatic step in cholesterol biosynthesis. The pharmaceutical agents used in the treatment of hyperlipidemia and cardiovascular disease can reduce serum concentrations of lycopene. Studies with cholestiramine showed that it lowered serum concentrations of lycopene by about 30% compared with baseline, whereas probucol decreased serum carotenoids, including lycopene, by 30% to 40% (128,129). Probucol, which has both lipid-lowering and antioxidant properties, may reduce circulating lycopene via reductions in lipoprotein particle size and by competition between the drug and carotenoids for incorporation into very-low-density (VLDL) lipoproteins (128).

Although CHD is the most common cause of death in the West, not every individual is destined to develop CHD. If it were possible to identify easily those individuals who are susceptible to atherosclerotic complications (mainly CHD), an individually targeted approach to this problem would be more logical and cost effective (Table 10). According to Havel (130), assessment of susceptibility is not simply a matter of determining the ambient level of LDL cholesterol but would require an inexpensive, safe (noninvasive) method to determine the presence and severity of atherosclerotic lesions. Alternatively, a simple and safe method to reduce the level of atherogenic lipoproteins (e.g., with a magic bullet to stimulate the synthesis of LDL receptors or to prolong their life span) could be used in all individuals with an LDL level above some defined set-

Table 10 The Individual (Genetic) and Population Approach to
Hyperlipidemia, Diet, and Coronary Heart Disease (CHD)

A. Individual (genetic) approach to hyperlipidemia and CHD
   1. Current
      a. Measurement of lipid levels:
         total serum cholesterol
         triglycerides
         HDL cholesterol
   2. Future
      a. Identification of major gene abnormalities and protein polymorphisms
      b. Noninvasive or minimally invasive evaluation of coronary lesions
      c. Prevention by a "magic bullet"
B. Population approach to diet and CHD
      a. Single diet is appropriate for almost all purposes
      b. Small reductions in LDL cholesterol can yield large overall benefits
      c. Compliance is enhanced by family and other social interactions
      d. Change in food supply is facilitated

Source: Ref. 130.

point. This possibility appears to be optimistic in view of current development of specific cholesterol synthesis inhibitors that in turn stimulate receptor synthesis (131). Safety would be of paramount importance in deciding the set-point above which such treatment can be justified. It appears unlikely that a drug that is safe for every individual will be developed.

The population approach to hyperlipoproteinemia and CHD has been predicted by extrapolating the results of intervention in hypercholesterolemic men for the general population (Table 10). Few studies to date have demonstrated the practicability of widespread modification of the diet. However, based on the current knowledge about the regulation of hepatic LDL receptors, the ingredients of an appropriate diet are reasonably simple and straightforward (130). The need for a population approach (Table 10) is based on the realization that treatment of only those individuals judged to be hypercholesterolemic (e.g., the upper 10% of the population) will not reduce the bulk of the burden of premature CHD in Western countries. The population approach is also based on the prediction that small reductions in LDL cholesterol will have substantial effects on the incidence of CHD, and it is necessarily confined to the use of dietary modification (130).

Connor and Connor (132) concluded that the dietary treatment and prevention of the atherosclerotic lesions underlying CHD have a logical and well-established rationale, developed over the past three decades. The low-fat, high-carbohydrate diet for these purposes is designed to prevent and treat hyperlipidemia and to have an antithrombotic action. The proposed low-cholesterol, low-fat diet is safe, inexpensive, and can become habitual through the process of gradual change, practice, and patience. It offers a practical means of dealing with some of the key risk factors in CHD, especially hyperlipidemia. The same dietary philosophy may also be applied to hyperlipidemia of differing severity, of different etiologies, and of different lipoprotein types. This dietary approach may be used with therapeutic benefit at any stage in the development of CHD. The nutritional changes instituted early in life will have the greatest impact. Since CHD is a familial disease, its control and treatment can be best approached on a family basis, by preventing diet-induced hyperlipidemia (132).

Garlic has been used for medicinal purposes since ancient times and is known to favorably influence a whole range of cardiovascular risk factors. In Germany, garlic preparations have been popularly used as drugs. However, much research is required to isolate the cholesterol-reducing factors from garlic. It seems that active ingredients of garlic may be lost in processing (133).

Evidence available indicates that the hypercholesterolemic effects of coffee may be related to its method of preparation. Boiled coffee, most frequently drunk in Nordic countries, may be more hypercholesterolemic than coffee prepared in other ways (134). These authors suggested that evidence may be strong enough to examine the coffee intake of people with high cholesterol levels and, where appropriate, recommend a switch in method of preparation.

It is now established that a modest intake of alcohol has a protective effect against CHD, perhaps via beneficial effects on HDL, fibrinogen, and platelet activity. However public health recommendations that emphasize the positive health effects of alcohol are likely to do more harm than good, in view of sharp increase in mortality from cerebrovascular disease, cancer, accidents, and violence associated with alcohol drinking (135).

Owing to the complex nature of the etiology of CHD, foods and nutrients other than those already investigated are likely to have either beneficial or deleterious effects. Nutritionists thus have an important role to play in the evaluation of and public commentary on new findings, in view of the powerful effects of advertising media by those with vested interests, and CHD being a highly emotive issue in many high-risk countries.

Although atherosclerosis in the cerebral and femoral arteries resembles pathological processes in the coronary arteries, the clinical features of stroke and peripheral arterial disease appear to be associated with risk factors that are not identical to those of CHD (1). Systolic blood pressure, cigarette smoking and heavy alcohol intake are the most important potentially modifiable risk factors for stroke. The raised fibrinogen levels also seem to confer risk (136,137). The lipoprotein-mediated risk and consequently the dietary determinants of LDL, VLDL, and HDL, so important in CHD, appear to be of less importance in strokes. The role of dietary factors in the etiology, prevention, and management of stroke has not been fully investigated. Epidemiological evidence suggested a protective effect of leafy green vegetables and fruits (138). In view of the importance of the latter in hypertension, dietary factors influencing this risk factor warrant further research. Patients with lipoprotein abnormalities should be advised accordingly, with general dietary advice given to the population at large. Although diet-related factors appear to be of less importance in the etiology of peripheral vascular disease, cigarette smoking is the most important risk factor in this regard (139).

Cardiomyopathy and cardiac failure occur as the result of specific nutrient deficiencies that are most commonly encountered in less affluent societies, e.g., beriberi resulting from thiamin deficiency in populations consuming highly milled rice as a staple food and Keshan disease, resulting from deficiency of selenium (140). Under such conditions, providing the required nutrient can both prevent and treat the clinical consequences of the deficiency. Alcohol intake in association with deficiencies of thiamin and other nutrients may result in a clinical syndrome similar to cardiomyopathy, usually characterized by cardiac failure. These conditions can be managed both by withdrawing or reducing alcohol and appropriate nutrient intakes. Anemia resulting from a range of nutrient deficiencies may also result in cardiac failure. According to Mann (1), CHD is rapidly overtaking the nutrition-related disorders of the heart and circulation in many developing countries. Thus, in addition to addressing the problems of undernutrition and malnutrition, nutritional recommendations in the less affluent countries must also ensure that CHD does not reach the epidemic proportions it has reached in many industrially developed Western countries (140).

CHD kills more people in the developed industrialized countries than any other disease and is responsible for considerable suffering and enormous expense to the health services. The principal focus of attention has been to encourage reduced consumption of fat, SFA, and cholesterol, the United States being in the forefront in this campaign. In the U.K., the authors of the COMA Report on Nutritional Aspects of Cardiovascular Disease (141) have concluded that diet is a major and modifiable cause of CHD, extending the concept to include prevention of the disease. SFAs were singled out as the major problem. This is because of the general preoccupation with the "lipid (or cholesterol) hypothesis":

Dietary SFA $\rightarrow$ raised LDL $\rightarrow$ atherosclerosis thrombosis $\rightarrow$ CHD mortatilty.

According to Gurr (142), this approach is not so simple to advocate that simple changes in diet alone could possibly achieve the desired objectives. Although public health strategies still focus principally on this approach, there is a need to expose its weaknesses. The U.K. Department of Health considers that the incidence and mortality from CHD could be substantially reduced if the British population were to reduce its consumption of total fat and SFA (141). The scientific evidence for links between SFA consumption and CHD has come mainly from three types of research studies:

Animal experiments
Epidemiological studies, and
Intervention trials with human subjects.

Applying a fresh look to the dietary recommendations, Gurr (142) has refuted the above-mentioned "lipid hypothesis," and concluded that CHD is not primarily caused by a high intake of saturated fatty acids (SFA), and major changes in SFA consumption are not likely to lead to greater benefits from CHD reduction. Gurr's arguments are based on the following deficiencies in the lipid hypothesis:

There is insufficient correspondence in vascular pathology between (a) animals and humans and (b) general atherosclerosis and lesions seen in familial hypercholesterolemia.
International epidemiology is flawed by confounding factors and selection biases. Within countries, epidemiology gives little support for a relationship between dietary fat and CHD. Fat intake does not explain total CHD, regional, sex, or social, class differences.
Trends in the CHD mortality are not coincident with changes in the amount and type of fat eaten.
The hypothesis cannot explain the greater risk in women compared with men, enhanced risk in post-menopausal women, or the consistent recent falls in mortality in women compared with more erratic changes in men in many countries. There have been no corresponding falls in CHD incidence.
Plasma total cholesterol is a weak predictor of CHD compared with hemostatic factors. Less than 50% of CHD risk is accounted for by known risk factors.
Extrapolations from drug trials in high-risk individuals to the general population are unwarranted.
Intervention trials have not demonstrated a major impact of dietary fat modification on CHD and none on total mortality. Only the most stringent diets achieve useful plasma cholesterol reductions.

REFERENCES

1. Mann, J., Disease of the heart and circulation: the role of dietary factors in aetiology and management, *Human Nutrition and Dietetics*, 9th ed. (J.S. Garrow and W.P.T. James, eds.), Churchill Livingstone, Edinburgh, London, 1993, p. 619.
2. Weatherall, D.J., D.A. Warrell, and J.G.G. Ledingham (eds.), *Oxford Textbook of Medicine*, 2nd ed., Vol. II (Sections 13.138 and 13.167), Oxford University Press, Oxford, 1987.

3. Keys, A., *Seven Countries: A Multivariate Analysis of Death and Coronary Heart Disease*, Harvard University Press, Cambridge, Mass., 1980.

4. Uemera, K., and Z. Pisa, Trends in cardiovascular disease mortality in industrialized countries since 1950, *World Health Status Quo 41*: 155 (1988).

5. Stamler, I., Population studies, *Nutrition, Lipids and Coronary Heart Disease* (R.I. Levy, B.M. Rifkin, B.H. Dennis, and N. Ernst, eds.) Raven Press, New York, 1979, p. 25.

6. Sytkowski, P.A., W.B. Kannel, and R.B.D'Agostino, Changes in risk factors and the decline in mortality from cardiovascular disease. The Framingham heart study, *N. Engl. J. Med. 322*: 1635 (1990).

7 Dwyer, T., and B.S. Hetzel, A comparison of trends of coronary heart disease mortality in Australia, USA and England and Wales with reference to there major risk factors—hypertension, cigarette smoking, and diet, *Intl. J. Epidemiol 9*: 65 (1980).

8. Beaglehole, R., D.R. Hay, F.H. Foster, and D.N. Sharpe, Trends in coronary heart disease mortality and associated risk factors in New Zealand, *New Zealand Med. J. 93*: 371 (1981).

9. Sigfusson, N., H. Sigvaldason, and L. Steingrimsdottir, Decline in ischaemic heart disease in Iceland and change in risk factor levels, *Br. Med. J. 302*: 1371 (1991).

10. Keys, A., A. Menotti, and M.J. Karvonen, The diet and 15-year death rate in the seven countries study, *Am. J. Epidemiol. 124*: 903 (1986).

11. Morris, J.N., J.W. Marr, and D.G. Clayton, Diet and heart: a postscrip, *Br. Med. J. 2*: 1307 (1977).

12. Shekelle, R.B., et al., Diet, serum cholesterol and death from coronary heart disease: the Western Electric study, *N. Engl. J. Med. 304*: 65 (1981).

13. Philips, R.L., J.W. Kuzma, W.L. Beeson, and T. Letz, Influence of selection versus lifestyle on risk of fetal cancer and cardiovascular disease among Seventh Day Adventists, *Am. J. Epidemiol. 112*: 296 (1980).

14. Burr, M.L., and B.K. Butland, Heart disease in British vegetarians, *Am. J. Clin. Nutr. 48*: (Suppl.): 830 (1988).

15. Miettinen, T.A., V. Nakkarinen, and J.K. Huttunen. Fatty acid compostion of serum lipid predicts myocardial infarction, *Br. Med. J. 285*: 993 (1982).

16. Riemersma R.A., F.A. Wood, and S. Butter, Linoleic acid content in adipose tissue and platelet fatty acids and coronary heart disease, *Br. Med. J. 292*: 1423 (1986).

17. Duthie, G.G., K.W.J. Wahle, and W.P.T. James, Oxidants, antioxidants and cardiovascular disease, *National Res. Rev. 2*: 51 (1989).

18. Truswell, A.S., and J.I. Mann, Epidemiology of serum lipids in southern Africa, *Atherosclerosis 16*: 15 (1972).

19. Martin, M.J., S.B. Hulley, and W.S. Browner, Serum cholesterol, blood pressure and mortality implications from a cohort of 36 / 662 men, *Lancet 2*: 933 (1986).

20. Parthasarathy, S., J.C. Kloo, and E. Miller, Low density lipoprotein rich in oleic acid is protected against oxidative modification: implications for dietary prevention in atherosclerosis, *Proc. Nat. Acad. Sci. USA 87*: 3894 (1990).

21. Mann, J.I., B. Lewis, and J. Shepherd, Blood lipid concentration and other cardiovascular risk factors: distribution, prevalence and detection in Britain, *Br. Med. J. 296*: 1702 (1988).

22. Keys, A., J.T. Anderson, and F. Grande, Prediction of serum cholesterol responses of man to changes in fats, in the diet, *Lancet 2*: 959 (1977).

23. Bonanome, A., and S.M. Grundy, Effect of dietary stearic acid on plasma cholesterol and lipoprotein levels, *N. Engl. J. Med. 318*: 1244 (1990).

24. Mensink R.P., and M.B. Katan, Effects of dietary *trans* fatty acids on high-density and low density lipoprotein cholesterol levels in healthy subjects, *N. Engl. J. Med. 323*: 439 (1990).

25. Ulbricht, T.L.V., and D.A.T. Southgate, Coronary heart disease: seven dietary factors, *Lancet 338*: 985 (1991).

26. Keys, A., J.T. Anderson, and F. Grande, Serum cholesterol response to changes in the diet. IV. Particularly saturated fatty acids in the diet, *Metabolism 14*: 776 (1965).

27. Edington J.D., M. Geekie, and R. Carter, Effects of dietary cholesterol concentration in subjects following reduced-fat high fiber diet, *Br. Med. J. 294*: 333 (1987).

28. Edington J.D., M. Geekie, and R. Carter, Serum lipid response to dietary cholesterol in subjects fed a low fat high fiber diet, *Am. J. Clin. Nutr. 50*: 58 (1989).

29. Anderson J.W., D.A. Deakins, and S.R. Bridges, Soluble fiber: hypocholesterolemic effects and proposed mechanisms, *Dietary Fiber—Chemistry, Physiology and Health Effects* (D. Kritchevsky, ed.), Plenum Press, New York, 1990, p. 339.

30. Swain, J.F., I.L. Rouse, C.B. Curley, and F.M. Sacks, Comparison of the effects of oat bran and low fiber wheat on serum lipoprotein levels and blood pressure, *N. Engl. J. Med. 322*: 147 (1990).

31. Leadbetter, J., M.J. Ball, and J.I. Mann, Effect of increasing quantities of oat bran in hypercholesterolaemic people, *Am. J. Clin. Nutr. 54*: 841 (1991).

32. Judd, P.A., and A.S. Truswell, Dietary fiber and blood lipids in man, *Dietary Fiber Perspectives: Reviews and Bibliography* (A. Leeds and A. Avenell, eds.) John Libbey, London 1985, p. 23.

33. Descovich, G.C., C. Ceredi, and A. Gaddi, Multicentre study of soybean protein diet for out-patient hypercholesterolaemic patients, *Lancet 2*: 709 (1980).

34. Van Raaij J.M.A., M.B. Katan, and C.E. West, Influence of diets containing casein, soy isolate and soy concentrate on volunteers, *Am. J. Clin. Nutr. 35*: 925 (1982).

35. Thorogood, M., R. Carter, and L. Benfield, Plasma lipids and lipoprotein cholesterol concentrations in people with different diets in Britain, *Br. Med. J. 295*: 351 (1987).

36. Sindhurani, J.A., and T. Rajamohan, Hypolipidemic effect of hemicellulose component of coconut fiber, *Indian J. Exp. Biol. 36*: 786 (1998).

37. Samochowiec, J., and B. Czerny, The influence of essential phospholipids (EPL) and allicin on lipid metabolism in man, *Herba Polonica 43*: 53 (1997).

38. Dwivedi, S., Putative uses of Indian cardiovascular friendly plants in preventive cardiology, *Ann. Nat. Acad. Med. Sci.* (India) *32*: 159 (1996).

39. Muriana, F.J.G., J. Villar, and V. Ruiz-Gutierrez, Intake of olive oil can modulate the transbilayer movement of human erythrocyte membrane cholesterol, *Cell. Mol. Life Sci. 53*: 496 (1997).

40. Reuter, H.D., H.P. Koch, and L.D. Lawson, Therapeutic effects and applications of garlic and its preparations, *Garlic: The Science and Therapeutic Application of Allium sativum L. and Related species* (H.P. Koch and L.D. Lawson, eds.), 2nd ed., Williams & Wilkins, Baltimore, 1996, p. 135.

41. Lau, B.H.S., M.A. Adetumbi, and A. Sanchez, *Allium sativum* (garlic) and atherosclerosis: a review, *Nutr. Res. 3*: 119 (1983).

42. Reuter, H.D., *Spektrum Allium, sativum L.*, Aesopusw GmbH., Basle, 1991.

43. Kourounakis, P.N., and E.A. Rekka, Effects on active oxygen species of allicin and *Allium sativum (garlic) powder*, *Res. Comm. Chem. Pathol. Pharmacol. 74*: 249 (1991).

44. Phelps, S., and W.S. Harris, Garlic supplementation and lipoprotein oxidation susceptibility, *Lipids 28*: 475 (1993).

45. Castelli, W.O., Cardiovascular disease in women, *Am. J. Obstet. Gynecol. 158*: 1553 (1988).

46. Verschuren, W.M.M., D.R. Jacobs, B.P.M. Bloemberg, D. Kromhout, A. Menotti, C. Aravains, H. Blackburn, R. Buzina, A.S. Dontas, F. Fidanza, M.J. Karvonen, S. Nedelikovic, A. Nissinen, and H. Toshima, Serum total cholesterol and long term coronary heart disease mortality in different cultures: twenty five year follow-up of the seven countries study *J. Am. Med. Asssoc. 274*: 131 (1995).

47. Brown, J., J.J. Albers, L.D. Fisher, F.M. Schaefer, J.T. Lint, C. Caplan, X.Q. Zhao, B.D. Bisson, V.F. Fitzpatrick, and H.T. Dodge, Regression of coronary artery disease as a result of intensive lipid lowering therapy in men with high levels of apolipoprotein B., *N. Engl. J. Med. 323*: 1289 (1990).

48. Ornish, D., S.E. Brown, L.W. Scherwitz, J.H. Billings, W.T. Armstrong, T.A. Ports, S.M. McLanahan, R.L. Kirkeeide R.J. Brand, and K.L. Gould, Can lifestyle change reverse coronary heart disease? *Lancet 336*: 129 (1990).

49. Tatami, R., N. Inone, H. Itoh, B. Kishino, N. Koga, Y. Nakashima, T. Nishide, K. Okamara, Y. Saito, T. Teramoto, T. Yasugi, A. Yamamoto, and Y. Goto, Regression of coronary atherosclerosis by combined LDL-apheresis and lipid-lowering drug therapy in patients with familial hypercholesterolemia: a multicenter study, *Atherosclerosis 95*: 1 (1992).

50. Watts, G.F., B. Lewis, J.N.H. Brunt, E.S. Lewis, D.J. Coltart, L.D.R. Smith, J.I. Mann, and A.V. Swan, Effects on coronary artery disease of lipid lowering diet, or diet plus colestyramine in the St. Thomas atherosclerosis study (STARS), *Lancet 339*: 563 (1992).

51. Chen J., and Y. Tang, Chemical constituents and antiatherosclerotic action of garlic, *Zhongguo Yaolixu Tangbao 7*: 88–91 (1990) (*Chem. Abstr. 115*: 269 (1991) (Chinese).

52. Castelli W.P., The triglyceride issue: a view from Framingham, *Am. Heart J. 112*: 432 (1986).

53. West, K.M., M.M.S. Ahuva, and P.F. Bennet, The role of circulating glucose and triglyceride concentrations and their interactions with other 'risk factors' as determinants of arterial disease in nine diabetic population samples from the WHO multinational study. *Diabetic Care 6*: 361 (1983).

54. Banaona, E., and C.S. Lieber, Effects of ethanol on lipid metabolism, *J. Lipid Res. 20*: 289 (1975).

55. Anonymous, Dietary sugars and human disease, Report on health and social subjects, No. 28, Department of Health, HMSO, London, 1989.

56. Anonymous, Fish oil (Editorial), *Lancet 2*: 203 (1988).

57. Lewis, B., Disorders of lipid transport, *The Oxford Textbook of Medicine* (D.J. Weatherall, J.G.G. Leadingham, and D.A. Warrel, eds), Oxford University Press, Oxford, 1987.

58. Junshi, C., T.C. Campbell, L. Junyao, and R. Peto, *Diet, Lifestyle and Mortality in China: A Study of the Characteristics of 65 Chinese Counties*, Oxford University Press, Oxford, 1990.

59. Gorden, T., W.B. Kannel, W.P. Castelli, and T.R. Dawber, Lipoproteins, cardiovascular disease and death. The Framingham study, *Arch. Intl. Med. 141*: 1128 (1989).

60. Gorden D.J., J.L. Prebstfield, and R.J. Garison. High-density lipoprotein cholesterol and cardiovascular disease. Four prospective American studies, *Circulation 79*: 8 (1989).

61. Grundy, S.M., Comparison of monounsaturated fatty acids and carbohydrates for lowering plasma cholesterol, *N. Engl. J. Med. 314*: 745 (1989).

62. Mann, J.I., Limes to legumes: changing concept of diabetic diets, *Diabetes Medicine 1*: 191 (1984).

63. Mattson, F.H., and S.M. Grundy, Comparison of effects of saturated, monounsaturated and polyunsaturated fatty acids on plasma lipids and lipoprotein in man, *J. Lipid Res. 26*: 194 (1985).

64. Mensink, R.P., and M.B. Katan, Effects of dietary trans fatty acids on high-density and low-density lipoprotein cholesterol levels in healthy subjects, *N. Engl. J. Med. 323*: 439 (1990).

65. Haskell, W.L., C. Camargo, and P.T. Williams, The effect of cessation and resumption of moderate alcohol intake on serum high-density lipoprotein fraction, *N. Engl. J. Med. 310*: 805 (1984).

66. Ball, M., and J.I. Mann, Apoproteins: Predictors of coronary heart disease? *Br. Med. J. 293*: 769 (1986).

67. Rosengren, A.L. Wilhelmsen, and E, Eriksson, Lipoprotein(a) and coronary heart disease: a prospective case control study in a general population sample of middle aged men, *Br. Med. J. 301*: 1248 (1990).

68. Maserei, J.R.C., I.L. Rouse, and W.J. Lynch, Effects of a lacto-ovo vegetarian diet on serum concentration of cholesterol triglyceride, HDL-C, HDL$_2$-C, HDL$_3$-C, apoprotein-B and Lp (a), *Am. J. Clin Nutr. 40*: 468 (1984).

69. Bang, H.O., J. Dyerberg and H.M. Sinclair, The composition of the Eskimo food in north western Greenland, *Am. J. Clin Nutr. 33*: 2657 (1980).

70. Fisher, M., P.M. Devine and P.H. Weiner, The potential clinical benefits of fish consumption, *Arch. Intl. Med. 146*: 2322 (1986).

71. Sinclair, H.M., Essential fatty acids in perspective, *Human Nutr. Clin Nutr. 38C*: 245 (1984).

72. Rao, G.H.R., E. Radha, and J.G. White, Effects of docosahexaenoic acid on arachidonic acid metabolism and platelet function, *Biochem. Biophys. Res. Commun. 117*: 549 (1983).

73. Lagarde, M., Metabolism of n-3/n-6 fatty acids in blood and vascular cells, *Biochem. Soc. Trans. 18*: 770 (1990).

74. MacIntyre, D.E., R.L. Hoover, and M. Smith, Inhibition of platelet function by *cis*-unsaturated fatty acids, *Blood 63*: 848 (1984).

75. O'Dea, K, M, Steel, and J. Nayghton, Butter enriched diets reduce arterial prostacyclin production in rats, *Lipids 23*: 234 (1988).

76. Meade, T.W., W.R.S. North, and R. Chakrabarti, Haemostatic function and cardiovascular death, *Lancet 1*: 1050 (1980).

77. Meade T.W., M.V. Vickers, and S.G. Thompson, The epidemiological characteristics of platelet aggregability, *Br. Med. J. 90*: 428 (1985).

78. Miller, G.V., J.K. Cruickshank, and L.J. Ellis, Fat consumption and factor VII coagulant activity in middle aged men. An association between a dietary and thrombogenic risk factor, *Atheroscerosis 78*: 19 (1989).

79. Meade, T.W., and W.R.S. North, Population based on distribution of haemostatic variables, *Br. Med. J. Bull 33*: 283 (1977).

80. Reddy D.S., Newer thrombolytic drugs for acute myocardial infarction, *Indian J. Exp. Biol. 36*: 1 (1998).

81. Cox, K.L., I.B. Puddley, and A.R. Morton, Controlled comparison of effects of exercise and alcohol on blood pressure and serum HDL cholesterol in sedentary men, *Clin. Exp. Pharmacol. Physiol. 17*: 251 (1990).

82. Glieberman, L., Blood pressure and dietary salt in human populations, *Ecol. Food Nutr. 2*: 143 (1973).

83. I.C.R.G., Intersalt: an international study of electrolyte excretion and blood pressure. Results for 24-hour urinary sodium and potassium excretion, Intersalt Cooperative Research Group, *Br. Med. J. 297*: 319 (1988).

84. Law, M.R., C.D. Fost, and N.J. Wald, By how much does dietary salt reduction lower blood pressure? *Br. Med. J. 302*: 811, 815, 819 (1991).

85. Cappucio, F.P., and G.A. MacGregor, Does potassium supplementation lower blood pressure? A meta-analysis of published results, *J. Hypertension 9*: 465 (1991).

86. Beilin, L.J., I.L. Rouse, and B.K. Armstrong, Vegetarian diet and blood pressure levels: incidental or causal association? *Am. J. Clin. Nutr. 48*: 806 (1988).

87. Swales, J.D., Salt substitutes and potassium intake, *Br. Med. J. 303*: 1084 (1991).

88. Holme, I., An effect of randomised trials evaluating the effect of cholesterol reduction on total mortality and coronary heart disease incidence, *Circulation 82*: 1916 (1990).

89. Dayton, S., M.L. Pearce, and S. Hashimoto, A controlled trial of a diet high in unsaturated fat in preventing complications of atherosclerosis, *Circulation 39/40* (Suppl. 2): 1 (1969).

90. Hjermann I, K. Byre, and I. Holme, Effects of diet and smoking intervention on the incidence of coronary heart disease, *Lancet 2*: 1303 (1981).

91. Hjermann, I., I. Holme, and P. Leren., Olso study diet and antismoking trial: results after 102 months, *Am. J. Med. 80* (Suppl 2A): 7 (1986).

92. Burr, M.L., J.F. Gilbert, and R.M. Holliday, Effects of changes in fat, fish and fiber intakes on death and myocardial reinfarction; Diet and Reinfarction Trial, *Lancet 2*: 757 (1989).

93. Ornish D., S.E. Brown, and L.W. Sherwitz, Can lifestyle changes reverse coronary heart disease? *Lancet 336*: 129 (1990).

94. Anonymous, Multiple Risk Factor Intervention Trial: risk factor changes and mortality results, *J. Am. Med Assoc. 248*: 1465 (1982).

95. WHO, Multifactorial trial in the prevention of coronary heart disease: 3. Incidence and mortality rates, WHO Collaborative Group World Health Organization, Rome, *European Heart J. 4*: 141 (1983).

96. Peto, R, S. Yusuf, and R. Collins, Cholesterol lowering trial results in their epidemiologic context, *Circulation 75* (Suppl 2): 451 (1987).

97. Oliver, M.F., Might treatment of hypercholesterolaemia increase noncardiac mortality? *Lancet 337*: 1529 (1991).

98. Muldoon, M.F., S.B. Mannicle, and K.A. Andrews, Lowering cholesterol concentrations and mortality: a quantitative review of primary prevention trials, *Br. Med. J. 301*: 309 (1990).

99. Lewis B., J. Mann, and M. Mancini, Reducing the risks of coronary heart disease in individuals and in the population, *Lancet 1*: 956 (1986).

100. WHO, Prevention of coronary heart disease, Technical Report Series, World Health Organization Expert Committee, 1982.

101. Anonymous, Dietary reference values for food, energy, and nutirents for the United Kingdom, Report on health and social subjects, No. 41, Dept. Of Health, HMSO, London, 1991.

102. N.T.F., The report of the Nutrition Task Force to the Department of Health, Shortcut Publishing, Wellington, 1991, p.1.

103. Watts, G.F., H. Ahmed, and J. Quing, Effective lipid-lowering diets including lean meat, *Br. Med. J. 296*: 235 (1988).

104. Farquhar, J.W., N. Maccaby, and P.D. Wood, Community education for cardiovascular health, *Lancet 1*: 1192 (1977).

105. Tuomilehto, J. Geboers, and T. Salonen, Decline in cardiovascular mortality in North Karelia and other parts of Finland, *Br. Med. J. 293*: 1068 (1986).

106. WHO/FAO, Fats and oils in human nutrition: Report of a Joint Expert Consultation (WHO/FAO) 1994, *Nutr. Rev. 53*: 202 (1995).

107. Merolli, A, Medium chain lipids: new sources, uses, *INFORM 8 (6)*: 597 (1997).

108. Gottschlich, M.M., Selection of optimal lipid sources in enteral and parenteral nutrition, *Nutr. Clin. Pract. 7*: 152 (1992).

109. Jandacek, R.J., J.A. Whiteside, B.N. Holcombe, R.A. Volpenhein, and J.D. Taulbee, The rapid hydrolysis and efficient absorption of triglycerides with octanoic acid in the 1 and 3 positions and long chain fatty acid in the 2 position, *Am. J. Clin. Nutr 45*: 940 (1987).

110. Ikeda, I., Y. Tomari, M. Sugano, S. Watanabe, and J. Nagata, Lymphatic absorption of structured glycerolipids containing medium chain fatty acids and linoleic acid and their effects on cholesterol absorption in rats, *Lipids 26*: 369 (1991).

111. Kinsella, J.E., B. Lokesh, S. Broughton, and J. Whelan, Dietary polyunsaturated fatty acids and eicosaniods: Potential effects on the modulation of inflammatory and immune cells: An overview, *Nutrition 6*: 24 (1990).

112. NRC. *Diet and Health Implications for Reducing Chronic Disease Risks*, National Academy Press, National Research Council, Food and Nutrition Board, Washington, DC, 1989.

113. Cater, N.B., H.J. Heller, and M.A. Denke, Comparison of the effects of medium-chain triacylglycerols, palm oil and high oleic acid sunflower oil on plasma triacylglycerols, fatty acids, lipid and lipoprotein concentrations in humans, *Am. J. Clin. Nutr. 65*: 41 (1997).

114. Kritchevsky, D., Fatty acids, triglyceride structure and lipid metabolism, *Nutr. Biochem 6*: 172 (1995).

115. Del Vecchio, A.J., High-laurate canola, *INFORM 7*: 230 (1996).

116. Bruckner, G., Fatty acids and cardiovascular disease, *Fatty Acids in Foods and Their Health Implications*, Marcel Dekker, New York, 1992 p. 735.

117. Lanza Jacoby S, H. Phetteplace, and R. Tripp, Enteral feeding, a structured lipid emulsion containing fish oil prevents the fatty liver of sepsis, *Lipids, 30*: 707 (1995).

118. Rickard, S.E., and L.U. Thomson, Health effects of flaxseed mucilage, lignans, *INFORM 8(8)*: 860 (1997).

119. Clark, W.F., A. Parbtani, M.W. Huff, E Spanner, H. De Salis, I Chin-Yee, D.J. Philbrick, and B.J. Holub, Flaxseed: a potential treatment for lupus nephritis, *Kidney Int. 48*: 457 (1995).

120. Clinton S.K., Lycopene: Chemistry, biology and implications for human health and disease, *Nutr. Rev. 56* (Suppl 1): 35 (1998).

121. Clinton S.K., and P. Libby, Cytokines and growth factors in atherosclerosis, *Arch. Pathol. Lab. Med. 116*: 1292 (1992).

122. Ross, R, The pathogenesis of atherosclerosis: a perspective for the 1990s, *Nature 362*: 801 (1993).

123. Frei, B., Cardiovascular disease and nutrient antioxidants: role of low-density lipoprotein oxidation, *Crit. Rev. Food Sci. Nutr. 351*: 83 (1995).

124. Mayne, S.T., Beta-carotene, carotenoids, and disease prevention in humans, *FASEB J. 10*: 690 (1996).

125. Kohlmeier, L., J.D. Kark, and E. Gomez-Garcia, Lycopene and myocardial infarction risk in the EURAMIC study, *Am. J. Epidemiol. 146*: 618 (1997).

126. Street, D.A., G.W. Constock, and R.M. Slkeld, Serum antioxidants and myocardial infarction. Are low levels of carotenoids and alpha-tocopherol risk factor for myocardial infarction? *Circulation 90*: 1154 (1994).

127. Fuhrman, B., A. Eils, and M. Aviram, Hypocholesterolemic effect of lycopene and beta-carotene is related to suppression of cholesterol synthesis and augmentation of LDL receptor activity in macrophages, *Biochem. Biophys. Res. Commun. 233*: 658 (1997).

128. Schafer Elinder, L., K. Hadell, and J. Molgaard, Probucol treatment decreases serum concentrations of diet derived antioxidants, *Arterioscler. Thromb. Vasc. Biol. 15*: 1057 (1995).

129. Gerster, H., The potential role of lycopene for human health, *J. Am. Coll. Nutr. 16*: 109 (1997).

130. Havel, R.J., Dietary and hereditary factors in coronary heart disease, *Diet, Nutrition & Health* (K.K. Carroll, ed.), McGill-Queens Univ. Press, London, 1989, p. 19.

131. Tobert, J., New developments in lipid-lowering therapy: the role of inhibitors of hydroxymethyl-glutaryl coenzyme A reductase, *Circulation 76*: 534 (1987).

132. Conner, S.L., and W.E. Conner, Coronary heart disease: prevention and treatment by nutritional change, *Diet. Nutrition & Health* (K.K. Correll, ed.), McGill-Queens Univ-Press, London, 1989, p. 33.

133. Mansell, P., and J.P.D. Reckless, Garlic: effects on serum lipids, blood pressure, coagulation, platelet aggregation and vasodilation, *Br. Med. J. 303*: 379 (1991).

134. Thelle, D.S.S. Heyden, and J.G. Foder, Coffee and cholesterol in epidemiological and experimental studies, *Atherosclerosis 67*: 97 (1987).

135. Marmont, M., and E. Brunner, Alcohol and cardiovascular disease: the status of the U-shaped curve, *Br. Med. J. 303*: 565 (1991).

136. Sharper, A.G., A.N. Philips, and S.J. Pocock, Risk factors for stroke in middle aged British men, *Br. Med. J. 302*: 1111 (1991).

137. Qizilbash, N., L. Jones, C. Warlow, and J.I. Mann, Fibrinogen and lipid concentrations as risk factors for transient ischaemic attacks and minor ischaemic strokes, *Br. Med. J. 303*: 605 (1983).

138. Acheson, R.M., and D.R.R. Williams, Does consumption of fruit and vegetables protect against stroke? *Lancet 1*: 1191 (1983).

139. Hughson, W.G., J.I. Mann, and A. Garrod, Intermittent claudication: prevalence and risk factors, *Br. Med. J. 1*: 1379 (1978).

140. Yang, G., J. Chen, Z. Wen, K. Ge, L. Khu, and X. Chen, The role of selenium in Keshan disease, *Adv. Nutr. Res. 6*: 203 (1988).

141. Anonymous, Report on Health and Social Subjects No. 46, Department of Health H.M.S.O., London, 1994.

142. Gurr, M., A fresh look at dietary recommendations, *INFORM 7(4)*: 432 (1996).

25
Diet, Nutrition, and Cancer

I. INTRODUCTION

The term *cancer* strikes great fear in the general population. For scientists, cancer refers to a disease process, carcinogenesis (1), which is thought to develop in more than one reversible and irreversible steps. These are characterized by the appearance of new types of cells, representing stages in the transformation from normal to malignant cells. Some of the reversible and irreversible steps may be influenced by dietary factors that can limit or protect the multistep developmental process of clinical cancer (2).

The methods of food production, processing, and distribution and related transformations brought about in the 20th century have significantly altered the eating patterns and lifestyle of the population, especially in the highly developed industrialized societies. The economic and social organizational changes in the developed world have greatly reduced the levels of physical activity, both at work and during leisure time, and have been accompanied by the widespread use of tobacco, alcohol, and other addictive substance. In addition, changes in sexual habits, methods of contraception, and family size have contributed to great changes in Western lifestyles. Diet and health in general must be viewed within this wider context (3).

With many of the so-called benefits of the modern lifestyle have come changes in the risk of several diseases such as cancer, coronary heart disease (CHD), AIDS, and many others. For over a half century, there has been conclusive proof of a close association between cigarette smoking and use of tobacco with increased levels of various forms of cancer (4). Similarly, alcohol drinking has now been shown to be a factor in increasing the risk of different forms of cancer (5), and coffee consumption is associated with increased risks of bladder cancer (6). Scientific evidence is accumulating to show that dietary factors may be linked to changes in the risk of many forms of cancers (2,7–11).

II. ROLE OF DIET IN CARCINOGENESIS

During the early part of the 20th century, several classic animal experiments have shown the potential effects of diet on carcinogenesis (12). Attempts were also made to identify preformed carcinogens and to assess their role in cancer formation. Metabolic changes induced by diet are currently thought to influence indirectly the risk of cancer, the carcinogens themselves being produced from certain dietary substances (8).

Earlier experimental designs used to obtain evidence of the association between cancer risk and dietary factors were correlation or ecological studies, wherein national cancer mortality rates were plotted against national food disappearance data, followed by calculation of the coefficient of correlation. Although a useful technique for generating scientific hypotheses and for testing

537

dietary associations obtained from other studies, with the mortality rate differences for broad agreement, correlation studies are a poor way of establishing that a dietary factor causes, promotes, or protects against cancer or for estimating the magnitude of the dietary link (2).

Thus, the etiological role of diet can be examined only by comparing the dietary exposure of persons with the disease under study with comparable healthy individuals. The case-control study is the most frequently used study design in cancer epidemiology; it involves identifying cases and choosing appropriate controls to compare their dietary experience. Questionnaires are used to build up a picture of the lifetime history of exposure to different dietary components, to see whether consistent differences emerge. In such retrospective studies, great care is required while analyzing lifetime habits related to diet to exclude bias, and minimize distortions of cases who have a "better" recall than controls.

Cohort (or prospective) is a more useful study design: disease-free individuals are identified and exposure information is collected. These individuals are then followed prospectively until groups of cases are identified, by comparing directly with the groups without the disease. Although exposure information is more unbiased in this design, large numbers of subjects with lengthy follow-up are needed, making the studies very expensive. The randomized clinical trial of diet as a preventive measure is the most ideal study design, though it is not a feasible alternative in epidemiological studies on diet and cancer, especially for the identification of dietary risk factors (2).

Approximately 80% to 90% of all human cancers may be attributable to environmental factors, including a wide range of lifestyle factors, such as diet, and social and cultural practices (7,13). The rates of cancer differ in different populations throughout the world and groups of migrants may acquire the cancer pattern of their new country or region (14), which may take within a few decades (as found in migrants to Australia) or even generations, as in case of breast cancers in Japanese migrants to the United States (15).

About one-third of human cancers may be directly related to some dietary components (7), meaning that 400,000 new cases of cancer each year may have a major dietary basis (16). Nutrition is thought to play a permissive role in enhancing the development of many cancers, at least about 80% having some link to nutrition. Within the European community alone, this represents around 1 million new cases of cancer each year. Because changes in nutritional intake could theoretically induce major alteration in cancer rates, this field is fast emerging as a topic of intensive research.

Apart from cancer quackery, a generally nutritious diet and other factors related to diet and lifestyle can reduce the risk of cancer initiation and promotion—e.g., maintaining a desirable weight and practicing a regular physical activity, since both obesity and physical inactivity are linked to an increased risk for many types of cancer. Obesity is related to all major forms of cancer, except lung cancer, especially breast cancer, endometrial cancer, colon cancer, and prostate cancer. The probable link is due to synthesis of estrogens by adipose tissue from other hormones in the bloodstream. High levels of estrogens in the bloodstream have been known to promote cancer. A long-standing excess energy intake can also promote cancer. The fat and kilocalories (kcals) are considered as promoters, rather than initiators of cancer, although the epidemiological evidence relating fat to cancer is not strong. A stronger link between diet and cancer concerns total kilocalories in the diet. Studies have shown that animals with a low kilocalorie intake have about 40% reduction in tumor yield, compared with those consuming a typical intake. The amount of fat in the diet is not important, as long as the low kcal diet is about 70% of the usual intake of energy. The mechanism behind this effect is probably hormonal. The energy-restricted animals have higher levels to inhibit tumor growth. The restricted diet may also lower serum estrogen levels.

Many single nutrients having antioxidant properties can act as anticarcinogens, preventing cancer, e.g., beta-carotene, vitamin E, vitamin C, and selenium. These antioxidants help to prevent the alteration of DNA by electron-seeking substances. Beta-carotene is strongly linked to a decrease in lung cancer risk in smokers. Also, vegetable and fruit intake may reduce risk of cancers of the G.I. tract, bladder, and cervix. Dietary fiber has a possible role in the prevention of colon cancer by decreasing transit time, so that stool is in contact with the colon for shorter period of time, which reduces the contact of carcinogens with the colon wall. Soluble fibers bind bile acids, blocking their recycling in the body. Bile acids may contribute to cancer risk by irritating the colon cells. Dietary fiber may also enhance the binding and excretion of the sex-linked hormones, testosterone and estrogen, from within the intestines, thus reducing the risks for prostate and colon cancers. However, the evidence regarding importance of dietary fiber in the prevention of colon cancer is still not conclusive. The possible carcinogenic agents in foods are fat (meats, milk, vegetable oils), alcohol (beverages), nitrites, nitrates (cured meats, ham, bacon, and sausages), aflatoxin (peanuts and other grains infected with mold), and benzo-a-pyrene (charcoal-broiled foods, especially meats).

A. Epidemiological Evidence

Willett (17) has reviewed nutritional/epidemiological studies made in the past decade. Dietary intake in terms of both food items and nutrients can now be assessed in the "usual diet" of very large numbers of individuals. Also, the epidemiologists are employing statistical techniques to separate the effects of its contribution to total energy intake. Analysis is difficult in such nutritional studies, because attempts are made to identify individuals at different levels of dietary exposure, whereas in "classic" epidemiology, one may find an unexposed group (e.g., of lifetime nonsmokers to compare with cigarette smokers).

Boyle (2) stated the following four simple criteria for the assessment of the quality of a study:

1. use of a validated method of estimating dietary and total energy intakes
2. adjusting the effect of each nutrient in the analysis, to take account of the energy intake
3. sufficient size of the study to detect the risk envisaged
4. sufficiently large range of dietary intakes in the population to allow the graded effects of dietary components or nutrients to be assessed.

Very few studies fulfil all these criteria, hence many early epidemiological studies have proved to be inconclusive. Boyle (2) has reviewed and summarized the evidence available and related to individual cancers in the order specified by the International Statistical Classification of Diseases, Injuries and Causes of Death (18).

1. Anticancer Drugs

Kulkarni (19) treated several malignant cases (10 patients) of advanced stages of cancer with Ayurvedic herbal drugs. These cases included squmous cell carcinoma, breast cancer, lung cancer, Hodgkins lymphoma, vocal cord cancer, multiple myeoloma, and edenocarcinoma. Ayurvedic preparations made from plant materials such as *Mesua ferrea*, *Asparagus racemosus*, *Adhatoda vasica*, *Tinospora cardifolia*, *Hemidesmus indicus*, *Withania somnifera*, *Smilar glabra*, *Piper cubeba*, *Piper longum*, *Glycyrrhiza glabra*, *Tribulus terrestris*, *Pterocarpus santalinus* and *Terminalia bererica*, when administered to these patients, were found to be an effective treatment in advanced, malignancies though not a total cure.

Hoffman (20) observed that aloe vera (*Aloevera barbadensis*) concentrations were able to stimulate the production of T-4 lymphocytes. Clinical studies showed an increase in T-4 lymphocytes (110 cubic millimeter in 4 weeks to 518 cubic millimeter in 18 weeks) thus protecting HIV patients. Administration of *Aloevera barbadensis* for a period of 4 months significantly decreased

'Karposi saroma', which was attributed to the production of T-4 lymphocytes, and subsequent production of cytokines, enhancing the anti-tumor activity. The less toxic nature of cesium chloride and *Aloevera barbadensis* make them excellent alternative drugs for the treatment of cancer and AIDS.

Kulkarni (21) discussed the role of diet in the treatment of cancer and AIDS. The products of Ayurveda Rashashala have been found to be useful adjuvant treatments for gaining self-confidence to fight cancers. Patients were treated with a herbal preparation such as *Chyavanprasha* and herbomineral preparations known as *Raktavardhak*. These *rasayanas* (chemicals) gave boost to various activities of body and mind. Change of lifestyle, mainly diet and meditation was advised, after the administration of the drug.

More than three decades ago, Burkitt (22) strongly supported the postulated protective role of a high fiber intake against cancer. Burkitt and other researchers suggested that native population in Africa had a lower incidence of colon cancer because they consumed fiber-rich diets. Willett et al. (23), more recently in a prospective study, examined the effects of dietary intake of fibers, as well as of other components, on colon cancer incidence in women over a six-year period. A dose-response decrease in the risk of colon cancer was observed with increasing intake of fruit fibers. Total dietary fibers, total crude fibers, and vegetable and cereal fibers were not clearly associated with a change in the risk. There are several micro nutrients (vitamin E and beta-carotene) associated with a high-fiber diet that might themselves be protective against cancer, e.g., in their combined analysis of 13 case-control studies, Howe et al (24) found that each of beta-carotene, ascorbic acid and fibers were individually significantly related to decreased cancer risk, but that after adjustment for one another, only the relationship with fibers remained strong and statistically significant. It is also likely that some of the apparent protective effect of various plant foods may be due to an inverse association of their intake with that of meat and animal fat. Most case-control studies (25–27) have shown a strong protective effect for dietary fruit and vegetables, but could not attribute the effect to fibers per se.

A following mechanism by which dietary fiber may be protective against colon cancer has been proposed: Insoluble fibers (e.g., wheat bran) increase fecal bulk and therefore dilute its contents, which decreases interactions between the intestinal mucosa and any carcinogens present in the feces. Furthermore, insoluble fibers reduce intestinal transit times, allowing less opportunity for fecal mutagens to interact with the intestinal epithelium. Fibers, as fermentative substrates, can also modify the activity of digestive microflora and lead to a modification or reduction in the production of mutagens (28). Some types of fibers can absorb mutagenic agents, leading to their excretion in the feces (29). A possible mechanism for the protective effect of fibers against breast cancer is that high-fiber intakes result in increased fecal losses of estrogens, which are associated with an increased risk of breast cancer, although experimental data on this relationship are unclear. A protective effect for fibers in the Nurses Health Study, even in the cohort that consumed 22 g fiber per day, was not evident (28). Willett et al. (29) also concluded that literature available does not support a protective effect for fibers in either colon cancer or breast cancer. However, the data require careful consideration. As to date, the evidence for a protective effect for fibers per se in carcinogenesis is inconclusive (30).

2. Fat and Fatty Acids

Ip and Marshall (31), reviewing the evidence for the carcinogenic effects of *trans* fatty acids, concluded that the available scientific data do not support this relationship. Seven studies of *trans* fatty acids and cancer represented the literature available on *trans* fat and cancer in animal models. Discounting the earliest reports because of poor experimental design, the remaining five studies showed that *trans* fat has the same effect on tumor development. Furthermore, increasing the intake of *trans* fat at the expense of *cis* fat does not produce an adverse outcome regarding cancer risk. Thus, to date there is no evidence to indicate that under properly controlled conditions, the intake of *trans* fatty acids is a risk factor for cancer.

The evidence that breast cancer is related to diet stems less from epidemiological evidence than from animal experimentation and from the analysis of ecologic data. The epidemiological evidence is that the impact of fat intake in general upon breast cancer risk is slight to negligible. There is at present no strong evidence that the intake of *trans* fatty acids is related to an increased risk of breast cancer.

However, there is a good and increasing evidence that diet is related to the risk of cancers of the colon and rectum. This evidence centers around the intake of saturated fat or animal fat as increasing risk, and the intake of fiber and vegetable products as decreasing risk. The clinical trials that are currently under way are evaluating dietary restriction of fat intake and supplementation of fiber and fruit and vegetable intake. No evidence indicates that the intake of *trans* fatty acids is related to increased risk of cancers of the colon and rectum.

According to Ip and Marshall (31), there is a good evidence that fat intake might be related to the risk of prostate cancer. Most of this evidence has focused on the consumption of saturated fat and on fats of animal origin. The intake of *trans* fatty acids, however, has not been correlated to prostrate cancer risk. One study that directly examined the relevance of *trans* fatty acids reported that they are not related to risk. Thus, it was summarized that there was little evidence to show that *trans* fatty acids are related to the risk of cancer at any of the major cancer sites (31).

Thorling (32) reviewed the recent information on obesity, fat intake, energy balance, and exercise with respect to cancer risk in humans. Animal experiments in the field are analyzed to find support for the epidemiological observations. Thorling (32) has discussed the problems involved in the interpretation of the human and animal data and attempted to extract the essence of the present body of knowledge. Obesity is undoubtedly associated with certain cancers, but its causal relationship is not fully established. Exercise to a moderate degree for prolonged periods of time evidently confers a decreased risk of some cancers. Causality is difficult to establish in human observations, but animal experimental results make such a relation appear very likely. Since a fat-rich diet in humans is often a diet relatively poor in fruits and vegetables, it is difficult to ascribe an increased cancer risk on a fat-rich diet to the intake of fat alone, because a shortage of the intake of fruits and vegetables may well be an important factor. Results of the animal experiments have generally supported the idea that fat is a promoter for a number of experimental cancers. The type of fat is probably important, although some controversies still exist concerning the relative effects of different types of fatty acids (32).

Kritchevsky (33) has clearly demonstrated that caloric restriction inhibits experimental carcinogenesis, whether spontaneous or induced by chemical carcinogens or by other means such as ultraviolet irradiation. In animal experiments (34), the effects of *ad libitum* feeding and 40% caloric restriction in rats were studied by treating them with 7,12-dimethylbenz (a) anthracene (DMBA) in order to induce mammary tumors. No tumors were found in the restricted rats, as against 58% tumor incidence in the control group fed with 3.9% fat (2.9% coconut oil and 1.0% corn oil). A similar experiment in rats treated with 1,2-dimethylhydrazine (DMH) to induce colonic tumors showed tumor incidence of 85% and 35% in *ad libitum* and calorie-restricted rats given DMBA, and 100% and 53% in rats given DMH, respectively (Table 1). The saturated fat was less carcinogenic than unsaturated fat (35). Kritchevsky and Klurfeld (36) also showed that restriction of calories by only 10% (fat intake equivalent to that of control) did not affect tumor incidence but reduced tumor burden (total tumor weight) by 47%. At 30% caloric restriction tumor incidence and burden were decreased by 42% and 95%, respectively (Table 2). In another study, Kritchevsky et al. (37) showed that compared to rats fed 5% corn oil *ad libitum*, the rats

Table 1 Effect of 40% Caloric Restriction and Fat Type on Chemical Carcinogenesis

Carcinogen	Rat strain	Dietary fat	Tumor incidence (%)	
			Ad libitum	Restricted
DMBA[a]	Sprague-Dawley	Coconut oil	58	0
		Corn oil	80	20
DMH[b]	F344	Butter oil	85	35
		Corn oil	100	53

[a]7,12-dimethylbenz (a) anthracene (DMBA).
[b]1,2-dimethylhydrazine (DMH).
Source: Ref. 33

fed 26.7% corn oil in the 25% calorically restricted diet exhibited 54% lower tumor incidence and tumor burden was 45% lower (Table 3). Thus, caloric restriction inhibited tumorigenesis even at high fat intake. Reviewing data from 82 studies, Albanes (38) concluded that tumor incidence decreased with increased caloric restriction. The mechanism (s) by which caloric restriction exerts cancer-inhibiting effect need to be elucidated (33).

Reviewing the epidemiological evidence for breast and colon cancer, Miller (39) concluded that although not all the finding are consistent, accumulated evidence indicates that both breast and colorectal cancers are associated with high fat intake. Perhaps most typically the pattern of high risk is associated with dietary consumption of high fat, possibly especially the saturated fat from animal sources, and low consumption of vegetables and possibly fiber, though the relevance of fiber as distinct from other potential protective factors from vegetables containing fiber remains to be established. The population-attributable risk from saturated fat for colo-rectal cancer is of the order of 42% with possibly 50% or more cases explained by dietary variables. For breast cancer the attributable risk from total fat is to the extent of 27% with an additional 12% from obesity. Thus, up to 40% of breast cancer may be preventable by dietary modification, although there is some concern that the effect of dietary modification for breast cancer could be delayed, as exhibited by the lack of change in breast cancer incidence in some religious groups that have adopted a low-fat diet (40). A fairly rapid impact of dietary modification of colon cancer rates has

Table 2 Effect of Graded Caloric Restriction on DMBA[a]-Induced Mammary Tumors in Sprague-Dawley Rats

Regimen	Tumor incidence (%)	Tumor multiplicity	Tumor burden (g)
Ad libitum	60	4.7 ± 1.3	10.1 ± 3.3
10% restricted	60	3.0 ± 0.8	5.4 ± 3.0
20% restricted	40	2.8 ± 0.7	4.7 ± 1.9
30% restricted	35	1.3 ± 0.3	0.9 ± 0.8
40% restricted	5	1.0 ± 0	—
P	0.005	NS	0.05

[a]7,12-dimethylbenz (a) anthracene
Source: Ref. 33.

Table 3   Effect of Fat Level and 25% Caloric Restriction on DMBA[a]-Induced Mammary Tumors in Sprague-Dawley Rats

Regimen	Tumor incidence (%)	Tumor multiplicity	Tumor burden (%)
Ad libitum			
5% corn oil	65	1.9 ± 0.3	4.2 ± 1.9
15% corn oil	85	3.0 ± 0.6	6.6 ± 2.7
20% corn oil	80	4.1 ± 0.6	11.8 ± 3.2
25% restricted			
20% corn oil	60	1.9 ± 0.4	1.5 ± 0.5
26.7% corn oil	30	1.5 ± 0.3	2.3 ± 1.6
P	0.005	0.0001	0.0001

[a]7,12-dimethylbenz(a)anthracene (DMBA).
Source: Ref. 33.

been postulated, with a possible delay of 40 or 50 years for breast cancer, especially if the full effect of dietary modification has to occur for women in their teens and twenties (39).

3.   Other Nutrients

According to Krishnaswamy (41), human diseases, including cancer, are closely linked to dietary habits. The health concerns in the field of human nutrition in the past about 3 decades have centered around deficiency disorders, with an emphasis on the role of nutrients in health and disease. Scientific developments are now highlighting the important role that diets can play in the prevention of chronic diseases such as cancer and cardiovascular disease, which are becoming more prevalent because of changing dietary patterns (42,43). Several functional foods have been known to either prevent or cure human diseases. Currently, such foods are of great public significance because they also promote positive health and nutrition.

Several institutes, such as WHO (42) and National Research Council (NRC) (44), have directed their attention to foods that have a positive role in maintaining health and in delaying age-related disorders such as cancer, cataract, and coronary artery disease. Debate, however, continues as to whether nutrients consumed in amounts above the RDAs can provide benefit beyond the traditional functional role of preventing deficiency disorders and associated biochemical or metabolic abnormalities. Several nonnutrient components appear also to be desirable components in the diet because they influence the pathogenetic mechanism that can either delay or decrease the sequential processes resulting in chronic disorders (45,46). It is important to document clearly the strength and consistency of functional food's association with health or disease, the magnitude of its effects and whether, as a lifestyle factor, it is practical to recommend the consumption of such food on a long-term basis. Krishnaswamy (41) has summarized the results of case-control studies on oral and esophageal cancers in India, with regard to their etiopathogenesis and prevention, and has provided an overview of the role that spices can play in modulating the process of carcinogenesis and precancerous events (47,48).

Poor dietary intake of vegetables and fruits coupled with low estimated intakes of beta-carotene, thiamin, riboflavin, folate, vitamin C, iron, and copper have been reported to increase the risk of cancers of the upper aereodigestive tract (49–51). The biological indicators of nutritional status, such as concentrations of vitamin A, vitamin E, red cell folate, and plasma zinc and selenium, were significantly decreased in subjects with oral or esophageal cancer, confirming low intakes of these nutrients from protective foods such as fruits, vegetables, and pulses. Epidemiological evidence strongly indicates that consumption of fruits and vegetables is important in the prevention of epithelial cancers, particularly those of the alimentary and respiratory tracts (52,53). Micronutrients in the diet, especially antioxidant vitamins, appear to play a vital role in reducing damage resulting from environmental exposure, and may act synergistically to enhance several protective mechanisms against carcinogenesis. Krishnaswamy (41) suggests that the antioxidant vitamins such as ascorbic acid can be considered candidates for chemoprevention of cancers.

Micronutrient intervention studies are gaining recognition as an approach in strengthening or refuting the existing evidence for a link between diet and cancer. Krishnaswamy et al. (54) conducted a randomized nutrient intervention study with a cocktail of antioxidant micronutrients in a placebo-controlled trial that focused on precancerous lesions in an area prone to palatal cancer. Antioxidant nutrients such as vitamin A, riboflavin, zinc, and selenium, the doses of which varied over a 4-month period, were given for one year on a biweekly basis. The study of premalignant lesions, which were epidemiologically to be associated with subsequent development of cancer, highlighted the preventive and therapeutic role of antioxidants in precancerous events. Risk of lesions was higher in those with low intakes of several protective foods, such as pulses, vegetables, fruits, milk, and milk products. Plasma vitamin A, iron, and folate status were also lower in those with lesions, reflecting the low intake of functional foods rich in micronutrients.

According to Krishnaswamy (41), the balance between prooxidants and antioxidants is critical in poorly nourished individuals, requiring public health action directed toward increasing the consumption of dark green and yellow vegetables, which possess several protective substances. A program can be envisaged in which the proscription and prescription of either dietary or chemopreventive substances result in making at-risk subjects resistant or tolerant to carcinogens in the environment. Such dietary modifications call for intensive nutrition education, with agricultural and horticultural interventions to increase the production and availability of foods rich in antioxidant nutrients.

Several nonnutrient components of plants act as detoxificants, immunomodulators, antioxidants, antimutagens, and anticarcinogens (55,56). Apart from known nutrients such as beta-carotene, ascorbic acid, vitamin E, and selenium, compounds such as phenols, flavonoids, isoflavones, isothiocyanates, diterpenes, methylxanthines, dithiols, and coumarins have been known to prevent cancer through their role in the inhibition of tumor production (57). These compounds in general act by quenching free radicals, inhibiting the activation of procarcinogens, and binding carcinogens to macromolecules. The functional components of the plant kingdom have diverse chemical structures and participate in many physiological and metabolic functions in the body, thus contributing to the promotion of health. These substances are present abundantly in yellow and green vegetables, *Allium* vegetables, fruits, and spices.

An induction of coordinated enzyme response in xenobiotic metabolism can effectively suppress carcinogenesis. The antineoplastic effects of inducing and inhibiting agents in various foods focus on specific monooxygenases, such as aryl hydrocarbon hydrolase (AHH), UDP-glucuronyl transferase (UDPGT), and glutathione-S-transferase (GST). Rajpurohit and Krishnaswamy (58) provided vegetables (e.g., spinach, amaranth, hibiscus, cabbage, and onion) and spices (turmeric and mustard) in amounts between 1% and 10% in the diet of rats and studied their effects on the induction potential of hepatic microsomal and cytosolic xenobiotic metabolizing enzymes. UDPGT and GST were significantly elevated in groups that received diets containing cabbage, onions, mustard, and turmeric. Turmeric significantly stimulated both liver and intestinal GST, with no effects on AHH (59). Enhancement of GST activity is associated with decreased response to chemical carcinogens and inhibition of tumors at several sites. The intake of these substances in adequate amounts keeps the enzyme detoxification system turned on to handle high concentrations of carcinogens, to inhibit damage to macromolecules, and to act as a scavenger of damaging free radicals (41).

The covalent binding of carcinogens to DNA is measured as an indicator of the highly reactive electrophilic intermediates formed during oxidative metabolism. Carcinogen-DNA adducts initiate carcinogenesis. The benzo(a)-pyrene binding to liver DNA indicated that green leafy vegetables, *Allium* vegetables (onion), and spices (mustard and turmeric) significantly inhibit the formation of carcinogen–DNA adducts in vivo in rats (58,60). Turmeric and its active component curcumin decrease the formation of benzo(a)-pyrene–DNA adducts. In very low concentrations, curcumin (a diferulyl methane in turmeric) inhibits benzo (a)-pyrene–DNA binding (41).

The antimutagenic potential of several nonnutrients has been evaluated on the basis of their GST-stimulating activity. Both turmeric and mustard at low levels (0.5–1%) significantly inhibited mutagenesis in a dose-response manner (61,62).

In Ayurveda, the classical Indian system of medicine, turmeric has been documented as a medicine for treating contusions, sprains, and bruises and as a carminative, astringent, and antiseptic. It also influences the blood lipid profile. Turmeric-based cosmetics such as skin creams and tooth powders are also used in India. The antimutagenic and anticarcinogenic properties of turmeric are being evaluated. Turmeric and its active component curcumin are potent antioxidants and can prevent nitrosamine formation from precursors and inhibit aflatoxin production (63). Curcumin is also a potent anti-inflammatory agent, and a peptide was isolated from turmeric that exhibits antioxidant properties against reactive oxygen species (64). Turmeric and curcumin were shown to inhibit tumors in skin (65), breast, oral cavity (66), and forestomach (67) in initiation and promotion models in several species of mice, rats, and hamsters. Turmeric's broad spectrum of action as an anti-initiator and antipromoter thus makes it an ideal medical food for prevention of cancer. The expected benefits of incorporating such functional foods liberally into routine diets may not only lower the risk of cancer but also reduce risk of other chronic disease, such as cardiovascular disease and cataract, and perhaps delay the aging process (41).

Willett et al. (68) examined epidemiological data from a variety of sources to assess the relationship between vitamin A intake and cancer risk. They also reviewed the evidence for an influence of vitamin A intake on the incidence of cancer at the three major sites accounting for a substantial portion of cancers in developed countries. The data available are compatible with a modest inverse association between intake of vitamin A and breast cancer, although it is not clear whether this effect may be due to preformed vitamin A, carotenoids, or both. The evidence that vitamin A protects against colon cancer is unconvincing. In the case of prostate cancer, early suggestions that vitamin A may increase incidence have not been confirmed by subsequent studies.

Prospective data from a large number of ongoing cohort studies in the United States and Europe are expected to be available within a couple of years, which will permit further assessment of potential correlations between vitamin A and cancer at various sites by analysis of much larger numbers of cases than are currently available. In addition to providing information on the overall associations, these studies are expected to provide data on interactions, latency, and dose-response. Over the next decade, intervention studies testing the effect of beta-carotene on the incidence of cancer at these sites will probably be reported. These intervention studies, with better control of bias, may leave open numerous questions on optimal dose and latency. Thus, even a null finding would not totally exclude the possibility that different doses of beta-carotene taken for a longer time might be effective. In the meantime, dietary recommendations to increase carotenoid intake by eating more fruit and green and yellow vegetables are not likely to be harmful but instead may offer a decreased risk of several cancers (68).

According to Astrog (69), large-scale intervention studies, with one exception, have failed to demonstrate any chemopreventive potency of beta-carotene supplementation in humans, revealing a lack of knowledge of the mechanisms involved. In addition to their antioxidant properties, which have long been thought to be the clue to their biological effects, carotenoids appear to have a variety of cellular actions that make them remarkable physiological modulators. Further research is needed before new chemoprevention trials can be undertaken on a strong scientific basis.

Carotenoids in general have been found to act on several cellular mechanisms, each involving one or more stages of carcinogenesis. Some of their actions on animal cells, such as the reduction of cell proliferation, suppression of cell transformation, induction of cellular differentiation, up-regulation of gap junctions, and immunostimulation, are strikingly similar to those of retinoic acid and other retinoids. The antioxidant properties of carotenoids may be responsible for some of their antigenotoxic and immunostimulating effects (70–72). The antioxidant effects of carotenoids do not appear to play any role in their actions on key mechanisms of carcinogenesis, such as xenobiotic-metabolizing enzymes, cell transformation, cell proliferation, or gap-junction cell communication (69).

Chung et al. (73) advised against ingesting large quantities of tannins (water-soluble polyphenols present in many plant foods) because they may possess carcinogenic and antinutritional activities, thereby posing a risk of adverse health effects. However, the intake of a small quantity of the right kind of tannins may be beneficial to human health. It is thus important to determine the right dose of the right kind of tannins to promote optimal health. A further systematic investigation of components of tannins is needed to evaluate their anticarcinogenic properties.

Reuter et al. (74) have reviewed the therapeutic effects and applications of garlic and its preparations. The only study in which garlic was used to treat patients with advanced stages of cancer was reported by Spivak (75). A garlic juice preparation was administered in doses of 0.2 to 2 ml intravenously or 1 to 5 ml intramuscularly daily for 3 to 7 days. Of 35 patients with cancer at various sites (lung, larynx; leukemia), 26 showed positive treatment results of differing degrees, though complete cure was not achieved in any case. Rainov and Burkert (76), however, reported the case of a man whose pituitary tumor shrank by 50% during the 5 months in which he ate 5 to 7 grams of fresh garlic daily. This was the first case ever reported of reduction of this type of tumor without chemotherapy or surgery (74).

Steinmetz et al. (77) reported an important epidemiological (prospective cohort) study in which the effects of the intake of 127 foods, including 44 vegetables and fruits, was determined in 41,378 American women (ages 55–69), followed by a 5-year monitoring of colon cancer incidence. The most striking result of this Iowa Women's Health Study was the finding that garlic was the only food that showed a statistically significant association with decreased colon cancer risk. For cancers anywhere in the colon, the modest consumption of one or more servings of garlic (fresh or powdered) a week resulted in a 35% lower risk, and a 50% lower risk was found for cancer of the distal colon (78). Although this study did not include onions, several other epidemiological studies have shown that onions and other *Allium* species are usually associated with decreased gastrointestinal cancer risk (52,53,79–82). However, in a series of epidemiological studies from the Netherlands, no association was found between supplemented garlic (pills) consumption and risk of stomach, colon, rectum, lung, or breast cancers (83–86). These studies should be viewed with caution, because the consumption of garlic supplements varies considerably with both type and brand (74).

Thompson (87) reviewed the potential health benefits of the antinutrients commonly found in plant foods. Although antinutrients such as phytic acid, phenolics (tannins), saponins, protease inhibitors, phytoestrogens and lignans have been shown to reduce the availability of nutrients and cause growth inhibition, they have been related to reduced cancer risks. The U. S. National Cancer Institute has identified a number of foods that are thought to be protective against cancer and on which research is currently being encouraged (88–90). Several of these substances found in plant foods may be responsible for the cancer-protective effect. According to Thompson (87), health benefits of these antinutrients are possible at a certain level of their intake without causing much adverse effects; e.g., Asian women who consume more soya products (containing phyto-estrogens and protease inhibitors) than American women are at lower risk of cancer and seem to have reduced rates of reproductive and pancreatic cancer (89). Several antinutrients appear to have similar beneficial effects, such as reduction in cancer risk or cardiovascular disease; thus, studies to determine the synergistic or antagonistic effects of mixtures of these antinutrients would be useful. The interaction of antinutrients with other components of the diet and the mechanism(s) of their action need to be elucidated to understand their role in health and disease (87).

Reviewing the chemistry, biology, and implications of lycopene for human health and disease, Clinton (91) concluded that most of the health benefits attributed to lycopene are derived from studies of estimated dietary intake or blood concentrations, reflecting the selection of tomato products for consumption rather than supplements. The availability of lycopene-enriched products in the market from the "health food" industry, even before the evidence has been developed to support the beneficial effects of these products, should be a matter of concern to nutrition scientists, dietitians, and medical practitioners. The information on potential risks, dose-response at stages of disease processes, pharmacokinetics, or mechanisms of action for purified lycopene preparations is not adequate. It is also not known which disease processes may be inhibited by pharmacologic lycopene supplements. Thus, complete fundamental studies concerning the biology of lycopene, including its absorption, metabolism, excretion, and biological functions in experimental models and humans, are imperative to undertake (91).

Evidence accumulating from various epidemiological studies around the world, however, suggests that a diet containing a diverse array of fruits and vegetables, including tomatoes, results in a lower risk of several types of cancer (92,93). Peto et al. (94) postulated that carotenoids, especially beta-carotene, present in several vegetables and fruits, may be the critical factor in these foods. This hypothesis was reinforced by rodent experiments and studies showing that higher blood concentrations of beta-carotene were correlated with lower risk of several cancers, particularly tobacco-related malignancies (95,96). No effects of beta-carotene were noted on skin cancer (97), colon adenomas (98), or overall cancer risk (99). Whereas two large, randomized, placebo-controlled trials in high-risk populations showed an increased rate of lung cancer in the groups receiving beta-carotene supplements (100,101), a protective effect against oral leukoplakia (102,103), and premalignant lesions of the cervix (104) has been suggested.

The results of these studies indicate that the simple extrapolation from fruit and vegetable intake to chemoprevention by a pure carotenoid will not be a panacea for cancer. Fruits and vegetables contain myriad chemical substances, some of which are nutrients—others that have potent biological activities are not nutrients by traditional classification. People who consume diets rich in fruits and vegetables often also consume more fiber, less fat, and fewer refined carbohydrates and demonstrate other health-conscious lifestyle behaviors.

According to Clinton (91), many of the direct effects of lycopene on developing tumors must be taken into consideration, along with indirect effects mediated through the host; e.g., lycopene could influence the cancer cascade by modulating hormone status, carcinogen metabolism, immune status, and angiogenesis (105–110).

III. EFFECTS OF DIET AND LIFESTYLE ON SPECIFIC CANCERS

A. Cancers of the Digestive Tract

1. Tongue, Mouth, and Pharyngeal Cancer

The majority of epidemiological studies combine these cancers together. Cigarette smoking and alcohol consumption have been reported to be independent risk factors for oral cancers, but their combined effects are often geometrically additive. Boyle et al. (111) reported that after stopping smoking for 10 years, the risk among ex-smokers fell to a level similar to that of lifelong non-smokers. An increased risk of oral cancer is linked to use of oral snuff (112) and fine homeground tobacco powder (113). Betel nut chewing is responsible for oral cancer in many parts of the world, including India (4). Poor dental hygiene has been regarded as an independent risk factor for oral cancer (114), which may be reduced by frequent consumption of fruits and vegetables (115,116).

2. Nasopharyngeal Cancer

Nasopharyngeal cancer has a pattern different from that of oral tumors and seems to involve Epstein-Barr virus (EBV) infections. There is a substantial risk of nasopharyngeal cancer among Chinese babies weaned on salted fish and preserved and fermented foods, and also among those who consume these foods during childhood (117). These foods are sources of volatile nitrosamines (carcinogens), some of which have been shown to induce nasal cavity tumors in experimental animals (118). Fong et al. (119) also noted that rats fed these salted fish produced urine containing mutagens.

3. Esophageal Cancer

Both cigarette smoking and alcohol intake are the most important risk factors for esophageal cancer in developed countries (5,120); the highest rates of this cancer prevail in France (121). About 85% of all cases of esophageal cancer in northwest France are attributable to the combined effects of cigarette smoking and alcohol consumption, closely linked behaviors that are difficult to separate. La Vecchia and Negri (122), however, showed that the risk of esophageal cancer has increased among nonsmokers who drink alcohol and among nondrinkers who smoke. Several other studies have shown a close association of esophageal cancer with a high prevalence of alcoholism, e.g., workers involved in the production and distribution of alcoholic beverages (123), Danish brewery workers (124), and men in the French department of Ille-et-Villaine (125). However, neither alcohol nor tobacco appears to be involved substantially in the high-incidence areas of many developing countries such as Iran and China, where drinking very hot drinks (126) or eating contaminated foods has been implicated as a risk factor. However, generalized dietary deficiencies of essential nutrients appear to be the major contributing factor to the carcinogenic process (127). Diet in the high-risk areas is often poor in vitamins A and C and several other micronutrients due to low intake of nutritious foods such as fruits and vegetables. Decarli et al. (128) suggested that these deficiencies and dietary patterns may be related to esophageal cancer risk in the developed countries. Negri et al. (129) estimated that about 90% of esophageal cancer in males of northern Italy could be attributed to cigarette smoking, high alcohol use, and low beta-carotene intake; the corresponding proportion of risk by these factors in females was 58%. A monotonous cereal-based diet (e.g., maize in northern Italy) can induce deficiency of many vitamins such as thaimin, riboflavin, niacin, and others, leading to pellagra, which is characterized by widespread inflammation of the upper digestive tract mucosa (2).

4. Stomach Cancer

Cancer of the stomach was the leading cause of mortality from cancer worldwide until the early 1980s and only recently has been overtaken by the "epidemic" form of lung cancer. Gastric cancer rates are still very high in China, Japan, and eastern European countries and northern Italy, but the incidence of stomach cancer in the West is declining. Epidemiological evidence suggests that a more affluent diet and improved food processing, especially refrigeration, are linked to these favorable trends, and that diet in early life may be very important in altering gastric carcinogenesis.

Diets rich in fresh fruits and vegetables (130) and especially garlic (117,131) are protective against stomach cancers, whereas diets rich in traditional starchy foods, mainly cereals, are positively associated with risk, which may serve as an index of poor diet. By combining the risks and benefits of high- and low-risk foods in a model, it is possible to predict a 5- to 10-fold variation in risk, which could account for much of the observed geographical variation in stomach cancer rates (132,133). The proposed links of stomach cancer with dietary salt and with salt nitrates or nitrites as well as the supposed protective effects of certain specific nutrients such as antioxidants, beta-carotene, and ascorbic acid, need further research to establish a firm association (134).

Joosens and Geboers (135) have presented the possible positive and negative etiological factors for stomach cancer and stroke (Table 4). The most important linking factors should be common to the two sets of factors (the intersection of the sets). It can be seen from Table 4 that dietary salt is the most obvious linking factor. Barring vitamin C, all the factors in the intersection of the sets are related to dietary salt. A high carbohydrate intake has been singled out as a possible factor promoting both stroke and stomach cancer. Salt intake may explain the higher prevalence of stomach cancer, stroke, and hypertension in lower socioeconomic classes, because cheap foods such as bread, potatoes, cheese, sausages, dried/smoked fish or meat, canned meats and vegetables, and fast foods are heavily salted (135). Table 5 gives the possible etiology of stomach cancer. All this evidence is consistent with clinical and epidemiological observations. Salt is caustic to the skin, as observed among workers in salt mines and among lobster fishermen, and also damages the taste buds. High blood pressure, which may be aggravated by salt, is the major contributor to strokes.

5. Colorectal Cancer

Colorectal cancer, the third most common form of cancer worldwide, has the its highest incidence rates in Western Europe and North America, intermediate rates in Eastern Europe and the lowest rates in sub-Saharah Africa (136); 166,000 new cases every year are reported in the European

Table 4 Possible Risk Factors for Stomach Cancer and Stroke

	For stomach cancer only	For stomach cancer & stroke[a]	For stroke only
Positive factors	Nitrates/nitrites	Salt (+)	Saturated fat (−)
	Nitroso-carcinogens	Pickled foods (+)	Low protein (+)
	Bracken fern	Smoked foods (+)	Alcohol
	Soil trace elements	Lard (+)	Lead
	Peaty soil	Soybean sauce (+)	The "Pill"
	Talcum in rice	Carbohydrate-rich foods (+)	Stress
	Atrophic gastritis (+)	Low socioeconomic class (+)	
		Salted fish or meat (+)	
Negative factors	Fat	Refrigeration of foods (−)	Polyunsaturated fat (−)
	Selenium	Fresh vegetables (−)	Treatment of hypertension
	Milk (−)	Vitamin C	Potassium
			Calcium
			Fiber

[a]The middle column is the intersection of the sets of risk factors for cancer and stroke.
(+) = positively related to salt intake; (−) = negatively related to salt intake
Source: Ref. 135.

Table 5   Possible Etiology of Stomach Cancer

High salt intake; hypertonic stomach content
Delayed emptying through duodenal osmoreceptors
Longer contact with caustic salt solution, especially in lower part of the
    stomach
Damaged gastric mucosa, increased DNA synthesis, ornithine decar-
    boxylase induction (proven in animals)
Atrophic gastritis, anacidity, bacterial overgrowth, nitrates to nitrites
Nitroso-carcinogens (salt is cocarcinogenic and promotes stomach can-
    cer in animals)
Stomach cancer, especially in lower part of the stomach

Source: Ref. 135.

Community alone (16). Very few specific risk factors of a nondietary origin have been established for colorectal cancer.

Although energy intake seems to be related to colorectal cancer, any proposed mechanism reflecting this is complex (137). Physically active individuals tend to consume more energy, but they also seem to have decreased colorectal cancer risk (138). Also, there is no consistent association between obesity and colorectal cancer risk and retrospective studies have to cope with the problems of weight loss from the disease. Thus, the positive effect of energy does not appear to be merely the result of overeating and may reflect differences in metabolic efficiency or body composition (2).

Epidemiological evidence has consistently shown that fat intake is positively related to colorectal cancer risk, based on results from ecological studies, animal experiments, and case-control and cohort studies; however, there have been meager systematic analytical studies involving human subjects. Many studies have failed to show an energy-independent effect of fat intake.

The prospective assessment of health of 88,571 female nurses in the United States, aged 34 to 59 years, followed for many years, indicated that after adjusting total energy intake, consumption of animal fat was associated with increased colon cancer risk (23). No association was found between vegetable fat and relative risk of colon cancer in women who ate beef, pork, or lamb as a main dish more than once per month. Willett et al. (23) suggested that high intake of animal fat increases the risk of colon cancer and supported the existing recommendations to substitute fish and chicken for meats with a high fat content. This study has provided the best epidemiological evidence, identifying increased meat consumption as a risk factor for colon cancer independently of its contribution to fat or to total energy intake. Laboratory studies have also shown that cooked meats may be carcinogenic due to production of amino imidazoazarenes (AIAs) during cooking (139,140). Evidence from animal feeding experiments has shown that AIAs are mammalian carcinogens that produce tumors in various anatomic sites of mice (141). Ha et al. (142), however, reported that fried ground beef can also produce certain anticarcinogenic substances; thus, we have a food with the potential to produce mixtures of both carcinogenic and anticarcinogenic compounds.

A case-control study involving Chinese in both North America and China, which have distinct differences in the risk of colorectal cancer, indicated that colorectal cancer risk in both areas increased with increasing total energy intake, especially from saturated fat (138), although no relationship was noticed with other sources of energy in the diet. Colon cancer risk was increased among men employed in sedentary occupations, and risk for colorectal cancer increased, for both sexes, with the time spent sitting, in both China and North America, the association of colorectal cancer risk with saturated fat was stronger among sedentary than active people. The risk among sedentary Chinese-Americans of either sex increased more than fourfold from the lowest to the highest category of saturated fat intake. Among the migrants to North America, the risk increased with increasing years spent in North America. Attributable risk calculations suggested that if these associations are causal, saturated fat intakes exceeding 10 g/day, especially in combination with physical inactivity, could account for 60% of colorectal cancer incidence among Chinese-American men and 40% among Chinese-American women (138).

The importance of specific fatty acids in the diet also has been recognized; some animal experiments have shown that linoleic acid (*n*-6 PUFA) promotes colorectal carcinogenesis (143,144), whereas a low-fat diet rich in eicopentenoic acid (*n*-3 PUFA) had an inhibitory effect on colon cancer (145). However, epidemiological studies have not been conducted to study the effects of *n*-3 and *n*-6 fatty acids on colorectal cancer.

The protective effect of dietary fiber against colorectal cancer was thought to be due to increased bulk and reduced transit time. This mechanism may not be as relevant to colorectal carcinogenesis as previously thought (146). The term *fiber* encompasses many components, each having specific physiological functions (see Chapter 3). Fiber is commonly classified into insoluble, nondegradable constituents (mainly present in cereal fiber) and soluble, degradable constituents, such as pectin and plant gums, present mainly in fruits and vegetables. Epidemiological studies have pointed out differences in the effect of these components. Although some case-control studies have reported a protective effect for total dietary fiber intake (147,148), as was also found in one prospective study (149), a large number of other studies could not find such a protective effect. Willett (137) has reviewed this topic in detail. Although a majority of studies in humans have found no protective effect from the fiber in cereals, the benefits of fiber from vegetables, and perhaps fruit sources, conceivably reflect an association with other nutrients present in fruits and vegetables, with fiber intake acting merely as an indicator of their consumption (2).

Alcohol consumption has been found to be positively associated with colorectal cancer (150), but it is not known whether the putative association is with alcohol per se or with the energetic effect of alcohol.

Some experimental evidence indicates that vitamin E and selenium may be protective against colon tumors (143) and that vitamin A and/or its precursor, beta-carotene, also have a protective effect (137). Eleven of 12 case-control studies found an inverse relation between coffee consumption and risk of colorectal cancer, suggesting that coffee drinking may be protective (6), but no association has been found with tea drinking or caffeine intake from all sources considered.

Thus, dietary factors seem to be important determinants of colorectal cancer risk. An effect of saturated fat appears to exist independently of energy intake, but meat intake may increase the risk. Whether the latter is independent of its fat content or its contribution to energy intake remains to be known. If it is independent, then it may relate to the mutagenic products formed in the cooking process. Vegetable fiber, directly or indirectly, appears to be protective, as does coffee consumption. Association of colorectal cancer with other dietary factors, such as calcium and cereal fiber, remains to be established fully.

B. Liver and Pancreatic Cancers

High alcohol intakes were found to be correlated with an increased frequency of primary liver cancer (5), although this remains to be established universally. Alcoholics in general have around 50% excess of liver cancer compared with non-alcoholics; this risk may, however, be quite underestimated, because the liver damage induced by alcohol may compel people to stop drinking well before the diagnosis of liver cancer is made in a patient (2). According to Boyle (2), part of the excess liver cancer risk in alcoholics may be attributed to dietary deficiencies, because a diet deficient in vitamin A and other micronutrients has been shown to increase the risk of hepatocellular carcinoma (151). The risk of primary liver cancer is significantly increased in people living in tropical areas of Africa and Asia who are infected with the hepatitis B virus and consume alcohol and are exposed to aflatoxin (*Aspergillus flavus*)-contaminated foods. Animal experiments have indicated that very early exposure to hepatitis B virus is particularly conducive to hepatonic development. Thus, the risk of primary liver cancer is increased greatly in people who are exposed to more than one factor (2).

Pancreatic cancer has been consistently found to occur more frequently in men than in women, in blacks than in whites, and in people living in urban than in people living in rural areas. Cigarette smoking has always been found to increase the risk of pancreatic cancer (120,152). The risk of pancreatic cancer dose not seem to be related to either coffee consumption (6) or to alcohol intake (153,154). However, certain specific dietary factors are likely to emerge as important determinants of pancreatic risk factor (155–160). A positive association between carbohydrate and cholesterol intake and an inverse relationship with dietary fiber and vitamin C intake have been reported. The consistency, strength, and specificity of these associations suggest underlying causal relationships between dietary factors and pancreatic cancer (157).

C. Lung and Laryngeal Cancers

A considerable body of evidence has accumulated to indicate that cigarette smoking is an overwhelming cause of lung cancer in humans (161). Lower risks associated with the regular consumption of one or more fruits and vegetables were reported in eight case-control studies. Steinmetz and Potter (162) reviewed the results of these studies and concluded that in each study a lower risk was observed with intakes of at least one vegetable high in beta-carotene, and in four of these eight studies, the lower risk was more evident in smokers than in nonsmokers.

Both tobacco smoking and alcohol consumption are major established risk factors for laryngeal cancer (5,120). Pipe and cigar smoking are especially strongly linked to laryngeal cancer, with a lower risk for filter, low-tar cigarettes. Some case-control studies have shown that a poor diet, especially one which is limited in fresh fruit and vegetables, (available vitamin A and C) is associated with the risk of laryngeal cancer (160,161,163,164).

D. Breast Cancer

Breast cancer is widespread, with over half a million new cases diagnosed worldwide each year (165). Despite many detailed epidemiological studies, however, the etiology of breast cancer remains to be firmly established (166).

Whereas the risk of breast cancer may increase with increasing body mass index among postmenopausal women (167), a number of other studies indicate that the same risk factor may reduce the risk of breast cancer at premenopausal ages. However, a number of biases, including the increased likelihood of finding a lump in thinner women, have complicated interpretation of these results (168). Former college athletes (169) and ballet dancers (170) were found to have reduced risk of breast cancer compared with non-athletes. This may be associated with physical activity or reduced body weight around menarche during adolescence or throughout one's lifetime.

The earlier hypothesis of association of breast cancer with dietary fat has remained very controversial (137). Although an increased risk of breast cancer with increasing saturated fat intake in postmenopausal women is a plausible conclusion, the evidence from detailed analytical studies in humans with breast cancer is unclear; both case-control studies (156), and prospective studies (171,172), provide little support for this association. The recent analysis of the U.S. Nurses Health Study also found no association between fat intake and intake of fiber and breast cancer risk in either pre- or postmenopausal women (173).

Lubin et al. (174) interviewed patients representing 854 biopsied cases of benign breast disease (BBD) and 755 matched surgical and 723 matched neighborhood control subjects between 1977 and 1980 in Israel, using a detailed food frequency questionnaire. Cases were classified according to degree of ductal atypia (Black-Chablon grading system). Women with atypic lesions (grades above 3) reported a higher intake of all types of foods compared with both control series. The increased consumption was due primarily to foods containing more than about 10% fat. Odd ratios associated with the highest fat consumption quartile were close to 3.0. There was a trend for increasing saturated fatty acid consumption with increasing ductal atypica. After adjusting for hormonal and demographic confounders, the association with fat intake was strengthened. Because atypic BBD is a precursor of breast cancer, the findings of this study lend support to the hypothesis that dietary fat is a risk factor for breast cancer (174).

Studies carried out in Greece and Italy indicated that green vegetable consumption is linked to low breast cancer (133,175), which may reflect low intake of fat or calories, or even suggest that some constituent of green vegetable may be protective (176). Even if such an association exists, current evidence suggests that it is weak (52,116,177).

A large number of studies have shown a modest increase in risk of breast cancer with increased alcohol intake (178,179), although no satisfactory biological explanation has been proposed. Although there is no conclusive proof that alcohol causes breast cancer, evidence available supports an association between breast cancer risk and alcohol consumption (2,179).

E. Cervical and Endometrial Cancers

The risk of cervical cancer is higher in the lower socioeconomic classes among long-term users of oral contraceptives as well as among cigarette smokers (120). Precursor of vitamin A (beta-carotene) and vitamin E or some other aspects of a vegetable-rich diet, appear to be protective (180); however, this association may simply reflect an index of a more health-conscious lifestyle (151). The key factor in cervical cancer appears be sexual behaviors; the younger the age at first intercourse, and the larger the number of sexual partners, the greater the risk of cervical cancer (181), which also increases in proportion to the number of pregnancies (182).

Endometrial cancer (gynecological malignancy) most readily correlates with hormonal changes, especially with increased estrogen levels (estrogen hormone use) and with low levels of progestogens. It thus relates to non-ovulation states in many women, to estrogen replacement treatment during menopause, and to obesity, which increases endogenous estrogen levels. Lew and Garfinkel (183) noted that the risks of long-term hormonal replacement therapy (HRT) use and of severe obesity are 5 to 10 times greater than normal. Ecological studies have shown positive correlations of endometrial cancer both with the nutritional status and diet, especially with meat, eggs, and milk consumption and with protein, fat, and total energy intakes. Few analytical studies have shown the protective effects of green leafy vegetables (184) or a positive association of endometrial cancer with total energy intake and with dietary carbohydrates, fats, and oils.

F. Ovarian and Prostatic Cancers

Epithelial ovarian cancer is the most common malignancy and the leading cause of death from gynecological cancer in most Western countries. The American Cancer Society One Million Study showed an elevated risk of ovarian cancer among obese women (183), though evidence from case-control studies is largely null. Loss of weight secondary to the cancer may complicate the analysis. The role of nutrition and diet are the major issues in ovarian cancer epidemiology; some ecological studies have shown correlations with fats, proteins, and energy intakes. Case-control studies also have shown a possible association of ovarian cancer with total fat intake, and some protective effect from green leafy vegetables (184).

The possible role of milk fat (185) and lactose (186–188) in increasing the risk of ovarian cancer has been debated. Cramer (186) proposed that galactose probably is toxic to the oocytes, whereas others claim that the real mechanism involves animal fat rather than milk sugar (189,190).

Prostatic cancer in men, like ovarian cancer in women, is one of the most frequent cancers world wide, with an estimated 235,000 cases occurring annually (166); its etiology is poorly understood. Because androgens are needed for the growth of the prostate, sex hormones are thought to be involved in the development of prostate cancer; however, both epidemiological studies and clinical observations provide little support to the hormonal theory (191). Although prostatic cancer rates have been linked to per capita fat intake (192), other aspects of diet are receiving increasing importance, viz., animal fat, beta-carotene, and milk intake. Whereas fat appears to increase the risk of prostate cancer, milk consumption may not be related to it, other than through its effects on fat intake. The precise nature of the dietary involvement, including the association of prostate cancer with vegetable intake, remains to be established.

G. Kidney and Bladder Cancers

Kidney cancer occurs more frequently in men than in women with a ratio of 2 to 1, renal cell adenocarcinoma accounting for around 85% of all kidney cancers in humans (2). Cigarette smoking has been found to be a high risk factor for kidney cancer, and a few case-control studies have indicated its positive association with obesity (193). However, there is no consistent evidence regarding obesity (194), the role of alcohol (5), or methylxanthine-containing beverages (6) on the risk of renal cell cancer. According to Maclure and Willett (193), significant trends in risk with increasing intake of animal protein, animal fat, and saturated fat (meat) and negative trends with markers of vegetable intake were noticed. The association of kidney cancer with meat intake was also confirmed by McLaughlin et al. (195), but not by McCredie et al. (196). The risk is also seen to be increased by kidney stones (193,195).

The association of bladder cancer with cigarette smoking is overwhelming (120,197). A number of other studies have also shown increased risks of bladder cancer with coffee consumption (6). Saccharine, used widely in the Western world, may be another potential risk factor, but the results of extensive investigations are largely reassuring (198). Some evidence indicates that a diet rich in fresh fruits and vegetables, and possibly in vitamin A, is protective for bladder cancer.

H. Thyroid Cancer

This is a rare and unusual form of cancer that occurs more commonly in women than in men, with a wide range of malignancy from the relatively benign to the rapidly fatal (199). Iodine deficiency was thought to be involved in the development of this disease, but this remains to be proved. A poor diet, especially if it contains natural goitrogens, is related to an increased risk of thyroid cancer (199,200).

IV. DIET AND CANCER: CAUSATIVE AND PREVENTIVE MECHANISMS

Diet may influence human carcinogenesis in the following six general ways (2,3,8):

1. Diet may provide the carcinogens or their immediate precursors
2. Diet may facilitate or inhibit the endogenous production of carcinogens

3. Dietary components may modify carcinogenesis by metabolic activation or inactivation
4. Dietary changes may increase or impede the delivery of carcinogens to their site of action
5. Diet may alter susceptibility of body tissues to cancer induction
6. Diet may alter the body's capacity to eliminate transformed (cancer) cells.

According to Boyle (2), the existence of each of the above six mechanisms in human studies can be demonstrated to some degree or another, but as yet no unifying theory has been proposed.

A. Cancer-Preventive Prospects of Diet and Nutrition

Identifying the risk factors is the first step in the process of cancer prevention, which can be begun right away despite the poorly understood underlying mechanism; e.g., lung cancer was thought to be linked to cigarette smoking and preventive policies started years before any plausible mechanism of action was identified.

Much scientific evidence indicates a consistent association between fat, especially saturated fat intake, and colon cancer. Thus, a reduction in colon cancer can be expected if a population reduces its intake of saturated fat, although it would be difficult to predict the magnitude of the effect and it is uncertain whether the effects of fat are mediated through certain precise biochemical mechanism, allowing another specific preventive strategy.

In view of the often reversible nature of the multistep carcinogenesis process, it would be vitally important if agents responsible for reversing these processes are identified. The most likely preventive factors appear to lie in fruits and vegetables and their constituents (162,177). Until 1991, a conclusion from 13 ecological studies, 9 cohort studies, and 115 case-control studies indicates that consumption of higher levels of fruits and vegetables is consistently associated, although not universally, with reduced risks of various types of cancer. This association is most marked for epithelial cancers, especially those of the intestinal and respiratory tracts, but these links are either weak or nonexistent for hormone-related cancers (162). Investigators have proposed that a large number of potentially anticarcinogenic agents are found in raw fruits and vegetables, such as carotenoids, vitamins C and E, selenium, dietary fiber, dithiolthiones, glucosinolates and indoles, isothiocyanates, flavanoids, phenols, protease inhibitors, plant sterols, allium compounds, and limonene. These agents have a very varied complementary and overlapping mechanisms of action, so it is unlikely that any one substance in these foods is responsible for the prevention of cancer.

After identifying the broad risk factor(s), it is necessary to identify the precise nutrient(s) or non-nutrient(s) responsible for the protective effects. However, it is still premature to estimate the level of intake of these foods, nutrients, or non-nutrients that confers protection. Nevertheless, a WHO group has proposed that intake of around 400g/day of fruits and vegetables (excluding potatoes) would be a reasonable goal, because this level corresponds to intakes in the Mediterranean areas, where cancer rates are in general lower than in North America or northern Europe (2). Hetzel and McMichael (3) have discussed several issues related to the effect of changing individual and population diets on the prevention of cancer and intervention trials for evaluating possible impact of dietary changes, including vitamin supplementation, to achieve reduction in cancers.

Sugimura et al. (201) have presented a proposal of 12 points for cancer prevention (Table 6). Diet, food, and nutrition are closely related to human cancer development. Some of these points are directly related to food, nutrition, and cancer, and others are recommendations for improvements in lifestyle. Diet and nutrition are also closely related to other factors such as smoking, alcohol intake, and exercise. Goel et al. (202) recently reported the antitumor and radio-

Table 6 Proposed 12 Points for Cancer Prevention

1. Eat a nutritionally balanced diet.
2. Eat a variety of foods.
3. Avoid excess calories, especially as fat.
4. Avoid excessive drinking of alcohol.
5. Don't use tobacco in any form.
6. Take vitamins in appropriate amounts; eat fiber and green and yellow vegetables rich in carotene.
7. Avoid drinking fluids that are too hot and eating foods that are too salty.
8. Avoid the charred parts of cooked food.
9. Avoid food with possible contamination by fungal toxins.
10. Avoid overexposure to sunlight.
11. Have an exercise program matched to your own condition.
12. Keep the body clean.

Source: Ref. 201.

protective action of a herb (*Podophyllum hexandrum*) thriving in the Himalayas. The radioprotective properties of *P. hexandoum* were found to be comparable to synthetic radioprotectors like diltiazem.

REFERENCES

1. Sporn, M.B., Carcinogenesis and cancer: Different perspective of the same disease, *Cancer Res. 51*: 6215 (1992).
2. Boyle, P., Nutritional factors and cancer, *Human Nutrition and Dietetics*, 9th ed. (J.S. Garrow and W.P.T. James, eds.), Churchill Livingstone, Edinburgh, London, 1993, p. 701.
3. Hetzel, B., and A.J. McMichael, *The LS Factor: Lifestyle and Health*, Penguin Books, Australia, 1987.
4. IARC, Monographs on the evaluation of carcinogenic risk of chemicals to humans. Tobacco habits other than smoking, betel-quid and areca-nut chewing and some related nitrosamines, No. 37, IARC, Lyon, 1985.
5. IARC, Monographs on the evaluation of carcinogenic risk to humans, alcohol drinking, No. 44, IARC, Lyon, 1988, p. 215.
6. IARC, Monographs on the evaluation of carcinogenic risk to humans, coffee, tea, mate, methylxanthines (caffeine, theophylline, thrombromine) and methlglyoxal, No. 51, IARC, Lyon, 1991.
7. Doll, R., and R. Peto, The cause of cancer: quantitative estimates of avoidable risks of cancer in the United States today, *J. Natl. Cancer Inst. 66*: 1191 (1981).
8. Armstrong, B.K., A.J. McMichael, and R. McLennan, Diet, *Cancer Epidemiology and Prevention* (D. Schottenfeld and J.F. Fraumeni, eds), W.B. Saunders, Philadelphia, 1982.
9. NAS. Committee on Diet, Nutrition and Cancer. National Academy of Science, National Academy Press, Washington, D.C., 1982.
10. Willett, W., and B. MacMahon, Diet and cancer—an overview, *N. Engl. J. Med. 310*: 633 (1984).
11. USSG, Report on Nutrition and Health, United States Surgeon General, US DHH Public Health Service Publication No. 88-50210, 1988.
12. Tannenbaum, A., Relationship of body weight to cancer incidence, *Arch. Pathol. 30*: 509 (1940).
13. Higginson, J., and C. Muir, Environmental carcinogenesis: misconceptions and limitations to cancer control, *J. Nat. Cancer Res. 63*: 1291 (1979).
14. Haenszel, W., Migrant studies, *Cancer Epidemiology and Prevention* (D. Schottenfeld and J.F. Fraumeni, eds.) W.B. Saunders, Philadelphia, 1982.

15. Boyle, P., and La Vecchia, Cancer aetiology, *Oxford Textbook of Oncology* (M.J. Peckman, R. Pinedo, and U. Veronesi, eds.), Oxford University Press, Oxford, 1993.

16. Jensen, O.M., J. Esteve, H. Moller, and H. Renard, Cancer in European community and its member states, *Eur. J. Cancer 26*: 1167 (1990).

17. Willett, W., *Nutritional Epidemiology, Monographs in Epidemiology and Biostatistics* 15, Oxford University Press, New York, 1990.

18. WHO, *International Statistical Classification of Diseases, Injuries and Causes of Death*, 9th rev., World Health Organization, Geneva, 1975.

19. Kulkarni, A.S., A ray of hope for cancer patient, *Proc. Intl. Seminar on Holistic Management of Cancer, Ayurveda Education Series 67*: (1998), *Med. & Aromat. Plants Abstr. 20(2)*: 143 (1998).

20. Hoffman, A.J., New protocol for the treatment of cancer and AIDS utilizing *Aloevera barbadensis* Miller and cesium chloride, *Proc. Intl. Seminar on Holistic Management of Cancer, Ayurveda Education Series, 67*: 44, (1998), *Med & Aromat Plants Abstr. 20(2)*: 148 (1998).

21. Kulkarni, P.H., Role of diet in treatment of cancer and AIDS, *Proc. Intl. Seminar on 'Holistic Management of Cancer', Ayurveda Education Series 67*: 23 (1998), *Med. & Aromat. Plants Abstr. 20(2)*: 148, 1998.

22. Burkitt, D.P., Some diseases characteristic of western civilization, *Br. Med. J. 1*: 274 (1973).

23. Willett, W.C., M.J. Stampfer, G.A. Colditz, B.A. Rosner, and F.E. Speizer, Relation of fat and fiber intake to the risk of colon cancer in a prospective study among women, *N. Engl. J. Med. 323*: 1664 (1990).

24. Howe, G.R., Dietary intake of fiber and decreased risk of cancers of the colon and rectum: Evidence from the combined analysis of 13 case-control studies, *J. Natl. Cancer Inst. 84*: 1887 (1992).

25. Trock, B., E. Lanza, and P. Grenwald, Dietary fiber, vegetables and colon cancer, *J. Nutr. Clin. Invest. 82*: 650 (1990).

26. Steinmetz, K.A., L.H. Kusho, R.M. Bostick, A.R. Folsom, and J.D. Potter, Vegetable, fruit and colon cancer in the Iowa Women's Health Study, *Am. J. Epidemiol. 139*: 1 (1994).

27. Steinmetz, K.A., and J.D. Potter, Vegetables, fruit and cancer. II Mechanisms, *Cancer Cause Control 2*: 427 (1991).

28. Roberton, A.M., and L.R. Ferguson, H.J. Hollands, and P.J. Harris, Adsorption of a hydrophobic mutagen to dietary fiber preparations, *Mutat. Res. 262*: 195 (1991).

29. Willett, W.C., Dietary fat and fiber in relation to risk of breast cancer, *J. Am. Med. Assoc. 268*: 2037 (1992).

30. Thebaudin, J.Y., A.C. Lefebvre, M. Harrington, and C.M. Bourgeois, Dietary fibres: Nutritional and technological interest, *Trends Food Sci. Technol. 8*: 41 (1997).

31. Ip, C., and J.R. Marshall, Trans fatty acids and cancer, *Nutr. Rev. 54*: 138 (1996).

32. Thorling, E.B., Obesity, fat intake, energy balance, exercise and cancer risk: a review, *Nutr. Res. 16*: 315 (1996).

33. Kritchevsky, D., Calories and cancer, *Diet, Nutrition & Health* (K.K. Carroll, ed.), McGill-Queen's Univ. Press, London, 1989, p. 250.

34. Kritchevsky, D., M.M. Weber, and D.M. Klurfeld, Dietary fat versus caloric content in initiation and promotion of 7,12-dimethylbenz (a) athracene-induced mammary tumorigenesis in rats, *Cancer Res. 44*: 3174 (1984).

35. Klurfeld, D.M., M.M. Weber, and D. Kritchevsky, Inhibition of chemically induced mammary and colon tumor promotion by caloric restriction in rats fed increased dietary fat, *Cancer Res. 47*: 2759 (1987).

36. Kritchevsky, D., and D.M. Klurfeld, Caloric effects in experimental mammary tumorigenesis, *Am. J. Clin. Nutr. 45*: 236 (1987).

37. Kritchevsky, D., M.M. Weber, C.L. Buck, and D.M. Klurfeld, Calories, fat and cancer, *Lipids, 21*: 272 (1986).

38. Albanes, D., Total calories, body weight and tumor incidence in mice, *Cancer Res. 47*: 1987 (1987).

39. Miller, A.B. Epidemiology of breast and colon cancer, *Diet, Nutrition & Health* (K.K. Carroll, ed.), McGill-Queen's Univ. Press, London, 1989, p. 243.

40. Kinlen, L.J., Meat and fat consumption and cancer mortality: A study of strict religious order in Britain, *Lancet 1*: 946 (1982).

41. Krishmnaswamy, K., Indian functional foods: Role in prevention of cancer, *Nutr. Rev.* **54**(S) 127 (1996).

42. WHO, Diet, nutrient and prevention of chronic diseases, Report of a World Health Organization Study Group, Who Tech. Rep. Ser. No. 797, 1990.

43. NRCC, National Research Council Committee on 'Diet and Health,' Implications for reducing chronic disease risk, National Academy Press, Washington, DC. 1989.

44. NRC, *Diet, Nutrition and Cancer*, National Research Council, National Academy Press, Washington, DC, 1982.

45. Huage, M.T., T. Osawa, C.T. Ho, and R.T. Rosen (eds.), *Food Phytochemicals for Cancer Prevention. I Fruits and Vegetables*, ACS Symp. Ser No. 546, American Chemical Society, Washington, DC, 1994.

46. Ho, C.T., T. Osawa, M.T. Huang, R.T. Rosen (eds.) *Food Phytochemicals for Cancer Prevention*, II. *Tea, Spices and Herbs*, ACS Symp. Ser No. 546, American Chemical Society Washington, DC. 1994.

47. Krishnaswamy, K., and M.P.R. Prasad, Diet and nutrition correlates of cancer, *Chemoprevention of Cancer* (S.V. Bhide and G.B. Maru, eds.), Omega Scientific Publishers, New Delhi, 1992, p. 83.

48. Krishnaswamy, K., Antimutagens and anticarcinogens in Indian diets, *Recent Trends in Nutrition* (C. Gopalan, ed.), Oxford University Press, New Delhi, 1993, p. 125.

49. Prasad, M.P.R., T.P. Krishna, S. Pasricha, M.A. Qureshi, and K. Krishnaswamy, Diet and oesophageal cancers—a case control study, *Nutr. Cancer 79*: 85 (1992).

50. Krishnaswamy, K., M.P.R.Prasad, T.P. Krishna, and S. Pasricha, Selenium in cancer: a case control study, *Indian J. Med. Res. 98*: 124 (1993)

51. Prasad, M.P.R., T.P. Krishna, S. Pasricha, M.A. Qureshi, and K. Krishnaswamy, Diet and oral cancer—a case control study, *Asia Pacific J. Clin. Nutr. 4*: 259 (1995).

52. Steinmetz, K.A., and J.D. Pottor, Vegetables, fruit and cancer: Epidemiology, *Cancer Causes Control, 2*: 325 (1991a).

53. Steinmetz, K.A., and J.D. Pottor, Food group consumption and colon cancer in the Adelaide case-control study. 1. Vegetables and fruits, *Int. J. Cancer 53*: 711 (1993).

54. Krishnaswamy, K., M.P.R. Prasad, T.P. Krishna, V.V. Annapurna, and G.A. Reddy, A case study by nutrient intervention of oral precancerous lesions in India, *Oral Oncol. Eur. J. Cancer 31*: 41 (1995).

55. Namiki, M., Antioxidants/antimutagens in food, *CRC Crit. Rev. Food Sci, Nutr. 29*: 273 (1990).

56. Clydesdale, F.M. (ed.), Special issue: Proceeding of the ILSI, NA Workshop on Substantiation of the impact of nutrient and non-nutrient antioxidants on health, *CRC Crit. Rev. Food Sci. Nutr. 35*: 1 (1995).

57. Wattenberg, L.W. Inhibition of chemical carcinogens by minor dietary components, *Molecular Interactions of Nutrition and Cancer* (M.S. Arnott, J. Van Eys and M. Wang, eds.), Raven Press, New York, 1982, p. 43.

58. Rajpurohit, R., and K. Krishnaswamy, Effects of common vegetables/spices on xenobiotic metabolism enzymes and in vivo carcinogen-DNA binding, *Indian J. Toxicol. 1-2*: 33 (1994).

59. Goud, V.K., K. Polasa, and K. Krishnaswamy, Effects of turmeric on xenobiotic metabolism enzymes, *Plant Foods Human Nutr. 44*: 87 (1993)

60. Mukundan, M.A., M. Chacko, V.V. Annapurna, and K. Krishnaswamy, Effect of turmeric and curcumin on BP-DNA adducts, *Carcinogenesis 14*: 493 (1993).

61. Polasa, K., B. Sesikeran, T.P. Krishna, and K. Krishnaswamy, Turmeric (*Curcuma longa*)-induced reduction in urinary mutagens, *Food Chem. Toxicol. 29*: 699 (1991).

62. Polasa, K., P.U. Kumar, and K. Krishnaswamy, Effect of *Brassica nigra* on benzo (a)-pyrene mutagenicity, *Food Chem. Toxicol. 32*: 777 (1994).

63. Krishnaswamy, K., Turmeric-a potential anticancer agent, *NFI Bull 14*: 1 (1993).

64. Srinivas, L., V.K. Salini, and M. Shylaja, Turmeric: a water soluble anti-oxidant peptide from turmeric (*Curcuma longa*), *Arch. Biochem. Biophys. 292*: 617 (1992).

65. Huang, M.T., R.C. Smart, C.O. Wong, and A.H. Conney, Inhibitory effects of curcumin, chlorogenic acid, caffeic acid, and ferulic acid on tumor promotion in mouse skin by 12-0-tetradecanoylphorbol-13 acetate, *Cancer Res. 48*: 5941 (1988).

66. Bhide, S.V., A.J. Amonkar, and M.A, Aziune, Use of oral, stomach, and mammary tumor models for testing of natural products as chemopreventive agents, *Chemoprevention of Cancer* (S.V. Bhide and G.B. Maru, eds.), Omega Scientific Publishers, New Delhi, 1992, p. 16.

67. Huang, M.T., Y.R. Lou, W. Ma, H.L. Newmark, K.R. Rehul, and A.H. Conney, Inhibitory effects of dietary curcumin on forestomach, duodenal and colon carcinogenesis in mice, *Cancer Res. 54*: 5841 (1994).

68. Willett, W.C., and D.J. Hunter, Vitamin A and cancers of the breast, large bowel and prostate: Epidemiological evidence, *Nutr. Rev. 52*(S): 53 (1994).

69. Astorg, P., Food carotenoids and cancer prevention: An overview of current research, *Trends Food Sci. Technol. 8*: 406 (1997).

70. Krinsky, N.I., Micronutrients and their influence on mutagenicity and malignant transformation, *Ann. New York Acad. Sci. 686*: 229 (1993).

71. Krinsky, N.I., Carotenoids and cancer: Basic research studies, *Natural Antioxidants in Human Health and Disease* (B. Frei, ed.), Academic Press, New York, 1994, p. 239.

72. Bendich, A., Antioxidant vitamins and human immune response, *Vitam. Horm. 52*: 35 (1998).

73. Chung, K.T., C.I. Wei, and M.G. Johnson, Are tannins a double-edged sword in biology and health? *Trends Food Sci. Technol. 9*: 168 (1996).

74. Reuter, H.D., H.P. Koch, and L.D. Lawson, Therapeutic effects and applications of garlic and its preparation, *Garlic: The Science and Therapeutic Application of Allium sativum L and Related Species* (H.P. Koch and L.D. Lawson, eds.), 2nd edn., Williams & Wilkins, Baltimore, 1996, p. 135.

75. Spivak, M.Y., On the use of phytoncides of garlic and onion for the treatment of tumorous patients, *Vopr. Onkol. (Problems in Onkology) 8*: 93 (1992) (Russian).

76. Rainov, N.G., and W. Burkert, Spontaneous shrinking of a macro prolactinoma, *Neurochirurgia 36*: 17 (1993).

77. Steinmetz, K.A., L.H. Kushi, R.M. Bostick, A.R. Folsom, and J.D. Pottor, Vegetables, fruit, and colon cancer in the Iowa Women's Health Study, *Am. J. Epidemiol. 139*: 1 (1994).

78. Steinmetz, K.A., and J.D. Potter, Two of the authors reply, *Am. J. Epidemiol. 141*: 85 (1995).

79. Shu, X.O., W. Zheng, N. Potischman, L.A. Brinton, M.C. Hatch, Y.T. Gao, and J.F. Fraumeni, A population-based case-control study of dietary factors and endometrial cancer in Shanghai, People's Republic of China, *Am. J. Epidemiol. 137*: 155 (1993).

80. Levi, F.S., S. Franceschi, E. Negri, and C. LaVecchia, Dietary factors and the risk of endometrial cancer, *Cancer 71*: 3575 (1993).

81. Levi, F.S., C. LaVecchi, C. Gulie, and E. Negri, Dietary factors and breast cancer risk in Vaud, Switzerland, *Nutr. Cancer 19*: 327 (1993).

82. Graham, S., J. Marshall, B. Haughey, A. Mittelman, M. Swanson, M. Zielezny, T. Byers, G, Wilkinson, and D. West, Dietary epidemiology of cancer of the colon in western New York, *Am. J. Epidemiol. 128*: 490, (1994).

83. Dorant, E., Onion and leek consumption, garlic supplement use, and the incidence of cancer, Ph.D. dissertation, Maastricht University, The Netherlands (Abstract), 1994.

84. Dorant, E., P.A. Vanden Brandt, R.A. Goldbohm, R.J.J. Hermus, and F. Sturmans, Agreement between interview data and self-administered questionnaire on dietary supplement use, *Eur. J. Clin. Nutr. 45*: 180 (1994a).

85. Dorant, E., P.A. Vanden Brandt, and R.A. Goldbohm, Allium vegetable consumption, garlic suppliement intake and female breast carcinoma incidence, *Breast Cancer Res. Treatment 33*: 163 (1995).

86. Dorant, E., P.A. Vanden Brandt, and R.A. Goldbohm, A prospective garlic supplement use, and the risk of lung carcinoma in the Netherlands, *Cancer Res. 54*: 6148 (1994b).

87. Thompson L.U., Potential health benefits and problems associated with antinutrients in foods, *Food Res. Int. 26*: 131 (1993).

88. Troll, W., and A.R. Kennedy, Workshop report for the Division of Cancer Etiology, National Cancer Institute, National Institute of Health. Protein inhibitors as cancer chemipreventive agents, *Cancer Res. 49*: 499 (1989).

89. Messina, M., and S. Barnes, The role of soy products in reducing risk of cancer, *J. Natl. Cancer Inst. 83*: 541 (1991).

90. Caragay, A.B, Cancer protective foods and ingredients, *Food Technol. 46*: 65 (1992).

91. Clinton, S.K., Lycopene: Chemistry, biology and implications for human health and disease, *Nutr. Rev.* (suppl. *1*): 35, (1998).

92. Block, G., B. Patterson, and A. Subar, Fruit, vegetables and cancer prevention: a review of the epidemiological evidence, *Nutr. Cancer 18*: 1 (1992).

93. Fund, W.C.R., *Food, Nutrition and the Prevention of Cancer: a Global Perspective*, American Institute for Cancer Research, Washington, DC, 1997.

94. Peto, R., R. Doll, J.D. Buckley, and M.B. Sporn, Can dietary beta-carotene materially reduce human cancer rates? *Nature 290*: 201, (1981).

95. Ziegler, R.G., A review of epidemiological evidence that carotenoids reduce the risk of cancer, *J. Nutr. 119*: 1162 (1989).

96. Mayne, S.T., Beta-carotene, carotenoids, and disease prevention in humans, *FASEB J. 10*: 690 (1996).

97. Greenberg, E.R., J.A. Baron, and T.A. Stukel, A clinical trial of beta-carotene to prevent basal cell and squamous cell cancers of the skin, *N. Engl. J. Med. 323*: 789 (1990).

98. Greenberg, E.R., J.A. Baron, and T. D. Tosteson, A clinical trial of antioxidant vitamins to prevent colorectal adonoma, *N. Engl. J. Med. 331*: 141, (1994).

99. Hennekens, C.H., J.E. Buring, and J.E. Manson, Lack of effect of long-term supplementation with beta-carotene on the incidence of malignant neoplasms and cardiovascular disease, *N. Engl. J. Med. 334*: 1145 (1996).

100. Omenn, G.S., G.E. Goodman, and M.D. Thornquist, Effects of a combination of beta carotene and vitamin A on lung cancer and cardiovascular disease, *N. Engl. J. Med. 334*: 1150 (1996).

101. Anonymous, The alpha-tocopherol, beta-carotene cancer prevention study group. The effect of vitamin E and beta-carotene on the incidence of lung cancer and other cancers in male smokers, *N. Engl. J. Med. 330*: 1029 (1994).

102. Toma, S., S. Benso, and E. Albanese, Treatment of oral leukoplakia with beta-carotene, *Oncology 49*: 77 (1992).

103. Garewal, H., Antioxidant in oral cancer prevention, *Am. J. Clin. Nutr. 62* (Suppl.):1417 (1995).

104. Meyskens, F.L., and A. Manetta, Prevention of cervical intra-epithelial neoplasia and cervical cancer, *Am. J. Clin. Nutr. 62* (Suppl.): 1417 (1995).

105. Stahl, W., and H. Sies, Lycopene: A biologically important carotenoid for humans? *Arch. Biochem. Biphys. 336*: 1 (1996).

106. Gerster, H., The potential role of lycopene for human health, *N. Engl. J. Med. 333*: 1757 (1995).

107. Folkman, J., Clinical applications of research on angiogenesis, *N. Engl. J. Med. 333*: 1757 (1995).

108. Bendich, A., Carotenoids and the immune response, *J. Nutr. 119*: 112 (1989).

109. Kobayashi, T., K. Lijima, and T. Mitamura, Effect of lycopene, a carotenoid on intrathymic T cell differentiation and peripheral CD4/CD8 ratios in a high mammary tumor strain of SHN retired mice, *Anticancer Drugs* (England) *7*: 195 (1996).

110. Geradelet, S., P. Astorg, and J. Leclerc, Effects of canthaxanthin, astaxanthin, lycopene and lutein on lower xenobiotic-metabolizing enzymes in the rat, *Xenobiotica* (England) *26*: 49 (1996).

111. Boyle, P., G.J. Macfarlane, T. Zheng, P. Maisonneuve, T. Evstifeeva, and C. Scully, Recent advances in epidemiology of head and neck cancer, *Curr. Opin. Oncol. 4*: 471 (1992).

112. Winn, D.M., W.J. Blot, C.M. Shy, L.W. Pickle, A. Toledo, and J.F. Fraumeni, Snuff dipping and oral cancer among women in the Southern United States, *N. Engl. J. Med. 304*: 745, (1981).

113. Sankaranarayan, R., S.W. Duffy, G. Padmakumary, N.E. Day, and T.K. Padmanabhan, Tobacco chewing, alcohol and nasal snuff in cancer of the gingiva in Kerala, India, *British J. Cancer 60*: 638 (1989).

114. Zheng, T.Z., P. Boyle, H.F. Hu, Dentition, oral hygiene, and risk of oral cancer: A case-control study in Beijing, China, *Cancer Causes Control 1*: 235 (1990).

115. McLaughlin, J.K., G. Gridley, G. Block, Dietary factors in oral and pharyngeal cancer, *J. Natl. Cancer Inst. 80*: 1237 (1988).

116. Steinmetz, K.A., and J.D. Pottor, Vegetable, fruits and cancer, I. Epidemiology, *Cancer Causes Control 2*: 325 (1991).

117. Yu, M.C., T.B. Huang, and B.E. Henderson, Diet and nasopharyngeal carcinoma: A case-control study in Guangzhou, China, *Int. J. Cancer 43*: 1177 (1989).

118. Delemarre J.F., and H.H. Themans, Adenocarcinoma of the nasal cavities, *Netherlands Tijdschrift voor Geneeskunde 115*: 688 (1971).

119. Fong., L.Y., J.H. Ho, and D.P. Huang, Preserved foods are possible cancer hazards, WA rats fed salted fish have mutagenic urine, *Intl. J. Cancer. 23*: 342 (1979).

120. IARC, Monographs on the evaluation of the carcinogenic risk of chemical to human, tobacco smoking, No. 38, IARC, Lyon, 1986, p. 279.

121. Levi, F., J.B. Ollyo, C. La Vecchia, P. Boyle, P., Monnier, and M. Savary, The consumption of tobacco, alcohol and the risk of adeno-carcinoma in Barrett's oesophagus, *Intl. J. Cancer 45*: 852 (1990).

122. La Vecchia, C., and E. Negri, The role of alcohol in oesophageal cancer in non-smokers and of tobacco in non-drinkers, *Intl. J. Cancer 43*: 784 (1989).

123. Clemmensen, J., Statistical studies in the aetiology of malignant neoplasms. I. Copenhagen Danish Cancer Registry, 1965.

124. Jensen, O.M., Cancer morbidity and causes of death among Danish brewary workers, IARC Non-serial publication, IARC, Lyon, 1980.

125. Tuyns, A., Cancer of the oesophagus in Ille-et Vilaine in relation to levels of consumption of alcohol and tobacco, *Bull. Du Cancer 64*: 45 (1977).

126. Victora, C.G., N. Munoz, N.E. Day, L.B. Barcelos, D.A. Peccin, and N.M. Braga, Hot beverages and oesophageal cancer in Southern Brazil: A case-control study, *Intl. J. Cancer 39*: 710 (1987).

127. Franceschi, S., E. Bidoli, A.E. Baron C. La Vecchia, Maize and risk of cancer of the oral cavity, pharynx and oesophagus in north-estern Italy, *J. Natl. Cancer Inst. 82*: 1407 (1990).

128. Decarli, A., P. Liati, E. Negri, S. Franceschi, and C. La Vecchia, Vitamin A and other dietary factors in the aetiology of esophageal cancer, *Nutr. Cancer 10*: 29 (1987).

129. Negri, E., C. La Vecchia, S. Franceschi, A. Decarli, and P. Bruzzi. Attributable risk of oesophageal cancer in northern Italy, *Eur. J. Cancer 28A*: 1167 (1992).

130. Risch, H.A., M. Jain, and N.W. Choi, Dietary factors and the incidence of cancer of stomach, *Am. J. Epidemical. 122*: 949 (1985).

131. Buiatti, E., D. Palli, and A. Decarli, A case-control study of gastric cancer and diet in Italy, *Intl. J. Cancer 44*: 611 (1989).

132. Trichopoulos, D., S. Yen, J. Brown, P. Cole, and B. Macmahon, The effect of westernization on urine estrogens, frequency of ovulation and breast cancer risk. A study of ethnic Chinese women in the Orient and the USA, *Cancer 53*: 187 (1984).

133. La Vecchia. C., A. Decarli, S. Franceschi, A. Gentile, E. Negri, and F. Parazzini, Dietary factors and the risk of breast cancer, *Nutr. & Cancer 10*: 205 (1987).

134. Buiatti, E., D. Palli, and A. Decarli. A case-control study of gastric cancer and diet in Italy. II Association with nutrients, *Intl. J. Cancer 45*: 896 (1990).

135. Joossens, J., and J. Geboers, Salt, stomach cancer and stroke, *Diet, Nutrition & Health* (K.K. Carroll, ed.), McGill-Queen's Univ. Press, London, p. 229.

136. Boyle, P., D.G. Zaridze, and M. Smans Descriptive epidemiology of colorectal cancer, *Intl. J. Cancer 36*: 9 (1985).

137. Willett, W., The search of causes of breast and colon cancer, *Nature 338*: 389 (1989).

138. Whittemore, A.F., A.H. Wu-Williams, and M. Lee, Diet, physical activity and colorectal cancer among Chinese in North America and China, *J. Natl. Cancer Inst. 82*: 915 (1990).

139. Sugimura, T., Past, present and future mutagens in cooked foods, *Environ. Health Persp. 67*: 5 (1986).

140. Felton, J.S., M.C. Kmize, and N.H. Shen, Identification of the mutagens in cooked beef, *Environ, Health Persp. 67*: 17 (1986).

141. Schiffman, M.H., and J.S. Felton, Fried foods and the risk of colon cancer, *Am J. Epidemiol. 131*: 376 (1990).

142. Ha, Y.L., N.K. Grimm, and M.W. Pariza, Anticarcinogens from fried beef: Heat altered derivatives of linoleic acid, *Carcinogenesis Inst. 8*: 1881 (1987).

143. Zaridze, D.G. Environmental aetiology of large-bowel cancer, *J. Natl. Cancer Inst. 70*: 389 (1983).

144. Sakaguchi, M., Y. Hiramatzu, and H. Takada, Effects of dietary unsaturated and saturated fats on azoxy-methane-induced colon carcinogenesis in rats, *Cancer Res. 44*: 1472 (1988).

145. Minoura, T., T. Takada, and M. Sakaguchi, Effect of dietary eicosapentaenoic acid on azoxy-methane-induced colon carcinogenesis in rats, *Cancer Res. 48*: 4790 (1988).

146. Kritchevsky, D., Diet, nutrition and cancer: The role of fiber, *Cancer 58* (Suppl. 8): 1830 (1986).

147. Tuyns, A.J., M. Haelterman, and R. Kaas, Colorectal cancer and the intake of nutrients: oligosaccharides are a risk factor, fats are not: a case-control study in Belgium, *Nutr. & Cancer, 10*: 181 (1987).

148. Kune, S., G.A. Kune, and L.F. Watson, Case-control study of dietary aetiological factors: The Melbourne colorectal cancer study, *Nutr. Cancer 9*: 21 (1987).

149. Heilbrun, L.K., J., H. Hankin, and A. Nornura, Colon cancer and dietary fat, phosphorus and calcium in Hawaiian-Japanese men, *Am. J. Clin. Nutr. 43*: 306 (1986).

150. Longencker, M.P., M.J. Orza, M.E. Adams, J. Vioque, and T.C. Chalmers, A meta-analysis of alcoholic beverage consumption in relation to risk of colorectal cancer. *Cancer Causes Control 1*: 59 (1990).

151. La Vecchia, C., A. Decarli., and M. Fasoli, Dietary vitamin A and the risk of infra-epithelial and invasive cervical neoplasia, *Gynecol. Oncol. 30*: 187 (1988).

152. Boyle, P., C.C. Hsieh, and P. Maisonneuve, Epidemiology of pancreas cancer, *Intl. J. Pancreatol. 5*: 327 (1989).

153. Velema, J.P., A.M. Walker, and E.B. Gold, Alcohol and pancreatic cancer. Insufficient epidemiological evidence for a causal relationship, *Epidemiol. Rev. 8*: 28 (1986).

154. Bouchardy, C., F. Clavel, C. La Vecchia, L. Raymond, and P. Boyle, Alcohol, beer and cancer of pancreas, *Intl. J. Cancer 45*: 842 (1990).

155. Bueno de Mesquita H.B., C.J. Moerman, S. Runia, and P. Maisonneuve, Are energy and energy providing nutrients related to carcinoma of the exocrine pancreas? *Intl. J. Cancer 46*: 435 (1990).

156. Howe, G.R., T. Hirohata, and T.G. Hislop, Dietary factors and risk of breast cancer: combined analysis of 12 case-control studies, *J. Natl. Cancer Inst. 82*: 561 (1990).

157. Howe, G.R., M. Jain, and A.B. Miller, Dietary factors and risk of pancreatic cancer: Results of a Canadian population-based case-control study, *Intl. J. Cancer 45*: 604 (1990).

158. Ghadirian, P., A. Simard, J. Baillargeon, P. Maisonneuve, and P. Boyle, Nutrition and pancreatic cancer in the Francophone community in Montreal, Canada, *Intl. J. Cancer 47*: 1 (1991).

159. Baghurst, P.A., A.J. McMchael, A.H. Slavolinek, K.I. Baghurst, P. Boyle, and A.M. Walker, A case-control study of diet and cancer of the pancreas, *Am. J. Epidemiol. 134*: 167 (1991).

160. Zatonski, W., K. Przewozniak, G.R. Howe, P. Maisonneuve, A.M. Walker, and P. Boyle, Nutritional factors and pancreatic cancer: A case-control study from south-west Poland, *Intl. J. Cancer 48*: 390 (1991).

161. La Vecchia, C., E. Biddi, and S. Barra, Type of cigarettes and cancer of the upper digestive and respiratory tract, *Cancer Causes Control 1*: 69 (1990).

162. Steinmetz, K.A., and J.D. Potter, Vegetables, fruit and cancer I. Epidemiology, *Cancer Causes Control 2*: 325 (1991).

163. Graham, S., C. Mettlin, J.R. Marshall, R. Priore, T. Rzepka, and D. Shedd, Dietary factors in the epidemiology of cancer of the larynx, *Am. J. Epidemiol. 113*: 675 (1981).

164. De Stefani, E., P. Correa, and E. Oreggia, Risk factors for laryngeal cancer, *Cancer 60*: 3087 (1987).

165. Parkin, D.M., E. Laara, and C. Muir, Estimates of the worldwide frequency of twelve common cancers in 1980, *Intl. J. Cancer 41*: 184 (1988).

166. Boyle, P., Epidemiology of breast cancer, *Bailliere's Clin. Oncol. 2*: 1 (1988).

167. De Waard, F., R.A. Baanders-van Halewijin, and J. Huizinga, The bimodal age distribution of patients with mammary carcinoma, *Cancer 17*: 141 (1964).

168. Swanson, C.A., D.Y. Jones, A. Schatzkin, L.A. Brinton, and R.G. Zeigler, Breast cancer risk assessed by anthropometry in the NHANESI epidemiological follow-up study, *Cancer Res. 48*: 5363 (1988).

169. Frisch, R.E., G. Wyshak, and N.L. Albright, Lower prevalence of breast cancers and cancers of the reproductive system among former college athletes compared to non-athletes, *Br. J. Cancer 52*: 885 (1985).

170. Warren, M.P., The effects of exercise on pubertal progression and reproduction function in girls, *J. Clin. Endocrinol. Metab 51*: 1150 (1980).

171. Willet, W.C., M.J. Stampfer, G.A. Colditz, B.A. Rosner, C.H. Hennekens, and F.E. Speizer, Dietary fat and the risk of breast cancer, *N. Engl. J. Med. 316*: (1987).

172. Jones, D.Y., A. Schatzkin, and S.B. Green, Dietary fat and breast cancer in the National Health and Nutrition Survey-1, Epidemiological follow-up study, *J. Natl. Cancer Inst. 79*: 465, (1988).

173. Willett, W.C., D.J. Hunter, and M.J. Stampfer, Dietary fat and fiber in relation to role of breast cancer, *J. Am. Med. Assoc. 268*: 2037 (1992).

174. Lubin, F., Y. Wax, E. Ron, M. Black, A. Chetrit, N. Rosen, E. Alfandary, and B. Modan, Nutritional factors associated with benign breast disease etiology: A case-control study, *Am. J. Clin. Nutr. 50*: 551 (1990).

175. Katsouyanni, K, D. Trichopoulos, and D. Boyle, Diet and breast cancer: a case-control study in Greece, *Intl. J. Cancer 38*:815 (1986).

176. Michnivicz, J.J., and H.L. Bradlow, Induction of estradiol metabolism by dietary indole-3 carbinol in humans, *J. Natl. Cancer Inst. 82*:947 (1990).

177. Steinmetz, K.A., and J.D. Potter, Vegetables, fruit and cancer. II Mechanisms, *Cancer Causes Control 2*:427 (1991).

178. Willet, W.C., M.J. Stampfer, G.A. Colditz, B.A. Rosner, C.H. Hennekens, and F.E. Speizer, Moderate alcohol consumption and risk of breast cancer, *N. Engl. J. Med. 316*:1174 (1987).

179. Longnecker, M.P., J.A. Berlin, M.J. Orza, T.C. Chalmers, A meta-analysis of alcohol consumption in relation to the risk of breast cancer, *J. Am. Med. Assoc. 260*: 652 (1988).

180. Cuzick, J., B. De Stavolo, and D. McCance, A case-control study of cervix cancer in Singapore, *Br. J. Cancer 60*:238 (1989).

181. Brinton, L.A., R.F. Hamman, G.R. Huggins, Sexual and reproductive risk factor for invasive squamous cell cervical cancer, *J. Natl. Cancer Inst. 79*:23 (1987).

182. Brinton, L.A., W.C. Reeves, and M.M. Brenes, Parity as a risk factor for cervical cancer, *Am. J. Epidemiol., 130*:486 (1989).

183. Lew, E.A., and L. Garfinkel, Variations in mortality by weight among 750,000 men and women, *J. Chronic Dis. 32*: 563 (1979).

184. La Vecchia, C., Nutritional factors and cancers of the breast, endometrium and ovary, *Europ. J. Cancer Clin. Oncol. 25*:1945 (1989).

185. Mettlin, C.J., and M.S. Piver, A case-control study of milk-drinking and ovarian cancer, *Am. J. Epidemiol. 132*:871 (1990).

186. Cramer, D.W., Lactase persistence and milk consumption as determinants of ovarian cancer risk, *Am. J. Epidemiol. 130*:904 (1989).

187. Cramer, D.W., B.L. Harlow, and W.C. Willett, Galactose consumption and metabolism in relation to the risk of ovarian cancer, *Lancet 2*:66 (1989).

188. Harlow, B.L., D.L. Cramer, J. Geller, W.C. Willett, D.A. Bell, and W.R. Welch. The influence of lactose consumption on the association of oral contraceptive use and ovarian cancer risk, *Am. J. Epidemiol. 134*: 445 (1991).

189. Mettlin, C.J., Progress in nutritional epidemiology of ovary cancer, *Am. J. Epidemiol. 134*: 457 (1991).

190. Cramer, D.W., and B.L. Harlow, A case-control study of milk drinking and ovarian cancer risk, *Am. J. Epidemiol. 134*:454 (1991).

191. Griffiths, K., C.L. Eaton, and P. Davis, Prostatic cancer: aetiology and endocrinology, *Hormone Res. 32*(Suppl.): 38 (1990).

192. Zaridze, D.G., and P. Boyle, Cancer of prostate: epidemiology and aetiology, *Br. J. Urol. 59*:493 (1987).

193. Maclure, M., and W. Willett, A case-control study of diet and risk of renal adenocarcinoma, *Epidemiology 1*:430 (1990).

194. Talamini, R., A.E. Baron, and S. Barra, A case-control study of risk factor for renal cell cancer in northern Italy, *Cancer Causes Control 1*:125 (1990).

195. McLaughlin, J.K., J.S. Mandel, W.J. Blot, L.M. Schuman, E.S. Mehl, and J.F. Fraumeni, A population-based case-control study of renal cell carcinoma, *J. Natl. Cancer Inst. 72*:275, (1984).

196. McCredie, M, J.M. Ford, and J.H. Stewart, Risk factors for cancer of the renal parenchyma, *Intl. J. Cancer 42*:13 (1988).

197. Lavecchia, C., P Boyle, and S. Franceschi, Smoking and cancer with emphasis on Europe, *Europ. J. Cancer 27*:94 (1991).

198. IARC, Overall evaluations of carcinogenicity: an updating of IARC Monographs, Vols. 1–42, IARC Monographs (Suppl. 7), IARC, Lyon 1987.

199. Franceschi, S., F. Levi, E. Negri, A. Fassina, and C. La Vecchia, Diet and thyroid cancer: a pooled analysis of four European case-control studies, *Intl. J. Cancer 48*:395 (1991).

200. Franceschi, S., P. Boyle, and P. Maisonneuve, The epidemiology of thyroid cancer, *Rev. Oncogenesis* (in press), (cited by Boyle, 1993 Ref. 2).

201. Sugimura, T., K. Wakabayashi, M. Nagao, and H. Ohgaki, Mutagens and carcinogens formed during cooking, *Diet Nutrition & Health* (K.K. Carroll, ed.) McGill-Queen's University Press, London, 1989, p. 207.

202. Goel, H.C., J. Prasad, and A. Sharma, Antitumor and radioprotective activity of *Podophyllum hexandrum, Indian J. Exp. Biol. 36*: 583 (1998).

26
Diet, Obesity, and Diabetes

I. INTRODUCTION

Both obesity and diabetes are closely related to diet and nutrition. Whereas diet can become the direct cause of obesity, diabetes can be treated and managed by regulating the diet. Obese diabetics are normally of the non–insulin-dependent (type II) variety, in whom weight loss can be of great advantage. However, caution is required if diabetics are taking insulin or hypoglycemic drugs, because a change in diet or weight loss will affect the dosage required to manage diabetes. The same applies to hypertensive patients, who will need to reduce medication during and after weight loss. Diabetes is closely related to cardiovascular disease, which can also be managed by the application of dietary and nutritional principles.

II. HEALTH RISK OF OBESITY

Obesity has been identified as one of the most important public health problems (1) and its prevalence has increased in recent years. The health hazards of obesity have been recognized even better in the affluent countries of the world. Cardiovascular disease is the main cause of increased mortality among obsese people. The mortality from coronary heart disease, congestive heart failure, stroke, and hypertension all increase with age, but within any age group, the mortality among obese persons is often greater than among lean ones (2).

A. Definition and Prevalence of Overweight and Obesity

The life insurance industry has known that people who are above a certain "desirable" weight for height are liable to die young and hence are less profitable to insure. Thus, these insurance companies publish tables of desirable weights, based on the mortality of people they have insured. This desirable range corresponds closely to the range of Quetelet's Index (QI), also known as body mass index (BMI), from 20 to 25. This index is calculated by dividing the individual's weight (kg) by the square of his/her height (m); e.g., a person who weighs 65 kg and who is 1.73 m tall would have a $QI = 65/1(1.73 \times 1.73) = 21.7$, which is in the desirable range of 20 to 25. More conveniently, a chart showing the boundaries of QI 20, 25, 30, and 40 are used in practice.

It is arbitrary to choose a value for QI above which an individual can be deemed to be obese. Mortality begins to increase significantly between QI 25 and 30, and increases rapidly at values above 30. Very thin people also show decreased longevity, so that below QI 20 there is increased mortality. Thus, an international consensus is that 20–24.9 is a desirable range, 25 to 29.9 is overweight; above 30 is obese, and over 40 is very obese. Garrow (3) employed the terms, grade

O, grade I, grade II, and grade III for the ranges of desirable, overweight, obese and, very obese, respectively.

A survey to assess the prevalence of overweight and obesity in the adult population of the United Kingdom was conducted in 1980 in a representative sample of 5,000 men and 5,000 women aged 16 to 64 years (Table 1). The proportion of men in grades I, II, and III was 34%, 6%, and 0.1%, respectively; for women it was 24%, 8%, and 0.3%, respectively. Prevalence was higher among the older subjects (4). Gregory et al. (5) reported the results of another survey done in 1987 using the same methodology, which showed an alarming increase in the prevalence of obesity (QI above 30), which overall increased from 6% to 8% in men and from 8% to 12% in women. Increase occurred in all age groups, but especially among women aged 25 to 34 years, in whom prevalence almost doubled over the 7-year interval (Table 1). In the developing countries, which are liable to food shortage due to famine and so on, obesity is in general rare, but in the relatively affluent and urbanized societies of these countries there is a rapidly increasing prevalence of obesity. In the affluent countries, the prevalence of obesity is often inversely related to the social class for reasons not well understood. Although grade I (QI 25–29.9) is usually more common among men than among women of the same age, obesity (QI above 30) is more common among women, and the preponderance of women increases with increasing severity of obesity. Whereas men tend to reach the maximum prevalence of obesity at about age 45, in women the prevalence seems to increase to age 65, after which it begins to decline. Also, cigarette smokers tend to be lighter than non-smokers and ex-smokers tend to gain weight. However, the fear of weight gain is not a good reason to start smoking, which leads to several health risk factors (see Chapter 25).

Heart disease is the main cause of premature death among obese people; hypertension, coronary thrombosis, and congestive heart disease are significantly more common among obese persons as compared with normal weight control subjects. The Seven Nations Study indicated that among men aged 45 to 60 years, allowing for age, blood pressure, plasma cholesterol, and smoking status, obesity made no further contribution predicting heart attack among men (6). This, however, should not be interpreted to mean that obesity per se is not a risk factor (2). Although both age and cigarette smoking are important contributors to the risk of heart disease in obese as well as nonobese people, obesity increases the risk (7). Despite the fact that high blood pressure, raised plasma level of LDL, and lower level of HDL cholesterol are all important risk factors, weight gain makes them worse, and weight loss makes them better.

A multivariate analysis of the data from the prospective community study from Framing-ham showed that obesity is related to the long-term risk of heart disease, even when the other major risk factors, such as age, blood pressure, plasma cholesterol, cigarette smoking, glucose tolerance, and left ventricular hypertrophy were allowed for. In women, obesity was one of the best predictors of cardiovascular disease, followed only by age and blood pressure in relative

Table 1   Prevalence (%) of Obesity (QI above 30) in a Representative Sample of Men and Women Aged 16–64 Years in the United Kingdom

Sex	Year	Age (Years)			
		16–24	25–34	35–49	50–64
Men	1980[a]	2.5	4.5	8.0	7.7
	1987[b]	3.0	6.0	11.0	9.0
Women	1980	3.5	4.5	9.0	14.3
	1987	6.0	11.0	10.0	18.0

Source: [a]Ref. 4, [b]Ref. 5.

importance (8). The Veterans Administration Normative Aging Study (9) also showed that weight change in both men and women was significantly related to change in cardiovascular risk factors. Whereas the weight gain was significantly found to be associated with increased blood pressure, cholesterol, triacylglycerol, fasting glucose, postprandial glucose, and uric acid, the weight loss was significantly associated with an improvement of all these factors.

Lapidus et al. (10), in a 12-year follow-up study, noted that Gothenburg (Sweden) people with a high waist-hip ratio (indicating that fat was largely in the abdominal cavity, rather than subcutaneously on the limbs) had a greater risk of heart disease and diabetes than people with a similar amount of fat distributed peripherally. This possibly relates to insulin insensitivity caused by a high flux of fatty acids in the portal circulation, as intra-abdominal fat cells release fatty acids very rapidly. Larsson (11) showed, however, that the increased mortality among men was not significantly linked to waist-hip ratio when the follow-up period was extended up to 20 years.

B. Effect of Obesity on Diabetes and Gallstone Formation

While type II (non–insulin-dependent diabetes mellitus, NIDDM) is not a major cause of death in normal-weight people, it can be an important contributor to morbidity and mortality in obese people. A man weighing 140% more than an average-weight person is 5.2 times more likely to die of diabetes than a normal-weight man, and for women the mortality ratio is 7.9 times higher for a similar degree of overweight (12). Sims et al (13) showed that the association between obesity and reduced insulin sensitivity (which is the primary problem in type II diabetes) is a causal one. Young male volunteers with no family history of diabetes or obesity who increased their weight by 21% (of which 73% was fat) showed significant biochemical changes in the direction of diabetes; after weight loss to normal values, these changes were found to revert to normal.

Obesity is an important risk factor for gallstone formation because the bile of obese people is super-saturated with cholesterol and hence liable to form gallstones. Excessive adipose tissue contains a large amount of cholesterol and is also a source of aromatase, the enzyme that converts androgens to estrogens, which probably explains the frequent menstrual problems of obese women. Obese men have an increased risk of colorectal and prostatic cancers; obese women have increased risk of cancers of breast, ovary, endometrium, and cervix (see Chapter 25). The latter may be associated with abnormal levels of sex hormones. Other health risks of obesity include osteoarthritis of the weight-bearing joints (especially back, hips, and knees) and problems with anesthesia and surgery, in addition to social discrimination (3). All these penalties of obesity decrease with weight loss, barring the risk of gallstone formation, because during weight loss in an obese person, the cholesterol in adipose tissue is mobilized and the bile may then become even more liable to form cholesterol stones.

Obesity and cigarette smoking, together with other risk factors, such as a high intake of saturated fat, salt, or alcohol, or lack of physical activity, all combined, can greatly increase the risk of many important human diseases, including diabetes (NIDDM). This tendency of obesity to increase risks of several diseases makes it a very important public health problem.

III. CAUSES OF OBESITY

Obese people in general have greater energy intake than their energy expenditure. Energy intake influences energy output in several ways: (a) when a person begins to eat more, dietary thermogenesis increases, accounting for about 10% of the excess intake, (b) the energy stored increases both the fat and fat-free mass, causing an increase in metabolic rate, and (c) the same adaptive or regulatory change in metabolic rate tends to oppose weight change. Thus, metabolic rate increases with overfeeding and decreases with underfeeding.

The thermodynamics of weight loss is simpler than that of weight gain, because although there is a substantial metabolic cost involved in storing excess dietary energy as body fat, protein, or glycogen, the mobilization of these energy stores requires little metabolic cost. It is a common experience that dieters lose weight rapidly at first and then more slowly, which is usually ascribed to metabolic adaptation of the body to the diet. The reasons for the decreasing rate of weight loss (2) include the following: (a) The initial weight loss accounts for a large proportion of glycogen, and 1 g glycogen binds about 3 g water, so that the glycogen loss is also accompanied by a corresponding loss of water and of weight in excess of the amount expected on the basis of 1 kg = 7000 kcal (average of values for fat, 1 kg = 9000 kcal, and fat-free tissue, 1 kg = 100 kcal). The excess weight in obese people is composed of 75% fat and 25% fat-free tissue, which is in turn about 75% water and 25% protein. (b) After the first few weeks, the dieter becomes less conscietious about keeping to the diet. (c) With substantial weight loss, metabolic rate is decreased, so that on a given diet the energy deficit is reduced, and the weight is lost move slowly. The average obese person has a higher metabolic rate than normal, and the decrease in metabolism on reduction to normal weight is the expected decrease from a high to normal level, and not to an abnormally low one (14).

The most obvious cause of overweight or obesity is the intake of excess energy, more than that required to maintain normal body composition. But there is no simple answer to the question, why do some people take much more energy than they require? Garrow (2) has described the following factors that predispose to obesity:

A. Genetics

Although obesity tends to run in some families, this does not prove that it is a genetically determined characteristic. Transmission of obesity within a family can also be cultural. Evidence indicates that the extent to which genetic factors may influence the risk of obesity can range from about 5% to 70%. It appears, however, that the characteristic that is inherited from parents is a tendency to overeat in certain circumstances, rather than a strictly governed genetic factor. If this tendency is resisted, it may be possible to resist development of obesity.

B. Age and Sex

The prevalence of obesity has been found increase with age in men up to age 50, and in women it continues to increase up to age 65 (Table 1). In every geographical region, the prevalence of obesity in the age group of 40–60 years is higher in women than in men (2).

C. Physical Inactivity

Severely obese people are in general physically inactive, because they are not fit to undertake much exercise. However, there is little evidence to show that inactivity either in children or adults is a cause of obesity (15). Most people in affluent countries lead sedentary lives, so it is rather difficult to show that an average obese person is physically more inactive than his/her lean equivalent.

D. Growth During Childhood

Most severely obese people were found to be fat babies, giving rise to a hypothesis that overfeeding in infancy causes an increase in the number of fat cells in the body, leading to obesity in adult life. However, prospective studies have failed to support this proposal. It is not possible to predict with accuracy which children will be overweight at age 7 years by analyzing birth weight or any other aspect of growth pattern during infancy (16). There is a significant correlation between the weight of a child in infancy at age 7 and adult weight assessed at age 28 (17,18), but children from obese families who become overweight also have been shown to grow taller and with an accelerated development and enter puberty earlier (2).

E. Socioeconomic Factors

An inverse relationship between the prevalence of obesity and socioeconomic status has been observed in the developed countries. A study in Finland by Rissanen et al. (19) showed that the risk of rapid weight gain (above 5 kg/5 years) was greatest for people with a low educational level, chronic disease, low physical activity during leisure hours, and high alcohol consumption and for those who stopped smoking cigarettes. The poorer and less well-educated people are thought to eat more fatty foods, rather than more expensive and nutritious fruits and vegetables, and to have many children, which is also associated with a high risk of weight gain. In the Finland study, high parity was found to be associated with high weight gain among women of low educational level, but with low weight gain in women of high educational level. Thus highly educated Finnish women who have many pregnancies appeared to be vigilant in preventing excessive weight gain, compared with the less educated ones.

IV. TREATMENT AND MANAGEMENT OF OBESITY

The primary treatment of obesity involves achievement of negative energy balance, either by increasing energy expenditure, decreasing energy intake, or by a combination of both. The best strategy depends on the ability, inclinations, and degree of obesity of the subjects. A severely obese person cannot be advised to significantly increase energy output by taking heavy physical exercise like aerobics, because the exercise tolerance of such people is generally very poor. On the contrary, a relatively sedentary person who is only marginally overweight would do well to take more exercise to help restore weight to normal. The exercise will also contribute to general fitness and confer other metabolic benefits that are not completely understood. While giving advice to obese patients, the following factors must be given consideration (3).

A. Factors Influencing Appropriate Advice

1. Age and Weight-for-Height of Patient

Weight loss is not appropriate for a patient who is in grade O (QI 20–24.9); the younger and more overweight the person, the greater will be the benefit obtained from weight loss.

2. Target Weight and Expected Benefit

It is reasonable to advise the patient to achieve target weight up to QI = 25 and not lower. Benefits can be expected from the realistic weight loss.

3. Previous Attempts at Weight Loss

It is necessary to take into consideration what methods were tried, for how long, with what result, and why were they thought unsatisfactory.

4. Domestic Factors

Domestic circumstances may limit dietary options, owing to patients' employment conditions— e.g., night shifts, catering or food handling business, or entertainment. It is also necessary that other members of the household are supportive to the patient's attempts at weight loss and cooperate in shopping and cooking.

5. Other Physical Disorders and Medication

It is necessary to emphasize that weight loss will affect the dosage required by patients on medication for hypertension or diabetes. Special considerations also apply in conditions such as pregnancy, epilepsy, gout and for certain psychotropic medication.

6. A Hidden Agenda

It may be helpful to find out whether the patient has any specific objective in seeking the help.

A doctor or dietitian thus can obtain a sound basis on which appropriate advice can be provided. Garrow (2) cautioned about the following two common pitfalls in obesity treatment, before providing specific advice:

a. Appropriate Rate of Weight Loss. Figure 1 shows the best practical range of rates of weight loss for most people; those who are younger, taller, and more overweight may aim for the higher limit, and those who are older, shorter, and less overweight should adopt the lower limit. The rate of weight loss is more rapid during the first month of dieting due to the glycogen/water effect (see above). Subsequently, the optimum rate of weight loss is about 0.5 to 1.0 kg per week, representing an average energy deficit of about 500 to 1000 kcal (2–4 MJ) day. There may be an excessive loss of lean tissue at energy deficit rates greater than 1000 kcal/day and it becomes difficult to provide the essential nutrients in such a restricted diet. Also, it is unnecessarily unpleasant, and there will have to be further large adjustments when the target weight is achieved to find a suitable weight maintenance diet. On the other hand, deficits less than 500 kcal/day take too long a time for the subject to reach the target weight, unless initial excess weight was very small (2).

b. Dieting Relationship Trap. Garrow (20) coined a term, dieting relationship trap, to describe hostility between obese patients and the health care professional, one who is trying to assist weight loss. Initially, the patient who comes for advice about losing weight is pleased to find a doctor or dietitian who is providing sensible dietary advice to obtain relief from the complications of obesity. If the patient is severely obese, both parties may underestimate the time which it will take to achieve adequate weight loss, and the difficulty of sustaining dietary compliance over a period of several months. The follow-up visits will go well so long as satisfactory weight loss has been achieved since the last visit, but inevitably the time comes when the patient returns having not lost weight, or even having regained some weight. Obese patients often suffer from low self-esteem, hence when they see that they have failed both themselves and the health care professional, they are likely to be precipitated into an agony of self-reproach. They apologize profusely for their weakness, confess their unworthiness for any further help or consideration, inviting the health carer to discharge them instantly, thus setting the trap.

The correct response of the health carer at this point is to agree that it is disappointing that weight loss has temporarily ceased, and to assure the patient that massive weight loss uninterrupted by setbacks is virtually unknown, and to get down to identifying the factors that precipitated the problem and how best they can be avoided in the future; i.e., encouragement must be provided, not criticism.

Obesity needs to be treated because the obese patient is liable to severe physical and social handicaps, which can be avoided by giving the patient a realistic estimate of the health hazards associated with the condition in that patient, a realistic target weight and rate of weight loss, and advice and encouragement to follow the specific treatment strategy that is most likely to achieve that target.

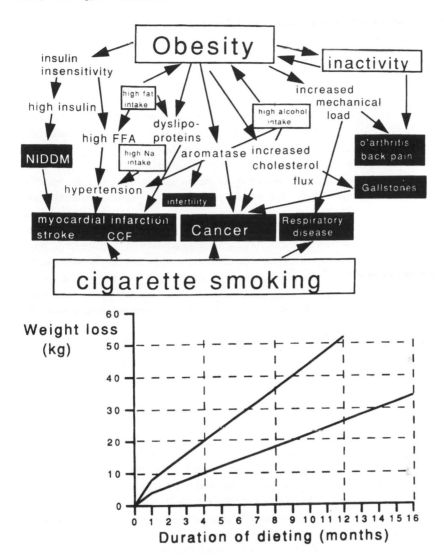

Figure 1 Desirable rates of weight loss in overweight and obese people. An average energy deficit of 1000 kcal/day will cause a weight loss at the upper limit of the zone, and 500 kcal/day at the lower limit. Younger, taller, male, and more overweight patients should aim at the upper line; the lower line is more appropriate for older, shorter, female, and less overweight patients. (From Ref. 2.)

B. Dietary Management of Obesity

Because the rate of weight loss with an energy deficit of 500 to 1000 kcal/day (Fig. 1) is ideal to achieve, it may seem logical to assess the present energy intake of the patient by means of a dietary history, and then prescribe a diet that provides 500 to 1000 kcal/day less, depending on the type of person. In practice, however, this is not useful, because it is very difficult to obtain a reliable estimate of habitual energy intake in obese patients (3). According to Garrow (2), a rule of thumb is to start with a diet supplying 1000 kcal/day for an average obese women, and to increase this upto 1500 kcal/day for men or younger, taller, or heavier women, or decrease to 800 kcal/day for older, shorter women. This estimate may be revised if the observed rate of weight loss is too high or too low, but a reducing diet should not be prescribed outside the range of 800 to 1500 kcal/day.

Because the diet must provide all the essential nutrients, food items that solely provide energy should be restricted, e.g., sucrose and alcohol. It is also desirable to restrict intake of fat, especially saturated fat. This can decease the risk of atheromatous heart disease, partly because fat has been shown to have a lower satiating capacity than isoenergetic quantities of carbohydrate or protein. Foods such as fruits, vegetables and whole-grain cereals should not be restricted, because these are important sources of micronutrients and non-starch poly-saccharides. It is important to ensure adequate protein intake to avoid the loss of lean tissue, but extremely high-protein diets are expensive and have not been shown to be particularly effective or acceptable. Within these guidelines one can construct an infinite variety of nutritionally sound reducing diets that can be adapted to the requirements of individual patients (2).

Commercial diets, such as very low-calorie diets (VLCD), which provide the recommended daily amounts of micronutrients with minimal calories are heavily advertised, and are quite popular in patients wishing to lose weight rapidly. However, the rapid weight loss may lead to excessive loss of lean tissue. Also, these products may be given to people for whom the weight loss is not appropriate, and the prospects for maintaining weight loss are not good for people who have not learnt the basic principles of weight reduction. Controversy exists among nutrition authorities regarding the place of VLCD in the treatment of severe obesity (21).

Patients should obtain clear instructions about a diet appropriate for their weight, tastes, and social circumstances, together with a realistic forecast of the rate of weight loss that this diet should produce. Skillful dietitians can provide this information, for there is much more than simply handling out a standard diet sheet.

Traditionally, patients are advised to take small meals evenly spaced throughout the day, which is probably sound advice, although there is no evidence of its efficacy based on randomized controlled trials. In a crossover trial in a metabolic ward, when obese patients were fed 800 kcal as either one or five meals a day, the patients were much hungrier, and lost more lean tissue, on the one-meal phase than when they received five meals a day (22). However, meal frequency has not been shown to influence total energy output. Booth et al. (23) suggested that it would be useful for patients to establish a formal pattern of eating meals at specified times, rather than continuous snacking or grazing, which makes if difficult to establish any control over total energy intake.

The understanding of human dietary behavior has shown that most of us eat more or less habitually or automatically. It is first necessary to be aware of what is being eaten and the circustances that tend to trigger inappropriate eating before the eating behavior of a patient can be changed. A mere recording of a food diary is associated with some weight loss in most people, suggesting that less food is eaten when one is attentive to what is being eaten. Food diaries are also useful for the dietitian to assess the patient's habitual diet. Recurrent domestic situations where one tends to participate in overeating must be avoided to increase the chance of compliance with the diet. Other members of the patient's family may provide intelligent cooperation with the patient's dieting efforts, especially by avoiding ignorant nagging or ridicule, which will defeat most dieters, unless they are very determined.

Eating behavior is not instinctive but learned, so obese people can be made to re learn inappropriate eating behavior. Although practitioners of behavior therapy are aware of the need to restrict energy intake, they have to make sure that restriction of energy intake is easier to achieve.

After having an initial assessment one-to-one with a dietitian to obtain the necessary information, it would be useful for the obese patient to work with a group of about 10 to 15 patients in follow-up session (24). The dietitian's time would be used more efficiently by talking to a group of patients than to repeat the same instructions many times to the members of the group individually. The patients can benefit from associating with other people in a similar situation and from hearing answers to problems raised by other members of the group, provided the group is skillfully and sensitively led. This is especially true for diffident patients who are not courageous enough to raise the problem themselves. However, group treatment is not a panacea, and may even prove disastrous if there is a particularly assertive or destructive personality within the group.

The results of the long-term effects of dietary treatment trials are inconsistent and rather poor (25). A trial conducted by Gilbert and Garrow (26) indicated that different obese patients probably have different requirements for dietary treatment.

Epidemiological studies have shown that people having stable weights tend to live longer, and have fewer cardiovascular disorders than those who have large variations in weight (27,28). It is not known how weight variation causes the ill health. It has been suggested that ill health or a particular type of personality associated with heart disease might cause the weight cycling. Also, alternating cycles of starvation and overeating are unhealthy, although weight cycling has not shown to significantly influence the metabolic rate or body composition (29).

C. Other Treatments/Therapies for Obesity

1. Drugs

Because hunger tends to make people on a low-energy diet eat more, drugs that decrease hunger should be useful in the control of obesity. Three types of drugs have this effect:

a. Bulk fillers, such as sugar gum, which decrease food intake if consumed in sufficient quantity, but discomfort is involved if taken in significant quantities.

b. Amphetamine and related drugs have a very significant anorectic effect and act as nerve stimulants, and hence are liable to be abused. Large doses of amphetamine can produce psychotic effects similar to schizophrenia.

c. The most widely used anorectic drug, D-fenfluramine, acts through the serotinergic system in the brain, and is a sedative rather than a stimulant. After testing its efficacy in a large long-term multicenter study, Guy-Grand et al. (30) concluded that to achieve the desirable range of weight-for-height, the average patient would have needed to lose about 36 kg, but at the end of the trial those who had taken the drug had about 26 kg still to lose, compared with controls (placebo) who had about 29 kg still to lose. Darga et al. (31) reported similar results from a long-term trial of fluoxetine given in a dosage of 60 mg/day. With a dropout rate of 41% and 27% for drug or placebo, respectively, after one year, the mean weight losses in completers on drug and placebo were 8.2 kg and 4.5 kg, respectively, but the mean starting weight of the group on the drug was 5.8 kg higher than those on placebo. According to Garrow (2), the benefits derived from the use of anoretic drugs probably do not outweight the disadvantages, and these drugs have not proved to be helpful to dieters in the long term.

Thermogenic drugs such as thyroids increase weight loss on a diet if given in a higher dose to override the effect of natural hormone. However, the extra weight loss is mainly of lean tissue. Efforts are being made to find a drug that will activate energy-wasting reactions (futile cycles) in the body without adverse effects.

Some drugs act by inhibiting digestion and absorption of food nutrients by the gut. Several substances block the action of digestive enzymes in vitro, but are not effective in preventing the digestion of a meal when taken orally. It is also necessary to demonstrate the safety of such drugs for long-term use, which is rather difficult. The nutrients that will not be absorbed in the small bowel will become available as substrates for anerobic oxidation by colon bacteria, leading to flatulence and other serious consequences.

Drugs that increase urine output cause a temporary decrease in weight but have no place in the treatment of obesity.

2. Exercise and Physical Activity

Physical activity increases energy expenditure, physical fitness, and sensitivity to insulin action, all of which have favorable effects on obesity. The maximum rate of work an average non-athlete person can put up is about 6 kcal (25 kJ)/min over 1 hour. The average resting metabolism is about 1 kcal (4 kJ)/min, so that after one hour the person doing exercise will have used about 360 kcal, while the person at rest used only 60 kcal. Thus, the net cost of an hour's exercise is approximately 300 kcal, which is probably the upper limit of an increase in energy expenditure to be achieved by an obese person by exercise.

No evidence has been found to support the claim that physical training selectively increases the fat-free mass of the body so that even though an obese person may not experience weight loss, some fat is being replaced by an equal weight of muscle (32). Obese patients should, however, be encouraged to exercise within their tolerance limits, which will increase physical fitness, although exercise alone will not achieve weight loss or alter the proportion of fat and lean tissue in the body to any significant extent.

3. Surgical Treatment

General physicians and dietians may consider surgical treatment as an option for severely obese patients. However, it must be emphasized that the surgical treatment of obesity (with one minor exception) is not an alternative to dieting but a method for trying to enforce dieting. The minor exception is apronectomy, cutting away fat hanging in a fold of the anterior abdominal wall, which is applicable only in very severely obese patients. Cutting (or sucking) fat from subcutaneous sites is advertised as a cosmetic procedure. However, the amount of fat thus removed is trivial in comparison to total excess fat in the obese patient, and in many cases the cosmetic result from an attempt to remove significant quantities of subcutaneous fat is not very satisfactory (2).

The gut may be cut and rejoined in an operation (gastric bypass surgery) to provide a relatively short exposure of food to the action of digestive enzymes, while the majority of the bowel is short-circuited. Thus, some of the food energy is not absorbed, and a large energy intake also provokes severe diarrhea. The weight loss caused by such operations depends more on the aversive consequences if the patient overeats, than on failure to absorb what is eaten.

Gastric stapling is a operation in which a line of staples closes off all but a small pouch at the fundus, which empties through a small stoma into the main stomach, so that only about 50 ml of food can be consumed at a time. Patients lose about one-third of their excess weight in one year after operation, after which there is tendency to gain weight. Weight loss in both gastric bypass and stapling operation is at the cost of greater metabolic complications, and a greater risk of nutrient deficiencies. Both the operations are technically reversible, and weight gain after reversal is rapid and almost universal (2).

4. Gastric Balloons and Jaw Wiring

Gastric balloons are inserted into the stomach to reduce its capacity, without the hazards associated with abdominal operations in obese persons. The weight loss thus obtained is small and not sustained, and the procedure carries a significant risk of gastric mucosal ulcers.

Jaw wiring, a standard orthodontic practice in which the upper and lower jaws are wired for the treatment of jaw fractures or to reset the jaws, often results in weight loss, because with this procedure the patient can drink but cannot chew, and liquid diets generally have a low energy density. When used as a treatment of obesity, a weight loss of about 36 kg was achieved in 9 months (33), but this could not be sustained after the removal of the wires. This procedure is not justified unless it is combined with some other method to help the patient to maintain weight loss.

D. Maintenance of Weight Loss in Obese People

The massive weight loss achieved through many months of diet and exercise cannot be maintained automatically after the intense dieting effort is over. On the contrary, the lost weight can be regained rapidly if efforts are not taken to maintain the weight loss. After weight loss, energy requirements are decreased, so if the patient begins to eat normally, the weight is regained to reestablish the equilibrium of the previous weight.

The weight can be controlled in part by noting unacceptable increases in weight and altering energy intake (or output) to compensate. Obese people who have lost weight can benefit from a "device" that warns them of weight gain, which may be a spouse, a housemate, or a favorite pair of jeans. Weight can also be monitored by a nylon cord fixed round the waist that becomes tight when excess weight is gained (3). Earlier versions of the waist cord were either too loose or too tight to monitor changes in weight accurately. In the newer versions, a monofilament nylon fishing line is secured to the end of a 35 mm long perspex rod by a knot in the hole. It is taken twice round the patient's waist, and the third turn passes through the hole and is secured by a knot in the hole, so that the maximum circumference is fixed. Some slack present in the cord is taken up as one or two loops around the right-hand end of the rod, which can be released to accommodate temporary periods of modest weight gain (2).

E. Prevention of Obesity

Special groups such as overweight children and obese expectant or lactating mothers should not try to lose weight. Weight loss in children is often associated with a decrease in height growth, and the best time for an expectant mother to lose weight is between pregnancies, although it is reasonable to aim for a constant weight during the pregnancy of a woman who starts to become obese, so that after childbirth she will weigh less than at the beginning of pregnancy. Both obese diabetics and hypertensive patients must be aware of the fact that weight loss will affect the dosage of the medications being used.

Because fatness at age 13 years is quite a strong predictor of adult fatness, the optimum time to prevent obesity would be between 7 and 12 years of age. People who have lost weight are very liable to regain it if after a period of dieting, they begin to "eat normally," necessitating secondary prevention. Garrow and Webster (34) have reviewed the effects of dieting and weight loss on metabolic rate in details. The weight lost after dieting incurs some metabolic costs and these costs are removed when the weight is lost, hence there is a reduction in metabolic rate after a weight loss; e.g., if a person who was stable at a weight of 100 kg achieves a weight of 70 kg and then goes back to his or her original diet, the weight will again be stabilized at 100 kg. To remain at 70 kg, this person will have to reduce energy intake by about 15%, which is the maintenance energy cost of the weight lost.

Although some studies have suggested that drinking in moderation may be beneficial for health, many of these studies do not address body weight. Evidence available suggests that consuming moderate amounts of alcohol is a risk factor for obesity, which is in turn a risk factor for several adverse health outcomes. According to Suter et al. (35), recommendations regarding alcohol intake should take into account a variety of factors, including baseline body weight, location of body fat, and overall diet. Moderate alcohol consumption enhances the development of positive energy balance, mainly because of alcohol-induced suppression of lipid oxidation.

Akoh (36) reviewed new developments in low-calorie fats and oil substitutes that are of value in the management of weight loss in obese people. Low-calorie fats and oil substitutes are intended to replace conventional fats and oils in the diet while retaining the required physical and organoleptic properties but with less than 9 kcal/g. Indeed, some of the fat substitutes may contribute zero calorie to the diet (36).

The most notable fat substitute is Olestra® (now Olean®), developed by Procter and Gamble Company. It is chemically a sucrose polyester or sucrose fatty acid polyester and was approved by the USFDA on January 24, 1996, for use in savory snacks. Other fat substitutes with potential to partially replace some, but not all, the calories from fat are either under development or are already on the market. Obviously, none of the fat substitutes, including Olestra, is free from possible side effects when consumed. However, the potential benefits may outweigh the problems when consumed in moderation.

According to Akoh (36), a new group of reduced-calorie fat substitutes gaining recognition is a family of structured or specialty lipids with the same triacylglycrol backbone as conventional fats and oils, but which contain short- or medium-chain fatty acids in addition to the long-chain fatty acids or contain poorly digestible fatty acids in amounts or at positions that do not occur naturally, e.g., Caprenin® Salatrim (Benefat™), developed by Nabisco Foods Group and marketed by Cultor Food Science, and several variants of these for specific nutritional pharmaceutical and physical properties and applications (36).

An exciting development from obesity research has been the observation that the thin rim of cytoplasm in the adipocyte does more than release and take up fatty acids. It also synthesizes proteins, such as lipoprotein lipase, the enzyme that breaks down triglycerides in the nearby capillary, which are deposited in the adipose tissue. The amount of this enzyme increases during abundant feeding and obesity, and tends to decrease during starvation. The role this enzyme plays in shuttling fat in and out of adipocytes and in the control of fat cell size is being elucidated. Another enzyme, adipsin, is made in fat cells and secreted into the bloodstream. It is not known if this enzyme plays any role in the production and perpetuation of obesity.

The puzzle of fat cells has not been resolved fully. They store fat and are always enlarged in obese persons and are more numerous in obese than in lean persons. The metabolic activity of fat cells and their influence on body weight regulation, and steps in their development, remain to be established.

V. DIET AND DIABETES

A. Forms of Diabetes

James and Pearson (40) have described different forms of diabetes mellitus (Table 2), all of which are characterized by a failure to maintain the concentration of blood glucose within the normal range. The old terms, "juvenile onset" and "maturity or adult onset," have now been replaced by type I and type II diabetes, respectively, because the age of onset is not the initial determinant of the form of diabets. The World Health Organization has defined borderline forms of high blood glucose as "impaired glucose tolerance" (IGT), formerly known as chemical diabetes; 2% to 5% of these patients each year progress to have higher glucose levels characteristic of diabetes. About a quarter of the IGT subjects respond normally 5 years later to a further test challenge of 75 g glucose, which is a standard oral glucose tolerance test to assess the ability of the pancreas to produce insulin, and for the tissues to respond to the circulating insulin.

Type I, or insulin-dependent diabetes mellitus (IDDM), is characterized by acute symptoms induced by a hyperglycemia, a high blood glucose level. Individuals with HLA tissue type DR3 and DR4 are highly susceptible to diabetes, and beta cell damage in them may be triggered by

Table 2   Different Forms of Diabetes Mellitus

Type I: Usually arises in childhood or young adulthood, associated with pancreatic damage. More likely in bottle-fed children than in breastfed. Susceptibility linked to specific blood group subtypes, e.g., HLA type DR 3 and DR 4 on chromosome 6. A condition of insulin deficiency.

Type II: Usually occurs in middle age or old age and is associated with insulin resistance and a high insulin output insufficient to cope with the demand for effective insulin action. Often precipitated by weight gain in genetically suceptible subjects. Associated with high secretion of proinsulin and amylin output.

Type II MODY (maturity onset diabetes of the young): A subgroup with distinct genetic characteristics presenting with modest diabetes.

Tropical diabetes mellitus: A condition linked to low-grade pancreatitis with pancreatic exocrine duct damage often accompanied by pancreatic calculi. Linked to the long-term effects of malnutrition.

Pancreatic insufficiency: Unusual disorder relating to pancreatic islet cell damage, e.g., from pancreatitis associated with alcoholism or from hemochromatosis. A condition of insulin deficiency.

Hormonal diabetes, e.g., Cushing's disease or in association with corticosteroid therapy which induces insulin resistance; acromegaly or glucagonomas or pheochromocytomas.

Genetic disease, e.g., receptor abnormalities, glycogen storage disease.

Source: Ref. 40.

viral infection or chemicals. An ongoing autoimmune process results in beta cell failure leading to eventual clinical symptoms of diabetes. The glucose in the blood fails to be absorbed by the tissues as the blood insulin level falls, leading to hyperglycemia. Antibodies to the pancreatic islet beta cells, which produce insulin, are found in the blood before and for 1 to 2 years after diagnosis. Some moderately overweight patients also have autoantibodies and can be misclassified as having NIDDM because they can be maintained on a diet and sulfonylureas for a time, before the autoimmune pancreatic damage and insulin dependence signifies their IDDM condition. The classic symptoms of IDDM at presentation include thirst, frequency of micturition, and weight loss, which can be explained biochemically. Once the kidney's threshold for glucose absorption exceeds the water is excreted with glucose by the kidney, leading to marked water loss and dehydration. Other symptoms are high glucagon secretion, low insulin output, and extreme ketosis because of excess acetone, acetoacetate, and beta-hydroxybutyrate production. Severe ketogenesis also dehydrates the patient, because organic acids such as ketone bodies and glucose spill into the urine and require water and cations such as K^+ to be excreted. The patient in a very ill, dehydrated, and semi-comatose state may have a sweet breath due to volatile acetone being expelled via the lungs.

Type II diabetes, also known as non–insulin-dependent diabetes mellitus (NIDDM), is characterized by the progressive development of insulin resistance. Around 2% to 3% of the population are known to have type II diabetes, but its rate appears to be increasing as adults become more overweight and live longer; the prevalence of diabetes is about 7% among those over 80 years of age.

The hormonal imbalance in the body of the diabetic person causes fat to accumulate in the liver cells, resulting in ketosis as the fat is metabolized into ketone. High blood and urine levels of ketones pull sodium and potassium with them, contributing to a chain of reactions leading to dehydration, ion imbalance, coma, and even death in people with poorly regulated insulin-dependent diabetes.

Non–insulin-dependent diabetes, which usually begins in adulthood, is often not accompanied by ketosis. It is linked to widespread inactivity and obesity and is commonly seen in countries such as the United States. Type II diabetes is also genetically linked, but the problem is not only with the beta cells of the pancreas but also with the insulin receptor on the cell surface of peripheral tissues, such as muscles. Thus, instead of insufficient insulin, there is an abundance of insulin in early stages of the disease, but it is used poorly. As the disease develops, pancreas function can later fail, leading to poor insulin output.

Many cases of type II diabetes are associated with obesity, but the hyperglycemia is not necessarily caused by diabetes. There is a growing number of lean people with type II diabetes. Obesity, with its large fat cells, simply increases the risk for a state of insulin resistance in the body, when the blood glucose is not readily transferred into cells leading to the development of hyperglycemia. Type II diabetes often disappears if the obesity is corrected. Thus, achieving a desirable weight should be a primary goal of treatment. Oral medicines that increase the ability of the pancreas to produce insulin are often prescribed, as well as occasional insulin injections. Regular exercise and regular meal patterns, with an emphasis on complex carbohydrates and dietary fiber, help to manage the disease effectively.

A clinical tool known as the glycemic index compares the total amount of glucose appearing in the bloodstream after eating a food with the total amount of glucose appearing in the bloodstream after eating the same amount of carbohydrate in the form of white bread or glucose. The glycemic index of a food is influenced by several factors, including the amount of dietary fiber in the food, the food's digestion rate, and its total fat content. Foods such as oatmeal that contain much soluble fiber increase blood glucose slowly after eating, in contrast to foods such as potatoes that are digested quickly, producing a rapid increase in blood glucose levels after eating. A diabetic person who eats many foods with a low glycemic index can manage to maintain normal blood glucose levels for prolonged times, after each meal.

The eventual complications of both types of unmanaged diabetes are blindness, loss of fingers and toes, kidney failure, and heart disease, which are linked to microscopic changes in the small blood vessels (capillaries). Nervous deterioration may also follow, resulting in lack of proper nerve stimulation, e.g., in the G.I. tract, where intermittent diarrhea and constipation can occur. High blood glucose levels may contribute to a rapid progression of fatty buildup in blood vessels, blocking the blood supply to nearby organs (atherosclerosis). The blood vessel and nerve complications of diabetes can be prevented, however, by effectively managing the blood glucose levels within the normal range.

The typical features of insulin-dependent and non–insulin-dependent diabetes as described by Wolever and Jenkins (37) are shown in Table 3. The recommended daily intakes in diabetes by the American Diabetic Association (ADA), 1986, are carbohydrate, 55% to 60% of energy; protein 0.8 g/kg body weight; fat, less than 30% of energy, PUFA, 6% to 8% calories; saturated fat, less than 10% of calories; cholesterol, less than 300 mg/day; and elemental sodium, less than 3

Table 3 Typical Features of Insulin-Dependent and Non–Insulin-Dependent Diabetes

Features	Insulin dependent	Non-insulin dependent
Percent of diabetic population	Less than 20%	Over 80% of total
Age of onset	Early (under 30)	Late (over 50)
Body weight	Normal weight	80% are overweight
Ketosis proneness	Ketosis prone	Not ketosis prone
Blood insulin level	Low or zero	Normal or raised
Treatment	Requires insulin	Diet ± oral agents ± insulin

Source: Ref. 37.

g/day. There is uncertainty on the use of dietary fiber, especially regarding its soluble and insoluble forms, which have quite different physiological effects. It is the soluble fibers that have the metabolic effects (colonic fermentation, cholesterol reduction, and reduced postprandial glycemia) that are desirable in diabetes. Examples of foods high in soluble dietary fibers are legumes, oats, barley, okra, and persimmon, whereas foods high in insoluble fibers are whole wheat, wheat bran, whole rye, brown rice, and millets. Recognizing these differences, the American Diabetic Association has advocated to double the intake of dietary fiber, using more soluble types, such as legumes, whole-grain cereals, root vegetables, tubers, and leafy vegetables, to improve carbohydrate metabolism and decrease blood lipids. The ADA has cautioned, however, about mineral deficiencies (e.g. Ca, Zn, and Fe) and gastric bezoars and abdominal discomforts arising from use of dietary fiber (37).

While both the ADA and the Canadian Diabetes Association (CDA) have recommended the use of some common starchy foods on the basis of their glycemic index (GI) (Table 4), the National Institutes of Health Consensus Development Conference Statement (38) has opposed this view, pointing out that there are many factors that alter glycemic effect, such as processing, cooking, food storage, mastication, diurnal variation in absorption, and racial and ethnic differences. Also, GI has no effect in mixed meals. Thus, an application of this concept remains a matter for debate, and studies of the longer-term effects of low-GI foods on metabolic control in diabetes are required. Individual physicians and dieticians, however, may try to apply the GI concept where it increases the variety of starchy foods acceptable to the diabetic patient.

Thus, the higher-fiber and low-GI foods offer some hope of filling the caloric void left by the reduction of saturated fat in diabetics. The fat is reduced to lower blood lipids and to minimize the risk of cardiovascular disease. At the same time, protein is held at a relatively low level to meet requirements at about 0.8 g./kg, but higher intakes are not recommended because of concerns over its possible effect in exacerbating preexisting or incipient renal damage. It is agreed that reduction in weight is very important in diabetic individuals who are overweight, because this may reverse the metabolic abnormalities of type II diabetes (39). Exercise would be a useful way to limit positive energy balance, providing that energy intake is also reduced or held constant. Exercise may also have possible independent benefits in terms of cardiovascular disease and bone and calcium metabolism. The use of n-3 fatty acids in diabetes remains to be clarified, as does the use of fructose to replace sucrose (37).

The prevalence of diabetes in a country can be predicted from the proportion of adults who are overweight, and particularly in those with a truncal fat distribution and a high waist/hip circumference ratio (40). The risk of developing diabetes in adults with a body mass index (BMI) of

Table 4 Glycemic Index (GI) Ranking Some Common Starchy Foods into Higher (Class I), Intermediate (Class II), and Lower (Class III) Groups

Class I GI > 90	Class II GI > 70–90	Class III GI < 70
Most breads	All bran	Pumpernickel bread
Plain crackers	Oatmeal	Most pasta
Most breakfast cereals	Most cookies or biscuits	Parboiled rice
Most potatoes	Buckwheat	Most dried legumes
Millet	Sweet corn	Nuts
Corn chips	Boiled new potatoes	Barley
	Yams	Bulgur (cracked wheat)
	Sweet potatoes	

Source: Ref. 37.

more than 30 is five times that of adults with a BMI of less than 25. According to Helmrich et al. (41), physically active individuals, e.g., those who jog, swim, dance, or engage in similar exercises for 20 minutes. three times a week, have only around 40% chance of developing diabetes, compared with inactive individuals.

The etiology of type II diabetes appears to involve both an impaired pancreatic secretion of insulin and the development of tissue resistance to insulin. The early phase of glucose intolerance in both normal and obese subjects is characterized by an abnormal early plasma glucose rise in response to carbohydrate intake. Because the early secretion of insulin is impaired and glycogen secretion is not suppressed, the rate of endogenous glucose production and release by the liver continues despite dietary inflow of glucose. Blood glucose rises excessively, which stimulates a prolonged surge in insulin secretion (42). The mechanisms in the tissues that respond to higher glucose and insulin levels, adjusting for the usual activation of the insulin receptor by insulin, become less effective, leading to the development of insulin resistance. Due to this insensitivity to insulin's action, glucose levels in the blood tend to rise further after a meal, which in turn stimulates insulin secretion.

As the human subjects gain weight, their insulin resistance increases, thus also increasing the demand for insulin secretion. Physical activity rapidly improves the tissue's sensitivity to insulin, independent of any effect on body weight. With the usual steady decline in physical activity and progressive weight gain with age, insulin resistance rises as adults age. Thus, there is an ever-increasing demand for more insulin. Eventually the pancreatic capacity for insulin output proves inadequate to maintain usual blood glucose levels, so both fasting and postprandial glucose levels increase excessively, resulting in diabetes.

The individual becomes aware of the problem when he or she develops blood glucose levels that exceed the kidney's capacity to reabsorb the filtered load in the renal tubules, leading to a spill-over of glucose into the urine. The glucose imposes an osmotic load that in turn leads to high urinary water loss and therefore thirst, the early symptoms of diabetes. Some other commonly observed symptoms include blurred vision, retinopathy, cataract, foot problems, and vascular disease. There is no such condition as mild diabetes, and asymptomatic patients are at risk for micro- and macrovascular complications, and hence need effective dietetic advice (2).

The capacity of pancreas to produce insulin varies among individuals and may be decreased in persons of low birth weight, suggesting that fetal nutrition influences early pancreatic cellularity and development (43).

Type II diabetes appears to have a strong familial genetic basis: the individual susceptibility to this disorder emerges from its subtype, with autosomal dominant inheritance showing a link to an abnormal glucokinase gene on chromosome 7p (44). This subtype, maturity-onset of diabetes of the young (MODY), presents in the second decade of life and can often be treated by diet or diet and sulfonylureas tablet. The glucokinase enzyme has been termed the pancreatic glucose sensor because it plays a key role in the regulation of glucose metabolism and the glucokinase gene is expressed both in the pancreatic beta cells and the liver. MODY is characterized by a subnormal beta cell secretion in response to glucose loading as in other forms of Type II diabetes. The latter also involves abnormalities in the secretion of a newly described protein, amylin, by the pancreatic beta cells. Amylin has 37 amino acids, and like insulin it is secreted in excess in people with glucose intolerance (45), but it is absent in the plasma of type I diabetics. Amylin acts as a potent stimulant of glycogenolysis and reduces the peripheral uptake of glucose by muscle. Long-term pancreatic overstimulation increases peripheral insulin resistance, further exacerbating diabetes, as the amylin polymerizes and accumulates between the beta cells of the pancreas, replacing the damaged beta cells; this explains why type II diabetic patients deteriorate progressively with time, as the capacity for insulin secretion by the damaged pancreatic islet cells falls (40).

B. Diabetes and Cardiovascular Disease

Diabetic patients are particularly likely to develop vascular disease, both microvascular and macrovascular types. The microvascular type is characterized by a thickening of the capillary basement membranes, in addition to increased capillary permeability, leading to hemorrhages, the leakage of exudates of fibrin and edema from the vessel wall, which then become thickened and blocked. In the eye tissues, these changes may lead to blindness, and in the kidney to severe renal failure. These microvascular complications appear to be proportional to the degree and duration to which blood glucose levels rise and become out of control.

Blindness and kidney failure are particular problems in the long-term management of type I diabetes. Cataracts can also form very rapidly in patients with poorly controlled diabetes and are ascribed to the excessive synthesis of sugar alcohol, sorbital, synthesized from glucose through hexose-6-phosphate pathway within the lens, leading to its damage. The high blood glucose levels are also thought to promote cataract development due to the diffusion of polysols into the lens.

Macrovascular disease involves the coronary, cerebral, and peripheral arteries and the aorta and appears to be a more severe form of the atherosclerotic disease in the industrially developed Western societies. The combination of vascular disease and sensory neuropathy appears to dramatically increase susceptibility to serious foot ulceration, infection, and ischemic damage. Cardiovascular disease is the major type of morbidity in both type I and type II diabetes (Table 5), and this finding has led to a very different approach to dietary management of diabetes (46).

The chronic elevation of blood glucose levels in diabetes causes glycosylation of a range of proteins, including those of endothelial surfaces and lipoproteins, which in turn induce the scavenger receptor–mediated uptake of low-density lipoproteins by the macrophages of the endothelium. These macrophages are now linked to stimulation of the atherosclerotic process. Additionally, the poor conversion of n-6 and n-3 essential fatty acids to their longer-chain metabolites via the insulin-desaturation step may also cause macrovascular disease. Prostaglandins, when in appropriate balance, function in normal platelet formation and the clearance of clots from the arterial walls, implicating the possible use of gamma-linolenic acid precursor to bypass the desaturation step in the linolenic acid metabolism. The use of substantial amounts of oily fish in the diet also seems to provide preexisting n-3 long-chain fatty acids and alpha-linolenic acid precursor. Higher intake of fish may be important in the long-term management of diabetes. The thrombotic tendency in diabetes is amplified by a high-fat, low-carbohydrate diet. Free radical and antioxidant mechanisms may also be involved in atherosclerosis and cardiovascular disease, which had become the principal cause of death in type I and type II diabetes during the 1950s and 1960s.

Claims have been made that simple sugars may have adverse effects on several metabolic conditions involved in the etiology of obesity, cardiovascular disease, and diabetes mellitus. On

Table 5   The Causes of Death (%) in Human Subjects With and Without Diabetes

	Diabetes		No diabetes	
	Men	Women	Men	Women
Cardiovascular disease	65	57	53	53
Coronary artery disease	46	35	35	28
Diabetes, e.g., coma	7	21		
Other causes	28	22	47	46

Source: Ref. 46.

the basis of available literature, Blaak and Saris (47) concluded that there was no consistent evidence to implicate differences in simple and complex dietary carbohydrates in the etiology of these human diseases. Moreover, there were indications that simple carbohydrates may have beneficial effects on glucose tolerance and blood lipid spectrum. These findings, however, need further research.

C. Dietary Management of Diabetes

Several revolutions in the dietary management of diabetes have not resolved all the dilemmas concerning balanced diabetic diets (Table 6), although prescribing the right amount of energy has always remained a central issue. Prior to the regular availability of insulin, starvation therapy was often used to manage type I diabetes to keep the patient alive, but after the discovery of insulin, it was possible to provide food and still control the blood glucose at reasonable levels by choosing the dose and timing for subcutaneous insulin injections. The problem of meeting the patient's energy needs and prescribing small precise amounts of carbohydrate still existed. Balancing the amount of carbohydrate fed with the insulin given was thought to be the key in controlling the immediate postprandial rise in blood glucose. A series of tests were conducted to monitor the response to food and to prescribe the correct amount of carbohydrate at different times of the day. After specifying the dietary amount of carbohydrate carefully, adequate quantities of fat and protein then could be prescribed to meet the patient's energy needs. This, in practice, led to the use of relatively low-carbohydrate, high-fat diets, unfortunately promoting the atherosclerosis and thrombosis to which diabetic patients are rather prone. The emphasis has now thus swung to ensuring control of both glucose and lipid levels to prevent micro- and macrovascular diseases (Table 7).

James and Pearson (40) have stated the following three practical approaches to dietary management, which are based on first assessing energy needs:

Table 6   Balancing the Diet in Diabetes

Food/Diet	Advantages	Disadvantages
Vegetables	Rich in: Soluble fiber Insoluble fiber Antioxidants	
Fruits	Rich in: Soluble fiber Antioxidants	High in simple sugar content
Fish	Rich in *n*-3 fatty acids	Heavy metal contamination (?)
Fat	Slows gastric emptying	Promotes thrombosis and atherosclerosis, depending on fatty acid
Protein	Modest glucose	Amplifies tendency to deteriorate renal function (?)
	Stimulating effect	
	Satiating	Often associated with saturated fat in meat and dairy products
Alcohol	Moderate intakes reduce cardiovascular morbidity and mortality	Induces weight gain
		Metabolized in preference to glucose

Source: Ref. 40.

Table 7 Different Approaches to Evaluating Diabetic Diets

Short-term[a]	Longer term
Glucose responses to a meal	Changes in body weight and composition
Diurnal glucose response to meals throughout the day	Blood HbA_{1c} levels for monitoring glycosylated hemoglobin levels
Fasting blood and urinary glucose levels after a special day's feeding	Monitoring blood lipid levels
24-hour urinary glucose output in first day	Repeated tests of retinal permeability or renal function, e.g., creatinine clearance, microalbuminuria

[a]Each of these options is also used as a test after feeding the patient a liquid formula or a normal diet over several weeks before testing.
Source: Ref. 40.

1. A pragmatic attempt to assess the patient's diet, using techniques such as 24-hour recall or simple dietary histories administered in the clinic, has often led to an underestimation of intake.
2. The dietary prescription is based on a crude assumption about the patient's energy needs, the figures being taken from tables based on age and sex, but without regard to the patient's weight. Thus, a crude value (e.g., 2000 kcal or 1500 kcal) was chosen for energy needs and the diet was then adjusted if the patient became too hungry, changed weight, or became more difficult to control.
3. With the recognition in 1973 by FAO that approximate energy needs could be expressed for adults simply on a weight basis, a new scheme evolved in the best clinics of prescribing, 46 kcal/kg for a moderately active male and 40 kcal/kg for a moderately active female, with subsequent adjustments for individual needs and daily variations in exercise patterns.

1. Appropriate Diabetic Diets

The progress in the evaluation of the most appropriate diet for diabetics has been rather slow, partly because of large variations among diabetics with regard to insulin resistance, body size, and pancreatic secretion of insulin. A variety of dietary manipulations, e.g., with fish, soluble fiber, or special dietary carbohydrates such as sorbital, need to be tested. All of these combinations may need to be evaluated in many different ways, with various evaluating techniques, either short-term (i.e., hours, days, or weeks), relating predominantly to glucose control, or larger term over months or years, relating to the development of microvascular or macrovascular disease (Table 8).

Interactions between dietary factors are also important and need to be recognized; e.g., fat delays gastric emptying and thus may modify the blood glucose response to a meal. Fat may also interact with glucose metabolism (47). Diabetic patients, when overfed, preferentially deposit the dietary fat despite a high glucose level. With an increase in fat depots, basal lipolysis rises, especially during insulin deficiency, and the resultant free fatty acids rise to compete with glucose as a metabolic fuel, further exacerbating the problem of diabetes. Thus, weight changes have a marked effect on diabetic control.

According to Blaak and Saris (48), the differences between simple and complex carbohydrates seems no longer clear-cut in terms of their glycemic responses. This is emphasized in several studies in which it has been shown that plasma insulin and free fatty acid responses to glucose saccharides were not influenced by chain length, and postprandial glucose and insulin curves

Table 8 Examples of Insulin Preparations Used in the United Kingdom

Insulin preparation	Species	Purity[a]	Retarding agent	Action (hours)		
				Initial	Maximum	Total
Short acting						
Neutral soluble	Beef	3	—	0.5	2–4	6–8
Human Actrapid (Novo)	Human	1	—	0.5	2–4	6–8
Intermediate						
Isophane	Beef	3	Protamine	1.2	5–8	18
Humalin I (Lilly)	Human	1	Protaminc	0.5–2	2–8	14–18
Long acting						
Humalin Zn	Human	3	Protamine + Zinc	3	8–12	30–40
Hypurin protamine Zinc (Weddel)	Beef	2	Protamine + Zinc	3	8–12	30–40

[a]1 = Highly purified; 2 = Purified; 3 = Conventional.
Source: Ref. 40.

were independent of the type of carbohydrate consumed in the meals. Blaak and Saris (48) generalized the effects of different types of carbohydrates and food-related factors on the postprandial glucose and insulin responses, as follows:

Carbohydrate type:	Amylose-amylopectin ratio
	Cooking time and procedure
	Physical form of the starch
	Differences in gelatinization time
	Particle size
Food-related factors:	Fat and protein
	Dietary fiber
	Antinutrients

2. *Dietary Management of Type I Diabetes (IDDM)*

Diabetic people need to be taught the practical skills of insulin administration and blood testing and acquire the knowledge to deal with different day-to-day situations, so that a healthy lifestyle to minimize the immediate and long-term impact of diabetes on health is achieved. Dietary counseling must complement the advice from other members of the diabetic team and the advice must be tailored to specific individual needs.

The amount of injectable insulin can be determined on the basis of (a) the extent of islet cell damage, (b) the magnitude of exercise taken, (c) whether the cellular response to insulin is normal or poor, leading to insulin resistance, and (d) the amount, type, absorption, and metabolism of food consumed.

The energy equivalence of the food should match the patient's energy needs, which in turn are determined by the individual's metabolic rate and the level of physical activity. Also, different types of injectable insulin act over different time scales, e.g., a subcutaneous injection of soluble insulin may last for 6 to 8 hours, but have a maximum impact at 2 to 4 hours (Table 8). Figures given in Table 8 are only guidelines and there can be considerable individual variation. Thus, an insulin regimen should be selected to suit the specific individual's needs.

According to James and Pearson (40), the immediate aim of dietary management of dia betes is to ensure that the blood glucose will not fall too fast or too low when a dose of insulin is given. Type I diabetics usually require soluble insulin 2 or 3 times daily, meaning that within 30 min of subcutaneous injection of insulin the blood glucose level may be falling as the hormone passes around the body. Insulin is therefore usually given about 30 min before meals.

The brain depends on glucose metabolism for its energy needs, unless the patient has turned ketotic, with elevated levels of blood ketone bodies. Therefore, it is necessary to prevent blood glucose levels from falling too rapidly and to a low level to avoid mental impairments. The vary ing susceptibility of different patients to hypoglycemia reflects adaptive changes in cerebral glu cose transporters responsible for controlling the uptake of glucose by brain. Some warning of hypoglycemia is given to most patients due to reflex increase in sympathetic nervous system activ ity, with a rise in pulse rate, pallor, sweating, fine muscle tremor, and occasionally an acute sense of hunger. Type I diabetic patients learn to recognize these symptoms and compensate by taking soluble carbohydrate, e.g. dextrose tablets (3 g each). Two such tablets are usually sufficient to limit a hypoglycemia episode. Taking larger doses of carbohydrate may lead to hyperglycemia, which may be misinterpreted as a need for more insulin. Dietary education programs for diabet ics and their relatives must include information about the recognition and management of hypo glycemia. A suitable carbohydrate for immediate ingestion should always be carried along with a diabetic identity card. Patients also need to be educated initially to recognize the problems caused by infection, alcohol drinking, delayed meal times, and exercise, along with legal requirements in relation to driving licenses. Multiple insulin injections with a dose of quick-acting, highly puri fied insulin to be taken before each of three meals together with an additional dose of intermedi ate insulin or long-acting insulin before dinner have now become popular. This system is further aided by the availability of portable multi-dose 'pen injectors' to handle insulin injections.

3. Dietary Management of Type II Diabetes (NIDDM)

The education and dietary management of type II diabetics depend on their individual needs, the approach for middle-aged overweight smokers differing from that for very elderly subjects. The basic aim in all patients is to relieve the symptoms of diabetes and to minimize its impact on micro- and macrovascular disease. All patients require dietary assessment and most of them need to modify their diet. All will need long-term ongoing education and screening for complications.

The traditional methods used a sequence of treatments to manage type II diabetes. Dieting is first used to reduce weight and the intake of quickly absorbed carbohydrates. Diet is aimed to limit the saturated fat intake to prevent cardiovascular disease associated with type II diabetes. If dietary measures recommended (Table 9) fail to control glycemia after a period of reasonable compliance, drug therapy is prescribed in addition to diet (49).

Two groups of oral hypoglycemia drugs are available. Sulfonlyurea is useful in normal-weight type II diabetics but may result in hypoglycemia if dosage is not accurate. Biguanide and sulfonylurea drugs are therefore often combined for maximum benefit, but around 30% of patients are eventually transferred to insulin within about 4 years of drug therapy (40). This fea ture may be ascribed to continuing amylin production in some patients with insulin resistance or type II diabetes, who then become dependent on insulin as their pancreatic insulin secretory capacity fails. Despite the additional treatment, diet is central to management in type II diabetics.

The diabetic diet can be planned in the following five stages (40):

1. Estimating the average daily energy need
2. Calculating the absolute intake of carbohydrate

Table 9 U.K. Dietary Recommendations for People with Diabetes

Energy	To maintain BMI = 22 kg/m^2
Carbohydrate (%) energy	50–55
Sucrose or fructose (added)	<25 g/day
Dietary fiber	>30 g/day
Total fat (% energy)[a]	30–35
Saturated fat[a]	<10%
Monounsaturated fat[a]	10–15%
Polyunsaturated fat[a]	<10%
Protein (% energy)	10–15
Salt	<6 g/day
Hypertensives	<3 g/day
Diabetic foods	Avoid

[a]These proposed fat intakes reflect the concern in the United Kingdom to advise diets that are considered practical. In countries with preexisting lower fat intakes, there should be no advice to increase them to these U.K. proposed levels. The dietary fiber is measured by the old method and 30 g corresponds to 18 g nonstarch polysaccharides.
Source: Ref. 49.

3. Specifying the type of dietary carbohydrate
4. Adjusting the pattern of intake to account for the timing and type of insulin injected, the patient's work schedule, and leisure activities, and for the diurnal variation in insulin sensitivity
5. Specifying intakes of *n*-3 fatty acids, vegetables, and fruits for metabolic, antioxidant, and non-starch polysaccharide (fiber) needs.

The energy needs of the diabetic patient can be estimated from sex, age, body weight, and general level of physical activity.

The energy needs of children less than 10 years of age are calculated on the basis of moderate activity. However, the energy needs of this group in the affluent societies may be 5% to 10% less than predicted because these children seem to be spending too much time watching television. Individual differences between children are also important and may vary about ± 25% of the average values; a very active child may need 20% to 30% higher energy than the calculated energy (see Chapter 8), which becomes obvious within 48 hours, if the child becomes hungry and hypoglycemic when exercising. Fasting blood glucose measurements will also be low (less than 4.5 mmol/l), or the child may complain of early morning headaches or have ketone bodies in the urine on waking due to hypoglycemia during the night. These features may not develop if the child is on a relatively low-carbohydrate, high-fat diet. Individual adjustments to the prescribed diet are done based on the child's appetite, which is the best guide to the child's energy needs for growth and physical activity.

For adolescents older than 10 years, energy needs are based on first estimating the basal metabolic rate (BMR) from set equations (see Chapter 8). The BMR value in MJ or kcal per day is then multiplied by the physical activity level (PAL) of the individual, as judged from a simple assessment of activity patterns. Adolescents go through their pubertal growth spurt at different ages and at different rates, so it is necessary to take into account their weight and to adjust to the changing body weights as puberty proceeds. Insulin requirements of adolescents increase significantly during their rapid growth phase, after which insulin requirements may decline, especially in teenage girls. Under these circumstances, if the dosage is not appropriately decreased, their insulin-driven appetite may lead to obesity problems. Dietary advice needs to be relevant and should also address issues such as smoking, junk food, sports, and exercise. The actual energy cost of pubertal growth is modest and far overweighed by the cost of sports and general physical activity undertaken, especially for boys.

The BMR of an adult diabetic patient can be estimated from the age, sex, and body weight. A suitable multiplier can then be found corresponding to the patient's estimated PAL. This preliminary guide is likely to be much more accurate than the estimation of energy needs from a simple dietary history or 24-hour recall. If the energy needs are being exceeded, the adults will complain of having to eat too much or they will begin to gain weight, hunger with weight loss becoming clear within 3 to 5 days.

Thus, diabetes is treated by having the person eat three regular meals and one or more snacks (including one at bedtime) of a precise carbohydrate to protein to fat ratio to maximize insulin action and minimize swings in blood glucose levels. A diet high in complex carbohydrates, along with ample dietary fiber, has been emphasized. Replacing the missing insulin either in the form of injections or oral tables, 1 to 6 times a day is very important. An insulin pump that dispenses insulin on a regular basis into the body and higher amounts after each meal has been developed. Supplied insulin requires a continuous source of glucose in the bloodstream on which to act. Physical activity and exercise enhance glucose uptake by muscle and reduce blood sugar. This is beneficial, provided the diabetics are aware of their blood glucose response to exercise and compensate appropriately.

Kuppu et al. (50) reported the hypoglycemic and hypotriglyceridemic effects of *methika churna* (fenugreek powder). Effects of fenugreek powder (a dose of 9 g given for 3 months) was examined on 15 people with diabetes type II. Significant decrease between final and initial blood glucose levels, serum cholesterol, and triglycerides values were observed; indicating that fenugreek (*Trigonellafoenum-graecum*) seed powder effectively controls blood glucose and triglycerides.

4. Carbohydrate Needs

It has been established that the disposal of absorbed carbohydrate is under immediate metabolic control provided insulin is available, whereas dietary fat is absorbed by different mechanisms. Fat is transported from the intestine via the lymph rather than the portal bloodstream and is readily deposited in adipose tissue by a pathway involving the non–insulin-sensitive enzyme lipoprotein lipase. Thus, feeding a high-fat diet to a diabetic patient bypasses the fine control of insulin metabolism and readily leads to fat storage and its side effects on lipoprotein metabolism and cardiovascular diseases. Diabetic patients are therefore currently advised to have 50% to 55% of dietary energy as carbohydrate, the total fat being limited to 30% to 35% of energy. Such a high-carbohydrate diet allows carbohydrate balance to be linked more readily with energy balance and insulin needs (40). The 55% value of carbohydrate energy needs can be readily converted to absolute carbohydrate allowances in grams/day by using a conversion factor, 16 kJ/g or 4 kcal/g, which can also be put in diagrammatically (51).

Because different carbohydrates are absorbed at different speeds, they have different effects on the blood glucose response to a meal. The smaller the response, the more favorable the food is considered for the diabetic patient. This response is expressed as glycemic index, the increase in blood glucose after a 50 g load of the food compared with an increase after consuming 50 g glucose; the response of the test food is expressed as a percentage of the standard glucose value. A few examples of the glycemic response of some foods are given in Table 10. The glucose from starchy foods tends to be absorbed more slowly, but there are marked variations between differ-

Table 10 The Glycemic Response of Different
Foods Expressed as a Glycemic Index[a]

Foods	Glycemic index
Fruit-derived foods	
Apple	39
Bananas	62
Orange juice	46
Pulses	
Lentils	29
Kidney beans	29
Haricot beans	31
Soya bean	15
Cereals	
White bread	69
Wholemeal bread	72
Oatmeal biscuits	54
Ryvita	69
Cornflakes	80
Oats porridge	49
All-Bran	51

[a]Glycemic index is a percentage of the response to an equivalent (50 g) weight of pure glucose in solution.
Source: Ref. 40.

ent starches (Table 10). Cereals have lower glycemic index because their starches are less readily hydrolyzed by the digestive enzymes. The complex starch structure is also influenced by the associated non-starch polysaccharides (NSP). Thus, the pectins, galactomannans, and other hemicelluloses in the soluble NSP fractions found in fruit, vegetables, cereals, and pulses restrict starch hydrolysis as well as producing gels in the intestine, retarding diffusion of glucose to the intestinal wall and the glycemic index further. The soluble NSPs in pulses effectively retard glucose uptake; thus, pulses are a useful source of slowly absorbed glucose. A readily absorbed carbohydrate is appropriate if soluble insulin is being injected before breakfast.

Pure glucose is rapidly absorbed in the fasting state with a clear rise in blood glucose occurring within 5 min; another manosaccharide, galactose, is absorbed quickly, but it has to be transformed into glucose within the liver before glucose levels rise. Fructose is absorbed more slowly and is metabolized via an insulin dependent pathway to acetyl CoA and thus can be utilized as a fuel in many tissues without much increasing blood glucose level, and without requiring insulin for its absorption by the tissues. Thus, fructose-containing diets have become popular in the management of diabetes, because it is possible to meet the energy requirements of patients without rapid fluctuations in blood glucose or an increase in insulin requirements. Use of fructose, however, can increase plasma triglycerides.

Disaccharides are also absorbed as rapidly as glucose, but their glycemic effects depend on the metabolic route of different constituent monosaccharides. Sucrose, providing half of its energy in the form of fructose, will comparatively have a lower glycemic effect. Glucose syrups, manufactured by hydrolyzing starches such as maize starch, are rapidly absorbed into circulating pool of glucose.

5. Eating Patterns and Physical Activity

Type I diabetic patients in the first few months of the disease may have some residual pancreatic function, but as islet damage progresses, they have almost no control over their tissue glucose uptake other than by use of insulin injections. Thus, the current trend in Western societies to eat one large meal a day is quite inappropriate for a diabetic patient. The standard approach of devising three meals plus three snacks a day that has evolved currently appears to reduce the daily fluctuations in blood glucose. A soluble insulin injection in the morning may be followed by a small breakfast 30 min later, containing cereals with low-fat milk and some fruit. Within about 2 hours, the surge in absorbed glucose will slow down but the soluble insulin will enter the bloodstream at a high rate, requiring a mid-morning snack, e.g. whole meal bread sandwiches with a tuna fish filling low in fat. This pattern may be followed by giving two further doses of soluble insulin injections, with two more meals and snacks to match the time of insulin action. Nocturnal hypoglycemia is a well-recognized problem with many insulin regimens and can be resolved with a suitable bed-time snack.

The doses of insulin and the quantity of food need to be adjusted in anticipation of physical activity and exercise. The latter promotes glucose uptake into muscle, even with only modest levels of circulating insulin. Extra carbohydrate may be taken in anticipation of the exercise to avoid a sudden hypoglycemic episode. The energy cost of the exercise may be estimated from published tables, with about 35% of the energy used being derived from carbohydrate (52). The type of carbohydrate supplement can be varied, depending on the type and time of exercise. The dose of insulin used and dietary carbohydrate can also be adjusted in the light of experience with multiple measures of blood glucose taken at intervals throughout the day, which is being seen as part of the normal assessment of the effectiveness of diabetic control.

A diurnal variation in the body's sensitivity to insulin has been recognized. About 2 to 3 hours before waking insulin resistance rises, resulting in blood glucose level around dawn. Certain physiological or pathological processes such as infections may also influence insulin requirements. It is vital that insulin dosage is tailored to individual needs and diabetic patients understand the factors that affect blood glucose control.

A daily regimen of six small meals or three meals and three snacks is appropriate for the insulin-dependent diabetic who has settled into a steady way of life. However, in those people who are liable to obesity, the exposure to food six times daily may be too much of a temptation to control. For the diabetic treated by diet alone, or a combination of diet and oral hypoglycemic agents, large meals must be avoided and four meals daily may be a suitable compromise (40).

The polyunsaturated characteristic of fish oils have probable beneficial effects on plasma lipids in people eating diets rich in fish. The seemingly beneficial traditional Eskimo diet has a high intake of long-chain, highly unsaturated fish fatty acids (*n*-3 fatty acids), in addition to about 50% less saturated fatty acids than the average European diet. Animal studies have indicated that the prothrombotic effects of saturated fatty acids may overweigh the antithrombotic effect of marine polyenes more readily than those of the terrestrial polyunsaturated fatty acids (53,54). The beneficial effects of *n*-3 fatty acids is probably to limit heart arrhythmias. The saturated animal fatty acids seem to promote cardiac arrhythmias after coronary occlusion (55).

6. Use of Very Low Calorie Diets in Diabetes

Very low calorie diets (VLCDs) can have marked metabolic improvement in type II diabetes (NIDDM), but they should not be used by diabetics who are not also very obese. If dieters are being treated with insulin, a marked reduction in the insulin dose would be essential. Sulfonylurea doses also need to be decreased proportionately. VLCDs can help NIDDM patients temporarily by decreasing fasting glucose by one-half, total plasma cholesterol by about 30% to 40% and bringing fasting plasma triglycerides levels to normal (56,57). Beyond 2 months on VLCD, patients usually no longer comply with the diet and the difficulty becomes one of restabilizing the patient on a normal diet that they can control without simply regaining the weight they had lost (58).

Concerned about the use of VLCDs at very low energy levels (e.g., less than 330 kcal/day), the UK Government has imposed a lower limit of 400 kcal/day for women and 500 kcal/day for men on diabetic regimens. The expert group also has indicated that only under clear medical supervision may these diets be prolonged for more than a month (59), especially in patients with diabetes. VLCDs may reduce risk, but without medical care unadjusted drug and insulin therapy can become catastrophic with profound hypoglycemia, hypotension, and dehydration with pre-renal failure. VLCDs do not sustain weight loss for longer periods and a beneficial fall in blood pressure in hypertensive diabetics may be no greater than with a similar weight reduction achieved by other means.

Failure to adhere to the dietary advice is widespread among diabetic patients. According to Turnbridge and Wetherill (60), less than about one-third of patients actually eat within 10% of their prescribed total carbohydrate allowance, and only about two-thirds manage to eat within 30% of the intended consumption. When specific amounts of carbohydrate are prescribed, it is not easy to assess in practice the patient's fat intake, so weight change is unpredictable, especially when a diet is used together with a hypoglycemic drug. Doctors often prescribe diets crudely and then attempt, unsuccessfully, to persuade patients to follow the diets by threatening them with diabetic complications or with the need for insulin injections if the patient does not comply with the diet. The failure of this approach has led to the recognition that a more sensitive behavioral approach is required (61).

The best management of the different forms of diabetics includes a scheme for monitoring blood glucose using a simple system where patients are taught to do their own tests of blood glucose during the day. A finger-prick is used to collect a drop of blood onto special enzyme-impregnated strips of paper that respond by changing color depending on glucose concentration in the collected blood drops. By monitoring diurnal fluctuation in glucose, a patient can adjust the regimen of insulin, even if there is little change in the urinary glucose output, because the renal threshold for glucose reabsorption is too high, varying between 7 and 12 mmol/l. If urinary glucose is present, it usually means that blood glucose levels are at least twice the normal level. Therefore, blood glucose monitoring undertaken at home is the best way of assessing the degree of control during the day.

Prolonged increases in blood glucose lead to the glycosylation of hemoglobin A at the terminal valine residue of the beta chain, producing HbAlc. The latter with two other minor forms of glycosylated hemoglobin, measured together, can provide another longer-term index of overall control of the diabetes.

Despite the optimum system set out as shown in Table 7, which includes the latest British Diabetic Association recommendations (49), it has been recognized that there is more than one diet composition that can be used with benefits, e.g., saturated fatty acids can be replaced by either complex carbohydrate or with poly- or monounsaturated fatty acids in different proportions to suit individual or local eating habits. It should be noted that the advice provided in Table 7 must not be pushed to extremes, e.g., an intake of 15 g/day of soluble fiber will produce about 10% improvement in fasting plasma glucose, glycosylated hemoglobin, and cholesterol, but huge doses up to 100 g/day may achieve little further improvement. Also, high intakes of polyunsaturated fatty acids are not advised, about 8% of the total dietary energy being appropriate. Although about 0.2 g/day of eicosapentaenoic acid from fish benefit the diabetic patients, intakes as high as 4 g/day may aggravate hyperglycemia and serum LDL concentration.

A European group for the WHO and the International Diabetes Federation have recently reassessed the problem of managing diabetes. Five-year targets to reduce diabetic complications have been developed, e.g., to reduce blindness and end-stage diabetic renal failure by a third or more, and to halve the rate of limb amputations for diabetic gangrene. This has presented the diabetic team and dietitians with an immense task, and will need newer and more vigorous approaches to clinical care and preventive work (40).

Shastri et al. (62) assessed the role of acetylation in the antiglycating and anticataract effects of aspirin (ASA) compared with that of sodium salicylate (SS), a nonacetyl analogue of ASA, on cataract development in diabetic rats. Streptozocin diabetic rats were provided with either ASA or SS, orally for 24 weeks. Appropriate drug control, normal control, and diabetic controls were run in parallel. Periodic estimations of blood glucose and glycated hemoglobin and assessments of cataract progession were done. Neither ASA nor SS influenced blood glucose levels. In the untreated diabetic groups, the onset and progression of cataract was quicker and complete within 16 weeks. Both ASA and SS delayed the onset and progression in diabetic rats, but ASA's effect was more pronounced than that of SS. The levels of glycated Hb and lens protein in diabetic rats were significantly reduced by ASA and not by SS for the same serum salicylate levels. ASA's anticataract potential far exceeded that of SS and ASA (not SS) inhibited protein glycation. These results thus favor the hypothesis that acetycation plays a major rote in ASA's anticataract effect via inhibition of glycation.

Noel et al. (63) discussed use of different types of alternative treatments for non–insulin-dependent diabetes mellitus in south Texas. Of 61 different plant medicines used, four most commonly reported were: nopal (*Opuntia streptacantha*) or the prickly pear cactus, chaya (*Cnidoscolus chayamansa*), mispero (*Eriobotrya japonica* or loquat, and savila (*Aloe vera*). Disease severity was not associated with the use of alternative treatments when controlling for other variables. Some of the identified plants had hypoglycemic properties.

According to Thompson (64), antinutrients found in plant foods, such as phytic acid, lectins, phenolic compounds, amylose inhibitors, and saponins, have been shown to reduce the blood glucose and insulin responses to starchy foods and/or plasma cholesterol and triglycerides. Thompson (64) further suggested that because these antinutrients can also be mitigating agents, they need reevaluation and perhaps a change in name in the future.

The observation that the addition of amylase inhibitor from wheat or microbial sources can reduce the blood glucose and raise insulin levels after raw starch intake by rats, dogs, and humans (65), has stimulated interest in the use of such antinutrients for therapeutic purposes in diabetes and for the control of obesity, followed by production of amylase inhibitor preparation (starch blockers) by several companies. Clinical studies, however, have shown that they do not influence the fecal calorie excretion, the postprandial plasma glucose levels, insulin, and starch metabolism. These were attributed mainly to the low purity and hence low anti-amylase activity of the starch blockers. Partial purification of the amylase inhibitors caused significant inhibition of amylase activity both in vitro and in vivo and reduction in postprandial plasma glucose and insulin levels (64). Lower blood glucose responses to antinutrient-containing test meals (e.g., cooked cereals, legumes, or starchy meals with added phytic acid or amylase inhibitors) were observed without causing much gastrointestinal discomfort (66,67). Undoubtedly, the physiological effects of antinutrients are related to their level of intake and the conditions under which they are taken, e.g., presence of other dietary constituents, nutritional and health status of the individual. There is a need to obtain information on the concentration of antinutrients in foods and their level of intake to balance their risks with benefits. Because several antinutrients appear to have the same mitigating effects, e.g. reduce cancer risk or cardiovascular disease, studies to determine the synergistic or antagonistic effects of mixtures of these antinutrients would also be of value. The interaction of antinutrients with other components of the diet and the mechanism of their action also need to be elucidated to understand the role of antinutrients in health and disease.

Rickard and Thompson (68) reported several beneficial health effects of flaxseed mucilage and lignans in humans. The viscous nature of soluble fibers such as flaxseed mucilage probably slows down the digestion and absorption of glucose, insulin, and other endocrine responses (69). Continuous stimulation of insulin by large rises in blood glucose is thought to precipitate insulin resistance, a predisposing factor for diabetes development. Food's ability to modulate glycemic response is tested by using a standard method where the effect of a test carbohydrate (50 g) is compared with 50 g of a standard carbohydrate (glucose or white bread). The addition of 25 g flaxseed mucilage to a 400 ml solution containing 50 g glucose was found to reduce the blood glucose response by 27% (70). Because similar blood glucose responses were also observed with 50 g of bread containing 25% flaxseed by weight (containing about 1.5–2 g mucilage), the mucilage content of flaxseed alone cannot explain the reduction in postprandial glucose response (68).

REFERENCES

1. James, W.P.T., Research on obesity: a report of the DHSS/MRC Group, HMSO, London, 1976.
2. Garrow, J.S., Obesity, *Human Nutrition and Dietetics*, 9th ed. (J.S. Garrow and W.P.T. James, eds.), Churchill Livingstone, Edinburgh, London, 1993, p. 465.
3. Garrow, J.S., Obesity and Related Diseases, Churchill Livingstone, Edinburgh, London, 1988.
4. Rosenbaum, S., R.K. Skinner, I.B. Knight, and J.S. Garrow, A survey of height and weights of adults in Great Britain, *Ann. Human Biol. 12*: 115 (1985).
5. Gregory, J., K. Foster, H. Tyler, and M. Wiseman, The dietary and nutritional survey of British adults, HMSO, London, 1990.
6. Keys, A., A. Menotti, Blackburn, et al., The seven countries study: 2289 deaths in 15 years, *Preventive Med, 13*: 141 (1984).
7. Manson, J.E., G.A. Colditz, M.J. Stamfer, et al., A prospective study of obesity and risk of coronary heart disease in women, *N. Engl. J. Med. 322*: 822 (1990).
8. Hubert, H.B., The nature of the relationship between obesity and cardiovascular disease, *Int. J. Cardiol. 6*: 268 (1984).
9. Borkan, G.A., D. Sparrow, C. Wisniei, and P.S. Vokonas, Body weight and coronary heart disease risk: Patterns of risk factor change associated with long-term weight change, *Am. J. Epidemiol 124*: 410 (1986).
10. Lapidus, L., C. Bengtsson, B. Larsson, K. Pennert, E. Rybo, and L. Sjostrom, Distribution of adipose tissue and risk of cardio-vascular disease and death; a 12 year follow-up of participants in the population study of women in Gothenburg, Sweden, *Br. Med. J. 289*: 1257, (1984).
11. Larsson, B., Regional obesity as a health hazard in men—prospective studies, *Acta Medica Scandinavica 723*(Suppl): 45 (1987).
12. Lew, E.A., and L. Garfinkel, Variations in mortality by weight among 750,000 men and women, *J. Chronic Dis. 32*: 563 (1979).
13. Sims, E.A.H., E. Danforth Jr, E.S. Horton, G.A. Bray, J.A. Glennon, and L.B. Salans, Endocrine and metabolic effects of experimental obesity in men, *Recent Progr. Hormone Res. 29*: 457 (1973).
14. Dore, C., R. Hesp, D. Wilkins, and J.S. Garrow, Prediction of energy requirements of obese patients after massive weight loss, *Human Nutr. Clin. Nutr. 36*C: 41 (1982).
15. Romanella, N.E., D.K. Wakat, B.H. Lloyd, and L.E. Kelly, Physical activity and attitudes in lean and obese children and their mothers, *Int. J. Obesity 15*: 407 (1991).
16. Mellbin, T., and J.C. Vuille, Physical development at 7 years of age in relation to velocity of weight gain in infancy, with special reference to incidence of overweight, *British J. Preventive Social Med. 27*: 225 (1973).

17. Garn, S.M., S.M. Bailey, and P.E. Cole, Continuities and changes in fatness and obesity, *Nutrition, Physiology and Obesity* (R. Schemmedl, ed.), CRC Press, Boca Raton, FL, 1980, p. 51.
18. Garn, S.M., D.C. Clark, and K.E. Guire, Growth, body composition, and development of obese and lean children, *Childhood Obesity* (M. Winik, ed.), John Wiley & Sons, London, 1975.
19. Rissanen, A.M., M. Heliovaara, P. Knekt, A. Reunanen, and A. Aromaa, Determinants of weight gain and overweight in adult Finns, *Europ. J. Clin. Nutr. 45*: 419 (1991).
20. Garrow, J.S., Treatment of obesity, *Lancet 340*: 409 (1992).
21. Garrow, J.S., Very low calorie diets should not be used, *Int. J. Obesity 13*(Suppl. 2): 145 (1989).
22. Garrow, J.S., M.L. Durrant, S. Blaza, D. Wilkins, P. Rayston, and S. Sunkin, The effect of meal frequency and protein concentration on the composition of the weight by obese subjects, *Br. J. Nutr. 45*: 5 (1981).
23. Booth, D.A., H.T. Campbell, and A. Chase, Temporal bounds of post-ingestive glucose-induced satiety in man, *Nature 228*: 1104 (1970).
24. Bush, A., J. Webster, G. Chalmers, et al., The Harrow Slimming Club: Report on 1090 enrolments in 50 courses, 1977–1986, *J. Human Nutr. Diet. 1*: 429 (1988).
25. Geppert, J., and P.L. Splett, Summary document of nutrition intervention in obesity, *J. Am. Diet. Assoc.* (Suppl): 31 (1991).
26. Gilbert, S., and J.S. Garrow, A prospective controlled trial of outpatient treatment for obesity, *Human Nutr. Clin. Nutr. 37*C: 21 (1983).
27. Wannamethee, G., and A.G. Shaper, Weight change in middle-aged British men: implications for health, *Europ. J. Clin. Nutr. 44*: 133 (1990).
28. Lissner, L., P.M. Odell, R.B. D. Agostino, et al, Variability of body weight and health outcomes in the Framingham population, *N. Engl. J. Med. 324*: 1639 (1991).
29. Jebb, S.A., G.R. Goldberg, W.A. Coward, P.R. Murgatroyd, and A.M. Prentice, Effects of weight cycling caused by intermittent dieting on metabolic rate and body composition in obese women, *Int. J. Obesity 15*: 367 (1991).
30. Guy-Grand, B., M. Apfelbaum, G. Orepaldi, A. Gries, P. Lefebvre, and P. Turner, International trial of long-term dexfenfluramine in obesity, *Lancet 2*: 1142 (1989).
31. Darga, L.L., L. Carrol-Michals, S.J. Borsford, and C.P. Lucas, Fluoxetine's effect on weight loss in obese subjects, *Am. J. Clin. Nutr. 54*: 321 (1991).
32. Forbes, G.B., Exercise and lean weight: the influence of body weight, *Nutr. Rev. 50*: 157 (1992).
33. Garrow, J.S., Dental splinting in the treatment of hyperphagic obesity, *Proc. Nutr. Soc. 33*: 29A (1974).
34. Garrow, J.S., and J.D. Webster, Effects on weight and metabolic rate of obese women on a 3.4 MJ (800 kcal) diet, *Lancet 1*: 1429 (1989).
35. Suter, P.M., E. Hasler, B and W. Vetter, Effects of alcohol on energy metabolism and body weight regulation: Is alcohol a risk factor for obesity?, *Nutr Rev 55*: 157 (1997).
36. Akoh, C.C., New developments in low calorie fats and oils substitute, *J. Food Lipids 3*: 223 (1996).
37. Wolever, T.M.S., and D.J.A. Jenkins, Diet and diabetes, *Diet, Nutrition and Health* (K.K. Carrol, ed), McGill Queens Univ. Press, London, 1989, p. 103.
38. Anonymous, Diet and exercise in noninsulin dependent diabetes mellitus, National Institutes of Health Consensus Development Conference Statement, *Diabetes Care 10*: 639 (1987).
39. Olefsky, J.M., and O.G. Kolterman, Mechanisms of insulin resistance in obesity and non insulin-dependent (Type II) diabetes, *Am. J. Med. 70*: 151 (1981).
40. James, W.P.T., and D.W.M. Pearson, Diabetes, *Human Nutrition and Dietetics*, 9th ed. (J.S. Garrow and W.P.T. James, eds.), Churchill Livingstone, Edinburgh, London, 1993, p. 521.
41. Helmrich, S.P., D.R. Ragland, R.W. Leung, and R.S. Paffenbarger, Physical activity and reduced occurrence of non-insulin-dependant diabetes mellitus, *N. England J. Med. 325*: 147 (1991).
42. Mirakou, A.D. Kelley, M. Mokan, et al., Role of reduced suppression of glucose production and diminished early insulin release in impaired glucose intolerance, *N. Engl. J. Med. 326*: 22 (1992).
43. Hales, C.N., D.J.P. Barker, P.M.S. Clark, et al., Fetal and infant growth and impaired glucose tolerance at age 64, *Br. Med. J. 303*: 1019 (1991).
44. Hattersley, A.J., R.C. Turner, M.A. Permutt, et al. Linkage of Type 2 diabetes to glucokinase gene, *Lancet 339*: 1307 (1992).

45. Koda, J.E., M. Fineman, T.J. Rink, G.E. Dailey, D.B. Muchmore, and L.G. Linarell, Amylin concentrations and glucose control, *Lancet 339*: 1179 (1992).

46. Kleinman, J.C., R.P. Donahue, M.I. Harris, F.F. Finucane, J.H. Madans, and D.B. Brock, Mortality among diabetics in national sample, *Am. J. Epidemiol. 128*: 389 (1988).

47. Randle, P.J., Fuel selection in animals, *Biochem. Soc. Trans 14*: 799 (1986).

48. Blaak, E.E., and W.H.M. Saris, Health aspects of various digestible carbohydrates, *Nutr. Res. 15*: 1547 (1995).

49. Lean, M.E., J.S. Brenchley, H. Conner, et al., Dietary recommendations for people with diabetes: an update for the 1990s, *J. Human Nutr. Diet. 4*: 393 (1991).

50. Kuppu, R.K., A. Srivastava, C.V. Krishnaswami, G. Vijaykumar, M. Chellamariappan, P.V. Ashabai, and O. BuchiBabu, Hypoglycemic and hypotriglyceridemic effects of methika churna (fenugreek), *Antiseptic 95*: 78 (1998).

51. Lean, M.E.J., and W.P.T. James, Diabetes: Prescription of diabetic diets in the 1980s, *Lancet 1*: 723 (1986).

52. Ahlboorg, G., P. Felig, L. Hagenfeldt, R. Hendler, and J. Wahren, Substrate turnover during prolonged exercise in man, *J. Clin. Invest. 53*: 1080 (1974).

53. Bang, H.O., J. Dyerberg, and H.M. Sinclair, The composition of the Eskimo food in North Western Greenland, *Am. J. Clin. Nutr. 33*: 2657 (1980).

54. Hornstra, G., Fish and the heart, *Lancet 2*: 1450 (1989).

55. Leaf, A., and P.C. Weber, Cardiovascular effects of n-3 fatty acids, *N. Engl. J. Med. 318*: 549 (1988).

56. Henefield, M., and M. Week, Very low calorie diet therapy in obese non-insulin dependent diabetes patients, *Int. J. Obesity 13* (Suppl. 2): 23 (1989).

57. Henry, R.R., O. Wallace, and J.M. Olefsky, Effects of weight loss on mechanism of hyperglycaemia in obese non-insulin dependent diabetes mellitus, *Diabetes 35*: 990 (1986).

58. James, W.P.T., Treatment of obesity: the constraints on success, *Clinics Endocrinol. Metab. 13*: 635 (1984).

59. Anonymous, Committee on Medical Aspects of Food Policy. The use of very-low-calorie diets in obesity, Department of Health, H.M.S.O., London, 1987.

60. Turnbridge, R., and J.H. Wetherill, Reliability and cost of diabetics diets, *Br. Med. J. 2*: 78 (1970).

61. Wing, R.R., and R.W. Jeffery, Outpatient treatments of obesity: a comparison of methodology and clinical results, *Int. J. Obesity 3*: 261 (1979).

62. Shastri, G.V., M. Thomas, A.J. Victoria, R. Selvakumar, A.S. Kanagasabapathy, K. Thomas and Lakshmi, Effect of aspirin and sodium salicylate on cataract development in diabetic rats, *Indian J. Exp. Biol. 36*: 651 (1998).

63. Noel, P.H., J.A. Pugh, A.C. Larme, and G. Marsh, The use of traditional plant medicines for non-insulin dependent diabetes mellitus in south Texas, *Phytotherapy Res. 11*: 512 (1997).

64. Thompson, L.U., Potential health benefits and problems associated with antinutrients in foods, *Food Res. Intl. 26*: 131 (1993).

65. Pulps, W., and U. Keup, Influence of an alpha-amylase inhibitor (Bay-d 7791) on blood glucose, serum insulin and NEFA in starch loading tests in rats, dogs and man, *Diabetologia 9*: 97 (1973).

66. Thompson, L.U., Antinutrients and blood glucose, *Food Technol. 42*: 123 (1988).

67. Boivin, M., B. Flourie, R.A. Rizza, V.L. Go, and E.P. DiMagno, Gastrointestinal and metabolic effects of amylase inhibition in diabetes, *Gastroenterology 94*: 387 (1988).

68. Rickard, S.E., and L.U. Thompson, Health effects of flaxseed mucilage, lignans, *INFORM 8(8)*: 860 (1997).

69. Jenkins, D.J.A., A.L. Jenkins, T.M.S. Wolever, V. Vuksan, A.V. Rao, L.U. Thompson, and R.G. Josse, Effect of reduced rate of carbohydrate absorption on carbohydrate and lipid metabolism, *Eur. J. Clin. Nutr. 49. (Suppl.)*: 68 (1995).

70. Cunnane, S.C., S. Ganguli, C. Menard, A.C. Liede, M.J. Hamaden, Z.Y. Chen, J.M. Wolever, and D.J. Jenkins, High alpha-linolenic and flaxseed (*Linum usitatissimum*): some nutritional properties in humans, *British J. Nutr. 69*: 443 (1993).

27
Diet and Health of Bones, Teeth, Skin, and Hair

I. INTRODUCTION

Calcium and phosphorus are closely related in the human body; both are found mostly in the bones and teeth in the form of hydroxyapatite $(Ca_{10}(PO_4)_6(OH)_2)$. Hydroxyapatite is arranged in a crystal structure around softer protein material in the bones, providing strength and rigidity. Skin, the largest single organ system in the body, provides an interface between the individual and the surroundings. The bones and teeth constitute the body's skeleton, but the ability to survive in a climatically hostile world relies on the integrity and normal functioning of skin and hair. The skin is divided into two interdependent but distinct layers; the outer epidermis (0.04–1.5 mm thick) provides a flexible waterproof barrier between internal and external environments and is pigmented to provide damage from ultraviolet radiation. Epidermis gives rise to the skin appendages such as hair, nails, sebaceous glands, and eccrine and apocrine sweat glands. Beneath the epidermis is the inner dermis (1.5–4 mm thick); both layers rely heavily for their integrity and normal function on adequate and balanced nutrition. Dietary imbalance, whether in the form of overall deficiency, specific shortage of vitamins such as vitamin A and D, excess of one component, or even food contamination can disturb the equilibrium of bones, teeth, skin, and hair. Extensive skin disease can stress the body and cause or reveal relative nutritional deficiencies (1).

Maiti and Singh (2) have recently reviewed bone morphogenetic proteins (BMPs), which have novel regulatory functions in bone formation. These are hydrophobic, non–species-specific glycoproteins and belong to the expanding transforming growth factor–beta (TGF-beta) superfamily. BMP has pleiotropic function, ranging from extraskeletal and skeletal organogenesis to bone generation and regeneration. It induces de novo bone formation in postfetal life through the process of direct (intramembranous) and endochondral ossification. BMP has been made available through recombinant gene technology in at least 10 forms for basic research and clinical trials.

Reid and New (3) reviewed the influence of nutrition on bone mass, examined initially the effects of bone mass with aging, defined the principal disease of bone mass (i.e. osteoporosis), considered the genetic and environmental factors influencing bone mass and summarized the methods of bone health assessment. The review also focused on the nutritional factors (from both dietary sources and in the form of supplementation) that may influence bone mass and fracture rates. These authors finally discussed examination of how our knowledge of nutrition factors can be used to target lifestyle changes in individuals at risk for future osteoporosis. According to Reid and New (3), bone is composed of an organic matrix of type I collagen associated with noncollagenous proteins and a large mineral component consisting of calcium hydroxyapatite. To date, measurement of bone mass takes into account only the mineral component of bone, while recognizing that the organic matrix is important in providing both structure and strength.

A large number of macro- and micronutrients, including mainly calcium, protein, fiber, potassium, and certain trace elements, influence bone health significantly. Calcium intake (and indeed Ca supplementation) is beneficial during peak bone mass development and has some effect at slowing bone loss in late postmenopausal women (particularly if Ca intakes are low). Growing evidence indicates that calcium may even help to prevent hip fracture. High protein intakes affect calcium balance and possibly acid-base status. However, long-term influences of high protein intakes are yet to be related to their possible detrimental effects on bone health. Increased fiber intake has been associated with decrease in Ca absorption. A decrease in the Ca absorption of about 20% to 30% was noted when fiber intake was raised from 0.1 to 30 g bran/day (4). The long-term lowering effects of high-fiber diets on circulating estradiol levels and bone health remain to be established. However, high Ca absorption from whole-wheat bread has been reported, similar to that measured for milk containing a comparable Ca load. High fiber intakes from a mixed diet do not appear to be detrimental to bone health. New et al. (5) noted the positive relationship between spine bone mass density (BMD) and fiber intake.

Growing evidence indicates beneficial effects of potassium ($KHCO_3$) on mineral balance and skeletal metabolism (3). A positive association has been reported between dietary intake of K and bone mass (5). Zinc, copper, and manganese are essential metallic cofactors for enzymes in the synthesis of various bone matrix constituents, but their role in bone health is not clear. Angus et al. (6), however, reported positive association between dietary intake of Zn and bone mass, and Strause et al. (7) have shown that bone loss in Ca-supplemented older postmenopausal women could be further arrested by concomitant increases in trace mineral intake. These trace elements (and vitamin C) may also function in an antioxidant capacity. A positive relationship between Mg intake and bone density also has been noted. Thus, prevention of osteoporosis might be possible by increasing dietary Ca, vitamin D, and possibly K, Mn, and vitamin K.

II. DIET, NUTRITION, AND BONE DISEASES

Both nutritional deficiency and excess may cause various bone diseases (Table 1). The peak bone mass and subsequent bone loss due to calcium intake seem to relate most of these bone diseases (8). However, the bone disorders most clearly related to nutrition are rickets in children and osteomalacia in adults, both caused by a deficiency or disturbance in vitamin D metabolism. Also, lack of copper, especially in small babies or in those on parenteral nutrition, can give rise to bone dis-

Table 1   Clinical Nutrition and Bone Diseases

Nutritional deficiency	Vitamin D	Rickets/Osteomalacia
	Vitamin C	Scurvy
	Copper	Fractures (premature infants, parenteral nutrition)
	Pyridoxine	Homocystinuria
Nutritional excess	Vitamin A	Hyperostosis, ligamentous ossification
	Vitamin D	Idiopathic hypercalcemia in infancy
	Aluminum	Aluminum osteodystrophy (dialysis and parenteral nutrition)
	Fluoride	Endemic, iatrogenic
	Cadmium	Fanconi syndrome, rickets/osteomalacia
Nutrition-related disorders	Calcium	Osteoporosis

Source: Ref. 9.

ease, which is attributed to the defective functioning of the copper-dependent amino acid oxidases, leading to failure of the collagen cross-linking.

Although bone diseases due to nutritional excess are rather uncommon, they can occur in the idiopathic hypercalcemia of infancy, in which hypervitaminosis A and D are implicated, causing generalized cortical hyperostosis in children. Occasionally, treatment of skin disease such as ichthyosis with vitamin A analogues can cause widespread ligamentous calcification. Excessive ingestion of fluoride, either in the diet (endemic fluorosis) or as a treatment for osteoporosis, may produce marked hyperostosis of bones and ligaments. Increased use of hemodialysis in chronic renal failure may lead to the accumulation of aluminum derived from tapwater in dialysis fluid, producing bone diseases collectively known as aluminum osteodystrophy. Prolonged parenteral nutrition in patients may similarly lead to a vitamin D–resistant bone disease due to aluminum excess. An excess of cadmium can also produce bone disease by causing multiple renal tubular abnormalities and generalized aminoaciduria (Fanconi syndrome) leading to rickets or osteomalacia (9–13).

A. Osteomalacia and Rickets

Smith (8) stated the following causes of rickets in childhood and osteomalacia in adults, attributable to a deficiency of vitamin D or disturbance in its metabolism:

1. Vitamin D deficiency
   Asian immigrants
   Elderly
2. Malabsorption
   Celiac disease
   Post-gastrectomy
   Intestinal bypass surgery
3. Renal disease
   Tubular: inherited hypophosphatemia
   Fanconi syndrome
   Glomerular: osteodystrophy
   Dialysis bone disease (aluminum excess)
4. Rare
   Vitamin D–dependent rickets
   Oncogenous rickets

Reichel et al. (14) have extensively reviewed the physiology of vitamin D. Nutritional rickets became common first in Asian immigrants, reflecting the rickets endemic in urban populations (15). After nutritional vitamin D deficiency, celiac disease is the next most frequent cause of rickets or osteomalacia. Inherited hypophosphatemia (vitamin D–resistant rickets) is also a significant cause of bone disease, one that provides a difficult clinical problem.

The causes of rickets are best understood, however, against the background of the current knowledge of vitamin D metabolism (Fig. 1). The significance of ultraviolet light in the vitamin D economy, and the widespread effect of this vitamin/hormone throughout the body have been reemphasized (16,17).

The clinical features of rickets and osteomalacia include bone deformity, bone pain, and tenderness and proximal muscle weakness (18). The biochemical changes associated with these symptoms are low plasma calcium, a reduction in plasma phosphate, an increase in the activity of the plasma alkaline phosphates, and a reduction in urine calcium excretion. The biochemistry of rickets and osteomalacia depends on its cause, as shown in Table 2; one or other of these bio-

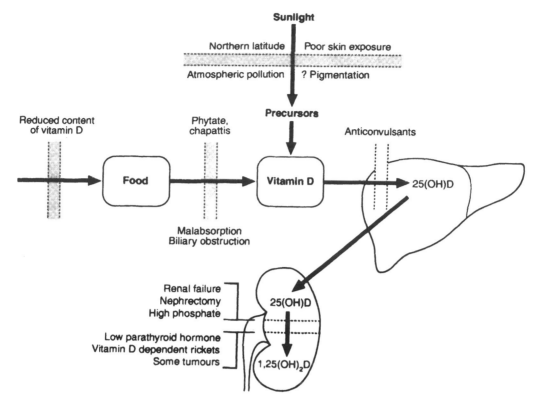

Figure 1   The known main causes of osteomalacia and rickets in relation to the sources and metabolic pathways of vitamin D. The shaded bars indicate factors that reduce the amount of vitamin D in the body (rectangle) or its subsequent conversion to 1, 25 (OH)$_2$D. (From Ref. 9.)

chemical changes may be used to diagnose osteomalacia, in addition to the measurement of 25(OH)D levels in the plasma to detect vitamin D deficiency. Patients with nutritional osteomalacia will have very low levels of 25(OH)D, although all patients with subnormal 25(OH)D may not develop bone disease. The presence of osteomalacia can be confirmed by transiliac bone biopsy (8).

"Nutritional rickets" occur especially in Asian immigrants in northern urban areas, and in elderly housebound people; the incidence is related to reduced exposure to ultraviolet light. Henderson et al. (15) showed that dietary factors become increasingly important, where ultraviolet light is limited. Among the Asian population, the contribution of a vegetarian diet rich in cereals (*chapattis*) to these disorders has been stressed. The possible relationship between dietary calcium deficiency and osteomalacia or rickets has not been resolved completely. It has been suggested that lack of dietary calcium and resultant hypocalcemia increase the circulating concentrations of 1,25(OH)$_2$D$_3$ and the breakdown of 25(OH)D$_3$ (19). A striking reduction in Asian rickets occurred when vitamin D supplements were made available to children up to 18 years of age (20). The frequency and importance of vitamin D deficiency is less well recognized in whites.

The malabsorptive causes of osteomalacia vary with surgical practice, celiac disease being the most common cause. The skeleton may be affected by Crohn's disease and ulcerative colitis, but these diseases produce osteoporosis rather than osteomalacia. These patients may also be taking corticosteroids.

Table 2 Biochemical Changes in Osteomalacia and Rickets

Cause	Plasma	Urine	Comments
Nutritional (vitamin D deficiency)	Ca, N or ↓ P ↓ P'ase ↑	Ca ↓	25-OHD ↓ 1, 25-(OH)$_2$D usually N (also biochemistry of underlying diseases)
Malabsorption	Ca N or ↓, P ↓, P'ase↑	Ca ↓	As for nutritional
Renal tubular	Ca N or ↓, P ↓ P'ase↑	Ca ↓ or N	Those with Fanconi syndrome have systemic acidosis
Glomerular	Ca ↓, P↑, P'ase↑	Ca ↓	Biochemistry of renal failure, 1, 25 (OH)$_2$D reduced.
Vitamin D deficiency			
Type I	Ca ↓, P↓, P'ase↑	Ca ↓	1,25(OH)$_2$D low
Type II	Ca ↓, P ↓, P'ase↑	Ca ↓	1,25(OH)$_2$D high
Oncogneous rickets/osteomalacia	Ca N, P ↓, P'se↑	Ca ↓ or N	1,25(OH)$_2$D low

↓ = decrease, ↑ = increase, N = Normal, P'ase = plasma alkaline phosphatase
Source: Ref. 9.

Many causes of osteomalacia are associated with renal disease, some of which are influenced by nutritional factors (tubular and glomerular causes). The major renal tubular cause of rickets is inherited hypophosphatemia, transmitted as an X-linked dominant character, with a persistent low plasma phosphate (13). There is probably an inborn abnormality in the exchange of phosphate between intra- and extracellular compartments. Renal glomerular osteodystrophy, with defective intestinal absorption of calcium due to a reduction in the production of 1,25(OH)$_2$D$_3$, is associated with an increase in bone resorption due to an excess of parathyroid hormone. Parathyroid hormone secretion is stimulated by hypocalcemia, caused by a progressive increase in plasma phosphate as renal inefficiency progresses. Defective mineralization and enhanced bone resorption both combine to produce catastrophic bone disease, especially in children. The accompanied changes in the bones of these patients include osteomalacia, osteoporosis, osteosclerosis, and osteitis fibrosa cystica (21).

Other rare forms of rickets include vitamin D–dependent rickets and rickets associated with mesenchymal non-malignant tumors that are not nutritional in origin.

In the absence of vitamin C, which is essential for the proper synthesis of collagen, the proline residues in collagen are insufficiently hydroxylated, the collagen not being formed into fibers. An infant with scurvy and periosteal hemorrhage has swollen and tender legs, with a widespread subperiosteal hemorrhage in the long bones, and cupped and fractured metaphyseal plates (18). In adults, vitamin C deficiency does not seem to affect the skeleton.

Copper is vital for the functioning of amino acid oxidases—e.g., lysyl oxidase is essential for the synthesis of the lysine aldehydes, which are intermediates in the cross-linking of collagen fibers. Copper-related bone disease may also occur in an X-linked recessive disorder of copper metabolism, Menkes' syndrome. Copper-deficiency bone disease can occur in premature infants and in those who have been on prolonged parenteral nutrition but is not reported in full-term or breast-fed infants (22). The syndrome in infants includes psychomotor retardation, hypopigmentation, sideroblastic anemia, and bone changes such as osteoporosis, subperiosteal bleeding, and fractures. The plasma copper concentration is normally less than 40 mcg/dl and ceruloplasmin level less than 13 mg/dl. The predisposing factors for copper deficiency syndrome include low birthweight and a dietary lack of copper, either in parenteral solutions or in copper-deficient (cow's) milk.

Skeletal abnormalities in which the bones become osteoporotic, the vertebrae are abnormal in shape, and the femoral heads turn too large can result from a disorder related to vitamin B_6 (pyridoxine). Pyridoxine is essential for the functioning of cystathione synthase. An inherited homocystinuria is a vitamin B_6–dependent disease (23).

Hypophosphatemia and whole-body phosphate deficiency may result from persistent treatment with phosphate-binding antacids such as aluminum hydroxide, leading to acquired hypophosphatemic osteomalacia. Bone disease and proximal myopathy are associated with elevated plasma levels of $1,25(OH)_2D_3$, secondary to low phosphate (8).

B. Bone Diseases Related to Nutritional Excess

A number of conditions associated with excessive intake of nutrients have been known to produce specific skeleton disorders (Table 1).

1. Hypervitaminosis A

Excess intake of retinoic acid can cause cortical hyperostosis (especially in children) and ectopic ossification of ligaments in adults. Prolonged overdosage with vitamin A in children increases cortical density, particularly of the long bones, and the bones become abnormally fragile and prone to fracture readily. The prolonged use of retinoic acid derivatives for skin diseases such as psoriasis and ichthyosis can lead to calcification of the ligaments, especially around the spine, with stiffness and reduced motility.

2. Hypervitaminosis D

Acute intoxication of vitamin D in the form of native vitamin D, $1,25(OH)_2D_3$ or 1-alpha-hydroxy vitamin D used therapeutically (24), have not been reported to produce skeletal abnormalities. Idiopathic hypercalcemia of infancy was thought to be related to excessive intake of vitamin D in early life. In the severe state of this disease, there is a characteristic appearance (elfin face syndrome), mental retardation, and occasional congenital heart disease (Williams' syndrome). The concentration of 25(OH)D may increase when the patients become hypercalcemiac (25), and radiographs of long bones show increased metaphysical density.

3. Excess of Aluminum, Fluoride, and Cadmium

Aluminum may accumulate in the skeleton under certain conditions, producing aluminum-osteodystrophy (26,27). This was first observed in patients on prolonged hemodialysis. The aluminum was found to accumulate from the dialysis fluid. Aluminum toxicity results in the excessive deposition of osteoid, with the histological appearance of osteomalacia. In the second type, bones appear to turn plastic, with little increase in osteoid but decreased osteoblastic activity (28). The higher aluminum accumulation probably produces a profound suppression of mineralization. In both these types of bone disease, aluminum appears to have a direct cellular effect on osteoblastic activity and bone formation.

High fluoride intake in the form of endemic fluorosis may result in progressive hyperostosis and ligamentous calcification, leading to reduced mobility and spinal cord and root compression. Fluoride given therapeutically for osteoporosis may increase vertebral trabecular bone density considerably. Administration of sodium fluoride is also associated with gastrointestinal disorders and with pain around the ends of long bones (8).

Cadmium excess, caused by industrial pollution, may result in osteomalacia and rickets. Cadmium is known to damage the renal tubules, producing Fanconi syndrome, leading to osteomalacia or rickets.

C. Osteoporosis

Osteoporosis is possibly related to dietary calcium, although this subject remains controversial. Osteoporosis is best thought of as a nutrition-related bone disease, leaving open the question of calcium. Thus, peak bone mass may be determined by other nutritional factors, particularly protein and energy during growth. Although in the past the importance of calcium intake has been emphasized for bone health, especially in elderly people, Kanis and Passmore (29) have forwarded evidence to suggest that calcium supplementation is neither necessary nor justified in otherwise healthy people.

Vitamin D deficiency in humans produces osteomalacia, and not osteoporosis, and only in experimental animals has it been shown that calcium deficiency causes osteoporosis. The possibility that in man malabsorption of calcium produces sufficient parathyroid overactivity to cause osteoporotic bone disease has not been established. A converse proposal that malabsorption of calcium is secondary to osteoporosis is an attractive alternative with many proponents. In this case, the rate of bone loss in osteoporosis would be independent of the calcium intake (8). There is no convincing evidence to relate calcium intake to bone mass, and any effect of supplemental dietary calcium in preventing bone loss is temporary and occurs only in the elderly (29).

There are several causes of osteoporosis (9,10,30), as classified in Table 3. Unlike in osteomalacia, in osteoporosis the amount of bone per unit volume decreases but without any change in its composition. There is no defect in mineralization and no excess of osteoid.

According to Smith (8), important in the definition of osteoporosis is that the amount of bone is sufficient to predispose to fracture, although more precisely osteoporosis can be defined as a condition in which the bone mineral density is more than 2 SD below the mean for young adults. Strictly, osteoporosis excludes those bone disorders associated with metastatic deposits and parathyroid bone disease (ostcitis fibrosa cystica), where the composition is abnormal.

Compared with men, women have a lower peak bone mass and a more rapid loss of bone related to the postmenopausal decline in estrogens, the most common cause of osteoporosis in females. Other risk factors that are common for both sexes include a strong family history of osteoporosis. Short stature and small bones, white or Asian race, inactivity, cigarette smoking, leanness, excessive alcohol consumption, possibly a low calcium intake, and early menopause in women. Most of these factors are related to each other.

Because bone loss in itself is symptomless, the symptoms and signs of osteoporosis are those associated with fractures; the main features include pain, deformity, and fracture, the latter mostly affecting the forearm, vertebrae, and femoral neck. Vertebral fractures are the most frequent and manifest early in osteoporosis, producing kyphosis and pain in the back with a loss of height. There is a significant reduction in bone mass density.

Among the rarer causes of osteoporosis (Table 3), at least three—viz., celiac disease, anorexia nervosa, and obsessional exercise—clearly relate to nutrition. Celiac disease, which is of common occurrence, may cause osteomalacia (or rickets), osteoporosis, or a combination of both. Recurrent iron-deficiency anemia, delayed puberty, and bone disease are predisposing factors for osteoporosis. Hormonal and physiological changes during growth and pregnancy may also relate to osteoporosis, although their etiology needs to be investigated. It has been suggested that osteoporosis may be related to deficiency of the calciotrophic hormones normally responsible for protecting the skeleton.

Table 3   Osteoporosis Classified According to Frequency
and Cause

Common	Old age
	Menopause
	Immobility
Less common	Endocrine
	Corticosteroid excess
	Hypogonadism
	Thyrotoxicosis
	Celiac disease (with osteomalacia)
Rare	Mastocytosis
	Anorexia nervosa
Topical	Space travel
	Obsessional exercise
Inherited	Osteogenesis imperfecta
	(brittle bone syndrome)
Chromosomal	Turner's syndrome
Idiopathic	Juvenile
	Pregnancy
	Young adult

Source: Ref. 9.

Controversies exist concerning the management of osteoporosis, the most common metabolic bone disease. There is divergent opinion on the role of calcium in its prevention and treatment. For pre- and postmenopausal women, hormone replacement therepay (HRT) with combined estrogen (and progesterone) is being increasingly prescribed because it has been shown that estrogen prevents subsequent bone loss in these women. HRT also appears to decrease overall mortality, although it may be associated with a slightly increased risk of breast cancer (31). However, barring certain circumstances, it is still not possible to identify and prediagnose women who will develop osteoporosis and structural failure with fracture.

Thus, in addition to nutrition, there are several factors that influence the growth, composition, and amount of skeleton and its subsequent decline. The nutritional component is clear only in some instances, especially those associated with specific vitamin deficiency and excess. In other bone diseases, such as osteoporosis, the changes in the skeleton depend as much on genetic, mechanical, and endocrine factors as they do on nutrition.

Recent investigations and clinical studies suggest that dietary lipids and antioxidant nutrients influence bone formation and cartilage biology. According to Seifert and Watkins (32), in animals, bone modeling appears to be optimal when *n*-3 fatty acids are supplied in the diet to moderate the metabolic and physiologic effects of *n*-6 fatty acids. In osteoporosis, greater osteoblastic activity results in excessive mineral loss and bone destruction. New evidence supports the idea that dietary fatty acids and antioxidants can attenuate osteoblastic activity to reduce the severity of osteolytic diseases of the bone and joint. Moreover, *n*-6 fatty acids may aggravate the deficiency of antioxidant enzyme protective systems in epiphyseal cartilage of long bones. For example, vitamin E was reported to increase in vivo trabecular bone formation rate and to restore collagen synthesis in chondrocytes enriched with ileinoleic acid. Seifert and Watking (32) have reviewed and presented new information that documents a role for dietary lipids and antioxidants in supporting bone formation and cartilage function for optimal health. It has been envisaged that decreasing bone resorption and stimulating bone formation with dietary *n*-3 fatty acids may afford a means to maximize bone mineral accretion in the young and minimize bone mineral loss in the elderly. Further research on dietary lipids and antioxidant compounds in bone biology may complement the current therapies for degenerative bone diseases.

Hodsman (33) concluded that the osteoporotic syndrome is so common in the aging population that it should not be regarded as a disease. Whether it is simply a phenomenon of senescence, or whether there is a district subgroup of female patients who lose bone mass faster than their peers, remains to be established. However, evidence clearly indicates that the factors leading to osteoporosis are multiple, and there is no convincing evidence that nutritional factors play a predominate role in the development of this syndrome. Given that the endocrine mechanisms leading to accelerated bone loss (apart from the occurrence of estrogen "lack" during menopause) are so controversial that the role of calcium deficiency in leading to osteoporosis and calcium supplementation should be viewed as an open question (33).

III.   DIET AND DENTAL HEALTH

Rugg-Gunn (34) has described the etiology of dental diseases and the dietary factors that can improve the health of teeth. Dietary sugars play an important role in dental caries, although conflicting evaluations and the desire of the sugar industry to maintain sugar intakes seem to mislead the common public and nutritionists and dietitians alike.

Teeth consist of three mineralized tissues, enamel, dentine, and cementum; the bulk of a tooth consists of dentine, which is mesodermal in origin. The dentine forms the root of the tooth and is covered by a thin layer of bone-like material called cementum; the outermost layer of the tooth crown consists of enamel—a hard substance of ectodermal origin. In older people, some of the root cementum may become exposed as the tooth's supporting tissues, consisting of the alveolar bone of the maxilla or madible, covered by epithelium, recede. Enamel has no cells, nerves, or blood vessels and is insensitive, but dentine is very sensitive to many stimuli. The nerves and blood vessels supplying nutrition to the dentine come from the pulp, forming the center of a tooth.

Dental caries (decay) and periodontal (gum) disease are the most common diseases of teeth (34). Dental caries begin on the tooth surface, usually in the enamel or in the cementum, and dentine of tooth roots in older people, progressively destroying the hard tissues of the teeth. The tooth becomes sensitive to cold drinks or foods when the dentine is involved, and when the caries reaches the pulp, the resulting pulpits may become painful. Infection then can spread into the alveolar bone, leading to an alveolar abscess.

Unlike dental caries, periodontal disease is more insidious and less painful. This disease is characterized by slow destruction of the periodontal ligament and adjacent bone, so that the tooth becomes loosened and may eventually fall out. Periodontal disease is characterized by inflammation of the gingivae, which lose their pink color and firm stippled appearance, become swollen and red, and tend to bleed (gingivitis). The latter can either be reversed (in favorable conditions) to a healthy state or progress to periodontal disease.

According to Rugg-Gunn (34), an essential factor in the etiology of dental caries and gingivitis is dental plaque, which is a white, slightly glutinous layer that builds up on the teeth surfaces if not cleaned. About 70% of the dental plaque consists of microorganisms; the rest is occupied by water, polysaccharides (mainly polyglucans), and, occasionally, shed epithelial cells. Dental plaque is often found in areas around the teeth that are least easily cleaned, especially in the pits and fissures of the occlusal surfaces, between the adjacent teeth. Irritants from the dental plaque permeate through the thin non-keratinized epithelium adjacent to the tooth surface, causing gingivitis.

The etiology of dental caries begins with the diffusion of dietary sugars into dental plaque, where they are metabolized by plaque microorganisms into organic acids, predominately lactic acid, with some acetic, formic, and propionic acids. The acids' production lowers the pH of dental plaque from a normal value of about 6.8 to as low as 4.5. The plaque acids tend to dissolve the mineral phase of the dental enamel, consisting of crystals of hydroxyapatite, and the process of dental caries begins. Around 5.5 is thought to be the critical pH below which the enamel hydroxyapatite will dissolve, and when the pH is above this value, remineralization or healing of the carious lesion takes place. A carious cavity in the tooth occurs when plaque pH is constantly low, i.e. when demineralization is greater than remineralization. After the surface of dental enamel is dissolved, dissolution occurs fastest just below the tooth surface, giving the appearance of a chalky white spot (precavitation carious lesion). This white spot eventually loses so much mineral that it breaks down to form a carious cavity. After this stage, remineralization will not occur and it is usual to fill or restore the tooth. However, cavities can be arrested if the local conditions improve. After seeing precavitation lesions, there is a chance to remineralize them by removing the overlying plaque and decreasing the amount and frequency of sugar ingestion. Use of fluorides through toothpastes, mouth rinses, or water may aid remineralization of teeth in children.

Factors other than dietary sugars and the presence of dental plaque may influence the occurrence of dental caries, e.g. the quantity and quality of saliva. Certain foods stimulate the salivary flow better than others. Saliva has buffering power (resists changes in pH) and contains calcium and phosphate required for remineralization. Diet appears to be more important in the cause and prevention of dental caries than in periodontal disease.

A. Diet and Dental Caries

Diet can influence teeth while they are forming, even before their eruption in the mouth as well as after the eruption, by a local direct effect. The post-eruptive effects of diet are considered to be more important in the health of teeth (34–36). The overwhelming evidence relating diet to dental caries shows that sugars are the most cariogenic (caries-inducing) foods in the diet. Experimental evidence relating diet and dental caries has been gathered from human observational studies (epidemiology), human interventional studies (clinical trials), animal experiments, enamel slab experiments, plaque pH studies, and in vitro laboratory experiments.

Epidemiological studies have shown a close relationship between sugar intake and dental caries on an intercountry basis. Sreebny (37), reporting data for 47 countries, found that the coefficient of correlation between sugar supply and caries experience in 12-year-olds was 0.7, and on a linear regression, for each rise in sugar supply of 20 g/person/day, caries increased by 1 DMFT (the number of decayed, missing, or filled teeth per person). For the 21 nations with a sugar supply of less than 50 g/person/day, caries development was consistently below 3 DMFT. In many developing countries, caries development is increasing in parallel with sugar consumption. Caries in Eskimos were very infrequent before the introduction of a high-sugar diet (38), but dental caries subsequently increased rapidly (39). The World Health Organization has collected data from many countries, including 20 developing countries, where surveys on the dental health of 12-year-olds were conducted. Of these 20 countries, 15 had shown marked increases in dental caries where per capita sugar consumption also had increased (40). In the island of Tristan da Cunha in the south Atlantic, sugar consumption rose between 1938 and 1966 from 2 to 150 g/person/day, and the percentage of dental caries rose, over the same period of time, from 4% to 42% in young children, from 1% to 33% in adolescents, and from 9% to 38% in adults (41).

Harris (42) reported the example of Hopewood House in Australia, where children received a lactovegetarian diet with virtually no sugar or white flour. Annual dental examinations and dietary surveys from 1947 to 1962 showed that 46% of 12-year-olds were free of caries, compared with only 1% in similarly aged schoolchildren living nearby. Newbrun (43) observed a very low caries rate in patients with hereditary fructose intolerance who avoid eating fructose or sucrose.

It has been shown that during wartime, countries usually experience a reduction in the availability of sugar. Reviewing 27 wartime studies from 11 European countries covering 750,000 children, Sognnaes (44) found that a reduction in caries was observed in all these studies. In Japan, where sugar consumption fell severely from 15 kg/person/year before the World War II to 0.2 kg/person/year in 1946, a close relation between annual sugar consumption and annual caries incidence was recorded (45). Rugg-Gunn et al. (46), in one better-designed study with a longitudinal analysis of diet and caries incidence together, showed that the weight of daily sugar intake was positively correlated with the incidence of caries in 12 to 14-year-old children, although the coefficient of correlation was low (+0.14), but 31 of 405 children eating the most sugar developed nearly one carious tooth surface per year more than the 31 children who had the lowest sugar intake. This study also indicated that the sugar-caries relation was independent of tooth-brushing frequency or the effectiveness of tooth cleaning.

In one of the biggest human interventional studies undertaken in the field of dental caries, Gustaffson et al. (47) examined 964 mentally deficient patients, 80% of whom were male, in the Uipeholm Hospital near Lund in southern Sweden in 1951. The patients were divided by wards into one control and six test groups, which were given high sucrose intakes at meals only or at and between meals, in nonsticky and sticky forms. It could be reasonably concluded that consumption of sugar even at high levels is associated with only a small increase in caries increment if taken upto four times a day as part of meals, and that consumption of sugar between meals as well as at meals is associated with a marked increase in dental caries. In a second important human interventional study conducted in Turku, Finland between 1972 and 1974 (48), with an objective of evaluating effect on dental caries of nearly total substitution of the sucrose in a normal diet with either fructose or xylitol. This study was restricted to adults to ensure full cooperation in adhering to the diet and included a wide range of biochemical and microbiological tests. The number of new carious lesions that developed during 2 years of study was 7.2 in the sucrose group, 3.8 in the fructose group, and 0.0 in the xylitol group. These figures include both precavitation carious lesions and carious cavities. When only cavities were counted, the result showed 56% fewer cavities in the xylitol group than in the sucrose group, with a similar number of cavities in the sucrose and fructose groups. Thus, the xylitol diet was less cariogenic than either the sucrose or the fructose diet, but fructose was no less cariogenic than sucrose. The persistent inability of plaque microorganisms to metabolize xylitol to organic acids probably explains this cariostatic effect. Xylitol thus appears to be a suitable substitute for sucrose from dental health point of view, with little evidence of osmotic diarrhea, even at daily intakes up to 200 g xylitol, and no other undesirable metabolic effects.

The effects of amount and concentration of sugars, the frequency of their use, and type of sugar have been tested in animal experiments. Kite et al. (49) fed two groups of rats the same high-sugar cariogenic diet, one group receiving their diet via stomach tube and the other in the conventional way. No caries was evidenced in the rats fed by stomach tube, whereas the rats fed in the normal way developed an average seven carious regions. Thus, sugar has to be present in the mouth for caries to occur. While there is a strong correlation between frequency of consumption of high-sugar diet and caries development (50), its relationship to total sugar intake is not always simple. Huxley (51) reported that whereas caries increased linearly with sugar concentration (0%, 15%, 30%, and 56%) in rats receiving one type of basic diet, no linerar increase was found in rats fed a different basic diet. Caries severity was found to increase with increasing sugar concentration, but the increase in severity declined when sugar concentration exceeded more than 40% (52). Both the amount and concentration of sugar eaten were found to be related to the severity of caries. According to Guggenheim et al. (53), among common dietary sugars (glucose, fructose, galactose, lactose, and maltose) sucrose is the most cariogenic sugar, which may be due to the superinfection or monoinfection of the experimental rats with streptococci, some strains of which utilize sucrose preferentially and do not thrive in its absence. All dietary sugars are thus cariogenic in rat experiments, and no studies have shown sucrose to be less cariogenic than other sugars.

Human enamel slab experiments have indicated that sucrose, glucose, and fructose induce caries-like lesions in the enamel slabs; lactose, sorbitol; and mannitol induce significantly fewer lesions than sucrose; and xylitol had no effect (54). Tehrani et al. (55) noted that increasing the concentration of sugars or the frequency of exposure to sugars enhanced the demineralization of the enamel slabs.

Plaque pH studies have shown that all sugar-containing foods lower plaque pH more than non-sugary foods, lactose and galactose producing lower pH drops than sucrose, glucose, fructose, or maltose. Many studies have shown that the sugar alcohols (xylitol, sorbitol, and mannitol) and related sweeteners (hydrogenated glucose syrup and isomalt) do not lower plaque pH; and indeed, chewing sugarless chewing gum actually raise plaque pH due to the increase in salivany flow, which is alkaline.

In vitro incubation experiments designed to test the ability of plaque microorganisms to metabolize a test food to acid have also shown that in general all sugar-containing foods are rapidly metabolized to acid, but starchy foods are metabolized more slowly, and xylitol is not metabolized at all; other sugars, such as sorbitol, mannitol, and hydrogenated glucose syrup, are broken down very slightly. These tests indicated that 5.5 was about the "critical pH" below which dental enamel dissolves in saliva or more importantly, in plaque fluid. Various incubation studies have shown that sucrose is very cariogenic. Lactose and galactose are less cariogenic than other common dietary mono- and disaccharides, but these small differences in the cariogenicity of dietary sugars are of little practical significance. The frequency of eating and quantity of food consumed are highly correlated, so it should not matter whether the dietary advice is to reduce the frequency or the amount of sugar consumed (34).

All carbohydrate foods including sugars and starches are considered cariogenic (56,57). Sreebny (37,57) correlated epidemiologically the caries status of 12-years-olds in 47 countries with availability of sugar and cereals in these countries. Cereal availability was quantified as (a) energy from cereal per day, and (b) energy from cereal as a percentage of energy intake (Table 4). The bivariate correlations between cereal availability and caries varied between –0.45 and +0.45, but were low and mainly negative when the data were controlled, by partial correlation, for sugar availability. In contrast, the bivariate correlation between sugar availability and caries was +0.70 and fell to only +0.67 and +0.60 when the data were controlled for total cereal and wheat availability, respectively (Table 4). These results suggest a much closer relationship between caries and sugar availability than between caries and the availability of starch cereal foods on a worldwide basis.

The extremely low caries incidence observed in people with hereditary fructose intolerance who eat starch in normal amounts (58) indicates that starchy foods are not cariogenic. Evidence obtained from various studies show that cooked staple starchy foods such as rice, potatoes, and bread have very low cariogenicity in humans; if finely ground, heat-treated, and eaten frequently, starch can cause caries, but the impact is less than that caused by a refined sugar such as sucrose. Because addition of sucrose increases the cariogenicity of cooked starchy foods, foods containing baked starch and substantial amounts of sucrose are as cariogenic as a similar amount of sucrose on its own (34).

Table 4 Correlations and Partial Correlations Between Caries Experience (DMFT) (for 12 year-olds) and Sugar or Cereal Availability in 47 Countries[a]

		Bivariate correlation	Partial correlation, controlling for sugar availability
Total cereals	Cal/day	−0.25	−0.03
	% of energy	−0.45[b]	−0.13
Wheat	Cal/day	+0.45[b]	+0.05
	% of energy	+0.29	−0.03
Rice	Cal/day	−0.07	+0.10
	% of energy	−0.09	+0.10
Maize	Cal/day	−0.37[c]	−0.24
	% of energy	−0.40[d]	−0.26
Sugar	g/day	+0.70[b]	
Controlling for total cereal (Cal/day)			+0.67[b]
Controlling for wheat (Cal/day)			+0.60[b]

[a]Raw data taken from Sreebny (37,57).
[b]$p < 0.005$
[c]$p < 0.02$
[d]$p < 0.05$
Source: Ref. 34.

1. Protective Foods Against Dental Caries

It was suggested that certain foods within the mouth provide substances that may actually protect teeth against dental caries (59). The direct protective effects in the mouth of some food compo nents such as phosphates have now been recognized. Other substances, such as fluoride, may be incorporated into teeth while they are forming, which helps protect the teeth. Inorganic phosphates protect teeth against dental caries by increasing availability of phosphate in plaque to encourage remineralization and resist demineralization. Sodium phosphates have been known to be more effective than calcium salts because of the lower solubility of calcium phosphates. Organic phosphates primarily act by binding to the tooth surface and reducing enamel dissolution, e.g., phytates.

Phosphates have proved to be less effective as anticaries substances in human experiments, although they have looked very promising in incubation and animal experiments, which can be ascribed to the higher salivary phosphate levels in humans than in rats. Because phytates reduce the absorption of certain micronutrients such as zinc in the gut, they are not suitable as food additives (34).

According to Edgar and Jenkins (60), honey contains esters and cations that could theoretically reduce caries development, although in animal experiments honey was found to be as cariogenic as sucrose or a mixture of fructose, glucose, and sucrose in the same proportions (45%, 35%, and 5%) as in honey (61). In the Vipeholm study, Gustaffson et al. (47) reported that patients in the chocolate group developed less caries than other groups receiving similar sugar levels at similar frequencies. This has led to speculation that chocolate might contain some protective factors, such as cocoa, which was confirmed in animal experiments (62). The active ingredient from cocoa has been isolated (63), but its extraction being expensive, it is likely to be much less effective than fluoride. Glycerrhizinic acid, a major constituent of liquorice also has anticaries properties, but is not likely to be used as food additive due to its other, undesirable properties.

Greenby (64) reviewed the literature on the cariogenicity of starches and starch-based foods, comparing starch with other carbohydrates and examining the effects of cooking, hydrolysis, and other methods of processing on its dental caries potential. Greenby (64) concluded that starch in its natural state is not cariogenic or of very low cariogenicity. Starch is not consumed in this form in Western diets. Cooking and processing denature starch and raise its potential cariogenicity. Mixtures of processed starches and sugars are more highly cariogenic than starches alone, providing the substrate for oral microorganisms to generate acids that can attack dental enamel. It has been suggested that dental caries attack may also be promoted by processed starches, contributing to the persistence or adherence of fermentable foods at susceptible sites on the teeth. Although carbohydrates in general have similar nutritional and physiological properties, major differences in dental caries potential appear to exist between starches and common dietary sugars, but the caries potential of the starches can be altered significantly by processing.

2. Intrinsic Sugar in Diets

Rugg-Gunn et al. (65) recorded the amount (gram weight) and percentage of free and intrinsic sugars consumed in the diets by Northumberland schoolchildren aged 11 to 14 years. About 69% of all sugars were free sugars, most of which came from confectionery, table sugar, and soft drinks (Table 5). Milk and fruits are the only important sources of intrinsic sugars. Lactose in cow's milk (about 4%) can be fermented to acid but has been found to be less cariogenic than other common dietary sugars. Milk also contains certain protective factors (e.g., calcium and phosphate) that can prevent dissolution of enamel. Proteins in milk also tend to be absorbed on to the enamel surface, preventing demineralization (66), and casein may have a specific anticaries effect, as indicated by enamel slab experiments (67,68) and animal experiments (69).

Human milk contains higher lactose levels (7%) and lower proportions of calcium, phosphate, and protein than cow's milk, indicating that human milk may give less protection against dental caries than cow's milk. However, there have been very few reports of caries development in infants receiving "on demand" breast-feeding (70). Given the importance of breast-feeding in

Table 5 Amount (g) and Percentage Contribution of Some Foods in the Free and Intrinsic Sugars Intake of 405 11- to 14-year-old Northumbrian Children (69% of Total Sugars Were Free Sugars)

Foods	Sugars			
	Free		Intrinsic	
	g	%	g	%
Confectionery	23	28	1	4
Table sugar	20	24	—	0
Soft drinks	14	17	2	6
Biscuits & cakes	10	12	3	8
Sweet puddings	7	9	6	15
Syrups & preserves	3	3	2	4
Breakfast cereals	2	3	1	1
Milk, butter, cheese	—	0	12	32
Other	3	3	6	15
Total	81	100	37	100

(Confectionery, Table sugar, Soft drinks Free % bracketed as } 69%)

Source: Ref. 65.

general and the very few reported cases of infantile caries, this should not discourage breast-feeding.

Cheese has anti-caries properties and its caries-protective effect has been supported by evidence from plaque pH studies (71), enamel slab experiments (72), and animal experiments.

Fruits contain soluble sugars (glucose, fructose, and sucrose) that can be fermented to organic acids by the plaque bacteria. However, apples, because of their crisp texture and fiber content, have emerged as a symbol of dental health, although there is little evidence of their effectiveness. Slack and Martin (74) recorded a very slightly lower caries incidence due to apple eating, whereas carrots had no effect on caries (75). Except for a report of Bibby (76), which showed an association of fruit-eating with caries, fruits in general have not shown to produce caries in a significant way. Thus, fruits can be considered less cariogenic, if not caries-protective. However, fruit juices have been found to be cariogenic (77), but it is not clear whether this depends on any added sugar or on the absence of salivary stimuli from the fiber-associated fruit components, or whether the natural enveloping of intrinsic sugars within the fruits' cell walls is crucial.

3. Other Sweeteners

Substances other than sugars that taste sweet are also used in foods and are grouped as either bulk sweeteners or intense sweeteners (artificial sweeteners), which provide little or no energy. Examples of bulk sweeteners that provide the same energy as sugars, include sorbitol, mannitol, xylitol, hydrogenated glucose syrup and isomalt, whereas commonly used intense sweeteners are saccharin, aspartame, acesulfame K, and thaumatin. Cyclamate, which is widely used in Europe is not permitted in the United Kingdom and the United States. The bulk sweetener lactitol was approved for use in 1988 (34).

Rugg-Gunn and Edgar (78) have reviewed the cariogenicity of the bulk and intense sweeteners. Evidence indicates that intense sweeteners are not likely to promote caries, which may be due to their composition. Whereas xylitol is hardly fermentable, other sugar alcohols such as sorbitol and mannitol are fermented to acids very slowly. Thus, these bulk sweeteners appear to have a low cariogenicity.

B. Periodontal Disease

Progressive destruction of the supporting alveolar bone and periodontal membranes, progressing from gingivitis, may result in tooth mobility and fall. The most important cause of periodontal disease is the persistent presence of plaque on teeth adjacent to the gingivae, dental calculus helping the plaque retention. In addition to these extrinsic factors, there may be intrinsic nutritional and hormonal (e.g., pregnancy) factors or those related to a wide variety of diseases, such as diabetes and blood dyscrasias (34).

Although sugar encourages the development of some plaque microorganisms, there is no evidence to show that this leads to the development of gingivitis or periodontal disease. There is also very little evidence that the general nutritional status modifies the progression of this disease (79). However, the most important determinant of periodontal disease appears to be age, which gradually decreases tooth support. The second most important factor is the quantity of plaque and calculus on the tooth. Some animal experiments have shown that vitamin A deficiency may cause gingival hyperkeratosis, destruction of the periodontal membrane, and resorption of alveolar bone; also vitamin B–complex deficiency may cause a nonspecific inflammatory change in response to local irritants. Vitamin D deficiency or an imbalance in the Ca/P intake may result in disturbance in the calcification of alveolar bone and teeth. Protein deficiency is also known to be related to osteoporosis of the alveolar bone and an enhanced inflammatory response to irritants.

C. Tooth Structure

In the 1930s dental caries was thought to be deficiency disease, vitamin deficiency being attributed as the primary cause for the development of carious cavities (80–82). After the 1940s, the post-eruptive effects of dietary sugar were accepted as the most important dietary factor in caries etiology. The vitamin D–deficiency hypothesis, however, may still have relevance in the developing countries, where dietary deficiency and illness have led to a high prevalence of hypoplastic teeth, which may be more caries susceptible when there is an increase in sugar availability. The deficiency of both vitamins A and D have been recognized as the cause of enamel hypoplasia, and protein deficiency in rats leads to dental hypoplasia and to impaired salivary gland development.

Despite the obvious significance of calcium in tooth development, there is very little evidence that dietary calcium influences caries susceptibility or resistance, probably because plasma calcium levels are precisely controlled, and teeth are much less susceptible to calcium deficiency than bones.

Development of caries tends to be lower in areas with hard water (83–84), but fluoride content of water is a more important determinant of caries severity than water hardness. There is an inverse relation between the fluoride concentration of drinking water and caries incidence (85). The optimum level of fluoride in temperate climates is 1.0 mg/l, whereas in warmer climates it might be nearer to 0.6 mg/l. Above these optimum limits in drinking water, fluoride may cause dental enamel to be imperfectly formed. These defects, known as enamel opacities or dental fluorosis, may range from small white diffused opacities to severe pitting and staining of the enamel. Fluoride prevents dental caries by being incorporated into the tooth structure while teeth are forming—the systemic effect—as well as by the local posteruptive action in the mouth—the topical action. Fluorides in toothpastes and mouth rinses provide a topical effect, and these products are not to be swallowed. Fluoride tablets that dissolve slowly in the mouth before ingestion and water fluoridation may act both systemically and topically. Fluoride may also be administered through salt and milk. Tea and fish are other dietary sources of fluoride. Whereas dietary molybdenum, strontium, boron, and lithium are related to a lower caries experience in humans, higher selenium is associated with increased caries prevalence. Although vegetables provide most of the trace elements, strontium, like fluoride, has only water as its main dietary source (86).

Tooth surfaces can become stained by certain foods and drinks, such as tea, coffee, curries, liquorice, and iron tonics, as well as by chewing beetlewine leaves.

D. Dental Erosion

Erosion of teeth can be defined as the progressive loss of tooth substance by a chemical process not involving microbial action, to distinguish it from dental caries (34). Dental erosion tends to occur in tooth surfaces not usually covered by plaque, dietary acids being the most important cause (87). Acidulated carbonated drinks, citrus fruit, vinegar, and iron tonics may be responsible for dental erosion (88). Dental erosion occurs most commonly in adolescents. The missing tooth tissue can usually be replaced by dentists.

E. Dietary Advice for Dental Health

The most important dietary advice for dental health would be to restrict the consumption of free (added) sugars. In view of strong pressures from the manufacturers of sugar and sugar-containing foods and drinks, it is a rather difficult advice to follow in practice. An excellent summary of dietary advice for dental health was published by the Health Education Authority (89).

Changing diet involves promoting healthy eating at several levels, e.g. central (government), local or district, and individual, for a country. At the central level, a government can introduce water fluoridation through legal action; e.g., in Ireland and Singapore, water fluoridation is mandatory. Uniform food labeling in a country can enable the informed consumer to choose foods selectively. Sugar labeling can be an essential part of this program. Restricting use of sugars in medicines like cough syrups also requires governmental regulation. Agricultural policy needs to be compatible with national health goals, e.g., the question of subsidizing sugar production. The changes in the nation's diet required for greater health need to be agreed on by all professional groups and accepted by the public. The advice to be given to the public then can be best coordinated by one of central agencies, such as the Health Education Authority in the United Kingdom. The objectives agreed on at the national level need to be implemented effectively at a local level. The state and district food policy and message for healthy eating also need to be agreed on and implemented by all professional groups, including health officials and dentists. Dietitians and dentists can cooperate to assist in the case of individual patients.

For infants and children, an adequate supply of fluoride is very important and if the fluoride level of water is less than optimal, dietary fluoride supplements may be recommended; these can be readily purchased in pharmacies as prescribed by a general practitioner or issued at community dental clinics. The current recommended dosages of fluoride in the United Kingdom are shown in Table 6.

For children and adolescents, restricting the confectionery, table sugar, and soft drinks that provide over two-thirds of the intake of free sugars would do much to reduce the high incidence of caries. It is important to provide positive advice with suggestions for healthier snack foods.

The incidence of dental caries is highest in young children, adolescents, and elderly people, and perhaps lowest in younger adults. Confectionery, table sugar, soft drinks, biscuits, cakes, and puddings are important sources of sugar and form the main target for dietary advice. The best advice for elderly people is still restriction of their sugar intake, which may also be important to improve the nutrient density of their diet with declining energy needs. It is also important that elderly people seek dental advice regularly to make eating as efficient and comfortable as possible.

Saliva has several vital functions in aiding eating, swallowing, and speaking and in preventing dental caries. Salivary flow decreases in old age due to atrophy and can be markedly reduced due to some diseases, e.g., Sjogren's syndrome, after radio-therapy to head and neck, and as a response to several drugs (34), followed by rampant dental caries. These circumstances may require severe sugar restriction with intensive topical fluoride therapy, although salivary substitutes available may also be useful to many patients (90).

Patients who suffer from phenylketonuria or cystic fibrosis may need to eat high-carbohydrate diets in the form of sugars. The patients' dentist must accept this and cooperate with the dietitian to ensure that caries is prevented as much as possible by means other than sugar restriction.

Several new types of oligosaccharides have been developed as bulking sucrose substitutes that have beneficial health effects. Although most of these oligosaccharides are constituents of

Table 6 Fluoride Dietary Supplements—Age-related Dosages (mg/day)

Age	Fluoride concentration in drinking water (ppm F)		
	<0.3	0.3–0.7	More than >0.7
2 weeks–2 years	0.25	0	0
2–4 years	0.50	0.25	0
4–16 years	1.00	0.50	0

Source: Ref. 85.

natural plant foods, they are currently mass-produced from sucrose, lactose, maltose, and starch derivatives by using specific bacterial enzymes. Sugar alcohols are produced by hydrogenation of oligosaccharides such as maltose, lactose, palatinose, and partly hydrolyzed starch derivatives. These newly developed oligosaccharides have some unique properties for digestion absorption, fermentation, and metabolism. Oku (91) classified sucrose substitutes into the following four groups, based on their beneficial health effects:

1. Those providing less available energy than that produced by sucrose. The available energy of sucrose substitutes is about 2 kcal/g.
2. Those having no effect on insulin secretion from the pancreas. Nondigestible oligosaccharides do not increase blood glucose level.
3. Those improving intestinal microflora. The beneficial bacteria increase and the harmful microbes decrease. As a result, putrefactive products decrease and the production of carcinogens also declines.
4. Those preventing dental caries. *Streptococcus mutans* cannot use nondigestible oligosaccharides, and these oligosaccharides do not produce insoluble glucans.

There are two types of noncariogenic sucrose substitutes (92): The first type is digested completely in the small intestine, e.g., coupling sugar and palatinit. The second type is not digested, e.g., reduced-energy oligosaccharides such as Neosugar®, maltitol, lactitol, and palatinit. Insoluble glucans and short-chain fatty acids (SCFA) are not produced from palatinose and coupling sugar, because these are not metabolized by *S. mutans*. The reduction in pH (which favors demineralization of tooth enamel) is not induced by the incubation of *S. mutans* in the presence of palatinose. The alpha-1,4 linkage between the glucose residues in the coupling sugar is first hydrolyzed by maltase, and then the sucrose unit obtained is further hydrolyzed by sucrase. The alpha-1,6 linkage of palatinose is hydrolyzed slowly by isomaltase and not by sucrase. Therefore, the ingestion of coupling sugar or palatinose increases the blood glucose level and stimulates insulin secretion, and availability of energy is similar to that of sucrose. These digestible noncariogenic sucrose substitutes are convenient sweeteners for growing children needing much energy (92). According to Oku (92), functional foods for specified health uses in Japan are regulated under the Nutritional Improvement Act. The health benefits of each such food product are judged based on comprehensive examination of the ingrediets and composition of the food product. Forty of these foods make use of oligosaccharides (e.g. Neosugar, xylo-oligosaccharides, soybean oligosaccharides, isomalto-oligosaccharides, glactosyl-sucrose, maltitol, palatinose) to improve the colonic environment and to prevent dental caries. Foods such as soft drinks, chocolate, cookies, gum, and candy that contain oligosaccharides for specified health uses are in great demand and will be developed with increasing frequency in the near future.

Many sugar alcohols such as xylitol, sorbitol, and mannitol are found naturally in plants and fruits (Table 7). However, most sugar alcohols are prepared commercially. Examples of some polyols developed at the Xyrofin Laboratories at Redhill, UK, the end-products, and their functional effects are given in Table 8 (93).

IV. DIET AND HEALTH OF SKIN AND HAIR

The barrier function of the epidermis of skin is localized in the stratum corneum or horny layer of skin, whose effectiveness depends on normal keratinization, and on epidermal lipids, constituting up to 10% of its dry weight. This lipid portion is derived from cell-wall phospholipid and is rich in essential fatty acids (EFA), the deficiency of which may result in a loss of the normal epidermal impermeability and an increase in water loss. Keratinization is primarily influenced by

Table 7 Natural Occurrence of Polyols

Polyol	Source	Level (g/liter juice)
D-Sorbitol	Apples	2.6–9.2
	Pears	11.0–26.4
	Cherries	14.7–21.3
	Sour cherries	13.1–29.8
	Plums	1.8–13.5
	Rowan	85.0
D-Mannitol		% dry weight
	Laminaria spp.	10
	Lactarius	15–20
	Agaricus	15–20
Xylitol	Yellow plums	0.93
	Straw berries	0.36
	Cauliflower	0.30

Source: Ref. 93.

Table 8 Some Xyrofin-supplied Polyols and Examples of Their Contribution to Product Development

Polyol	End-product example	Effect of Polyol
Xylitol	Chewing gum	Unique dental benefits and refreshing cooling effect
Lactitol	Baked goods	Part or full sugar replacement and reduction in calories
Malitol	Confectionery	Replacement of sugar in confectionery, reduction in calories
Sorbitol	Toothpastes	Sugar-free sweetness and retention of moisture

Source: Courtesy of Xyrofin Laboratories at Redhill, U.K.

the essential dietary nutrients, vitamins, and minerals. The inner dermis allows these nutrients to pass to the epidermis and provides tough structural support for the protection of the body against physical and mechanical injuries (1); the deficiencies of vitamin C, copper, or protein cause defects in collagen formation, rendering the skin more vulnerable to injury.

A. Role of Vitamins in the Health of Skin and Hair

1. Vitamin A

Vitamin A may be taken either in the form of retinol or its precursor, beta-carotene, which is split in the intestine to vitamin A. Along with its vital role in vision, growth, reproduction, and embryonic development, vitamin A also has an important physiological function in the maintenance of differentiated epithelia, although the precise molecular mechanisms of its role are not yet known (94). The development of synthetic analogues of vitamin A (retinoids), which have reduced toxicity compared with the natural vitamin, are now being used in pharmacological doses to treat certain skin diseases, e.g. all-trans retinoic acid, which was used both topically and systematically in acne, psoriasis, ichthyosis, and actinic keratoses, although its toxicity remained high. Newer, less toxic, and more effective vitamin A derivatives such as isotretinoin, etretinate, and acetretin have been introduced into clinical practice (95).

Vitamin A was thought to act on epithelial surfaces as an "antikeratinizing" agent. When retinal is absent, goblet mucous cells disappear from mucosal surfaces, to be replaced by basal keratinocytes, which then gradually convert the original epithelium into stratified keratinized epithelium. As the normal lubricating mucus is lost, infection, irritation and sloughing of the surface occur. With an increased keratinization, the hyperplastic skin has reduced the number of sebaceous glands and blockage of sweat glands. A classic vitamin A deficiency in the form of plugging of the follicular openings with spiny horns (phrynoderma) then sets in. Cod liver oil can cure this disorder and it has been suggested that the disorder is caused by the deficiency of EFAs (96).

Among various caroteroids found in plants, beta-carotene is the most potent provitamin A, found in leafy green vegetables and yellow, orange fruits. Approximately one-half of the vitamin A in people on mixed diet is supplied through beta-carotene. Beta-carotene appears to be nontoxic, unlike retinal, and when taken in large amounts is absorbed unchanged from the gut. As a result, there is some carotene in normal skin, and excess amount may produce yellow discoloration, especially when blood carotene levels reach about four times normal. The hypothesis that carotenes play a role in photosynthesis by absorbing wavelengths that are lower than those absorbed by chlorophyll, and that they provide a photoprotective action against damage, has led to the investigation of carotenes as a photoprotective drug. The only condition in which this has proved to be unequivocally effective is erythropoietic protoporphyria (97).

A number of skin diseases produce pathological changes in keratinization, including congenital and hereditary diseases (e.g., ichthyosis, Darier's disease, and commonly acquired psoriasis and acne), where follicular keratin is altered. The administration of high doses of vitamin A is limited by its toxicity; e.g., 500 mg in an adult, 100 mg in a small child, and 30 mg in an infant can result in an acute syndrome of raised intracranial pressure, followed by extensive peeling of skin after 24 hours. Chronic administration of lesser amounts (doses over 7.5 mg/day are not recommended) may result in similar but milder cerebral symptoms, together with pain and tenderness of bones, with bony overgrowth. The skin may become dry and pruritic (palms and soles) with considerable tenderness. Disturbed hair growth is accompanied by dry lips and nasal mucosa, which may crack, become irritable, and begin to bleed. Vitamin A may either prevent or even reverse the early changes of malignancy. Vitamin A influences cellular differentiation and its deficiency appears to enhance the effects of carcinogens (98); the basal cells of many epithelia show decreased differentiation and enhanced DNA synthesis; these changes can be reversed by giving vitamin A (1).

2. Vitamin D

Dietary calciferol (D_2) is formed by the solar irradiation of plant sterols: cholecalciferol (D_3) in the human skin is synthesized by ultraviolet irradiation of 7-dehydrocholesterol. Vitamin D is not associated with any cutaneous disorders, but the recent finding that vitamin D can interfere with keratinocyte proliferation has led to the development of synthetic vitamin D derivatives (e.g. calcipotriol), which have shown only a slight influence on calcium metabolism but have useful effects when applied topically in psoriasis (99).

3. Vitamin C

Because they lack 1-gulono lactone oxidase, humans and some other primates are not able to synthesize vitamin C, and it must be obtained through fruits and vegetables in the diet. Vitamin C deficiency produces a major metabolic defect in the form of impairment of the hydroxylation of proline and lysine in collagen synthesis. Insufficiently hydroxylated collagen has a lower melting point and cannot form normal fibers, resulting in structural changes of bones, mucous membrane, and skin, which have collagen content.

Experimental vitamin C deficiency in humans was found to result in cutaneous changes, such as enlargement and keratoses of the hair follicles, especially on the upper arms (100,101). Plugging of follicles was followed by coiling of the hairs into the typical corkscrews. The next change to occur was capillary dilatation, followed by hemorrhage around follicles, especially on the lower limbs, as a result of high gravitational pressure in the defective capillaries. The capillaries around the follicles appear to proliferate and have decreased amounts of collagen both within and around the vessel walls (1).

4. B Complex Vitamins

a. Niacin. Nicotinic acid (pyridine 2-carboxylic acid) and its derivatives, collectively called niacin, are required for the synthesis of two coenzymes of oxido-reductases, viz., nicotinamide adenine dinucleotide (NAD) and nicotinamide adenine dinucleotide phosphate (NADP). These are widely distributed in foods and can also be formed from tryptophan, 60 mg of which is equivalent to 1 mg of niacin. In maize, which is also low in tryptophan, niacin is highly protein-bound and not readily available without roasting or alkali pre-treatment. Niacin deficiency can lead to pellagra in people consuming maize as a staple food. Pellagra is characterized by three Ds: diarrhea, dementia, and dermatitis. The cutaneous eruption is a consistent, typical and almost diagnostic symptom of pellagra. The rashes develop on the skin, with a sensation of burning or irritation in light-exposed areas. Edema becomes apparent, followed by blistering or development of thick brown scales. In the chronic state, scaling increases and the skin begins to fissure, followed by hemorrhage.

Histologically, early lesions show a chronic inflammatory infiltrate in the upper dermis, followed by hyperkeratosis, with patchy retention of the cell nuclei and thickening of the epidermis. The amount of melanin increases as the skin becomes darkened. In chronic cases there may be hyalization of the dermal collagen, followed by fibrosis and epidermal atrophy (102).

b. Riboflavin. Riboflavin deficiency often occurs in association with other B complex vitamin deficiencies. Sebrell and Butler (103) noted that the oral, flexural and genital lesions that were originally included in the clinical manifestation of pellagra were actually due to riboflavin deficiency. After a period of 1 to 2 years on a deficient diet, a moist angular cheilitis develops, associated with a seborrheic dermatitis–like eruption in the nasolabial folds and eylids, glossitis, and fissuring of the vermilion of the lips. There may also be maceration of skin on the genitalia (1).

c. Pyridoxine. Symptoms similar to those of riboflavin deficiency are seen in people with pyridoxine deficiency, which appear within a few weeks if a diet poor in B complex vitamins is given together with the pyridoxine antagonist, desoxypyridoxine. The lesions on the skin are rapidly cleared when pyridoxine is administered (104).

d. Biotin. Avidin of raw egg white binds biotin, preventing its absorption. Biotin deficiency causes a severe exfoliative dermatitis in animals. A similar but milder dermatitis has been produced in humans fed large amounts of raw egg white and has been described in patients on total parenteral nutrition deficient in biotin (105).

B. Role of Minerals in the Health of Skin and Hair

1. Zinc

Of the total amount of adult body's zinc (1.4–2.3g), about 20% is present in the skin. The epidermis contains 70.5 µg/g dry weight and the dermis has 12.6 µg/g. Scalp hair from schoolchildren was found to have 125 to 225 µg/g of zinc (106). Zinc-deficient animals show retardation in

Table 9 Cutaneous Manifestations of Zinc Deficiency

Skin Surface
    Weeping dermatitis (around the body orifices of the extremities)
    Secondary infection
    Poor wound healing
    'Eczema craquele'
Hair
    Excessive fragility
    Sparse scalp hair
    Absent pubic hair
Nails
    Paronychia
    Nail deformities

Source: Ref. 1.

growth and testicular atrophy, together with loss of hair and thickening and hyperkeratosis of the epidermis. The cutaneous manifestations of zinc deficiency have now been recognized [Table 9]. However, zinc being present ubiquitously in foods, its deficiency is unlikely but can occur in association with certain disease conditions (Table 10).

Greaves and Boyd (107) showed decreased circulating levels of zinc in patients with extensive skin disease, but these changes were secondary to the skin problem, rather than the cause of it. Moynahan and Barnes (108) demonstrated that dietary supplements of zinc could completely cure *acrodermatitis enteropathica*, an otherwise miserable and usually fatal skin disease.

Acrodermatitis enteropathica (AE) is a rare congenital disease characterized by alopecia, diarrhea, and an exudative dermatitis affecting the skin around the body orifices and on the

Table 10 Causes of Zinc Deficiency

Acrodermatitis enteropathica
Total parenteral nutrition
Intestinal disease
    Crohn's disease
    Jejunoileal bypass
    Steatorrhea
    Chronic diarrhea
Pancreatic disease
    Alcoholic pancreatitis
    Cystic fibrosis
Liver disease
    Alcoholic cirrhosis
    Primary biliary cirrhosis
Renal disease
    Chronic renal failure
Fetal alcohol syndrome
Penicillamine therapy
Phytate-rich diet

Source: Ref. 1.

extremities. Hair is lost diffusely and extensively, and the hair becomes hypopigmented and fragile. In the 1950s, the antifungal agent diadoquin was regularly and successfully used to treat AE, and it is known that drug enhances intestinal zinc absorption (109). AE rapidly responds to zinc supplements, even in adults in whom the condition has been present since infancy. It is now established that the manifestations of AE are due solely to a shortage of zinc (110). In normal adults, a recommended intake of zinc may be 15 mg Zn per day, whereas patients with AE can be relieved of their symptoms by receiving one 220 mg tablet of zinc sulfate per day, which provides 55 mg of zinc.

Zinc deficiency has been shown to worsen preexisting facial acne (111). Also, zinc-deficient patients have poor wound-healing ability; as a result, zinc supplements have been recommended in the management of chronic gravitational ulcers (112). Some elderly patients with bedsores may be zinc-deficient (113).

2. *Iron*

Apart from iron's vital role in the hemopoietic system, chronic iron deficiency may result in spoon-shaped nails (koilonychia), hair loss, glossitis with loss of papillae, angular cheilitis, and pruritus. Although diffuse hair loss has been described in iron deficiency, an exact relationship between the two remains to be established. Any debilitating illness may cause diffuse hair loss. Itching is now accepted as a feature of iron deficiency and occurs in 7% to 14% of patients. Angular cheilitis has also been attributed to iron deficiency (114).

Iron overloads may occur through repeated blood transfusions, wherein iron in cutaneous macrophages may cause the skin to turn dusky gray in color. Excessive iron deposition in tissues such as liver may result in serious dysfunction. Pancreatic damage and the skin changes may lead to a condition known as bronze diabetes. According to Milder et al. (115), in hemochromatosis, 82% of patients showed skin pigmentation due to increased melanin formation. Other cutaneous signs included the loss of body hair and gynecomastia, both probably a consequence of testicular atrophy.

Patients suffering from cutaneous hepatic porphyria present with photosensitivity and increased fragility of light-exposed skin, such as on the backs of the hands, where even the slightest trauma, such as rubbing against clothing, may damage the skin surface. In more severe condition, bullae develop after exposure to sun and there may be scarring, hyperpigmentation, and an increase in hair growth, evident in both sexes. This disorder results from a reduction in the activity of the hepatic enzyme uroporphyrinogen decarboxylase. In nearly every case there is an evidence of a prolonged positive iron balance, with hepatic siderosis and cirrhosis. Among the Bantus of South Africa, siderosis is a consequence of drinking beer with a low pH brewed in iron pots and is associated with a high frequency of cutaneous hepatic porphyria (116).

3. *Copper*

Most of the approximately 100 µg/100 ml of human serum copper is tightly bound to ceruloplasmin, and exchangeable copper is bound to albumin. The importance of copper in the skin lies in its role in collagen and elastin formation. The enzyme lysyl oxidase requires copper as a cofactor. This enzyme catalyzes the formation of cross-linkages in collagen, giving the skin its tensile strength.

Lack of copper causes Menkes' disease (117), in which there is copper deficiency in both ceruloplasin and albumin-bound copper, due to a block in intestinal absorption of copper (118). This is a recessive disorder characterized by deficient lysyl oxidase, which is copper-dependent. Cutaneous features include pallid skin, horizontal tangled eyebrows, a change in the appearance of the upper lip to produce a Cupid's bow, and hypopigmented brittle and twisted hair. In affected children, the hair is normal at birth, but it is gradually replaced with hair that is light in color, brittle, and has peculiar twists. The skin is paler than normal. The abnormal hair has about ninefold increase in free SH-groups, a change that is also seen in copper-deficient sheep (119). A syndrome similar to Menkes' disease was described in infants fed for a prolonged period by total parenteral nutrition; symptoms rapidly responded to introduction of copper (120).

4. Manganese

The human body has about 15 mg of manganese, mostly present in the nuclei and liver mitochondria. Manganese deficiency is rare in humans but may cause weight loss, dermatitis, and slowing of hair and nail growth. The hair may become reddish (121).

5. Selenium

Selenium is a constituent of glutathione peroxidase, which breaks down in the presence of reduced glutathione, potentially damaging reactive peroxides. Dietary deficiencies in China are endemic and may produce cardiomyopathy and inflammatory joint disease, with a cutaneous symptom of whitening of the nails in children on total parenteral nutrition, which could be reversed by administering selenium (122).

Reilly (123) has recently reviewed the information on the nature and biological role of selenium, its levels in the diet, and the pros and cons of its use in functional foods. Evidence available indicates that selenium deficiency may be related to a variety of degenerative diseases, including cancer, and that protection against such conditions can be conferred by increasing intake of selenium.

Dietary deficiency, whether primary or conditioned, can be associated with dermatological lesions that can respond to specific therapy with vitamins, minerals, or unusual diets. Dermatoses are also associated with obesity, and therapies directed at weight reduction may provide the best management of dermatological problems. Dermatological disorders associated with undernutrition and/or malnutrition can be managed by increasing protein intake in the diet. Food allergies producing dermatoses should be ruled out if they are suspected on the basis of family history or by history of the patient's food intake. Every patient presenting a dermatological disorder should have a careful nutritional history and physical examination. Biochemical studies may be carried out to rule out any evidence of nutritional abnormality. The underlying defects related to skin disorders of unknown etiology may be the result of improper nutrition and metabolic error endured for long periods of time. Their correction by diet or improved metabolism may require long and intensive therapy (123).

6. Toxic Trace Elements

Lead may be consumed in toxic quantities, through environmental pollution. A blue line on the gums is characteristic, but not diagnostic, and may occur with other metallic poisons such as mercury, bismuth, iron, silver, and thallium. The blue is due to the interaction of hydrogen sulfide from anerobic organisms and circulating lead compounds. Cutaneous involvement is not a recognized feature of chronic lead ingestion, despite its profound effect on porphyrin metabolism, possibly causing blistering of the skin (124).

Arsenic has been used as a therapeutic agent for ages to treat (with some success) inflammatory skin diseases like psoriasis. High arsenic intakes may also result from contaminated drinking water and foods polluted with pesticides and herbicides. A prolonged exposure to arsenic may produce pigmented skin with characteristic "raindrop" hypopigmented macules on a diffusely bronzed background. The palms and soles often show punctate hyperkeratosis and development of carcinomata, which may take as long as 13 years after exposure (1).

Thallium-containing pesticides may pollute foods. Thallium is highly toxic and if the patient survives the acute phase, an extensive characteristic alopecia may develop about 2 weeks later.

Lithium is abundant in alkaline springwater and lithium salts are used therapeutically to treat manic-depressive states. In toxic quantities, lithium may worsen psoriasis.

Allergic contact to nickel may cause dermatitis, especially in women, in whom prevalence is higher (10%). It is thought that a low-nickel diet will help to control the dermatitis, which may persist, however, especially on the hands, long after exposure to topical nickel has ceased.

Chronic mercury poisoning from environmental pollution may produce vague symptoms that are difficult to diagnose (125). Its association with "pink disease" in children remains to be established (1).

C. Essential Fatty Acids in Health of Skin and Hair

Fats are necessary components of the diet. It has been shown that rats reared on a fat-free diet developed a deficiency disease that could not be corrected by adding fat-soluble vitamins A and D to the diet. In addition to kidney failure, the animals had a high fluid intake not accounted for by increased urinary output. The animals had a high transepidermal water loss (TEWL) resulting from a defective epidermal barrier. This disorder could be corrected by adding fat to the diet and the unsaturated fraction of the fat was found to be responsible. The action of unsaturated fraction was competitively inhibited by saturated fat. The name essential fatty acid (EFA) has now replaced the original term, vitamin F. All EFAs are now known to be polyunsaturated fatty acids (PUFA), although not all PUFAs are essential.

Two groups of EFAs are known, the n-3 group, derived from alpha-linolenic acid, and the n-6 group, derived from linoleic acid (18:2, n-6). The n-3 EFAs are formed in marine plankton and reach human diet through fish or flesh of marine animals, whereas n-6 EFAs are found in vegetables and red meats. These two groups are entirely separate and cannot be metabolized one from the other.

According to Basnayake and Sinclair (126), when rats were placed on a diet lacking in EFAs immediately after weaning, the first cutaneous change, evident after 1 week, was a rapid reduction in linoleic and arachidonic acids. After 5 weeks, skin scaliness developed and animals drank more. By 10 weeks on the diet, TEWL was about 10 times higher than normal. As the available linoleic acid level falls further, the enzymes that normally convert linoleic acid into arachidonic acid act on oleic acid to form $\Delta 5, 8, 11$-eiocosatrienoic acid (n-9). This abnormal fatty acid is detectable only in traces in normal skin and is a marker for EFA deficiency. Allen (1) stated the following effects of experimentally produced EFA deficiency in rats:

Hair loss
Scaling dermatitis
Sebaceous-gland hyperplasia
Increased transepidermal water loss
Poor wound healing
Stunted growth
Renal failure
Atrophy of exocrine glands
Fatty atrophy of the liver
Reproductive failure

The essentiality of the n-3 group is still controversial. In experimental EFA deficiency, the cutaneous changes can be reversed either by the n-3 or the n-6 group, although sensitivity to the n-6 group is higher (127).

Dried epidermis is about 10% lipid by weight. Its structural integrity and barrier function depend on both "bricks" provided by the stratum corneum cells and the "mortar" provided by the lipid between the cells. Structural failure results from the incorporation of more saturated or monounsaturated fats into the phospholipids of cell walls, resulting in a fluid loss. Defective intercellular lipid also results in increased water loss (128). Because linoleic acid (18:2, n-6) is absent in EFA deficiency, oleic acid (18:1, n-9) is incorporated into ceramides in its place, resulting in failure to form normal lamellar granules. Thus, the water barrier becomes defective (129). In EFA-deficient skin, the epidermis thickens, with the development of a granular layer but without the parakeratosis, a marked feature of certain scaling diseases of skin such as psoriasis (130).

Using eicosatrienoic acid (n-9) as a marker of EFA deficiency, EFA deficiency in patients following extensive bowel resection could be induced. Although there was scaling of the skin, there was no increase in TEWL, unlike in rats (131). EFA deficiency can be corrected by the topical application of linoleic acid and by using derivatives of EFAs such as prostaglandin E_2 (132). The n-3 EFAs are much less potent in reversing cutaneous changes than the n-6 series.

The eicosanoid metabolism is most probably disturbed in psoriasis, with high levels of leukotrienes B_4 and C_4, 12-hydroxy eicosatetranoic acid (12 HETE), and free arachidonic acid all being described in the skin (133). Similar changes are not seen in other inflammatory skin diseases such as atopic eczema. It is not known whether these disturbances are primary or the consequence of other preceding phenomena. Research into the possibility that dietary supplements of fish oil might be beneficial in psoriasis was stimulated by the observation that the prevalence of psoriasis was low in Eskimos (134), whose natural diet is rich in n-3 fatty acids.

Trials on dietary supplements with fish oil in treating psoriasis have shown beneficial results (135,136). It was found that daily therapy with 50 ml of fish oil to provide about 9 g EPA led to clinical improvement in more than 50% of the patients treated. Bittiner et al. (137) confirmed these results in a double-blind trial. After 8 weeks' treatment there was a significant reduction in the itching, erythema and scaling of the active group, with a decrease in the area of skin affected by psoriasis.

Urticaria lesions consisting of pruritic areas of redness and dermal swelling are variable in size, shape, and distribution and may affect deeper tissues, giving rise to angioedema. These lesions may be caused by local release of histamine from mast cells. The mast cells are induced to degranulate through the binding of IgE (immunoglobulin E) to the cell surface. An immunological cause is throughout in all cases of urticaria, food usually being blamed in the absence of any other obvious provoking factor. Milk, egg, fish, and nuts are most likely foods to cause the problem (138). Food allergies of this type are usually acquired during childhood and are rarely seen for the first time in adults. Breast-feeding commonly prevents the development of food allergy in children, but allergies have been known to occur in children initally fed breast, soy, or cow's milk (139).

Urticaria may be triggered pharmacologically by certain chemical agents in the diet, such as salicylates, yeast products, benzoate derivatives, and the dye tartrazine. These substances lower the threshold at which mast cells are triggered to release histamine. Foods such as shellfish and srawberries may also act in a similar way to cause urticaria, although clinically the condition is identical to IgE-mediated food allergy (1).

Atopic children show a high incidence of true food allergy and may have eczema (138), although evidence is insufficient to show that food allergy plays a direct role in producing eczema (140). In a study of 541 patients with atopic dermatitis, 84 were found to have histories of cutaneous symptoms related to diet, but in the urticaria group, there was a good correlation in those who believed that their eczema was made worse (141).

Dietary manipulation in skin diseases is often made on the assumption that the disorder is caused by a food allergy. Claims of food-associated diseases have usually been unsubstantiated, a misuse of the term allergy, which should be restricted to describing only those reactions in which an immune response can be demonstrated. The only immunological reaction that has been shown to occur unequivocally from food is a Type I IgE–mediated reaginic response, characterized by immediate onset, angioedema-like swelling around lips, burning of the mouth and throat, and widespread urticaria.

Dermatitis herpertiformis, a relatively uncommon skin disease, is characterized by the development of intensely itchy blisters, especially over the knees, elbows, and sacral area, with no symptoms of malabsorption. Patients usually have subtotal villous atrophy in the small intestine as in celiac disease (142). Despite lack of symptoms, patients also show slight folate and iron deficiency and impaired D-xylose absorption. As with celiac disease, the gastrointestinal changes respond to the exclusion of gluten from the diet. This disease responds dramatically to treatment with dapsone, but the drug needs to be continued indefinitely; however, after the exclusion of gluten from the diet, the dosage of dapsone may be decreased (1).

REFERENCES

1. Allen, B.R., Skin and hair, *Human Nutrition and Dietetics*, 5th ed., (J.S. Garrow and W.P.T. James, eds.), Churchill Livingstone, Edinburgh, London, 1993, p. 668
2. Maiti, S.K., and G.R. Singh, Bone morphogenetic proteins—novel regulators of bone formation, *Indian J. Exp. Biol. 36*: 237 (1998).
3. Reid, D.M., and S.A. New, Nutritional influences on bone mass, *Proc. Nutr. Soc. 56*: 977 (1997).
4. Heaney, R.P., C.M. Weaver, and M.L. Fitzsimmons, Soybean phytate content: effect on calcium absorption, *Am. J. Clin. Nutr. 53*: 741 (1991).
5. New, S.A., C. Bolton-Smith, D.A. Grubb, and D.M. Reid, Nutritional influences on bone mineral density: A cross-sectional study in pre-menopausal women, *Am. J. Clin. Nutr. 65*: 1831 (1998).
6. Angus, F.M., P.N. Sambrook, N.A. Pocock, and J.A. Eisman, Dietary intake and bone mineral density, *Bone & Mineral 4*: 265 (1988).
7. Strause, L., P. Saltman, K.T. Smith, M. Bracker, and M.B. Andon, Spinal bone loss in post-menopausal women supplemented with calcium and trace mineral, *J. Nutr. 124*: 1060 (1994).
8. Smith, R., Clinical nutrition and bone disease, *Human Nutrition and Dietetics*, 9th ed., (J.S. Garrow and W.P.T. James, eds.), Churchill Livingstone, Edinburgh, London, 1993, p. 556.
9. Smith, R., Disorders of the skeleton, *Oxford Textbook of Medicine*, 2nd ed. (D.J. Weatherall, J.G.G. Ledingham, and D.A. Warrell, eds.) Oxford University Press, Oxford, 1987, p. 1.
10. Stevenson, J.C., Osteoporosis: Pathogenesis and risk factor, *Bailliere's Clinical Endocrinology and Metabolism*, Vol. 2, No. 1 Metabolic Bone Disease (T.J. Martin, ed.), Bailliere Tindall, London, 1988, p. 87.
11. Lindsay, R., Management of Osteoporosis, *Bailliere's Clinical Endocrinology and Metabolism* (Vol. No. 1, 2). Metabolic Bone Disease (T.J. Martin, ed.) Bailliere Tindall, London, 1988, p. 103.
12. Eisman. J.A., Osteomalacia, *Bailliere's Clinical Endocrinology and Metabolism*, (Vol. No. 1, 2) Metabolic Bone Disease, Bailliere Tindall, London, 1988, p. 125.
13. Thakker, R.V., and J.L.H. O'Riordan, Inherited forms of rickets and osteomalacia, *Bailliere's Clinical Endocrinology and Metabolism* (Vo. No. 1, 2). *Metabolic Bone Disease*, Bailliere Tindall, London, 1988, p. 157.
14. Reichel, H., H.P. Koeffler, and A.W. Norman, The role of the vitamin D endocrine system in health and disease, *N. Engl. J. Med 3230*: 980 (1989).
15. Henderson, J.B., M.G. Dunnigan, and W.B. McIntosh, The importance of limited exposure to ultraviolet radiation and dietary factors in the aetiology of Asian rickets: a risk factor model, *Quart. J. Med. 63*: 413 (1987).
16. Holick, M.F., Photosynthesis of vitamin D in the skin: effect of environment and lifestyle variables, *Fed. Proc. 46*: 1876 (1987).

17. Webb, A.R., and M.F. Holick, The role of sunlight in the cutaneous production of vitamin D_3, *Ann. Rev. Nutr. 8*: 375 (1988).

18. Behrman, R.F., and V.C. Vaughan, *Nelson Textbook of Paediatric*, 13th ed., W.B. Saunders, Philadelphia, 1987.

19. Clements, M.R., L. Johnson, and D.R. Fraser, A new mechanism for induced vitamin D deficiency in calcium deprivation, *Nature 325*: 62 *(1987)*.

20. *Dunnigan, M. G., B. M. Glekin, J. B. Henderson, et al, Prevention of rickets in Asian children: assessment of Glasgow campaign, Br. Med. J. 291*: 239 (1985).

21. Kanis, J.A., T.F. Cundy, and N.A.T. Hamdy, Renal osteodystrophy, *Bailliere's Endocrinology and Metabolism* (Vol.No. 1,2) Metabolic Bone Disease (T.J. Martin, ed.), Bailliere Tindall, London, 1988, p. 193.

22. Shaw, J.C.L., Copper deficiency and non-accidental injury, *Arch. Dis. Childhood 63*: 448 (1988).

23. Mudd, S.H., and H.L. Levy, Disorders of transulfuration, *The Metabolic Basis of Inherited Disease* 4th ed. (J.B. Stanbury, J.B. Wyngaarden, and D.S. Fredrickson, eds.), McGraw-Hill, New York, 1978, p. 459.

24. Davis, M., and P.H. Adams, The continuing risk of vitamin D intoxication, *Lancet 2*: 621 (1978).

25. Stern, P.H., and N.H. Bell, Disorders of vitamin D metabolism—toxicity and hypersensitivity, *Metabolic Bone Disease: Cellular and Tissue Mechanisms* (C.S. Tam, J.N.M. Heersche, and T.M. Murrary, eds.) CRC Press, Boca Raton, 1989, p. 203.

26. Alfrey, A.C., Aluminum intoxication, *N. Engl. J. Med. 310*: 1113 (1984).

27. Nebeker, H.G., and J.W. Coburn, Aluminium and renal osteodystrophy, *Ann. Rev. Med. 37*: 79 (1986).

28. Andress, D.L., A.A. Maloney, J.W. Coburn, et al., Osteomalacia and aplastic bone disease in aluminium related osteodystrophy, *J. Clin. Endocrinol. Metab 65*: 11 (1987).

29. Kanis J.A., and R. Passmore, Calcium supplementation of the diet, *Br. Med. J. 298*: 137, 205 (1989).

30. Riggs, B.L., and L.J. Melton, *Osteoporosis: Aetiology, Diagnosis and Management*, Raven Press, New York, 1988.

31. Barrett-Conner, E., Postmenopausal oestrogen replacement and breast cancer, *N. Engl. J. Med. 321*: 319 (1989).

32. Seifert, M.F., and B.A. Watkins, Role of dietary lipid and antioxidants in bone metabolism, *Nutr. Res. 17*: 1209 (1997).

33. Hodsman, A.B., Diet in relation to osteoporosis, *Diet, Nutrition & Health* (K.K. Carroll, ed.), McGill-Queeris Univ. Press, London, 1989, p. 188.

34. Rugg-Gunn, A.J., Dietary factors in dental diseases, *Human Nutrition and Dietetics*, 9th ed. (J.S. Garrow and W.P.T. James, eds.), Churchill Livingstone, Edinburgh, London, 1993a, p. 567.

35. Rugg-Gunn, A.J., Diet and dental caries, *The Prevention of Dental Disease*, 2nd ed. (J.J. Murray, ed.), Oxford University Press, 1989, p. 4.

36. Rugg-Gunn, A.J., *Nutrition and Dental Health*, Oxford University Press, Oxford, 1993b.

37. Sreebny, L.M., Sugar availability, sugar consumption and dental caries, *Community Dentistry: Oral Epidemiol. 10*: 1 (1982).

38. Zitzow, R.E., The relationship of diet and dental caries in the Alaskan eskimo population, *Alaska Med. 212*: 10 (1979).

39. Moller, I.J., S. Poulson, and V. Orholm Nielsen, The prevalence of dental caries in Godhavn and Scoresbysund districts, Greenland, *Scand J. Dental Res. 80*: 168 (1972).

40. Sheiham, A., Changing trends in dental caries, *Int. Dental J. 13*: 142 (1984).

41. Fisher, F.J., A field study of dental caries, periodontal disease and enamel defects in Tristan da Cunha, *Br. Dental J. 125*: 447 (1968).

42. Harris, R., Biology of the children of Hopewood House, Bowral, Australia. 4. Observations on dental caries experience extending over 5 years (1957–61), *J. Dental Res. 42*: 1347 (1963).

43. Newbrun, E., *Cariology*, Williams & Wilkins, Baltimore, 1978.

44. Sognnaes, R.F., Analysis of wartime reduction of dental caries in European children, *Am. J. Dis. Childhood 75*: 792 (1948).

45. Takahashi, K., Statistical study on caries incidence in the first molar in relation to the amount of sugar consumption, *Bull. Tokyo Dental College 2*: 44 (1961).

46. Rugg-Gunn, A.J., A.F. Hackett, D.R. Appleton, G.N. Jenkins, and J.E. Eastoe, Relationship between dietary habits and caries increment assessed over two years in 405 English adolescent school children, *Arch Oral Biol. 29*: 983 (1984).

47. Gustaffson, B.E., C.E. Quensel, L.S. Lanke, et al., The Vipeholm dental caries study. The effect of different levels of carbohydrate intake on caries activity in 436 individuals observed for five years, *Acta Odontol. Scandinavica 11*: 232 (1954).

48. Scheinin, A., and K.K. Makinen, Turku sugar studies. I–XXI, *Acta Odontol. Scandinavica 33* (Suppl. 70): 1 (1975).

49. Kite, O.W., J.H. Shaw, and R.F. Sognnaes, The prevention of experimental tooth decay by tube-feeding, *J. Nutr. 42*: 89 (1950).

50. Konig, K.G., P. Schmid, and R. Schmid, An apparatus for frequency-controlled feeding of small rodents and its use in dental caries experiments, *Arch. Oral Biol. 13*: 13 (1968).

51. Huxley, H.G., The cariogenicity of dietary sucrose at various levels in two strains of rat under unrestricted and controlled frequency feeding conditions, *Caries Res. 11*: 232 (1977).

52. Hefti, A., and R. Schmid, Effect on caries incidence in rats of increasing dietary sucrose levels, *Caries Res. 13*: 298 (1979).

53. Guggenheim, B., K.G. Konig, E. Herzog, and H.R. Muhlemann, The cariogenicity of different dietary carbohydrates tested on rats in relative gnotobiosis with a streptococcus producing extracellular polysaccharide, *Helvetica Odontol. Acta 10*: 101 (1966).

54. Koulourides, T., R. Bodderi, S. Keller, L. Manson-Hing, J. Lastra, and T. Housch, Cariogenicity of nine sugars tested with an intraoral device in man, *Caries Res. 10*: 427 (1976).

55. Tehrani, A., F. Brude Vold, F. Attarzadeh, J. van Houte, and J. Russo, Enamel demineralization by mouthrinses containing different concentrations of sucrose, *J. Dental Res. 62*: 1216 (1983).

56. Rugg-Gunn, A.J., Starchy foods and fresh fruits: their relative importance as a source of dental caries in Britain: A review of the literature. Occasional paper No. 3, Health Education Authority, London, 1988.

57. Sreebny, L.M., Cereal availability and dental caries, *Community Dent. Oral Epidemiol. 11*: 148 (1983).

58. Nubrun, E., C. Hoover, G. Mettraux, and H. Graf, Comparison of dietary habits and dental health of subjects with hereditary fructose intolerance and control subjects, *J. Ani. Dental Assoc. 101*: 619 (1980).

59. Osborn, T.W.B., and J.N. Noriskin, The relationship between diet and dental caries in South African Bantu, *J. Dental Res. 16*: 431 (1937).

60. Edgar, W.M., and G.N. Jenkins. Solubility-reducing agents in honey and partially refined crystalline sugar, *Br. Dental J. 136*: 7 (1974).

61. Shannon, I.L., E.J. Edmonds, and K.O. Madsen, Honey: Sugar content and cariogenicity, *J. Dentistry Children 46*: 29 (1979).

62. Stralfors, A., Inhibition of hamster caries by cocoa, *Arch. Oral Biol. 11*: 323 (1966).

63. S-Gravenmade E.J., and G.N. Jenkins, Isolation, purification and some properties of a potential cariostatic factor in cocoa that lowers enamel. solubility, *Caries Res. 20*: 433 (1986).

64. Greenby, T.H., Summary of the dental effects of starch, *Int. J. Food Sci. Nutr. 48*: 411 (1997).

65. Rugg-Gunn, A.J., A.F. Hackett, D.R. Appleton, and P.J. Moynihan, The dietary intake of added and natural sugars in 405 English adolescents, *Human Nutr. Appl. Nutr. 40A*: 115 (1986).

66. Jenkins, G.N., and D.B. Ferguson, Milk and dental caries, *Br. Dental J. 120*: 472 (1966).

67. Bibby, B.G., C.T. Huang, D. Zero, S.A. Mundorff, and M.F. Little, Protective effect of milk against 'in vitro' caries, *J. Dental Res. 59*: 1556 (1980).

68. Thompson M.E., J.G. Dever, and E.I.F. Pearce, Intraoral testing of flavoured sweetened milk, *New Zealand Dental J. 80*: 44 (1984).

69. Reynolds, E.C., and I.H. Johnson, Effect of milk on caries incidence and bacterial composition of dental plaque in the rat, *Arch. Oral Biol. 26*: 445 (1981).

70. Hackett, A.F., A.J. Rugg-Gunn, J.J. Murray and G.J. Roberts, Can breast feeding cause dental caries? *Human Nutr Appl. Nutr. 38A*: 23 (1984).

71. Rugg-Gunn, A.J., W.M. Edgar, D.A.M. Geddes, and G.N. Jenkins. The effect of different meal patterns upon plaque pH in human subjects, *Br. Dental J. 139*: 351 (1975).

72. DeASilva, M.F., G.N. Jenkins, R.C. Burgess, and H.J. Sandham, Effects of cheese on experimental caries in human subects, *Caries Res. 20*: 263 (1986).

73. Edgar, W.M., W.H. Bowen, S. Amsbaugh, S. Monell-Torrens, and J. Brunelle, Effects of different eating patterns on dental caries in the rat, *Caries Res. 16*: 384 (1982).

74. Slack G.L., and W.J. Martin, Apples and dental health, *Br. Dental J. 105*: 366 (1958).

75. Reece J.A., and J.N. Swallow, Carrots and dental health, *Br. Dental J. 128*: 535 (1970).

76. Bibby, B.G., Fruits and vegetables and dental caries, *Clin. Preventive Dentistry 5*: 3 (1983).

77. Winter, G.B., Problems involved with the use of comforters, *Int. Dental J. 30*: 28 (1980).

78. Rugg-Gunn, A.J., and W.M. Edgar, Sweetners and dental health, *Comman Dental Health 2*: 213 (1985).

79. Russell, A.L., International nutritional surveys, a summary of preliminary dental findings, *J. Dental Res. 42*: 233 (1963).

80. Mellanby, M., The relation of caries to the structure of teeth, *Br. Dental J. 44*: 1 (1923).

81. Mellanby, M., The role of nutrition as a factor in resistance to dental caries, *Br. Dental J. 62*: 241 (1937).

82. Young, M., The role of nutrition as a factor in resistance to dental caries, *Br. Dental J. 62*: 252 (1937).

83. Dean, H.T., F.A. Arnold, and E. Elvolve, Domestic water and dental caries. (V), *Public Health Rep. 57*: 1155 (1942).

84. Ockerse, T., Relation of fluoride content, hardness and pH values of drinking water and incidence of dental caries, *South African Med. J. 18*: 255 (1944).

85. Murray J.J., A.J. Rugg-Gunn, and G.N. Jenkins, *Fluorides in Caries Prevention*, 3rd ed., Butterworth-Heinemann, Oxford, 1991.

86. Curzon, M.E.J., and T.W. Cutress, *Trace Elements and Dental Disease*, John Wright, Boston, 1983.

87. Asher, C., and M.J.F. Read, Early enamel erosion in children associated with excessive consumption of citric acid, *Br. Dental J. 162*: 384 (1987).

88. Eccles, J.D., Erosion affecting the palatal surfaces of upper anterior teeth in young people, *Br. Dental J. 152*: 375 (1982).

89. H.E.A., The scientific basis of dental health education: a policy statement, Health Education Authority, London, 1986.

90. Rugg-Gunn, A.J., Practical aspects of diet and dental caries in the elderly, *The Dental Annual* (D. Derrick, ed.), John Wright, Bristol, 1985, p. 159.

91. Oku, T. Special physiological functions of newly developed mono- and oligo-saccharides, *Functional Foods* (I. Goldberg, ed.) Chapman & Hall, New York, 1994, p. 202.

92. Oku, T. Oligosaccharides with beneficial health effects: A Japanese perspective, *Nutr. Rev. 54(5)*: 59 (1996).

93. Sicard, P.J., and Y. Le Bot, Manufacturing opportunities with non-sugar sweeteners, *Sugarless Towards the Year 2000*, Royal Society of Chemistry, 1994.

94. Elias, P.M., and M.L. Williams, Retinoid effects on epidermal differentiation, *Retinoids: New Trends in Research and Therapy* (J.H. Saurat, ed.), Karger, Basel, 1985, p. 138.

95. Saurat, J.H. (ed)., *Retinoids: 10 years on*, Karger, Basel, 1991.

96. Ramalingaswami, V., and H.M. Sinclair. The relation of deficiency of vitamin A and of essential fatty acids to follicular hyperkeratosis in the rat, *Br. J. Dermatol. 65*: 1 (1953).

97. Frain-Bell W., *Cutaneous Photobiology*, Oxford Medical Publications, Oxford Univ. Press, Oxford, 1985.

98. Bjelke, E., Dietary vitamin A and human lung cancer, *Int. J. Cancer 15*: 561 (1975).

99. Kragballe, K., B.T. Gjertsen, G.de Hoop, et al., Doubleblind, right/left comparison of calcipotriol and betamethasone valerate in treatment of psoriasis vulgaris, *Lancet 337*: 193 (1991).

100. Bartley, W.M., A. Krebs, and J.R.P O.Brien, Medical Research Council Special Report Series No. 280, HMSO, London, 1953.

101. Hodges, R.E., E.M. Baker, J. Hood, et al., Experimental scurvy in man, *Am. J. Nutr. 22*: 535 (1969).

102. Moore, R.A., T.D. Spies, and Z.K. Cooper, Histopathology of the skin in pellagra, *Arch. Dermatol. Syphiol., 46*: 100 (1942).

103. Sebrel, W.H., and R.E. Butler, Riboflavin deficiency in man: preliminary note, *Public Health Report No. 53*: 2282 (1938).

104. Mueller, J.F., R.W. Vilter, Pyridoxine deficiency in human beings induced with desoxypyridoxine, *J. Clin. Invest. 29*: 193 (1950).

105. Innis, S.M., and D.B. Allardyce, Possible biotin deficiency in adults receiving long-term parenteral nutrition, *Am. J. Clin. Nutr. 37*: 185 (1983).

106. Weismann, K., Zinc metabolism and the skin, *Recent Advances in Dermatology* (5) (A. Rook and J. Savin, eds.), Churchill Livingstone, Edinburgh, London, 1980, p. 109.

107. Greaves, M., and T.R.C. Boyd, Plasma zinc concentrations in patients with psoriasis, other dermatoses and venous leg ulceration, *Lancet 2*: 1019 (1967).

108. Moynahan, E.J., and P.M. Barnes, Zinc deficiency and a synthetic diet for lactose intolerance, *Lancet 1*: 676 (1973).

109. Cousins, R.J., and K.T. Smith, Zinc-binding properties of bovine and human milk in vitro: influence of changes in zinc content, *Am. J. Clin. Nutr. 33*: 1083 (1980).

110. Gartside. J.M., and B.R. Allen, Treatment of acrodermatitis with zinc sulphate. *Br. Med. J. 3*: 521 (1975).

111. Baer, M.T., J.C. King, T. Tamura, and S. Margen, Acne in zinc deficiency, *Arch. Dermatol. 114*: 1093 (1978).

112. Husain, S.C., Oral zinc sulphate in leg ulcers, *Lancet 2*: 1069 (1969).

113. Thomas, A.J., V.W. Bunker, L.J. Hinks, et al., Energy, protein, zinc and copper status of 21 elderly inpatients: analysed dietary intake and biochemical indices, *Br. J. Nutr. 59*: 181 (1988).

114. Dreizen, S., and B.M. Levy, *Handbook of Experimental Stomatology*, CRC Press, Boca Raton, Florida, 1981.

115. Milder, M.S., J.D. Cook, S. Stray, and C.A. Finch, Idiopathic hemochromatosis, an interim report, *Medicine 59*: 34 (1980).

116. Dean, G., *The Porphyrias: A Study of Inheritance and Environment*, 2nd ed. Pitman Medical, London, 1971.

117. Menkes, J.H., M. Alter, G.K. Steigleder, et al., A sexlinked recessive disorder with retardation of growth, peculiar hair and focal and cerebral and cerebellar degeneration, *Pediatrics 29*: 764 (1962).

118. Lott, I.T., R.D. Paolo, D. Schwartz, et al., Copper metabolism and steely hair syndrome, *N. Engl. J. Med. 292*: 197 (1975).

119. Gillespie, J.M., The isolation and properties of some soluble proteins from wool. VIII. The proteins of copper-deficient wool, *Aust. J. Biol. Sci. 17*: 282 (1964).

120. Bennani-Smiers, C.J. Medina, and L.W. Young, Infantile nutritional copper deficiency, *Am. J. Dis. Childhood 134*: 1155 (1980).

121. Doisy E.A., Manganese homeostasis in humans and its role in disease states. *Essential and Toxic Trace Elements in Human Health and Disease* (A.S. Prasad, ed.) Alan R. Riss, New York, 1972, p. 253.

122. Kein, C.L., and H.E. Ganther, Manifestations of chronic selenium deficiency in a child receiving total parenteral nutrition, *Am. J. Clin. Nutr. 37*: 319 (1983).

123. Reilly, C., Selenium: A new entrant into the functional food arena, *Trends Food Sci. Technol. 9*: 114 (1998).

124. Allen, B.R., M.R. Moore, and J.A. A. Hunter, Lead and skin, *Br. J. Dermatol. 92*: 715 (1975).

125. Gesterner, H., and J. Huff, Clinical toxicology of mercury, *J. Toxicol. Environ. Health. 2*: 491 (1977).

126. Basnayake, V., and H.M. Sinclair. The effect of deficiency of essential fatty acids upon the skin, *Biochemical Problems of Lipids* (G. Popjak and E. LeBreton, eds.), Butterworths, London, 1956.

127. Ziboh, V.A., and R.S. Chapkin, Biologic significance of polyunsaturated fatty acids in the skin, *Arch. Dermatol. 123*: 1686 (1987).

128. Landmann, L., The epidermal permeability barrier, *Anatomy & Embryol. 178*: 1 (1975).

129. Elias, P.M., and B.E. Brown, The mammalian cutaneous permeability barrier: defective barrier function in essential fatty acid deficiency correlates with the abnormal intercellular lipid deposition, *Laboratory Invest. 39*: 574 (1978).

130. Prottey, C., Essential fatty acids and the skin, *Br. J. Dermatol. 94*: 579 (1976).

131. Prottey, C., P.J. Hartop, and M. Press, Correction of the cutaneous manifestations of essential fatty acid deficiency in man by the application of sunflower seed oil to the skin, *J. Invest. Dermatol. 64*: 228 (1975).

132. Ziboh, V.A., and S.L. Hsia, Effects of prostaglandin E$_2$ on rat skin: inhibition of sterol ester biosynthesis and clearing of scaly lesions in essential fatty acid deficiency, *J. Lipid Res. 13*: 458 (1972).

133. Camp, R.D.R., Role of arachidonic acid metabolism in psoriasis and other skin diseases, *New Perspectives in Anti-Inflammatory Therapies. Adv. in Inflammation Res.* Vol. 12 (A. Lewis, N. Ackerman, and I. Offernes, eds.), Raven Press, New York, 1988, p. 163.

134. Kromann, N., and A. Green, Epidemiological studies in the Uppernarvik district of Greenland, *Acta Medica Scandinavica 200*: 401 (1980).

135. Ziboh, V.A., K.A. Cohen, C.N. Ellis, et al., Effects of dietary supplementation with fish oil on neutrophil and epidermal fatty acids, *Arch. Dermatol. 122*: 1277 (1986).

136. Maurice, D.D., P.C. Bather, and B.R. Allen, Arachidonic acid metabolism by polymorphonuclear leukocytes in psoriasis, *Br. J. Dermatol. 114*: 57 (1986).

137. Bittiner, S.B., W.F.G. Tucker, I. Cartwright, et al., A double blind, randomised, placebo-controlled trial of fish oil in psoriasis, *Lancet 1*: 378 (1988).

138. Lessof, M.H., D.G. Wraith, and T.G. Merrett, Food allergy and intolerance in 100 patients local systemic effects, *Quart. J. Med. 195*: 259 (1980).

139. Halperen, S.R., W.A. Sellars, R.B. Johnson, et al., Development of childhood allergy in infants fed breast, soy or cow's milk, *J. Allergy Clin. Immunol. 51*: 139 (1973).

140. Allen, B.R., Role of diet in treating atopic eczema: dietary manipulation has no value, *Br. Med. J. 297*: 1459 (1988).

141. Bonifazi, E., L. Garofalo, A. Monterisis, and C.L. Meneghini, History of food allergy, RAST and challenge tests in atopic dermatitis, *Acta Dermatol. Venereol. 92*: 91 (1980).

142. Shuster, S., A.J. Watson, and J. Marks, Coeliac syndrome in dermatitis herpetiformis, *Lancet 1*: 1101 (1968).

28
Diet and Diseases of the Liver and Kidneys

I. INTRODUCTION

The liver is a vitally important organ of the human body, constituting about 5% of the body weight in the infant, and 3% in the adult; it receives around 28% of the total blood flow and consumes 20% of the oxygen used by the body (1). The liver performs special functions as a guardian interposed between the digestive tract and rest of the body. Absorbed dietary nutrients of the diet pass directly to the liver via the portal blood system or through the lymphatic system (long-chain fatty acids). The liver handles nutrients such as carbohydrates, amino acids, fats, vitamins, and minerals as well as toxic pollutants such as alkaloids, xenobiotics, endotoxins, and all other potentially harmful antinutrients of the diet. These are stored, metabolized, and excreted by the liver into the blood or bile. The liver also has an important role in the synthesis of specialized transport proteins of the blood plasma and those needed to maintain the integrity of the circulation, e.g., blood clotting factors.

The kidney is the primary organ of excretion, especially for small water-soluble, non–protein-bound molecules, whereas the liver removes and excretes lipid-soluble, protein-bound, and other longer molecules that must be catabolized to smaller water-soluble products prior to their excretion. The kidneys maintain many aspects of the internal chemical environment of the body by removing waste products of nitrogen metabolism, such as urea, uric acid, and creatinine, as well as hydrogen ions and sulfates arising from the degradation of sulfur-containing amino acids and surplus quantities of water, sodium, potassium, phosphate, magnesium, chloride, and other ions. The liver, in contrast, serves to metabolize endogenous hormones, metabolic end-products such as bilirubin and urea, and tissue breakdown products as well as dietary pollutants.

As a major guardian of the body, the liver's sinusoidal lining cells have considerable pinocytic and phagocytic activity (2). Thus, the liver is the most important site for removing solid foreign material such as bacteria and their endotoxins absorbed from intestine. It is also a principal site for the coordination of the integrated metabolic changes occurring in response to infection, trauma, or injury (acute-phase response). Thus, both the liver and kidney play a central role in almost every aspect of nutrition and of the excretion of toxicants and the body's waste products. They also function together in the activation of vitamin D. Whereas 25 –(OH) D is formed in the liver, it is converted by the tubular cells of the kidney to 1, 25 $(OH)_2$ D_3, the most active form of vitamin D.

II. DIET, NUTRITION, AND LIVER DISEASES

A. Carbohydrate Status During Liver Disease

Normal glucose homeostasis can be maintained with even about 20% of the normal hepatic parenchymal mass and the normal kidney can synthesize glucose (gluconeogenesis) when the liver is diseased, with no significant hypoglycemia. The latter, may, however, occur in fulminant hepatic failure, or secondary to toxic overdose of drugs such as acetaminophen or alcohol.

Patients with cirrhosis of the liver often have glucose intolerance that is more marked after an oral rather than an intravenous load. Advanced liver disease is characterized by high insulin levels due to reduced hepatic uptake, and fasting glucagon levels are 2 to 3 times higher than normal (3) and do not decrease in response to glucose. Levels of growth hormone, 90% of which is cleared by the liver, are also markedly raised during liver abnormalities and fail to be suppressed by feeding (4). High growth hormone levels do not stimulate the liver to produce more insulin-like growth factors (IGF-I); indeed, their levels in liver disease are subnormal (5). Also, basal somatostatin levels are raised and may increase further after meals (6).

Lactic acidosis results in liver disease due to an increase in fasting blood gluconeogenic precursors and decreased capacity for gluconeogenesis (7). Approximately 60% of patients with lactic acidosis are prone to liver disease (8). Lactic acidosis may be precipitated by feeding fructose, sorbitol, or ethanol (9).

Liver disease influences several other hormones in addition to those related to carbohydrate metabolism, e.g., prolactin and thyroid-stimulating hormone increase, whereas pituitary hormones such as gonadotropins, FSH, and LH are not affected. However, there is an increase in T4 and reverse T3 levels, with a decrease in the active hormone T3 (10–12). In humans, circulating T4 is converted to T3 mainly in the liver by the selenium-containing enzyme thyroxin 5′ deiodinase I. Liver abnormalities are accompanied by decreased activity of this enzyme, accounting for the observed changes.

Gross changes in sex hormones in liver disease include about an eight-fold increase in sex-hormone–binding globulin, with 50% reduction in testosterone and a universal decrease in free testosterone. Also, there is a marked increase in the conversion rate of the weak androgen androstenedione to estrone and estradiol by the liver. Young athletes who abuse anabolic steroids may experience benign hepatic tumors (adenomas) and occasionally hepatocarcinoma, especially when exogenous 17 alpha-alkylated androgens lead to dilation of the biliary canaliculi, loss of villi, and decreased excretion of bromosulphalein and organic anions (13). These changes, including those related to adenomas, are revessible on stopping the steroids.

B.   Changes in Osmolality and Blood Coagulation

Parenchymal hepatic disease is manifested as impaired renal handling of sodium (14). This abnormality is mainly of sodium, and not water, metabolism. Most patients excrete urine of low osmolality when given excess water, and when sodium is given it is retained (15). Liver disease is thought to be characterized by decreased effective blood volume, with a reduced albumin concentration and diminished peripheral vascular resistance, due to both anatomic arteriovenous shunts and an undefined circulating vasodilator. Under these circumstances, renal retention of sodium is seen as a secondary event. Lieberman et al. (16) proposed that liver disease is characterized by inappropriate sodium retention by the kidney and an increase in total plasma volume.

The liver synthesizes most of the blood coagulation factors, such as antithrombin III. Bleeding is a common problem in patients with malabsorption of fat-soluble vitamins due to reduced bile salts. Patients with hepatitis and cirrhosis are not able to carboxylate the vitamin K–dependent clotting factors, even after vitamin K supplcments (17). In liver disease, portal hypertension appears to affect platelet number and function significantly. Thus, decreased platelets, clotting factors, and increased fibrinolysis due to decreased clearance of plasminogen activators lead to bleeding disorder in liver disease (2).

C. Metabolism of Vitamins A and D in Liver Disease

The liver stores around 90% of the body's store of retinyl esters. Liver parenchymal cells take up chylomicron remnants and retinyl esters, and they also synthesize retinol-binding protein (RBP). These cells are thus responsible for the mobilization of retinol from the liver. However, nearly all the vitamin A in the liver is transferred to specialized cells localized in the perisinusoidal space where vitamin A is principally stored (Ito or stellate cells or fat-storing cells). Retinol bound to RBP is released from the liver; it then binds to transthyretin (prealbumin), which also binds the thyroid hormones. In liver disease, the levels of retinol, RBP, and transthyretin decrease considerably. Affected patients often show abnormal dark adaptation (18).

Osteodystrophy may deveop in patients with a variety of liver diseases affecting the main hepatic cells (parenchymal liver disease) as well as obstructive cholestatic jaundice (19,20). Children with liver disease show retarded growth with adversely affected bone metabolism. In cholestatic disease, bite salt deficiency with malabsorption of vitamins D and K and fat predominates. The unabsorbed fat forms insoluble calcium soaps in the intestine, the degree of calcium malabsorption being directly related to the degree of steatorrhea (21). Many patients with this type of liver disease have osteomalacia, which responds to vitamin D therapy (22). However, some patients with long-standing intrahepatic cholestasis with osteoporosis-like syndrome may not respond to vitamin D (20).

The liver converts vitamin D to its first metabolite, 25-hydroxy cholecalciferol, which in turn forms the precursor for its second hydroxylation in the kidney to the active hormone 1.25-dihydroxycholecalciferol.

Cholestasis or drugs such as cimetidine can experimentally decrease the activity of the hepatic 25-hydroxylase enzyme. Subnormal levels of 24, 25-dihydroxy vitamin D, also produced by the kidney, have been found in patients with normal levels of 25-hydroxy vitamin D and 1,25-dihydroxy vitamin D, indicating that the control of vitamin D metabolite formation may be defective in some forms of liver disease (23). The bone disease may complicate liver disease in the absence of vitamin D deficiency and with adequate levels of 25-hydroxy vitamin D. The bone loss may produce frequent severe spontaneous fractures, especially of the axial skeleton. Skeletal abnormalities may involve secondary hyperparathyroidism (24), liver being more closely involved in the peripheral metabolism of parathyroid hormone into biologically active metabolites (25). In both children and adults, the decreased production of stomatomedin (IGF-I) may have profound effects on growth and maintenance of skeletal mass (5,26).

D. Water-soluble (B-Group) Vitamins and Liver Disease

The adult liver, which weighs about 2 kg, serves as a store of riboflavin, niacin, folate, cobalamin (B_{12}), and pantothenic acid, and contains between 10 and 200 times the RNI values (Table 1). However, thiamin and vitamin B_6 are not preferentially stored in the liver. Liver disease can be expected to be associated with vitamin deficiency, especially those vitamins for which liver is the major repository in the body (2). Baker et al. (27) in an extensive study of patients with mild fatty liver, severe fatty liver, and cirrhosis, as compared to biopsies from normal subjects, found decreased levels of most of B-group vitamins (Table 2)

Patients with cirrhosis do not have reduced levels of thiamin, nor does the lack of dietary thiamin impair the liver's pentose phosphate pathway, although development of fatty liver does reduce the liver's thiamin content (Table 2) (28). Thiamin deficiency, which is not common in other forms of liver disease, is often seen in alcoholic liver disease (29).

Deficiency of riboflavin leads to accumulation of triglycerides in the liver (30) decreased

Table 1 Vitamin (B Group) Content of Tissues in Relation to the RDAs of Adults

Vitamin	RNI Female (mg/day)	RNI Male (mg/day)	Liver (mg/kg)	Kidney (mg/kg)	Heart (mg/kg)	Muscle (mg/kg)	Brain (mg/kg)	Whole body (mg/kg)
Thiamin	0.4	0.4	2.2	2.8	3.6	1.2	1.6	0.02–0.08
Riboflavin	1.1	1.3	16.0	20.0	8.0	2.0	2.5	0.1–0.5
Nicotinic acid	13	17	58	37	41	47	20	3–7
B_6	1.4	1.2	2.5	1.1	0.8	0.9	0.7	0.03–0.08
B_{12}	1.5[b]	1.5[b]	500[b]	200[b]	—	8[b]	10[b]	0.2–0.8[b]
Folate	0.2	0.2	9.5	2.1	1.0	0.8	1.1	0.005–0.020
Biotin	0.2	0.2	0.7	0.7	0.2	0.004	0.6	0.0002–0.0005
Pantothenic acid	3–7	3–7	43	19	16	12	15	0.15–0.50

[a]Quantities are expressed in mg/kg wet weight.   RNI = UK-recommended nutrient intake.
[b]Quantities are in micrograms.   — = Not known.
Source: Ref. 2.

Table 2 Hepatic Levels of Water-Soluble Vitamins in Liver Disease

Vitamins (µg/g)	Normal biopsy	Normal autopsy	Steatosis Mild	Steatosis Severe	Cirrhosis
Vitamin B_{12}	1.7	1.6	1.2	0.34	0.45
Folic acid	11.2	9.8	6.7	3.0	3.1
Folinic acid	3.9	3.8	3.2	1.8	1.7
Vitamin B_6	12.4	9.7	4.6	1.6	3.7
Thiamin	8.8	7.3	2.8	1.7	7.7
Nicotinic acid	144	125	89	21	24
Biotin	386	405	76	27	222
Pantothenic acid	62	59	52	23	25

Source: Ref. 27.

fatty acid dehydrogenation, and diminished levels of linoleic, linolenic, and arachidonic acids (31). Patients with chronic alcoholism show frequent evidence of riboflavin deficiency (32), with accumulation of liver fat. Stanko et al. (33) showed that riboflavin administration to alcoholic rats can experimentally reverse the accumulation of free fatty acids and esterified fat, although there is no such evidence in humans.

There is a marked reduction in the hepatic concentration of nicotinic acid in cases of alcoholism and cirrhosis, and as with riboflavin, niacin treatment can prevent the increase in liver lipid caused by alcoholism (34). This is ascribed to the inhibition of the peripheral release of free fatty acid and inhibitory action of niacin on liver alcohol dehydrogenase. Both riboflavin and niacin are required for the maintenance of reduced glutathione in the liver, and thus to protect the liver against oxidative stress.

Although the liver does not store pyridoxine (B_6), it is intimately involved in its metabolism, because it plays an important role in the conversion of pyridoxine to pyridoxal and pyridoxal phosphate, more active forms of B_6 used by other tissues. Intravenous injections of pyridoxine substantially raise the plasma levels of vitamin B_6 in healthy individuals, but there is little or no rise in patients with hepatits, cirrhosis, or cholestasis (35). Unlike pyridoxal phosphate, plasma levels of pyridoxal itself appear to be raised in cirrhosis (36), indicating that there is more rapid dephosphorylation of pyridoxal phosphate in liver disease. It has been estimated that around 30% to 50% of alcoholics without liver damage and 80% to 100% of alcoholics with liver damage may have vitamin B_6 deficiency.

Leevy et al. (37) reported an approximately 60% decrease in total liver folic acid content in alcoholics. Chronic alcoholics given a low-folate diet may develop megaloblastic changes within about 5 weeks, whereas healthy people given a folate-free diet may take about 22 weeks to develop similar changes (38). Alpers et al. (39) also noted that ingestion of about 80 g of alcohol per day was associated with low serum folate and megaloblastic changes in about 80% of subjects. In addition to that seen in alcoholics, folate deficiency commonly occurs in other forms of liver disease, and an onset of viral hepatitis may be associated with an excessive excretion of urinary folic acid (40).

Deficiency of cobalamin (B_{12}) is not common in liver disease, unless it is complicated by gastric or ileal dysfunction. Acute liver damage will cause a release of vitamin B_{12}, the increase in serum levels of B_{12} being directly proportional to the liver damage (41). Whereas patients with acute hepatitis have an increase in free B_{12}, bound B_{12} increases in patients with chronic disease because of the increase in the plasma concentration of the trans cobalamins (viz., transcobalamin-I) (42), so that vitamin B_{12} passes from the liver to the plasma. The major circulating form of vitamin B_{12} in healthy subjects is methyl-cobalamin, which is metabolized to 5-deoxy-adenosyl-cobalamin in the plasma of patients with liver disease (2).

E. Copper and Iron Nutrition in Liver Disease

The liver stores copper in the form of metallothionein, the excessive copper being excreted in the bile. Copper may accumulate in the liver in diseases in which there is excessive copper absorption or in which copper cannot be excreted adequately, increasing hepatic copper levels considerably (Table 3). The uncomplexed copper undergoes a redox cycle between its cuprous and cupric states in the presence of reducing equivalents, and this one-electron redox cycle can be very damaging because each cycle gives rise to a free radical. When copper accumulates to a level where it cannot be tightly bound to metallothionein, the resultant free radical damage leads to liver damage and cirrhosis. In Wilson's disease, there is a congenital defect in the export of cop-

Table 3 Hepatic Copper Levels in Various Liver Diseases

Condition	Liver copper (µg/g dry wt.)
Normal	
Healthy adult	9–17
Fetus	80–146
Newborn baby	206–413
Pathological	
Wilson's disease	152–1828
Childhood cholestasis	52–1082
Primary biliary cirrhosis	29–1008
Extrahepatic biliary obstruction	111–226
Indian childhood cirrhosis	1367–4788
Idiopathic copper toxicosis	708–3255

Source: Ref. 2.

per from liver to the plasma, leading to its accumulation, whereas in Indian cirrhosis there is excessive absorption of copper metabolized from the brass jugs used to store milk. In biliary disease, the patient is not able to excrete copper in the bile, exacerbating the cirrhosis (2).

Approximately 10% of the body's iron is present in the liver as protein ferritin. The liver also secretes the iron-transporting protein, transferrin, which has a very high affinity for iron, thus preventing iron from undergoing redox cycling and depriving the invading organisms of the required iron. Iron is primarily maintained in the ferric state, bound to transferrin by the plasma ferroxidase, ceruloplasmin. Cells and tissues requiring iron use specific receptors, binding transferrin to make the iron available.

Although the liver is spared any serious ill-effects of iron-deficiency, it is vulnerable to disorders of iron overload, because, like copper, iron undergoes a redox cycle between its ferrous and ferric states, giving rise to radical injury if it is not tightly bound and kept in the ferric state. Free radical damage may occur when the binding proteins are saturated or powerful reductants are available. Excessive use of vitamin C (ascorbic acid), normally thought to be without any side effects, may exacerbate the condition of patients with iron overload. The latter may occur either due to increased iron absorption or through multiple blood transfusions.

Hemochromatosis, an inherited disease is characterized by an excessive absorption of iron, which is deposited in the liver parenchyma. Similarly, absence of transferrin is a rare human disorder (atransferrinemia) in which the liver takes up but does not release the administered iron (43).

Zellweger syndrome, once thought to be a variant of hemochromatosis, is characterized by wider spread iron deposition in the body and is caused by the absence of peroxisomes (44). It is not known in what way peroxisomes are required for normal iron metabolism in the body. Kwashiorkar is also characterized by an absence of peroxisomes (45) and an accumulation of iron in the liver (46).

Hepatic iron overload is frequently encountered in alcoholic cirrhosis; about 7% of patients experience severe siderosis that mimics hemochromatosis (47). Also, most patients who suffer from porphyria cutania tarda have hepatic siderosis with elevated serum iron levels (48).

In addition to blood transfusional iron overloads, which causes iron accumulation in the Kupffer cells, dietary iron overload has been reported in the South African Bantu, who brew sorghum beer in empty iron drums, resulting in high levels of bioavailable iron that leads to siderosis in those who drink such beer. In this form of siderosis, the iron is reticuloendothelial, whereas in experimental dietary iron overloads the iron is parenchymal; this indicates that the iron in Bantu siderosis is absorbed in a form that is not associated with transferrin transport to the liver parenchyma, perhaps due to the yeast siderophores present in the beer. The abnormal iron distribution may also be related to concurrent vitamin C deficiency (49).

Deshpande et al. (50) recently studied the protective effect of turmeric extract (TE) in diet on carbon tetrachloride (CCl_4)-induced liver damage in rats. Rats were divided into five groups: (a) untreated, (b) CCl_4-treated, (c) pre-TE for 2 weeks followed by CCl_4, (d) TE+CCl_4 given concurrently, and (e) 5% TE as positive control. The serum levels of bilirubin, cholesterol, aspartate aminotransferase (AST), alanine amino transferase (ALT), and alkaline phosphatase (AP) were estimated after 1, 2, and 3 months. CCl_4 caused a maximum increase (two to threefold) in all above parameters. As compared with the CCl_4 group, the group receiving a short pretreatment of TE showed reduction in cholesterol, bilirubin, AST, ALT, and AP activity; concurrent treatment of TE + CCl_4 reduced to a greater extent the levels of all parameters, except ALT. It was concluded that concurrent treatment of TE provided a significant protection against CCl_4, though the values did not reach normal levels (50).

Although the normal liver has considerable ability to regenerate, advanced liver disease can significantly reduce this ability. According to Corish (51), in compensated liver disease all efforts should be made to maintain nutrition status. In decompensated liver disease, symptoms of decompensation may require therapeutic dietetic intervention. Early nutrition assessment and dietetic intervention in the management of malnutrition, ascites, encephalopathy, and esophageal varices are mandatory and have shown reduced morbidity and mortality in these patients.

Nutrient intake, weight changes, appetite, nausea, diarrhea or steatorrhea, and biochemical measurements of vitamin and mineral levels can all provide information that can form the basis for a treatment plan. Across-the-board enforced restrictions of protein, fat, and sodium may adversely affect overall nutrient intake.

A patient with liver disease is already at risk of infection and malnutrition and should not be prescribed a diet that could result in long-term negative nitrogen balance. With the use of lactulose to maintain regular bowel function, a protein intake of 1.0 to 1.5 g/kg/day should be encouraged (52,53). Kearns et al. (54) reported that resolution of encephalopathy in a group of patients with alcoholic liver disease who were aggressively fed via nasogastric tube was significantly faster than the group of control patients given oral diet and nutrition supplements. Restriction of dietary fat is justifiable only in patients with symptomatic steatorrhea. Restriction in fat intake is rarely needed.

A diet very low in sodium helps to resolve ascites more quickly than a less strict salt restriction. However, this should not be instituted at the expense of overall nutritional status. A diet containing approximately 40 mmols Na$^+$ is appropriate for patients at home. Fluid restriction is generally required only when serum sodium falls below 125 mmol/liter. Restriction can vary from 500 to 1500 ml, which can severely limit nutrition support. Patients need to be educated in managing their fluid restriction and encouraged not to "waste" their fluid allotment on low-calorie beverages (51). Corish (51) recommended the following amounts of nutrients for patients with liver disease:

1. Energy intake should be 1.2 to 1.4 times basal energy expenditure.
2. Proteins should be consumed at the rate of 1.0 to 1.5 g/kg body wt.
3. Sodium and fluid are to be restricted in accordance with the patient's clinical condition and electrolyte status.
4. Nutrition requirements should be met orally with the use of nutrition supplements as appropriate or enterally via a fine-bore feeding tube. Peripheral and total parenteral nutrition should be used only as a last choice when gut failure exists.
5. It is imperative that all patients have early nutrition assessment and regular monitoring of their nutrition status.

Reuter et al. (55) have reviewed the antihepatotoxic effects of garlic in animals. Adequate liver protection by several defined constituents of garlic was shown with freshly prepared rat hepatocytes treated with carbon tetrachloride, a strong liver toxicant. At the concentration of 0.5 µg/ml, S-allylcysteine completely neutralized cytotoxicity. Allicin was also effective (56).

According to Huh et al. (57), two enzymes that control the detoxification of xenobiotic agents in rat liver, viz., glutathione-S-transferase and glutathione peroxidase, are activated by pressed garlic juice.

Kagawa et al. (58) gave garlic extract 6 hours after liver poisoning with carbon tetrachloride at doses of 10, 100, and 500 mg/kg and vitamin E (25 mg/kg) as a positive control. The high amount of lipid peroxides and accumulation of triglycerides in the liver observed in the afflicted animals was significantly decreased in animals treated with garlic extract. Vitamin E inhibited lipid peroxidation but not fat deposition.

According to recent reports, S-allylcysteine and S-allylmercaptocysteine, which are proposed to be the main active constituents of an aged garlic extract, are also effective in controlling hepatopathy and liver damage induced by hepatotoxins during acute hepatitis (59–62).

The antitoxic effects of garlic can also be tested by using a model in which the pathologic change in organs of rats poisoned by cadmium is tested. Lee and associates fed rats 100 ppm Cd with or without garlic addition (6.67%) in the feed over a 12-week period. The group fed with garlic had significantly fewer lesions in the testes, liver, and kidneys. It was suggested that certain components of garlic chelated the metal (63,64). Park and Cha (65) noticed a similar detoxifying effect of garlic in rats exposed to methyl mercuric acetate (66).

Fields et al. (66) ascertained whether a reduction in hepatic lipogenesis would be beneficial to ameliorate copper deficiency. Garlic oil extract was found to ameliorate the severity of copper deficiency, although hepatic lipogenesis was not influenced. Huh and associates noted that activities of hydroxylase, glutathione peroxidase, and the hepatic xanthine oxidase were enhanced by the constituents of garlic oil (diallyl disulfide) (67–69).

II. ROLE OF DIET IN GALLSTONE FORMATION

Gallstones (cholelithiasis) or biliary calculi is the most common disease of bile and gallbladder. Calculi form within the gallbladder and usually stay there, in which case they generally do not cause problems. Why some stones cause symptoms and others do not is not known, and there is no relation to size, shape, density, number, or composition of gallstones. Most gallstones occur in multiple numbers and may be up to 2 cm in diameter and grow at the rate of about 1 to 2 mm per year (2).

Gallstones may be rich in cholesterol (more than 70% w/w), as found in industrially developed societies, and they may also contain calcium salts, mainly carbonate, phosphate, palmitate, or bilirubinate. The proportion of calcuim-rich stones increases with patient age.

A. Cholesterol-rich Gallstones

Pathogenesis of cholesterol-rich gallstones involves both physical and chemical factors (70). Three major factors include supersaturation of the bile with cholesterol, imbalance of nucleating and antinucleating factors, and stasis within the gallbladder. Diet and nutrition appear to influence these factors.

Bile is supersaturated when its cholesterol content exceeds its ability, at equilibrium, to suspend cholesterol in mixed micelles (4–8 nm), stable particles in which discs of a phospholipid cholesterol bilayer are surrounded by a negatively charged ring of bile acids. In addition, there are other cholesterol carriers in bile, viz., 40 to 80 nm unilamellar vesicles containing phspholipid and cholesterol. When the cholesterol content of these metastable vesicles rises too high, they fuse and form large, unstable, multilamellar vesicles (liquid crystals). When nucleating factors are dominant, these liquid crystals turn into crystals of cholesterol. The latter then turn into macroscopic stones in the presence of mucus to trap the crystals and glue them together. Biliary sludge is an early stage in this process; it may disappear, stay the same, or turn into one or more stones (2).

Epidemiological studies have shown that gallstones are common in all industrially developed countries, women being affected twice as often as men; the prevalence of gallstones rises with age to a peak of 30% to 60% in elderly women (71,72). According to Jensen and Jorgensen (73), about one in 150 people among the middle aged may develop gallstones each year. Gallstones have been rarely noted in the rural areas of developing countries but have been more common in Europe in the past 100 years.

Although genetic factors are involved, as shown by family incidence and twin studies (74,75), environmental factors seem to be preeminent; e.g., in the United Kingdom, gallstones are one-half as common as expected in vegetarians (76). Genetic susceptibility and unfavorable environment appear to combine in North American Indians to give them the highest prevalence of gallstones in the world; about 70% of young Pima women have gallstones by the age of 30 years (77).

Golden and Heaton (2) listed the following conditions and treatments that are associated with gallstones, obesity and hypertriglyceridemia being the most important that operate through hypersecretion of cholesterol into the bile. However, other conditions such as liver cirrhosis and resection or terminal ileum disease may operate through hyposecretion of bile salts. Constipation may alter the composition of the bile salt pool. Multiparity, abdominal surgery, and treatment with total parenteral nutrition and octreotide may be factors in gallbladder stasis. Hormonal treatments with estrogens, progestogens, and fibrates cause hypersecretion of cholesterol and gallbladder bile to become supersaturated with cholesterol, leading to the lithogenic process.

B. Diet, Obesity, and Gallstones

In a huge prospective study in American nurses, MacLure et al. (78) noted a close association between obesity (weight gain since maturity) and the risk of gallstones; thinness protects against the disease. Teenage girls rarely develop gallstones, and those who do are nearly always obese (79). Scragg et al. (80) reported that obesity is not a risk factor in older people (above 50 years), at least not in men, when obesity is expressed as body mass index. On the contrary, abdominal obesity, measured as a raised waist-hip circumference ratio, is a risk factor in both men and women (81,82). Obesity perhaps operates through associated metabolic disturbances, especially insulin resistance and hyperinsulinemia, which are in turn associated more with abdominal than with general obesity. Lack of physical exercise or loss of muscularity may also be a risk factor, because unfitness has similar metabolic penalties as obesity (83), and men who develop a paunch are more prone to develop gallstones, even if they are not obese (81).

Insulin is most probably involved in the pathogenesis of cholesterol-rich gallstones, besides its link with obesity and abdominal fat, because hypertriglyceridemia is strongly associated with gallstones, independent of obesity (84), and also with supersaturated bile (85). Laakso et al. (86) noted that plasma triglycerides co-vary with plasma insulin levels.

Adult-onset diabetics who are treated with insulin have bile that is more saturated with cholesterol (87). Insulin promotes the secretion of cholesterol into bile by activating the receptors on liver cells, which enables LDL cholesterol to be transferred from blood into bile (88). Insulin also seems to activate the rate-limiting enzyme for cholesterol synthesis (89). According to Heaton et al. (81), plasma insulin tends to be high in people with gallstones, both in the fasting state and after meals. The insulin hypothesis thus explains why gallstones are related to obesity, especially abdominal obesity, and to hypertriglyceridemia. A moderate intake of alcohol seems to protect against gallstones (90). Alcohol also makes people more sensitive to insulin so that their fasting level is lower (91).

A substantial amount of cholesterol (300–500 mg/day) is metabolized to bile acids, which are excreted into the bile, holding cholesterol in solution. Like dietary cholesterol, biliary cholesterol is also poorly absorbed in the small intestine, but the bile acids, chenodeoxycholic and cholic acid, are readily absorbed by passive diffusion by the small intestine. This bile acid pool recycles about 20 times per day. Bile acids escaping intestinal absorption enter the colon, where they are metabolized by anerobic bacteria, which convert cholate to deoxycholate in the cecum. Because the colon has no special transport system for absorbing bile salts (unlike the ileum), deoxycholate (DCA) is absorbed slowly and incompletely. With slowing down of colonic transit time, more DCA is absorbed, expanding its circulating pool (92). The latter leads to gallstone formation because the more DCA there is in bile, the more the bile is likely to precipitate cholesterol, increasing the risk of gallstones (93). In otherwise healthy subjects, constipation, at least in nonobsese people, seems to promote gallstones (94). Thus, anything, dietary or otherwise, that promotes colonic stasis is likely to increase the risk of gallstones (2). The bacterial formation of DCA is pH-dependent, so at pH values below 6.0, the enzyme 7-alphadehydroxylase, which catalyzes formation of DCA, is inhibited. When bacteria in the colon ferment carbohydrates to short-chain fatty acids, the pH tends to be lower. Thus, anything that increases the concentration of short-chain fatty acids in the colon will reduce the risk of gallstones by reducing biliary DCA levels (2).

C. Diet, Lifestyle, and Gallstones

Diet and eating habits may promote gallstones in many ways. Younger women with gallstones tend to have a longer overnight fast than control subjects matched for body mass index (95) that favors gallstone formation. Fasting induces gallbladder stasis, allowing time for the formation and growth of cholesterol crystals. As an overnight fast lengthens, the bile in the gallbladder increases, thus the bile becomes more saturated with cholesterol (96).

Overeating also appears to be a key factor in gallstone formation, as indicated by its link with obesity. Some case control studies have indicated higher energy intakes in people with gallstones than in controls, whereas most other studies have not shown such a relationship (80,97). In one well-conducted case-control study, Scragg et al. (80) found that high energy was associated with gallstones in women up to 49 years, but not in older women or men. None of these studies assessed energy output and they used crude methods for assessing energy intake. Energy imbalance is possibly a factor in people of all ages, but appears to be more related to low energy output due to lack of physical activity or a genetic cause.

Extrinsic (added or refined) sugars, which are usually blamed for promoting obesity, may also promote gallstones indirectly (80,97). However, the role of sugar in gallstone formation remains to be established firmly. Sugars have been known to raise fasting plasma triglycerides (98) and enhance plasma insulin response (99), both of which are associated with gallstone formation. Reiser et al. (100) also reported that a high intake of sugars induces fasting hyperinsulinemia in about 20% of healthy people. If hyperinsulinemia indeed promotes gallstones, then all rapidly digested carbohydrates, such as starch in finely ground flour or cooked potatoes, may also be as important as refined sugar. Pastides et al. (101) noted that women with gallstones in Athens were found to consume potatoes and cereal products more often than control subjects.

Heaton (102) proposed that dietary fiber deficiency promotes gallstones, because lack of cell wall material in ileal effluent entering colon enhances DCA absorption in the following ways: (a) when less polysaccharide is available for fermentation to short-chain fatty acids, cecum pH rises so bacterial enzymes form DCA more actively; (b) less particulate material is available to which DCA can bind hydrophobically to make more DCA available for absorption; and (c) when the colon contents are less bulky and are transported more slowly, this allows more time for the absorption of DCA.

Evidence available shows that addition of wheat bran to a Western-type diet decreased the DCA content of bile, making it less saturated with cholesterol (103). However, epidemiological evidence for a low intake of dietary fiber as a causative factor is lacking, case-control studies generally being negative (80,97,104). Hood et al. (105) also reported that adding bran to the diet of people whose gallstones had been dissolved medically did not prevent their stones from re-forming.

Three case-control studies have shown that vegetable fiber, or at least high vegetable intake, has a protective role against gallstones (101,106,107) as was also shown by a large prospective study (108). MacLure et al. (108) suggested that beans probably have protective effects on gallstones. If vegetables and beans are protective, their mode of action is unknown.

Although in laboratory animals gallstones can be induced by feeding cholesterol, there is little evidence that a high intake of cholesterol promotes gallstones in humans (109). Alcohol consumption, however, protects against gallstones (80,101). McLure et al. (78) reported that women showed a dose-related decrease in the risk of gallstones as alcohol intake increased, but as little as 5 g alcohol daily reduced the gallstone risk by about 40%, probably due to decreased secretion of cholesterol; it was noted in one experiment that drinking half a bottle of white wine daily reduced the cholesterol saturation of bile (110).

From the above review, it can be concluded that obesity promotes gallstones, it being a dominant risk factor in younger women; and in men (and possibly in women), it is the abdominal fat distribution that influences gallstone pathogenesis. Obesity may operate through insulin resistance and hyperinsulinemia. Refined sugars and rapidly digestible starch may cause gallstones, via hyperinsulinemia, and dietary fiber appears to have a role in the prevention of gallstones. Drinking alcohol in moderation is also protective (2).

III. DIET AND DISEASES OF THE KIDNEYS AND URINARY TRACT

A. Renal Pathophysiology and Function

The kidneys are each composed of about one million functional units, termed nephrons, each nephron consisting of a glomerulus, a tuft of capillaries invaginated into an epithelial sac (Bowman's capsule) from which arises tubule. The blood flow through kidneys is large, about one-fourth of the cardiac output at rest (1300 ml/min). Renal arteries are branched into arterioles, which divide to constitute the glomerular capillaries. These unite to form the efferent arterioles, supplying blood to the renal tubules. The hydrostatic pressure within the glomerular capillaries results in the filtration of fluid into Bowman's capsule. The fluid is similar in its composition to that of plasma, except that it normally contains no fat and very little protein. The filtrate thus formed in the glomerulus (at about 125 ml/min) passes into the proximal convoluted tubule and from there through the loop of Henle and distal convoluted tubule to the collecting ducts. Of the approximately 180 liters of water and 22.5 mol of sodium filtered through the glomerular capillaries per day, only about 1.5 liters of water and 100 to 200 mmol of sodium are excreted in the urine (111).

The kidneys thus maintain both the volume of the body fluids and their electrolyte composition within narrow limits by modifying urine composition. Extreme responses to dehydration and overhydration in healthy adults are produced by a change in either direction of only around 2% in the body's water content; the daily urine volume may vary from the usual 1500 ml to 500 ml under stress and can increase to about 20 liters in overhydration.

Kidneys release renin in response to low blood pressure or lack of adequate blood flow (ischemia) to the kidneys, which converts the liver-derived angiotensinogen to angiotensin 1, which is activated in the lungs to angiotensin 2. The latter is a potent vasoconstrictor, directly increasing the systemic blood pressure. It also stimulates release of aldosterone from the adrenal glands, which aids in salt and water conservation. Kidneys degrade several polypeptide hormones, such as parathyroid hormone, calcitonin, insulin, and gastrin.

Thirst, polyuria, and polydipsia are the clinical features of diabetes mellitus and diabetes insipidus, as well as of renal failure, wherein kidneys are not able to conserve water. Consequently, the patient has an increased water requirement to maintain the fluid balance of the body. In peripheral and pulmonary edema, there in an increase in the extracellular fluid volume and total body sodium. Water and sodium overloads result from a renal failure to regulate sodium metabolism, as seen in cardiac failure and intrinsic renal disease. Under these conditions, patients seem to benefit from measures designed to promote the loss of body sodium. Excessive renal sodium loss may also occur due to defective tubular reabsorption of sodium. This condition often responds to sodium supplementation with a restoration of total body sodium, an improvement in renal blood flow glomerular filtration rate (GFR).

Blood hemoglobin concentration, and plasma levels of urea, creatinine, sodium, potassium, biocarbonate, calcium, inorganic phosphate, albumin, and alkaline phosphatase are convenient biochemical indices monitored serially. Plasma concentration of urea and creatinine change significntly due to defective renal excretory function. These metabolites are therefore measured to assess the progression of renal failure. Patients' muscle mass, meat intake and GFR influence serum creatinine concentration in people with kidney disease. Diagnostic radiological and radionucleotide imaging tests have become important tools in assessing renal function. Noninvasive ultrasound screening allows rapid assessment of renal size and is useful for excluding urinary tract obstruction.

GFR falls lead to increases in the serum concentration of potassium and phosphate ions, and metabolic acidosis is caused by the failure of the renal tubules to conserve bicarbonate ions. The changes in plasma calcium and alkaline phosphatase concentrations are signs of the secondary effects of renal dystunction on vitamin D and bone metabolism. Sodium being an important determinant of extracellular and plasma volumes, changes in sodium are more reliably assessed clinically by the presence or absence of peripheral edema as well as by the measurement of blood pressure. The excretary capacity of the kidney varies at different stages of acute and chronic renal failure and with different types of renal diseases, e.g., in tubulo-interstitial disease urinary volumes are larger than in glomerulonephritis. Abnormal urinary constituents such as blood and protein do not necessarily show the presence of kidney disease and need further investigation (111).

B. Dietary Management of Renal Diseases

Dietetics has greatest significance in the management of kidney disease when renal function is impaired. There is no need to alter eating habits and lifestyle of patients as long as kidneys continue to maintain ionic balance and sodium excretion, as they do in urinary tract infections, asymptomatic glomerulonephritis, mild proteinuria, and hypertension. Tubular disorders such as Fanconi syndrome may result in abnormal losses of sodium, potassium, magnesium, and phosphate ions, which can be treated by providing supplements of the appropriate salts in addition to a normal diet.

Dietary intervention in renal disease can help to promote the patient's health through regulation of protein intake and control of fluid, sodium, potassium, and phosphate intake as well as by maintaining plasma levels of urea and electrolyte within normal limits. Severely restricted diets (e.g., very low protein diets), however, may not be required, because these may minimize changes in plasma urea concentration but lead to severe muscle wasting. Adequate energy, minerals, and vitamins should be provided, considering the nutritional status of the patient, especially in children, to promote growth.

1. Acute Glomerulonephritis

Acute glomerulonephritis (GN) is characterized by inflammation of the glomeruli, with congestion, cellular proliferation, and infiltration of leukocytes and other cells. Clinical symptoms include hypertension, oliguria, hematuria, and often peripheral and pulmonary edema. Development of acute renal failure may rarely require dialysis.

The medical treatment of post-infectious GN aims at dealing with the symptoms rather than the cause, although antimicrobial treatments are given to cure the infection. The use of salt and water restriction and diuretics is useful in the treatment of acute nephritis. Protein restriction is often not necessary unless the patient is uremic. On the contrary, protein supplements may be required if protein intake is low. The salt and fluid restriction will depend on the level of fluid retention. Oliguric patients are asked to restrict their fluid to 500 ml plus the volume of the previous day's urine output, the sodium intake being restricted to 80 to 100 mmol/day.

The nephrotic syndrome is characterized by heavy proteinuria (over 3.5 g/1.73 m^2 body surface area per 24 hr), edema, and hypoalbuminemia. Hepatic albumin synthesis may increase nephrotic syndrome (112), as the absolute plasma concentration of high-molecular-weight proteins rises in this condition (113). The liver compensates by overproducing its export proteins. The hyperlipidemia and hypercoagulability of the nephrotic syndrome are caused by enhanced hepatic secretion of lipoproteins and coagulation factors. The syndrome also increases susceptibility to infection.

With the fall in plasma albumin levels, the balance of hydrostatic and colloid osmotic pressures across capillaries in the body is changed, which favors movement of water and solute from the blood plasma to the interstitial fluid. The fall in the plasma volume is then compensated by sodium being avidly reabsorbed from the renal tubules. The sodium is retained in the body, and the plasma volume restored at the expense of a greatly increased extracellular volume, manifesting as peripheral edema.

A wide variety of renal and systemic disorders result in a nephrotic syndrome, especially in children, known as minimal change disease because of a loss of foot processes in the glomerular epithelial cells. It is usually benign but may lead to renal impairment or hypertension.

Patients with minimal change disease often respond to steroids with or without other immunosuppressive agents, such as cyclophosphamide or cyclosporin A. The nephrotic syndrome can be managed by removal of salt and water and avoidance and treatment of complications such as thrombosis and hyperlipidemia. Salt and water are restricted and appropriate diuretics are used. In severely hypoalbuminemic patients with gross fluid overload, salt-poor albumin may be given intravenously to promote and augment diuresis. Over-enthusiastic diuretic therapy may lead to a risk of intravascular volume depletion and acute renal failure through hypoperfusion. Daily fluid loss should not generally exceed 1 kg, to avoid the problem of hypovolemia.

Because of the heavy proteinuria and the resultant fall in serum albumin levels, the high-protein diet (80–100 g protein) prescribed in the past has not shown beneficial result (114) and indeed may have detrimental effects on the hepatic synthesis of albumin (115). Also, the consumption of a high-protein diet by patients with glomerulonephritis may promote the progression of renal insufficiency (116). Frequently, anorexic patients may have difficulty in complying with a high-protein diet. According to Khan et al. (111), at present intake of 1 g of protein/kg ideal body weight is recommended.

The patients' nitrogen balance needs to be maintained by providing an adequate intake of energy for the appropriate utilization of protein, about 200 kcal (840 KJ)/g of dietary nitrogen being usually sufficient. Sodium should be restricted to 80 to 100 mmol/day if edema has not been controlled successfully with diuretics.

Serum lipid concentrations increase in the nephrotic syndrome (117); the most frequently reported abnormalities are increases in total, LDL, and VLDL cholesterol, which can be reversed after remission (118). Appel (119) also noticed increased levels of total, LDL, and VLDL cholesterol but normal levels of HDL cholesterol in the majority of nephrotic patients. Berlyne and Mallick (120) found an increase in ischemic heart disease in patients with nephrotic syndrome; Waas and Cameron (121) did not.

Because a majority of nephrotic patients undergo remission, there is no consensus on treatment of hyperlipidemia. The risk to an individual patient depends on factors such as genetic predisposition, the duration of unremitting nephrotic syndrome, hyperlipidemia, concurrent hypertension, diabetes, and the use of steroids. Dietary interventions such as substitution of PUFA for some of the saturated fat in the diet, reduction of total fat intake, and weight reduction in the obese have been recommended. Lipid-lowering drugs may be useful in the majority of patients with unremitting nephrotic syndrome and hyperlipidemia. Appel and Appel (122) have reviewed the usefulness of drugs such as bile-acid sequestrants (cholestyramine), fibric acid derivative (gemfibrozil), and HMG-CoA reductase inhibitors.

2. Acute Renal Failure

Acute renal failure (ARF) results from a variety of insults to the kidneys, and its causes may be grouped into pre-renal, renal, and post-renal types (Table 4). Classical features of ARF are those due to the precipitating underlying disorder in addition to those of uremia. ARF begins with a phase of very low urinary output (oliguria), followed by a recovery phase characterized by diuresis. In oliguria, the body accumulates nitrogenous waste products, water, potassium, sodium, inorganic acids, and phosphate. The fatal features of ARF include pulmonary edema, hyperkalemia, and acidosis. The underlying disorder may be complicated by septicemia and failure of liver, heart, or lungs. Nitrogenous waste products accumulate rapidly as the result of tissue breakdown, with catabolic response to trauma and infection. The recovery (diuretic) phase of ARF may be delayed for several weeks, when renal tubutes cannot concentrate urine effectively and there is a risk of fluid and electrolyte depletion during dialysis. Hypokalemia and hyponatremia are

Table 4   Causes of Acute Renal Failure

Type	Cause
Pre-renal	Fluid loss
	Diarrhea and vomiting
	Heat injury
	Burns
	Excessive diuretics
	Blood loss
	Gastrointestinal
	External bleeding
	Surgery
	Hypotensive states
	Cardiogenic shock
	Heart failure
	Sepsis
Renal	Acute glomerulonephritis
	Vasculitis
	Disseminated intravascular coagulation
	Nephrotoxic agents
	Sepsis
	Untreated pre-renal causes
	Bilateral renal infarction
	Obstetric complications (e.g., eclampsia)
	Hypercalcemia
Post-renal	Prostatic enlargement
	Bilateral ureteric stones
	Urethral strictures
	Postoperative bladder dysfunction
	Carcinoma of the cervix

Source: Ref. 111.

common with a urinary output of 3 to 5 liters/day. The latter, however, may cease (anuria) or alternate with high outputs (polyuria) in obstruction of the urinary tract. High-output renal failure may occur with substantial urinary water losses, but poor excretion of nitrogenous compounds, which in turn accumulate in blood. Measurement of plasma and urine sodium, creatinine, and osmolality may aid in the distinction of pre-renal and renal causes of ARF, provided diureties are not given. Radiological investigations are invaluable tools in evaluating patients with ARF, e.g., a plain abdominal x-ray may reveal calculi causing obstruction to both ureters. Ultrasonography and renal biopsy may also be used for further investigations.

The extra-renal causes of ARF, such as infection and trauma, as well as uremia must be treated medically. Loss of body fluids may lead to "pre-renal" ARF, which should be treated promptly by appropriate fluid replacement to prevent the development of tubular necrosis. In the oliguric phase, patients should be given a volume of fluid equal to the previous 24-hour urine output plus extra-renal fluid losses from the gut, drains, and fistulae, and an estimated 500 ml should be added for the fluid losses from the skin and respiratory tract. In catabolic patients, renal replacement therapy should be instituted earlier. The indications for dialysis include fluid overload, hyperkalemia, and severe acidosis. Hemodialysis is employed on a daily basis to remove toxic waste products and fluid prior to infusing blood products or parenteral nutrition. Hemofiltration (a continuous blood purification method) may suit patients with cardiovascular instability better than intermittent daily hemolysis.

Renal replacement therapy has improved the prognosis of ARF patients, preventing deaths due to uremia. However, there is a greater risk of death from infection and poor wound healing when there is inadequate nutritional support. Lee (115) grouped ARF patients according to their underlying diagnosis and degree of catabolism: (a) non-catabolic, resulting from non-traumatic medical causes (e.g., drug overdose), (b) moderately catabolic, which usually develops after surgery, and (c) severely catabolic, occurring with major trauma, burns, and sepsis. These three groups have different nutritional requirements (111).

The dietary needs of non-catabolic patients are determined by serum biochemistry, assessed daily. If serum creatinine concentration is less than 400 μmol/l, dietary protein restriction is not usually necessary. However, the provision of adequate protein and energy to these patients is often not easy because of their anorexia. The choice of acceptable protein supplements may be determined by the electrolyte status and fluid needs. A minimum energy intake of 1.4 × BMR (basal metabolic rate) is required. Daily recording of the patient's weight is important, and daily food intake can be assessed and changes made if necessary. If tube-feeding is required, fluid and electrolyte restriction must be considered. In edematous anuric or oliguric patients, sodium restriction is often needed, and high sodium foods causing thirst should be avoided. Normally, a diet containing 80 to 100 mmol of sodium is recommended, but occasionally a lower (40 mmol) sodium may be necessary with severe fluid restriction.

Severe hyperkalemia (above 5 mmol/l) can be controlled by giving cation exchange resins (e.g., calcium resin), administered either orally or rectally. Glucose and insulin given intravenously can also rapidly reduce serum potassium concentration.

Aggressive dietary treatment should be started early in moderately and highly catabolic patients with restricted protein, potassium, and fluid intake. However, the present policy is to feed the patient and then dialyze as necessary, which reduces the severe muscle wasting due to catabolism and inadequate nutrition. Moderately and severely catabolic patients require 9 to 14 g (60–90 g protein) and 14 to 18 g (90–115 g protein) N, respectively, with 30 to 50 g of N loss per day. In orally fed catabolic patients with renal failure, the energy intake varies according to the underlying disease.

The daily energy requirement may be 1.25 × BMR, approximately; the factor may vary from 1.4 to 1.6 for severe infections and 1.85 to 2.05 for severe burns. The fluid volume to be given is about 2.5 liters/day, which may be restricted to 1 to 1.5 liters/day, limited to the amount of fluid that is removed during a single dialysis session. The remaining fluid allowance is required for the continuous infusion of crystalloid fluid to maintain the potency of catheters to monitor central venous and pulmonary arterial pressures and to administer other drugs.

Wherever possible, feeding should be via the gut, and when enteral feeding is not tolerated because of diarrhea or vomiting, parenteral nutrition may be preferred via a central venous catheter. The requirements for parenteral nutrition are estimated using the same criteria as enteral feeding (123). A solution of pure crystalline amino acids is used as the preferred source of nitrogen in total parenteral nutrition (TPN). A more concentrated solution such as Aminoplex can be used where fluid restriction is necessary. The electrolyte-free solutions are usually preferred in ARF. Patients' requirements for electrolytes and minerals may vary greatly. Potassium phosphate and mangesium are often required to be restricted and can be omitted from the TPN formulation and then added in small quantities as per individual needs. Vitamins and minerals are usually provided in standard doses from special ready-to-use vials. All the dietary restrictions can cease, as dialysis treatment is phased out and the patients' plasma biochemistry returns to normal, the patient being encouraged to eat normally with dietary supplements, if necessary.

3.   Chronic Renal Failure

The clinical symptoms of chronic renal failure (CRF) depend on the degree of renal inefficiency. Asymptomatic patients may be incidently diagnosed when serum urea and creatinine concentrations are requested. CRF patients often present to the non-nephrologist, and investigations for anemia, dyspnea, pruritus, bone pain, and neuropathy may all lead to a diagnosis of CRF. Because of the kidneys' large functional reserves, sumptoms may not occur until the GFR falls below 20 ml/min; and below 10 ml/min, symptoms of uremia are usually present. Patients with GFR below 5 ml/min often need renal replacement therapy, but patients with diabetic nephropathy or cardiac failure may become symptomatic even at higher levels of GFR. Anemia is commonly seen in CRF as the result of insufficient erythropoietin production. As the GFR declines, the serum phosphate levels rise. Lack of active vitamin D causes impaired calcium absorption by the intestine, leading to hypocalcemia. The high phosphate and low serum calcium levels stimulate the secretion of parathyroid hormone, resulting in bone demincralization. These changes result in renal bone disease with a range of bone disorders such as osteoporosis, osteomalacia, and osteitis fibrosa. Continued hyperphosphatemia may result in bone pains and fractures, and soft tissue calcification in the eyes, skin, and muscles.

Specific clinical features of CRF for the underlying renal disorder may include rash and arthropathy in systemic lupus erythematosus and lung symptoms in sarcoidosis and the vasculitides, with further decline in renal function; nocturia and polyuria develop, which are secondary to a loss of the kidneys' concentrating ability, resulting in an acute exacerbation of chronic renal failure if there are abnormal fluid losses (e.g., gastroenteritis or infection (111)).

Because the course of chronic renal insufficiency cannot be predicted with certainty, some patients may remain in a state of chronic stable renal failure for long, whereas other may progress steadily toward the end-stage disease. CRF patients have a decreased renal reserve and are thus susceptible to acute deterioration of renal function due to fluid depletion from gastroenteritis or blood loss. Hypotensive episodes such as myocardial infarction and catabolic states such as infections and trauma are also importantly involved. Obstruction of the urinary tract is a common reversible cause of deterioration of renal function in stable CRF and is sought in all acute or chronic cases.

The patient needs to be followed regularly to control high blood pressure, to treat urinary tract infection, and to monitor serum electrolyte and creatinine concentration, because uncontrolled hypertension will accelerate the CRF progression. Most nephrologists use serum creatinine concentration and initiate dialysis when it approaches 1000 µmol/l or earlier if the patient develops severe acidosis, marked fluid retention, hyperkalemia, or uremic symptoms (111).

Dietary phosphate should be restricted when the serum phosphate levels exceed 2.0 mmol/l, because intestinal phosphate absorption is not reduced in renal failure and a phosphate-free diet is not practical. Hypocalcemic patients benefit from a rise in serum calcium when calcium carbonate is given between meals. These patients are also given 1-hydroxy vitamin D or 1,25 $(OH)_2$ vitamin D to suppress parathyroid overactivity (activated form of vitamin D). Renal failure almost invariably leads to anemia, requiring treatment of iron deficiency with iron supplements.

Animal experiments have shown that dietary protein restriction, antihypertensive agents, and limiting hyperlipidemia and phosphorus intake decrease the progressive renal failure in partially nephrectomized rats. There are certain difficulties in designing and conducting studies to assess the role of dietary protein restriction in human subjects (124,125). Locatelli et al. (126), in a prospective multicenter trial, concluded that protein restriction did not retard the progression of CRF, although compliance for the group that was assigned the low-protein diet was found to be poor. According to Mitch (127), the goals of CRF before the patient must be treated by dialysis or transplantation are (a) to minimize the mineral and electrolyte disturbance, (b) to lower or reduce the pool of accumulated waste products, (c) to maintain adequate protein nutrition, and (d) to retard or, in some cases, halt the progression of renal insufficiency. Low-protein diets can be used safely and can have a major impact on the course of disease, at least for some kidney failure patients.

Protein intake in both diabetic and nondiabetic individuals should not be reduced below 0.6 g of protein/kg IBW (initial body weight), because the intake of essential amino acids may become insufficient to maintain nitrogen balance (128), and a further reduction in total protein intake will require the addition of essential amino acids or keto acids to the basic diet (129). Both protein and energy intake need to be assessed regularly to ensure that malnutrition and muscle wasting do not occur.

Blood transfusions and treatment with drugs such as angiotensin-converting enzyme inhibitors may lead to hyperkalemia, which may be precipitated by infection, trauma, or surgery, as found in severely acidotic patients with only moderately impaired renal function. Normal potassium intake (about 80 mmol/day) varies according to culture and food habits; vegetarians and vegans may have problems of potassium control because foods such as pulses, nuts, and fruits are rich sources of potassium. Serum potassium levels reach the upper limit of normal at 5.0 mmol/l; a restriction to 50 mmol/day should be adopted by removing high-potassium foods like meat, fish, milk, eggs, nuts, pulses and dried fruits.

As plasma phosphate rises, oral calcium carbonate or magnesium carbonate may be given to reduce phosphate absorption and to maintain plasma levels within a normal range of 0.7 to 1.2 mmol/l. Dietary phosphate should be controlled at 600 to 700 mg/day, by avoiding dairy products and cereals, especially bran.

CRF patients lose about 60 to 100 mmol/day of sodium even when salt intake is restricted, and dehydration occurs if sodium losses are excessive. A moderate salt intake of 80 to 100 mmol of sodium is required in cases of severe hypertension and edema. An intake of 500 ml of fluid plus the equivalent of the previous day's urine output has been recommended (111).

C. Renal Replacement and Therapy

1. *Hemodialysis and Peritoneal Dialysis*

Patients with end-stage renal failure need dialysis for their survival. Although dialysis cannot substitute for healthy normal kidneys, it does allow patients to avoid the dangers of fatal uremia. Dialysis does not relieve all symptoms of renal damage, and dietary and fluid restrictions must continue. The principles of the two options, viz., hemodialysis and peritoneal dialysis, are the same. A semipermeable membrane acts as a filter, separating the blood from the dialysate compartment. Diffusion of solutes across the dialyser membrane enables removal of uremic toxins from the blood, retaining the high molecular weight components of blood such as proteins. The dialysate concentration of electrolyte is controlled to allow diffusion of excess electrolytes and urea from the blood. Acetate or bicarbonate is used to correct the dialysate acidosis. The ultrafiltration of water in hemodialysis is achieved by generating hydrostatic pressure across the membrane and in peritoneal dialysis by osmosis, using variable concentration of glucose in the dialysate fluid.

Whereas hemodialysis requires blood and dialysate circuits, peritoneal dialysis uses human peritoneal membrane for blood purification. In hemodialysis, blood and dialysate are brought into the dialyser, which has an artificial membrane made of cellulose or a like material. The dialyser may be either "flat-bed," with membrane sheets to separate blood and dialysate, or "hollow fiber," in which blood flows through microscopic lumina in a bundle of thousands of hollow fibers while the dialysate circulates around the fiber. The blood flow required for adequate dialysis is around 200 to 300 ml/min, while dialysate flows at 500 ml/min. Such high blood flow rates can be obtained by creating a system that gives access to a substantial blood vessel. An arteriovenous fistula is created surgically by anastomosing an artery (often in the forearm) to an adjacent vein. An anticoagulant, heparin, is added before the blood passes into the dialyser to prevent clotting. The blood passes through the dialyser while the dialysate flows in the opposite direction. The dialysate drains out, and the purified blood returns to the vein within about 3 to 6 hours. Most patients with end-stage disease on hemodialysis are given 12 hours of dialysis weekly in two or three 4 to 6 hourly sessions.

The vascular peritoneal membrane consists of mesothelial cells; in humans this is about one square meter in surface area and the peritoneal cavity is a potential space with no fluid. In peritoneal dialysis, dialysate is poured from a collapsible bag and tubing into the peritoneal cavity via a catheter and allowed to equilibrate for 6 to 8 hours. The dialysate is then drained out and fresh dialysate is instilled. Removal of fluid relies on creating an osmotic gradient across the peritoneal membrane. Glucose is used for ultrafiltration as an osmotic agent, concentrations varying according to the amount of ultrafiltration. Acetate or lactate is used as a buffer instead of bicarbonate. Long-term peritoneal dialysis, termed continuous ambulatory peritoneal dialysis (CAPD), can be self-administered by the patient, usually 3 to 4 times/day, using 1500 to 2000 ml of dialysate in each exchange. CAPD is especially useful in those who have difficulty with vascular access, e.g., diabetics or patients with heart disease who cannot tolerate hemodialysis. Infection is the main problem with CAPD: totally aseptic conditions are needed during handling of the fluids and catheters.

Dietary resistrictions have become less severe thanks to the technical advances in dialysis, thus improving the quality of the patient's life. However, an adequate protein intake is necessary because dialysis is a catabolic process—catabolic hormones such as glucagon, glucocorticoids, and adrenaline are released during hemodialysis. Peptides (2–3 g) and amino acids (as much as 7 g) are lost into the dialysate (130), which must be replaced.

Khan et al. (111) recommended a high-fiber, low-fat, and low-sugar diet during hemodialysis to limit the risk of hyperlipidemia. An energy intake of about 35 kcal/kg/day is generally recommended; weight loss in obese patients may be achieved by restricting the intake to a level of 500 kcal below their current needs, which will change as they lose weight.

Serum potassium levels of 3.5 to 4.9 mmol/1 should be maintained following a dialysis session, with an intake of 30 to 60 mmol. Other factors, such as constipation, the potassium content of the dialysis fluid, acidosis, infection, tissue damage, and drugs will also influence the serum potassium level. In acidosis, there is a release of potassium from the intracellular to the extracellular space which cannot be excreted in renal failure. Potassium intake can be reduced by restricting high-potassium foods.

Hyperphosphatemia may lead to secondary hyper-parathyroidism and bone disease (renal osteodystrophy), which can be prevented by restricting phosphate intake to 0.8 to 1.1 g/day; by decreasing high phosphate containing foods, such as cheeses, milk, eggs, high-protein foods, whole meal bread, bran, nuts, and yeasts; and by using oral phosphate binders.

The urinary output generally diminishes the longer a patient remains on dialysis; around 500 ml/day of fluid is allowed in addition to the equivalent volume of the urine passed. Fluid accumulation can be measured by weighing the patient (1 kg wt = 1 liter of body water) and a maximum of 2 liters of fluid may be gained between dialysis, and less if cardiac failure is present. Dietary sodium should be restricted to 80 to 100 mmol/day, because excessive salt intake will result in increased thirst and will make fluid restriction more difficult. Salt restriction also aids in the control of hypertension.

Dialysis patients require supplementation with water-soluble vitamins, especially folic acid and vitamins that are destroyed by prolonged cooking, as well as by dialysis per se to remove potassium. Excessive vitamin C intake, however, may lead to accumulation of oxalic acid and deposition of calcium oxalate in the soft tissues and bones (131).

Vitamin A, being bound to retinol (a high-molecular-weight protein) is not dialysable. Supplementary vitamin A is therefore not necessary and should not be prescribed, to avoid its possible toxic accumulation in bone. Iron supplements, however, are given to make up for blood losses during hemodialysis (5 liters/year).

Fluid and dietary restrictions are less severe in peritoneal dialysis. The protein intake recommended for CAPD patients is at least 1.1 g/kg/day. The consumption of the recommended amount of protein may be difficult if the patient's appetite is poor. A low-phosphate, low-electrolyte protein supplement may therefore be required, e.g., protein forte, which may be discontinued if the appetite improves. A large energy intake is not required in CAPD, as around 70% of the glucose in the CAPD bags is absorbed through the peritoneum. Patients should thus be encouraged to restrict high-fat and high-sugar diets. Obesity can be a major problem in the CAPD patient because of absorption of sugar from the dialysate (400–900 kcal/day). Diabetics are especially at risk and need guidance and regular monitoring. A high-fiber diet to prevent constipation will be useful. Because CAPD patients consume larger quantities of protein, larger doses of phosphate binders may need to be prescribed. A fluid intake of 1000 ml plus the equivalent of the previous day's urinary output is generally recommended. An increase in the weight of most anuric patients often indicates fluid retention (111).

Hypertriglyceridemia is the most common abnormality in patients with renal failure and those on dialysis, leading to accelerated atherosclerosis and cardiovascular deaths. The efficacy of low-saturated-fat diets in patients with dialysis has been established. Dietary restriction of fat, exercise, and correction of other risk factors such as smoking have been advised.

Anthropometry is employed to assess the nutritional status of patients on dialysis, by measuring height, weight, and body proportions, which provide useful data in the initial assessment of a patient with end-stage renal failure. For those initiating dialysis, baseline measurements of body mass index (BMI) indicate the presence of obesity or undernutrition. The mid-upper arm circumference (MUAC) and triceps skin fold (TSF) are also useful in monitoring changes in body composition and response to any dietary supplymentation that may be necessary.

The mid-arm muscle circumference (MAMC) can be computed from the following formula (111):

MAMC (cm) = MUAC(cm) – 3.14 × TSF (cm)

The measurement should be recorded post-dialysis and in the non-fistula arm, which is useful for assessing the body protein stores and thus the degree of undernutrition. Dietary intake needs are estimated at regular intervals to ensure adequacy of the patient's diet within the recommended guidelines.

D. Erythropoietin Therapy

The advances in recombinant human erythropoietin therapy have revolutionized the treatment of anemia in renal failure, replacing the need for blood transfusions for dialysis patients with anemia. Evidence available shows that erythropoietin treatment is safe and effective when used carefully, and many symptoms of CRF previously thought to be of uremia can be reversed by correcting anemia.

Erythropoietin is given either intravenously or subcutaneously, twice or thrice weekly, the dose varying with individuals. Patients with hemoglobin levels below 80 g/l should be treated to meet a target of 100 g/l. Erythropoietin treatment increases utilization of iron through a rapid erythrocytosis for which iron supplements are required. Hypertension is the most frequently encountered side effect (132), the cause of which is not clear. Occasionally, it may also produce clotting due to enhanced platelet stickiness, resulting in an increased need for heparin in hemodialysis patients (133). The subsequent increases in plasma potassium and phosphate after the correction of anemia with erythropoietin therapy will need anticipatory management. Patients with iron deficiency, continuing blood loss, aluminum intoxication, infection, and malignancy do not often respond to erythropoietin treatment.

E. Kidney Transplantation

Transplantation of healthy kidneys is the optimum treatment for end-stage renal failure. The kidney may be obtained from a cadaver or from a living relative. The donor's and recipient's blood groups must be compatible. Some patients, such as those who have received transplants in the past or those who have been given multiple blood transfusions, may develop antibodies to HLA antigents, making them highly sensitized to antigens from a broad spectrum of donors.

After a successful transplantation, the patient requires immunosuppressive drugs to prevent rejection, such as prednisolone, azathioprine, and cyclosporin A. These drugs may cause certain undesirable side effects such as leukopenia, susceptibility to infection, weight gain, renal dysfunction, hypertension, osteoporosis, and hyperlipidemia. Transplant rejection is also treated with high doses of steroids or monoclonal antibodies (111).

The patient with a renal transplant may pose unique medical and nutritional problems, with a range of recurrence of the primary renal diseases. After the dietary and fluid restrictions of renal replacement therapy, the new transplantation patient may need to increase fluid and nutritional intake. Steroid-induced increase in appetite may lead to obesity and hyperlipidemia. Hypertensive patients should be advised to continue salt restriction. Steroid drugs may induce diabetes in some patients and drugs such as cyclosporin A may cause hyperkalemia on a long-term basis. Immunosuppressive drugs, diabetes, use of beta blockers, and obesity all may lead to hyperlipidemia, which is commonly observed in transplant patients. Thus, a diet low in fat and sugar and high in nonstarch polysaccharides has been recommended to maintain the ideal body weight. Lipid-lowering drugs should be used with care because many produce side effects in conjunction with immunosuppression (111).

IV. KIDNEY AND BLADDER STONES

About 95% of renal and bladder calculi are made up of calcium salts, around 3% are uric acid salts, and 1% are cystine. Most stones contain a mixture of mainly calcium oxalate, calcium phosphate, and magnesium ammonium phosphate, although about one-third of stones may be pure calcium oxalate. The process of stone formation is favored in infected urine in which bacteria have converted urea into ammonia, making the urine more alkaline. The solubility of salt in urine depends on the product of its ionic activities, which are also influenced in part by the presence of other ions in the urine. Calcium oxalate crystals present in all urines are precipitated from a supersaturated solution of calcium oxalate. These are small crystals and normally washed out through urine. However, these crystal may grow as influenced by other chemical constituents of urine as well as by disease and diet. Substances such as citrate, pyrophosphate, nephrocalin, and glycosaminoglycans that are present in the urine inhibit the crystal growth.

Most stones remain in the kidneys, without producing symptoms (silent stones), but they may grow, sometimes to a very large size. Repeated infection may lead to chronic pyelonephritis, a common cause of chronic renal failure. Renal colic (the excruciating pain caused by a stone passing down the urinary tract) is well known. This pain stops after the stone is passed either naturally or removed surgically. Some patients may never have another attack, but others may have frequent attacks of passing many small (gravel) stones.

Bladder stones normally occur in males and in adults and they are often associated with prostatic obstruction or other causes of urinary stagnation. Stagnation and infection of urine and prolonged confinement to bed may predispose the person to stone formation.

The epidemiological evidence shows that a single-cereal diet (wheat, rice, or millet) can be a predominant causative factor of endemic bladder calculi (134). This theory probably explains the so-called bladder stone belt extending from the Middle East across India and the Far East from Thailand to Indonesia. Although maize is the staple food of Africa, it does not seem to be associated with bladder stones (111). Milk consumption may have a protective role against bladder stone formation. Valyasevi et al. (135) reported that in one Thai community where infants are weaned early, often on the first day after birth, bladder stones are hyperendemic.

Hypercalciuria, hyperoxaluria, hyperuricosuria, and cystinuria are the conditions that most predispose to kidney and bladder stone formation. Hypercalciuria implies that the 24-hour urinary calcium level on a free diet is higher than normal. Hypercalciuria is generally defined as the excretion of more than 7.5 mmol/day in women, 10 mmol/day in men, and over 0.1 mmol/kg/day of calcium in either sex when the patient is examined on a defined 50 mmol/day calcium intake (136).

Khan et al. (111) grouped idiopathic hypercalciuria into absorptive, renal, and resorptive types. Secondary hypercalciuria may occur with primary hyperparathyroidism sarcoidosis via vitamin D excess, immobilization, and medullary sponge kidneys that are associated with increased incidence of stone formation. Dietary hypercalciuria is rare and can be readily controlled by diet. Persistent hypercalciuria (over 200 mg/day after a week on a 400 mg calcium diet) is indicative of type 1 absorptive hypercalciuria, and a calcium excretion of less than 200 mg/day of type 2. Type 1 can be managed by using calcium-binding resin such as sodium cellulose phosphate and dietary changes, whereas type 2 can be controlled by diet alone.

About 50% of the patients forming calcium stones have hypercalciuria; there is increasing evidence that a low urinary citrate output may occur, especially in women. Coe et al. (137) have assessed the use of citrate therapy. Hypercalciuria with enhanced risk of stone formation also occurs in hyperparathyroidism, which causes calcium stones in 5% to 10% of people. A low-calcium diet, restricting the intake of foods such as milk, yogurt, and cheese, has been recommended for patients with calcium stones.

In addition to calcium, urinary oxalate may contribute to about 70% of stones in the Western population. Around 10% of the urinary oxalates are dietary in origin; however, a greater part of the oxalate excreted in the urine is of endogenous origin, often coming from tissue metabolism of glycine (111). According to Khan et al. (111), hyperoxaluria commonly results from gastrointestinal malabsorption, which paradoxically increases absorption of dietary oxalates. Malabsorption of fatty acids in the gut leads to calcium binding and production of calcium soaps of fatty acids, leaving the oxalates free (unbound) to be absorbed. A low-calcium diet also exaggerates enteric hyperoxaluria. The treatment aims at reducing dietary oxalate and increasing calcium intake to ensure precipitation of calcium oxalates in the intestinal lumen. Cholestyramine may be given to absorb some of the malabsorbed bile salts and improve diarrhea.

A rare inherited (autosomal recessive) error of glycine metabolism gives rise to primary hyperoxaluria due to enzymatic defects. Stone formation occurs in childhood and recurrent episodes often damage kidneys, leading to chronic renal failure.

A typical U.K. diet contains about 120 mg of oxalic acid, of which about 75 mg may come from five cups of tea. Thus, it is advisable for anyone who has passed a stone containing oxalate to avoid high-oxalate foods such as tea, rhubarb, and spinach (250 to 800 mg/100 g). A very restrictive low-oxalate diet (30 mg/day) should be tried only by those who have formed stones repeatedly at short intervals and have marked hyperoxaluria.

Around one-fourth of patients with uric acid stones show hyperuricosuria; an excessive dietary intake of purines is the cause in most cases. Sources of purine include liver, kidney, sweetbreads, anchovies, sardines, and brains. The volume, pH, and uric acid concentration of urine are the determinants of uric acid stone formation. At low urinary pH, uric acid is less soluble and five-sixths of uric acid is dissolved when the pH is 6.5. Thus, alkalis such as potassium citrate may be given daily, with an adequate fluid intake.

Cystinuria is the result of an inborn metabolic error wherein the renal tubules fail to reabsorb the amino acids cystine, lysine, arginine, and ornithine, which pass in urine in large amounts. Cystine, being least soluble in the urine, tends to precipitate out, forming stones.

The most important measure to be used in the prevention of all types of stones is an adequate fluid intake. A good flow of urine washes out particles of gravel. The urine flow being lowest during the night, enough water should be drunk before going to bed. Patients with kidney or bladder stones should drink sufficient water to produce at least 2.5 liters of urine daily. The fluid intake is especially important for those living in the tropics or working in hot environments, because urinary output is diminished by the amount of water lost in sweating.

Drugs such as bendrofluazide decrease urinary calcium by abut 30%, probably by a renal tubular mechanism. Pyridoxine given to patients forming oxalate stones is thought to divert glycine metabolism toward serine and away from oxalate. Oral penicillamine administration has been found to be useful in cystinuria, because it combines with cystine, which can be excreted in a more soluble form.

The calcium and oxalate content of the diet should be monitored because the excess of both of these is associated with stone formation. Thus, foods rich in oxalate and calcium (Table 5) should be avoided. A high-fiber diet should be encouraged to reduce calcium absorption, because the phytate present in cereal fiber (bran) binds calcium in the gut (111).

According to Massey (138), both salt-loading studies and reports of free-living populations find that urinary calcium excretion increases approximately 1 mmol (40 mg) for each 100 mmol (2300 mg) increase in dietary sodium in normal adults. Renal calcium stone-formers with hypercalciuria thus appear to have greater proportional increases in urinary calcium (approximately 2 mmol) per 100 mmol increase in salt intake. Therefore, reduction of dietary NaCl may be a useful strategy to decrease the risk of forming calcium-containing kidney stones. As dietary factors influencing the development of kidney stones are being re-evaluated, more research is needed to determine the long-term effects of a diet high in sodium chloride, because this is a modifiable risk factor. Evidence available suggests that calcium oxalate stone-formers with hypercalciuria may benefit from decreasing NaCl intake to 100 mmol/day. It remains to be demonstrated, however, that limiting NaCl intake will prevent reoccurrence of calcium stone formation (138).

Table 5 Foods Rich in Oxalate and Calcium

Food	Oxalate (mg/100 g)
Beetroot	500
Chocolate	117
Rhubarb	600
Peanuts	187
Tea infusion	55–78 (mg/100 ml)
Food group	*Foods rich in calcium* (>200 mg/100 g)
Dairy products	Dried skimmed milk Cheddar cheese Yogurt
Cereals	Muesli
Meat and fish	Pilchards, sardines

Source: Ref. 111.

REFERENCES

1. Baldwin, R.L., and N.E. Smith, Molecular control of energy metabolism, *The Control of Metabolism* (J.D. Sink, ed.), Pennsylvania State University Press, University Park, 1974. p. 17.
2. Golden, M.H.N., and K.W. Heaton, Nutrition and the liver, *Human Nutrition and Dietetics*, 9th ed. (J.S. Garrow and W.P.T. James, eds.), Churchill Livingstone, Edinburgh, London, 1993, p. 507.
3. Marco, J., J. Diego, M.L. Villaneuva, et al., Elevated plasma glucagon levels in cirrhosis of liver, *N. Engl. J. Med. 289*: 1107 (1973).
4. Penerai, A.E., P. Salemo, M. Menneschi, et al., Growth hormone and prolactin responses to thyrotrophin releasing hormone in patients with severe liver disease, *J. Clin. Endocrinol. Metab. 45*: 140 (1977).
5. Wu, A., D.B. Grant, J. Hambley, and A.J. Levi, Reduced somatomedin activity in patients with chronic liver disease, *Clin. Science 47*: 359 (1974).
6. Verrillo, A., A. de Teresa, C. Martino, et al., Circulating somatostatin concentrations in healthy and cirrhotic subjects, *Metabolism 35*: 130 (1986).
7. Conner, H., H.F. Woods, J.D. Murray, and J.G. Ledingham. The utilization of L.(+) lactate in patients with liver disease, *Ann. Nutr. Metab. 26*: 308 (1982).
8. Mulhausen, R., A. Eichenholz, and A. Blumentals, Acid-base disturbances in patients with cirrhosis of liver, *Medicine 46*: 185 (1967).
9. Cohen, R.D., Disorders of lactate metabolism, *J. Clin. Endocrinol. Metab. 5*: 613 (1976).
10. Nomura, S., C.S. Pitman, J.B. Cambers, et al., Reduced peripheral conversion of thyroxine to triiodothyronine in patients with hepatic cirrhosis, *J. Clin. Invest. 56*: 643 (1975).
11. Sheridan, P., C. Chapman, and M.S. Losowsky, Interpretation of laboratory tests of thyroid function in chronic active hepatitis, *Clinica Chim. Acta 86*: 73 (1978).
12. Chopra, I.L., U. Chopra, and S.R. Smith, Reciprocal changes in serum concentrations of 3,3,5- triiodothyronine (reverse T3) and 3,3,5- triiodothyronine (T3) in systemic illness, *J. Clin. Endocrinol. Metab. 41*: 1043 (1975).
13. Lowdell, C.P., and I.M. Murray Lyon, Reversal of liver damage due to long-term methyltestosterone and safety of non-17 alpha-alkylated androgens, *Br. Med. J. 291*: 637 (1985).
14. Epstein, M. (ed). *The Kidney in Liver Disease*, Elsevier, New York, 1992, p. 35.
15. Vaamonde, C.A., Renal water handling in liver disease, *The Kidney in Liver Disease* 2nd ed. (M. Epstein, ed.), Elsevier, New York, 1983, p. 55.

16. Lieberman, F.L., E.K. Denison, and T.B. Reynold, The relation of plasma volume, portal hypertension, ascites and renal sodium retention in cirrhosis: the overflow theory of ascites formation, *Ann. N. Y. Acad. Sci. 170*: 202 (1970).

17. Blanchard, R.A., B.C. Furie, and M.J. Jorgensen, Acquired vitamin K-dependent carboxylation deficiency in liver disease, *N. Engl. J. Med. 305*: 242 (1981).

18. Goodman, D.S., Plasma retinol binding protein, *The Retinoids*, Vol. 2 (M.B. Sporn. A.B. Roberts, and D.S. Goodman, eds.), Academic Press, New York, 1984, p. 41.

19. Mobarhan, S.A., R.M. Russell, R.R. Recker, et al., Metabolic bone disease in alcoholic cirrhosis: a comparison of the effect of vitamin D_2, 25-hydroxy vitamin D or supportive treatment, *Hepatology 4*: 266 (1984).

20. Kaplan, M.M., Primary biliary cirrhosis, *N. Engl. J. Med. 316*: 521 (1987).

21. Whelton, M.J., A.K. Kehayoglou, J.E. Agnew, et al., Calcium absorption in parenchymatous and biliary liver disease, *Gut 12*: 978 (1971).

22. Kooh, S.W., G. Jones, and B.J. Reilly, Pathogenesis of rickets in chronic hepato biliary disease in children, *J. Paediatrics 94*: 870 (1979).

23. Kaplan, M.M., M.J. Goldberg, D.S. Matloff, et al., Effect of 25-hydroxy vitamin D_3 on vitamin D metabolism in primary biliary cirrhosis, *Gastroenterology 81*: 681 (1981).

24. Dibble, J.B. P. Sheridan, R. Hampshire, et al., Evidence for secondary hyperparathyroidism in the osteomalacia associated with chronic liver disease, *Clinical Endocrinol. 15*: 373 (1981).

25. Martin, K.J., K.A. Hruska, and J.J. Freitag. The peripheral metabolism of parathyroid hormone, *N. Eng. J. Med. 301*: 1092 (1979).

26. Bennett, A.E., H.W. Wahner, B.L. Riggs, and R.L. Hintz, Insulin-like growth factors I and II: aging and bone density in women, *J. Clin. Endocrinol Metab. 59*: 701 (1984).

27. Baker, H., O. Frank, H. Ziffer, et al., Effects of hepatic disease on vitamin B complex vitamin titres, *Am. J. Clin. Nutr. 14*: 1 (1964).

28. Frank, O., A. Luisada Opper, and M.F. Sorrell, Vitamin deficits in severe alcohol fatty liver of man calculated from multiple reference points, *Exp. Mol. Pathol. 15*: 191 (1971).

29. Camilo, M.E. M.Y. Morgan, and S. Sherlock, Erythrocyte transketolase activity in alcoholic liver disease, *Scand. J. Gastroenterology 16*: 273 (1981).

30. Sugioka, S., E.A. Porta, P.N. Corey, and W.S. Hartroft. The liver of rats fed riboflavin at two levels of protein, *Am. J. Pathol. 54*: 1 (1969).

31. Mookerjea, S., and W.W. Hawkins, Some anabolic aspects of protein metabolism in riboflavin deficiency in the rat, *Br. J. Nutr. 14*: 231 (1960).

32. Rosenthal, W.S., N.F. Adham, R. Lopez, and J.M. Cooperman, Riboflavin deficiency in complicated chronic alcoholism, *Am. J. Clin. Nutr. 26*: 858 (1973).

33. Stanko, R.T., H. Medelow, H. Shinozuka, and S.A. Adibi, Prevention of alcohol-induced fatty liver by natural metabolites and riboflavin, *J. Lab. Clin. Med. 91*: 228 (1978).

34. Baker, H., O. Frank, and M.F. Sorrell, Nicotinic acid and alcoholism, *Bibliotheca Nutr. et Diet 24*: 32 (1976).

35. Spannuth, C.L., D. Mitchell, J. Stone, et al., Vitamin B_6 nutriture in patients with uremia and liver disease. *Human Vitamin B_6 Requirements*, National Academy of Sciences, Washington, D.C., 1978, p. 180.

36. Henderson J.M., M.A. Codner, B. Hollins, et al. The fasting B_6 vitamin profile and response to a pyridoxin load in normal and cirrhotic subjects, *Hepatology 6*: 464 (1986).

37. Leevy, C.M., A. Thompson, and H. Baker, Vitamins and liver injury, *Am. J. Clin. Nutr. 23*: 493 (1970).

38. Eijhner, E.R., and R.S. Hillman, The evolution of anaemia in alcoholic patients, *Am. J. Med. 50*: 218 (1971).

39. Alpers, D.H., R.E. Clouse, and W.F. Stenson, *Manual of Nutritional Therapeutics*, Little Brown, Boston, 1983.

40. Retief, F.P., and Y.J. Huskisson, Serum and urinary folate in liver disease, *Br. Med. J. 2*: 150 (1969).

41. Wiss, O., and F. Weber, The liver and vitamins, *The Liver: Morphology, Biochemistry, Physiology*, vol. 2 (C.H. Rouiller, ed.), Academic Press, New York, 1964, p. 145.

42. Linnell, J., The fate of cobalamins in vivo, *Cobalamin Biochemistry and Pathophysiology* (B.M. Babior, ed.), Wiley, New York, 1975. p. 287.

43. Goya, N., S. Miyazaki, S. Kodate, and B. Ushio, A family of congenital atransferrinaemia, *Blood 40*: 239 (1972).

44. Goldfischer, S., Peroxisomes in disease, *J. Histochem. Cytochem. 27*: 137 (1979).

45. Doherty, F., M.H.N. Golden, and S.E.H. Brooks, Peroxisomes and the fatty liver of kwashiorkor: an hypothesis, *Am. J. Clin. Nutr. 54*: 674 (1991).

46. Golden, M.H.N., and D.D. Ramdath, Free radicals in the pathogenesis of kwashiorkor, *Proc. Nutrition Soc. 46*: 53 (1987).

47. Jakobivits, A.W., M.Y. Morgan, and S. Sherlock, Hepatic siderosis in alcoholics, *Digestive Dis. Sci. 24*: 305 (1979).

48. Grossman, M.E., D.R. Bickers, M.B. Poh-Fitzpatrick, et al., Porphyria cutania tarda: Clinical features and laboratory findings in 40 patients, *Am. J. Med. 67*: 277 (1979).

49. Lipschitz, D.A., T.H. Bothwell, H.C. Seftel, et al., The role of ascorbic acid in the metabolism of storage iron, *Br. J. Haematol. 20*: 155 (1971).

50. Deshpande Usha R., S.G. Gadre, A.S. Raste, D. Pillai, S.V. Bhide, and A.M. Samuel, Protective effect of turmeric (*Curcuma longa* L.) extract on carbon tetrachloride-induced liver damage in rats, *Indian J. Exp. Biol. 36*: 573 (1998).

51. Corish, C., Nutrition and liver disease, *Nutr. Rev. 55*: 17 (1997).

52. Shronts, E.P., M.S. Teasley, S.L. Theole, et al., Nutrition support of the adult liver transplant candidate, *J. Am. Diet. Assoc. 87*: 441 (1987).

53. Porayko, M.K., S. Dicecco, and S.J.D. O'Keefe, Impact of malnutrition and its therapy on liver transplantation, *Sem. Liver Dis. 11*: 305 (1991).

54. Kearns, P.J., H. Young, et al., Accelerated improvement of alcoholic liver disease with enteral nutrition, *Gastroenterology 102*: 200 (1992).

55. Reuter, H.D., H.P. Koch, and L.D. Lawson, Therapeutic effects and applications of garlic and its preparations, *Garlic: The Science and Therapeutic Application of Allium sativum L. and Related Species.* (H.P. Koch and L.D. Lawson, eds.), 2nd ed., Williams and Wilkins, Baltimore, Maryland, 1996, p. 135.

56. Nakagawa, S., S. Yoshida, Y. Hirao, S. Kasuga, and T. Fuwa, Cytoprotective activity of components of garlic, ginseng and ciuwjia on hepatocyte injury induced by carbon tetrachloride in vitro, *Hiroshima J. Med. Sci. 34*: 303 (1985).

57. Huh, K., S.H. Nam, J.M. Park, and U.K. Chang, Effect of garlic on liver microsomal aniline hydrolase activity in mouse, *J. Resource Dev. Veungnam Univ. 4*: 71 (1985).

58. Kagawa, K., H. Matsutaka, Y. Yamaguchi, and C. Fukuhama, Garlic extract inhibits the enhanced peroxidation and production of lipids in carbon tetrachloride-induced liver injury, *Japn. J. Pharmacol. 42*: 19 (1986).

59. Nakagawa, S., S. Kasuga, and H. Matsuura, Prevention of liver damage by aged garlic extract and its components in mice, *Phytother. Res. 3*: 50 (1989).

60. Naito, S.N., N. Yamaguchi, and Y. Yokoo, Studies on natural antioxidant. III. Fractionation of antioxidant activity from garlic extract (Nippon Shokuhin Kogyo Gakkaishi) *J. Japn. Soc. Food Sci. Technol. 28*: 465 (1981) (Japanese).

61. Kodera, Y., Method for preparing an S-allylcysteine-containing composition, *Europ. Patent No. 429 080*, 1991.

62. Blakely, S.R., D.L. Mislo, E.D. Brown, M.Y. Jenkins, and G.V. Mitchell, Gender differences in the induction of hepatic detoxification enzymes in garlic-fed hypercholesterolemic or iron loaded mature rats. *FASEB J. 7*: A864 (1993).

63. Lee, H.S., E.S. Bae, and C.W. Cha, The effect of garlic on pathological damage of testis due to cadmium poisoning, *Korea Univ. Med. J. 21*: 39 (1985). [*Chem. Abstr. 102*:144325 (1985) (Korean).]

64. Lee, D.G., J.G. Min, and C.W. Cha, A study on the effect of garlic in the inhibitory action of cadmium on ALAD activities in human blood in vitro, *Korea Univ. Med. J. 22*: 135 (1985). [*Chem. Abstr. 103*: 191016 (1985) (Korean).]

65. Park, J.S., and C.W. Cha. A study on the effect of garlic on the toxicity of phenyl mercury acetate in rats, *Korea Univ. Med. J. 21*: 49 (1984). [*Chem. Abstr. 102*: 144326 (1985) (Korean).]

66. Fields, M., C.G. Lewis, and M.D.L. Ure, Garlic oil extract ameliorates the severity of copper deficiency, *J. Am. Coll. Nutri. 11*: 334 (1992).

67. Huh, K., C.W. Choi, S.Y. Cho, and S.H. Kim, Effect of *Allium sativum* L. on the hepatic xanthine oxidase activity in rat, *J. Resource Dev. Yeungnam Univ. 2*: 111 (1983).

68. Huh, K., S.I. Lee, J.M. Park, and S.H. Kim, Effect of diallyl disulfide on the hepatic glutathione-S-transferase activity in rat: diallyl disulfide effect on the glutathione-S-transferase, *Arch. Pharmacol. Res.* (Seoul) *9*:205 (1986), [*Chem. Abstr. 106*: 131525 (1987).]

69. Huh, K., S.I. Lee, J.M. Park, and S.H. Kim, Effect of garlic on the purine metabolic pathway, *J. Pharm. Soc. Korea 30*:62 (1986) [*Chem. Abstr. 105*: 132751 (1986).]

70. Paumgartner, G., and T. Sauerbruch, Gallstones: pathogenesis, *Lancet 338*: 1117 (1991).

71. Diehl, A.K., Epidemiology and natural history of gallstone disease, *Gastroenterol. Clinic North America 20*: 1 (1991).

72. Heaton, K.W., F.E.M. Braddon, R.A. Moutford, et al., Symptomatic and silent gallstones in the community, *Gut. 32*: 316 (1991).

73. Jensen, K.H., and T. Jorgensen, Incidence of gallstones in a Danish population, *Gastroenterology 100*: 790 (1991).

74. Jorgensen T., Gallstones in a Danish population: familial occurrence and social factors, *J. Biol. Sci. 20*: 111 (1988).

75. Kesaniemi, Y.A., M. Koskenvuo, M. Vuoristo, and T.A. Miettinen, Biliary lipid composition in monozygotic and diazygotic pairs of twins, *Gut 30*: 1750 (1986).

76. Pixley, F., D. Wilson, K. McPherson, and J. Mann, Effects of vegetarianism on development of gallstones in women, *Br. Med. J. 291*: 11 (1985).

77. Sompliner, R.E., P.H. Bennett, L.J. Comess, et al., Gallbladder disease in Pima Indians: Demonstration of high prevalence and early onset by cholecystography, *N. Engl. J. Med. 283*: 1358 (1970).

78. MacLure, K.M., K.C. Hays, G.A. Colditz, et al., Weight, diet and risk of symptomatic gallstones in middle-aged women, *N. Engl. J. Med. 321*: 563 (1989).

79. Lee, S.S., B.K. Wasiljew, and M.J. Lee, Gallstones in women younger than thirty, *J. Clin. Gastroenterol. 9*: 65 (1987).

80. Scragg, R.K.R., A.J. Michael, and P.A. Baghurst, Diet, alcohol and relative weight in gallstone disease: a case-control study, *Br. Med. J. 288*: 1113 (1984).

81. Heaton, K.W., F.E.M. Braddon, P.M. Emmett, et al, Why do men get gallstones? Role of abdominal fat and hyperinsulinaemia, *Eur. J. Gastroenterol. Hepatol. 3*: 745 (1991).

82. Hartz, A.J., D.C. Rupley, and A.A. Rimm, The association of girth measurements with disease in 32 856 women, *Am. J. Epidemiol. 119*: 71 (1984).

83. Houmard, J.A., W.S. Wheeler, M.R. McCammon, et al., Effects of fitness level and the regional distribution of fat on carbohydrate metabolism and plasma lipids in middle to older-aged men, *Metabolism 40*: 714 (1991).

84. Thijs, C., P. Knipschild, and P. Drombacher, Serum lipid and gallstones; a case-control study, *Gastroenterology 99*: 843 (1990).

85. Alvaro, D., F. Angelico, A.F. Attili, et al., Plasma lipid lipoproteins and biliary lipid composition in female gallstone patients, *Biomedica Biochem Acta 45*: 761 (1986).

86. Lakso, M., K. Pyorala, E. Voutilainen, and J. Marniemi, Plasma insulin and serum lipids and lipoproteins in middle-aged non-insulin-dependent diabetic and non-diabetic subjects, *Am. J. Epidemiol. 125*: 611 (1987).

87. Kajiyama, G., K. Oyamada, S. Nakao, and A. Miyoshi, The effect of diabetes mellitus and its treatment on the lithogenicity of bile in man, *Hiroshima J. Med. Sci. 30*: 221 (1981).

88. Chait, A., E.L. Bierman, and J.J. Albers, Low-density lipoprotein receptor activity in cultured human skin fibroblasts—mechanisms of insulin-induced stimulation, *J. Clin. Investigation 64*: 1309 (1979).

89. Lakshmanan, M.R., C.M. Hepokroeff, and C.C. Ness, Stimulation by insulin of rat liver hydroxymethylglutaryl coenzyme A reductase and cholesterol-synthesizing activities, *Biochem. Biophys. Res. Commun. 50*: 704 (1973).

90. La Vecchia, C., E. Negri, B.D. Avanzo, et al., Risk factors for gallstone disease requiring surgery, *Int. J. Epidemiol. 20*: 209 (1991).

91. Razay, G., K.W. Heaton, C.H. Bolton, and A.O. Hughes, Alcohol consumption and its relationship to cardiovascular risk factors in British women, *Br. Med. J. 304*: 80 (1992).

92. Marcus, S.N., and K.W. Heaton, Intestinal transit deoxycholic acid and the cholesterol saturation of bile—three inter-related factors, *Gut 27*: 550 (1986).

93. Marcus, S.N., and K.W. Heaton, Deoxycholic acid and the pathogenesis of gallstones, *Gut. 29*: 522 (1988).

94. Heaton, K.W., P.M. Emmett, C.L. Symes, et al., Gallstones in people who are not obese may be explained by slow colonic transit, *Gut 32*: A1210 (1991).

95. Capron, J.P., J. Delamarre, and M.A. Herve, Meal frequency and duration of overnight fast: a role in gallstone formation? *Br. Med. J. 283*: 1435 (1981).

96. Bloch, H.M., J.R. Thornton, and K.W. Heaton, Effects of fasting on the composition of gallbladder bile, *Gut 21*: 1087 (1980).

97. Pixley, F., and J. Mann, Dietary factors in the aetiology of gallstones, a case control study, *Gut 29*: 1511 (1988).

98. Werner, D., P.M. Emmett, and K.W. Heaton, The effect of dietary sucrose on factors influencing cholesterol gallstone formation, *Gut 25*: 269 (1984).

99. Mazzaferri, E.L., G.H. Starich, and S.T. St. Jeor, Augmented gastric inhibitory polypeptide and insulin response to a meal after an increase in carbohydrate (sucrose) intake, *J. Clin. Endocrinol. Metab. 58*: 640 (1984).

100. Reiser, S., E. Bohn, and J. Hallfrisch, Serum insulin and glucose in hyperinsulinemia subjects fed three different levels of sucrose, *Am. J. Clin. Nutr. 34*: 2348 (1981).

101. Pastides, H., A. Tzonon, and D. Trichopoulos, A case-control study of the relationship between smoking, diet and gallbladder disease, *Arch. Intern. Med. 150*: 1409 (1990).

102. Heaton, K.W., The role of diet in the aetiology of cholelithiasis, *Rev. Clin. Nutr. 54*: 549 (1984).

103. Heaton, K.W., Effect of dietary fiber on biliary lipids, *Nutrition in Gastrointestinal Disease* (L. Barbara, G. Bianchi Porro, R. Cheli, and M. Lipkin, eds.), Raven Press, New York, 1987, p. 213

104. Jorgensen, T., and L.M. Jorgensen, Gallstones and diet in a Danish population, *Scand. J. Gastroenterol. 24*: 821 (1989).

105. Hood, K., D. Gleeson, D. Ruppin, and H. Dowling, Can gallstone recurrence be prevented? The British/Belgium post-dissolution trial, *Gastroenterology 94*: A 548 (1988).

106. Alessandrini, A., M.A. Fusco, E. Gatti, and P.A. Rossi, Dietary fiber and cholesterol gallstones: a case control study, *Italian J. Gastroenterol. 14*: 156 (1982).

107. Attili, A.F., and the Rome Group for the Epidemiology and Prevention of Cholelithiasis, 1987, Diet and gallstones: results of an epidemiological study performed in male civil servants, *Nutrition in Gastrointestinal Disease* (L. Barbara, G. Bianchi Porro, R. Cheli, and M. Lipkin, eds.), Raven Press, New York, 1987, p. 225.

108. MacLure, K.M., K.C. Hayes, G.A. Colditz, et al., Dietary predictors of symptom-associated gallstones in middle-aged women, *Am. J. Clin. Nutr. 52*: 16 (1990).

109. Scragg, R.K.R., Aetiology of cholesterol gallstones, *Gallstone Disease and Its Management* (M.C. Bateson, ed.), MTP Press, Lancaster, 1986, p. 25.

110. Thornton, J., C. Symes, and K. Heaton, Moderate alcohol intake reduces bile cholesterol saturation and raises HDL cholesterol, *Lancet 2*: 879 (1983).

111. Khan, I.H., P. Richmond, and A.M. MacLeod, Dieseases of the kidneys and urinary tract, *Human Nutrition and Dietetics*, 9th ed., (J.S. Garow and W.P.T. James, eds.), Churchill Livingstone, Edinburgh, London, 1993, p. 597.

112. Ballmer, P.E., B.A. Weber, and P.B. Roy-Chaudhury et al., Elevation of albumin synthesis rates in nephrotic patients measured with (1^{13}C) leucine, *Kidney Intl. 41*: 132 (1992).

113. Cameron, J.S., Clinical consequences of the nephrotic syndrome, *Oxford Textbook of Clinical Nephrology* (J.S. Cameron, A.M. Davison, J.P. Grunfeld, D. Kerr, and E. Ritz, eds.), Oxford Univ. Press, Oxford, 1992, p. 276.

114. Keysen, G.A., R.W. Davies, and F.N. Hutchison, Effect of dietary protein intake and angiotensin-converting enzyme inhibition in Heyman nephritis, *Kidney Int. 36* (Suppl. 27): 154 (1989).

115. Lee, H.A. Nutritional support in renal and hepatic failure, *Practical Nutritional Support* (S.J. Karran and K.G.M. Alberti, eds.), Pitman Medical, London, 1980, p. 275.

116. El. Nahas, A.M., A. Masters-Thomas, and S.A. Brady, Selective effect of low protein diets in chronic renal diseases, *Br. Med. J. 289*: 1337 (1984).

117. D'Amico, G., and M.G. Gentile, Pharmacological and dietary treatment of lipid abnormalities in nephrotic patients, *Kidney Int. 39* (Suppl.): 65 (1991).

118. Joven, J., C. Villabona, and E. Vilella, Abnormalities of lipoprotein metabolism in patients with the nephrotic syndrome, *N. Engl. J. Med. 323*: 579 (1990).

119. Appel, G., Lipid abnormalities in renal disease, *Kidney Int. 39*: 169 (1991).

120. Derlyne, G.M., and N.P. Mallick, Ischaemic heart disease as a complication of nephrotic syndrome, *Lancet 2*: 399 (1969).

121. Waas, V.J., and J.S. Cameron, Cardiovascular disease and the nephrotic syndrome: The other side of the coin, *Nephron 27*: 58 (1981).

122. Appel, G.B., and Appel, A.S., Lipid lowering agents in proteinuric disease, *Am. J. Nephrol. 10* (Suppl. 1): 110 (1990).

123. Forest, C.E., and G.H. Hartley, Parenteral nutrition in acute renal failure, *J. Human Nutr. Diet. 4*: 361 (1991).

124. El Nahas, A.M., and G.A. Coles, Dietary treatment of renal failure: ten unanswered questions, *Lancet 1*: 597 (1986).

125. Giovannetti, S., Answers to ten questions on the dietary treatment of chronic renal failure, *Lancet 2*: 1140 (1986).

126. Locatelli, F., D. Alberti, and G. Graziani, Prospective randomized, multicentre trial of effect of protein restriction on progression of chronic renal inefficiency, *Lancet 337*: 1299 (1991).

127. Mitch, W.E., Diet and kidney diesease, *Diet, Nutrition, and Health* (K.K. Carroll, ed.), McGill-Queen's Univ. Press, London, 1989, p. 130.

128. Mitch, W.E., Dietary protein restriction in patients with chronic renal failure, *Kidney Int. 40*: 326 (1991).

129. Mitch, W.E., M. Walser, T.I. Steinman, S. Hill, S. Zeger, and K. Tungsanga, The effect of a ketoacid-amino acid supplement to a restricted diet on the progression of chronic renal failure, *N. Engl. J. Med. 311*: 623 (1984).

130. Wolfson, M., M.R. Jones, and J.D. Kopple, Amino acid losses during haemodialysis with infusion of amino acids and glucose, *Kidney Int. 21*: 500 (1982).

131. Yamauchi, A., M. Fujii, and D. Shirai, Plasma concentration and peritoneal clearance of oxalate in patients on continuous ambulatory peritoneal dialysis (CPAD), *Clin. Nephrology 25*: 181 (1986).

132. Winearls, C.G., D.O. Oliver, M.J. Pippard, C. Reid, M.R. Downing, and P.M. Cotes, Effect of human enythropioetin derived from recombinant DNA on the anaemia of patients maintained by haemodialysis, *Lancet 2*: 1175 (1986).

133. Bommer, J., C. Alexiou, U. Muller-Buhl, J. Eidfert, and E. Ritz, Recombinant human erythropoietin therapy in haemodialysis patients: dose determination and clinical experience, *Nephrol. Dialysis and Transplantation 2*: 238 (1987).

134. Halstead, S.B. Cause of bladder stones in England: a retrospective epidemiological study, *Urolithiasis: Clinical and Basic Research* (L.H. Smith, W.G. Robertson, 2nd, P.B. Finlayson, eds.), Plenum, London, 1981, p. 325.

135. Valyasevi, A., S.B. Halstead, and S. Dhanamita, Studies in bladder stone disease in Thailand. 6. Urinary studies in children, 2–10 years old, resident in a hypo- and hyperendemic area, *Am. J. Clin. Nutr. 20*: 1362 (1967).

136. Sharman, V.L., Hypercalciuria, *New Clinical Applications in Nephrology. Calculas Disease* (G.R.D. Catto, ed.), Kluwer Academic, Lancaster, 1988, p. 35.

137. Coe, F.L., J.H. Parks, and J.R. Aspin, The pathogenesis and treatment of kidney stones, *N. Engl. J. Med. 327*: 1141 (1992).

138. Massey, L.K., Dietary salt, urinary calcium and kidney stone risk, *Nutr. Rev. 53*: 131 (1995).

29
Diet and Gastrointestinal Diseases

I. INTRODUCTION

The principal fatal diseases of the stomach and bowel include acute diarrhea; cancers of the large bowel, stomach, esophagus, liver, and pancreas; peptic ulcer; and liver disease (hepatitis and cirrhosis). Food poisoning or infection is the major cause of fatal acute diarrhea, the most commonly found malady in the malnourished societies of developing countries. In the industrially developed countries, cancer is the principal cause of gut-related deaths, of which cancer of the large bowel (colon and rectum) has the highest cumulative incidence worldwide, followed by stomach cancer. The increase in large bowel cancer in Japan has been shown to be related to a transition from a traditional low-fat, high-starch diet to one containing more fat, meat, and sugar (1). Diet is implicated in the etiology of both large bowel and stomach cancer (see Chapter 25).

Cummings (2) listed the following major gastrointestinal (G.I.) causes of morbidity:

1. Acute diarrhea and vomiting
2. Peptic ulcer and dyspepsia (including heatburn and hiatus hernia)
3. Constipation and abdominal pain (including irritable bowel)
4. Hemorrhoids and fissure
5. Hernia
6. Gallstones
7. Appendicitis
8. Malabsorption syndromes (including celiac disease and sprue)
9. Diverticular disease of the colon
10. Ulcerative colitis and Crohn's disease
11. Pancreatitis
12. Liver disease (hepatitis, alcohol-induced disorders and cirrhosis)
13. Food intolerance

Although most of these gut diseases are not fatal, they are significant causes of poor health. Surgical operations related to the gut include repair of hernias, appendectomy, treatment of hemorrhoids and anal fissure, removal of gallstones, and surgery for peptic ulcer.

Diet and nutrition play a major role in the management of actue diarrhea through the use of oral rehydration therapy in celiac disease (gluten-free diets) and malabsorption (low-fat and nutritional supplements) as well as in constipation and diverticular disease (high non-starch polysaccharide and resistant starch diets). In all other G.I. disorders, diet and nutritional therapy can become useful adjuncts to the medical treatment.

The use of garlic for stomach and intestinal troubles has been known since ancient times. The consumption of garlic by the people of the Balkans is considered to be the reason for their exceptional resistance to all kinds of intestinal diseases (3,4). According to Reuter et al. (4), the stimulating effect of garlic oil on the mucous membranes of the stomach causes a stimulation of the glands, which then secrete an increased amount of hydrochloric acid and digestive enzymes into the gastric juice. The antibacterial property of garlic is highly effective in the intestines, especially on pathological intestinal flora; suppressing the foreign organisms and favoring the normal coli vegetation (5,6). This explains the repeatedly observed effects of garlic against pathogenic organisms causing typhus, paratyphus, cholera, dysentery, and the like. The simultaneous antiseptic and fermentative inhibitory effects of steam-distilled garlic oil reduce or prevent G.I. autointoxication, especially by phenols and indoles. The clinical efficacy of garlic for G.I. problems has been reported by many researchers (7–9). Fresh garlic and steam-distilled garlic oil have been found to be highly effective in the therapy of G.I. catarrh in horses, cattle, and goats and are equally effective in the treatment of atony and hypertony of the forestomach of ruminant animals (4).

II. ESOPHAGEAL DISORDERS: DYSPHAGIA AND HEARTBURN

Both dysphagia and heartburn arising from esophageal disorders are associated with chest pain. Dysphagia (swallowing difficulty) is accompanied by reduced food intake, leading to rapid weight loss. Oral dysphagia may arise from inability to initiate swallowing by emptying the mouth and is often due to neuromuscular problems such as Parkinson's disease, motor neuron disease, and muscular dystrophy. The principal causes of oropharyngeal and esophageal dysphagia are shown in Table 1 (2). Pharyngeal dysphagia is associated with failure to coordinate closure of the entry to the trachea adequately, with the result that food is inhaled, causing choking and coughing on swallowing. Fluids may be regurgitated through the nose. Among the major causes of oropharyngeal dysphagia are stroke, head injury, and physical obstruction of the pharynx due to an enlarged thyroid (goiter), or head and neck cancers. Acute tonsillitis can also commonly cause dysphagia. A psychological disorder in which the patient may sometimes complain of something permanently sticking in the throat (no physical abnormality), often known as globus hystericus, has also been reported.

Oropharyngeal dysphagia is difficult to manage, and proper assessment of the patient's swallowing ability requires various medical skills. Maintenance of body weight is important, if necessary, by resorting early to enteral feeding via a fine-bore nasogastric tube or gastrostomy.

In addition to stricture, neuromuscular disorders such as achalasia and scleroderma are common causes of esophageal dysphagia. Esophageal strictures may be malignant, gradually causing dysphagia for solid food. Chronic benign strictures due to acid-pepsin disease are often preceded by heartburn. The initial intermittent dysphagia becomes more difficult with both liquid and solid foods. The esophagus may become more cold-sensitive than usual.

Malignant strictures can be managed by surgery, and benign strictures may be treated with endoscopic dilatation, requiring attention to diet to maintain reasonable nutritional status. Patients with esophageal narrowing may require protein and energy supplements in the form of liquid feeds. The particle size of the diet should be commensurate with the degree of esophageal narrowing. Patients with esophageal stricture rarely choke, unlike persons with pharyngeal disorders (2).

Heartburn is characterized by an irritating sensation (hot or burning) that occurs retrosternally, often accompanied by the rise of acid into the mouth, and pain (gripping) that may radiate into the arm and throat and through the back. The burning sensation is due to reflux into the lower esophagus of acid and pepsin from the stomach, which may lead to inflammation (esophagitis). The reflux of gastric contents into the esophagus is normally prevented by an efficient valve at the gastro-esophageal junction. Most reflux occurs as the result of lowering of the pressure in the

Table 1 Principal Causes of Dysphagia

Type	Causes
Oropharyngeal	
Neuromuscular	Stroke
	Head injury
	Muscular disorders
	Motor neuron disease
	Parkinson's disease
Physical obstruction	Pharyngeal pouch
	Goiter
Psychological	Globus hystericus
Infections	Acute tonsillitis
Esophageal	
Neural	Achalasia
	Multiple sclerosis
	Diffuse esophageal spasm
Muscular	Scleroderma
	Dystrophia myotonica
Physical obstruction	Stricture
	Cancer
	Chronic esophagitis
	Diverticulum
	External compression
	Postoperative
Infections	Monilia

Source: Ref. 2.

lower esophageal sphincter (LES), which becomes hypotonic in heartburn, relaxing inappropriately. Reflux is thought to occur mainly at night, although Gudmundsson et al. (10) showed that
during the period from 5 pm to midnight, the esophagus was most exposed to acid. LES pressure
is raised by protein and lowered by fat, alcohol, smoking, and coffee (11–14). Pregnancy as well
as variation in the estrogen and progesterone levels during the normal menstrual cycle may also
lower LES pressure, giving a greater tendency to heartburn during the luteal phase (15,16). Also,
physical pressure on the abdomen (during bending) and straining (due to constipation) may
aggravate reflux, as may anatomical disruption of the gastro-esophageal junction after surgery or
in hiatus hernia (2).

Some people are very susceptible to heartburn, the gnawing pain in the chest caused by the
reflux of acid from the stomach into the esophagus. Unlike the stomach, the esophagus has no
mucous lining to protect it. The acid quickly erodes the esophageal lining, causing pain. An
important dietary measure for avoiding heartburn is to eat smaller meals, and especially meals
that are low in fat, because fatty meals remain in the stomach longer than low-fat meals. Observing the recommendations for prevention of ulcer also helps, viz., stop smoking if one smokes and
avoid foods and other substances that can specifically contribute to heartburn, such as chili powder, onions, garlic, peppermint, caffeine, alcohol, and chocolate. It is best not to lie down after
eating.

Certain physical conditions such as pregnancy and obesity result in increased production of
estrogen and progesterone, which in turn relax the lower esophageal (cardiac) sphincter to accentuate heartburn. Adipose (fat) tissue turns circulating hormones into estrogens. Obese persons

should slim down to a more healthy weight. Long-term heartburn may require aggressive medical therapy because it may lead to alteration in esophageal cells, increasing the risk of a rare form of cancer.

Weight reduction, avoiding tight clothing around the abdomen, and cessation of smoking help to manage heartburn, which can usually be controlled by following the checklist given below (2):

1. Decrease weight to ideal
2. Avoid constricting clothes and bending
3. Elevate head of bed or pillows
4. Stop smoking
5. Avoid alcohol, coffee, and fatty foods, especially in the evening
6. Review drugs
7. Combat gastric acid
8. Consider surgery

Hamilton et al. (17) reported that elevation of the pillow on a 10-inch wedge was most beneficial in reducing acid exposure in the lower esophagus. It is advisable to avoid coffee, alcohol, and fat intake and large meals at night. These general measures have been found to be successful in the majority of heartburn cases. Another effective therapy aims at neutralizing or reducing gastric acid secretion by using anti-secretary drugs such as cimetidine, ranitidine, or omeprazole and antacids. In severe cases, such as in hiatus hernia, surgery may be beneficial.

III. DISORDERS OF STOMACH AND DUODENUM

A. Gastric and Duodenal Ulcers and Dyspepsia

Gastric and duodenal ulcers are the most common disorders of the G.I. tract, duodenal ulcer being more common than gastric ulcer. Deaths may occur through the complications of bleeding and perforation. An increase in the consumption of nonsteroidal anti-inflammatory drugs such as aspirin, indomethacin, diclofenal, ibuprofen, ketoprofen, naproxen, and so forth has been found to be associated with occurrence of bleeding peptic ulcer (18).

An unfortunate sign of so-called success can be an ulcer; because in many "successful" people, stress and tension greatly excite the nerves that control the stomach, which in turn increases acid secretion by the stomach's parietal cells. The acid erodes through the mucous layer into the stomach tissue, resulting in gastric ulcer. The acid can also erode the tissue lining of the duodenum to give rise to a duodenal ulcer. A peptic ulcer generally refers to either of these types of ulcers.

Some people are more susceptible to ulcers than others because of a decreased ability of their stomach and intestinal cells to protect themselves from acid. Research indicates that an infection by bacteria, especially by *Helicobacter pylori*, is a possible provoker of ulcers in humans.

Most ulcers in younger people occur in the duodenum; they occur mostly in the stomach in elderly people. The typical symptom of an ulcer is pain 2 hours after eating, when the digestive acids that work on a meal irritate the ulcer after most of the meal has moved to the jejunum of the small intestine.

In the past, milk and cream therapy (the Sippy diet) was used to help cure ulcers. Today, it is known that milk and cream are both the worst foods for an ulcer, because the calcium in these foods stimulates gastrin, the hormone that in turn increases stomach acid secretion. Thus, this therapy actually inhibits ulcer healing.

Antacid medications are a first line of medical treatment for ulcers, along with the medicines called H_2 blockers, including cimetidine (Tagamet), ranitidine (Zantac), famotidine (Pepcid), and others. They prevent histamine-related acid secretion in the stomach and gastrin release. By preventing histamine from increasing acid secretion, the H_2 blockers greatly speed up ulcer healing, thus reducing the need for surgical treatment. Coating agents, such as sucralfate, that coat the ulcer are also commonly used.

Patients with ulcer are advised to stop smoking if practiced and minimize the use of aspirin and other aspirin-like drugs. These practices reduce the mucus secreted by the stomach. These therapies, combined with use of antacids as needed, have so revolutionized ulcer therapy that changing one's diet is of minor importance today. The current diet therapy, however, recommends that foods that increase ulcer symptoms be avoided (e.g., coffee, tea, alcohol, pepper, chili and other spices). It is also advocated to eat nutritious meals on a regular schedule, chew foods well, and lose weight, if one is overweight.

Peptic ulcer seems to involve acid secretion in the stomach; the other factors that are associated include the integrity of the mucus layer, gastric emptying and duodenal motility, bicarbonate secretion in the stomach, gastric blood flow, prostaglandin production in the mucosa, and infection with *Helicobacter pylori*. Diet has little proven role in either cause or management of peptic ulcer.

The cardinal symptom of peptic ulcer is pain felt in the epigastrium, which is burning or nagging in quality and relieved by suppressing gastric acid. Peptic ulcer pain is one of a number of gastroduodenal systems collectively called *dyspepsia*, which is any type of discomfort affecting the upper abdomen or lower chest and is associated with meals. Dyspepsia is synonymous with indigestion, whose symptoms may include pain, heartburn, nausea, abdominal distension, discomfort, flatulence, and regurgitation. Dyspepsia is caused by a number of conditions, including peptic ulcer, esophagitis, gallbladder disease, pancreatitis, irritable bowel and other colonic disorders, and hepatitis.

Peptic ulcer can be managed by suppressing acid and eliminating its secretion, strengthening mucosal resistance by drugs and eliminating *Helicobacter pylori*. Stopping smoking speeds up the healing of ulcers (19). Dietary restrictions of alcohol and coffee are not of proven benefit and thus not mandatory. Some studies (20) have indicated that a moderate alcohol intake promotes ulcer healing. Excessive milk intake is thought to promote gastric secretion, leading to hypercalcemia. There is no evidence to show that avoiding eating of spicy foods or acidic foods like citrus fruits is of any help in healing of peptic ulcer. One clinical trial, however, has shown that a high-fiber diet delays relapse after ulcer healing (21).

Peptic ulcers can be effectively controlled by drug therapy, e.g., drugs inhibiting gastric acid secretion, gastric acid neutralizers (antacids), drugs inhibiting gastric acid and pepsin secretion, those which increase mucus defense, prostaglandin analogues that inhibit gastric secretion, and antibiotics eliminating *Helicobacter pylori*.

B. Gastric Surgery

Surgery is performed in cases of peptic ulcer for which prolonged medical treatment has failed, for bleeding and perforation of pyloric stenosis, and in suspicious malignant gastric ulcer. Whereas selective (proximal) vagoctomy is the most favored operation because it is associated with a less than 10% complication rate, partial gastrectomy may be required in some circumstances and is combined with various drainage procedures. The normal stomach controls emptying of its contents most effectively, through pancreatic biliary secretions. Some breakdown (grinding) of larger particles takes place in the gastric antrum. Gastric surgery disrupts this regulation. Cummings (2) listed the following major problems following gastric surgery:

1. Early dumping
2. Diarrhea
3. Bile vomiting
4. Small stomach syndrome
5. Weight loss
6. Anemia
7. Rare sequelae: hypoglycemia (late dumping), bone disease, and B_{12} deficiency.

The most common postsurgical problem is early dumping, characterized by a feeling of fullness and abdominal distension within about 30 minutes of starting a meal, often accompanied by nausea, vomiting, sweating, faintness, and palpitations. Gastric surgery almost always leads to accelerated gastric emptying, which occurs both for solids and liquids after partial gastrectomy and after truncal vagotomy with pyloroplasty. Accelerated gastric emptying leads to the "dumping" into the duodenum of large amounts of hypertonic fluid, which is normally held back by the intact stomach.

Early dumping can be managed by preventing hypertonic material from entering the upper gut by avoiding sugary foods, milk, and low-molecular-weight carbohydrates. Starch is preferable in small frequent meals. Alcoholic beverages, being hypertonic, should be cut down. Soluble dietary fiber such as pectin aids in slowing gastric emptying (22).

Total removal of stomach (gastrectomy), an occasional surgical measure, almost always causes epigastic discomfort, fullness, and nausea, usually accompanied by dumping and unpleasant bile vomiting. Patients are often malnourished and require supportive dietary management. Frequent 2-hourly meals without any hypertonic foods are useful. The patient must chew food thoroughly and should not swallow indigestible material, which may obstruct the small bowel. Dietary supplements may be required, especially in the early months, to maintain adequate caloric intake. Vitamin B_{12} and iron deficiency are most common and must be treated.

Gastric surgery also frequently leads to diarrhea (post-vagotomy diarrhea) due to failure to control gastric emptying and denervation of the small bowel. The result is rapid passage of food through the gut, increased bile acids in the colon, and mild malabsorption. Dietary treatment is similar to that for early dumping, together with anti-diarrheal drugs (codeine and loperamide).

Late dumping is a rare condition, comprising the onset of sweating, palpitations, weakness, and occasional unconsciousness, 2 to 3 hours after a meal. These symptoms are readily recognized as those produced by hypoglycemia. The entry of hypertonic sugary foods into the duodenum is thought to lead to high levels of insulin secretion, which in turn causes hypoglycemia. Late dumping can be managed by giving glucose or sugar orally and by providing an early dumping diet regimen.

Nutritional complications related to weight loss, iron-deficiency anemia, B_{12} deficiency, and osteomalacia may also follow gastric surgery. Weight loss occurs as the result of reduced food intake as a consequence of the development of postsurgical syndrome. Iron-deficiency anemia, although mild in others, may be severe in menstruating women. This can be treated with liquid iron preparations. Vitamin B_{12} deficiency can be managed with regular hydroxycobalamin injections. Osteoporosis and osteomalacia, which occur commonly after gastric surgery, can be managed by maintaining vitamin D levels and exercise (2).

C. Diarrhea and Vomiting

Diarrhea is defined as the frequent passage of loose, watery stools. Acute diarrhea, which is often a short-lived, self-limiting condition, may be caused by bacterial infection (*Escherichia coli*, *Campylobacter jejuni*, *Vibrio cholerae*, *Staphylococcus aureus*, *Clostridium perfringens*, *Bacillus cereus*, *Vibrio parahemolyticus*, *Shigella* sp., *Salmonella* sp., *Yersinia* sp.) and a number of viruses. These can produce acute gastroenteritis, food poisoning, and traveler's diarrhea. The diarrhea-causing bacteria either secrete an enterotoxin (toxigenic) or invade the bowel wall (invasive). Whereas cholera and *E. coli* are toxigenic, *Shigella* (dysentery) and *Salmonella* (typhoid) are of invasive types.

Chronic diarrhea may occur in malabsorption syndromes (celiac disease, tropical sprue, and pancreatic insufficiency), inflammatory bowel disease (ulcerative colitis and Crohn's disease), following gut resection, chronic parasitic and other infections (Giardia and tuberculosis), drugs (laxative abuse), irritable bowel, and diverticular disease (2).

There is a massive fecal loss of water and electrolytes in acute diarrhea which is made worse if accompanied by vomiting and sweating. Normal stool contains very little sodium and is high in potassium. As stool weight increases, sodium concentration rises and potassium falls. At about 500 g of stool/day, sodium and potassium are equimolar (55 mmol/kg), approaching plasma levels thereafter (130 mmol/l for sodium and 4 mmol/l for potassium) at stool outputs of over 5 kg/day. With stool weights of up to 1000 g day, losses of sodium and potassium are not greater than normal dietary intakes found in Western populations (i.e., about 150 mmol/day for sodium and 75 mmol/day for potassium). Beyond this, replacement of electrolytes is essential and is advisable at much lower stool outputs if there is accompanying fever, anorexia, and vomiting (Table 2) (23,24).

Acute diarrhea quickly gives rise to salt and water depletion, especially in the very young, as shown by fatigue, irritability, drowsiness, muscle cramps, thirst, loss of appetite, nausea, headache, and faintness. Urine volume decreases and salt depletion may lead to vomiting. Moderate dehydration is difficult to diagnose unless the patient is weighed daily.

Severe diarrhea may need rapid intravenous fluid and electrolyte replacement. In recent years, the advent of oral rehydration therapy (ORT) has been a very useful and effective way of treating diarrhea. First used to treat cholera in the Philippines (25), ORT has been applied to all causes of acute diarrhea and for all age groups. ORT is based on the observation that the capacity of the gut to absorb salt and water, in the presence of glucose or amino acids, remains relatively intact despite pronounced sodium secretion induced by binding of enterotoxin to gut epithelial cells (26). ORT solutions thus combine the maximum tolerable amounts of salt within an absorbable carbohydrate.

Table 2 Electrolyte Losses in Adult Feces

Daily stool amount (g)	Losses (mmol/day)	
	Sodium	Potassium
200	6	13
400	20	23
600	37	31
800	56	38
1000	76	45
2000	190	70
3000	316	88
4000	452	101
5000	595	111
6000 or > 6000	130 mmol/kg	20 mmol/kg

Source: Ref. 2.

Table 3   Electrolyte Concentrations (mmol/l) of Some Oral Rehydration Therapy (ORT) Solutions

Name	Sodium	Potassium	Glucose/sucrose	Made to recommended volume of (ml)
WHO-ORT[a]	90	20	111	1000
Dioralyte	35	20	200	200
Electrolade	50	20	111	200
Electrosol	35	20	200	200
Glucolyte	35	20	200	200
Paedialyte	75	20	139	250
Rehidrat	50	20	187[c]	230
Oxo	140	5	0	200
Home brew[b]	34	14	280[b]	500

[a]WHO-recommended solution.
[b]Home brew recipe: dissolve 1/4 teaspoonful salt and 4 heaped teaspoonsful sugar in 150 ml boiling water. Add 150 ml fresh orange juice and make up to 500 ml with tapwater. Sugar all present as sucrose.
[c]Glucose + sucrose.
Source: Ref. 2.

Cummings (2) provided a list of available powders for formulating ORT and a recipe for homemade solutions (Table 3). A variety of electrolyte concentrations are found, with the WHO-ORT being the highest for sodium (except for Oxo). The WHO mixture has been targeted at the mild to moderate diarrhea of the tropics, whereas other solutions are used in non-tropical countries, where the wide variation in the electrolyte content has been found to be safe and effective in treating modestly dehydrated people (27).

Glucose-based ORTs need good (microbiologically safe) water. The high osmolarity of glucose itself may perpetuate diarrhea and mixing errors may cause hypernatremia. Thus, the use of soluble starch (rice or cereals) has replaced a part or all of the glucose (28,29). Gore et al. (30) also found that rice-based solutions decreased the severity of diarrhea in chloera and were more palatable and reduced vomiting (31,32). Cereal starches are well digested in the gut and provide some protein.

D.   Malabsorption

Malabsorption may result from impaired digestion and absorption of carbohydrate, protein or fat, and is classically termed *steatorrhea*, the passage of excessive amount of fat in the feces. It is encountered commonly in pancreatic insufficiency, celiac, and Crohn's disease. In all these conditions, there is also variable malabsorption of carbohydrate and protein in addition to fat. The principal causes of malabsorption observed in clinical practice are shown in Table 4. Celiac disease and tropical sprue are the most commonly encountered causes of malabsorption; patients usually pass stools that are bulky and porridgy, foul-smelling, greasy, and difficult to flush away. There may be loss of appetite and weight, although in some forms of malabsorption, such as pancreatic insufficiency, the appetite is increased. Symptoms such as abdominal distension, increased gas, and pain may lead to anemia and bone disease as later complications.

Malabsorption may be clinically assessed by measuring fecal fat or fat absorption and screening blood for specific nutritional deficiencies such as iron, B_{12}, and folic acid. Anatomical examination of the stomach and small bowel by x-ray may also be used, followed by mucosal biopsy (2).

Table 4 Principal Causes of Malabsorption

Type	Causes
Anatomical	Surgical resection (short bowel syndrome)
	Fistula
	Gastric surgery
	Blind loop and stricture
	Jejunal diverticulosis
Enzymatic deficiencies	Pancreatic disease
	Biliary obstruction
	Disaccharidase deficiencies
Mucosal defects	Celiac disease
	Tropical sprue
	Crohn's disease
	Radiation
Systemic causes	Scleroderma
	Diabetes
	Lymphoma
	Thyroid disease
	Severe skin disorders
Drugs	Cholestyramine
	Antibiotics (Neomycin)
	Excess laxatives
Infections	Giardia and parasitic infestation
	Tuberculosis
	Bacterial overgrowth
	Whipple's disease

Source: Ref. 2.

Nutritional supplements to be given on prescription have been developed for specific disorders such as bowel fistula, disaccharide intolerance, celiac disease, cystic fibrosis, dysphagia, gastrectomy, and other intestinal surgery and malabsorption; these are also available for several other more general health problems such as cancer cachexia, anorexia nervosa, liver disease, hypercholesterolemia, and inherited metabolic disorders. The problem of weight loss thus can be managed in patients who lose their appetite.

Low-fat diets are useful in the management of diarrhea but reduce energy intake significantly. Nutritional supplements can be used to counteract steatorrhea while keeping energy intake high. Medium-chain triglycerides (MCT) are more readily hydrolyzed by pancreatic lipase than long-chain fat. Also, they do not require micelle formation for their absorption, being taken up directly into the portal vein. They aid in the absorption of fat-soluble vitamins. However, MCTs provide less energy than long-chain fat (8.3 vs. 9.0 kcal) and cause diarrhea. They are generally given in a dose of 15 ml four times a day to provide 350 to 400 kcal.

In malabsorption, partly digested carbohydrate and protein enter into the large bowel where they are fermented by the colon bacteria to produce gases (carbon dioxide and hydrogen). Gas problem can be minimized by attention to the type of carbohydrate in the diet, e.g. omitting foods containing nonabsorbable sugars such as raffinose and stachyose (peas and beans), avoiding lactose if there is lactase deficiency, and ensuring that dietary starch is in a readily digestible form (33). Fermentation of dietary fiber (nonstarch polysaccharides, NSP) is also a source of gas production in the colon, although it is less of a problem with poorly digested NSP sources (e.g.,

Table 5 Diet to Reduce Gas Formation

Sugars	Avoid nonabsorbable sugars such as raffinose and stachyose, present mostly in peas and beans. Lactose—avoid milk if evidence of lactase deficiency
Oligosaccharides	Fructans are not digested in small bowel. Present in artichokes, onions, leeks, chicory, salsify
Starch	Most starch should be freshly cooked and eaten hot, or as white bread Rice starch is readily digestible
	Avoid unmilled grains and seeds, unripe banana, and incompletely cooked potato and maize; cooked and cooled starches other than cereal starches
NSP (fiber)	Do not encourage consumption of high-fiber foods. Keep intake of fruit, vegetables and pulses to average or below average amounts. Soluble fiber is potentially worse than insoluble

Source: Ref. 2.

wheat bran). A rapidly fermented material will produce gas at a rate that the colon cannot absorb fast enough (34), causing discomfort. Examples of some low-gas diets are given in Table 5.

Vitamins and minerals are often required to treat anemia and bone disease in malabsorption or to prevent development of deficiency. Supplements of individual vitamins and minerals are preferred to mixed preparations and allow the doses to be tailored to the patient's needs and monitored using hematological and biochemical indices.

E. Celiac Disease

Celiac disease is a common cause of malabsorption, with a morphologically abnormal jejunal mucosa that improves when gluten is withdrawn from the diet and relapses on gluten challenge (35,36). Dicke (37) first established a link between cereals and celiac disease and showed that it was a protein, gluten, which damaged the intestine. Celiac disease, more appropriately termed gluten-induced enteropathy, is most prevalent in Galway, Ireland, and occurs in all societies where wheat is a staple food.

Gluten consists of an insoluble fraction, glutenin, and a soluble fraction containing a series of gliadins (alpha, beta, gamma, and omega) that are toxic. Gliadins are thought to damage mucosa through an immune mechanism. Celiac mucosa contains increased numbers of immunocytes, secreting mainly IgM, IgA, and IgG. Serum levels of IgA are raised and plasma antibodies to gluten fraction are found in blood (38).

Flat jejunal mucosa is the characteristic lesion of celiac disease. Both the anatomical and functional digestive ability of the intestine are affected by decreased activities of disaccharidases. Cummings (2) listed the following causes of a flattened jejunal mucosa:

1. Celiac disease (gluten enteropathy)
2. Tropical sprue
3. Acute gastroenteritis
4. Milk and soya protein intolerance (infants)
5. Kwashiorkor
6. Hypogammaglobulinemia
7. Bacterial overgrowth

8. Dermatitis herpetiformis
9. Drugs (e.g., mefenamic acid)

Clinical features in children include abdominal distension and wasting around buttocks, loss of apptetite, and bulky, pale stools. Adult celiac disease is characterized by diarrhea, anemia, and weight loss. Anemia is caused by folate and iron deficiency (39). The diarrhea is characterized by steatorrhea. About 60% of patients show weight loss, and approximately 40% have abdominal pain, oral ulceration, and anemia. Rarely, bone pain may occur with skin lesions, vitamin K deficiency, ankle edema, amenorrhea, and depression. Jejunal biopsy helps diagnosis.

Diet is the key to the management of celiac disease. Toxic protein gluten being present in wheat, barley, rye, and oats, these foods must be excluded from the patient's diet for life. Rice, maize, and soya products are safe. Some patients are sensitive to oat gluten, whereas others are not. Obvious foods such as breakfast cereals, bread, cakes, pastry, biscuits, and pies can be easily omitted from the diet, but hidden sources of gluten are difficult to exclude, because wheat flour is added to many products. Food labeling often makes this clear, and patients should learn to look at it. Skerritt and Hill (40) have made available a simple home test kit for gluten in foods for celiac patients.

Because diet without the major cereals is quite restricting, a large number of gluten-free food products have been developed. The U.K. Coeliac Society provides information about diet, gluten-free food brands and other aspects. Iron and folate supplements may be useful in the beginning. Bulk laxatives help in relieving constipation. A gluten-free diet reduces the risk of intestinal malignancy. Around 15% of patients who do not respond to gluten withdrawal may be managed with corticosteroids. Many patients with dermatits herpetiformis (blistering and irritating eruption) also have a flat jejunal mucosa and respond to gluten withdrawal (2).

F. Tropical Sprue

Tropical sprue is characterized by morphological changes in the intestinal mucosa similar to those of celiac disease. It is a chronic intestinal disorder that occurs in the tropics, characterized by villous atrophy leading to malabsorption of fat, vitamin B_{12}, and folate; it can be treated by using broad-spectrum antibiotics (41). The morphology of the normal small-bowel mucosa of people living in the tropics varies from that of people in the temperate regions. In the tropics, normal finger-like villi are rarely present; instead, the mucosa appears flattened, with leaves and ridges (42). In tropical sprue, which is a distinct entity, there is progressive failure of bowel function that requires specific treatment. Tropical sprue occurs solely in those who have lived in, or have traveled to, India, southeast Asia, northern South America, and Africa. It is characterized by chronic diarrhea, often followed by an acute episode, with weight loss, anorexia, anemia, and edema. The condition may become fatal if it remains untreated. A persistent enteric bacterial or viral infection affects both jejunum and ileum. Malabsorption of fat, vitamin B_{12}, folate, and xylose are followed by megaloblastic anemia and secondary lactose intolerance. Specific treatment includes broad-spectrum antibiotics and folate. Diet therapy is supportive rather than therapeutic. Patients need to correct weight loss.

G. Short Bowel Syndrome (SBS)

Sometimes a portion of small bowel must be removed surgically after mesenteric embolism or thrombosis, intestinal strangulation, trauma, Crohn's disease, or lymphoma. Removal of 50 to 100 cm segments of small bowel is usually without any nutritional consequence, unless it is in the terminal ileum. However, larger resections leaving less than 1 m bowel will result in severe, acute, and long-term problems.

The management of SBS depends on the amount of bowel resected, the site of resection (i.e., jejunum or ileum), the amount of any associated colonic resection, and presence or absence of an ileocecal valve. A massive ileocolonic resection is hardest to manage, mid-jejunal being best. Survival is possible with as little as 30 to 60 cm of small bowel because the patients adapt after the initial episode in the residual small and large bowels. The intestinal adaptation may include an increase in the mass of remaining bowel, hypertrophy of the mucosal surface, and lengthening of the villi, resulting in significant increase in the absorptive surface (43), which occurs as a result of the exposure of the remaining bowel to nutrients, bile, and pancreatic enzymes, and the tropic effect of gut hormones and short-chain fatty acids (44,45). A converse of this adaptation occurs during starvation in the form of atrophy (46).

The ileum is responsible for absorption of B_{12}, bile acid, salt, and water; short resections of the terminal ileum (less than 100 cm), which often include the ileocecal valve, result in bile malabsorption and consequent diarrhea and mild steatorrhea and eventual B_{12} deficiency. Gallstones are also more common.

SBS can be effectively managed by using the bile-acid-binding resin cholestyramine, given in a single morning dose, when bile acid concentrations are high in the duodenum. Vitamin B_{12} may be provided prophylactically. A reduced-fat diet, though not essential, may help to decrease diarrhea.

Diarrhea and weight loss are common after ileal resection of over 100 cm, giving rise to substantial steatorrhea due to chronic bile acid deficiency. A low-fat diet is effective in controlling diarrhea but may not help to maintain weight. Vitamin B_{12} injections are essential. The gastric hypersecretion in SBS patients may impair pancreatic enzyme activity and thus it should be suppressed with H_2 blockers.

Massive resection of jejunum and ileum produce an acute problem of watery diarrhea, weight loss, and malabsorption, necessitating total parenteral nutrition (TPN), which may prove to be life saving until recovery. Oral feeding can be introduced as soon as the patient can tolerate it, to encourage growth and adaptation of the remaining bowel mucosa. Starchy foods have lower osmolarity than sugars and are less likely to aggravate diarrhea. A low-fat diet of 30 g/day is a standard practice, but its use has been challenged (47). Fat-soluble vitamins as well as iron and zinc are essential. The essential fatty acids may be provided through topical application (skin-rub).

Patients with short bowel syndrome who retain most of their large intestine after massive small bowel loss may get oxalate renal stones, which are caused by precipitation of calcium salts and increase in oxalate solubility by the excess fat in the colon. Also, lactic acidosis may arise as the result of microbial fermentation of excess carbohydrate reaching the cecum. These conditions may be treated with a low-fat and low-oxalate diet and antibiotics, respectively (2).

H. Lactose Intolerance

The universal presence of lactose, a disaccharide of glucose and galactose, in all mammalian milks necessitates that the newborn mammals have the required enzyme, lactase (beta-1, 4-galactosidase), to utilize this milk sugar. However, after weaning, lactase activity has been found to decline rapidly in all species, including humans. In the absence of lactase, milk consumption may produce diarrhea, abdominal pain, and distension because the unabsorbed lactose exerts an osmotic effect in the small intestine, resulting in large amounts of fluid and sugar entering the large bowel, where lactose is rapidly fermented to produce gas, and osmotic diarrhea ensues (48,49). Certain traditional milk-drinking populations appear to retain the ability to digest lactose into adulthood, e.g., the so-called Aryan peoples in the Middle East, northern India, northern Europe, and whites from North America, Australia, and New Zealand, although even among these pople about 5% to 10% may have lactase deficiency (2). In addition to these genetic factors, lac-

Table 6 Causes of Lactase Deficiency (Lactose Intolerance)

Genetic	Absent at birth (rare)
	Declines after weaning (common)
Acquired	Protein-calorie malnutrition
	Celiac disease
	Tropical sprue
	Small-bowel resection
	Crohn's disease
	Acute gastroenteritis
	Chronic alcoholism
	Immunodeficiency syndrome
	Cow's milk protein intolerance

Source: Ref. 2.

tose intolerance may also be acquired as the result of gastrointestinal disease affecting mucosa (Table 6).

Although lactose intolerance can be diagnosed with certainty by jejunal biopsy and lactase assay, it can be assessed indirectly by recording a blood glucose rise of less than 20 mg/100 ml of blood after a standard dose of 50 g of lactose to adults or by a breath hydrogen increase over fasting of more than 20 ppm. The latter test is subject to a number of potential errors.

Dietary management of lactose intolerance includes a low-lactose diet, with reduced intake of milk, ice cream, and other milk products. Most cheeses are low in lactose, although milk is added back in the manufacture of certain soft cheeses, which may contain small amounts of lactose. Although naturally prepared yogurts are virtually lactose-free, many yogurts today are made by adding milk and milk solids, giving lactose levels similar to that of fresh milk (around 5 g/100 ml). However, symptoms ascribed to lactose intolerance, secondary to gastrointestinal disease, are often caused by intolerance to other components of diet than lactose, and treatment of the primary cause is essential. According to Bayless et al. (48) and Havenberg et al. (50), most people with low lactase activity can tolerate moderate amounts of lactose in their diet (around 10–15 g/day), provided it is taken in small amounts.

I. Crohn's Disease

This is a chronic inflammation affecting any part of the gut from mouth to anus; it typically occurs in the ileocecal region and colon and is discontinuous. Crohn's disease frequently recurs after surgical resection of the affected areas of gut. The bowel becomes thickened, with ulceration of the mucosa, stricturing, and fistula formation. The following factors may contribute to malnutrition in Crohn's disease (2): anorexia (fear of provoking abdominal pain, effect of drugs, zinc deficiency leading to loss of taste, and salt deficiency in severe diarrhea), malabsorption (mucosal inflammation, gut resection or bypass, blind loop syndrome, and fistula), enteric losses (protein-losing enteropathy, bleeding into gut), and other factors (psychological depression, stress, drugs, and self-imposed diets).

Crohn et al. (51) described this condition, calling it regional ileitis. The cause of this disease is not known (52), although a familial tendency is known to exist. Clinical features of the disease include abdominal pain and diarrhea, which occur in 80% to 90% of cases. Other symptoms are weight loss, anorexia, fever, nausea and vomiting, tiredness, intestinal obstruction, and fistula. In the colonic type, rectal bleeding occurs in about 50% of patients with perianal disease. Systemic manifestations include arthritis, iritis, and, more rarely, liver and skin disorders.

Retarded growth and sexual development in children due to Crohn's disease respond to adequate treatment.

Anemia and weight loss, which are commonly associated with Crohn's disease, are usually caused by iron or folate deficiency or a combination of both. B_{12} deficiency may occur after ileal resection or in extensive ileal disease, and drugs such as sulfasalazine may cause hemolysis and aggravate folate deficiency. The cause of anemia can be known by examining blood iron, ferritin, folate, and B_{12} levels. After the underlying problem is treated, appropriate hematinics may be prescribed. Maintenance of weight in patients with Crohn's disease can be managed by attempting to improve appetite and reducing malabsorption, by correcting micronutrient deficiencies, especially that of zinc, avoiding appetite-depressing drugs, prescribing corticosteroids, and encouraging consumption of a wide range of foodstuffs.

"Bowel rest" may be provided to the patients with Crohn's disease through various enteral and parenteral regimens when patients do not respond to conventional treatment. Due to the absence of nutrients and potential antigens and digestive activity in the bowel, mucosa has a chance to heal itself. Parenteral nutrition is designed to cope with nutritional deficiencies and ensure an adequate intake of protein and energy. Various options and combinations, such as total parenteral nutrition (TPN), TPN plus some oral nutrition, and formula diets through nasogastric tubes, may be tried. Intravenous feeding to replenish water and electrolyte losses and provide nutritional support can be life saving in acutely ill patients. Enteral feeding with elemental diets is less taxing for the patient and is as effective as the conventional steroid treatment (53) for inducing remission and thus can be used as an alternative to steroids and their side effects. According to Giaffer et al. (54), elemental, not polymeric, diets must be used. Jones et al. (55) suggested that the benefit of elemental diet lies in the avoidance of dietary allergens, which needs to be confirmed. Patients with Crohn's disease may develop osteomalacia and deficiencies of fat-soluble vitamins, magnesium, and zinc, which can be dealt with by conventional therapy.

J. Constipation

The carbohydrates that have not been digested in the small intestine are passed on to the large bowel, where through bacterial activity energy is salvaged from carbohydrates, such as resistant starch, nonstarch polysaccharides (dietary fiber), dextrins, oligosaccharides (raffinose, stachyose, fructans), lactose in lactase-deficient people, and commercial preparations such as polydextrose, palatinit, lactulose, and the bulk laxatives isapgol and sterculia. According to MacFarlane and Cummings (56), around 10 to 60 g of carbohydrate enter the colon in people eating Western-style diets; the amount may be much higher in Asian societies where the diet in rich is cereal carbohydrates. Some protein (6–12 g/day from western diets) may also escape digestion in the small intestine, depending on its physical form.

Carbohydrate and protein are broken down in the large bowel by the action of anerobic microorganisms, giving a range of fermentation products (56). Through fermentation, diet plays a role in the metabolism of colonic epithelial cells, liver, muscle and microflora, as well as influencing fecal output, breath gases, and urine and blood composition. The principal products of fermentation and their fate are shown in Table 7.

Constipation, difficult or infrequent evacuation of the bowels, is caused by a slow movement of fecal material through the large intestine. The stool becomes dry and hard, as fluids are increasingly absorbed during their extended time in the large intestine. Inhibition of normal bowel reflexes and ignoring normal urges for long periods of time can result in constipation. Muscle spasms of an irritated large intestine can also slow the movement of feces. Certain drugs, such as antacids, can also cause constipation.

Table 7 Principal Products of Fermentation and Their Fate

Substrate	Product	Main fate
Carbohydrate	Short-chain fatty acids	Absorbed by blood
	Acetate	Metabolized by muscle
	Propionate	Cleared by liver
	Butyrate	Metabolized by colonic epithelial cells
	Lactate, ethanol	Absorbed by liver
	Gases (H_2, CO_2, CH_4)	Expelled via breath or per rectum
	Bacterial growth	Feces
Protein	Short-chain fatty acids	As above
	Branched-chain fatty acids	Absorbed by liver
	Ammonia	Either absorbed or used by bacteria for protein synthesis
	Amines, phenols, carboxylic acids	Absorbed-metabolized in liver or mucosa, excreted in urine

Source: Ref. 2.

Constipation is difficult to diagnose. Normal stool frequency may range from 3 to 12 times a week, and definitions of "normal" can vary from person to person. The presence of unusually hard, dry stools at infrequent intervals may be the best guide to recognize constipation. Any sudden and prolonged changes in stool frequency need to be evaluated by a physician.

Constipation can be treated by eating dietary fiber in the form of whole grain cereals, pulses, and leafy vegetables. Dietary fibers stimulate persistalsis by drawing water into the colon to form a bulky, softer stool. A person with constipation should also drink more fluids along with dietary fiber. Eating dried fruits also stimulates the bowel. Development of more regular bowel habits by allowing the same time each day for a bowel movement can help to train the large intestine to respond routinely. Also, relaxation facilitates regular bowel movements, as does regular exercise.

Constipation is a disorder of motor activity of the bowel, characterized by the infrequent and difficult passage of small amounts of hard feces. Transit times of feces, which correlate closely with stool weight and are determinant of constipation, were found to be 58 h for men and 70 h for women in the U.K. population (2). Low stool weight may be associated with an increased risk of certain "Western diseases" such as bowel cancer, diverticular disease, appendicitis, and various anal conditions (57). Stool weights below around 150 g/day and slow transit (more than 4–5 days) are generally associated with greater risk of bowel disease. Marcus and Heaton (58) noted that experimentally induced constipation led to irritable bowel–like symptoms.

Transit time (probably an inherited characteristic) and diet (the major environmental variable) control stool weight. There are very few experimental data to support the suggestion that exercise, stress, and hormones may alter the bowel habit. However, it has been well established (in over 100 studies) that nonstarch polysaccharide (NSP) (dietary fiber) increases the amount of stool passed and influences bowel habit in other ways (59). NSP is not the only dietary component to influence bowel habit: any carbohydrate that reaches the colon will have a laxative effect, including resistant starches and poorly absorbed ions such as sulfate.

Fiber and other carbohydrates have now been shown to be extensively metabolized by local bacteria. Fecal weight may increase through a variety of mechanisms, including increased bacterial growth and excretion and unmetabolized NSP (such as bran) that hold water and increase bulk. Stool volume is also increased by gas trapped in the matrix, which in turn stimulates motor activity, resulting in faster transit, and allows less time for dehydration of stool (60,61).

In addition to inadequacy of fiber intake, other important causes of constipation include (2):

1. Diverticular disease
2. Irritable bowel syndrome
3. Megacolon
4. Central nerous system disorders (multiple sclerosis and Parkinson's disease)
5. Colorectal diseases (cancer, hemorrhoids, and anal fissure)
6. Drugs (antacids, opiates, anticholinergics, and many others)
7. Endocrine disorders (hypothyroidism, diabetes)
8. Inactivity (due to travel or confinement to bed)
9. Self-imposed or thereapeutic diets in slimmers and anorexia nervosa
10. Pregnancy and menstrual cycle

Thus, it is important to dignose first the correct cause of constipation prior to its management. Certain general measures include allowing time for unhurried visits to the toilet and prompt attention to the stool call, because neglecting the call to stool may be the real cause of constipation. The general advice to drink more fluid and take more exercise has not proved to be of value in relieving constipation.

Laxatives are a valuable adjacent to the management of constipation. Bulk laxatives are chemically NSP and are most favored. For example, isapgol, a seed mucilage from the plantago family (Isogel, Fybogel, Regulan); sterculia, a plant gum (Normacol); methycellulose (Celevac); and dephytenized bran (Trifyba). These laxatives are best taken along with meals, starting with a dose of 3.5 to 7.0 g/day and increasing up to 10.5 to 14.0 g/day, if needed, to produce one soft motion three or more times weekly. The British National Health Service has approved stimulants such as Senokot and Bisocodyl, magnesium sulfate (Epsom), sodium sulfate salts, fecal softeners (Docusate), and lactulose as laxatives.

Laxatives work either by irritating the intestinal nerve junctions to stimulate the peristaltic muscles or by drawing water into the intestine to enlarge the stool. A larger stool stretches the peristaltic muscles, making them rebound and then constrict, which helps the bowel movement. Regular use of laxatives, especially of the irritating types, may decrease muscle action in the large intestine, causing more future constipation. The G.I. tract may then become dependent on laxatives for its function. Thus, it is unwise to use laxatives routinely.

Dietary management of constipation includes meals high in NSP, although there is no universal dose. The amount required is that which will produce a satisfactory bowel habit. This may be achieved by increasing the patient's NSP intake from 12 to 18–24 g/day. Patients with lifelong constipation of moderate severity respond rather poorly to bulk stimulants. The whole-grain cereal sources rich in NSP are the most effective bulking foods (59). Rapidly fermentable carbohydrates, such as low-molecular-weight sugars, oligosaccharides, and soluble dietary fiber, are less effective and tend to produce excess gas. NSP intake may be increased by increasing bread intake (up to 200 g/day) and resorting to 100% wholemeal, eating a whole-wheat breakfast cereal or one with added bran (50 g/day), increasing intake of fruit and vegetables (to 400 g/day), eating more legumes (peas and beans), and using bulk laxatives. Use of pulses can produce flatulence due to oligosaccharide fermentation.

High NSP diets may produce abdominal distension, bloating, pain, and increased flatus in patients who increase their NSP intake too quickly. A slow change in diet allows the gut to adjust to these changes. Also, the high phytate content of raw bran and bran products may result in mineral imbalance, especially in the elderly, young women, and the unemployed (62). High-fiber diets are also not suitable for the treatment of constipation due to neurological disorders or to obstructive lesions of the gut.

K. Irritable Bowel Syndrome (IBS)

IBS (or irritable colon, mucous colitis, spastic colon) is one of the most common disorders seen in the hospital gastroenterology clinic. It is a disorder of motor activity of the whole bowel, though colonic symptoms often predominate. It is more common in women. The clinical features of IBS include abdominal pain and altered bowel habit. The pain may be anywhere in the abdomen but usually in the left or right iliac fossa and is related to either meals or defecation. The bowel disturbance can be in the form of diarrhea, constipation, or a combination of both. Two types of syndromes have been recognized: (a) abdominal pain and constipation (usual), and (b) painless diarrhea (less common). Other symptoms of IBS are abdominal distension, bloating, excess wind, passage of mucus, a sensation of incomplete rectal emptying, and fleeting rectal pain.

Patients with IBS appear to have a greater frequency of high-amplitude pressure waves during interdigestive periods, which may be associated with the abdominal pain. These patients also show exaggerated motility responses to meals and to pharmacological stimulation of the gut. Increased frequency of psychological disorders is a major feature of IBS: patients become more anxious, depressed, and generally neurotic (63); stress is the major factor precipitating these symptoms. Smooth muscle dysfunction, urinary difficulties, dyspareunia, and dysmenorrhea are some of other complaints in IBS. Physical examination and investigations often do not reveal any significant organic abnormality, about which the patient needs to be reassured during the management of IBS. Antispasmodics and antidepressants are the most widely used drugs to provide psychological relief to the patient. Wheat bran and other bulk laxatives are also often given, whose results have been variable. They may even aggravate IBS symptoms through gas production, although in patients who are acutely constipated they are of some benefit (64).

Exclusion diets in IBS are not advisable unless specific food intolerances are suspected. The patient should be encouraged to eat a prudent diet, with enough NSP and resistant starch to ensure a regular bowel habit (2).

L. Diverticular Disease

A diverticulum is a pouch protruding outwards from the bowel wall; it may occur anywhere in the gut. However, the term diverticular disease is often restricted to condition that affects only the large intestine, especially the sigmoid colon. Diverticular disease emerged in the twentieth century and is most commonly seen in industrially developed societies. It is rare in people under age 40 but affects more than about 30% of people over the age of 65. It is also rare in the developing countries.

The essential pathological features of this disease are sigmoid muscular hypertrophy and diverticula. The bowel wall becomes greatly thickened due to changes in the circular muscle and taeni coli, which results in apparent shortening of the bowel, making the mucosa concertina up in folds over the hypertrophied muscle. The bowel lumen is narrowed considerably.

Approximately 80% of patients with diverticula do not have any symptoms. Some complain of pain in the left iliac fossa, which may be colicky, and of alteration in bowel habit. In about 5% of patients, complications may develop as the result of infection in a diverticulum (diverticulitis), which may proceed to perforation, abscess formation, and bleeding.

Painter (65) suggested that diverticular disease is caused by lack of fiber in the diet; it is more common in omnivores than in vegetarians (66). The cause of muscular hypertrophy is thought to be the need to propel the hardened bowel contents that result from diets low in fermentable carbohydrates such as fiber. After the muscular thickening, the bowel lumen becomes narrowed, thus closing off small chambers where high pressures build up and force herniation of diverticula through the bowel wall (65). The motility pattern may be very similar to that seen in IBS, leading to a suggestion that diverticular disease is a later development of IBS. According to Cummings (2), these two conditions are currently considered to be separate entities. The bacterial production in the lumen of an agent active on the neuromuscular components of the bowel wall has been suggested but needs confirmation.

The uncontrolled trials of wheat bran (67) and subsequent controlled trials (68) have shown substantial improvements in the symptoms of most of patients with diverticular disease. In one controlled study, patients were given a bran crispbread providing an additional 6.1 g dietary fiber per day, which increased the fiber content of the diet by about a third and was equivalent to about 4 g of NSP. Wheat bran was found to be more effective than other sources of NSP or bulk laxatives for diverticular disease, and coarse bran better than fine. Bran, however, may aggravate flatus production, abdominal distension, and incomplete emptying of the rectum (69). Other treatments include antispasmodics for the pain and, occasionally, antibiotics to control infection. Surgery may be needed in life-threatening complications.

M. Ulcerative Colitis

Ulcerative colitis is a chronic inflammation of mucosa of large bowel leading to bloody diarrhea. At present, diet is not thought to have any role in the etiology of ulcerative colitis. Like diverticular disease, ulcerative colitis is also a disease of modern civilization, predominantly affecting industrialized societies. Affecting both sexes equally, the disease usually presents in patients between the ages of 20 and 40 years.

The mucosa of the colon becomes inflamed in ulcerative colitis, the inflammation always involving the rectum and extending proximally toward the cecum in a continuous manner. While distal (sigmoid-rectal) disease is fairly benign, involvement of the white colon carries a cumulative risk of developing bowel cancer with time. Clinical symptoms include diarrhea and passing both blood and mucus per rectum. The severity of an attack can be gauged by the frequency of bowel actions, presence of fever, pulse rate, anemia, and toxic megacolon.

Ulcerative colitis can be managed medically, largely through use of corticosteroids, sulfasalazine, or the more recently developed 5-amino-salicylic acid preparations. Surgery may be required in severe or complicated cases, involving total colectomy with either an ileostomy or ileorectal pouch construction. Low-residue diets prescribed in the past have not proved to be beneficial. Patients should be encouraged to eat a normal diet. Patients with lactase deficiency can benefit from a diet free of milk. Bowel-rest regimens have not proved to be effective in managing the inflammation of the colon.

IV. ANAL DISORDERS

Hemorrhoids and anal fissure are two major anal disorders that respond to dietary management.

A. Hemorrhoids (Piles)

Hemorrhoids are vascular cushions of the anal canal that have prolapsed through the external sphincter, presenting as a tender swelling of the anal margin (pile). These are thought to be due to constipation and straining at stool and are more common in Western societies. An epidemiological study (70) did not show association of hemorrhoids with constipation. Hemorrhoids cause local pain and bleeding. Avoidance of constipation, by use of bulking agents, is a valuable adjunct to various surgical treatments (71,72).

Hemorrhoids, also known as piles, are swollen veins of the rectum and anus. The blood vessels in this area are subject to intense pressure, particularly during bowel movements. Physiological conditions such as pregnancy, obesity, violent coughing or sneezing, or strain during prolonged sitting and bowel movement can add stress to the vessels, leading to a hemorrhoid. This condition may develop unnoticed until a strained bowel movement precipitates symptoms. The pain is often aching and steady, and bleeding appears in the form of a streak in the feces. Pressure from prolonged sitting or exertion can bring on symptoms, although diet, lifestyle, and possibly heredity also play a role. Rectal bleeding may also indicate other problems, such as cancer, for which it is necessary to consult the physician. The physician may suggest numerous self-care measures to treat hemorrhoids. Pain can be reduced by warm, soft compresses or sitting in a tub of warm water for 15 to 20 minutes. Dietary therapy to treat constipation also helps to cure piles.

B. Anal Fissure

Anal fissure is a linear ulcer at the end of the anal canal that may be related to local trauma (2). They are more common in the young and in women and cause intense pain on defecation. Anal fissure often coexists with hemorrhoids and is usually managed surgically. Jensen (73) reported that bran given three times a day was beneficial in preventing recurrence of anal fissure.

V. GASTROSTOMY, JEJUNOSTOMY, ILEOSTOMY, AND COLOSTOMY

A. Gastrostomy, Jejunostomy, and Ileostomy

Frequently an opening (stoma) needs to be made in the gut in order to feed the patient (gastrostomy, jejunostomy) or as a part of the treatment of ulcerative colitis (ileostomy). Both gastrostomy and jejunostomy are common routes for administering enteral feeds in patients having problems of swallowing or nutritional support in addition to their diet. Gastrostomy tubes are now placed by percutaneous puncture. Nausea and vomiting are the major problems that occur due to delayed gastric emptying, fat intolerance, sudden large boluses of feed, drugs, psychopathology, and infection. Diarrhea is caused by intolerance to high osmolar load of feed, inappropriate hormonal release, antibiotic and laxative therapies, bacterial infection, and lactose intolerance. An ileostomy involves the end of the ileum brought out through the abdominal wall as a permanent fistula. It is an exclusive necessity for patients with total colectomy for ulcerative colitis or Crohn's disease. The patients should be encouraged to eat a normal diet. However, because of the absence of large intestine, salt and water conservation are affected and the patient is not able to derive any energy from unabsorbed carbohydrate through fermentation.

According to Bingham et al. (74), most patients with ileostomies can eat a normal diet without suffering nutritional deficiencies, although they may experience digestive problems with some foods. Based on a survey of 79 ileostomy patients, Bingham et al. (74) have given the following general dietary advice:

1. Eat a full and varied diet, trying everything.
2. Foods high in fiber will increase effluent output, others will be visible in the effluent and may cause occasional discomfort.
3. Chew all food thoroughly, especially nuts.
4. Beware of salt and water depletion during ileostomy diarrhea (extra salt may be needed).

5. Some foods cause more odor than others, e.g. fish, onion, leaks, and garlic. Peas and beans will cause excessive gas.

6. Patients with established ileostomies should eat more in the morning and at midday and less in the evening to reduce the need to empty their bags at night.

7. Eat refined carbohydrate and protein rather than fat and fiber, in case of difficulty gaining weight after surgery, especially due to malabsorption.

Ileostomy patients can obtain help through the Ileostomy Association of Great Britain and Ireland, Mansfield, Notts., U.K.

B. Colostomy

Colostomy refers to the opening of the large intestine as a fistula onto the anterior abdomen wall. Temporary or loop colostomy is often performed in adults to relieve more distal obstruction or abscess after abdominal wounds. Permanent colostomy may follow surgery for bowel cancer and diverticular disease.

Dietary management of colostomy is simpler than that of ileostomy (75). Constipation is more of a problem than diarrhea. The major causes of constipation are low intakes of NSP and resistant starch, drugs, and, rarely, a mechanical obstruction. Low fluid intake may lead to constipation only where dehydration is common (hot, tropical, and desert regions). Constipation can be treated in the same way as is normal constipation, except that suppositories of and enemas are less easily retained.

Colostomic diarrhea is more common in right-sided stomas and can be caused by food poisoning, antibiotics, dietary anomalies, or disease recurrence high up in the bowel. Electrolyte replacement may be necessary if colostomy outputs exceed 1 kg/day. Bowel rest with a low-residue diet decreases output and anti-diarrheal drugs may be useful in noninfectious causes (2).

REFERENCES

1. Bingham, S.A., Mechanisms and experimental and epidemiological evidence relating dietary fibre (non-starch polysaccharides) and starch to protection against large bowel cancer, *Proc. Nutrition Soc.* *49*: 35 (1990).

2. Cummings, J.H., Nutritional management of diseases of the stomach and bowel, *Human Nutrition and Dietetics*, 9th ed. (J.S. Garrow and W.P.T. James, eds.), Churchill Livingstone, Edinburgh, London, 1993, p. 480.

3. Petkov, V., Bulgarian traditional medicine: a source of ideas for phytopharmacological investigations, *J. Ethnopharmacol. 15*: 121 (1986).

4. Reuter, H.D., H.P. Koch, and L.D. Dawson, Therapeutic effects and applications of garlic and its preparations, *Garlic: The Science and Therapeutic Application of Allium sativum L. and Related Species* (H.P. Koch and L.D. Lawson, eds.), 2nd ed., Williams & Wilkins, Baltimore, Maryland, 1996, p. 135.

5. Noda, K., S. Isozaki, and H. Taniguchi, Growth promoting and inhibiting effects of spices on *Escherichia coli*, *J. Japn. Soc. Food Sci. Technol. 32*: 791 (1985). (Japanese)

6. Shashikanth, K.N., S.C. Basappa, and V. Sreenivasmurthy, Effects of feeding raw and boiled garlic (*Allium sativum* L.) extracts on the growth, caecal microflora, and serum proteins of albino rats, *Nutr. Rep. Int. 33*: 313 (1986).

7. Barowsky, H., and L.J. Boyd, The use of garlic (Allisatin) in gastrointestinal disturbances, *Rev. Gastroenterol. 11*: 22 (1944).

8. Singh, S.C., A note on some home remedies available from kitchen stock in Eastern Uttar Pradesh, *J. Econ. Tax. Bot. 5*: 149 (1984).

9. Zimmermann, W., Der obere Dunndarm. Eine Phytotherapiestudie, *Therapiewoche 35*: 1592 (1985).

10. Gudmundsson, K., F. Johnsson, and B. Joelsson, The time pattern of gastro-esophageal reflux, *Scand. J. Gastroenterol. 23*: 75 (1988).

11. Dennish, G.W., and D.O. Castell, Inhibitory effect of smoking on the lower oesophageal sphincter, *N. Engl. J. Med. 284*: 1136 (1971).

12. Hogan, W.J., S.R.T. Viegas de Andrade, and D.H. Winship, Ethanol-induced acute oesophageal motor dysfunction, *J. Appl. Physiol. 32*: 755 (1972).

13. Nebel, O.T., and D.O, Castell, Inhibition of the lower oesophageal sphincter by fat a mechanism for fatty food intolerance, *Gut. 14*: 270 (1973).

14. Cohen, S., Pathogenesis of coffee-induced gastro-intestinal symptoms, *N. Engl. J. Med. 303*: 122 (1980).

15. Fisher, R.S., G.S. Roberts, C.J. Grabowski, and S. Cohen, Altered lower esophageal sphincter function during early pregnancy, *Gastroenterology 74*: 1233 (1978).

16. Van Thiel, D.H., J.S. Gavaler, and J.F. Stremple, Lower esophageal sphincter pressure during the normal menstrual cycle, *Am. J. Obstet. Gynecol. 134*: 64 (1979).

17. Hamilton, J.W., R.J. Boisen, and D.T. Yamaoto, Sleeping on a wedge diminishes exposure of the oesophagus to refluxed acid, *Digestive Dis. Sci. 33*: 518 (1988).

18. Kurata, J.H., and E.D. Corboy, Current peptic ulcer time trends: an epidemiological profile, *J. Clin. Gastroenterol. 10*: 259 (1988).

19. Okada, M., T. Yeo, and K. Maeda, Predictors of duodenal ulcer healing during treatment with cimetidine, *Gut 31*: 758 (1990).

20. Sonnenberg, A., S.A. Muller-Lissner, and E. Vogel, Predictors of duodenal ulcer healing and relapse, *Gastroenterology 81*: 1061 (1981).

21. Rydning, A., A. Berstad, E. Aadland, and B. Odegaard, Prophylactic effect of dietary fibre in duodenal ulcer disease, *Lancet 2*: 736 (1982).

22. Leeds, A.R., F. Edied, and D.N.L. Ralphs, Pectin in the dumping syndrome: reduction of symptoms and plasma volume changes, *Lancet 1*: 1075 (1981).

23. Gleibermann, L., Blood pressure and dietary salt in human populations, *Ecol. Food Nutr. 2*: 143 (1973).

24. I.C.R.G., Intersalt: an international study of electrolyte excretion and blood pressure: Results from 24-hour urinary sodium and potassium excretion, Intersalt Cooperative Research Group, *Br. Med. J. 2*: 319 (1988).

25. Phillips, R.A., Water and electrolyte losses in cholera, *Fed. Proc. 23*: 705 (1964).

26. Field, M., D. Fromm, Q. Al-Awqati, and W.B. Greenough, Effect of cholera enterotoxin on ion transport across isolated ileal mucosa, *J. Clin. Invest 51*: 796 (1972).

27. Cutting, W.A.M., M.R. Belton, and R.P. Brettle, Safety and efficacy of three oral rehydration solutions for children with diarrhoea (Edinburgh, 1984–85), *Acta Paediatr. Scand. 78*: 253 (1989).

28. Patra, E.C., D. Mahalanabis, and K.N. Jalan, Is oral rice electrolyte solution superior to glucose electrolyte solution in infantile diarrhoea? *Arch. Dis. Children 57*: 910 (1982).

29. Molla, A.M., S.A. Sarkar, and M. Hossain, Rice powder electrolyte solutions as oral therapy in diarrhoea due to *Vibrio cholerae* and *Escherichia coli*, *Lancet 1*: 1317 (1982).

30. Gore, S.M., O. Fontaine, and N.F. Pierce, Impact of rice-based oral rehydration solution on stool output and duration of diarrhoea: meta-analysis of 13 clinical trials, *Br. Med. J. 304*: 289 (1992).

31. Carpenter, C.C.J., W.B. Greenough, and N.F. Pierce, Oral rehydration therapy—the role of polymeric substrates, *N. Engl. J. Med. 319*: 1346 (1988).

32. Molla, A.M., A. Molla, J. Rohide, and W.B. Greenough, Turning off the diarrhoea: the role of food and ORS, *J. Pediatr. Gastroenterol. Nutr. 8*: 81 (1989).

33. Englyst, H.N., and J.H. Cummings, Resistant starch, a 'new' food component: a classification of starch for nutritional purposes, *Cereals in a European Context, First European Conference on Food Science and Technology* (I.D. Morton, ed.), Ellis Horwood, Chichester, 1987, p. 221.

34. Christl, S.U., P.R. Murgatroyd, G.R. Gibson, and J.H. Cummings, Production, metabolism and excretion of hydrogen in the large intestine, *Gastroenterology 102*: 1269 (1992).

35. Dawson, A.M., and P. Kumar, Coeliac disease, *Disorders of the Small Intestine* (C.C. Booth and G. Neale, eds.), Blackwell Scientific Publications, Oxford, 1986, p. 153.

36. Davidson, A.G.F., and M.A. Bridges, Coeliac disease: a critical review of aetiology and pathogenesis, *Clinica Chim. Acta. 163*: 1 (1987).

37. Dicke, W.K., Coeliac disease: Investigations of harmful effects of certain types of cereal on patients with coeliac disease, Doctoral Thesis, University of Utrecht, The Netherlands, 1950.

38. Levenson, S.D., R.K. Austin, and M.D. Dietler, Specificity of antigliadin and body in coeliac disease, *Gastroenterology 89*: 1 (1985).

39. Fotherby, K.J., E.P. Wriaght, and G. Neale, ^{51}(Cr) EDTA/^{14}C-mannitol intestinal permeability test: Clinical use in screening for coeliac disease, *Scand J. Gastroenterol. 23*: 171 (1988).

40. Skerritt, J.H., and A.S. Hill, Self-management of dietary compliance in coeliac disease by means of ELISA 'home test' to detect gluten, *Lancet 337*: 379 (1991).

41. Tomkins, A.M., Tropical malabsorption: recent concepts in pathogenesis and nutritional significance, *Clin. Sci. 60*: 131 (1981).

42. Wood, G.M., J.C. Gearty, and B.T. Cooper, Small bowel morphology in British Indian and Afro-Caribbean subjects: evidence of tropical enteropathy, *Gut 32*: 256 (1991).

43. Weser, E., Nutritional aspects of malabsorption: Short gut adaptation, *Am. J. Med. 67*: 1014 (1979).

44. Polak, J.M., S.R. Bloom, N.A. Wright, and M.J. Daly, Basic science in gastroenterology: structure of the gut, Glaxo Group Research, Royal Postgraduate Medical School, 1982.

45. Sakata, T., Stimulatory effect of short-chain fatty acids on epithelial cell proliferation in the rat intestine: a possible explanation for trophic effects of fermentable fibre, gut microbes, and luminal trophic factors, *Br. J. Nutr. 58*: 95 (1987).

46. Atmann, G.G., Influence of starvation and refeeding on mucosal size and epithelial renewal in rat small intestine, *Am. J. Anatomy 133*: 391 (1972).

47. Simko, V., A.M. McCarrol, and S. Goodman, High-fat diet in a short bowel syndrome: intestinal absorption and gastroentero-pancreatic hormone responses, *Digestive Dis. Sci. 25*: 333 (1980).

48. Bayless, T.M., B. Rothfield, and C. Massa, Lactose and milk intolerance: clinical implications, *N. Engl. J. Med. 292*: 1156 (1975).

49. Tandon, R.K., Y.K. Joshi, and D.S. Singh, Lactose intolerance in North and South Indians, *Am. J. Clin. Nutr. 34*: 943 (1981).

50. Haverberg, L., P.H. Kwon, and N.S. Scrimshaw, Comparative tolerance of adolescents of differing ethnic backgrounds to lactose-containing and lactose-free dairy drinks. I. Initial experience with a double-blind procedure, *Am. J. Clin. Nutr. 33*: 17 (1980).

51. Crohn, B.B., L. Ginzburg, and G.D. Oppenheimer, Regional ileitis: A pathologic and clinical entity. Description of 14 cases, *J. Am. Med. Assoc. 99*: 1323 (1932).

52. Mendeloff, A.I., The epidemiology of inflammatory bowel disease, *Clin. Gastroenterol. 9*: 259 (1980).

53. O'Morain, C., A.W. Segal, and A.J. Lavi, Elemental diet as primary treatment of acute Crohn's disease: a controlled trial, *Br. Med. J. 288*: 1859 (1984).

54. Giaffer, M.H., G. North, and C.D. Holdsworth, Controlled trial of polymeric versus elemental diet in treatment of acute Crohn's disease, *Lancet 335*: 816 (1990).

55. Jones, V.A., R.J. Dickinson, and E. Workman, Crohn's disease: maintenance of remission by diet, *Lancet 2*: 177 (1985).

56. MacFarlane, G.T., and J.H. Cummings, The colonic flora, fermentation and large bowel digestive function, *The Large Intestine: Physiology, patho-physiology and Diseases* (S.F. Phillips, J.H. Pemberton, and R.G. Shorter, eds.), Raven Press, New York, 1991, p. 51.

57. Burkitt, D.P., and H. Trowell, *Western Diseases*, Arnold, London, 1981.

58. Marcus, S.N., and K.W. Heaton, Irritable bowel-type symptoms in spontaneous and induced constipation, *Gut 28*: 156 (1987).

59. Cummings, J.H., The effect of dietary fiber on fecal weight and composition, *CRC Handbook of Dietary Fiber in Human Nutrition* (G.A. Spiller, ed.), CRC Press Florida, 1986, p. 211.

60. Stephen, A.M., and J.H. Cummings, Mechanism of action of dietary fibre in the human colon, *Nature 284*: 283 (1980).

61. Cummings, J.H. Constipation. *Diseases of the Gut and Pancreas* (J.J. Misiewicz et al., eds.), Blackwell Scientific, London, 1987, p. 59.

62. Gregory, J., K. Foster, H. Tyler, and M. Wiseman, The dietary and nutritional survey of British adults, OPCS Social Survey Division, HMSO, London, 1990.

63. Drossman, D.A., D.C. McKee, and R.S. Sandler, Psychosocial factors in the irritable bowel syndrome. A multivariate study of patients and non-patients with irritable bowel syndrome, *Gastroenterology 95*: 701 (1988).

64. Cann, P.A., N.W. Read, and C.D. Holdsworth, What is the benefit of coarse wheat bran in patients with the irritable bowel? *Gut 25*: 168 (1984).

65. Painter, N.S., *Diverticular Disease of the Colon—A Deficiency Disease of Western Civilization*, William Henimann Medical Books, London, 1975.

66. Gear, J.S.S., A. Ware, and P. Fursdon, Symptomless diverticular disease and intake of dietary fibre, *Lancet 1*: 511 (1979).

67. Painter, N.S., A.Z. Almedia, and K.W. Colebourne, Unprocessed bran in treatment of diverticular disease of the colon, *Br. Med. J. 2*: 137 (1972).

68. Brodribb, A.J., and D.M. Humphreys, Diverticular disease: three studies. Part II—Treatment with bran, *Br. Med. J. 6*: 425 (1976).

69. Brodribb, A.J., Treatment of symptomatic diverticular disease with a high-fibre diet, *Lancet 1*: 664 (1977).

70. Johanson, J.F., and A. Sonnenberg, The prevalence of haemorrhoids and chronic constipation: an epidemiologic study, *Gastroenterology 98*: 380 (1990).

71. Wood, C. (ed.), *Haemorrhoids—Current Concepts on Causation and Management*, Royal Society of Medicine, Academic Press, London, 1979.

72. Moesegaard, F., M.L. Nielsen, J.B. Hansen, and J.T. Knudsen, High-fiber diet reduces bleeding and pain in patients with hemorrhoids, *Dis. Colon Rectum 25*: 454 (1982).

73. Jensen, S.L., Maintenance therapy with unprocessed bran in the prevention of acute and anal fissure recurrence, *J. Royal Soc. Med. 80*: 296 (1987).

74. Bingham, S., J.H. Cummings, and N.I. McNeil, Diet and health of people with an ileostomy—1. Dietary assessment, *British J. Nutr. 47*: 399 (1982).

75. Elcoat, C., *Stoma Care Nursing*, Bailliere Tindall, London, 1986.

30
Diet and Inherited Metabolic Disorders

I. INTRODUCTION

Of the over 3000 inherited metabolic disorders described in the literature (1,2), many are very rare, but because these disorders are numerous, they contribute significantly to morbidity and mortality, especially during childhood. Dietetic treatment plays an important role in the management of at least a few of these diseases. Therapeutic diets used with varying degree of success act by (3):

1. preventing the accumulation of a substrate and its derivative, as in a low-phenylalanine controlled diet for phenylketonuria
2. providing a metabolite that becomes rate-limiting as a result of a metabolic block, e.g., the administration of arginine in children with argininosuccinase deficiency
3. providing a metabolite whose deficiency can be dangerous, as in a diet to prevent hypoglycemia in glucose-storage disease
4. providing a cofactor or precursor, e.g., large doses of pyridoxine for a variant of homocystinuria.

The dietitian, physician, and hospital staff must cooperate closely in educating the patient and/or parents. Industry support in making available suitable synthetic foods is also essential. In the United Kingdom, the Advisory Committee on Borderline Substances provides advice on those conditions in which "foods" may be classified as National Health Service (NHS) drugs and are prescribed as such. A scientifically excellent diet will be useless unless it is taken by the patient—and most of the patients being young, presentation of substitutes for everyday items of food is a real task for the dietitians.

The diagnosis of a congenital error can be very difficult to make in some cases. The patients with some metabolic disorders may respond to the administration of a specific cofactor given on a trial basis. Both cofactor and a diet may be given if the patient is very ill. Nutritionists are divided in their opinions on whether to try a mixture of cofactors before an accurate diagnosis has been made (3).

II. DISORDERS OF AMINO ACID METABOLISM

A. Phenylketonuria

Cotton (4) reported the heterogeneity of phenylketonuria (PKU) at the clinical, protein, and DNA levels. PKU is one of the few causes of mental handicap for which there is a reasonably effective treatment. Early definitive diagnosis and commencement of treatment must be pursued with urgency to avoid deterioration. In the United Kingdom, neonates are screened between the 6th and 14th days after birth. Populations differ in incidence of hyperphenylalaninemia and carry different alleles. According to Smith et al. (5), about 1 in 10,000 (445 subjects) had levels of blood phenylalanine persistently above 240 μmol/l, resulting from gene maturation for phenylalanine hydrolase in majority of cases (273 had classic PKU). Three were found to have defects in the metabolism of the cofactor. In the classic form of PKU, the blood phenylalanine levels exceed 1200 μmol/l. Also, the plasma tyrosine levels are low or low normal, with large amounts of abnormal metabolites appearing in the urine (Fig. 1). PKU results when less than 1% of normal activity of phenylalanine hydrolase is present in the liver, which converts phenylalanine to tyrosine (Fig. 1). With around 1% to 5% of the normal activity, it produces a milder form of the disease (variant or atypical PKU), and with reduced but more than 5% activity of the enzyme, there will be mild hyperphenylalaninemia. In around 1% to 3% of patients with defective hydroxylation of phenylalanine, deficiency of a cofactor, tetrahydrobiopterin, leads to brain damage that cannot be prevented by dietary treatment.

Hyperphenylalaninemic infants are responsive to diet and are customarily treated when plasma levels exceed 600 μmol/l. Maintenance blood levels of phenylalanine aimed for during treatment are between 180 and 480 μmol/l. Smith and her colleagues have shown that treated children with PKU, although they appeared to have normal IQs, showed certain cognitive defects, such as educational problems, and behavior disorders, such as hyperactivity. According to Smith et al. (6) the desirable blood levels of phenylalanine should be revised and maintained between 120 and 130 μmol/l. A practical and social difficulty for achieving such a tight control is the complicating factor that the failure to provide the essential requirement of the amino acid, phenylalanine, itself leads to brain damage. Clayton (3) suggested that the policy of not usually treating children with untreated levels between 240 and 600 μmol/l may also need revision.

The higher levels of blood phenylalanine cause alterations in myelin and amine metabolism that may interfere with the integrity of the nervous system permanently, necessitating lifelong

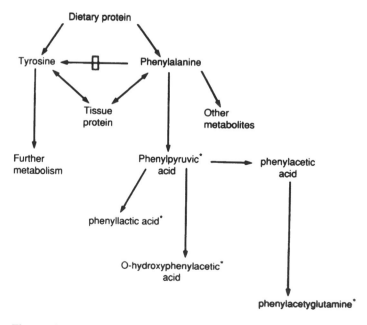

Figure 1   Phenylketonuria (PKU) = Impairment of phenylalanine activity in PKU. * = Major urinary metabolites in untreated PKU. (From Ref. 3.)

treatment (7). A low-phenylalanine controlled diet requires regular monitoring of blood phenylalanine levels. The recommended intake of nutrients, apart from phenylalanine and tyrosine, is similar to that for the normal infant. However, the controlled use of protein-containing conventional foods requires that amino acid supplements (except phenylalanine), protein-free energy, and a comprehensive range of macro and micro vitamins and minerals must be supplied. Phenylalanine being essential, it also needs to be supplied in controlled amounts (1 g of natural protein has around 50 mg phenylalanine).

The essential requirement must be ingested each day; an aliquot of total daily requirement is given with each meal. To restrict the phenylalanine levels within the range of 180 to 480 µmol/l plasma, only one-third to one-tenth of the normal protein intake is required, necessitating use of synthetic protein containing all essential amino acids. For infants and very young children, cysteine, histidine, arginine and probably proline are also required as dietary essentials. In addition, tyrosine may also become essential because of the metabolic block. The protein substitute may be a mixture of amino acids without phenylalanine or an enzymatic or acid hydrolysate of protein that still contains some phenylalanine.

The protein substitute must be given in divided portions at meals during the day, especially to infants and young children. Affected infants often do not tolerate more than 70 to 90 mg phenylalanine per kg body weight per 24 h, although in the first month of life and during periods of rapid growth the patient may tolerate upto 110 mg/kg/24 h. Preparations of amino acids without fat but including carbohydrate are recommended for older children and adults. Essential macro and trace elements may be given as separate supplements or included in the commercial protein substitute. All required vitamins should be supplied either separately or as part of the manufacturer's formulation of a low-phenylalanine protein substitute.

Practical management of diet includes regular (weekly) monitoring of blood levels of phenylalanine on nonfasting specimens taken 3.5 to 4 h after a feed or main meal, using a capillary sample in a micromethod. The recommended frequency of monitoring is weekly in infants during the first months of life, fortnightly after weaning and during the toddler age after adjusting the diet, every 3 to 4 weeks in preschool children, and monthly thereafter until the teens, when the frequency may be reduced to only 2 or 3 months or even less. More frequent monitoring and a chemical method of measuring phenylalanine will be needed if the stricter limits suggested by Smith et al. (6) are adopted. Clayton (3) has described the detailed low-phenylalanine infant feeding plan, a weaning menu, and the diet for a school child. A high-energy drink is recommended if an affected child does not eat, to prevent catabolism and a rise in phenylalanine level. Breastfeeding of a newly diagnosed infant may be continued because human milk is lower in phenylalanine per unit of nitrogen than cow's milk. Also, the breast milk can be combined with the use of a protein substitute.

The dietitian should educate and encourage the patient and the parents, providing adequate interpretation regarding how a scientifically correct diet can be made into one that the patient will relish and eat. The dietition can also provide low-phenylalanine cooking hints and numerous recipes for suitable ice creams, gravy, apple cake, and so on. Lists of the phenylalanine contents of many manufactured foods and their composition should be made available through useful leaflets and booklets published regularly by the National Society for Phenylketonuria and Allied Disorders.

Recurrent infections may adversely affect the child's appetite, in which case one should not attempt to force-feed the low-phenylalanine protein substitute, which may be stopped for a few days if necessary. The patient should be given fluids containing carbohydrates such as fruit juices with sugar or glucose polymer and whichever foods contain phenylalanine exchanges of his or her liking. The protein substitutes should not be recommended until the patient is taking phenylalanine exchanges. The sweetener aspartame, used widely in several manufactured foods, contains phenylalanine and should not be given to PKU patients of any age, although saccharin is suitable for use.

If a PKU mother consumes a normal diet during pregnancy her offspring is likely to have a number of severe congenital abnormalities, including microcephaly, mental subnormality, and heart defects. The infant will not have PKU unless the father is a carrier. If a PKU women desires to have a child and is not already receiving a low-phenylalanine controlled diet, such treatment should commence a few weeks before contraception is stopped, and the diet should be continued throughout the pregnancy. The strict diet should aim to control blood phenylalanine levels between 60 and 180 μmol/l, which should be monitored frequently. It is necessary to treat even milder forms of the disease with untreated phenylalanine levels above 300 μmol/l. During pregnancy, adequate amounts of a low-phenylalanine protein substitute must be given, together with additional tyrosine (4–9 g) to maintain the plasma tyrosine levels within the range of 30 to 80 μmol/l. Careful monitoring of plasma levels of phenylalanine is very important because after about the 20th week of pregnancy the requirement for this amino acid increases rapidly, and the diet will have about three times the amount of phenylalanine given in the early part of the pregnancy. The energy intake should be sufficient for the mother to gain weight at the appropriate level and overweight women planning to become pregnant should be encouraged to reduce weight while they are still practicing contraception because it is difficult to maintain satisfactory phenylalanine levels while losing weight without causing possible harm to the fetus when slimming is undertaken during pregnancy (3).

B. Homocystinuria

Classic homocystinuria is caused by deficient formation of cystathionine synthetase, required to convert homocysteine to cystathionine in the metabolism of methionine. This impaired conversion results in the accumulation of homocystine, methionine, and other sulfur-containing metabolites, and a low level of plasma cystine. The disorder is characterized by mental subnormality (usually not severe), lens displacement, skeletal abnormalities, and thrombotic problems.

Althogh dietary treatment is of value, the variable course of the condition, even among siblings, makes the assessment rather difficult. In some families, patients have shown a clear biochemical response to large doses of pyridoxine with clinical benefits. For patients who do not respond to pyridoxine or show only a partial biochemical response, a diet that is low in methionine and supplemented with cystine is recommended. Several commercial protein substitutes low in or free of methionine are available. Pulses, soya lentils, and gelatin are also relatively low in methionine and can be included in the diet. Lists of foods that provide 25 mg methionine exchanges are available.

Because cystine is not synthesized properly, a supplement of 150 to 200 mg/kg body weight/24 h is needed for infants; this should be increased to 1 to 2 g/24 h in children and adults, unless cystine is incorporated in the proprietary protein substitute. Cystine provides at least some cysteine, which is probably an essential amino acid in homocystinuria (3).

Although the administration of choline (the precursor of methyl donor betaine or of betaine itself) reduces the plasma levels of homocysteine, it also increases the level of methionine. The rate of homocysteine methylation is thought to increase through betaine-homocysteine methyltransferase. If betaine is prescribed, a large accumulation of methionine should not be allowed. Some patients with homocystinuria require folate but this too may lead to methionine accumulation, requiring monitoring of its levels.

C. Tyrosinemia Type I

This rare hereditary condition arises from a deficiency of fumarylacetoacetate hydrolase, which catalyzes the final step in the breakdown of tyrosine (8). It presents early in life with progressive liver failure. Even if diagnosed and treated early, it carries a poor prognosis, and many patients will die of liver failure; those who do survive may have a high risk of developing a hepatoma. Highly variable clinical presentation and the acute form in infancy often lead to death in the first year of life. Some more chronic forms do respond to a diet low in phenylalanine and tyrosine and often methionine. Vitamin D supplements are required. A liver transplant is the only successful treatment of the disease.

D. Branched-Chain Amino Acid Disorders and Maple Syrup Urine Disease

Many congenital errors of branched-chain amino acid (BCAA) metabolism are known, some of which are vitamin-responsive, e.g., a rare form of maple syrup urine disease (MSUD) that responds to thiamin, and some forms of propionic acidemia responding to biotin. Some pediatricians prescribe an empirical trial of large doses of vitamins. Many of these conditions are very rare and often go unrecognized as the true cause of death in infancy.

Often, these disorders present as emergencies during infancy, with relatively nonspecific symptoms and signs that include lethargy or irritability, hypotonia, failure to feed, acidosis (which may not be present), hypoglycemia, convulsions, vomiting, and diarrhea. The diagnosis is usually difficult, and sepsis in infancy may exhibit similar clinical features (3).

There is an urgent need to arrest catabolism and promote anabolism by providing a high-energy protein-free supplement that may be administered as a continuous nasogastric feed or as frequent feeds. A very low protein diet may be introduced gradually to provide 0.5 g protein per kilogram of body weight per 24 h, along with a comprehensive vitamin supplement to provide the recommended intake for any infant (9,10).

Those patients who do not respond to treatment with a cofactor vitamin, or those who respond only partially, will require a permanent protein-restricted diet to prevent accumulation of metabolites. The amount of protein tolerated by the patient will have to be determined by trial and error and may be around 0.75 to 1.5 g/kg body weight/24 h, the higher amounts being required by the younger patients during the growth period. If the amount of protein tolerated is too low to not hinder growth, supplementary amino acids that are appropriate for the specific metabolic block should be provided.

Sodium overload and hypoglycemia must be avoided. Clayton (3) suggested the following therapies to correct acidosis: keeping urine alkaline to increase excretion of methylmalonate, use of glycine to reduce accumulation of some organic acids such as isovaleric acid, and carnitine to prevent accumulation of propionyl-CoA. It is advisable to transfer the patient to a center with special expertise in managing the high-energy low-protein regimen for feeding.

In the classic form of MSUD, there is a failure of oxidative decarboxylation of alpha-ketoacids derived from the branched-chain amino acids (leucine, valine, and isoleucine). These amino acids and their alpha-keto-acids increase in blood, cerebrospinal fluid, and urine. Dietary management consists of measuring the branched-chain amino acids in the blood plasma. This condition (MSUD) is named after the odor of the urine, which is similar to that of maple syrup.

Classically, MSUD may present acutely in an apparently normal infant in the neonatal period, with feeding difficulties, vomiting, irregular respiration, and severe neurological degeneration. The infant often dies if left untreated, with brain damage in the rare survivor. Prompt treatment is therefore essential.

Dietary management includes restricting the intake of leucine, valine, and isoleucine, which requires severe restriction of natural protein and supplementation with amino acid mixture free of branched-chain amino acids (around 2–3 g mixture per kg/24 h). Appropriate vitamin and mineral macro and micro-nutrients must be provided as in PKU, as well as adequate energy from carbohydrate and fat. It is necessary to monitor the plasma levels daily during the early introduction of the synthetic branched-chain amino acids. Natural proteins may be introduced through modified milk formulas to replace synthetic branched-chain amino acids after stable blood levels are achieved. Weaning onto restricted quantities of some normal foods may be possible by use of food tables. Diet management is difficult in view of the involvement of three branched-chain amino acids. Early diagnosis and treatment in the neonate stage is vital but even so, if the patient survives, the prognosis for normal neurological development is poor (3).

E. Disorders of the Urea Cycle

Disorders of the urea cycle include:

1. Carbamylphosphate synthetase deficiency
2. Ornithine transcarbamylase deficiency
3. Arginosuccinic acid synthetase deficiency (citrullinemia)
4. Arginosuccinic acid lyase deficiency (argininosuccinic aciduria)
5. Arginase deficiency (argininemia)

Although these disorders may present at any age, the neonatal period is most likely. Patients even with milder forms may have acute episodes of hyperammonemia, which is mainly responsible for the clinical symptoms such as vomiting, focal neurological signs, convulsions, and fetal coma. Headache, ataxia, and confusion are seen in older patients. The onset of coma carries a poor prognosis. In neonates, the levels of ammonia may rise to over 400 μmol/l plasma, and in acute encephalopathy in older children to above 250 μmol/l.

Hemodialysis or peritoneal dialysis is essential in severe ammonia intoxication. Dietary treatment should aim to limit the total nitrogen intake by providing a low-protein diet of 0.7 g/kg body weight/24 h, with a supplement of 0.7 g/kg body weight of all essential amino acids. In urea cycle defects, specific supplements with 1-arginine or 1-citrulline is used because of relative insufficiency of these amino acids. Drugs may be used to enhance the renal excretion of nitrogen (precursor of ammonia), e.g., sodium benzoate conjugates with glycine to form hippuric acid that is excreted in the urine. Diet efficiency may be moitored by determining plasma levels of ammonia and essential amino acids and by watching growth. A high-energy protein-free regimen is necessary during periods of food refusal and when ammonia levels are high as catabolism worsens the clinical state. It is not easy for these children to obtain adequate growth, because of poor appetites and frequent refusals to eat (3).

III. DISORDERS OF CARBOHYDRATE METABOLISM

A. Glycogen Storage Disorder

Several inherited disorders affect glycogen metabolism, requiring dietary therapy. Glucose-6-phosphatase deficiency is also often referred to as type 1a glycogen storage disease or Von Gierke disease. The enzyme is normally present in liver, renal tubular cells, and enterocytes. The endogenous glucose formed either by glycogenolysis or gluconeogenesis is not released by the liver if glucose-6-phosphatase is deficient, and the condition will lead to severe hypoglycemia, hyperlacticacidemia, hyperuricemia, hyperlipidemia, and hepatomegaly. Patients fail to grow or develop normally. During childhood, intensive dietary therapy is needed. The patient may become more tolerant of the condition after the growth has ceased (3).

Dietary management consists of oral supplements of glucose and/or glucose polymers given to the infant to provide 0.5 g of carbohydrate/kg body weight/h. The concentrations of solutions stronger than 15% to 20% may cause diarrhea. The required glucose drinks can be reduced in amount as the child grows. The adolescent may need around 0.1 g of carbohydrate/kg/h, which can be achieved by increasing the concentration of the solution to 25%. Use of a continuous naso-gastric feed in prepubertal patients with severe disease is more practical at night. Patients who are being well treated become very vulnerable to falls in the blood glucose level, needing constant attention.

Older patients can do well with uncooked corn starch, about 2 g/kg body weight made up 1:3 with water at room temperature and given every 4 to 6h in addition to normal meals. Both lac-tose and fructose in the diet should be avoided, as galactose and fructose are metabolized to lac-tic acid. For infants, a lactose (and therefore galactose) + sucrose + fructose-free milk substitute should be given. Older children and adults should avoid drinking ordinary milk, avoid cane sugar, and eat fruit in small quantities, sweetened with glucose.

A similar dietary treatment is needed for patients with type 1b, in which there is defective transport of glucose-6-phosphate across the microsomal membrane of hepatocytes and leukocytes.

Patients with deficiency of the debranching enzyme, amylo-1,6-glucosidase, have hepatomegaly and fasting hypoglycemia, which may be asymptomatic. Patients improve markedly at puberty and the condition carries a better prognosis than glucose-6-phosphatase deficiency. Patients with hepatic phosphorylase defect also have hepatomegaly, but growth retardation is slight and symptoms are milder. Both these groups may be treated with a diet with a protein intake dou-ble the normal for age and frequent meals and snacks. A high-protein snack containing some starch is usually sufficient at bedtime, although patients with the debrancher deficiency may require another snack during the night or even a nocturnal drip feed. The long-term complications in most patients may include retarded growth, adenomas, and hyperlipidemia (6).

A deficiency of galactose-1-phosphate uridyl transferase, which metabolizes galactose to glucose, leads to galactosemia, producing accumulation of galactose-1-phosphate in tissues and erythrocytes. This condition usually presents when the infant begins to receive milk, though indi-viduals vary greatly in the rate of development of symptoms and signs. An acute fulminating dis-order may be associated with an infective organism such as *E. coli*, in which case death can occur within 24 hours without a diagnosis being made. More often there is failure to thrive, with vom-iting, diarrhea, jaundice, and hepatomegaly. If the patient survives without treatment, which is very unusal, the child will be mentally retarded and have liver cirrhosis and cataracts (3).

It is important to exclude diagnosis of galactosemia in a jaundiced infant. If the condition is suspected it is advisable to treat the child emperically for a day or two until the diagnosis is confirmed or excluded by the laboratory. Lactose-free milk will not harm a sick infant who has no galactosemia.

Early dietary treatment can prevent renal and hepatic damage and cataracts. Although severe mental retardation can often be prevented, unfortunately these patients can achieve intel-ligence only in the low normal range and have visual problems and ovarian dysfunction. The diet should necessarily exclude galactose, and therefore lactose or mammalian milk.

A galactose-lactose free milk substitute should be used to replace normal milk for infants. It should be noted that milk is added to many manufactured foods and lactose is used in tablets. An up-to-date list of suitable foods must be made available to patients and their parents. Clayton (3) has described a suitable diet that should be monitored by determining galactose-1-phosphate in erythrocytes.

Hereditary fructose intolerance can lead to a serious condition caused by a deficiency of fructose-1-phosphate aldolase B, manifesting in the infant when fructose or sucrose is given as a cane sugar or fruit juice. It is a potentially fatal disorder, with development of liver failure, if the condition is not recognized and treated in time. The infant fails to thrive, feeds badly, and devel-ops lethargy, hepatomegaly, and possibly jaundice.

Dietary treatment consists of excluding all fructose, sucrose, and sorbitol from the diet. These patients develop phobia toward anything that is sweet. Even very small amounts of fructose can be harmful and lead to hypoglycemia and liver damage.

A condition characterized by deficiency of fructose-1,6-biphosphatase affects gluconeognesis, presents the infant with hypoglycemia and symptoms of acidosis due to accumulation of acetate and ketones. Patients who do not dislike sweet foods should receive regular meals, preferably using glucose or its polymers, especially during infections. The diet may include small amounts of fruit and added cane sugar, avoiding fructose and honey.

Favism, well recognized in southern Italy and Greece, is associated with a deficiency of the B variant of erythrocyte glucose-6-phosphatase enzyme. In this condition, acute hemolytic anemia follows the ingestion of broad beans (fava), which must be excluded from the diet. This disorder has been reported even in breast-fed infants whose mothers have eaten the beans (3).

Marked lactosuria together with aminoaciduria, proteinuria, and renal tubular acidosis may be found in patients who do not lack intestinal lactase activity. Affected infants develop severe diarrhea, vomiting, and acidosis early in life (first few days), the condition becoming life threatening. Patients respond well to a lactose-free diet. This is a transient disorder from which the child recovers between 12 and 18 months of age.

Normally, infants of all races are born with intestinal lactase activity. Congenital lactase deficiency may present during the first few days of life as profuse watery diarrhea and failure to thrive. The acidic stool may contain lactose, with some lactosuria. Intestinal lactase deficiency is usually detected with the hydrogen breath test or by a jejunal biopsy. A lactose-free proprietary milk constitutes the treatment, followed by weaning to a lactose-free diet. Macro- and micro-vitamins and minerals must be supplied in appropriate quantities, depending upon the composition of the proprietary preparations being used.

Congenital sucrose-isomaltase deficiency is a rare condition that causes severe diarrhea in infants or occasional bouts in older children. The disorder can be diagnosed by determining enzyme activity on a jejunal biopsy. Treatment consists of excluding sucrose from the diet. The condition often improves with age.

Glucose-galactose malabsorption is a condition caused by the absence of an intestinal transport system. Only around 10% of glucose may be absorbed, perhaps due to the presence of another transport system. The disorder is characterized by profuse watery diarrhea (appearing soon after the infant receives the first feed), severel dehydration, and acidosis.

Because fructose has a separate carrier mechanism for its absorption, treatment consists of the removal of all glucose and galactose (sucrose and lactose) from the diet and replacing them with fructose. Fructose solution has a high osmolality and should be introduced gradually, while the infant is still on an intravenous drip. Sole-fructose proprietary feed may be given. The variety of foods used at the time of weaning is very limited. The patient may be gradually able to tolerate a little glucose and later on eat small amounts of starchy foods like potatoes. With such a restricted diet, supplementation of macro- and micro-nutrients becomes vitally important.

IV. CYSTIC FIBROSIS

Cystic fibrosis is a hereditary disorder the affecting exocrine glands that is characterized by abnormal composition of exocrine secretions (3). It can lead to pancreatic insufficiency during childhood. The patient may have higher energy requirement (20–50% or more) than normal, although this is debated. There are repeated respiratory infections, with varying degrees of steatorrhea, emphasizing the need for high-energy foods. Thus, fat intake should not be limited and diet may have whole milk, full-fat cheese, full-cream yogurt, butter, and margarine, fried foods, and chocolates. Glucose polymers and sugar, sweets, jam, honey, and concentrated glucose drinks and supplemented flavored milk shakes are also used.

In infants, breast-feeding should be combined with a pancreatic supplement. Weaning may commence at about 3 months of age in order to boost energy intake. It is necessary to take pancreatic enzymes along with every meal and snack, unless the latter consists of only such items as squash, fruit, or boiled sweets. Clayton (3) has mentioned some modern preparations of pancreatic enzymes in the form of enteric-coated pH-sensitive microspheres. Pancreatic powder is used for infants. The diet should include at least two good portions of protein along with fruits and vegetables, with supplements of 8000 IU vitamin A, 800 IU of vitamin D, and 100 to 200 mg of vitamin E daily.

V. GENETIC DISORDERS OF CELLULAR ORGANELLES

Clayton (3) has described the following three inborn errors of intracellular organelles:

1. lysosomal storage disorders
2. mitochondrial disorders
3. peroxisomal disorders

These conditions may arise from mutations in the structural genes for the proteins in an organelle, and from mutations in the gene coding for components required to transport proteins into the organelles. Dietary treatment is not available for lysosomal storage disorders.

The mitochondrial disorders and fat oxidation defects can arise from dysfunctions in transport system (e.g., carnitine deficiency), substrate utilization in TCA cycle, oxidative-phosphorylation, and respiratory electron-transport chain, which may together present as a myopathy or an encephalomyopathy, with hypoglycemic episodes. The diagnosis of these disorders is complex, requiring elaborate biochemical facilities such as in a teaching hospital (11). Przyrembel (12) prescribed the following dietary treatment for mitochondrial disorders:

Defect	Diet
Carnitine deficiency	Low fat, high carbohydrate
Carnitine deficiency, carnitine palmitoyl transferase	MCT fat, high carbohydrate
Pyruvate carboxylase	High protein, high carbohydrate
Acyl-CoA dehydrogenases	
	High carbohydrate, frequent meals
Phosphoenolpyruvate carboxykinase	
Pyruvate dehydrogenase	High fat, low carbohydrate

Fasting periods should be avoided, and such diets may include trials of megadoses of a variety of vitamins and/or carnitine, around 50 to 200 mg/kg body weight/24 h (3).

Two diseases affecting peroxisomal functions (13) that respond to dietary treatment are Refsum disease–adult type and adrenoleukodystrophy. In Refsum disease there is a disorder in the oxidation of phytanic acid (PA), a 20-C acid that is impaired as the result of deficiency of phytanic acid alpha-hydrolase. PA is derived either from food or from the conversion of free phytol in food. Normally, only a trace of PA is present in serum, which increases greatly in amount in Refsum disease. The symptoms of the disorder include cerebral ataxia, peripheral neuropathy, retinitis pigmentosa with night blindness, and cardiomyopathy, which usually appear before the age of 20 years. Dietary treatment aims at maintaining the serum PA levels below 10 mg/100 ml. The predominant sources of PA in the diet are dairy products, fats, and meats of ruminants and other fats. Phytol occurs in a variety of foods such as corn oil, nuts, and spices. It is not known whether chlorophyll-bound phytol also should be restricted. A practical diet severely restricts fat and prohibits ruminant meat but allows skimmed milk and vegetables. During periods of loss of appetite, a high-carbohydrate intake should be adminstered (14).

Andrenoleukodystrophy is a group of degenerative neurological disorders characterized by demyelination and an accumulation of saturated, very long chain fatty acids in body fluids and tissues. Use of a diet in which these acids are restricted along with a supplement of oleic acid may reduce X-linked leukodystrophy. The disease presents at about 8 years of age. Moser et al. (15) have reviewed peroxisomal disorders.

REFERENCES

1. Mckusick, V.A., *Mendelian Inheritance in Man*, 8th ed., Johns Hopkins University Press, Baltimore, 1988.
2. Scriver, C.R., A.L. Beaudet, W.S. Sly, and D. Valle (eds.), *The Metabolic Basic of Inherited Disease*, 6th ed., McGraw-Hill, New York, 1989.
3. Clayton, B., Dietetic treatment of inherited metabolic disease, *Human Nutrition and Dietetics*, 9th ed. (J.S. Garrow and W.P.T. James, eds.), Churchill Livingstone, Edinburgh, London, 1993, p. 723.
4. Cotton, R.G., Heterogeneity of phenylketonuria at the clinical, protein and DNA levels, *J. Inherit Metab. Dis. 13*: 739 (1990).
5. Smith, I., B. Cook, and M. Beasley, Review of neonatal screening programme for phenylketonuria, *Br. Med. J. 303*: 333 (1991).
6. Smith, I., M.G. Beasley, and A.E. Ades, Intelligence and quality of dietary treatment in phenylketonuria, *Arch. Dis. Childhood 65*: 472 (1990).
7. Thompson, A.J., I. Smith, and D. Brenton, Neurological deterioration in young adults with phenylketonuria, *Lancet 336*: 602 (1990).
8. Kvittingen, E.A., Tyrosinaemia type I—an update, *J. Inherit. Metab. Dis. 7*: 13 (1991).
9. Collins, J.E., and J.V. Leonard, The dietary management of inborn errors of metabolism, *Human Nutr: Appl. Nutr. 39A*: 255 (1985).
10. DHSS, Present-day practice in infant feeding: Third report, Report of Health and Social Subjects No.32, Dept. of Health and Social Security, HMSO, London, 1988.
11. Pollitt, R.J., Disorders of mitochondrial beta-oxidation: Prenatal and early postnatal diagnosis and their relevance to Reye's syndrome and sudden infant death, *J. Inherited Metab. Dis. 12*(Suppl. 1): 215 (1989).
12. Przyrembel, H., Therapy of mitochondrial disorders, *J. Inherit. Metab. Dis. 10*: 129 (1987).
13. Monnens, L., and H. Heymans, Peroxisomal disorders: Clinical characterisation, *J. Inherit. Metab. Dis. 10*(Suppl. 1): 23 (1987).
14. Dickson, N., J.G. Mortimer, and J.M. Faed, A child with Refsum's disease: successful treatment with diet and plasma exchange, *Develop. Med. Child Neurol. 31*: 81 (1989).
15. Moser, H.W., A. Bergin, and D. Cornblath, Peroxisomal disorders, *Biochem. Cell Biol. 69*: 463 (1991).

31
Dietary Management of Underweight Babies

I. INTRODUCTION

Aggett (1) categorized underweight babies in to the following three types:

1. Low birthweight (LBW), weighing less than 2.5 kg
2. Very low birthweight (VLBW), below 1.5 kg
3. Extremely low birthweight (ELBW), weighing less than 1.0 kg

LBW infants are often small because they are born preterm, i.e., before the completion of 37 weeks of gestation; their weight may then be appropriate for gestational age (AGA). However, those showing intrauterine growth retardation are small for dates (SFD). A baby is said to be SFD if its birthweight is below the 10th centile of expected weight for its gestational age; 2.5 kg is the 10th weight centile for a fetus of about 31 weeks gestation.

It has been estimated that around 16% of the world's live births are of LBW, 90% of which are born in the developing countries, and of these around 75% are SFD. The SFD babies are, in general, relatively mature, having been delivered late in pregnancy and as such do not face difficulties arising from the loss of intrauterine development of metabolic functions. However, AGA infants of similar weight are characterized by immaturity problems and are vulnerable to cardiopulmonary disorders and other metabolic stresses. Although modern advances in the care of LBW AGA infants have improved the chances of their survival, meeting their nutritional requirements has emerged as a major challenge (1).

The fetus trebles its body weight at a rate of 15 to 20 g/kg/day between 24 and 36 weeks postconceptional age; the AGA infant is deprived of this phase of development. The LBW AGA infants also have problems with protein, energy, and mineral supply and are susceptible to infections and metabolic disorders arising from stress, such as surgery.

During the last trimester of gestation, the fetus accumulates about 550 g fat, increasing its body fat from 1% to 16%, which is an important source of energy reserve. LBW infants weighing between 1.0 and 2.0 kg would survive for only 4 to 12 days, compared to 30 days for a starved term infant weighing 3.5 kg (2). Both AGA and SFD-type LBW infants are especially vulnerable to hypoglycemia because of their limited supply of glycogen and fat stores. Also, VLBW infants have impaired gluconeogenesis and limited fat oxidation. There is a surge in the capacity for gluconeogenesis and fatty acid oxidation in full-term babies that matches the loss from transplacental supply of nutrients such as glucose and amino acids. This switch allows the newborn child to metabolize a lipid-rich diet. Fatty acid oxidation inhibits glucose oxidation and stimulates formation of gluconeogenic substrates, such as lactic acid, pyruvic acid, and alanine. These essential adjustments are slower to develop in preterm infants (3). Thus, LBW infants need a nutrient inflow to match their specific requirements. They need glucose as the main oxidative substrate for the brain, their overall glucose consumption being higher (5–6 mg/kg/min) than that of the full-term infant (3–5 mg/kg/min) (4). Even moderate hypoglycemia (plasma glucose below 2.6 mmol/1) in LBW infants may lead to subsequent impaired neurodevelopment (5). A range of appropriate nutrients is required during the fetal and postnatal periods to bring about desired change in brain-cell division, migration, and organization.

II. NUTRITIONAL MANAGEMENT OF LBW INFANTS

The nutritional management of LBW infants has been reviewed in detail (6–9). Ideal critieria to evaluate nutritional requirements of LBW babies are not known. LBW infants can be very different from normal babies and their problems can be unique. Preterm infants rapidly lose extracellular fluid after delivery, with 8% to 10% weight loss, and have different metabolic demands ex utero than in utero.

The adequacy of supplying appropriate nutrients in required quantities is being evaluated on the basis of both short-term (systematic biochemical, anthropometric, and metabolic) and long-term studies of the development and performance of children later in life. The recommended intakes of nutrients for the oral feeding of LBW infants (6,7), are only a basis for current feeding systems until more refined recommendations are available. For certain nutrients, the recommended intakes have been empirically derived from calculating the amount that would be supplied by human breast milk, which may not be suitable for nutrients such as energy, protein, calcium, and sodium (1).

A. Energy

LBW infants have higher energy needs than normal full-term babies because they have higher resting metabolic rates (RMR), inefficient intestinal absorption, less efficient thermal regulation, and enhanced growth rates. The RMR increases during the neonatal period and is directly related to energy intake and the rate of weight gain. Thus, RMR is highest in babies who are growing fast or those who are recovering from starvation. Also, the RMR of SFD infants is generally higher than AGA infants, who require nutrients to support their developmental changes. The estimated energy intake of LBW neonates, assuming 80% absorptive efficiency, is 90 to 170 kcal/kg body weight/day and that recommended in practice is 120 to 130 kcal/kg/day (1).

Essential amino acids and intracellular cations such as Mg and Zn are required for the synthesis of lean tissue (7), the overall growth of the child depending upon supply of all needed nutrients. The amount of feed and its composition as well as the efficiency of intestinal absorption influence the energy intake lost in feces. Appropriate quantity and quality of fat and carbohydrate enhance the energy absorption up to 80% or more in stable LBW infants, amounting to a daily fecal loss of 10 to 30 kcal/kg (10). Up to 10 kcal/kg/day should be allowed for thermoregulatory activity.

Human breast milk with an energy density of 65 to 70 kcal/day can meet an intake of 120 to 130 kcal/kg/day, with a volume of 180 to 200 ml/kg/day. The proprietary formulas with an energy density of 65 to 85 kcal/day can meet these requirements at volumes of 200 to 250 ml/kg/day. Pasteurization of human milk will denature the enzymes present in raw human milk and will not support growth. SFD infants grow faster than AGA ones and do this with a low energy deposition, i.e., predominated by protein and water deposition (11), and do not necessarily benefit from increased energy intakes. The AGA babies also become fatty on higher energy intakes.

B. Protein, Carbohydrate, and Fat

A daily net protein accumulation of 1.6 to 2.0 g/kg increases the nitrogen content of the fetus from 14.6 to 18.6 g/kg between 24 and 36 weeks of gestation. Around 90% of the digested and absorbed dietary protein nitrogen is incorporated into the infants' tissues. Protein constitutes about 10% of the energy intake. The supply of essential amino acids, energy, and other nutrients such as Mg, Zn, and P required for the synthesis of lean tissue determine the overall efficiency of incorporation and tolerance of dietary protein. The child's immature protein metabolic pathways and inability of the kidney to handle unused amino acids pose problems in specifying the mixture of amino acids required by LBW infants. Also, there is a specific need for amino acids such as glycine, cysteine, and taurine, which are not thought to be essential for adults (12). These amino acids are required for tissue synthesis and cannot be synthesized by the infant's body in sufficient amounts because of to immature development of metabolic pathways.

Inadequate protein intakes may lead to poor growth, hypoalbuminemia, and edema, and protein intakes higher than 4 g/kg/day may not be utilized efficiently (13). Intakes above this level lead to acidosis, high blood ammonia concentrations and enhanced plasma levels of phenylalanine, tyrosine, and methionine as the result of nondevelopment of catabolic liver enzymes. The increased renal solute load causes dehydration, and the problem is exacerbated by the disrupted amino acid metabolism.

Human breast milk may not supply all the estimated requirements of the LBW child even at daily intake rates of 80 to 200 ml/kg, especially when the child is gaining weight rapidly. Under these circumstances, supplementation of the feed with other protein sources such as whey-based formula, hydrolyzed casein, or human milk protein would be required (14).

Carbohydrates constitute around 40% of breast milk energy, lactose being the predominant carbohydrate in the milk. The LBW child can assimilate other disaccharides and polysaccharides through intestinal enzymes. Polymeric carbohydrates thus formed decrease the osmolality of the feeds, minimizing the risk of osmotic diarrhea in some immature neonates who cannot use lactose.

Lactose per se is not essential but its constituent, galactose, is required for cerebroside and glycosaminoglycan synthesis. It is not known whether the LBW child's liver is able to synthesize galactose from glucose. Galactose is also an important precursor for glycogen synthesis. Thus, inclusion of lactose or galactose in the LBW child's feed is advisable. Lactose increases the absorption of minerals and promotes the growth of intestinal lactobacilli, which tend to reduce intestinal infection.

Fat constitutes about 50% of breast milk energy and is the main source of energy for the neonate. Its digestion and absorption depend on the child's pancreatic, gastric, and lingual lipases and on bile salts. In preterm LBW babies, lipase activity is low, but this can be compensated for by lipase activity in the breast milk and by the type of milk fat from breast milk that can be absorbed by the LBW child, although lipase activity is lower in more preterm babies and in infants given formula feeds, and in infants fed pasteurized human milk.

The unsaturated fatty acids present in human milk (linoleic, linolenic, arachidonic, and docosahexanoic acids) are absorbed more efficiently than the saturated fatty acids of the same chain length. Human milk has around 60% to 70% of the long-chain unsaturated fatty acids.

The LBW child may show clinical, biochemical, and histological evidence of deficiency of the essential fatty acids if the intake of linoleic acid is less than 1% of the energy intake. Thus, formula-fed LBW babies should receive at least 4.5% and 0.5% of their energy intake as linoleic and linolenic acids, respectively. The marine fish oils are better sources of the long-chain polyenoic acids than vegetable oils. Fetal brain rapidly accumulates polyenoic acids during the last trimester of pregnancy, which the LBW infants miss. These infants fed a formula with a fatty acid content simulating that of human milk can achieve retinal function similar to that of infants fed breast milk (15,16).

The medium-chain fatty acids (C 8–12) are absorbed more easily than the long-chain fatty acids and can enter the mitochondria for oxidation without requiring the carnitine transfer system. Some LBW babies may not be able to synthesize carnitine from lysine. Larsson et al. (17) noted that carnitine supplementation improved the fatty acid oxidation transiently in preterm neonates.

Inositol has a fundamental role in phospholipid metabolism, in intracellular signaling, and in the stimulation of the normal development of the child. Inositol supplementation in preterm babies tends to decrease the incidence of pulmonary and retinal damage. Hallman et al. (18) have proposed that LBW infants should receive an intake of inositol equivalent to that present in breast milk.

C. Water and Electrolytes

Around 50% to 70% of the weight gain in the growing, well-fed LBW child consists only of water. Water loss occurs through kidney, skin, lungs, and gut. The extrarenal water loss through skin and lungs amounts to 30 to 60 ml daily. The water loss via skin is increased by activity, respiratory stress, low humidity, and high environmental temperature. The transepidermal water loss in the first 3 days of life of an infant of 32 weeks gestation is around 2 to 6 ml/kg/h, which is higher in infants of shorter gestations (19). However, the water loss becomes similar to that of full-term infants within 1 to 2 weeks when the skin becomes keratinized rapidly postnatally. The extrarenal water loss can be decreased by maintaining humidity above 80% and using heat shields to increase local humidity. Fecal water loss is about 5 to 20 ml/kg body weight daily.

The urinary volume depends on the osmotic load to be excreted. Whereas normal neonates born at 40 weeks gestation do not have a urinary osmolality of greater than 500 mmol/kg, VLBW infants normally have a urine osmolality of 60 to 200 mmol/kg (20). Most LBW infants can achieve a urinary osmolality of only 170 mmol/kg, thus excreting more water with any solutes or osmolar loads than usual. The customary renal solute loads of 14 to 15 mmol/kg daily need to be excreted in 90 ml/kg/day. Adding all these losses, the daily water requirement amounts to 150 to 200 ml/kg body weight, and some of this water can be produced metabolically in the body (about 12 ml/100 kcal). Thus, with a daily energy intake of 120 to 130 kcal/kg, about 15 ml of water/kg will be produced. The adequacy of an infant's water intake has to be monitored by clinical evaluation, by regular weighing, and by measuring changes in plasma sodium and urine specific gravity or osmolality.

Water overloads can be caused by stresses such as asphyxia or respiratory distress (21), in which water excretion may be limited inappropriately by the secretion of arginine-vasopressin (AVP). Water intake then may be required to be restricted, along with a risk of restricting the intake of other nutrients (1).

A 25-week preterm fetus has 94 mmole of sodium/kg body weight, which falls to 74 mmol/kg at term. Sodium accumulates daily at 0.5 to 1.1 mmol/kg in the second half of gestation. During the first 4 to 5 days of life, the LBW infant may lose about 12% of body weight and 6 to 16 mmol of sodium/kg, representing the loss of extracellular fluid and the acquisition of body water compartmentation similar to full-term infants (22).

Most LBW babies will achieve a positive sodium balance during the second week of life with approximately 1.6 mmol of sodium/kg/day. The sodium intake needs to be adjusted to maintain normal plasma sodium levels of 130 to 135 mmol/l. Preterm infants under 30 weeks gestation with immature renal tubular sodium reabsorption may need as much as 8 to 12 mmol/kg/day. After 32 to 34 weeks, most LBW infants can maintain normal plasma sodium levels.

Potassium deficiency is very rare, even during rapid growth when potassium is required for new tissue. Daily intakes of around of 2.0 to 3.5 mmol/kg are provided by mature breast milk (10–17.5 mmol/l), meeting the needs of most LBW infants.

D. Minerals

The normal fetus will accumulate around 120 to 150 mg (3.0–3.25 mmol) of calcium/kg/day between 26 and 36 weeks gestation, with 60 to 75 mg (1.94–2.42 mmol) of phosphorus/kg/day. About 99% of the calcium and 80% of the phosphorus are deposited in bone. Breast milk or proprietary formulas can hardly meet these rates. Early neonatal calcium deficiency can lead to asymptomatic hypocalcemia, stimulating the release of parathyroid hormone and mobilization of skeletal calcium. The latter can be prevented or its incidence reduced by early introduction of feeds or calcium in parenteral nutrition. Late neonatal hypocalcemia (3–15 days of age) may present initially with convulsions.

Almost all infants weighing less than 1.5 kg will have reduced bone mineralization; around 57% of ELBW infants develop severe changes (23). Adequate deposition of skeletal calcium depends on the supply of phosphorus, in the absence of which metabolic bone disease may occur even with adequate supplies of vitamin D. Hypomineralization and metabolic bone disease are more common in infants fed human milk (24). Thus, adequate supplies of both calcium and phosphorus are essential to prevent silent early bone disease leading to retardation of subsequent linear growth (25). The supplies of both calcium and phosphorus need to be carefully balanced because calcium cannot be utilized effectively for bone formation in the absence of phosphorus. The use of large calcium intakes (more than 140 mg/kg/day) will not only be ineffective in improving bone mineralization but detrimental, leading to impaired absorption of fat, intraluminal precipitation of calcium, hypercalcemia, metabolic acidosis, and phosphorus depletion (1).

A fetus weighing 1 kg has around 0.2 g of magnesium, which increases to 0.8 g in a full-term infant weighing 3.5 kg. About 65% of the body's magnesium is present in the skeleton. LBW babies weighing 1 kg may accumulate magnesium at 10 mg/kg/day; at 1.5 kg body weight, the rate would be 8.5 mg/kg/day. VLBW infants may require as much as 20 mg/kg/day of magnesium to approximate fetal accretion rates (26). Human breast milk provides only about 3.0 mg/day of Mg. Incorporation of mangesium into tissue during rapid weight gain results in a low plasma Mg concentration in preterm infants, as evidenced clinically with convulsions and a persistent low plasma calcium level (1).

A fetus weighing 1 kg has about 65 mg of iron, which is increased at the rate of 1.8 mg/kg/day during the last trimester. The iron stores of LBW infants weighing less than 1.4 kg may be exhausted after 6 to 8 weeks of postnatal life without iron intakes. Frequent blood sampling also depletes the infant's iron stores (3.4 mg Fe/g of hemoglobin). A total iron intake of 2.0 to 2.5 mg/kg/day, including that supplied by feeds, is adequate for most LBW infants. Some proprietary formulas contain sufficient iron to achieve this intake without any supplement. Excessive iron supplements may cause enhanced lipid peroxidation and hemolytic anemia, may alter intestinal flora, and may increase the risk of gram-negative septicemia. Blood transfusions can supply significant amounts of iron.

The fetus can accumulate copper at the rate of 51 μg/kg/day, to have 14 mg at full term. Around one-half of this amount is present in the liver. Sporadic copper deficiency may occur in artificially fed LBW infants, but it is rare in breast-fed infants.

E. Vitamins

Vitamin deficiencies in LBW infants are rare. However, LBW infants may be at risk for inadequate intake of the fat-soluble vitamins. Low plasma levels of retinol are usually found with metabolic evidence of vitamin A deficiency (27). Vitamin E is thought to decrease the risk of pulmonary damage and also possibly prevents retinal damage and brain hemorrhages. However, these benefits have not been clearly demonstrated. Before 32 weeks of gestation, the intestinal response to vitamin D [1, 25(OH)$_2$ calciferol] is poor, and such preterm infants may require extra vitamin D to optimize calcium and phosphorus metabolism.

LBW infants need vitamin K supplementation because of their rapid systemic utilization of vitamin K, low dietary intake, and limited intestinal production of this vitamin. Infants may be given 0.5 to 1.0 mg of vitamin K intramuscularly on the first day of life; the dose should be repeated weekly until the baby starts feeding orally, providing 2 to 3 μg/kg/day of vitamin K.

Deficiencies of water-soluble vitamins are also rare. Thiamin, vitamin C, and folate are heat-sensitive, so they are likely to be lost from heat-processed formula feeds and pasteurized milk. Ascorbic acid influences iron absorption and possibly reduces the transient hypertyrosinemia and hyperphenyl-alaninemia in LBW infants.

Riboflavin, being photolabile, is lost when human milk is exposed to light. LBW infants occasionally experience pyridoxine deficiency, and biotin deficiency is seen in infants fed intravenously. Deficiency of cobalamin (B$_{12}$) and thiamin is seen in infants being breast-fed by mothers deficient in these vitamins (1).

The immaturity of the gut and other organs of LBW infants creates difficulty in feeding them, which may lead to cardiopulmonary and other systemic disorders. The fetus can swallow at 16 weeks, and gut motility appears at 28 weeks gestation, although effective sucking, intestinal motility, and protection of the airways are not present until 34 weeks (28).

Enteral feeding of critically ill LBW infants is very difficult, and most are routinely fed intravenously. However, small amounts of enteral feeds are beneficial because they stimulate a physiological hormonal surge and a bile flow and induce maturation of the intestinal mucosa. Large volumes of enteral feeds may predispose infants to apnea, ileus, and enterocolitis (29).

Infants are fed gradual increases of volumes during the first week of life, although they can tolerate intakes of 90 to 260 ml/kg/day from third day of life (20). Human milk may not provide some preterm infants with enough nutrients, such as energy, protein, calcium, phosphorus, iron, sodium, vitamin C, and folate, but breast milk does confer improved immune function and protection (30) as well as a better lipid profile and better developmental progress (31). SFD infants are clearly benefited by breast milk. LBW babies can also progress well on specific formula feeds designed for them.

Hinds et al. (32) reviewed the effect of caffeine on pregnancy outcome variables. Evidence available suggests that heavy caffeine use (≥300 mg/day) during pregnancy is associated with small reductions in infant birth weight that may be especially detrimental to premature or low-birth-weight infants. Some researchers have also documented an increased risk of spontaneous abortion associated with caffeine consumption before and during pregnancy. Overwhelming evidence, however, indicates that caffeine is not a human teratogen and that caffeine has no effect on preterm labor and delivery.

Low birthweight (<2500 g or 5.5 lb) of an infant may be the result of a shortened gestational period (prematurity) or the result of intrauterine growth retardation (IUGR), resulting in a small for gestational age (SGA) infant. Total consumption of more than about 300 mg/day of caffeine during pregnancy has been found to be associated with reduced birth weight, increased risk of LBW infants, and/or IUGR in case-control (33), prospective (34–38), and retrospective (39–43) studies. Two studies failed to show associations between coffee or caffeine intake and LBW (44,45) after controlling for maternal smoking and length of gestation.

In a prospective study of 414 smokers, Peacock et al. (38) observed a 6% reduction in birth weight that could be attributed to a caffeine intake of 1,400 mg/week, after making statistical adjustment for smoking and alcohol drinking. In another prospective study of 9,921 healthy pregnant women, 53 women having fetuses with a gestational age of at least 24 weeks consumed more than 5 cups of coffee daily. These women had a significantly higher prevalence (13.2%) of fetuses who were small for gestational age (SGA) (36).

A Yale–New Haven Hospital study of 3,981 women demonstrated a dose-response of caffeine intake to increased risk of LBW babies in single deliveries after 36 weeks. The adjusted relative risk of an LBW delivery was 1.4 for mothers consuming 1 to 150 mg of caffeine/day, 2.3 for mothers consuming 151 to 300 mg/day, and 4.6 for those consuming more than 300 mg daily. The corresponding decreases in birth weight were 6, 31, and 105 g, respectively (34). The value of 105 g represented a significant decrease in birthweight. Because gestational age was not related to caffeine consumption in this study, Hinds et al. (32) postulated that maternal caffeine consumption probably had an effect on birthweight through IUGR. Caffeine being structurally similar to adenine and guanine, it may possibly interfere with cell division and metabolism. Also, caffeine has a vasoconstrictive effect on placental intervillous blood flow that may also contribute to the potential risk of IUGR (46).

Fenster et al. (40) showed that women who decreased their caffeine intake to 300 mg/day within 6 weeks of their last menstrual period also reduced their risk of delivering LBW infants, compared with women who did not reduce their caffeine intake early in their pregnancies. The former women also had a lower risk of delivering infants with IUGR.

A consistent negative correlation between infant singleton birthweight and caffeine consumption above 300 mg/day shows that women should limit their daily intake to less than 300 mg. More research is required to understand the mechanism(s) that allow caffeine to exert an effect on fetal growth (32).

REFERENCES

1. Aggett, P.J., The low-birthweight infant, *Human Nutrition and Dietetics*, 9th ed., (J.S. Garrow and W.D.T. James, eds.), Churchill Livingstone, Edinburgh, London, 1993, p. 714.
2. Heird, W.C., J.M. Driscoll, and J.N. Schullinger, Intravenous alimentation in pediatric patients, *J. Pediatrics 80*: 351 (1972).
3. Girard, J., Metabolic adaptations to change of nutrition at birth, *Biol. Neonate 58* (Suppl.1): 3 (1990).
4. Kalhan, S., D. Bier, and Savins, Estimation of glucose turnover and 13C recycling in the newborn by stimulations (1–13C) glucose and (6, 62 H_2) glucose tracers, *J. Clin. Endocrinol. Metab. 50*: 456 (1980).
5. Lucas, A., R. Morley, and T.J. Cole, Adverse neurodevelopmental outcome of moderate neonatal hypoglycaemia, *Br. Med. J. 297*: 1304 (1988).
6. AAP, Committee on Nutrition, 1985, Nutritional needs of low birthweight infants, American Academic of Pediatrics, *Pediatrics 75*: 976 (1985).
7. ESPGAN, Committee on the Nutrition of the Preterm Infant, 1987, *Nutrition and Feeding of Preterm Infants* (B. Wharton, ed.), Blackwell Scientific Publications, Oxford, 1987.
8. Shaw, J.C.L., Growth and nutrition of the very preterm infant, *Br. Med. Bull. 44*: 984 (1988).
9. Cowett, R.M. (ed.), *Principles of Perinatal-Neonatal Metabolism*, Springer-Verlag, London, 1991.
10. Reichaman, B.L., P. Chessex, and G. Putet, Partation of energy metabolism and energy cost of growth in the very low-birthweight infant, *Pediatrics 69*: 446 (1982).
11. Chessex, P., B. Reichman, and G. Verellen, Metabolic consequences of intrauterine growth retardation in very low-birthweight infants, *Pediatric Res. 18*: 709 (1984).
12. Chesney, R.W., Taurine: Is it required for infant nutrition? *J. Nutr. 118*: 6 (1988).
13. Kashyap, S., K.F. Schulze, and M. Forsynth, Growth, nutrient retention, metabolic response in low-birthweight infants fed varying intakes of protein and energy, *J. Pediatrics 113*: 713 (1988).
14. Putet, G., J. Rigo, B. Salle, and J. Senterre, Supplementation of pooled human milk with casein hydrolysate: energy and nitrogen balance and weight gain composition in very low-birthweight infants, *Pediatric Res. 21*: 458 (1987).
15. Uauy, R.D., D.G. Birch, and E.E. Birch, Effect of dietary omega-3 fatty acids on retinal function of very low-birthweight neonates, *Pediatric Res. 28*: 485 (1990).

16. Koletzko, B., Fats for brains, *Europ. J. Clin. Nutr. 46*(S): 51 (1992).

17. Larsson, L.E., R. Olegard, and B.M. Ljung, Parenteral nutrition in preterm neonates with and without carnitine supplementation, *Acta Anaesthesiologica Scandinavica 34*: 501 (1990).

18. Hallman, M., K. Bry, and K. Hoppu, Inositol supplementation in premature infants with respiratory distress syndrome, *N. Engl. J. Med. 326*: 1233 (1992).

19. Rutter, N., The immature skin, *Br. Med. Bull. 44*: 957 (1988).

20. Coulthard, M., and E.N. Hey, Effect of varying water intake on renal functions in healthy preterm babies, *Arch. Dis. Childhood 65*: 614 (1985).

21. Rees, L., Hyponatraemia in the first week of life in preterm infants. 1. Arginine-vasopressin secretion, *Arch. Dis. Childhood 59*: 414 (1984).

22. Bauer, K., G. Bovermann, and A. Roithmaier, Body composition, nutrition and fluid balance during the first two weeks of life in preterm neonates weighing less than 1500 grams, *J. Pediatrics 118*: 615 (1991).

23. Koo, W.W., and R.C. Tsang, Mineral requirements of low-birthweight infants, *J. Am. College Nutr. 10*: 474 (1991).

24. Abrams, S.A., R.J. Schanler, and C. Garza, Bone mineralization in former very low birthweight infants fed either human milk or commercial formula, *J. Pediatrics 112*: 956 (1988).

25. Lucas, A., R. Morley, and T.J. Cole, Breast milk and subsequent intelligence in children born preterm, *Lancet 339*: 261 (1989).

26. Giles, M.M., I.A. Laing, and R.A. Elton, Magnesium metabolism in preterm infants: effects of calcium, magnesium and phosphorus and of postnatal and gastational age, *J. Pediatrics 117*: 147 (1990).

27. Woodruff, C.W., C.B. Latham, H. Mactier, and J.C. Hewett, Vitamin A status of preterm infants: correlation between plasma retinol concentration and retinol dose response, *Am. J. Clin. Nutr. 46*: 985 (1987).

28. Milla, P.J., and W.M. Bisset, The gastrointestinal tract, *Br. Med. Bull. 44*: 1010 (1988).

29. Anderson, D.M., and R.M. Kliegman, The relationship of neonatal alimentation practices to the occurrence of endemic necrotizing enterocolitis, *Am. J. Perinatology 8*: 62 (1991).

30. Lucas, A., and T.J. Cole, Breast milk and neonatal necrotising enterocolitis, *Lancet 336*: 1519 (1990).

31. Lucas, A., R. Morley, and T.J. Cole, Breast milk and subsequent intelligence in children born preterm, *Lancet 339*: 261 (1992).

32. Hinds, T.S., W.L. West, E.M. Knight, and B.F. Harland, The effect of caffeine on pregnancy outcome variables, *Nutr. Rev. 54*: 203 (1996).

33. Caan, B.J., and M.K. Goldhaber, Caffeinated beverages and low birth weight: a case-control study, *Am. J. Public Health 79*: 1299 (1989).

34. Martin, T.R., and M.B. Bracken, The association between low birth weight and caffeine consumption during pregnancy, *Am. J. Epidemiol. 126*: 813 (1987).

35. Godel, J.C., H.F. Pabst, P.E. Hodges, K.E. Johnson, G.J. Froese, and M.R. Joffres, Smoking and caffeine and alcohol intake during pregnancy in a northern population: effect on fetal growth, *Can. Med. Assoc. J. 147*: 181 (1992).

36. Furuhashi, N., S. Sinzi, M. Suzuki, M. Hiruta, M. Tanaka, and T. Takahashi, Effects of caffeine ingestion during pregnancy, *Gynecol. Obstet. Invest. 19*: 187 (1985).

37. Munoz, L.M., B. Lonnerdal, C. Keen, and K.G. Dewey, Coffee consumption as a factor in iron deficiency anemia among pregnant women and their infants in Costa Rica, *Am. J. Clin. Nutr. 48*: 645 (1988).

38. Peacock, J.L., J.M. Bland, and H.R. Anderson, Effects on birth weight of alcohol and caffeine consumption in smoking women, *J. Epidemiol. Commun. Health 45*: 159 (1991).

39. Watkinson, B., and P.A. Fried, Maternal caffeine use before, during and after pregnancy and effects upon offspring, *Neurobehav. Toxicol. Teratol 7*: 9 (1985).

40. Fenster, L., B. Eskenazi, G.C. Windham, and S.H. Swan, Caffeine consumption during pregnancy and fetal growth, *Am. J. Public Health 81*: 458 (1991).

41. McDonald, A.D., B.G. Armstrong, and M. Sloan, Cigarette, alcohol and coffee consumption and prematurity, *Am. J. Public Health 82*: 87 (1992).

42. Fortier, I., S. Marcoux, and L. Beaulac-Baillargeon, Relation of caffeine intake during pregnancy to intrauterine growth retardation and preterm birth, *Am. J. Epidemiol. 137*: 931 (1993).

43. Berkowitz, G.S., T.R. Hoflord, and R.L. Berkowitz, Effects of cigarette smoking, alcohol, coffee, and tea consumption on preterm delivery, *Early Human Dev. 7*: 239 (1982).

44. Linn, S., S.C. Schoenbaum, R.R. Monson, B. Rosner, P.G. Stubblefield, and K. Ryan, No association between coffee consumption and adverse outcomes of pregnancy, *N. Engl. J. Med. 306*: 141 (1982).

45. Shu, X.O., M.C. Hatch, J. Mills, J. Clemens, and M. Susser, Maternal smoking, alcohol drinking, caffeine consumption, and fetal growth: results from a prospective study, *Epidemiology 6*: 115 (1995).

46. Kirkinen, P., P. Jouppila, A. Koivula, J. Vuori, and M. Puukka, The effect of caffeine on placental and fetal blood flow in human pregnancy, *Am. J. Obstet. Gynecol. 147*: 939 (1983).

32
Diet and Alcoholic Disorders

I. INTRODUCTION

Chronic alcoholism has been regarded as a psychosomatic disease with both psychological and physiologic determinants. Better understanding of the "agent (ethyl alcohol)-host-environment" triangle is necessary to elucidate the etiology and pathogenesis of the chronic alcohol-related disorders. Chronic alcoholism is thus a disease of multiple etiology, the agent (alcohol) being only one of the causes. Other causes related to nutrition, metabolism, and genetic endowment of the host may be more critical in the pathogenesis of alcoholism than the agent.

The ingested ethanol distributes in total body water present in blood, body tissues, and body secretions. Most persons are drunk at blood levels of ethanol greater than 150 mg percent (a level signifying medico-legal evidence of intoxification) and in danger of respiratory arrest at 400 to 500 mg%. Cytoplasmic NAD-linked alcohol dehydrogenase is the principal enzyme oxidizing alcohol, which is saturated at about 10 mg% (2 mM) alcohol level in the body. Two other enzymes in the liver are also capable of oxidizing alcohol, viz., H_2O_2-dependent catalase, which oxidizes alcohol to acetaldehyde, and a microsomal ethanol-oxidizing (MEO) system. Pyruvate is converted to acetyl CoA by pyruvate dehydrogenase, which also metabolizes acetaldehyde to hydroxyethylthiamin pyrophosphate. The acetaldehyde group is then transferred to lipoic acid to form acetyl lipoate, whose acyl group is finally transferred to CoA. This system probably accounts for about 10% of the oxidation of acetaldehyde and has been demonstrated in rat liver systems. The second pathway involves aldehyde dehydrogenase producing acetic acid, which is further metabolized to acetyl CoA with ATP and a thiokinase.

Vitamin-containing coenzymes are involved in the oxidation of alcohol in the body, so vitamin deficiency may impair the rate of alcohol oxidation, increasing the retention of alcohol in the blood of malnourished alcoholics. However, there is little evidence for this assumption either in man or in animals. The effects of nutrition on alcohol metabolism appear to be relatively small because of the highly limiting effect of alcohol dehydrogenase on the overall oxidation of alcohol. The two opposite effects of alcohol on the nutritional status include a metabolic sparing action that delays the onset of symptoms and a diuretic effect that enhances vitamin loss, leading to depletion of stores. A chronic alcoholic, in the long run, may turn to be either more or less susceptible to deficiency disease when subsisting on suboptimal diets.

The readily oxidizable, hydrogen-rich ethanol increases the NADH/NAD ratio in the cytoplasm of liver, having significant effects. Pyruvate is reduced to lactate, whose levels after ethanol ingestion may rise higher than after glucose administration. The increased NADH/NAD (and NADPH/NADP) ratio in the liver cells leads to the generation of reduced synthetic products of acetate, e.g., fatty acids and cholesterol. Also, increased reduction of dihydroxy-acetone phosphate promotes triglyceride synthesis through production of alpha-glycerophosphate. These changes in lipid metabolism are associated with the alcohol-induced pathogenesis of fatty liver.

The ethanol-induced rise in blood lactate affects renal function by markedly reducing the excretion of urate, which may account for the classic association of gouty attacks with alcohol drinking. Ethanol may also markedly decrease galactose tolerance, which is thought to be due to the inhibitory effect of the enhanced liver cell NADH/NAD ratio.

Several case studies have indicated that chronic alcoholics are most prone to deficiency diseases of protein; water-soluble vitamins, especially those of the vitamin B group such as thiamin, niacin, riboflavin, pyridoxine, and folic acid; and minerals, such as magnesium, potassium, and zinc.

Thiamin levels matching the biochemical criteria of thiamin deficiency have been observed in chronic alcoholics in proportion to the severity of thiamin deficiency, and alcoholic pellagra results from a lack of nicotinic acid and/or its precursor, tryptophan. Manifestations of protein deficiency in alcoholics include the appearance of fatty liver, hypoalbuminemia, hypocholesterolemia, edema, and normocytic anemia, which are not as severe as those seen in kwashiorkor. General dehydration is associated with mineral deficiencies, especially sodium, chloride, potassium, magnesium, and zinc, and mild to severe acidosis may also be present as evidence of a deficit in total body base.

Chronic alcoholism can lead to cardiac failure associated with a cardiomyopathy different from that seen in beriberi and not responsive to thiamin therapy. Chronic alcohol intake in some patients also induces serious forms of cardiac and skeletal myopathy that respond only to withdrawal of alcohol, and in advanced cases even the withdrawal of alcohol may not reverse the process.

Intravenous and oral fluids, tranquilizing drugs, high protein, and polymineral and multivitamin therapy is traditional for hospitalized chronic alcoholics. It is vital to encourage these patients to seek appropriate dietary advice in a clinical setting during the sober states. A preventive approach to the inevitable depletion of essential nutrients during the drinking bout can thus be planned.

According to Suter et al. (1), despite the apparent negative effects of alcohol on the function of various biochemical systems, including energy metabolism, there is no need to completely avoid alcohol consumption. The recommendations for sensible drinking are based on evidence other than body weight issues (2). "Sensible drinking" limits would probably enhance the development of weight gain and these recommendations should be interpreted and implemented with caution (3,4). Nevertheless, people who want to maintain their body weight without sacrificing their moderate alcohol intake should reduce their consumption of fat-derived energy to well below their requirements. Fat intake should be kept as low as possible, especially in subjects with a higher baseline fatness or in obese subjects (5–8). The reduction in fat intake should be at least equal to the energy content of the consumed alcohol (6, 9–10).

Alcohol consumption is often associated with higher fat intake. Also, alcohol is metabolized more slowly than it is absorbed from the intestinal tract. The higher the fat content of the consumed diet, the more restrictive alcohol consumption should be to minimize the risk of a positive fat balance. It is important to know how much alcohol calories count. The effect of alcohol on body weight may vary considerably. What is moderate for one person may be too much for another, which also applies to the effects of alcohol on body weight (7). In moderate consumers, alcohol energy counts considerably as long as no adjustments in substrate intake (especially fat intake) occur. With increasing amounts of alcohol, alcohol calories count less, but they count more with regard to overall toxicity (e.g., carcinogenesis).

The biphasic effect of alcohol on many body functions, including body weight, is nicely represented in the classical engravings of Beer Street and Gin Lane by the 18th century artist William Hogarth. The people in Beer Street are overweight, with the characteristic beer belly. They are moderate to heavy regular alcohol consumers who add alcohol to their usual food intake.

If they increase their alcohol intake, they find themselves sooner or later in Gin Lane, where people are typically malnourished and emaciated (1). Major strategies to control body weight should focus on the primary prevention of obesity.

II. DIETARY MANAGEMENT OF ALCOHOL-RELATED DISORDERS

Although alcoholism has been suggested as a major cause of malnutrition in the developed Western world, in practice malnutrition has been noticed only in patients with alcoholic pancreatitis and liver cirrhosis. Alcohol intakes of 11% to 12% of energy are not unusual in people with one or another nutritional disorder, such as hyperlipidaemia (11).

In the majority of nutritional studies of alcoholic liver disease, one or a number of tests are performed (Table 1), which constitute a more sensitive index of malnutrition than body weight. An apparently overweight, "healthy" looking chronic drinker may still be suffering from underlying nutritional deficiencies; e.g., Bunout et al. (12), in a study of 100 consecutive chronic alcoholic patients without obvious liver disease, noted that around two-thirds had abnormal liver biopsies, but normal anthropometric measurements. By the time patients develop clinical liver disease, they often develop hematological, biochemical, and immunological indications of protein-energy malnutrition (PEM) (13). Many of the blood tests, such as albumin and transferrin, are influenced by liver damage per se as well as by malnutrition and thus should be interpreted with caution (14). Although older patients are likely to exhibit more evidence of PEM in the absence of clinical liver disease, alcoholic hepatitis is particularly associated with the presence of adult kwashiorkor or marasmus. Schneeweiss et al. (15) observed that the percentage of total calories derived from protein in cirrhotics was 12%, compared to 17% in normal control. The severity of PEM may correlate with the degree of liver damage, and patients with significant alco-

Table 1 Nutritional Assessment in Liver Disease

Assessment of dietary intake
Anthropometric measurements
   Arm muscle circumference—skeletal muscle
   Skin-fold thickness—fat stores
Biochemistry
   Creatinine/height index—lean body mass
Intradermal skin testing for energy-generalized malnutrition
Tests for specific deficiencies
   RBC folate
   Serum vitamin levels
   Assessment of trace mineral deficiency
Energy balance—indirect calorimetry
   Compared to dietary caloric intake
Studies of nitrogen status and metabolism
   Serum amino acid levels
   Ratio of branched-chain to aromatic amino acids (BCAA/AAA)
   Nitrogen balance
   Total body nitrogen—capture of neutron activation
   Nitrogen index
   Labeled amino acid kinetic studies—^{13}C, ^{14}C-leucine

Source: Ref. 11.

holic liver disease tend to have a lower protein intake than usual, but still may remain above the minimum amount needed for health (16).

Alcoholism is considered one of the principal causes of nutritional disturbance in the adult population of North America and of other developed countries. A chronic alcoholic is often grossly undernourished and suffers from numerous nutritional disorders, such as beri-beri, peripheral neuropathy, macrocytic anemia, and Wernicke-Korsakoff syndrome (17). According to Kalant (17), the term "empty calories" as applied to alcohol is potentially misleading. If it is intended to convey the idea that ethanol provides calories without a corresponding content of vitamins or other essential nutrients, then the term is just as correct with respect to ethanol as it is with respect to sucrose, refined fat, or various other sources of calories. However, if it is meant to imply that the calories generated by the oxidation of alcohol are dissipated as heat and are not available metabolically in biosynthetic reactions, then the term "empty calories" is being used quite incorrectly. Animal experiments have shown that normal growth can be sustained on a diet in which a substantial portion of the carbohydrate has been replaced equicalorically by ethanol. Kalant (17) has reviewed the effects of alcoholism on intestinal malabsorption, impaired storage after absorption, impaired activation of vitamins, impaired tissue utilization, and increased excretion, and the interaction between dietary deficiency and direct effects of ethanol.

A.   Acute Alcoholic Hepatitis

Patients are often anorexic and wasted, with a negative nitrogen balance. Unable to tolerate oral food, these patients frequently have encephalopathy, necessitating protein restriction, and suffer from maldigestion or malabsorption of protein (18). Thus, AAH patients may require enteral feeding through polyurethane tubes. Protein intakes of more than 80 g/day could be tolerated through enteral feeding and positive nitrogen balance can be achieved without exacerbating the encephalopathy (19). Although some trials of enteral feeding have not shown a clear benefit for enteral nutrition over a routine hospital diet with abstinence from alcohol, it is difficult to achieve positive nitrogen balance consistently without the enteral use of energy-rich diets, with 9.4 g N/l given as a continuous infusion (20). Blendis (21) has reviewed trials using corticosteroid treatment and possible protection by propylthiouracil in severe AAH patients.

Parenteral nutrition (PN) has been restricted because it is feared that infused amino acids, especially the aromatic amino acids (AAA) and methionine, may cause portosystemic encephalopathy (PSE), although infusions of 50 to 77 g of protein at 21g/day via a peripheral vein were not known to induce PSE in AAH patients (22). Forbes et al. (23) also demonstrated that even patients with fulminant hepatic failure could tolerate PN very well. Thus, both enteral and PN in AAH appear to promote improvement in both nutrition and liver function, though with no significant improvement in mortality (11).

B.   Liver Cirrhosis

According to Watson (24), cirrhosis due to high, prolonged alcohol intake is clearly immunosuppressive, which may account for increased disease. It is, however, less clear that more moderate intakes of alcohol profoundly influence immune systems. Significant changes do occur in lymphocyte sensitivity to alcohol in vitro and cell development, as shown by decreased natural killer (NK) cells.

Cirrhotic patients without alcoholic hepatitis show elevated plasma levels of aromatic amino acids (AAA) but a decrease in the level of branched-chain amino acids (BCAA) (25). Skeletal muscle biopsies show that only valine is depleted. Cirrhotic patients have an average minimum protein requirement of 0.74 g/kg/day, whether natural or BCAA-enriched protein is used. Swart et al. (26) noted that at 0.93 g/kg/day, a positive nitrogen balance could be maintained, with an average gain of 1.2 g N/day. Whole-body protein synthesis rates in cirrhosis may remain unchanged, increased, or decreased, based on the severity of the disease or on the presence of glucose intolerance or insulin resistance. Malnourished patients show greater nitrogen retention on the same nitrogen intake. Cirrhotic patients seem to maintain a positive nitrogen balance on only modest increases in protein intake equivalent to the RNI levels, i.e., 0.75 g/kg/day (11).

Smith et al. (19) found that 9 out of 10 cirrhotic malnourished patients tolerated a high-energy (2000 kcal), low-protein (40g), low-salt (1 g Na) formula with significant increases in albumin and ferritin levels as well as increases in the creatine/height ratio and in mid-arm muscle and fat areas when fed enterally, although these were all short-term improvements.

Parenteral nutrition in cirrhosis has proved to be problematic (27). Weber et al. (28) confirmed the failure of intravenous BCAA-enriched solutions to affect nitrogen balance, though they did decrease the plasma ammonia levels, indicating a possible therapeutic role for such solutions in the management of encephalopathy.

Portal systemic encephalopathy (PSE) is a brain disorder characterized by adverse changes in mental function and neuromuscular movement. It occurs acutely in fulminant liver failure; it may be episodic in cirrhotics before becoming a chronic condition. PSE is associated with the shunting of blood from the portal system directly into the systemic circulation, thereby passing the liver. Patients show apathy, irritability, drowsiness, and coma. The central role of nitrogenous material in the gastrointestinal tract in the pathogenesis of PSE has been established (29), although other factors, such as infection, electrolyte imbalance, and intravascular volume depletion, are thought to be involved. Several nitrogen-containing materials such as ammonia, methionine and its metabolites, and the mercaptans have been implicated, including disturbances in serum amino acid metabolism.

Levels of aromatic amino acids, phenylalanine and tyrosine, rise markedly in severe liver disease. These amino acids compete for the transport carrier process across the blood-brain barrier, which also transfers the BCAAs. An excess phenylalanine level in the brain will saturate the phenylalanine-catecholamine pathway, resulting in excessive production of the sympathomimetic amines, tyramine and octopamine, which interfere with normal neurotransmission. Thus, amino acid solutions rich in BCAA, in addition to protein restriction, were proposed as a treatment for both acute and chronic PSE (30). Evidence available indicates that intravenous BCAA solutions may result in rapid improvement in PSE, but no change in mortality compared with conventional therapy (31,32). The oral feeds with BCAA mixtures also have not shown any consistent results.

Alternatively, the use of amino acids as the alpha-keto analogues has been tried. The administration of five essential amino acids—valine, leucine, isoleucine, methionine, and phenylalanine—as their calcium salts in gelatin capsules was found to improve the behavior of patients significantly, both clinically and psychologically (33). The ornithine salts of branched-chain keto acids produced a significant improvement over the BCAA (68 mmol/day) in a double-blind crossover study (34), although calcium salts of branched-chain keto acids had little effect and ornithine alpha-keto glutarate induced mental deterioration.

Lactulose, a synthetic nonabsorbable disaccharide, is widely used to manage constipation. It is valuable in PSE, because it provides substrate for colon microflora, which divert N-containing compounds from ammonia and other metabolites to provide substrate for bacterial protein synthesis. The latter causes a rise in fecal nitrogen. Lactulose fermentation decreases colonic pH, which alters absorption of ammonia or aromatic amino acids by the colon. The rapid introduction of this therapy may lead to cramps and flatulence. Combined with oral neomycin, a nonabsorbable antibiotic, there is tendency to decrease intestinal fermentation (11).

Because dietary protein intake is implicated in the pathophysiology of PSE, protein restriction has been considered a standard part of the therapy. Use of a dairy protein (e.g., milk, cheese) in the treatment of PSE has been found to be better than animal (meat) protein, possibly because of changes in colonic bacterial flora—from urease-containing bacteria on a meat diet (with ammonia produced from urea) to predominantly lactobacilli on a milk-rich diet (35). With the advent of highly successful oral therapy for PSE, such as lactulose and neomycin, the need for a special diet has now diminished. However, PSE patients do need protein and yet are being treated with protein restriction. Protein requirements in these patients may vary from 0.7 to 1.0 g/kg body weight, so that intake of 40 g of protein daily or less may be well below the requirements. Greenberger et al. (36) first suggested that vegetable protein might be beneficial. Vegetable proteins are richer in arginine and both basic amino acids, arginine and ornithine, are involved as intermediates in the hepatic urea cycle. Thus, they increase the uptake of blood ammonia, whose levels fall as urea production rises. Also, animal proteins have a higher content of methionine, which could be detrimental to the formation of mercaptans. Vegetable protein diets decrease the net absorption of nitrogen as a result of the increased fiber content of diet, which leads to enhanced bacterial synthesis in the colon, with greater endogenous protein losses and an increase in fecal nitrogen excretion on vegetable diets (37). This is followed by a significant decrease in urinary urea and total nitrogen excretion.

Portal hypertension is characterized by salt and water retention, leading to the development of massive ascites with or without peripheral edema. Even cirrhotic patients without ascites experience the problem of sodium handling and compensate with an increase in levels of atrial natriuretic peptide (ANP). With an increase in dietary sodium intake, plasma ANP levels rise, and in cirrhotic patients with ascites, plasma ANP levels do not compensate with increased sodium intake, which therefore must be restricted (38) together with fluid intake and diuretic therapy. Sodium intake may be 2 g or 100 meq daily in patients with moderate ascites. In addition, they also require potassium-sparing diuretics acting at the distal nephron site. As patients become more resistant to these drugs and require additional diuretics, sodium intake must be further restricted to 1 g of sodium or 50 meq per day. The patients non-responsive to such a regimen will need hospitalization with bed rest and sodium intake restricted to the lowest level of 20 meq per day, with one liter of fluid.

Massive ascites may be associated with the loss of muscle mass from the limbs and trunk, resulting in a cachetic appearance. The total body nitrogen is a useful measure in the assessment of lean body mass. The state of ascites affects nitrogen metabolism in the liver and other tissues, in addition to its effects in diminishing food intake.

Cirrhosis is also associated with an increased incidence of diabetes; up to 70% of cirrhotic patients may have impaired carbohydrate tolerance, and around 30% are clinically diabetic. Early normal glucose and insulin levels may be associated with hyperglucagonism and glucagon resistance (39). The high fasting and postprandial serum insulin levels and down-regulated insulin receptors mimic obese patients with non–insulin-dependent diabetes (40).

The recommended increase in the intake of carbohydrate to 50% of dietary calories in the form of high-fiber foods for noncirrhotic diabetics also applies equally well to cirrhotic patients with diabetes. Legumes, in contrast to bread-based meals, induce lower postprandial glucose as well as insulin and gastric inhibitory peptide (GIP) responses, due to slower absorption of these foods. Uribe et al. (41) reported that when 40 g of vegetable protein in the form of legumes was included in the diets of insulin-dependent diabetic cirrhotic patients, there was a reduction in their insulin requirements and an increase in hypoglycemic episodes. Uribe et al. (42) further observed that patients with chronic encephalopathy and diabetes given equicaloric diets of vegetable and animal protein, supplemented with 35 g fiber daily, had significantly decreased fasting blood glucose levels on the vegetable protein diet. Thus, slowly digestible carbohydrate, high-fiber, and vegetable-rich diets have been found to be beneficial in treating cirrhotic patients with "hepatogenous diabetes", because such diets improve carbohydrate tolerance and decrease insulin requirements.

There is an increase in the contribution of fat to the total metabolic requirement in cirrhosis that is associated with greater turnover of free fatty acids, and increased production of ketone bodies. Impaired fat absorption has been noted in patients with alcoholic cirrhosis, especially in the presence of chronic pancreatitis or in response to neomycin therapy. A reduced bile salt pool size in cirrhosis also affects fat absorption, though the effect is small. Also, the lower concentration of luminal bile salts impairs the absorption of fat-soluble vitamins (43). A therapy with bile acids such as ursodiol was found to decrease fecal fat excretion from 14 to 10 g per day (44). Modest fat malabsorption may also occur when skin irritation (pruritus) arises due to the accumulation of bile acids in skin, as in primary biliary cirrhosis treated with the bile salt–binding agent cholestyramine. Medium-chain triglycerides may be given in doses of 5 ml, 3 to 4 times daily, providing 350 to 450 kcal in the form of emulsified milk shakes, if oral lipid supplementation is believed necessary (45).

C. Alcoholic Pancreatitis

According to Mezey et al. (46), alcohol is responsible for two syndromes affecting the pancreatic gland that develop because of diminished protein, carbohydrate, and fat intake, viz., acute and chronic pancreatitis. In acute pancreatitis, the patient experiences acute abdominal pain. This syndrome is characterized by the development of small-intestine paralysis (ileus) and an acute rise in the serum levels of the pancreatic enzymes amylase and lipase. The illness may last about 5 to 10 days. A few patients may develop hemorrhagic pancreatitis with a bloody peritoneal exudate with development of pancreatic pseudocyst, abscess, or formation of fistula. Life-threating complications include hypocalcemia, hyperglycemia, and hypoxia. Dietary management requires fasting to induce bowel rest and parenteral nutrition in prolonged states. Intravenous calcium and insulin may be needed to treat hypocalcemia and hyperglycemia (11).

Chronic pancreatitis is characterized by pancreatic inflammation induced by alcohol, one of the earliest lesions being the formation of plugs in the small pancreatic ducts due to protein precipitation of glycoproteins and calcium (47). Alcohol alters pancreatic secretion in humans (48) and indirectly acts via the autonomic nervous system or by stimulating gastrointestinal hormones, with an involvement of pancreatic metabolism of alcohol, altering the redox state or acetaldehyde production.

Western diets high in protein and fat, along with alcoholism, have been found to be closely associated with chronic calcific pancreatitis. A form of chronic alcoholism is also correlated with malnutrition (49). Patients suffer mainly from fat malabsorption with steatorrhea when pancreatic secretion and enzyme output fall below 10% of normal (50); nitrogen malabsorption is much less severe and vitamin deficiencies are uncommon.

Dietary treatment involves a low-fat diet, e.g., 25 g fat daily, together with pancreatic enzyme replacement. For efficient lipolysis, about 8000 units of lipase must be delivered to the duodenum. Thus, about equivalent amount of pancreatic enzyme capsules should be given every 4 hours. Gastric acidity can be reduced to increase enzyme activity by creating alkaline duodenal pH, using an H_2 blocker such as cimetidine 800 mg, ranitidine 300 mg, or omeprazole 20 mg. This also reduces steatorrhea significantly.

The classic alcoholic cirrhotic patient has a hyperkinetic circulation with a high cardiac output and occasional high-output heart failure. Alcoholic cardiomyopathy is clinically similar to a typical beriberi cardiomyopathy; only a minority of patients will respond to thiamin supplementation (50 mg thiamin daily) (51). Although chronic alcoholism is commonly associated with thiamin deficiency, the assessment usually depends on measurement of transketolase activity in vitro, which may exaggerate the deficiency. The more sensitive measurement of thiamin phosphate ester levels (52) indicates that only about 8% of patients with alcoholic liver disease have thiamin deficiency. The cardiomyopathy and the proximal myopathy of chronic alcoholism result from chronic muscular damage from alcohol, rather than from an acute vitamin deficiency (53).

Deficiencies of all four fat-soluble vitamins occur in patients with chronic liver disease (54), the most common being that of vitamin K, found both in cases of chronic obstructive jaundice and in hepatic insufficiency. Vitamin K injections can correct an abnormal prothrombin time in obstructive liver disease; in other liver diseases, a pure fatsoluble vitamin deficiency is rare. Osteomalacia from vitamin D deficiency is less common than osteoporosis in patients with primary biliary cirrhosis (55). Also, clinical vitamin E deficiency is found only in patients with biliary atresia and rarely in primary biliary cirrhosis.

Significant deficiencies of water-soluble vitamins are usually confined to thiamin and folate deficiency. Folate deficiency may be a rare cause of macrocytic anemia associated with liver disease, and Wernicke's encephalopathy is the only neurological disorder corrected by thiamin therapy (56). Iron deficiency is common, but it is often related to chronic blood loss rather than deficient intake, and zinc deficiency is rarely a clinical problem (11).

Rajashree and Rajamohan (57) reported that rats fed ethanol (3.76 g/kg body wt/day) for 45 days exhibited high levels of tissue malondialdehyde, hydroperoxide, and diene conjugates. Activity of tissue superoxide dismutase, catalase, and glutathione content decreased. Administration of water-soluble proteins of garlic (500 mg/kg body wt/day) to alcohol-fed rats resulted in significant increase in antiperoxide activity and decrease in the activity of glutathione peroxidase and glutathione S transferase as compared to a standard drug, gugulipid (50 mg/kg body wt/day).

Kalant (17) presented numerous implications with respect to the treatment of alcoholics showing nutritional deficiencies associated with use of alcohol, as also noted by Ryle and Thomson (58). The impairment of intestinal absorption by ethanol may markedly decrease the value of the water-soluble vitamins taken up by the carrier-mediated processes; and alcohol-induced pancreatitis and its resultant steatorrhea, on the other hand, may decrease the absorption of fat-soluble vitamins. In both these cases, it may be necessary to use parenteral administration until the absorption defects have been corrected. Alcoholic liver damage may also decrease vitamin storage and lead to a large loss of vitamins in the urine. These patients, on admission, would require considerably larger doses of vitamins for the correction of their deficiency than their normal requirements in the diet. Under such circumstances, it is best to use the parenteral forms of the vitamins. The therapy can be changed to oral administration of lower doses later, when gastrointestinal mucosal functioning has been normalized. It may be prudent to use activated forms of vitamins if activation of vitamin is impaired by alcohol, e.g., thiamin pyrophosphate instead of thiamin.

Also, there is a need for awareness of possible nutritional deficiencies even when gross nutrition, as reflected in body weight and muscle mass, appears to be normal. An apparently normal dietary history is not necessarily a guarantee in all subjects that alcohol has not produced a significant nutritional deficiency. The clinical state of the patient, and the necessary and relevant laboratory tests, must still be assessed in each case individually to decide whether vigorous treatment of dietary deficiency is necessary (17).

REFERENCES

1. Suter, P.M., E. Hasler, and W. Vetter, Effects of alcohol on energy metabolism and body weight regulation: Is alcohol a risk factor for obesity? *Nutr. Rev. 55*: 157 (1997).

2. Anonymous, Royal College of Physicians, Alcohol and the heart in perspective: sensible limits reaffirmed, Report of Councils of the Royal Colleges of Physicians, Psychiatrists and General Practioners, Royal Colleges, London, 1995, p. 1–36.

3. Colhoun, H., Y. Ben-Shlomo, and W. Dong, Ecological analysis of collective alcohol consumption in England: importance of average drinking, *British Med. J. 314*: 1164 (1997).

4. Chenet, L., M. Mckee, M. Osler, and A. Krasnik, Alcohol policy in the Nordic countries: Why competition law must have a public health dimension (editorial), *Br. Med. J. 314*: 1142 (1997).

5. Clevidence, B.A., P.R. Taylor, M.S. Campbell, and J.T. Judd, Lean and heavy women may not use energy from alcohol with equal efficiency, *J. Nutr. 125*: 2536 (1995).

6. Crouse, J.R., and S.M. Grundy, Effects of alcohol on plasma lipoproteins and cholesterol and triglyceride metabolism in man, *J. Lipid Res. 25*: 486 (1984).

7. Lands, W.F., Alcohol and energy intake, *Am. J. Clin. Nutr. 62* (Suppl.): 1101 (1995).

8. Suter, P.M., Y. Schutz, and E. Jequier, The effect of ethanol on fat storage in healthy subjects, *N. Engl. J. Med. 326*: 983 (1992).

9. Sonko, B.J., A.M. Prentice, and P.R. Murgatroyd, Effect of alcohol on postmeal fat storage, *Am. J. Clin. Nutr. 59*: 619 (1994).

10. Suter, P.M., How much do alcohol calories count? *J. Am. Coll. Nutr. 16*: 105 (1997).

11. Blendis, L.M., Nutritional management of alcohol-related disease, *Human Nutrition and Dietetics*, 9th ed. (J.S. Garrow and W.P.T. James, eds.), Churchill Livingstone, Edinburgh, London, 1993, p. 738.

12. Bunout, D., V. -Gattas, and H. Iturriaga, Nutritional status of alcoholic patients: its possible relationship to alcoholic liver damage, *Am. J. Clin. Nutr. 38*: 469 (1983).

13. O'Keefe, S.J.D., A. El Zayadi, and T. Carrahet, Malnutrition and immune competence in patients with liver disease, *Lancet 2*: 615 (1980).

14. Merli, M., A. Romiti, O. Riggio, and L. Capocaccia, Optimal nutritional indexes in chronic liver disease, *J. Parent. Ent. Nutrition 11* (Suppl.): 130 (1987).

15. Schneeweiss, B., W. Graninger, and P. Ferenci, Energy metabolism in patients with acute and chronic liver disease, *Hepatology 11*: 387 (1990).

16. Gabuzda, G.J., and L. Shear, Metabolism of dietary protein in hepatic cirrhosis, Nutritional and clinical considerations, *Am. J. Clin. Nutr. 23*: 479 (1970).

17. Kalant, H., Alcohol use and nutrition, *Diet, Nutrition and Health* (K.K. Carroll, ed.), McGill-Queen's Univ. Press, London, 1989, p. 176.

18. Soberon, S., M.P. Pauley, and R. Duplantier, Metabolic effects of enteral formula feeding in alcoholic heapatitis, *Hepatology 7*: 1204 (1987).

19. Smith, J., J. Horowitz, and J.M. Henderson, Enteral hyperalimentation in undernourished patients with cirrhosis and ascites, *Am. J. Clin. Nutr. 35*: 56 (1982).

20. Rees, R.G.P., T.M. Cooper, and R. Beetham, Influence of energy and nitrogen contents of enteral diets on nitrogen balance, *Gut. 30*: 123 (1989).

21. Blendis, L.M., Review article: the treatment of alcoholic liver disease, *Alimentary Pharmacol. Therapeutics 6*: 541 (1992).

22. Galambos, J.T., T. Hersh, and T. Fulenwider, Hyperalimentation in alcoholic hepatitis, *Am. J. Gastroenterol. 72*: 535 (1979).

23. Forbes, A., C. Wicks, and W. Marshall, Nutritional support in fulminant hepatic failure: the safety of liquid solutions, *Gut 28*: 1347 (1987).

24. Watson, R.R., Alcohol and cellular immune response, *Nutrition, Disease Resistance and Immune Function* (R.R. Watson, ed.), Marcel Dekker, New York, 1984, p. 313.

25. Blendis, L.M., and D.J.A. Jenkins, Nutrition and diet in the management of diseases of the gastrointestinal tract, nutritional support in liver disease, *Modern Nutrition in Health and Disease* (M.E. Shils, V. Young, eds.), 7th ed., Lea & Febiger, Philadelphia, 1988, p. 1182.

26. Swart, G.R., J.W.O. Van den Berg, and J.L.D. Wattimena, Elevated protein requirements in cirrhosis of the liver investigated by whole-body protein turnover studies, *Clin. Sci. 75*: 101 (1988).

27. Silk, D.B.A., Parenteral nutrition in patients with liver disease, *J. Hepatology 7*: 269 (1988).

28. Weber, F.L., B.S. Bagby, L. Licate, and S.G. Kelson, Effects of branched-chain amino acids on nitrogen metabolism in patients with cirrhosis, *Hepatology 11*: 942 (1990).

29. Conn, H.O., and M.M. Lieberthal, *The Hepatic Coma Syndrome and Lactulose*, Williams & Williams, Baltimore, 1984.

30. Fisher, J.E., H.M. Rosen, and A.M. Ebeid, The effect of normalization of plasma amino acids on hepatic encephalopathy in man, *Surgery 80*: 77 (1976).

31. Eriksson, L.S., and H.P. Conn, Branched-chain amino acids in the management of hepatic encephalopathy: an analysis of variants, *Hepatology 10*: 291 (1990).

32. Vilstrup, H., C. Gluud, and F. Hardt, Branched-chain enriched amino acid versus glucose treatment of hepatic encephalopathy: A double-blind study of 65 patients with cirrhosis, *J. Hepatology 10*: 291 (1990).

33. Maddrey, W.C., F.L. Weber, and A.W. Coulter, Effects of keto analogues of essential amino acids in portosystemic encephalopathy, *Gastroenterology 71*: 190 (1976).

34. Herlong, H.F., W.C. Maddrey, and M. Walser, The use of ornithine salts of branched-chain ketoacids in portal systemic encephalopathy, *Ann. Intern. Med. 93*: 545 (1980).

35. Fenton, J.C.B., E.J. Knight, and P.L. Humpherson, Milk and cheese diet in portosystemic encephalopathy, *Lancet 1*: 164 (1966).

36. Greenberger, N.J., J.E. Carley, and S. Schenkers, Effect of vegetable and animal protein diets in chronic hepatic encephalopathy, *Am. J. Digestive Dis. 22*: 845 (1977).

37. Weber, F.L., D. Minoo, K.M. Fresard, and J.G. Banwell, Effects of vegetable diets on nitrogen metabolism in cirrhotic subjects, *Gastroenterology 89*: 538 (1985).

38. Warner, L.C., P.J. Campbell, and G.A. Morali, The response of a trial natriuretic factor and sodium excretion to dietary sodium challenges in patients with chronic liver disease, *Hepatology 12*: 460 (1990).

39. Silva, G., R. Gomis, and J. Bosctz, Hyperglucagonism and glucagon resistance in cirrhosis, *J. Hepatology 6*: 325 (1988).

40. Blei, A.J., D.C. Robbins, and E. Drobney, Insulin resistance and insulin receptors in hepatic cirrhosis, *Gastroenterology 83*: 1191 (1982).

41. Uribe, M., M.A. Marquez, and G.G. Ramos, Treatment of chronic portal systemic encephalopathy with vegetable and animal protein diets: A controlled crossover study, *Dig. Dis. Sci. 27*: 1109 (1982).

42. Uribe, M., M. Debilodox, and G. Malpica, Beneficial effect of vegetable protein diet supplemented with psyllum plantago in patients with hepatic encephalopathy and diabetes mellitus, *Gastroenterology 88*: 901 (1985).

43. Jenkins, D.J.A., M.A. Gassull, and A.R. Leeds, The relation of impaired vitamin A and E tolerance to fat absorption in biliary diversion, *Int. J. Vitamin Nutr. Res. 2*: 226 (1976).

44. Salvivoli, G., L. Carati, and R. Lugli, Steatorrhoea in cirrhosis: effect of ursodeoxycholic acid administration, *J. Int. Med. Res. 18*: 289 (1990).

45. Munoz, S.J., Nutritional therapies in liver disease, *Nutrition and the Liver, Seminars in Liver Disease*, Vol. 11(4) (A.J. McCullough and A.S. Tavill, eds.), Thieme Medical Publishers, New York, 1991, p. 278.

46. Mezey, E., C.J. Kolmari, and A.M. Dietzl, Alcohol and dietary intake in the development of chronic pancreatitis and liver disease in alcoholism, *Am. J. Clin. Nutr. 48*: 148 (1988).

47. Nakamura, K., H. Sarles, and H. Payan, Three-dimensional reconstruction of the pancreatic ducts in chronic pancreatitis, *Gastroenterology 62*: 942 (1972).

48. Mott, C., H. Sarles, and O. Tiscornia, Inhibitory action of alcohol on human exocrine pancreatic secretion, *Am. J. Digestive Dis. 17*: 902 (1972).

49. Sarles, H., An international survey on nutrition and pancreatitis, *Digestion 9*: 389 (1973).

50. Dimagno, E.P., J.R. Malagelado, and V.L.W. Go, Relationship between alcoholism and pancreatic insufficiency, *Ann. N. Y. Acad. Sci. 252*: 200 (1975).

51. Ikram, H., A.H. Maslowski, and B.L. Smith. The haemodynamic, histopathological and hormonal features of alcoholic cardiac beriberi, *Quart. J. Med.* (NS) *50*: 359 (1981).

52. Dancy, M., J.M. Bland, and G. Leech, Preclinical left ventricular abnormalities in alcoholics, *Lancet 1*: 1122 (1985).

53. Urbano-Marquez, A., R. Estruch, and F. Navarro-Lopez, The effect of alcoholism on skeletal and cardiac muscle, *N. Engl. J. Med. 320*: 409 (1989).

54. Leevy, C.M., and H. Baker, Introduction: vitamins and alcoholism, *Am. J. Clin. Nutr. 21*: 1325 (1968).
55. Eastell, R., E.R. Dickson, and S.F. Hodgson, Rate of vertebral bone loss before and after liver transplantation in women with primary biliary cirrhosis, *Hepatology 14*: 296 (1991).
56. Diamond, I., Alcoholic myopathy and cardiomyopathy, *N. Eng. J. Med. 320*: 458 (1989).
57. Rajasree, C.R., and T. Rajamohan, Antiperoxide effect of garlic protein in alcohol fed rats, *Indian J. Exp. Biol. 36*: 60 (1998).
58. Ryle, P.R., and A.D. Thomson, Nutrition and vitamins in alcoholism, *Clinical Biochemistry of Alcoholism* (S.B. Rosalki, ed.), Churchill Livingstone, Edinburgh, London, 1984, p. 188.

33
Diet and Some Minor Disorders

I. TRAUMA

Trauma causes a generalized response in the body, and body tissues far removed from the site of injury may be affected. D.P. Cuthberson first clearly defined the body's integrated physiological and metabolic response to trauma and showed that the environment influenced the response, which was also affected by the patient's nutritional status and dietary intake before, during, and after the trauma. Francis Moore extended these investigations, concentrating on surgical trauma (controlled injury), and developed fluid and electrolyte therapy to maintain physiological homoestasis in the immediate postoperative periods (1). The tissue-loss analysis after the trauma provided an in-depth study of the association between protein and energy metabolism (2–4).

Cuthbertson and Zagreb (5) classified metabolic response to trauma into two main phases: the ebb phase and the flow phase (Fig. 1). Oxygen consumption falls in the first ebb phase, lasting up to 1 to 2 days, and then it rises, remaining elevated until the stimulus to the hypermetabolism of tissues is decreased. The flow phase may last 3 to 10 days, depending on the severity of the response to injury. The unclear distinction between the ebb and flow phases can be shown more precisely by measuring changes in the glucose flux: there is a switch from glycogenolysis (glucose breakdown) to gluconeogenesis (glucose synthesis) as patients move from the ebb to the flow phase (Fig. 1). The oxygen uptake may not recover from the ebb phase and a further decline in a "necrobiotic phase" would be irreversible, with eventual occurrence of death.

A. Ebb (Shock) Phase

The early neuroendocrine response to the injury is characterized by a marked stimulation of the sympathetic nervous system, with an upsurge in adrenaline output from the adrenal medulla and a rise in cortisol production and secretion from the adrenal cortex in response to a rise in adrenocorticotropic hormone (ACTH) production from the anterior pituitary gland. There is also a rise in antidiuretic hormone (ADH) due to stimulation of the posterior pituitary gland. The ADH increase may reflect the acute cardiovascular changes, involving pronounced sequestering of fluid in the extravascular space and a decreased venous return, with an eventual fall in cardiac output. The stimulated parasympathetic output is not compensated for by an increase in heart rate as venous return falls. With a decline in cardiac output, tissue perfusion falls and oxygen uptake is reduced. However, the tissues are not inhibited metabolically, thus the ebb phase may not be associated with low uptake of O_2, provided the circulatory perfusion of tissues is maintained (4).

The enhanced activity of sympathetic nervous system also increases secretion of glucagon hormone and inhibits insulin secretion within a few minutes of an incision during surgery carried out with anesthesia. In trauma and surgery, the release of tissue factors such as cytokines in response to pain alters the central neuronal responses to produce hormones. Local anesthesia or

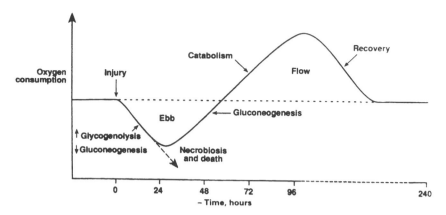

Figure 1 Diagrammatic representation of the ebb and flow phases in the metabolic response to injury. (From Ref. 5.)

use of spinal anesthetics can decrease the activities of sympathetic and parasympathetic nervous systems and subsequent hormonal responses, although some response persists because of the release of tissue factors. The latter may directly influence vasculature to produce peripheral vasodilation and shock. Fluid therapy with electrolytes (0.9% saline) and colloid (e.g., plasma) given immediately after the traumatic shock, will increase the patient's blood volume to boost the cardiac output and maintain tissue perfusion. These treatments prevent the necrobiotic phase, leading to the patient's survival. The chance of survival and rapid recovery depend on the effectiveness with which blood volume is restored and pain is relieved during this "golden hour" phase. Providing food or enteral or parenteral nutrition at this time is of little significance as compared with the urgent need for anesthesia and expansion of blood volume (4).

In addition to decreasing urinary output, the ADH response directly influences energy metabolism. Depressed insulin and increased secretion of glucagon, catecholamine, and cortisol stimulate ketogenesis. Ketogenesis at this early stage in very ill patients influences or predicts survival; i.e., the patients with blood ketone body levels of more than 2.0 mM have a lower morbidity and mortality. The development of ketosis at this stage is associated with a decreased loss of tissue protein and a low negative nitrogen balance. Compared with men, women are known to develop ketosis far better and survive major trauma better. Induction and maintenance of ketogenesis thus has been therapeutic in decreasing the tissue protein loss after trauma (6). Other changes in energy metabolism during the ebb phase include a rise in blood glucose level from hepatic glycogenolysis, lactic acidemia in proportion to tissue anoxia, rise in plasma alanine due to an increase in peripheral protein catabolism, peripheral lipolysis with increased plasma glycerol and free fatty acids, marked rise in ketogenesis, and rise in the synthesis of acute-phase proteins. Gluconeogenesis in the early stages of the ebb phase is not stimulated until some recovery from the shock. Because of insufficient glycogen stored in the liver and muscle to maintain adequate blood glucose for longer than 24 hours, and because gluconeogenesis cannot be stimulated soon after the injury, there may be a need to provide glucose intravenously to maintain adequate blood glucose concentration. When blood glucose levels fall, tissues such as brain, red cell, and renal medulla must depend on ketone bodies for energy, which explains the importance of early ketosis. The ketogenesis, in turn, depends on the increased supply of free fatty acids (FFA) from lipolysis of adipose tissue (7). The glycerol released during lipolysis is also used to make glucose in the liver. The FFA may be directly oxidized to produce energy. The poor tissue perfusion and stimulated lipolysis in the ebb phase may cause high serum lipid levels after major injury or sepsis, when administration of extra fat intravenously may be dangerous.

The ebb phase also coincides with the beginning of "the acute-phase response," wherein the synthesis of acute-phase proteins by the liver is stimulated by the production of cytokines such as interleukin-6 (IL-6). There is a marked fall in the plasma levels of albumin, transferrin, and other export proteins, such as retinol-binding protein (RBP). This negative acute-phase response is also cytokine-related and depends more on the transfer of these proteins to the extravascular space through membrane changes that depend on cytokines (IL-2). Macrophases and damaged tissue release proteolysis-inducing factor, leading to early responses in muscle protein metabolism induced by a circulating protein. During muscle breakdown, the carbon-skeletons of the branched-chain amino acids are utilized by the muscle as energy substrates and the keto acids thus derived are released into the blood for use as ketogenetic substrates for the liver. Alanine released from proteolysis also serves as a nitrogen carrier, as muscle takes up substantial amounts of pyruvate. This enables transfer of nitrogen from the deamination and transamination of some of the amino acids released by muscle proteolysis for gluconeogenesis (4).

B. Flow Phase

The transition from the ebb to flow phase of the response to physical injury to the body is accompanied by a gradual increase in oxygen uptake, associated with a switch from glycogenolysis to gluconeogenesis. This progression depends on the magnitude of severity of the injury as well as the effectiveness of the remedial measures taken during the early period of shock. Broom (4) divided the flow phase into two distinct parts: catabolism and recovery (Fig. 1). The rate of O_2 uptake increases dramatically from the minimum seen in the ebb phase to a level well above the normal for the noninjured state during the catabolic phase, which then falls once again to normal in the recovery phase. The extent of trauma determines the magnitude of resting O_2 uptake and time taken for its return to normal after injury.

The increase in O_2 uptake is closely related to the enhanced metabolic activity of tissues, except in major burn injury, which is associated with a dramatic increase in energy expenditure to compensate for the large evaporative loss. The extent of injury is reflected in the protein metabolic response: the larger the injury, the greater will be the loss of lean body mass, as evidenced by an increase in urinary nitrogen excretion (5).

The metabolic response to the flow phase of injury (Table 1) involves all aspects of intermediary metabolism and all tissues; the rise in blood glucose is proportional to the extent of the injury. There is a marked increase in hepatic gluconeogenesis in response to cytokine secretion. The drive to make new glucose from amino acids and glycerol is not hindered by the oral or intravenous supply of glucose. Thus, infusion of substantial amounts of glucose to these patients will merely exaggerate the marked hyperglycemia, producing fluid and electrolyte imbalances, which are made worse by the development of a post-traumatic insulin-resistant state (8).

The nutritional input during the flow phase markedly influences the negative nitrogen balance. Providing exogenous amino acids at this time stimulates protein synthesis, limiting the protein loss from the body. The urinary nitrogen losses, however, continue to be high because amino acid catabolism is sustained and rate of proteolysis is much less sensitive than normal to being inhibited by infused amino acids. The extravascular albumin and other proteins return to the bloodstream, as fluid exchange between the blood and the extravascular compartment returns to normal. Also, there is a rise in hepatic secretion of albumin that compensates for the plasma protein losses in the injured or burn tissues. The protein loss into the burn can be enormous, and despite marked increases in hepatic protein synthesis and the provision of extradietary protein or intravenous amino acids, the plasma levels of many proteins such as albumin remain low (4).

Table 1   Metabolic Response to the Flow Phase of Injury

Duration
From 1 to 3 days after injury, depending on the severity of the injury and measures taken to
    counteract the shock

Characteristics
Increased oxygen uptake
Increased gluconeogenesis and hepatic glucose output, independent of exogenous glucose input
Increased lipolysis and FFA utilization
Development of "controlled" ketosis and increased ketone body utilization, if not suppressed by
    exogenous glucose administration
Increased protein breakdown and increased urinary nitrogen excretion
Protein synthesis variable depending on decreased circulating albumin and other hepatic export
    proteins
Acute-phase protein response with increased hepatic secretion of fibrinogen, ferritin, alpha-
    macroglobulin, and many others

Summary
Loss of lean body mass

Source: Ref. 4.

II. SEPSIS

In addition to being an exaggerated response to trauma, sepsis has varied effects on energy metabolism. There are differences in oxygen consumption, urinary nitrogen losses, circulating protein levels, and carbohydrate and fat metabolism between trauma, starvation, and sepsis. The metabolic alterations observed in a patient with major sepsis are given in Table 2. There may be marked decrease or increase in resting O_2 uptake, depending on the phase of sepsis. In a severe infection with a cavitating abscess, O_2 uptake may be decreased as during ebb or shock phase, and after the abscess is drained, the O_2 uptake will increase in response to the fall in the toxin and cytokine leakage into the bloodstream, as in the normal flow phase of injury.

Sepsis is often characterized by a large increase in hepatic glucose production, though this effect is variable and sometimes disputed. Poor aerobic tissue metabolism is reflected in poor utilization of glucose by the tissue and an insulin resistance state, which explains the marked hyper-

Table 2   Metabolic Responses to Sepsis

Marked increase in glucose synthesis, poor peripheral glucose utilization, poor aerobic metabolism
Decreased plasma free fatty acids, lipolytic changes unknown
No ketosis, ketone metabolism rates unknown
Marked rise in protein breakdown rates, large increases in urinary nitrogen
Increased visceral and acute-phase protein synthesis
Marked fall in plasma albumin concentration, with sequestration in the extravascular space
Probable glucose substrate or futile cycling accounting for ineffective use of high rates of protein break-
    down
Variable effects on oxygen uptake

Source: Ref. 4.

glycemia. In sepsis there is disappearance of the ketonic response normally seen in the post-traumatic state. The ketone bodies may increase in blood only for a short period of time, which may be due to defective ketogenesis. There is disruption in the mitochondrial structure in the livers of septic patients and the conformation of the adenosine triphosphatase (ATPase) protein is also disrupted with loss of the inner mitochondrial membrane structure and ATPase activity. There is a block in three specific sites in the energy metabolism: pyruvate dehydrogenase, citrate synthase, and isocitrate dehydrogenase, decreasing the overall aerobic metabolism of glucose and fatty acids. In this situation, the infused lipid or glucose also may not be utilized efficiently. The anerobic glycolytic breakdown of glucose therefore becomes more important, which explains the substantial increase in the production of lactic acid in septicemia. Liver biopsies of septic patients show increases in phosphofructokinase-II activity necessary during glycolysis that seems to continue for some considerable time after sepsis begins. Fructose-2,6-biphosphate appears to regulate glycolysis by stimulating activity of phosphofructokinase-I and glycosis. Glucose supply through gluconeogenesis is essential for glycolysis. An impaired gluconeogenesis may lead to hypoglycemia (as in injury), indicating total system failure and impending death. "Futile" (substrate) cycles may be stimulated in septicemia, with production of heat and inefficient use of glucose, which probably explains rapid loss of lean body mass in severe sepsis. The body protein is being utilized to make glucose, which in turn is wasted to produce heat in futile cycles (4).

After the source of infection in sepsis is isolated and drained, the body begins to use fat as a preferred fuel when insulin resistance limits peripheral glucose uptake, dropping the respiratory exchange ratio to about 0.7 (4).

The loss of protein is associated with an increase in the rate of muscle proteolysis and an increase in plasma levels of amino acids, especially alanine. The released amino acids are transported to the liver for gluconeogenesis and visceral protein synthesis as well as toward the immune system for specific host defense mechanism. The loss of albumin in the acute-phase response is also greatly increased. The macrophages and damaged tissues produce a variety of prostaglandins and leukotrienes, which play a role in inducing cytokine secretion; e.g., leukotriene B_4 induces the secretion of the cytokine interleukin-1 (IL-1) by macrophages. The cytokines are low-molecular-weight (15–30 KD) specialized proteins synthesized by many types of cells, including the activated macrophages. The damaged tissue or lipopolysaccharide (LPS) associated with the cell walls of bacteria invading host tissue provide the required activation. The cytokine release generally promotes recovery during sepsis as also in trauma or inflammatory situations. Such cytokines have powerful effects on a variety of body tissues and may either promote or inhibit certain specific enzyme(s). Cytokines are thought to act through specific protein receptors at the cell surface and through various signal transduction pathways at the cellular level (9). The signal-transduction pathways include tyrosine kinase and protein phosphorylase, G proteins and receptor-enzyme coupling, adenylate cyclase and cyclic AMP, phospholipases, inositol phosphates, and prostaglandins/leukotrienes. The cytokines have been classified according to their amino acid sequence homology and physiological functions. Large quantities of IL-1 and tumor necrosis factor (TNF) are produced during the flow phase of injury or sepsis, which induces a hyperglycemic response via gluconeogenesis in the liver, whereas TNF-alpha and IL-2 produced during the ebb or shock phase tend to lead to hypoglycemia. TNF is a 17-KD protein having a range of metabolic effects in animals; it may interact with other cytokines to induce the release of prostaglandin E_2 (PGE$_2$) from the endothelial wall by stimulating the release of arachidonic acid from membrane phospholipids. Archidonic acid is rapidly metabolized to produce PGE$_2$, which in turn produces a variety of effects, depending on its site of synthesis.

The fatty acid profile of endothelial membrane phospholipids influences both the amount of prostaglandins released and their effects on hormone systems and on other tissues. Thus, the previous fatty acids and nutrition may affect the patient's response to infection or trauma. It is known that the major sepsis syndrome is characterized by exaggerated cytokine response and a disruption in the balance between the cytokines released, especially TNF-α, with consequent multiple end-organ failure. Monoclonal antibodies to TNF-α are now being used to combat the major tissue effects of TNF-α and to prevent the organ failure that is a major problem in severely injured or septic patients (10,11). With the introduction of anti-TNF drugs based on monoclonal antibody synthesis, it should now be possible to promote host tissue responses that lead to wound healing and bactericidal action controlled by specific cytokines while repressing those cytokines that are responsible for tissue destruction and undesirable host responses.

A. Dietary Management of Trauma and Sepsis

Nutritional support in trauma and sepsis is best provided by the oral or by the enteral route with a nasogastric tube or a tube specially inserted by surgery into the stomach or duodenum. Glucose supplied to the gut lumen is rapidly passed via the portal circulation to the liver as glucose, but glucose presented to the intestine via the mesenteric arterial system is primarily metabolized to lactic acid. The intestinal route for providing the body with nutrients is always preferred to that fed to the gut.

The management of acute trauma and sepsis requires the rapid restoration of the blood volume with saline, other electrolyte solutions, albumin, and plasma. Tissue perfusion falls without an adequate circulation, leading to pronounced metabolic changes; e.g., body temperature may fall markedly as metabolism is inhibited. Anesthesia can prevent neurogenic response to the shock syndrome, and rapid and effective surgery may limit tissue destruction and removes the tissue where blood supply is cut off. In sepsis, it is vital to localize the infection and identify the organism to provide an appropriate antibiotic (4).

The loss of water, electrolytes, and plasma proteins in the damaged tissue and the rest of the body must be made up by restoring blood volume and circulating output. However, high rates of glucose and fat infusion can be hazardous at this time, and both hyperglycemia and hypertriglyceridemia should be avoided.

After dealing with the ebb phase, the patient often displays an increase in body temperature with a rise in metabolism when entering the flow phase. Nutrition at this critical stage is very important. Amino acid input is especially important in septic and severely traumatized patients, who also require modest glucose supply (180 g/day). Fluid and electrolyte balance continue to be crucial, especially in burn cases, where the losses are remarkable. These losses may also be reduced by use of artificial skin grafting. Nursing of burned patients at around 30°C is important because of the higher temperature of the burn skin. The relatively anoxic burned tissue is dependent almost entirely on glucose, so the demand for glucose may be substantial (6–10 liters of fluid/day and up to 30 MJ of energy). Part of this energy may be replaced by fat after cytokine inhibition of lipoprotein lipase has passed. Except for patients with major burns, the energy requirements of traumatized and septic patients are not large, and their O_2 uptake rises only minimally above the usual resting levels; the provision of around 10 to 12 MJ energy/day may be enough in these cases. Amino acids needs may double to around 25% of total energy needs in severe injury (4).

III. HEMOPOIESIS AND ANEMIAS

Hemopoietic cells have the same nutritional requirements of other normally growing cells. However, the rate of renewal of blood cells is much greater than that of any other body tissue, which makes the hemopoietic system especially vulnerable to deficiencies of folate and cobalamin, which have an important role in nucleotide synthesis. Iron is an essential component of the hemoglobin molecule, so the supply of iron may become an important limiting factor in the production of red blood cells (RBCs). Except for iron, folate, and cobalamin, the deficiencies of other nutrients, e.g., ascorbic acid, vitamin E, vitamin A, riboflavin, and copper rarely affect hemopoiesis (12). A vegetarian diet is often associated with adverse effects on hemopoiesis. Cobalamin is entirely absent in the vegetable kingdom and a strictly vegetarian diet has no cobalamin other than that arising by contamination of water supply or bacteria. Also, iron is only poorly available for intestinal absorption from a vegetarian diet, making nutritional iron deficiency common among vegetarians.

A. Iron Deficiency Anemias

Most of the body's iron (3–4 g in adults) is present in circulating hemoglobin in RBCs, with smaller amounts in myoglobin and various heme and non-heme enzymes (cytochromes). The remaining iron is stored in the form of ferritin and hemosiderin in the liver, spleen, and bone narrow (12).

Modest iron deficiency in asymptomatic subjects can be detected by blood tests; signs of severe anemia increase as the level of hemoglobin falls. Anemia is characterised by lack of energy, tiredness, shortness of breath, palpitations, headache, weakness, dizziness and irritability. Epithelial surfaces may show a sore mouth and tongue, angular stomatitis, and a sensation of a lump in the throat with difficult swallowing. Pallid appearance of mucous membranes, irregular or broken nails, and splenomegaly occur in severe anemia.

Iron deficiency is manifested by a fall in hemoglobin below the normal level (13 g/dl in men and 12 g/dl in women). There is a decrease in the size of the red cells, the smaller red cells having less hemoglobin. The serum iron level (normal, 11–28 μmol/l) is below 11 and iron-binding capacity (normal, 47–70 μmol/l) increases above 70. The serum ferritin level falls below 11 μg/l and stainable iron is absent from aspirated marrow particles (12).

Thalassemic anemia is also characterized by small red blood cells, as is anemia of chronic disorders, which must be differentiated from iron deficiency anemia. Thalassemias result from a reduced rate of production of one or more of the globin chains of hemoglobin and are characterized by relatively high red-cell counts, with normal serum iron and ferritin levels. Anemias of chronic disorders closely resemble iron deficiency, but unlike iron deficiency, the iron-binding capacity is either normal or low.

Iron deficiency can be firmly diagnosed by knowing serum iron and ferritin levels and iron-binding capacity. Iron deficiency anemia is indicated by a low serum iron level with an increase in iron-binding capacity or a low serum ferritin level. Nutritional iron deficiency can be established by assessing the subject's diet and by the exclusion of blood loss, mainly via menstruation and the G.I. tract. Intestinal malabsorption due to gluten sensitivity, gut resection, or gastroctomy can also be the cause of iron deficiency anemia. A careful history and the examination of feces samples for hookworm ova and occult blood aid in diagnosis.

Oral iron salts, usually ferrous sulfate, as tablets supplying 200 mg of iron are often satisfactory. The tablets are best taken without food. Ascorbic acid, such as in orange or lime juice, enhances iron absorption. Response is usually accompanied by clinical benefit and a rise in the hemoglobin level of about 1 g/dl/week. The treatment should aim to replenish iron stores in addition to correcting the anemia, which may require 6 months of therapy (12).

Many studies reported in the International Conference on Iron Deficiency and Behaviorial Development showed an association between iron deficiency anemia (IDA) and less than optimal behavior in infants and children, as demonstrated by lower scores on tests of development, learning, and school achievement. A problem with the interpretation of these studies is that IDA is associated with other adverse environmental and nutritional conditions that may independently affect behavior. However, new studies using randomized designs with appropriate controls presented in this conference have shown that iron therapy in preschool and school-aged children with IDA resulted in improvements in certain behavioral tests. The research on children and a number of animal studies suggest that IDA is causally associated with less than optimal behavior. Therefore, it is important that IDA be prevented and treated in all children. Because the specific mechanism and functional significance of these behavioral changes are not completely understood, further studies are essential to clarify the effects of IDA itself and to determine the importance of lesser degrees of ID in children (13).

B. Nutritional Cobalamin Deficiency

Cobalamin originates from bacterial synthesis. Herbivorous animals obtain their cobalamin via bacterial flora in their foregut and carnivores obtain it from animal products in their diets. Strictly vegetarian diets supply no cobalamin. Populations on mixed diets get between 3 and 7 µg cobalamin per day (Europe, America). Calculations based on food intakes indicate an intake of 0.49 to 2.8 µg cobalamin/day in Africa, 0.46 µg in India, 0.3 µg in Bangladesh, 1.36 µg in Pakistan, 0.72 µg in Indonesia, 1.02 µg in Burma, and 1.24 µg in China.

FAO/WHO (14) recommended the following safe levels of intake (µg/24 h) of cobalamin:

Adults	1.0
Pregnant women	1.4
Breast-feeding women	1.3
Infants	0.1
Children (1–10 years)	0.4 µg/kg
Children (11–16 years)	1.0

These data show that average Western diets supply more cobalamin than is required whereas vegetarian diets supply lower than safe limits. A cobalamin intake of up to 0.5 µg/24 h is not safe, and a minimum safe level of cobalamin intake is one that maintains the serum cobalamin level above the range associated with megaloblastic anemia, i.e., above 170 pg/ml, corresponding to between 0.5 and 1.0 µg cobalamin/24 h (12). Absolutely strict vegetarians are rare and most take some form of animal product, the most commonest being cow's milk, which contains around 3.6 µg cobalamin/liter. Yogurt has about 0.8 µg cobalamin/liter and cheddar cheese has 10 µg/kg, whereas whole eggs supply about 30 µg cobalamin/kg.

Chanarin et al. (15) reported results of a study of 95 patients with nutritional cobalamin deficiency in Hindu Indians who were lifelong vegetarians. Typical cobalamin deficiency symptoms included tiredness (33%), shortness of breath (25%), loss of appetite (23%), loss of weight (22%), general aches (19%) due to associated osteomalacia and calcium and vitamin D deficiency, vomiting (19%), paresthesias (11%), change in skin pigmentation (8%), sore mouth and/or tongue (7%), diarrhea (6%), and headache (5%). Loss of hair color was seen in a 19-year-old male with a hemoglobin level of 3.6 g/dl. Oral cobalamin therapy restored the normal jet black color of the hair. Other physical symptoms include pallor of the mucous mebranes and a smooth tongue, which was common. One severely anemic patient had a 3-cm splenomegaly that disappeared after cobalamin therapy (15).

The hemoglobin level at diagnosis in these patients ranged from 3.0 to 16 g/dl; all had macrocytic anemia with megaloblastic marrow. Serum cobalamin levels were low in all and red-cell folate was low in 31 out of 78 patients, but no patient required folate to achieve a response.

Nutritional cobalamin deficiency can be suspected in a vegetarian patient with a macrocytic blood picture, though macrocytosis may be absent in patients with thalassemia trait or iron deficiency. In the latter case, iron therapy will bring out macrocytosis. Marrow examination may be necessary for diagnosis, which will show megaloblastic hemopoiesis. Measurement of the serum cobalamin level is not helpful to distinguish those who have a megaloblastic anemia, but a normal level excludes such deficiency. Other causes of megaloblastic anemia, such as pernicious anemia, carcinoma of the stomach, pregnancy, and nutritional folate deficiency generally associated with alcoholism, must be excluded.

To establish that nutritional megaloblastic anemia is caused by cobalamin deficiency, it is necessary to confirm that the patient responds fully to oral cobalamin therapy in a mixed diet—about 5 µg daily. Such responses are not as dramatic as those seen with a large injection of cobalamin.

In older patients, pernicious anemia is the common alternative diagnosis and a cobalamin absorption test at an early stage may be sensible. This is carried out by the urinary excretion method, which consists of an injection of 1000 µg of cyanocobalamin to restore a normal blood picture. Nutritional cobalamin deficiency is diagnosed if the cobalamin absorption test is normal and the patient responds to cobalamin.

In the short term, oral or parenteral cobalamin treatment can restore the blood to normal, and patients treated initially with oral cobalamin will benefit in the long term by one or more injections of hydroxo-cobalamin to restore the cobalamin stores. Patients should be persuaded to include foods of animal origin (dairy products, fish, poultry) in their diets to avoid relapses. Young patients are quite amenable to changes in diet. Food supplements can successfully provide cobalamin to restore deficiencies. Cobalamin supplements are available in various prepacked cereal products, such as cytocon (50 µg cobalamin per tablet) or in liquid form as a multivitamin preparation. A 50 µg dose allows about 2 µg to be absorbed and larger doses of oral cobalamin (about 1%) are absorbed by passive diffusion. Strict vegetarians should take a daily dose of oral cobalamin to meet their normal requirements.

Severe nutritional cobalamin deficiency may be associated with infertility in women, although pregnancy can occur successfully. Under these circumstances, only minimal cobalamin stores are passed on to the fetus and the infant can present with megaloblastic anemia due to cobalamin deficiency. Cobalamin deficiency in the mother, either nutritional or due to undiagnosed pernicious anemia, results in low fetal cobalamin stores. The cobalamin levels of breast milk are about the same as that in maternal plasma, and a low maternal plasma cobalamin level leads to cobalamin deficiency in the neonate.

Jadhav et al. (16) described a disorder in the breast-fed infants of cobalamin-deficient vegetarian mothers in India. The infants had retarded development, abnormal skin pigmentation, and a megaloblastic anemia. The infants responded to cobalamin therapy. Supply of cobalamin to the mothers would restore the level in breast milk and provide cobalamin for the infant. Reports of a similar disorder in the offspring of white mothers who had been strict vegetarians for between 5 and 12 years are available. The infants of these mothers developed normally for the first 4 months of life and presented clinically between 6 and 12 months of age. They were lethargic, hyperirritable, and weak and could not support their heads or turn over. They also became inactive and withdrawn. One infant had marked hyptonia, exaggerated reflexes, and partial atrophy and was in a coma on presentation. Most of the affected infants were underweight and had increased pigmentation on the backs of the hands, especially over the knuckles and feet. One child had a cardiac failure. The hemoglobin level ranged from 2.2 to 7.3 g/dl in five infants, and was 13 g/dl in the sixth child. All infants had low serum cobalamin levels and bone marrows were severely megaloblastic; all responded dramatically and completely to cobalamin injections.

C. Folate Deficiency

Folate analogues are present in all fresh foods. The tetrahydrofolates and analogues differ from each other in their glutamate chain length and in whether they carry a substituent, which may be either a formyl or a methyl. All natural folates are reduced and require reducing agents to prevent their oxidation during collection, storage, and assay; this is usually done by adding ascorbic acid. Natural folates are heat labile and may be lost during cooking and food processing. Cooking may destroy about 40% to 50% of folate (16,17). Table 3 shows the distribution of folates in different foodstuffs. All foods contain folates, although some (such as vegetables, milk, and liver) have relatively higher values.

Physical folate analogues (reduced forms) with one glutamic acid residue (monoglutamates) are virtually completely absorbed from the gut, but there is uncertainty regarding the absorption of polyglutamates (about 70%). All resulting folate monoglutamates are converted to 5-methyl H_4, the form of folate found in the enterocyte and in portal blood.

Folate deficiency can be detected by assaying folate levels in appropriate tissue samples, e.g., red cell, serum, or liver. Red cell folate levels are the most satisfactory means of measuring tissue folate stores. The microbiological assay with *Lactobacillus casei* or the isotope dilution method of whole blood hemolyzed in 1% fresh ascorbic acid is employed, the result being expressed in nanogram of folate per unit of packed red cells. Healthy subjects have red cell folate levels of 145 to 400 ng/ml. Folate is incorporated into red cells during erythropoiesis. A young red cell population, as indicated by a raised reticulocyte count, has a higher red cell folate level than mature red cells. The folate is locked in the red cell until its demise after about 110 days. A low red-cell folate level is unequivocal evidence of folate deficiency.

Serum folate levels fall after only a few days of low intake and are thus less satisfactory as a test for folate deficiency. A low serum folate is best looked upon as indicative of a negative folate balance, but this will have to continue for several months to deplete folate stores. The normal serum folate range is between 3 and 20 ng of folate/ml. The normal range of folate in the liver tissue varies from 4 to 17 µg/g of wet liver, with a mean of 7.0.

Table 3 Distribution of Folate Analogues in Different Foodstuffs Over 24 Hours

Foodstuff	Folate (µg)
Meat	13.9
Liver	26.6
Milk	34.0
Eggs, cheese, yogurt	18.3
Vegetables	64.1
Fruit	24.6
Bread	19.5
Cereal, cake, sweets	24.1
Beer	?

Source: Ref. 18.

The recommended daily allowances for folate are shown in Table 4. The RDAs given by FAO/WHO are similar to those used in Canada and the United States, i.e., 3.1 µg folate/kg body weight/24 h. Basal estimated folate requirements are around 50 to 70 µg/24 h, which are based on the daily loss of folate and are partly assessed by liver biopsy. Thus, the total folate content of a normal adult human liver ranges from 7.5 to 22.5 mg, which may fall to 1.5 mg in folate-deficient patients with megaloblastic anemia. The folate loss over the period before megaloblastic anemia appears may range from 48 to 158 µg/24 h (17), and an optimal hematological response in a folate-deficient patient with megaloblastic anemia may require 200 µg folate daily. Further dietary folate intakes are correlated with folate status, largely red cell folate. Populations with a mean folate intake of 150 to 200 µg/24 h usually have around 8% of the people showing evidence of folate deficiency. The folate intake on a Western-type mixed diet just meets the requirements of around 95% of the people, with a daily intake of 3.1 µg of folate/kg body weight.

Folate deficiency due to inadequate dietary intake is more frequent in developing countries and unusual in the developed countries. The frequency of folate deficiency in pregnancy is the best test for folate deficiency in all populations. Folate is required for the synthesis of the basic components of DNA and for an increase in cell division, as in the developing fetus, so its requirement is increased during pregnancy. A woman's capacity to cope with the increased folate requirement in pregnancy depends on folate stores of the body and folate intake during pregnancy. At term, 24% to 34% of women on mixed diets in London had low red cell folate levels, indicating folate deficiency (18), whereas in Nigeria 85% of women had low red cell folates at term (19). Presence of megaloblasts in bone marrow examination is another way of assessing the frequency of folate deficiency in pregnancy.

Clinically, folate deficiency causes megaloblastic anemia, whose features are similar to those noticed in patients with cobalamin deficiency. Depression and weakness are more common in folate-deficient megaloblastic anemia, but neuropathy as found in cobalamin deficiency is rare (20).

Folate-deficient patients are usually anemic, with abnormally large red blood cells, i.e., a raised MCV. In severely anemic patients, total white cells and platelets are both low. Marrows are always megaloblastic, with low serum and red cell folate levels. If the serum cobalamin level is normal in a patient with a megaloblastic anemia, the diagnosis is folate deficiency, although a low serum cobalamin level does not necessarily mean cobalamin deficiency. Around 30% of patients with primary folate deficiency have low serum cobalamin levels that rise to normal range after 1 week of folate therapy.

Folate deficiency can cause marked growth retardation and delay the onset of puberty, as was shown in subjects with sickle-cell anemia, which further increases folate requirement. Folate thereapy resulted in dramatic growth spurts, and women over 20 years of age who had been amenorrheic started having regular mensus thereafter (21).

Smithells et al. (22) and Laurence et al. (23) reported a reduction in the incidence of neural tube defects when either folate or a multivitamin including folate was given before and after conception to women who had previously given birth to an affected child. These reports have been confirmed in a large study involving 1,817 women with a history of neural tube defect (24). In a group given 4 mg of folate daily, six neonates had a neural tube defect as compared to 21 in the group of women not receiving folate. This difference was highly significant. There is probably a relatively high folate requirement by the fetus at a stage of development when vascularization is such that nutrients may not reach the developing cells in adequate amounts. Abnormally high plasma folate levels may overcome this physiological failure by allowing folate to diffuse to reverse this localized deficiency (12).

In the Western countries, groups at risk of nutritional folate deficiency are premature infants, pregnant women, and elderly people. Lower red cell folate levels were found in 12% of elderly patients admitted to the hospital, among 10% of elderly in homes in Norway, and in 8% of the elderly living at home in Wales. Poverty or disability, including depression, has been found to be the cause. The folate deficiency in the elderly is generally subclinical and rarely appears as megaloblastic anemia, unless associated with other factors, such as alcoholism.

In the developing countries, clinically overt folate deficiencies are far more common, especially in pregnant women; the frequency of low red cell folate levels in Africa ranges from 26% to 37%. Folate deficiency in premature infants leads to anemia that is not corrected by oral iron, and failure to gain weight, requiring folate supplements (Table 4).

The folate and cobalamin contents of goat and human milk are 6 and 52 μg/l and 0.1 and 4 μg/l, respectively. The very low folate content of goat's milk may lead to folate-deficient megaloblastic anemia in children (3–5 months) receiving mainly goat's milk as their diet. It is necessary to provide folate supplements if only goat's milk is used (25).

An increased folate requirement during pregnancy that is not met from the diet may lead to megaloblastic anemia. Folate in pregnancy is required for the increase in cell division that is associated with expansion of the maternal red cell mass, development of the placenta, growth of the uterus and fetus, and supply of fetal stores of folate in the last weeks of pregnancy. Increased folate requirement is evident by the 20th week of pregnancy, as indicated by a decline in serum and red cell folate levels. There is an altered renal threshold for folate in pregnancy, with an average folate loss of 14 μg/24 h as compared to 4.2 μg/24 h in the nonpregnant state. In some women, the daily folate loss in urine during pregnancy may reach as high as 50 μg (26). Megaloblastic marrow changes in pregnancy indicating manifestation of folate deficiency range from 25% to 60% of all women near term.

Iron deficiency being the major cause of anemia in pregnancy, it is difficult to recognize early evidence of folate deficiency because of the dominance of iron deficiency in the blood picture. Failure to respond to oral iron supplements may indicate folate deficiency. Diagnosis is easier when megaloblastic anemia is more pronounced, although an increase in the MCV is one of the physiological changes in pregnancy that by itself does not suggest megaloblastic anemia. The latter can be confirmed, however, by marrow aspiration. Diagnosis is almost always made either in the last weeks of pregnancy or in the puerperium. The incidence of megaloblastic anemia in pregnancy has been found to have its peak frequency at the end of the part of the year when fresh vegetables and fruits are least available in various countries. The frequency of anemia is around

Table 4 Dietary Requirements for Folate

Group	Safe level of intake (μg/24 h)
Adult males	200
Adult females	170
Pregnant women	370–470
Lactating women	270
Children	
1–6 years	50
7–12 years	102
13–16 years	170
Infants	
0–0.25 year	16
0–.26-0.5 year	24
0.6–1.0 year	32

Source: Ref. 12.

10 times greater in twin pregnancies and recurs in further pregnancies, indicating higher folate requirement with twins and continued folate deficiency.

The provision of once-daily oral iron and folate supplements throughout pregnancy has been found to alleviate anemia most successfully. Megaloblastic anemia in pregnancy is therefore a rare occurrence in countries where such prophylactic measures are undertaken. The amount of folate supplement required during pregnancy has been debated. One approach is to determine the amount of additional folate needed to maintain the red cell folate level during pregnancy and another is to determine the amount of folate required to the prevent appearance of megaloblastic anemia. Fifty µg of folate/24 h had no significant effect on the red cell folate level and 100 µg/24 h raised the red cell folate level in the first half of pregnancy, followed by a plateau in the second half. Higher doses of folate were associated with a marked elevation of red cell folate that continued throughout pregnancy (27,28). These data led to the recommendation of a total daily folate intake of 370 µg/24 h (Table 4). According to Chanarin (12), the folate should be supplied at 200 µg of pteroylglutamate per 24 h, so that even those on a poor diet will receive adequate folate, and those on a reasonable or good diet will get more than they need. Excess folate is excreted through the urine or degraded, with its breakdown products appearing in the urine. Assessment of folate requirement by the amount needed to prevent the emergence of megaloblastic anemia is less satisfactory because of the difficulty in recognizing blood changes and in interpreting marrow aspiration in the presence of iron deficiency. Folate should be combined with iron in a single tablet, giving the least amount of iron that is effective and safe, to avoid the side effects of excess iron, such as gastrointestinal upsets (12). Chanarin and Rothman (29) reported that 30 mg of iron (present in 90 mg of ferrous fumarate) taken once daily both prevents anemia and maintains the serum iron level throughout the pregnancy, although most iron and folate preparations contain more iron than this. Supply of excess iron may lead to poor compliance.

In addition to neural tube defects, prematurity also has been shown to be associated with folate deficiency. A high frequency of low-birthweight infants was noted among South African Bantu women on a staple diet of boiled maize. In this study, the effects of iron alone, iron and folate, and iron, folate, and cobalamin were investigated in both African and white women on a mixed Western diet. The doses of iron, folate, and cobalamin were 200 mg, 5 mg, and 50 µg/24 h, respectively. These supplements had no effects on birthweight or duration of pregnancy in the white group. However, in the African group given only iron, 19 out of 63 neonates weighed less than 2.27 kg, and the number fell to 4 of 65 in the folate-supplemented group. Cobalamin had no effect. Folate was found to be associated with an increase in birthweight from 2.466 to 2.798 kg (30). The folate supplements prolonged the duration of gestation by 1 week and increased size of placenta from 456 to 517 g (31).

Alcoholism can complicate nutritional folate deficiency, especially when alcohol is substituted for food (18). It may also complicate disorders such as hemolytic anemia with an increased requirement of folate and some exfoliative skin disorders.

D. Other Nutrient Deficiencies Influencing Hemopoiesis

Chronic vitamin A deficiency is often associated with an anemia, sometimes a severe anemia that resembles the anemia of chronic disorders. It has features similar to those of iron deficiency, including low serum iron level, but the iron-binding capacity is normal or low and storage iron is present. Anemia can be developed by experimentally inducing vitamin A deficiency in humans, with hemoglobin levels falling from 15 to 12 g/dl (32).

Lane and Alfrey (33) reported that volunteers on riboflavin-deficient diets given a riboflavin antagonist developed pure red cell aplasia. This is occasionally also observed in nutritional deficiencies associated with alcoholism, when a smooth, cherry-red tongue is said to be one of the manifestations.

Around 80% of the patients with vitamin C deficiency suffering from clinical scurvy are anemic. This deficiency is thought to be related to folate deficiency, because both ascorbic acid and folate are water-soluble vitamins, occurring in similar foods. Both are also labile and susceptible to oxidative destruction. A hematologic response is obtained with oral ascorbate when anemia is normocytic and the marrow is normoblastic. In many patients, the marrow is megaloblastic and most of these patients also respond only to ascorbate, although such response will not occur if the diet lacks folate. Other patients with scurvy and megaloblastic marrow respond well to folate alone and there may be a second response when ascorbate is added (12,17). The folate and ascorbate deficiencies tend to coincide because a diet lacking in one will certainly lack the other. The suggestion that reducing properties of ascorbate are required to maintain folate analogues in the reduced state applies only to the in vitro situation, and there is no evidence that ascorbic acid is required for folic acid metabolism in vivo (12).

IV. ASTHMA AND FOOD ALLERGY

Asthma is a chronic inflammatory disease of the airways and is associated with recurrent episodes of branchoconstriction and enhanced bronchial hyperresponsiveness (34). Recurrent bouts of wheezing, chest tightness, and cough, occur in susceptible individuals, especially during night and early morning times. Asthma patients often have IgE-mediated responses to common aeroallergens, which is an important predisposing factor for the development of asthma. Rumsaeng and Metcalfe (35) have recently described the association between food allergy and asthma. Respiratory responses, such as bronchoconstriction and increased airway hyperresponsiveness, have been investigated in asthma patients, following positive double-blind, placebo-controlled food challenges (DBPCFCs). It is expected that the recognition of food-induced asthma and appropriate concomitant management will help to improve asthmatic control and bring relief to asthmatics. Assuming a 3% asthma prevalence and 2% food-induced wheezing in asthma patients, a prevalence of food-induced asthma has been estimated to be 6 out of 10,000 individuals (35).

A. Pathogenesis and Clinical Manifestations

Mast cells, food-specific IgE, and basophils are vital factors in the pathogenesis of symptoms during immediate food hypersensitivity. Increased plasma concentrations of histamine appear to be associated with the development of urticaria, laryngeal edema, wheezing, vomiting, diarrhea, and hypertension after blinded food challenges (36). Food antigens interact with surface-bound IgE on mast cells, as evidenced by an immediate wheal and erythema response in the skin, or by elevated histamine levels (37,38). Sampson et al. (39) have detected elevated serum tryptase levels (a marker of mast cell degranulation) in patients with fatal food-induced anaphylaxis. Basophils from food-hypersensitive children are associated with high rates of spontaneous histamine release, especially after challenge with specific food antigens (40). According to Rumsaeng and Metcalfe (35), relatively few antigens cause allergic reactions. Most patients are allergic to a single food, multiple food allergies being uncommon. Infants and children are often allergic to milk, eggs, soy, peanuts, or wheat (41). Milk and eggs are particularly associated with asthma in most children, whereas adults are commonly allergic to peanuts, tree nuts, fish, shellfish, and eggs. Major food antigens are proteins or glycoproteins of molecular weights between 10,000 and 40,000 daltons, which are relatively resistant to denaturation by heat and acid or to enzymatic degradation (35).

Major cross-reactive allergens have been implicated in pollens, fruit, and vegetables, with highly prevalent IgE to food allergens (42,43). Food allergy caused by crustacea and mollusks has also been reported in patients allergic to house dust mites (44–46). Van Ree et al. (46) reported a group of 28 house dust mite allergic patients who showed asthmatic symptoms after eating snail, the cross-reactive allergens being confirmed by radioallergosorbent test (RAST).

Clinical manifestations of food allergy include allergen-specific IgE-mediated hypersensitivity reactions, which develop rapidly after ingestion of the inciting antigen (47). Target organs are exposed to food antigens sequentially in a logical manner; oropharyngeal reactions appear first, with characteristic pruritus, urticaria, and angioedema of the lips, tongue, palate, and throat. After the allergen reaches the stomach and intestine, nausea, cramping, abdominal pain, flatulence, abdominal distension, and diarrhea result, followed by systemic anaphylaxis with the involvement of several target organ responses.

Respiratory manifestations in food-hypersensitive patients during DBPCFC include allergic symptoms of the upper respiratory tract, e.g., rhino-conjunctivitis and laryngeal edema, as evidenced by itchy, watery eyes and nose, sneezing, hoarseness, dry cough, and a "lump in the throat." The pulmonary response of bronchospasm usually manifests in the form of chest tightness, shortness of breath, and repetitive coughing and wheezing (35).

Systemic anaphylaxis resulting from a systemic IgE-mediated hypersensitivity reaction may develop within minutes to often no more than an hour after exposure to a food allergen. Clinical symptoms include pruritus, urticaria, angioedema, laryngeal edema, bronchospasm, abdominal cramping, diarrhea, cardiac dysrrhythmias, hypotension, and vascular collapse. Fatal reactions may develop quickly, or the initial milder symptoms may progress to overt cardiorespiratory arrest and shock over several hours. Exercise in conjunction with food ingestion (shrimp, wheat, eggs, or celery) has been found to provoke reactions in some patients.

B. Food-Induced Asthma

Most common food allergens have been found in house-dust samples that eventually enter the food chain. Ingestion of such food or even inhalation of aerosolized food allergen may provoke asthmatic symptoms. IgE specific to foods has been commonly noticed in food-sensitive asthmatics, the diagnosis being confirmed by DBPCFCs.

Food-induced asthma generally occurs within minutes to one hour of food ingestion; symptoms include itchy, watery eyes and nose, and itching in the mouth, which may then progress to deep, repetitive coughing, shortness of breath, and wheezing. Acute asthma attacks may be severe and progress to systemic anaphylaxis and even death. Respiratory reactions from food allergens may be subtle, presenting only with cough, chronic asthma, or enhanced bronchial hyperreactivity.

Not all asthmatics who are food-allergic have food-induced asthma, and specific food elimination in such patients may not prevent asthma. In some who develop symptoms after meals or consumption of acidic foods, gastroesophageal reflux may be a predisposing factor for asthma. Exercise-induced anaphylaxis may be diagnosed in patients who develop asthma and systemic anaphylaxis with exercise and ingestion of specific food. Also, not all that wheezes is asthma; e.g., children with cystic fibrosis may have wheezing and G.I. symptoms that mimic asthma and food allergy (35).

Food preservatives, additives, and colorants, such as sulfites, monosodium glutamate (MSG), tartrazine, and other dyes, have been reported to cause urticaria and asthmatic symptoms in a few sensitive patients. Whereas sulfite-containing foods may cause bronchospasm and severe asthmatic attacks, MSG has been reported to cause "Chinese restaurant syndrome," consisting of symptoms such as paresthesias; burning sensations of the neck, chest, and limbs; palpitations; and weakness.

Occupational asthma is a reversible airway obstruction induced by inhaled agents found in the workplace, e.g., exposure to shelfish during seafood processing (48,49), to wheat and rye (baker's asthma), to green coffee beans and tea by factory workers, and to grain storage mites by grain workers (35).

C. Diagnosis of Food Allergy

Food allergy may be diagnosed by knowing the patient's history, physical examination, skin testing, or in vitro antigen-specific IgE tests. The results of an appropriate exclusion diet and blinded provocation, performed when it is safe, aid in the dignosis of food allergy. A careful history is very useful in identifiying the food(s) that cause allergic symptoms. A skin prick test with food extracts is a simple and reliable method of demonstrating food allergen–specific IgE antibodies. Intradermal skin testing for foods carries a higher risk of a systemic reaction and hence is not recommended. In vitro food antigen–specific IgE determinations help in evaluating patients with extensive skin disease. Elimination of suspected food is usually tried as a part of a diagnostic approach. If symptoms resolve, confirmation by food challenge is recommended (35).

Many physicians use oral food challenge as the diagnostic technique to evaluate various food-related complaints. Open food challenges and single-blinded challenges do help in the diagnosis of food allergy. However, DBPCFCs are more desirable for confirming the diagnosis, especially in an academic research setting. Patients with a convincing history of systemic anaphylaxis to a specific food are not challenged with that food. A randomized challenge with an equal number of placebo and food antigen exposures is used to control a variety of confounding factors. DBPCFCs are performed in a clinic or hospital setting only if trained personnel and equipment for treating systemic anaphylaxis are available.

D. Dietary Management of Food Allergy and Asthma

Suspect foods are eliminated for 10 to 14 days before the oral challenge, and antihistamines are discontinued and other medications are minimized. Inhaled beta-agonists are often withheld for at least 6 hours. The challenge may occasionally be conducted with a patient receiving beta-agnoists and/or theophyllinc. In these patients, the medications should be identical on placebo and test days. Pulmonary function tests are serially conducted for up to 8 hours to study late asthmatic reactions. Oral food challenges are often performed on an empty stomach, starting with a dose unlikely to provoke symptoms. The dose is then doubled every 30 to 60 minutes or more, depending on the type of reaction suspected and length of time needed to produce symptoms. After the patient has tolerated 10 grams of lyophilized food blinded in capsules or liquid, the food is given openly in usual amounts under observation to prevent alteration of the allergenic epitomes during food preparation and/or digestion. A positive oral challenge test shows the cause-and-effect relationship of the foods and patients' symptoms (50).

After identifying the allergic food, strict elimination of that food is the most effective treatment to prevent allergic reactions. Patients need to be educated on how to read and understand food labels to detect hidden food allergens. Patients who accidently eat a food to which they are sensitive and who develop laryngeal or pulmonary symptoms should be treated immediately with epinephrine and/or inhaled or nebulized beta-agonists. Hypotensive episodes also call for an epinephrine injection. Patients who may potentially develop anaphylactic reactions can be taught how to self-administer epinephrine whenever there is a need. However, such self-medication should immediately be followed by professional medical help.

Besides food antigens, a range of aerollergens, food preservatives, and chemical additives trigger asthma (chronic inflammatory condition of the airways); affected patients should be treated appropriately for bronchial inflammation and advised to avoid aeroallergens and foods to which they are specifically sensitive. Patients are often allergic to a single, common, allergenic food, and it is unnecessary to eliminate several foods, which may lead to malnutrition. The use of oral desensitization, prophylactic medications, or immunotherapy remains to be established in well-designed studies for efficient management of food allergies (35).

REFERENCES

1. Moore, F.D., Homeostasis: bodily changes in trauma and surgery. The responses to injury in man as the basis for clinical management, *David-Christopher Textbook of Surgery* (D.C. Sabiston, ed.), 11th ed., Saunders, Philadelphia, 1977, p. 26.

2. Cuthbertson, D.P., The metabolic response to injury and other related explorations in the field of protein metabolism: an autobiographical account, *Scottish Med. J. 27*: 158 (1982).

3. Kinney, J.M., Weight loss, calorimetry and malnutrition, *Perspectives in Clinical Nutrition* (J.M. Kinney and P.R. Borum, eds.), Pall Urban and Schwarzenberg, Baltimore 1989, p. 3.

4. Broom, J., Sepsis and trauma, *Human Nutrition and Dietetics*, 9th ed. (J.S. Garrow and W.P.T. James, eds.), Churchill Livingstone, Edinburgh, London, 1993, p. 456.

5. Cuthbertson, D.P., and H.C. Zagreb, The metabolic response to injury and its nutritional implications, *J. Parenteral Enteral. Nutr. 3*: 108 (1979).

6. Blackburn, G.I., J.P. Flatt, G.H.A. Clowes, and T.F. O'Donnell, Peripheral intravenous feeding with isotonic amino acid solutions, *Am. J. Surgery. 125*: 447 (1973).

7. Newsholme, E.A., and C. Start, *Regulation in Metabolism*, J. Wiley & Sons, Chichester, 1973, p. 315.

8. Cahill, G.F. Jr., Insulin resistance in critically ill patients, Proc. 5th European Congress on Parenteral and Enteral Nutrition, Sir David Cuthberton Lecture, 1984.

9. Clemens, M.J., Cytokine, *Medical Perspective Series* (A.P. Read and T. Brown, eds.), Bios Scientific Publishers, London, 1991.

10. Billiau, A., and F. Vandekerckhove, Cytokines and their interactions with other inflammatory mediators in the pathogenesis of sepsis and septic shock, *Europ. J. Clin. Investigation 21*: 559 (1991).

11. Dinarello, C.E., Interleukin-1 and interleukin-1 antagonism, *Blood 77*: 1627 (1991).

12. Chanarin, I., Nutritional management of diseases of blood, *Human Nutrition and Dietetics*, 9th ed. (J.S. Garrow and W.P.T. James, eds.), Churchill Livingstone, Edinburgh, London, 1993, p. 584.

13. Haas, J.D., and M.W. Fairchild, Summary and conclusions of the International Conference on Iron Deficiency and Behavioral Development, Oct. 10–12, 1988, *Am. J. Clin. Nutr. 50*: 703 (1989).

14. FAO/WHO Expert Consultation 1988. Requirements of Vitamin A, Iron, Folate and Vitamin B_{12}, Food and Agriculture Organization of the United Nations, Rome and World Health Organization, 1988.

15. Chanarin, I., V. Malkowska, A-M O'Hea, M.G. Rinsler, and A.B. Price, Megaloblastic anaemia in a vegetarian Hindu community, *Lancet 2*: 1168 (1985).

16. Jadhav, M., J.K.G. Webb, S. Vashaava, and S. Baker, Vitamin B_{12} deficiency in Indian infants, a clinical syndrome, *Lancet 2*: 903 (1962).

17. Chanarin, I., *The Megaloblastic Anaemias*, 2nd ed., Blackwell, Oxford, 1979.

18. Chanarin, I., *The Megaloblastic Anaemias*, 3rd ed., Blackwell, Oxford, 1990.

19. Fleming, A.F., J.D. dev. Hendriks, and N.C. Allan, The prevention of megaloblastic anaemia in pregnancy in Nigeria, *J. Obstr. Gynaec. British Commonwealth 75*: 425 (1968).

20. Shorvon, S.D., M.W.P. Carney, I. Chanarin, and E.H. Reynolds, The neuropsychiatry of megaloblastic anaemia, *Br. Med. J. 281*: 1036 (1980).

21. Watson-Williams E.J., Folic acid deficiency in sickle-cell anaemia, *East African Med. J. 39*: 213 (1962).

22. Smithells, R.W., S. Sheppard, and C.J. Schoralo, Apparent prevention of neural tube defects by preconceptional vitamin supplementation, *Arch. Dis. Childhood 56*: 911 (1981).

23. Laurence, K.M., N. James, M.H. Miller, G.B. Tennant, and H. Campbell, Double-blind randomized controlled trial of folate treatment before conception to prevent recurrence of neural tube defects, *Br. Med. J. 282*: 1509 (1981).

24. MRC, Prevention of neural tube defect: results of the Medical Research Council, Vitamin Study Research Group, *Lancet 338*: 131 (1991).

25. Chanarin, I., *The Megaloblastic Anaemias*, Blackwell, Oxford, 1969.

26. Landon, M.J., and F.E. Hytten, The excretion of folate in pregnancy, *J. Obstr. Gynaecol. British Commonwealth 78*: 769 (1971).

27. Hansen, H., and G. Rybo, Folic acid dosage in prophylactic treatment during pregnancy, *Acta Obstr. Gynaecol. Scandinavica 46* (Suppl.7): 107 (1967).

28. Chanarin, I., D. Rothman, A. Ward, and J. Perry, Folate status and requirement in pregnancy, *Br. Med. J. 2*: 390 (1968).

29. Chanarin, I., and D. Rothman, Further observations on the relation between iron and folate status in pregnancy, *Br. Med. J. 2*: 81 (1971).

30. Baumslag, N., T. Edclstcin, and J. Metz, Reduction of incidence of prematurity by folic acid supplementation in pregnancy, *Br. Med. J. 1*: 1161 (1970).

31. Chanarin, I., Folates and cobalamins, *Clin. Haematol. 14*: 629 (1985).

32. Majia, L.A., R.E. Hodges, G. Arroyave, F. Viteri, and B. Torun, Vitamin A deficiency and anaemia in Central American children, *Am. J. Clin. Nutr. 30*: 1175 (1977).

33. Lane, M., and C.P. Alfrey, The anaemia of human riboflavin deficiency, *Blood 22*: 811 (1963).

34. National Asthma Education and Prevention Program. Expert Panel Report II: Guidelines for the diagnosis and management of asthma, February, 1997.

35. Rumsaeng, V., and D.D. Metcalfe, Asthma and food allergy, *Nutr. Rev. 56* (S II): 153 (1998).

36. Sampson, H.A., and P.L. Jolie, Increased plasma histamine concentrations after food challenges in children with atopic dermatitis, *N. Engl. J. Med. 311*: 372 (1984).

37. Grazanka, A., J. Domaniewski, and M. Swiatkowski, Ultrastructural evaluation of mast cells in food allergy, *Patol Pol. 40*: 235 (1989).

38. Reimann, H.J., J. Ring, and B. Ultsch, Intragastral provocation under endoscopic control (IPEC) in food allergy: mast cell and histamine changes in gastric mucosa, *Clin. Allergy 15*: 195 (1985).

39. Sampson, H.A., L. Mendelson, and J.P. Rosen, Fatal and nearfatal anaphylactic reactions to food in children and adolescents, *N. Engl. J. Med. 327*: 380 (1992).

40. Sampson, H.A., K.R. Broadbent, and J. Bernhisel-Broadbent, Spontaneous release of histamine from basophils and histamine-releasing factor in patients with atopic dermatitis and food hypersensitivity, *N. Engl. J. Med. 321*: 228 (1989).

41. Burks, A.W., and H.A. Sampson, Food allergies in children, *Curr. Probl. Pediatr. 23*: 230 (1993).

42. Bircher, A.J., G. Van Melle, and E. Haller, IgE to food allergens are highly prevalent in patients allergic to pollens, with and without symptoms of food allergy, *Clin. Exp. Allergy 24*: 367 (1994).

43. Heiss, S., S. Fischer, and W.D. Muller, Identification of a 60 kd cross-reactive allergen in pollen and plant-derived food, *J. Allergy Clin. Immunol. 98*: 938 (1996).

44. Witteman, A.M., S. Vanden Oudenrijin, and Van Leeumen, IgE antibodies reactive with silverfish, cockroach, and chironomid are frequently found in mite-positive allergic patients, *Int. Arch. Allergy Immunol. 108*: 165 (1995).

45. Van Ree, R., L. Antonicelli, and J.H. Akkerdaas, Possible induction of food allergy during mite immunotherapy, *Allergy 51*: 108 (1996).

46. Van Ree, R., L. Antonicelli, and J.H. Akkerdaas, Asthma after consumption of snails in house-dust-mite-allergic patients: a case of IgE cross-reactivity, *Allergy 51*: 387 (1996).

47. Rumsaeng, V., and D.D. Metcalfe, Food allergy, *Semin. Gastrointest. Dis. 7*: 134 (1996).

48. Desjardins, A., J.L. Malo, and J.L. Archeveque, Occupational IgE-mediated sensitization and asthma caused by clam and shrimp, *J. Allergy Clin. Immunol. 96*: 608 (1995).

49. Lemiere, C., A. Desjardins, and S. Leher, Occupational asthma to lobster and shrimp, *Allergy 51*: 272 (1996).

50. Bousquet M., Mechanisms in adverse reactions to food: The lung, *Allergy 50*: 52 (1995).

34
Diet and Nervous System Disorders

I. INTRODUCTION

Certain nutrients are essential for the development and functioning of the nervous system, and the absence of these dietary elements may influence the brain's neurochemistry and even human behavior. Diet also influences the progress of neurological and neuropsychiatric disorders, both genetic and environmental factors being involved in the etiology and pathogenesis of these neurological disorders (1).

II. DEVELOPMENT AND METABOLISM OF THE BRAIN

A vast number of cells are produced in the brain of a normally developing fetus, the cell division coming to a halt after the birth. The brain, however, continues to develop, as the cells migrate, organize, and myelinate. The proliferation of neurons is completed by mid-pregnancy, whereas cellular migration can continue until the infant is 5 months of age. Neuronal organization begins in mid-pregnancy and continues for several years postnatally.

The neurons produce cellular extensions or neurites, as axons of great length. In addition to these, multiple small extensions or dendrites also grow for the interaction with other neural cells. Continued development of dendrites depends both on the availability of nutrients and different stimulation of the brain. Intense neuronal development and interaction occurs from mid-gestation to about 2 years of age, although general brain maturation may continue until the age of 20 years in women and 25 years in men (1).

An adult human brain has around 100 billion neurons, with an equal number of supporting glial cells. Brain cortex alone contains about 20 billion neurons and 40 billion glial structural cells, which control most of the functions of the central nervous system. Each neuron develops 1,000 to 10,000 connections or synapses with other cells and receives input from around 1,000 other neuronal synapses.

Glial structural cells have no axons or synapses. These are of two types: the macroglia, including astrocytes and oligodendrocytes, and the smaller microglia, acting as macrophages in the brain (2). The astrocytes are located close to the blood vessels, their projections surrounding the vessel. Thus, they control the nutrient supply to the brain through the blood vessels. The oligodendrocytes synthesize and maintain the myelin sheath in the brain (white matter) and serve as neuronal satellite cells within the brain (gray matter). The myelination process involves the secretion of up to 40 layers of lipid-rich membrane that surround each axon. This sheath electrically insulates the axons, thus allowing neuronal stimulus to pass to the axon. The myelin has higher proportion of white matter and about 30% protein, the remainder consisting of phospholipid, some cholesterol, and glycolipids, e.g. galactocerebroside, a sphingoglycolipid important in myelin metabolism. The *n*-3 and *n*-6 fatty acid content of both myelin and the other brain membranes is high, placing unusual demands on the supply of these long-chain (C24 and C26) polyunsaturated fatty acids during the development of the fetus and in the first one or two years of postnatal life. The structure and function of cerebral membranes also need an adequate supply of dihomo-gamma-linolenic acid (C20:3) and arachidonic acid (C20:4) derived from linoleic acid (C18:2).

Myelin and the neuronal and glial cells are rich in protein, requiring its appropriate supply during fetal cell proliferation and postnatal brain maturation. Nutrients are also required to provide energy for cellular metabolism and to synthesize neurotransmitters needed for the neuronal activity of the brain.

The metabolic activity of the brain accounts for about 20% to 30% of the body's resting metabolic rate. The brain's energy requirement and blood flow vary from birth to old age; the newborn brain withstands hypoxia for a longer time than in adulthood. The cerebral blood flow and oxygen uptake are highest at the age of 6 years, when the brain consumes over 60 ml O_2/min, more than 50% of total body basal oxygen consumption. The oxygen uptake of an adult human brain weighing 1,400 g is around 49 ml O_2/min (1).

Mature neurons require a continuous supply of energy to maintain their function. Neurons have a limited store of glycogen, because they have a high turnover rate. Glucose is the main energy substrate for the synthetic and functional activities of the central and peripheral nervous system; about one-fifth of the glucose in the arterial flow to the brain is taken up for metabolism. Around 50% of the glucose metabolized by the brain during the first month of life uses a hexose monophosphate shunt to supply ribose sugar for the synthesis of nucleic acids and reduced nicotinamide adenine dinucleotide phosphate (NADPH) for lipid biosynthesis.

Amino acid catabolism contributes less than 10% of the total energy supply of the brain. Although nervous tissue can synthesize some amino acids, all essential amino acids must be supplied through the blood across the blood-brain barrier.

Around 8% of the brain by weight is protein, which accumulates linearly from 6 months of gestation until the second postnatal year and then slows down. A continued supply of almost all amino acids is needed for the biosynthesis of brain proteins. The amino acid composition of the blood plasma is primarily determined by the protein content of the feed in the first few months of life. The amino acids of human milk protein are present in approximately the same proportions as needed for tissue synthesis, although cysteine, taurine, and tryptophan are often present in higher concentrations. Also, higher levels of glutamine, aspartate, *N*-acetylaspartate, and gammabutyric acid are seen in the brain than in the plasma. Especially, the transmitters glutamate, gamma-butyrate, and glycine are released at about 90% of the synapses in the mammalian brain. Nicholls (3) adduced that the dominant excitatory neurotransmitter, glutamate, is involved in the postsynaptic receptor function and its presence is implicated in pathways of memory and learning as well as the mechanisms of ischemic brain damage.

The significance of nutritional factors is being increasingly recognized in brain function, especially during fetal and early postnatal periods. The vulnerable period may extend throughout gestation and infancy. The effects of extrinsic harmful factors, such as teratogenic drugs, fetal hypoxia, or malnutrition, depend largely on the timing of damage in relation to the stage of brain development, e.g., there may be a vulnerable period for myelination when the fetus is more sensitive to external factors such as maternal malnutrition and placental insufficiency. Nutritional deprivation may particularly affect brain development from the last trimester of gestation until the second year of postnatal life. Higher cortical functions are in immature form at birth, but the subcortical functions are mature by this time. Defective brain growth may result in a reduced rate of growth of the head and in a small head circumference. Microcephaly (small head) resulting from a prenatal disorder is often obvious at birth but may also become evident later (1).

III. NUTRITIONAL DISORDERS OF THE BRAIN

A prenatal nutritional disorder during brain development may lead to general functional defects of varying severity, such as subnormal intelligence or other cognitive deficits, with the preservation of normal general intelligence. Serious intellectual defects such as mental deficiency are often obvious during the first year of life; cognitive development depends on brain maturation, which may continue until young adult life.

Specific nutrient deficiencies in the mother have been known to produce a range of disorders in the development and function of fetal brain; e.g., the early impact of a folate deficiency leads to the development of neural tube defects (NTD) (4). NTDs include spina bifida, in which the neural tube fails to close at 4 weeks of fetal life, and anencephalus, in which the forebrain fails to develop properly. Other conditions such as encephalocele (hernial protrusion of the brain) and iniencephaly (brain matter protruding through a fissure in the occiput) also exist. Zinc deficiency is thought to play a role in these conditions. These disorders probably arise as a complex interplay between genetic and environmental factors. For reasons not known, female children are especially affected by anencephaly. Poorer populations have the highest incidence of NTDs, although the prevalence rate of NTDs is falling worldwide, with evidence suggesting that the availability of dietary folate plays a dominant role in NTD incidence. Environmental influences are also seen by variations in incidence of these disorders, especially spina bifida and anencephaly; e.g. in Britain and Ireland, anencephalus and spina bifida show an excess incidence in babies conceived in the spring.

Maternal illness may affect the incidence of NTD, diabetic mothers being particularly susceptible to NTD. This is thought to result from a delayed switch from anaerobic to aerobic glucose metabolism in early uterine life due to the high prevalence of glucose levels, which explains the failure of normal cell development and an induction of NTD.

Animal experimental studies have shown the importance of an appropriate micronutrient intake. Rats fed folate-deficient diets that are supplemented with antifolates produce NTDs. Similarly, hydrocephalus can be shown to be caused by vitamin B_{12} deficiency and NTD by pyridoxal and pantothenic acid deficiency. Vitamin E deficiency may cause NTDs in some species, and zinc deficiency has been shown to increase the rate of hydrocephalus, but not NTDs (4).

Excess of certain fat-soluble vitamins such as vitamin A may lead to major disorders in fetal development. This teratogenic effect of excess vitamin A has led to advice for pregnant women in the United Kingdom to avoid eating livers rich in vitamin A.

Neuringer et al. (5) reviewed the essentiality of n-3 fatty acids for the development and function of retina and brain. Docosahexenoic acid (22:6, n-3 or DHA) is synthesized either by the mother or the fetus from alphalinolenic acid (18:3, n-3) by competing with desaturase and elongation enzymes involved in the conversion of linoleic acid (18:2, n-6) to arachidonic acid (20:4, n-6 or AA). Both DHA and eicosapentenoic acid (20:5, n-3 or EPA) are present abundantly in fish, and smaller amounts are present in leafy vegetables and some plant seeds (soy and rapeseed). Evidence available has shown that the fetus in later pregnancy depends on the placental uptake of these long-chain n-3 fatty acids because of the limited capacity of the fetal liver or brain to produce enough DHA from alpha-linolenic acid. Despite the lower plasma levels of alpha-linolenic and linoleic acids, the fetus has higher DHA, and AA levels of the cerebral gray matter are very high, constituting around one-third of the total fatty acid content of ethanolamine and serine phospholipids. DHA is also concentrated in the synaptosomes and synaptic vesicles and is found in high concentrations in the retina. Around one-half of the adult DHA content of the brain and retina is deposited during fetal life. The DHA and arachidonic acid content of the cerebrum and cerebellum increase 3 to 5 times during the last trimester of pregnancy and in the first 3 months of infancy. Thus, provision of these long-chain fatty acids in the diet or from their precursors is crucial for the mental development of the fetus and infant.

Human milk provides a preformed source of DHA after birth; it is not present in most artificial milk formulas made from bovine fat. Animal experiments have shown that diets deficient in essential fatty acids (EFAs) tend to affect n-6 more than n-3 metabolism. Prematurely born babies who have missed their late-pregnancy phase of DHA and other EFA accumulation in the brain have been found to respond to feed supplements of fish oils rich in DHA (1), as evidenced by changes in electro-retinograms, an enhanced head circumference, and accelerated functional development (6). Studies of nonhuman primates have shown that DHA rapidly accumulates in the brain at 1 to 2 years of age in previously deficient young animals, although this delayed therapy does not restore retinal function.

Simeon and Grantham-McGregor (7) have reviewed children's behavior and mental development as influenced by diet and nutrition. Even short-term food deprivation, such as missing breakfasts, was thought to lead to a deterioration in classroom behavior. Recent studies, however, have shown that for well-nourished children, missing breakfast on a single occasion has only modest effects on school performance, although there are changes in the responses of both the central and autonomic nervous systems. These effects were more evident in mildly malnourished children, with a deterioration in verbal fluency and in the efficiency of arithmatic problem-solving.

Marked mental changes are evident in the acute phase of severe protein-energy malnutrition (PEM), with early changes in mood and responsiveness after the first few days of successful therapy. However, malnourished children show very slow development even after the recovery, the long-term effects of PEM being marked. Grantham-McGregory et al. (8) reported that a substantial portion of the effect was seen in the children's siblings who had not been severely malnourished, suggesting that familial or social factors are also important.

Mild to moderate malnutrition in schoolchildren is clearly associated with the degree of stunting in height and poor mental development, which can be treated by providing both nutritional supplements and training for mothers in simple play therapy as a social stimulus (8). Although the food supplement mostly improves locomotor development, both mental stimulation and food supplements are required to produce the greatest benefit. Such improvement may be sustained for many years after only 1 to 2 years intervention and training. Thus, brain function appears to be very plastic in early childhood and the critical period for brain development is not confined only to fetal life and early infancy.

The brain is most sensitive to iron deficiency during the first 2 years of life, which may produce long-term consequences. Experimental evidence indicates that children over 2 years of age with moderate iron deficiency in the developing countries improved their mental function and school achievements when their anemia was corrected by iron supplementation. Pollitt et al. (9) also showed that prophylactic iron supplements in early infancy improved subsequent mental performance in children of the developing countries. These studies strongly support the public health importance of ensuring an adequate iron status during infancy and childhood (7).

Singh and Dhawan (10) identified the chemical constituent responsible for the facilitatory effect of *brahmi* (*Bacopa monniera* L.) on learning schedules, as a mixture of two saponins, designated bacosides A and B. The bacosides significantly improved acquisition, consolidation, and retention in the shock-motivated brightness, discrimination response, and active-conditioned avoidance response and produced a dose-dependent facilitation of discretion between aversive (Lici) and palatable fluid (sucrose) in the conditioned taste aversion (CTA) response. Bacosides also attenuated the retrograde amnesia produced by immobilization-induced stress, ECS, and scopolamine. They also enhanced protein kinase activity and increased hippocampus. A single dose of 20 to 200 mg and multiple doses of 100 to 200 mg were found to be safe for administration up to 4 weeks with healthy male volunteers in a double-blind placebo-controlled and non-cross-over regulatory phase clinical trials.

A. Amino Acid Metabolism and Brain Function

Some amino acids, such as glycine, aspartate, and glutamate, function as neurotransmitters (Table 1). Amino acids can influence brain function in the following manner: abnormalities of some amino acid metabolism may lead to the accumulation of a specific amino acid or its metabolite, which may cause brain damage and mental defects. It is possible to alter human behavior by manipulating the diet to alter the transport of individual amino acids into the brain. It can be shown experimentally that this change in behavior is preceded by altered synthesis rates of neurotransmitters from the precursor amino acids. Wurtman (11) adduced that the rate of cerebral amino acid uptake modulates neurotransmitter responses.

Tryptophan, phenylalanine, and tyrosine as well as valine, leucine, and isoleucine are taken up through a special transport system required for the absorption of large neutral amino acids. Stimulation of insulin secretion in response to ingestion of carbohydrates, produces a selective fall in the plasma concentration of these branched-chain amino acids as they are transferred into muscle. This fall allows the enhanced uptake of tryptophan and tyrosine into the brain. This change, along with the induced synthesis of 5-hydroxytryptamine (5-HT) from tryptophan, is thought to produce increased dowsiness and mood changes after a carbohydrate-rich meal. 5-HT is also linked to the selective appetite drive for carbohydrate. Drugs for appetite control (e.g. fen-fluramines and fluoxetenes) have been developed to inhibit 5-HT reuptake and thus induce

Table 1 Amino Acid Precursors of Neurotransmitters

Precursor amino acids	Neurotransmitters
As in transmitter	*Amino acids*
	Gamma-amino butyrate
	Glycine
	Aspartate
	Glutamate
	Acetylcholine
	Monoaminergic
Tyrosine	Dopamine
	Adranaline
	Noradrenaline
Tryptophan	Serotonin
	Purinergic
	Adenosine
	ADP
	ATP
	AMP
Arginine	*Nitric oxide*
As in transmitter	N-acetyl amino acids
	N-acetyl peptides

Source: Ref. 1.

anorexia, especially for carbohydrate-rich foods. Protein-rich meals, on the contrary, lower brain tryptophan levels, although brain tyrosine levels and catecholamine formation rise (11). Patients with sleep disorders or depression, when treated with large doses of tryptophan, were found to have enhanced serotonin and depressed catecholamine synthesis. According to Wurtman (11), patients with a low ratio of plasma tryptophan to large neutral amino acids benefit most from this treatment.

A series of amino acid metabolic disorders have been found to cause brain damage or mental disturbances. The fetus normally has plasma concentrations of amino acids 1.5 to 3 times higher than those of the mother. The placenta has active transport systems for all the amino acids expect cysteine, taurine, glutamate, and aspartate. When the mother fasts, the fetal concentrations of amino acids change, with a fall in the essential amino acids and a rise in glycine concentrations. This has been likened to the pattern seen in kwashiorkor. In utero, fetal amino acids are mainly used for protein synthesis and because fetal tissues cannot metabolize amino acids well, the fetus is protected from high concentrations of amino acids (e.g. phenylalanine). Any rise in amino acid concentrations will be buffered by exchange of amino acid across the placenta.

1.   Phenylketonuria (PKU)

It is a standard practice now to screen newborns for PKU, which makes it possible to prevent the microencephaly and mental retatrdation associated with this condition. Babies and children are maintained on special diets with restricted intake of phenylalanine. Without such a treatment, permanent damage may occur within about 2 to 3 months. The blood levels of phenylalanine must be maintained between 180 and 600 μmol (30 to 100 mg/l), at the same time ensuring that phenylalanine deficiency is not induced, which occurs if plasma levels fall below 60 μmol. The clinical features of phenylalanine deficiency include reduced weight gain, feeding difficulties, and happy rash. Dystrophic changes in the skin, hair and nails develop, with frequent infections, followed by convulsions, mental retardation, and death if the condition is not treated. Maintenance of correct phenylalanine levels is thus crucial to avoid mental retardation during infancy and childhood. Dietary control is less important once brain development is complete.

Adult women with PKU who conceive may have either spontaneous abortions or babies with mental retardation, microencephaly, congenital heart disease, and other organ defects. Maternal plasma levels of phenylalanine should be maintained below 250 μmol/l to prevent fetal values rising above 400 μmol/l (12). Congenital heart disease can be avoided if dietary restriction is reinstituted pre-conceptually but not 2 to 3 months after conception. Head circumference and birthweight are linked to the mother's phenylalanine concentration at conception and a good dietary control from the time of conception allows normal fetal growth with little or no evidence of mental impairment in the offspring (12).

2.   Tyrosinemia

In this inborn error, there is a defect in the catabolism of tyrosine with elevated tyrosine blood levels and, occasionally, increased phenylalanine concentrations. The babies often fail to thrive and become mentally retarded with behavioral abnormalities. Dietary restriction and use of ascorbic acid have been advocated for the neonate.

3.   Abnormalities of Other Amino Acids

Serine is an important precursor of glycine in the brain. Glycine deficiency may lead to spastic babies who may respond to dietary glycine supplementation. The condition appears to affect glycine-responsive receptors in the spinal cord. In patients with the fetal disease amyotrophia lateral sclerosis, there is a decreased number of glycinergic receptors. Some improvement occurs with 2 to 4 g/day of threonine because the latter experimentally increases the glycine content of the spinal cord (13).

A range of amino acid precursors serve as neutrotransmitters (Table 1). Thus, there is an increasing interest in manipulating diet to assess their usefulness in a variety of mental disorders. Around 60% of patients with epilepsy have decreased ability to synthesize gamma-aminobutyric acid in those regions of the brain responsible for the seizures. Gamma-aminobutyrate has been known to be an inhibitory neurotransmitter.

B. Vitamins and Brain Function

In addition to their role in normal brain development and function, vitamins are specifically required for their free radical scavenging role in the brain, metabolically a highly active organ. Thus, vitamin C concentrations are about 4 to 10 times higher in the brain than in plasma and may have an important antioxidant role in the retina and lens, preventing or delaying the development of age-related retinal atrophy and cataract. Other vitamins play a crucial role in the synthesis of neurotransmitters in the brain. Vitamin C is also required for the binding of serotonin to its receptors.

Human and animal experiments have shown that severe deficiencies of thiamin, niacin, pyridoxine, folate, or vitamin B_{12} may impair memory, which can be restored to normalcy by providing the deficient vitamin (14). There is some evidence of a relationship between vitamin C intake and mental health. Poor vitamin C status observed in patients in mental hospitals (15,16) may have been the consequence, in part at least, of low dietary intake. Maas et al. (17), however, noted that schizophrenic and neurotic patients with anxiety had lower plasma ascorbate levels than those without anxiety. Furthermore, reports of high ceruloplasmin levels together with a low ratio of free ascorbic acid to ascorbate metabolites in the urine of schizophrenics (18,19) has led to the hypothesis that the fundamental biochemical lesion in schizophrenia might be a disorder in ascorbate metabolism coupled with a defect in copper metabolism. Briggs (18) suggested that the condition in its early stages might possibly be controlled by high (about 500 mg/day) intakes of vitamin C. Milner (20) provided corroborating evidence, in a controlled blind study with 40 psychiatric patients: there were significant improvements in depressive, manic, and paranoid symptom-complexes, after saturation with vitamin C. Milner (20) suggested that psychiatric patients probably have an unusually high demand for vitamin C.

Studies on experimental scurvies in humans (21–23) showed that one of the four prison inmate subjects, during a period of intense anxiety, excreted more ascorbic acid in his urine than he was ingesting. When the cause of anxiety was removed, this man began to retain the vitamin. These investigators, in subsequent studies (24,25), depleted five prison inmates of ascorbic acid and then repleted them by feeding varying levels of vitamin C. Psychological testing was done near the beginning, at midpoint, and at the end of the depletion period, at midpoint of the repletion period, and after 15 days of load dosing (26). The tests included four behavioral areas: mental function, psychomotor performance, physical fitness, and personality. The most significant changes were observed in personality, as measured by the Minnesota Multiphasic Personality Inventory (MMPI). During the depletion course, four MMPI scales (Hypochondriasis, Hysteria, Depression, and Social Introversion) showed significant increases, the changes occurring when the body ascorbate pool (normally about 1,500 mg) was depleted to levels ranging from 761 to 562 mg, with blood plasma ascorbate levels of 1.21 to 1.17 mg/100 ml. These personality changes were reversed during the repletion stage. In two subjects, intakes of 6.5 mg ascorbic acid/day were sufficient to effect the reversal. Grosz (27) also reported the lack of a statistically significant response in serum ascorbic acid levels to hysteria. These investigations have shown the importance of ascorbic acid in the maintenance of mental health.

Thiamin deficiency adversely affects synthesis of the neurotransmitter amino acids, glutamate and aspartate. Also, thiamin is crucially involved in the glucose metabolism on which brain development and function depend. Infantile beriberi in breast-fed babies from mothers on a thiamin-deficient diet may be acute and occurs in association with cardiac failure. The clinical symptoms, such as irritability, vomiting, and convulsions, simulate meningitis; a less severe form simulates Wernicke-Korsakoff syndrome. Rarely seen in the developed countries, thiamin deficiency may take the form of a subacute encephalomyelopathy (28). In older children and in adults, there may be a progressive loss of the sense of vibration with paresthesia and a burning sensation in the feet as the first symptom of peripheral neuritis, followed by motor paralysis and loss of tendon reflexes.

Alcoholism often leads to thiamin deficiency, severe cases leading to a range of Wernicke-Korsakoff disorders. Epileptic patients treated long term with phenytoin develop a substantial risk of thiamin deficiency not related to alcohol, with a prevalence of about 25% (29). Thiamin therapy in children may help to correct some of their metabolic features (1).

Pyridoxine is required both for the synthesis and metabolism of almost all neurotransmitters and is also critically involved in the synthesis of several hormones, such as insulin and growth hormone. Clinical symptoms of pyridoxine deficiency include fatigue, nervousness, irritability, depression, insomnia, and difficulties in walking. In adults dizziness, peripheral neuritis, neuralgia, and carpal tunnel syndrome induced by connective-tissue swelling at the wrist are more evident. Infants fed milk substitutes deficient in pyridoxine were shown to develop irritability and convulsive seizures that can be successfully treated with pyridoxine. It is thus important to ensure dietary pyridoxine sufficiency during early infancy.

Infantile spasms, or West's syndrome, is characterized by a sudden brief flexion of neck or trunk and raising of both arms. It is a rare genetic disorder leading to seizures and mental retardation in infancy, boys being more frequently affected than girls. These children respond rapidly to a high therapeutic dose of 500 mg pyridoxine. However such higher doses of pyridoxine may induce hypotonia in neonates because a child usually requires 0.3 to 0.9 mg pyridoxine/day. Long-term anticonvulsive therapy with phenytoin or succinimide has been reported to be associated with decreased plasma levels of pyridoxine and requires only modest pyridoxine supplements.

A deficiency of cystathione synthase leads to an inborn error of methionine utilization, known as homocystinuria, resulting in mental retardation with convulsions in about 10% to 15% of cases. The administration of 50 to 500 mg of pyridoxine per day leads to marked biochemical and clinical improvement in some patients. Low-methionine diets should be adopted if the child fails to respond to pyridoxine therapy.

A number of hydrazine-induced drugs used on a long-term basis may induce pyridoxine deficiency even in adults, with symptoms such as irritability, peripheral neuropathy, and convulsions, e.g., antidepressant drugs, iproniazid, nialamide, and isocaroxazid; and the antituberculosis drug isonicotylhydrazine (INH). Penicillamine and cycloserine may also bind and inactivate pyridoxine. Thus, patients taking these drugs and alcohol may have higher requirements for vitamin B_6. Isoniazid treatment to patients with tuberculosis results in marked pyridoxine deficiency. Isoniazid pyridoxine hydrazone is excreted in the urine in amounts sufficient to deplete body stores of pyridoxal phosphate, leading to peripheral neuropathy. These patients respond to oral pyridoxine supplements. The vitamin supplement does not reduce the pharmaceutical effect of INH, and pyridoxine doses of 10 mg/day may be needed during long-term treatment with isoniazid.

Oral contraceptives with a high progesterone content may induce depression because of disturbed tryptophan metabolism. Dickerson (30) observed that excretion of tryptophan metabolites can be normalized by administering 20 mg of pyridoxine. Tryptophan pyrrolase, the rate-limiting enzyme in the niacin pathway, utilizes pyridoxine to synthesize nicotinic acid at the expense of serotonin pathways, thus interfering with the synthesis of this neurotransmitter. Only those women showing evidence of a disturbance in tryptophan metabolism respond to pyridoxine supplements. The depression induced by long-term treatment with corticosteroids also can be prevented by vitamin B_6 supplementation.

Overdoses of pyridoxine (100–1000 mg/day) have been reported to impair memory and nullify the beneficial effect of L-dopa in the control of Parkinson's disease. This effect appears to depend on pyridoxine accelerating the decarboxylation of L-dopa to dopamine in extracerebral tissues, which then reduces the amount of L-dopa entering the brain to replenish striatal dopamine, found deficient in Parkinson's disease.

In addition to interacting with folate metabolism, vitamin B_{12} is also needed as a coenzyme for the conversion of methylmelonyl coenzyme A to succinyl coenzyme A in the TCA cycle, the deoxyadenosyl vitamin B_{12} being needed for the last step. Thus, the plasma levels of the potentially toxic methylmalonate are reduced by this reaction.

Vitamin B_{12} is also required to maintain myelin in the nervous system, and inadequate myelin synthesis results in neurological damage, emphasizing the role of methionine. The decrease in methylene tetrahydrofolate leads to depressed synthesis of DNA, affecting cell division in the growing brain. Deficient remethylation of homo-cysteine to methionine also causes decreased availability of S-adenosylmethionine, thus interfering with essential methylation reactions. Deficient methylmalonyl-CoA mutase then leads to an increase in the content of odd fatty acids (15- and 17-carbon fatty acids), and branched fatty acids in the myelin of the nervous tissue (31). The consequences of vitamin B_{12} deficiency can be serious; breast-fed infants whose mothers consume a strict vegan diet are especially at high risk of serious infantile neurological disorders, which can be irreversible. B_{12} deficiency may lead to brain atrophy, myoclonic seizures, microcephaly, and cortical blindness after birth. More subtle effects of B_{12} deficiency are evident in patients with pernicious anemia, in whom dementia may develop. Some of the decline in cognitive function associated with aging can be prevented or reversed by improving vitamin B_{12} and folate status (32).

Because nitrous oxide inactivates vitamin B_{12}, N_2O anesthesia may lead to post-operative B_{12} deficiency, causing neurological deterioration due to myeloneuropathy in marginally B_{12}-deficient patients (33).

Lack of folic acid has an important role in precipitating neural tube defects. It is also seen in alcoholic patients and in patients treated with phenytoin and phenobarbital drugs. Folate deficiency can lead to depression and even dementia (30).

Whereas milder niacin deficiency may produce weakness, tremor, anxiety, depression, and irritability, patients with more severe cases may experience delirium; chronic severe deficiency of niacin may lead to dementia, with patients needing to be admitted to mental hospitals. The possibility of pellagra should be considered in any unexplained delirium or dementia in a person on poor diet for prolonged periods. The condition may also be accompanied by signs of PEM, anemia, and other deficiencies, e.g., of thiamin and other vitamins. Decreased sensation in the feet and loss of vibration and position sense may give rise to ataxia, and spasticity and exaggerated tendon reflexes are signs of involvement of the pyramidal tracts. These are features of subacute combined degeneration of the cord and may be associated with vitamin B_{12} deficiency.

Infants and children suffering from trisomy 21, prematurity, and zinc deficiency, and patients treated with anticonvulsant drugs, are at risk for low serum vitamin A concentrations, leading to infantile hydrocephalus, raised intracranial pressure, and headache and nausea in adults. These effects may also occur in patients suffering from hypervitaminosis A, with drowsiness, vertigo, and vision problems. Alcoholics may be more sensitive to vitamin A overdose. Vitamin E supplementation can limit vitamin A toxicity by decreasing plasma retinol-binding protein and retinol concentrations (34).

Vitamin E has been thought to be involved in various neurological disorders such as epilepsy, intracranial hemorrhage, Parkinson's disease, multiple sclerosis, myotonic dystrophy, and Alzheimer's disease. It is adduced that oxygen-derived free radical species are involved in neurological conditions such as cerebral ischemia, Down syndrome, muscular dystrophy, and mental retardation. Free radicals may be induced by free transition metals such as iron and copper. Lipid hydroperoxides may be decomposed to form peroxyl and alkoxyl radicals in the nervous system. Excess free radical activity has been reported in some neurological disorders that have been treated with vitamin E supplementation alone or in combination with other antioxidants (35,36).

According to Muller (36), vitamin E supplements can increase stores of this vitamin and prevent the complications of periventricular hemorrhage and retinopathy in premature babies. In Down syndrome, the cytoplasmic Cu:Zn-superoxide dismutase activity increases by about 50% without change in brain glutathione peroxidase activity, suggesting that brain is likely to be more susceptible to oxygen free radical stress. Acceleration of oxidative processes in Down syndrome may explain the clinical and biochemical symptoms of rapid aging and the early occurrence of clinical dementia.

Vitamin E is thought to prevent the epilepsy induced after brain hemorrhage, when forced-out iron is likely to produce secondary damage to tissue from free radical activity. Vitamin E therapy has been reported to be successful in a number of brain disorders.

In geographical areas such as Finland, where selenium intakes were low until Serich fertilizers were used, selenium therapy in conjunction with vitamin E was found to be beneficial in a variety of brain disorders, such as neuronal ceroid lipofuscinosis. The best responders to antioxidant therapy showed no neurological dysfunction except deteriorated vision (37,38).

Multiple sclerosis is thought to result from a disorder involving the demyelination and scarring of brain and spinal cord. It is a chronic disabling, fluctuating neurological condition, with a peak onset between 25 and 35 years of age. It is characterized by impairment of vision, coordination, sensation, intellect, and sphincter control, with ensuing death. It is more prevalent in people living in cold countries and consuming diets rich in animal fats containing saturated fatty acids (39). Vitamin E with selenium and vitamin C and a balanced intake of n-6 and n-3 polyunsaturated fatty acids has been used to treat multiple sclerosis, because enhanced peroxidation rate has been thought to be a pathological factor in this disease.

Antioxidant treatment with vitamin E may postpone the need for L-dopa in Parkinson's disease, a degenerative neurological disorder with progressive degeneration of the pigmented nuclei in the brainstem and a loss of the neurotransmitter dopamine in the basal ganglia (40,41).

Dementia is frequently observed in elderly patients with Alzheimer's disease. Decrease in cerebral blood flow, glucose utilization, and oxygen consumption are common to many dementias, which result from abnormalities in brain structure. Reduced blood flow and oxidative metabolism lead to loss of balance between pro-oxidants and antioxidants. Aluminum toxicity may be one of the causal factors, because aluminum is found in higher concentrations in the brains of some patients. Simultaneous reductions in the cortical contents of selenium and zinc may indicate reduced antioxidant activity.

Vitamin K is involved in a number of plasma coagulation factors and proteins, and its deficiency results in coagulation defects in newborns, e.g., the early hemorrhagic form, the classic type, and late neonatal vitamin K deficiency. These disorders are characterized by vomiting, lethargy, hemorrhage, convulsions, loss of appetite, unconsciousness, dyspnea, and intracranial bleeding. Most infants suffering from late neonatal hemorrhage disease had no vitamin K pro-phylaxis at birth, and their mothers were often treated with drugs affecting vitamin K metabolism (41).

C. Minerals, Trace Elements, and Brain Function

Iron is vital for brain development and function (see Chapter 7). Beard et al. (42) reviewed the information on the location and function of iron in the central nervous system (CNS), with par-ticular emphasis on human biology. Iron is distributed to different cell types in the brain in a het-erogeneous fashion through the action of transferrin, transferrin receptors, and the metabolic needs of those cells. The function of this iron and its storage is documented in states of growth and development as well as during pathological states associated with aging. According to Beard et al. (42), available evidence suggests that abnormally low levels of iron interfere with an organ-ism's interaction with its environment, altering affective behavioral systems in subtle ways. In addition, it appears that there may be one or more critical developmental periods during which insufficient iron availability can produce deficits in neural functioning and behavior that may be impossible to remedy by iron replenishment. Assessing the effects of iron deficiency on brain and related functions in animal models has important implications for understanding behavioral dis-orders in humans.

Dobbing (43) reviewed the growing research relating iron nutrition to cognition and behav-ior. Several reports have shown that iron-deficient children have altered attention spans, lower intelligence scores, and some degree of perceptual disturbance. Similar data do not exist for adult humans, although there is no clear indication that this relationship is developmentally interlinked, except for a few studies in which nutritional insult could have interfered with the structural organ-ization of the brain (44,45). Two reports of adult human subjects with serum ferritin levels within the normal range suggested that cortical electro-encephalogram patterns showed greater asym-metry as ferritin concentrations decreased (46,47). These studies indicated that the biochemical alterations that occur in the brain with chronic iron deficiency should occur similarly in adults and children if the severity of iron deficiency is similar. A UNESCO conference held in 1990 focused on the relationship between iron deficiency and cognitive performance and human behavior. It was concluded that the blinded clinical trials indicated that cognition is altered by iron deficiency (48), although the causal mechanism(s) remain unknown. Anemia has significant impact on affec-tive behavior (49,50). Lozoff (51) suggested that iron deficiency may also profoundly influence affect (emotions) in infants. Pollitt (48) reported that emotions may significantly mediate the rela-tionship between iron deficiency and cognitive deficits.

A number of neurological disorders, such as Parkinson's disease (52), multiple sclerosis (53), Alzheimer's disease (54), and Hallervorden-Spatz disease (55), have been reported to be associated with disruptions in iron homeostasis in the brain. Normal neurological function depends on normal iron homeostasis. The brain has the highest rate of oxidative metabolism of any organ in the body, reflected in the higher levels of iron in the brain than any other organ except the liver (56).

Magnesium activates most enzymes involved in phosphorus metabolism and mitochondr-ial oxidative metabolism. Magnesium and calcium interdependently influence the excitability of neuromuscular activity. The blood-brain barrier limits the uptake of magnesium from blood into the central nervous system.

Hypomagnesemia can induce tetany in newborns, and neonatal tetany due to magnesium deficiency is usually characterized by hypocalcemia resistant to calcium therapy. Magnesium deficits in children can produce restlessness and psychomotor instability, though not mental retardation. Hypomagnesemia in adults causes nervousness, muscular twitchings, an unsteady gait, salivation, and muscular tetany leading to convulsions. Acute symptomatic hypomagnesemia may produce carpopedal spasm, facial muscle twitching, apathy, anorexia, tremors, convulsions, delirium, hallucinations, coma, and death. Rogers (57) reported that magnesium deficiency is involved in disorders such as organic brain syndrome, Alzheimer's disease, intestinal spasms, migraine, chronic fatigue, depression, and panic attacks.

Miners of manganese ore, such as those in Chile, may develop 'manganese madness' (locura manganica) due to toxic excessive intakes of Mn, which is deposited in the basal ganglia and produces some features similar to that of Parkinson's disease. Mn deficiency, however, may rarely be a risk in hospitalized patients.

Experimentally, copper has been shown to result in marked morphological and functional changes in the brain, pancreas, heart, and adrenals of animals. Major endocrine alterations in Cu deficiency are changes in catecholamines, opiates, and opiate receptors in the brain, as well as in the opiates and neuropeptides of the pituitary and hypothalamus. Decreases in noradrenaline and dopamine in some regions of the brain have been implicated in neurological disorders resulting from Cu deficiency. According to Bhathena et al. (58), feeding fructose can produce a severe Cu deficiency in humans. Cerebeller ataxia is known to occur in humans as the result of nutritional deficiency of Cu (1).

Defective intestinal absorption leading to copper deficiency may cause Menkes' disease, with features such as extensive brain damage, convulsive seizures, and mental retardation. Patients often fail to thrive and have poor psychomotor development, seizures, a tendency to hypothermia, distinctive facial features, and very characteristic kinky or "steel" hair. Nadal and Baerlocher (59) reported that parenteral copper-histidine supplemented by oral D-penicillamine was beneficial in one case study.

Wilson's disease is a rare inherited defect characterized by excess copper accumulation that leads to progressive fatal copper toxicity, wherein brain copper levels rise 10 times the levels found in normal brain and cornea. These patients may also present with liver disease or with neurological symptoms without mental retardation.

Patients suffering from alcohol withdrawal seizures may present with low cerebrospinal fluid zinc levels; increased values are present in patients on estrogen thereapy. Henkin et al. (60) showed that acute severe zinc deficiency causes neurophysiological impairment in humans, especially impairment of dark adaptation. Zinc influences appetite, taste, smell, and vision in the central nervous system, and zinc deficiency may cause neuropsychiatric alterations such as anorexia, apathy, irritability, jitteriness, and mental lethargy. Zinc deficiency may also affect cone-mediated vision, associated with optic neuropathy (61). A few patients with acrodermatitis enteropathica who are mentally handicapped may respond rapidly to oral zinc supplementation (1).

Zinc deficiency is thought to be involved in the etiology of anorexia nervosa. Sauna users may lose zinc by sweating, and the catabolic of starvation may release tissue zinc into the plasma, leading to hyperzincuria (62). Safai-Kutti (62) noted that a daily ingestion of 45 mg of zinc (as zinc sulfate) resulted in weight gain in 17 young female patients with long-term anorexia nervosa.

Selenium has been hypothesized to be related to various neurological disorders, such as epilepsy, PKU, maple syrup urine disease, Parkinson's disease, amyotrophic lateral sclerosis, neuronal ceroid lipofuscinoses, myotonic dystrophy, multiple sclerosis, Down syndrome, Alzheimer's disease, and neurotoxicity of mercury. Selenium supplementation alone or in combination with other antioxidants have been found to benefit the patients with these disorders clinically. Selenium toxicosis, although very rare, can affect gastrointestinal tract, skin, hair, and nails; some patients may suffer from lassitude. Selonis reported from China had features such as peripheral anesthesia, pain in the extremities with subsequent numbness, convulsions, paralysis, motor disturbance, and hemiplegia. Other factors, such as fluorosis and heavy metal toxicity may also contribute to the toxic symptoms. Afflicted residents evacuated from the affected areas were found to improve as their diets changed (1).

D. Other Nutritional Disorders of the Nervous System

1. Favism

Favism is an inherited sex-linked recessive disorder causing red-cell fragility, the expression of a mutation of the glucose-6-phosphate dehydrogenase (G-6-PD) gene, which has over 300 variants. The deficiency of G-6-PD influences the pentose phosphate pathway that produces NADPH required for glutathione reduction. The reduced glutathione protects red cells from oxidative stress and production of enhanced oxygen-derived free radicals. Thus, individuals with favism are not able to regenerate glutathione to prevent hemolysis arising from exposure to hemolytic agents such as naphthalene (moth balls), oxidant drugs, and faba (fava) bean. Risk of exposure also includes breast-feeding, if the mother is eating the *Vicia faba* bean. Favism causes an acute hemolytic anemia due to ingestion of faba bean or inhalation of pollen from the plant. Glycosides, vicinin, and agglucon inhibit G-6-PD. A versatile diet rich in antioxidant vitamins and minerals has been recommended for mothers breastfeeding their babies. Drugs that should be avoided in favism include antimalerial drugs, sulfonamides, sulfones, nitrofurans, antihelminthics, analgesics, dimercaprol, phenylhydrazine, naphthalene, vitamin K, and its water-soluble analogues, methylene blue, toluidine blue, and faba bean.

2. Spinal Ataxia

This disorder is characterized by a principal lesion in the dorsal column of the spinal cord, with a unsteady gait due to loss of proprioceptive sensation. The patient sways while standing upright with eyes closed. The vibration sense in the legs is also often lost. Long-term nutritional conditions caused by unbalanced diets have been described, such as the nutritional amblyopia of strict vegetarians in Malaysia, and the tropical ataxic neuropathy found in Africa.

Lack of vitamin B_{12} appears to be the essential dietary abnormality, although in some forms of tropical ataxia, vitamin B_{12} plays a secondary role. Consumption of large amounts of cassava, which contains the glyceride linamarin in its leaves and roots, has been found to be associated with this disorder. Linamarin is cyanogenic, i.e., it is broken down to yield free hydrogen cyanide by plant enzymes when crushed or left standing in water. However, the ingested cyanide can be detoxified by sulfur-containing amino acids, which convert it to thiocyanate, and by hydroxycobalamin to form cyanocobalmin. The latter limits the availability of vitamin B_{12} for normal neuronal function. Thiocyanate overload resulting from the consumption of the poorly detoxified cassava may worsen any iodine deficiency, because thiocyanate decreases the secretory capacity of the thyroid gland. Cassava eaters thus have an increased risk of developing goiter.

Clinically, tropical ataxia is characterized by tingling, coldness, and numbness in the extremities due to peripheral neuropathy, followed by motor weakness and ataxia, which become severe with involvement of the spinal cord. Severe cases present ataxia with loss of reflexes, especially in the lower limbs, amblyopia, and hearing disturbances. There may be organic psychosis (sign of B_{12} deficiency) if the brain is affected.

Malabsorption of vitamins and deficiencies of B group vitamins such as folate are seen in many cases. Dumas et al. (63) noted a causal link with folate deficiency in Senegal, with B_1 and B_2 deficiency in Nigeria, and with B_{12} deficiency in Senegal and South Africa.

3. Neonatal Jaundice and Kernicterus

Hemoglobin degradation produces bilirubin leading to neonatal jaundice. This condition must be diagnosed and treated early, because bilirubin is toxic to the brain. Severity of the disorder may be assessed by measuring total serum bilirubin; patients with values over 175–210 μmol/l by the third post-term day are thought to have pathological jaundice.

If neonatal jaundice is not treated early, bilirubin toxicity leads to brain damage and the affected infant becomes irritable or lethargic, sucks poorly, vomits its feed, and may later develop neurological symptoms of kernicterus, including hypertonia, paralysis of upward gaze, a typical high-pitched cry (opisthotonus), fever, apnea, and convulsions. Many babies survive with deafness and mental retardation (64).

A routine use of 450 to 460 nm phototherapy has been recommended, effective therapy requiring a minimum irradiance of 1 mW/cm^2 of skin. In phototherapy, neonates require additional fluid, about 10% to 15% extra daily. A daily dose of 0.5 mg/kg of riboflavin decreases the need for phototherapy by stimulating the photolysis of bilirubin (65).

4. Lathyrism

Certain excitary amino acids have been suggested to be involved in the pathogenesis of some neurological disorders, such as Alzheimer's disease, epilepsy, and Parkinson's disease. Ingestion of the excitotoxin, beta-N-oxalylamino-L-alanine (BOAA), a constituent of *Lathyrus sativus* pulse, has been found to result in lathyrism in India and Ethiopia. Lathyrism is characterized by muscle cramps, weakness, and stiffness or an acute onset of paraplegia. The toxin can be destroyed by boiling. A related compound to BOAA, namely beta-N-methylamino-alpha-alanine (BMAA) found in *Cycas circinalis* palm, has been linked to Guamian amyotrophic lateral sclerosis, a form of amyotrophic lateral sclerosis seen in various Pacific islands. BMAA in primates produces changes suggestive of pyramidal and extrapyramidal tract dysfunction (63).

IV. EXERCISE, PHYSICAL ACTIVITY, AND BRAIN FUNCTION

The supply of blood to the human brain during muscular work was thought to be constant, owing to autonomous regulation of brain circulation. This view was brought into question by the use of combined position emission tomography (PET) examinations together with radioactive isotopes (66). Significant increases in blood circulation in regional cerebrum sections could be demonstrated during directed hearing, seeing, speaking, and index finger movements (67). It is not known whether a raised substrate supply of free fatty acids, ketone bodies, lactate, and ammonia is metabolized by brain cells during muscular exertion. Static (isometric) exercise apparently causes no increase in brain blood flow. The observable blood flow increase during dynamic work could be explained by movement-dependent mechanoreceptors (67).

During physical exercise, the psyche can be influenced biochemically in different ways. Using an artificial tooth crown and electric irritation of the dental pulp, it has been experimentally demonstrated that before and after exercise, and before and after a blockade of the opioid effect with Naloxon, there was a rise in pain tolerance and a highly significant mood improvement (67).

Conlay et al. (68) reported a reduction of plasma choline of about 40% in trained athletes running a distance of 26 km. The reduction in plasma choline associated with strenous exercise thus may decrease acetylcholine release, thereby affecting endurance performance.

The neurotransmitters acetylcholine, catecholamine, and serotonin are synthesized from precursors normally obtained from the diet. The levels of these nutrients in the brain control the rates at which the neurotransmitter products are synthesized. A diet can thus control the synthesis of neurotransmitters in the brain, because the biochemical precursors of these neurotransmitters readily enter the brain tissue, and the rate-limiting enzymes of the neurotransmitter synthesis pathway are not saturated with precursor substrate at their physiological concentrations. These neurotransmitters have no feedback mechanism to inhibit their own synthesis. Therefore, the consumption of additional precursors, such as choline, tyrosine, or tryptophan, can generate more of the respective neurotransmitter products (i.e., acetylcholine, catecholamine, or serotonin). The concentration of these substances is known to influence blood pressure, sleep, memory, pain, and mood. An appropriate diet thus could influence the athlete's performance, his or her response to stress, decision-making ability, and fatigue. Conlay et al. (68) pointed out that the choline requirement for highly trained athletes has not yet been defined. A highly intensive training program may use up large quantities of choline for the synthesis of acetylcholine, potentially depleting membrane stores. Conlay et al. (68) hypothesized that supplemental choline may improve endurance or performance by increasing acetylcholine release, by improving signal transmission, or by enhancing the athlete's thought processes as well. Hollmann and Struder (67) concluded that differing quality and quantity of physical exercise as well as nutrition certainly influence human brain function, although many questions without answers remain as a challenge for further research work.

Scientific support for many observed associations between food intake and mood is sparse. Of particular interest are issues surrounding food intake, food cravings, and mood in women throughout the menstrual cycle (69). Research is needed to support or disprove current hypotheses about the relationship between food intake and mood, and to elucidate the complexity of factors that influence this relationship. Food intake appears to increase in premenstrual women, although the causes of food cravings or the usefulness of foods or nutrients to improve mood are not known. Some evidence indicates that a high-carbohydrate, low-protein meal will improve mood in women with premenstrual syndrome (PMS), but there are few data to demonstrate similar effects in healthy women or those with psychologic disorders such as depression. Women most likely crave foods such as carbohydrate and chocolate for their sensory properties (taste), rather than for the nutrient or bioactive compounds they contain (69).

REFERENCES

1. Westermarck, T., and E. Antila, Diet in relation to the nervous system, *Human Nutrition and Dietetics*, 9th ed. (J.S. Garrow and W.P.T. James, eds.), Churchill Livingstone, Edinburgh, London, 1993, p. 651.
2. Davidson, A.N., Biochemistry of the nervous system, *The Molecular Basis of Neuropathology* (A.N. Davidson and R.H.S. Thompson, eds.), Edward Arnold, London, 1981, p. 1.
3. Nicholls, D., A bioenergetic approach to nerve terminal, *Biochim. Biophys. Acta 1101*: 264 (1992).
4. Scott, J.M., P.N. Kirke, and D.G. Weir, The role of nutrition in neural tube defects, *Ann. Rev. Nutr.*, *10*: 277 (1990).
5. Neuringer, M., G.J. Anderson, and W.E. Connor, The essentiality of *n*-3 fatty acids for the development and function of the retina and brain, *Ann. Rev. Nutr. 8*: 517 (1988).
6. Anonymous, The nutritional role of fat, Marabou Symposium, *Nutr. Rev. 50* (Part II): 1 (1992).
7. Simeon, D.T., and S.M. Grantham-McGregor, Nutritional deficiencies and children's behaviour and mental development, *Nutr. Res. Rev. 3*: 1 (1990).
8. Grantham-McGregor, S.M., C.A. Powell, S.P. Walker, and J.H. Himes, Nutritional supplementation, psychosocial stimulation and mental development of stunted children: The Jamaican study, *Lancet 338*: 1 (1991).
9. Pollitt, E., J. Haas, and D. Levitsky, International conference on iron deficiency and behavioural development, *Am. J. Clin. Nutr. 50*: 565 (1989).

10. Singh, H.K., and B.N. Dhawan, Neuro-psychopharmacological effects of the ayurvedic noortropic *Bacopa monniera* L. (Brahmi), *Indian J. Pharmacol. 29*: 5359 (1997).

11. Wurtman, R.J., Nutritional control of brain tryptophan and serotonin, *Biochemical and Medical Aspects of Tryptophan Metabolism* (O. Hayaishi, Y. Ishimura and R. Kido, eds.), Elsevier Science Publications, Amsterdam, 1980, p. 31.

12. Krywawych, S., M. Haseler, and D.P. Brenton, Theoretical and practical aspects of preventing fetal damage in women with phenylketonuria, *Inborn Errors of Metabolism* (J. Schamb, F. Van Hoof, and H.L. Vis, eds.), Nestle Nutrition Workshop, Series Vol. 24, Raven Press, New York, 1991, p. 125.

13. Roufs, J.L., L-threonine as a symptomatic treatment for amyotrophic lateral sclerosis (ALS), *Hypotheses 34*: 20 (1991).

14. Cherkin, A., Interaction of nutritional factors with memory processing, *Nutrients and Brains Functions* (W.B. Essman, ed.), Karger, Basel, 1987, p. 72.

15. Horwitt, M.K., Ascorbic acid requirement of individuals in a large institution, *Proc. Soc. Exp. Biol. Med. 49*: 248 (1942).

16. Leitner, Z.A., and I.C. Church, Nutritional studies in a mental hospital, *Lancet 1*: 565 (1956).

17. Maas, J.W., G.C. Gleser, and L.A. Gottschalk, Schizophrenia, anxiety and biochemical factors, *Arch. Gen. Psychiatr. 4*: 109 (1961).

18. Briggs, M.H., Possible relations of ascorbic acid, ceruloplasmin and toxic aromatic metabolites in schizophrenia, *New Zeal. Med. J. 61*: 229 (1962).

19. Briggs, M.H., E.D. Andrews, G.B. Kitto, L. Segal, V. Graham, and W.J. Baillie, A comparison of the metabolism of ascorbic acid in schizophrenia, pregnancy and in normal subjects, *New Zeal. Med. J. 61*: 555 (1962).

20. Milner, G., Ascorbic acid in chronic psychiatric patients—a controlled trial, *Br. J. Psychiatr 109*: 294 (1963).

21. Baker, E.M., R.E. Hodges, J. Hood, H.E. Sauberlich, and S.C. March, Metabolism of ascorbic-1-^{14}C acid in experimental human scurvy, *Am. J. Clin. Nutr. 22*: 549 (1969).

22. Hodges, R.E., The effect of stress on ascorbic acid metabolism in man, *Nutr. Today 5*: 11 (1970).

23. Hodges, R.E., E.M. Baker, J. Hood, H.E. Sauberlich, and S.C. March, Experimental scurvy in man, *Am. J. Clin. Nutr. 22*: 535 (1969).

24. Baker, E.M. III., R.E. Hodges, J. Hood, H.E. Sauberlich, S.C. March, and J.E. Canham, Metabolism of ^{14}C-and ^{3}H-labeled l-ascorbic acid in human scurvy, *Am. J. Clin. Nutr. 24*: 444 (1971).

25. Hodges, R.E., J. Hood, J.E. Canham, H.E. Sauberlich, and E.M. Baker, Clinical manifestations of ascorbic acid deficiency in man, *Am. J. Clin. Nutr. 24*: 432 (1971).

26. Kinsman, R.A., and J. Hood, Some behavioral effects of ascorbic acid deficiency, *Am. J. Clin. Nutr. 24*: 455 (1971).

27. Grosz, H.J., The relation of serum ascorbic acid level to adrenocortical secretion during experimentally induced emotional stress in human subjects, *J. Psychosom. Res. 5*: 253 (1961).

28. Haas, R.H., Thiamin and the brain, *Ann. Rev. Nutr. 8*: 483 (1988).

29. Keyser, A., and S.F.T.M. De Brujin, Epileptic manifestations and vitamin B$_1$ deficiency, *Europ. Neurol. 31*: 121 (1991).

30. Dickerson, J.W.T., Nutrition and disorders of the nervous system, *Nutrition in the Clinical Management of Disease* (J.W.T. Dickerson and H.A. Lee, eds.), 2nd ed., Edward Arnold, London, 1988, p. 326.

31. Kuhne, T., R. Bubl, and R. Baumgartner, Maternal vegan diet causing a serious infantile neurological disorder due to vitamin B$_{12}$ deficiency, *Europ. J. Pediatrics 105*: 205 (1991).

32. Rosenberg, I.H., and J.W. Miller, Nutritional factors in physical and cognitive functions of elderly people, *Am. J. Clin. Nutr. 55* (Suppl. 6): 1237 (1992).

33. Holloway, K.L., and A.M. Alberico, Postoperative myeloneuropathy: a preventive complication in patients with B$_{12}$ deficiency, *J. Neurosurgery 72*: 732 (1990).

34. Garrett-Laster, M., L. Oaks, R.M. Russel, and E. Oaks, A lowering effect of a pharmacological dose of vitamin E on serum vitamin A in normal adults, *Nutr. Res. 1*: 559 (1981).

35. Sokol, R.J., Vitamin E and neurologic function in man. *Free Radical Biol. Med. 6*: 189 (1989).

36. Muller, D.P.R., Antioxidant therapy in neurological disorders, *Adv. Exp. Med. Biol. 264*: 475 (1990).

37. Santavuori, P., H. Heiskala, T. Westermarck, K. Sainio, and R. Moren, Experience over 17 years with antioxidant treatment in Spielmeyer-Sjogren disease, *Am. J. Med. Genet. 5* (Suppl.): 265 (1988).

38. Santavuori, P., H. Heiskala, T., Autti, E. Johansson, and T. Westermarck, Comparison of the clinical courses in patients with juvenile neuronal ceroid lipofuscinosis receiving antioxidant treatment and those without antioxidant treatment, *Adv. Exp. Med. Biol. 266*: 273 (1989).

39. Bates, D., Dietary lipids and multiple sclerosis, *Uppsala J. Med. Sci. 48* (Suppl.): 173 (1990).

40. Anonymous, DATATOP, deprenyl and tocopherol antioxidant therapy of Parkinsonism, Parkinson Study Group, *Arch. Neurol. 46*: 1052 (1989).

41. Fahn, S., An open trial of high-dosage antioxidants in early Parkinson's disease, *Am. J. Clin. Nutr. 53*(S): 380 (1991).

42. Beard, J.L., J.R. Conner, and B.C. Jones, Iron in the brain, *Nutr. Rev. 51*: 157 (1993).

43. Dobbing, J., Vulnerable periods in the developing brain, *Brain Behaviour and Iron in the Infant Diet* (J. Dobbing, ed.), Springer-Verlag, London, 1990, p. 1.

44. Dallman, P.R., M.N. Slimes, and E.C. Manies, Brain iron: persistent deficiency following short term iron deprivation in the young rat, *Br. J. Haematol. 31*: 209 (1975).

45. Dallman, P.R., and R.A. Spirito, Brain iron in the rat: extremely slow turnover in normal rat may explain the long-lasting effect of early iron deficiency, *J. Nutr. 107*: 1075 (1977).

46. Tucker, D.M., and H.H. Sandstead, Spectral electroencephalographic correlates of iron status: tired blood revisited, *Physiol. Behav. 26*: 439 (1981).

47. Tucker, D.M., H.H. Sandstead, R.A. Swenson, B.G. Sawler, and J.G. Penland, Longitudinal study of brain function and depletion of iron stores in individual subjects, *Physiol. Behav. 29*: 737 (1982).

48. Pollitt, E., Iron deficiency, *The Impact of Poor Nutrition and Disease on Educational Outcomes*, UNESCO Conf., Paris, 1990.

49. Lozoff, B., G.M. Brittenham, F.E. Viteri, A.W. Wolf, and J.J. Urrutia, Developmental deficits in iron deficient infants: effects of age and severity of iron lack, *J. Pediatr. 100*: 351 (1982).

50. Lozoff, B., G.M. Brittenham, A.W. Wolf, Iron deficiency anemia and iron therapy: effects on infant developmental test performance, *Pediatrics 79*: 981 (1987).

51. Lozoff, B., Behavioural aspects of iron deficiency in infancy, *Am. J. Clin. Nutr. 50* (Suppl.): 641 (1989).

52. Olanow, C.W., D. Marsden, D. Perl, and G. Cohen (eds.), Iron and oxidative stress in Parkinson's disease, *Ann. Neurol. 32* (Suppl): 1 (1992).

53. Drayer, B., P. Burger, B. Hurwitz, D. Dawson, and J. Cain, Reduced signal intensity on MR images of thalamus and putamen in MS, *Am. J. Neuroradiol. 8*: 413 (1987).

54. Connor, J.R., Proteins of iron regulation in the brain in Alzheimer's disease, *Iron and Human Disease* (R.B. Lauffer, ed.), CRC Press, Ann Arbor, 1992, p. 365.

55. Swaiman, K.F., Hallervorden-Spatz syndrome and brain iron metabolism, *Arch. Neurol. 48*: 1285 (1991).

56. Hallgren, B., and P. Sourander, The effect of age on the nonhaem iron in the human brain, *J. Neurochem. 3*: 41 (1958).

57. Rogers, S., Chemical sensitivity: breaking the paralyzing paradigm: how knowledge of chemical sensitivity enhances the treatment of chronic disease, *Internal Med. World Rep. 7*: 13 (1992).

58. Bhathena, S.J., L. Recant, N.R. Voyles, M. Fields, B.W. Kennedy, and Y.C. Kim, Interactions between dietary copper and carbohydrates on neuropeptides and neurotransmitters in CNS and adrenals, *Trace Elements in Man and Animals* (C. Momcilovic, ed.), 7: IMI, Zagreb, 1991, p. 13.

59. Nadal, D., and K. Baerlocher, Menke's disease: long-term treatment with copper and D-penicillamine, *European J. Pediatrics 147*: 621 (1988).

60. Henkin, R.I., B. Patten, P. Re, and D.A. Bonzert, A syndrome of acute zinc loss: Cerebellar dysfunction, metal changes, anorexia and taste and smell dysfunction, *Arch. Neurol. 32*: 745 (1975).

61. Dreosti, I.E., Zinc and the central nervous system, *Neurobiology of the Trace Elements*, Vol. 1. (I.E. Dreosti and R.M. Smith, eds.), Humana Press, Clifton, N.J., 1983, p. 135.

62. Safai-Kutti, S., Oral zinc supplementation in anorexia nervosa, *Acta Psychiatrica Supplementum 361* (82): 14 (1990).

63. Dumas, M., C. Giordano, and I.P. Ndiaye, African tropical myeloneuropathies, *Advances in Neurology* (J.S. Chopra, K. Jagannathan, and I.M.S. Sawney, eds.), Elsevier Science Publications, Amsterdam, 1990, p. 343.

64. Chan, M., Neonatal jaundice, *Diseases of Children in the Subtropics and Tropics*, 4th ed. (P. Stanfield, M. Brueton, M. Chan, M. Parkin, and T.E. Waterson, eds.), Edward Arnold, Sevenoaks, 1991.

65. Rivlin, R.S., Hormones, drugs and riboflavin, *Nutr. Rev. 37*: 241 (1979).
66. Ingvar, D.H., and L. Philipson, Distribution of cerebral blood flow in the dominant hemisphere during motor ideation and motor performance, *Ann. Neurol. 2*: 230 (1977).
67. Hollmann, W., and H.K. Struder, Exercise, physical activity, nutrition and the brain, *Nutr. Rev. 54* (Suppl.): 37 (1996).
68. Conlay, L.A., L.A. Sabounjian, and R.J. Wurtman, Exercise and neuromodulators: choline and acetyl-choline in marathon runners, *Int. J. Sports Med. 13* (Suppl. 1): 141 (1992).
69. Kurzer, M.S., Women, food and mood, *Nutr. Rev. 55*: 268 (1997).

35
Diet and Mental Health

I. INTRODUCTION

During the past couple of decades, researchers have demonstrated that the adult (developed) human brain is sensitive to normal variations in diet and nutrient intake; such variations, however, produce no clinical or biochemical evidence of malnutrition. Significant changes in macronutrient (protein and carbohydrate) and micronutrient (B vitamins and iron) intakes have been found to influence the synthesis of brain neurotransmitters, the chemical messengers of the brain. The functional and behavioral significance of such diet-induced changes in brain chemistry remain to be established fully. The current research is examining the association between marginal intakes of the micronutrients and poor cognitive performance in humans as well as the effectiveness of nutrients in the treatment of neurological disorders (1).

Hypotheses are being developed that sugar (sucrose) causes hyperactivity and that milk or sucrose causes juvenile delinquency. However, no plausible mechanisms by which these effects are brought about have been forwarded to support these hypotheses. Appropriate trials conducted to test the hypothesis that sucrose causes hyperactivity have shown quite the opposite results. Thus, although distinct and predictable biochemical changes in brain appear to be associated with dietary variations, their behavioral significance is at present unknown (1).

II. EFFECTS OF NUTRITION ON BRAIN BIOCHEMISTRY AND METABOLISM

A. Brain Metabolism

Malnutrition has been known to cause morphological and biochemical changes in the developing brain, the magnitude of such changes depending on both the timing and severity of the nutritional insult. However, the developed brain is much less likely to suffer permanent effects from nutrient deficiencies. The biochemistry of the adult (developed) brain is directly influenced by normal variations in nutrient availability, such as those occurring with the consumption of normal food (2–4). It is necessary to know whether or not these biochemical changes have any meaningful effects on brain functions such as behavior.

The fully developed human brain has around 100 billion nerve cells (neurons) and about an equal number of supporting or glial cells. Although the human brain weighs only 2% of total adult body weight, it receives 15% of cardiac output and accounts for 20% to 30% of the resting metabolic rate. The high energy requirement of the brain has not been related to protein synthesis, a high-energy-requiring process that occurs in the brain at an overall rate similar to that in muscle cells. The constant chemical processes required to release electrical energy of the brain probably account for most of the high energy needs of the brain. Despite its high energy requirements, the brain does not store energy-producing nutrients, and it heavily depends on a continuous supply of glucose and oxygen. Glucose permeates the blood-brain barrier readily, enabling influx of glucose to the brain in excess of its needs (see Chapter 34).

In addition to glucose, other nutrients required by the brain include fat, amino acids, vitamins, and minerals. Fat, taken up more slowly, supplies essential fatty acids and other lipids required to maintain the normal structure and composition of the brain, but it provides little energy, except during periods of the food deprivation, when metabolic adaptation takes place. Amino acids, taken up by specific mechanisms, play key roles in the brain as neurotransmitters as well as the precursors of proteins. Amino acids also serve as a small (10%) source of energy. The concentration of vitamins and minerals in the brain is influenced by their plasma concentrations (1).

Brain function primarily relies on active and effective communication among nerve cells and is relatively sensitive to the availability of various nutrients from the diet. Also, brain neurons use several substances as the chemical link for communication. Around 30 to 40 such substances have been identified as neurotransmitters, which are amino acids, monoamines, or peptides (see Table 1, Chapter 34).

Diet influences neuron function of the brain because the synthesis of most of the neurotransmitters depends on enzyme systems using nutrients as substrates and cofactors (1).

B. Brain Neurochemistry

Several food nutrients serve as precursors for the formation of neurotransmitters; e.g., consumption of relatively small quantities of the amino acids tryptophan or tyrosine or the vitamin choline enhances synthesis of the neurotransmitters serotonin, the catecholamines, and acetylcholine, respectively. Neurochemical changes in the brain occur especially after a meal of carbohydrate or of protein. Carbohydrate-rich meals preferentially enhance tryptophan uptake and serotonin synthesis, whereas high-protein meals tend to raise tyrosine levels and promote catecholamine synthesis, but reduce tryptophan levels and serotonin synthesis (2–4).

Many nutrients, such as pyridoxine, vitamin C, iron, copper, and zinc, act as coenzyme or cofactors of enzymes in the synthesis of neurotransmitters. It is not known whether the brain is more sensitive than other body tissues to fluctuations in dietary and plasma concentrations of these nutrients. Pollitt et al. (5) have related iron deficiency to cognitive test performance in preschool children and shown that some behaviors are altered (See Chapter 34).

It is known that amino acids, carbohydrates, vitamins, and minerals favorably influence synthesis of neurotransmitters and function of neuron systems. Newer evidence also indicates that the composition of dietary fat influences these factors. According to Foot et al. (6), dietary fat was reflected in the composition of neuron membranes when experimental animals were fed with varying quantities of polyunsaturated and saturated fatty acids. The physiochemical properties of the neuron membrane changed as its chemical composition altered. The function of certain proteins embedded in the neuron membrane depends on the lipid environment in which they exist. Thus, both membrane-bound enzymatic activities and the availability of receptor molecules are thought to be influenced by alterations in membrane composition and hence dietary fat.

III. DIET AND BEHAVIOR

Dietary substances most probably influence human behavior through their action in brain neurochemistry. After eating a sumptuous meal, one does not feel hungry, which has been accepted as a normal behavioral response. Sleepiness also has been recognized as a consequence of the consumption of a large meal. Researchers are now attempting to find out whether diet can be used to treat certain abnormal behaviors, such as affective disorders or criminal (aggressive) behaviors. There is a need to establish a relationship between diet and abnormal behavior.

The pharmacological loads of nutrients such as tryptophan, tyrosine, or choline, under certain circumstances, have been known to affect brain functions regulated by the neurotransmitters synthesized from these nutrients; e.g., tryptophan reduces appetite and causes sleepiness, and tyrosine may cause depression or mild Parkinson's disease in some people, whereas choline has shown beneficial effects in a condition known as tardive dyskinesia, wherein the use of neuroleptic drugs to treat schizophrenia induces a facial movement disorder (2,3).

The use of neurotransmitter precursor nutrients to treat neurological disorders has been promoted because these nutrients have relatively fewer side effects than the drugs. Also, the quantity of precursor nutrients needed to influence the behavior is within the range of usual consumption (1); e.g., 1 g tryptophan (the normal dietary intake) increases sleep (7), but a dose of 2 g tryptophan decreases appetite in healthy young adult males (8). However, the applications and benefits of neurotransmitter precursor therapy in the treatment of diseases of the central nervous system (CNS) or in the management of human behavior need to be established fully.

The effects of carbohydrate or protein in single meals on human brain serotonin and catecholamine synthesis have been studied. Spring et al. (9), noting differences in mood scales, reported that the response to high- versus low-carbohydrate diets differed with the age and sex of the individual and the time of the day the meal is consumed.

Deficiencies of micronutrients, the vitamins and minerals, have been well known to alter human behavior, although it is not known to what extent variation in nutrient intake, usually judged to be consistent with adequate diets, influences behavior. Oski et al. (10) and Pollitt et al. (5) studied effects of variations in body iron status, within ranges accepted as normal, on brain function in infants and children, respectively. It was shown that brain function in individuals with marginal iron deficiency, but without anemia, could be improved by iron supplements.

Goodwin et al. (11) obtained an indirect evidence of subtle relationships between nutrient status and brain function in the elderly population. These authors noted that individuals performing most poorly on IQ and memory tasks had the lowest intake and plasma levels of several vitamins of the B group, although biochemical and clinical evidence of vitamin deficiencies was absent. The effects of dietary improvement or nutrient supplementation on either IQ or memory of these individuals, to establish cause and effect, were not studied. It would be important to determine whether the nutrient adequacy of the brain is compromised by present standards of nutritional adequacy (1).

B. F. Feingold (12) hypothesized that the artificial food additive (colors and flavors) and naturally occurring salicylates in foods are associated with behavior disorders such as hyperactivity and learning disabilities in children. This publication steamed up interest in the relationship between diet and human behavior disorders. Based on Feingold's hypothesis, many hyperactive children were given additive (salicylate)- free diets. The initial compelling effects of the diets were that 50% to 70% of hyperactive children showed dramatic improvement in behavior; more elaborate, well-controlled double-blind studies, however, showed only marginal effects of additive-free diets, a small minority of children being benefitted. When hyperkinetic children who had shown improvement on the exclusion diet were challenged with a composite of artificial food dyes, they did not respond by behavioral changes (13,14).

According to the report of the Council for Agricultural Science and Technology (CAST) on Diet and Health (1), some investigators believe that the North American diet is probably negatively affected by food processing, supporting Feingold's hypothesis that sugar consumption causes hyperactivity and/or aggression in children. The data obtained in a study by Lester et al. (15) seem to support the hypothesis, indicating that the dietary proportion of refined carbohydrate foods negatively influence intellectual functioning in children. The CAST report has pointed out methodological flaws related to the inadequacy of 24-hour food records used to define habitual intake of individuals in this study. The use of associative data to suggest cause and effect also has been criticized. Because correlated data cannot identify cause and effect, the reported data could be interpreted to suggest that children with lower IQs eat a poorer diet than the children with higher IQs (16). Kruesi (17), in appropriate double-blind trials, disproved the hypothesis that sucrose causes hyperactivity. Behar et al. (18) noted that children given sucrose were less active than those given placebo. Thus, there are no research data to support the hypothesis that sugar causes hyperactivity and learning disabilities.

Rapoport and associates (19,20) reported that food substances other than nutrients, such as caffeine (5 mg/kg body weight twice a day), caused behavioral changes in children and adults (19). The behavioral effect of caffeine is modified by both the amount of caffeine that is consumed habitually as well as by individual personality characteristics (20).

Although many of the current postulations regarding relationships between abnormal human behavior and diet remain to be established, Pollitt et al. (21) demonstrated that learning ability and performance in children, measured midmorning, was improved after a breakfast meal, as compared with fasting. The results of a study by Gray and Gray (22), however, did not support the often-promoted view that food additives or sucrose (sugars) cause hyperactivity, and that milk or sucrose causes juvenile delinquency.

In an attempt to reduce antisocial behavior, several penal institutions have recently changed the diets fed to their inmates, focusing primarily on a reduction in sucrose consumption. Such dietary changes have not been supported with plausible mechanisms by which positive effects could be brought about and advocates have failed to conduct appropriate trials. Gray and Gray (22) have extensively reviewed the literature on the role that reactive hypoglycemia, food additives, food allergies, or dietary inadequacies and excesses may play in the etiology of juvenile delinquency and abnormal human behaviors. Meager evidence was found to support the theories that any of these factors play a role in delinquent behavior (22), and inadequate evidence is available to suggest that dietary changes or megavitamins therapy are effective in the treatment of antisocial behaviors.

Despite the ample evidence to indicate that normal diet and dietary substances have subtle effects on human behaviors, the significance of the association between diet and behavior, to either the etiology or treatment of central nervous system disease or of abnormal behaviors remain to be established (1).

IV. DIET AND DISEASES OF THE NERVOUS SYSTEM

The incidence of senile dementia, especially Alzheimer's disease, has caused serious health problems in the industrially developed countries of the Western world, including the United States, with large social and economic effects. It has been estimated that around 50% of all nursing home patients are affected by senile dementia (23), and about one-half of all the patients with senile dementia who have undergone autopsy suffered from Alzheimer's disease (24). Another estimate indicated that 22% of all individuals over 80 years of age in the United States have senile dementia of the Alzhimer's type, and that these individuals constitute the majority of the patients staying in nursing homes for extended periods of time (25). According to a report of the Select Committee on Aging 1984, the United States spends over $6.5 billion under Medicare for patients with Alzheimer's disease, the total cost to families being around $24 billion (26).

Despite the modern improvement in diagnostic techniques, it has not been possible to definitely diagnose a live patient as having Alzheimer's disease instead of some other form of dementia (27). The incidince of senile dementia in general, and of Alzheimer's disease in particular, is difficult to assess. The latter is generally characterized by progressive abnormalities in memory, behavior, and cognition, and is diagnosed upon autopsy by a distinctive type of structural degeneration in the brain cells.

Among the several etiologies proposed for Alzheimer's disease are included a deficit in the brain levels of choline acetyltransferase (the enzyme that synthesizes acetylcholine), deposition of aluminum in the brain, synthesis of abnormal brain proteins, and viral agents (23). Congenital factors may also be important in the etiology of senile dementia. The first two hypothesized causes of Alzheimer's disease, viz, choline acetyltransferase deficiency and aluminum toxicity, could theoretically be related to diet and nutrition, although the evidence relating diet to either of the incidence or treatment of Alzheimer's disease is very meager (24).

It has been established that the activity of choline acetyltransferase in the cerebral cortex and hippocampus formations of the brains of patients who died with Alzheimer's disease is reduced by 60% to 90%, compared with that of age-matched controls who died of unrelated causes (28). Several researchers have also found that increasing plasma and ultimately brain levels of choline increased the synthesis of acetylcholine in the brains of animal models and reduced memory impairment in old mice (29).

Bartus et al. (30), in 14 feeding trials, noted that feeding large doses of choline or lecithin (a dietary form of choline) had little or no effect on the memories or cognitive skills of patients with Alzheimer's disease. It is not likely that even pharmacologic doses of choline or lecithin will aid in the treatment of Alzheimer's disease, but cholinomimetic drugs may possibly help in the treatment of some patients with this condition (30).

Some investigators have suggested that excessive exposure to aluminum may influence the development of Alzheimer's disease, based on production of a neuro-fibrillar degeneration similar to that observed in patients with Alzheimer's disease in the brains of experimental animals by injecting (not feeding) aluminum salts (31–33). Also, several researchers have recorded elevated levels of aluminum in the brains of patients who died of Alzheimer's disease (34–36), although McDermott et al. (37) and Merkesbery et al. (38) could not confirm these observations.

It is known that many renal patients who accidently receive aluminum in dialysate fluids may develop symptoms of aluminum toxicity, including dementia. King et al. (39) and Sedman et al. (40) demonstrated that children receiving large oral doses of aluminum in pharmaceutical products developed symptoms of aluminum toxicity. According to Lione (41) and Greger (42), the amount of aluminum in the diets of Americans is manyfold smaller (20–40 mg/day) than the amounts consumed in pharmaceutical products such as antacids (840–5000 mg/day) and analgesics-buffered aspirin (126–728 mg/day). Dietary levels of aluminum (120 mg/day) appear to have little effect on the metabolism of young adults in a controlled study (43,44). This finding is not surprising, because aluminum consumed orally is rather poorly absorbed. The use of large doses of aluminum-containing pharmaceutical products by children who have renal problems appears to be contraindicated. Further research is needed to establish etiology and treatment of senile dementias, including Alzheimer's disease. There is little evidence to indicate that diet and nutrition are major factors in these conditions (24).

REFERENCES

1. Anonymous, Diet and behavior, Diet and Health, Report of the Council for Agricultural Science and Technology, No. 11, 51–54, March 1987.
2. Anderson, G.H., and J.L. Johnson, Nutrient control of brain neurotransmitter synthesis and function, *Can. Physiol. Pharmacol. 61*: 271, 1983.
3. Wurtman, R.J., Behavioral effects of nutrients, *Lancet 1*: 1145–1147, 1983.
4. Leprohon-Greenwood, C.E., and G.H. Anderson, An overview of the mechanisms whereby diet affects brain function, *Food Technol. 40*: 132–139, 1986.
5. Pollitt, E., R.L. Leibel, and D.B. Greenfield, Iron deficiency and cognitive performance in preschool children, *Nutr. Behav. 1*: 137, 1983.

6. Foot, M., T.F. Cruz, and M.T. Clandinin, Influence of dietary fat on the lipid composition of rat brain synaptosomal and microsomal membranes, *Biochem. J. 208*: 631, 1982.

7. Hartman, E., and D. Greenwood, Tryptophan and human sleep: An analysis of 43 studies, *Progress in Tryptophan and Serotonin Research* (H.G. Schlossburger, W. Kochen, B. Linzen, and H. Steinhard, eds.), de Gruyter, New York, 1984, pp 297–304.

8. Hrboticky, N., L.A. Leiter, and G.H. Anderson, Effects of L-tryptophan on short term food intake in lean men, *Nutr. Res. 5*: 595, 1985.

9. Spring, B., O. Maller, J. Wurtman, and L. Digman, Effects of protein and carbohydrate meals on mood and performance: Interactions with sex and age, *J. Psychiatr. Res. 17*: 155, 1983.

10. Oski, F.A., A.S. Honig, B. Helu, and P. Howanitz, Effects of iron therapy on behavior performance in nonanemic iron-deficient infants, *Pediatrics 71*: 877, 1983.

11. Goodwin, J.S., J.M. Goodwin, and P.J. Garry, Association between nutritional status and cognitive functioning in a healthy elderly population, *J. Am. Med. Assoc. 249*: 2917, 1983.

12. Feingold, B.F., *Why Your Child is Hyperactive?* Random House, New York, 1975.

13. Lewis, M.H., and R.B. Mailman, Development disorders and defined diets, *Cereal Foods World 29*: 152, 1984.

14. Taylor, E., Diet and behavior, *Arch. Dis. Child. 59*: 97, 1984.

15. Lester, M.L., R.W. Thatcher, and L. Monroe-Lord, Refined carbohydrate intake, hair cadmium levels, and cognitive functioning in children, *Nutr. Behav. 1*: 3, 1982.

16. Anderson, G.H., and N. Hrboticky, Approaches to assessing the dietary component of the diet-behavior connection, *Nutr. Rev. (Suppl.) 44*: 42, 1986.

17. Kruesi, M.J.P., Carbohydrate intake and children's behavior, *Food Technol. 40*: 150, 1986.

18. Behar, D., J.L. Rapoport, A.J. Adams, C.J. Berg, and M. Cornblath, Sugar challenge testing in children considered behaviorally "sugar positive," *Nutr. Behav. 1*: 277, 1983.

19. Rapoport, J.L., M. Jensvold, R. Elkins, M. Buchsbaum, H. Weingartner, C. Ludlow, T. Zahn, C. Berg, and A. Neims, Behavioral and cognitive effects of caffeine in boys and adult males, *J. Nerv. Ment. Dis. 169*: 7, 1981.

20. Rapoport, J.L., Effects of dietary substances in children, *J. Psychiatr. Res. 17*: 187, 1983.

21. Pollitt, E., R.L. Leibel, and D.B. Greenfield, Brief fasting, stress and cognition in children, *Am. J. Clin. Nutr. 34*: 1526, 1981.

22. Gray, G.E., and L.K. Gray, Diet and juvenile delinquency, *Nutr. Today 18(3)*: 14, 1983.

23. Thal, L.J., Senile dementia in the 1980's: Current concepts of the pathogenesis of senile dementia of the Alzheimer type, *Geriatr. Med. Today 3*: 86, 1984.

24. Anonymous, Diet and senile dementia, Diet and Health: Report of the Council for Agricultural Science and Technology, No. 11, 55–56, March, 1987.

25. Brody, E.M., M.P. Lawton, and B. Liebowitz, Senile dementia: Public policy and adequate institutional care, *Am. J. Public Health 74*: 1381, 1984.

26. Anonymous, Select Committee on Aging, Alzheimer's disease. Committee Publ. No. 98–402, U.S. Govt. Print. Office, Washington, D.C., pp 1–61, 1984.

27. Massey, E.W., and C.E. Coffey, Senile dementia in the 1980's: Modern therapeutic approaches, *Geriatr. Med. Today 3*: 104, 1984.

28. Coyle, J.T., D.L. Price, and M.R. DeLong, Alzheimer's disease: A disorder of cortical cholinergic innervation, *Science 219*: 1184, 1983.

29. Blusztajn, J.K., and R.J. Wurtman, Choline and cholinergic neurons, *Science 221*: 614, 1983.

30. Bartus, R.T., R.L. Dean III, B. Beer, and A.S. Lippa, The cholinergic hypothesis of geriatric memory dysfunction, *Science 217*: 408, 1982.

31. DeBoni, V., A. Otvos, J.W. Scott, and D.R. Crapper, Neuro-fibrillary degeneration induced by systemic aluminum, *Acta Neuropathol. 35*: 285, 1976.

32. Crapper, D.R., S. Quittkat, S.S. Krishnan, A.J. Dalton, and V. DeBoni, Intranuclear aluminum content in Alzheimer's disease, dialysis encephalopathy, and experimental aluminum encephalopathy, *Acta Neuropathol. 50*: 19, 1980.

33. Troncoso, J.C., D.L. Price, J.W. Griffin, and I.M. Parhad, Neurofibrillary axonal pathology in aluminum intoxication, *Ann. Neurol. 12*: 278, 1982.

34. Crapper, D.R., S.S. Krishnan, and S. Quittkat, Aluminum neurofibrillary degeneration and Alzheimer's disease, *Brain 99*: 67, 1976.

35. Perl, D.P., and A.R. Brody, Alzheimer's disease: X-ray spectrometric evidence of aluminum accumulation in neurofibrillary tangle-bearing neurons, *Science 208*: 297, 1980.

36. Crapper, D.R., R. McLachlan, B. Farnell, H. Galin, S. Karlik, G. Eichhorn, and V. Deboni, Aluminum in human brain disease, *Biological Aspects of Meals and Metal-Related Diseases* (B. Sarkar, ed.), Raven Press, New York, pp 209–218, 1983.

37. McDermott, J.R., I.A. Smith, K. Iqbal, and H.M. Wisniewski, Brain aluminum in aging and Alzheimer's disease, *Neurology 29*: 809, 1979.

38. Markesbery, W.R., W.D. Ehmann, T.I.M. Hussain, M. Alauddin, and D.T. Goodin, Instrumental neutron activation analysis of brain aluminum in Alzheimer's disease and aging, *Ann. Neurol. 10*: 511, 1981.

39. King, S.W., J. Savory, and M.R. Wills, The clinical biochemistry of aluminum, *CRC Crit. Rev. Clin. Lab. Sci. 14*: 1–20, 1981.

40. Sedman, A.B., G.N. Wilkening, B.A. Warady, G.M. Laum, and A.C. Alfrey, Encephalopathy in childhood secondary to aluminum toxicity, *J. Pediatr. 105*: 836, 1984.

41. Lione, A., The prophylactic reduction of aluminum intake, *Food Chem. Toxicol. 21*: 103, 1983.

42. Greger, J.L., Estimated aluminum content of typical diets in the United States, *Food Technol. (Suppl.) 39*:73, 76, 78–80, 1985.

43. Greger, J.L., and M.J. Baier, Excretion and retention of low or moderate levels of aluminum by human subjects, *Food Chem. Toxicol. 21*: 473, 1983.

44. Greger, J.L., and M.J. Baier, Effect of dietary aluminum on mineral metabolism of adult males, *Am. J. Clin. Nutr. 38*: 411–419, 1983.

36

Human Dietetics and Health:
An Integrated Approach

I. A BRIEF HISTORY OF WORLD AGRICULTURE

The health of a human population in a society depends not only on the supply of hygienic food with a high nutritional quality but also on several environmental factors, such as social and economic conditions, women's educational status, the implementation of immunization programs, availability of uncontaminated water, and overall agricultural development. In addition, clean housing and a pollution-free environment, as well as individual behavior relating to smoking and the use of alcohol and drugs, contribute to the health of the people. Food and nutrition influence the body's immunity through multiple complex mechanisms, and unspecified improvements in diet have contributed to the better health of people, as evidenced by the more affluent societies throughout the world in the 1950s. Life expectancy has increased substantially and progressively, with a remarkable fall in the death rates of children. In the undeveloped countries, however, improvements in diet, hygiene, and immunization have been less effective in decreasing childhood mortality.

Medical science has provided new understanding of the causes of disease, and the introduction of the germ theory of disease and the need for public hygiene created demands on national governments for public work based on hygienic principles and a concern for the evils of uncleanliness, foul air, and poor sanitation. Thus, public health professionals were able to force changes in medical education to emphasize the teaching of sanitary science (1).

Malnutrition was identified as a cause of ill health and poor physical and mental performance among the poor working classes of Britain in 1900, the extent of malnourished children in different areas ranging from 30% to 60%. A subsidized school meals service, started in 1906, provided needed protein and energy. By the 1920s, the dairy industry and the government promoted the consumption of milk, and cod-liver oil was added to prevent rickets. The use of milk was seen to be a suitable alternative to a whole meal and its growth-promoting properties were well recognized by the 1930s.

The amazing impact of the discovery of the vitamins on clinical medicine was evident soon, although the development of modern nutrition had to wait until the basis of meeting energy needs was established by Atwater and Benedict in the United States. The modest need for protein and essential amino acids was also reassessed by Chittenden. It the late 1920s, McCollum classified fruit, vegetables, and milk as "protective foods," animal dietary studies having provided the basis for establishing vitamin requirements. McCarrison, then head of India's National Institution of Nutrition, linked rat studies to human growth and deficiency disease. The discovery of vitamins and their benefits to growth and health of children fed with supplements of milk, meat, and other protective foods reemphasized the significance of diet for health.

In Britain, Fletcher and Mellanby, who were in charge of the British Medical Research Council from 1919 to 1949, were prominent in public health. Carefully thought out national nutrition policy was established, and nutrition education on protective foods was thought essential to improve children's health. The link between poverty, a poor diet, and poor health, emphasized by Boyd Orr in the 1930s, led to the provision of free milk to the vulnerable groups in society, i.e., to infants, schoolchildren, and pregnant and lactating mothers.

During and after World War II, all the national governments recognized the importance of having enough high-quality food for their peoples. Widespread starvation and concern for food supplies in Russia, Poland, and Germany in the 1930s dominated agricultural and food policies worldwide.

The combination of intensive nutrition education, a rationing system based on scientific principles, and the development of agriculture and food distribution policies ensured a balanced diet and the conquest of deficiency diseases in the 1940s. Massive American aid after the war and eventual food rationing in Europe helped the food industry ensure widespread availability of food with enough energy, protein, and micronutrients at the cheapest possible cost. Agricultural research and production being a priority, the production of meat, milk, and butter was enhanced substantially throughout Europe. With increased food supplies, food legislation and health policy were geared to ensure that the vulnerable groups in society received special attention (1).

During the 1950s, the emphasis on nutritional deficiency switched to the tropical world, where famine and specific deficiency diseases such as beriberi and pellagra were problems. Research into the nutritional basis of kwashiorkor and marasmus and the conquest of nutritional deficiency desease became an international priority. Postwar human nutritional research slowed down, but research into animal production was boosted. The United Nations Food and Agriculture Organization was established by Boyd Orr.

Food production became a priority in Europe and North America, with the proliferation of agricultural research institutes, the boosting of government subsidies to the farmers, and the development of free national agricultural advisory services. Marketing boards and farming cooperatives and price support schemes provided the needed incentive to increase production of milk, butter, and meat. Eventually there was an enough food for everybody to choose an enjoyable, balanced, and cheap diet with sufficient energy, protein, vitamins, and minerals.

New seeds of crops, use of fertilizers and mineral supplements, growth regulators, pesticides, and improved management techniques revolutionized agricultural production throughout the world. The steady fall in food prices came through a major success in the farming industry. Conversion of cereals to animal protein was adopted in the Western countries where agriculture proliferated. This process was found to be more expensive in ruminants such as cattle and sheep than in pigs. Thus, cheaper pork and bacon could be produced by improved management techniques. Chickens proved to be even more efficient converters of cereals into meat protein. Egg and chicken production also increased dramatically, with a fall in their prices.

Farm productivity was enhanced remarkably from 1945 to 1980, especially in Western Europe and the United States. Mountains of unsold food had to be stored before being disposed of in some way. The United States of America and EEC began to compete on the world market, selling cereals, butter, beef, and other foods below world prices to the Soviet Union and eastern Europe. The farmers in the developing countries had little incentive to produce crops for export. Thus, the affluence of European and North American farmers was preserved by the taxpayer at the cost of the rural poor in the developing countries. In the 1990s, Europeans were trying to adjust their subsidy policies, as a part of the long-standing international trading adjustment of the European Community's Agriculture Policy (CAP) to the General Agreement on Tariffs and Trade (GATT) (1).

II. CHANGING DIETARY PATTERNS WITH AFFLUENCE

A nation's state of affluence appears to determine the principal components of its diet, as evidenced by the fall in the consumption of starchy foods and the rise in animal fats and sugars. Simple sugars (sucrose and glucose) constitute over 50% of the total dietary carbohydrates in very affluent societies compared to 5% to 10% in many communities with a low income. Part of this change in the diet probably comes from the widespread cultural perception that freedom and affluence is part of the enjoyable Western lifestyle, so any affluent subsection in a developing country seeks to adopt a similar affluent lifestyle, which is promoted by the intense marketing of multinational companies of the West (e.g., Coca-Cola, MacDonald's, and Kentucky Fried Chicken). Despite their traditional diet, with a fat content of only 13% in 1963, (2), the Japanese increased their fat intake to 28% by the 1980s (3). Western snack foods and soft drink companies and tobacco firms have established their marketing strategies throughout the developing world by influencing international organizations, government ministers, and trade policies.

Food policies and diets in Eastern Europe and the developing countries have been based on the same nutritional principles developed in Western Europe and the United States of America, i.e., to provide enough energy, protein, and other nutrients to permit children to grow and adults to work. With the collapse of the Communist system, policy makers of Eastern Europe still perceive the people's needs in old-fashioned terms, with an emphasis on animal protein and fat production. With vegetables and fruits becoming scarce commodities in Eastern European countries, there were high rates of diabetes, hypertension, hypercholesterolemia, CHD, and diet-related cancers. Despite the well-established links between saturated fatty acid intake, elevated blood cholesterol, and heart disease, the dietary patterns of urban and rural dwellers in the same country showed marked differences, with higher intakes of fat, sugar, and salt in urban than in the rural areas. The latter often depend on the locally available staple cereals, tubers, vegetables, and fruits.

III. FOOD SAFETY AND SECURITY

The postwar emphasis on improving agriculture and food supplies for a balanced, nutritious diet also meant ensuring that foods were safe from toxic and antinutritional factors; this required development of complex regulatory procedures and food laws for compositional standards, nutritional needs, and food labeling. It was the responsibility of national governments to ensure toxicological and microbiological food safety; a balanced diet depended more on the consumer's choice, which in turn depended on general nutritional education. Food technologists and toxicologists financed by food industries soon dominated the advisory processes, nutritional issues being considered less important in the affluent societies. Food availability was thought to be based on a free market, despite large variation in food prices and sales resulting from agricultural subsidies and unscrupulous strategies. The FAO and WHO established a standing committee (Codex Alimentarius) to agree on internationally binding regulations for analytical methods, food labeling issues, and toxicological problems. Modern concepts of nutrition and dietetics were mostly ignored or were seen as a matter of the consumer's discretion not to indulge in the enjoyable foods rich in fat, sugar, and salt.

A common basis of food labeling includes standard displays of the absolute amounts of nutrients per 100 g of food product. However, the WHO, United States, United Kingdom and EC have produced different values for the RDA or other reference values, leading to consumer confusion. The issues of food labeling are perceived as the basis of nutrition policies in countries that emphasize health and nutrition education. In the Western countries concerned with reducing the fat and saturated fat content of the diet, foods are increasingly being labeled for their fat, carbo-hydrate, and protein content—although it is difficult to purchase foods according to individual need without knowledge of one's BMR and physical activity pattern. Food labels often fail to dis-play the real significance of the fat, sugar, or salt content in an understandable way. The food industry is reluctant to label food products in a manner that emphasizes their undesirable nutri-tional qualities.

Compositional standards were thought to provide a form of consumer protection; e.g., food products could be guaranteed to have a minimum content of meat, fat, or fruit, as well as to have enough protein, energy, and other nutrients to prevent adulteration of good-quality products. Leg-islation was required to specify standards for producing certain traditional food products such as cheeses and to protect special foods and drinks from being copied.

A growing consensus prevails that the food standards are old-fashioned and that there should be less regulation and a greater emphasis on nutrient declaration and education. However, many food companies compete on price by decreasing the more expensive ingredients, such as protein.

In northern Europe and the United States, over 70% of the food consumed has been processed, preserved, and/or packaged in one way or other. This has substantially increased the consumption of fat, sugar, and salt. New processing techniques have improved the flavor of food products by adding sugars, fats, salt, and spices to enhance their texture, crispness, and taste. Meats, salamis, and pies are manufactured from soya or other vegetable products to resemble any meat by adding special flavors, chemical binders, preservatives, and additives. With the avail-ability of low-priced foods, the poorer sections of the community had access to readily available and attractively packaged cheap foods.

In northern Europe and the United States, supermarkets provided cheaper food, often of high quality and in a far greater variety than available at a small local shop. During the 1970s and 1980s, the distribution and selling of food products by these supermarkets have been revolution-ized, taking over three-quarters of all food sales in the United Kingdom. In the 1990s, these super-markets realized that they can sell more profitably by concentrating on the quality of the product. In the West, there is a change from a cheap food policy based on earlier concepts of food being chosen as a social and enjoyable feature of life to new concerns for health. According to James (1), eating for health is once more on the national agenda of the Western countries for almost the first time since World War II.

International committees have been able to draw together evidence from all over the world on what constitutes a healthy diet. These committees now recommend the optimum range of nutrient intake to sustain the health of individuals of different ages. The modern nutritional approaches specify nutrient goals to limit the development of chronic diseases of adult life rather than prevention of deficiency diseases. These developments have been rather slow and have only emerged since the early 1960s (4).

Keys (5), in the Seven Country Study, for the first time established the nutritional basis for coronary heart disease (CHD). In volunteer medical students, Keys (5) demonstrated that stan-dard amounts of a specific type of saturated fatty acid increased total blood cholesterol to vary-ing degrees in different individuals, and that switching to diets rich in polyunsaturated fatty acids lowered blood cholesterol levels.

Keys and associates in public health soon began to advocate major changes in the eating pattern of Americans. The American Heart Association also then advocated a new diet based on reduction in total fat and saturated fatty acid intakes. This action was planned by a voluntary organization for the benefit of the public, leading to intense personal interest in health, with a fear that illness in middle and old age could become financially crippling.

In the United States and Canada, public health concerns have not resulted in coherent public policy as reflected in governmental action. According to James (4), Americans respond more readily to new ideas on the promotion of healthy living than Europeans, who remain passive, with government taking responsibility for policy-making for providing health care and for protecting the consumer.

Cannon (6) reviewed 100 different reports published on diet in relation to the chronic diseases of affluent societies. Norway was the first country to establish a national policy, the government taking steps through its many departments to promote all measures necessary to encourage its people to eat a healthy diet. Thus, Norwegians in 1974 changed agriculture, retail, tax, and food policies to reduce prevalence of CHD. Most other governments also have introduced schemes to rectify their original policies geared to promote animal products after the World War II. Cannon (6) showed that the many committee reports consistently distinguished between advice suitable for individuals and policies suitable for implementation at a population level. The new reports specify the ideal amounts of nutrients required by individuals, rather than advising people to eat less or more of a particular food. It has now been possible to integrate preventive programs aimed at controlling a range of diseases, such as obesity, cancer, and heart disease.

The developing countries still remain concerned with the problems of both undernutrition and malnutrition, with rapid increases in contagious diseases, obesity, heart disease, and cancers. Many countries are required to deal with the dual problems of malnutrition in the rural areas and chronic diseases of CHD and cancer in the urban communities. Despite these problems of hunger and diseases, the estimated life expectancies in Asia, Latin America, and Africa have increased from the 1950s to the 1980s and are expected to increase markedly over the next 30 years (Table 1). With a decrease in infant and childhood mortality, there is an increase in the proportion and total numbers of people living into old age. Many of these people who acquired immunity to prevalent infectious diseases may become susceptible to cardiovascular diseases and cancers if their dietary patterns are not appropriate, i.e., by excluding infant mortality, cardiovascular diseases and cancers account for a very high proportion of deaths in the developing world (Table 2) (7).

Table 1   Life Expectancy Trends at Birth for Different Regions of the World (Both Sexes Combined)

Region	1950–1955	1980–1985	2020–2025 (projected)
North America	69.0	74.6	79.7
Europe	65.3	73.2	79.1
Oceania	60.8	68.0	75.6
The former U.S.S.R.	64.1	67.9	76.7
Latin America	51.2	64.5	72.8
Asia	41.1	59.3	72.8
Africa	38.0	49.9	65.2
Developed countries	65.7	72.3	78.7
Developing countries	41.0	57.6	70.4
World total	45.9	59.6	71.3

Source: Ref. 7.

Table 2 Causes of Death in 1980 in the Developed and Developing Countries and World Total

Causes of death	Developed countries	Developing countries	World total
Diseases of circulatory system	54	19	26
Neoplasms	19	5	8
Infectious and parasitic diseases	8	40	33
Injury and poisoning	6	5	5
Perinatal mortality	2	8	6
All other causes	12	23	21

Source: Ref. 7.

IV. NUTRITIONAL GOALS AND DIETARY GUIDELINES

Nutrient goals are the average values of nutrient intakes that are appropriate to ensure optimum health. Intermediate targets may first be set before achieving the optimum nutrient goals, which may be far removed from the prevailing intakes in the society. The United Kingdom, the Netherlands, and Europe have developed such pragmatic policies. It is thought appropriate to consume complex carbohydrates to the extent of 50% of total energy intake by eating starchy foods of a wide variety (potato, bread, pasta, rice, or other cereals). The nutrient goals set on a scientific basis may be specified through dietary guidelines. Thus, there may be many culinary ways of achieving a nutrient goal. James and Ralph (8) described a scheme for converting goals into guidelines for the consumption of specific foods.

According to WHO (9), total fat intake should be 20% to 30% of energy, restricting saturated fatty acids below 10% (national average intake), although individual intake may vary. A population strategy is distinguished from prescribing diets for individuals, requiring a very different approach to policy-making, and the need to specify populations at risk. The average level of weight, blood pressure, serum cholesterol, fecal weight, or alcohol intake in a population are often seen as inappropriate because there is a close correlation between the mean body mass index (BMI) and proportion of the population that is obese. For most conditions of public health significance, the whole population tends to shift up or down, as the behavioral, eating, and drinking patterns change; this suggests that government strategies should consider the lifestyle of the whole population and not only the high-risk groups who can see their doctors for specific problems such as diabetes or hypertension.

More lives may be saved by tackling the modest risk that applies to a very large number of people with elevated blood pressure or serum cholesterol levels rather than by treating a small number of people at very high personal risk. An individual may take a small risk by being overweight, mildly hypertensive, or having a total blood cholesterol level of 5.5 mmol/l, but the government cannot provide huge resources for coronary care units and rehabilitation services for strokes or type II diabetes.

Taking a global view of diet in relation to health, WHO (7) produced a lower and an upper nutrient goal (Table 3). The lower fat intakes of the peoples of China, Indonesia, or southern India have been taken into account, because there is no perceived benefit from an intake of as high as 30%. The lower values for these populations seem reasonable, there being either no or only modest evidence of harm from changes in consumption between the lower and upper limits. Data given in Table 4 show an intermediate goal proposed by the WHO European office, signifying that the UK and Scandinavian countries would find a large-scale change in fat intake too daunting for immediate policy development (10).

Table 3 Population Nutrient Goals

	Limits for population average intakes	
	Lower	Upper
Total energy[a]		
Total fat (% total energy)	15	30[b]
Saturated fatty acids (% total energy)	0	10
Polyunsaturated fatty acids (% total energy)	3	7
Dietary cholesterol (mg/day)	0	300
Total carbohydrate (% total energy)	55	75
Complex carbohydrate (% total energy)[c]	50	70
Dietary fiber (g/day)[d]		
As non-starch polysaccharides	16	24
As total dietary fiber	27	40
Free sugars (% total energy)[e]	0	10
Protein (% total energy)	10	15
Salt (g/day)	[f]	6

[a]Energy intake should be sufficient to allow for normal childhood growth, for the needs of pregnancy and lactation, and for work and desirable physical activities and to maintain appropriate body reserves of energy in children and adults. Adult population on average should have a BMI of 20 to 22 [BMI = weight in kg/(height in m)^2].
[b]An interim goal for nations with high fat intakes; further benefits would be expected by decreasing fat intake toward 15% of total energy.
[c]A daily minimum intake of 400 g of vegetables and fruits, including at least 30 g of pulses, nuts, and seeds, should contribute to this component.
[d]Dietary fiber includes the nonstarch polysaccharides (NSP), the goals for which are based on NSP obtained from mixed food sources.
[e]These include monosaccharides, disaccharides, and other short-chain sugars.
[f]Not defined.
Source: Ref. 7.

The lower fat intake goal of 15% was chosen because too low a fat content often signifies a bulky diet with inadequate energy intakes for young children in the developing countries (Africa, Asia) and for very active adults, e.g., cane cutters of Central America. The average fat intake in China is about 14%, with only about 13% of the people having even first-degree chronic energy deficiency, i.e., with a BMI of 17.0 to 18.4. Also, on these fat intakes, a very small proportion of people is obese. The upper fat intake goal was chosen on a pragmatic basis to combat CHD, although Keys (5) recognized that total fat intakes in Greece and Crete were about 40%, with a substantial number of obese people having a very low rate of CHD. However, it was thought that in practice, reducing the total fat intake could also decrease saturated fatty acid consumption. Thus, an upper fat goal was specified in an attempt to decrease the prevalence of obesity with its many complications, in addition to any effect on CHD. The upper goal for total fat was also established because of concerns about the prevalence of cancers in many societies with high-fat diets. Animal experiments have shown that fat intake promotes carcinogenesis, and cancer epidemiologists have advocated lowering of fat intakes, even below 30%. This level is, however, not based on detailed assessment in case-control, prospective, or metabolic studies of the graded effects of fat on the risk of carcinogenesis. Thus, the upper level may be seen as one chosen pragmatically (4).

The proposed upper limit for saturated fatty acids (10% of energy intake) has been chosen arbitrarily. There is a gradient of risk from levels of 1% to 2% in rural China to those of 20% or

Table 4   Intermediate and Ultimate Nutrient Goals for Europe

	Intermediate goals		
	General population	Cardiovascular high-risk group	Ultimate goals
Energy[a] (%) derived from:			
Complex carbohydrates[b]	>40	>45	45–55
Protein	12–13	12–13	12–13
Sugars	10	10	10
Total fat	35	30	20–30
Saturated fat	15	10	10
P:S ratio[c]	<0.5	<1.0	<1.0
Dietary fiber (g/day)[d]	30	>30	>30
Salt (g/day)	7–8	5	5
Cholesterol (mg/4.18 MJ)	—	<100	<100
Water fluoride (mg/l)	0.7–1.2	0.7–1.2	0.7–1.2

Alcohol intake should be limited. Iodine prophylaxis should be applied when necessary and nutrient density should be increased: A BMI of 20 to 25 is both an intermediate and an ultimate goal, although this value is not necessarily appropriate for the developing world, where the average BMI may be around 18 (4).
[a]All the values given refer to alcohol-free energy intakes.
[b]The complex carbohydrate figures are implications of the other recommendations.
[c]This is the ratio of polyunsaturated to saturated fatty acids.
[d]Dietary fiber values are based on analytical methods that measure nonstarch polysaccharide and the enzyme-resistant starch produced by food processing or cooking methods.
Source: Ref. 4.

more in Scotland in the 1970s and in Eastern Europe in the 1990s. For this reason, WHO (7) has specified 0% as the lower limit, signifying that there was no lower limit below which there was no further reduction in risk.

The proposed goals for polyunsaturated fatty acid (PUFA) intakes, however, are difficult to justify. A minimum intake of essential fatty acids is thought to be about 1% of total energy, so the chosen 3% value is in keeping with this. The originally chosen upper limit of 10% involved a concern regarding the possible free radical inducing effect of high PUFA levels, although the latter are often associated with higher intakes of antioxidants like alpha-tocopherol. The P to S ratio is not considered at present a suitable index, because the primary benefit derived is essentially from a lower saturated fatty acid intake.

A recent report of a Joint Expert Consulation (11) on Fats and Oils in Human Nutrition has provided minimum desirable intakes of fats and oils for adults, infants, and young children, giving upper limits of fat/oil intakes. This report has also given recommendations for saturated and unsaturated fatty acids and cholesterol, isomeric fatty acids, and substances associated with fats and oils, such as antioxidants, carotenoids, and essential fatty acids (see Chapter 22 for details).

With no need for refined sugar in the diet and its adverse effects on dental caries well established, WHO (7) has set the lower goal for sugar at 0% of energy intake. The upper goal of 10% of total energy was chosen from epidemiological studies, with several authorities suggesting goals corresponding to 7.5% to 15% of energy, despite the original claims made for the role of sucrose in inducing hypertriglyceridemia, CHD, and diabetes.

Recently, attempts have been made to establish goals for intakes of dietary fiber, which is now defined to be the nonstarch fraction of the dietary polysaccharides (NSP) that resists digestion by alpha-amylases in the intestine. This fraction is found in the plant cell wall, its intake having profound effects on both the small and large intestine. There is a great interest in the role of dietary fiber in the prevention of colonic diverticular disease and large bowel cancer and the effects of NSP in prevening constipation by increasing fecal bulk. A large number of physiological feeding studies, in which mean daily fecal weight was the measured effect, has shown that constipation occurs at fecal weights below 100 g and transit times lengthen at fecal weights below 150 g. So a goal of 150 g daily, correponding to an NSP intake of about 22g/day, was used. A value of 32 g of NSP was chosen as the upper limit beyond which no further benefit could be derived. These values of 22 and 32g of NSP were obtained from northern European and American adults and had to be modified to take account of the shorter, lighter, populations of the world. Thus the lower and upper values of 16 g and 24 g of NSP have been set as nutrient goal (Table 3).

The values for complex carbohydrates are obtained by subtracting the specified fat and protein values from the total energy intake, because there are few studies specifying how much starch is required for health. Starchy foods are often rich in micronutrients and have other effects in terms of bulking the food and slowing the passage and diffusion of nutrients.

It is unusual to find societies not complying with the protein intake limits of 10% and 15% of the energy intake. However, the requirements of essential amino acids are now thought to be higher in adults than were proposed earlier. With tacit support from FAO/WHO (12), Young et al. (13) have revised the FAO/WHO/UNU values for the essential amino acids, which were too low. New nutrient goals for protein may emerge in due course from detailed physiological and nutritional studies. The latest proposal—that adults should have the same amino acid ratios as children at the minimum protein intake—may trigger the need for a profound change in agricultural production to ensure that enough animal protein is consumed by the people.

Quantitative goals are often more useful than the vague suggestion that "moderation in everything" or "choosing a variety diet" is the key to health. The WHO committee has now suggested that a dietary as well as nutrient goal could be developed, with a healthy population eating on average 400 g of vegetables (excluding potatoes) plus fruit daily and 30 g of pulses; these values were taken and developed from data on Mediterranean food patterns because the protective role of vegetables and fruit in relation to many diseases is difficult to assign to any specific nutrient.

After setting the nutrient goals, nutritionists and dietitians should interpret them in relation to prevailing nutrient intakes and dietary patterns. Migrant studies have shown that people of different racial and cultural groups respond rather uniformly to diet, though the nutrient goals set can be achieved in different ways. Thus, these goals need not specify the dietary changes required. However, appropriate dietary guidelines are needed, which can be developed as general national targets or as individual guidelines (4).

Governments are responsible for implementing national starategies for changes in the dietary patterns of their peoples. In addition to the Department of Agriculture, Fisheries and Food, the education for nutrition and health in the United Kingdom involves responsibilities of several other government departments, such as Employment, Environment, Foreign Affairs, Health and Safety Commission, Information, Trade and Industry, Education and Science, Energy, Finance, Health, Home Office, Social Security, and Transport. Thus, social policy will influence the purchasing power of the poor, and differential tax rates on food may make some food products costly. Import/export regulations limit or extend the variety of food products available in a country. Even within the Ministries of Agriculture and Health, a range of policies may influence the production, processing, distribution, and retailing of food in different ways. The promotion of fluoridation, for example, can have a marked influence on dental caries.

Postwar food policies in most countries have distorted the marketplace by allowing food marketing monopolies and cooperatives to develop. Such vested interests often promote the sales of individual food products rather than appropriate government policies for influencing dietary patterns.

James (4) suggested that governments should influence food patterns by establishing standards for catering in official institutions, such as government offices, schools, hospitals, prisons, and the armed forces. Health service can provide information, advice, and practical help in changing diets, because a majority of the population attends a primary health care unit each year.

The health departments are often overwhelmed by Ministries of Finance, Trade, Foreign Affairs, and Agriculture, which have a profound influence on food prices and policies. The health promotion aims at the development of institutional changes, but the health departments usually end up promoting health education alone. WHO (7) proposed the active involvement of voluntary and nongovernmental organizations (NGOs) by the Ministry of Health for the effective stimulation of government action.

The U.K. government has stimulated an effective action by setting targets for changes in dietary behavior and reductions in disorders such as obesity and premature deaths from heart disease and some cancers. A new approach to nutrition policy making was taken in 1991 by accepting that many government departments are involved in the nutrition education of the public. The cabinet-approved White Paper (14) adjusted and extended the targets by newly analyzing public health policy changes. It has been envisaged that the next decade will bring astonishing changes in the social food patterns for the overall health of the people.

In his keynote address given at the Symposium on Diet, Nutrition and Health: An update, held at The University of Western Ontario, June 16 to 19, 1996, Dr. W.P.T. James, Director of the Rowett Research Institute in Aberdeen, Scotland, stated that nutrition research was entering a new era because of the recognition of the nutritional basis of several public health problems. Current initiatives in the United Kingdom, The Netherlands, France, Denmark, and Germany have been supported by the agricultural research sector, stemming from concern for the food supply. Surveillance systems in Europe continue through the MONICA (monitoring of CVD) programs run by WHO centers. The epidemiological evidence of the changing mortality rates for coronary heart disease (CHD) has implicated new factors, such as antioxidants, specific fatty acids, nutrient-gene interactions, fetal nutrition, and syndrome X. Dr. James emphasized the importance of establishing public health policies that recognize the interplay of agricultural, industrial, and governmental sectors in addition to food and health sectors (15).

In addition to the above remarks by Dr. James, the following significant observations were noted in the symposium (15):

1.   The cardiovascular mortality rates in Hungary are among the highest in the world, and health indices are declining in Russia. Substantial improvements are occurring in the Czech Republic and the former East Germany, while Poland, Bulgaria, and Romania display little change. The CVD rates are associated with risk patterns that shift with food prices, food availability, and prevention programs.

2.   A dramatic decrease in coronary mortality rates has occurred in Denmark, Finland, Iceland, Norway, and Sweden since 1970, which is associated with decreased fat intake and increased intake of fruit and vegetables. Other factors include improved treatment of CHD; promotion of lower salt intake; addition of selenium to fertilizer since 1985, leading to increased antioxidant effect; and availability of phytoestrogens in rye and soy.

3.   The decreasing rate of CHD in the European population, in contrast to the increasing rate in indigenous peoples, appears to be related to acculturation. In the European population that settled in New Zealand about 150 years ago, the decreasing CHD rate is related to reductions in smoking, blood pressure, total cholesterol, and saturated fat intake. In the Maori, who have resided in New Zealand for a thousand years, syndrome X prevails and, CHD mortality is more than double the rate in the European population. The Pacific Islanders who migrated recently to

New Zealand have switched their diet from a diet high in coconut oil (53% fat and 45% saturated fat) to a diet lower in total fat, but containing hydrogenated vegetable oils. The result: the total cholesterol, low-density lipoproteins, BMI, and blood pressure of these people have all increased. The favorable effects of coconut oil and safflower oil on blood lipids compared to the adverse effects of butter and fats containing *trans* fatty acids have been demonstrated. For the Maori and Pacific Islanders, weight loss, physical activity, and increased intake of *cis* monounsaturated fats are very important, whereas New Zealand's national recommendation to decrease fat intake to 20% is most applicable to the European population.

4.   The diets of four population groups with low CHD rates have been described: traditional Japanese, Greenland Eskimos, Tarahumara Indians, and Mediterranean people. The protective factors in the diets of these populations are polyunsaturated fat, both *n*-6 and *n*-3, monounsaturated fat, soluble fiber, antioxidants, especially vitamin E, saponins, folic acid, and vegetable protein. The pathogenic nutritional factors for CHD are dietary cholesterol, saturated fat, *trans* fatty acids, total fat, total calories, and alcohol. To quantitate the main harmful dietary factor, Dr. William E. Conner of the Division of Endocrinology, Department of Medicine, Oregon Health Sciences University, Portland Oregon, has developed a cholesterol–saturated fat index (CSI = 1.01 × g saturated fat + 0.05 × mg cholesterol) which is 14 for a serving of beef and 3 for a serving of fish. An average American diet has a CSI of 23; the Japanese diet, 13; and clinical diets for treatment of hypercholesterolemia, 8. Dr. Conner's "Alternative American Diet" recommends 20% to 25% fat, 15% protein, and 60% to 65% carbohydrate as starch, not refined sugars. Dietary therapy should be the mainstay for prevention and treatment of hyperlipidemia and CHD.

5.   Hypertension has a high prevalence, contributing about 30% to the risk of CVD. While it is essential to control hypertension with medication, the interplay between dietary, genetic, and lifestyle factors that influences the development of hypertension and syndrome X has been emphasized. Excessive consumption of fat and alcohol contributes to abdominal obesity, insulin resistance, and high blood pressure, which are linked to type II diabetes mellitus, hyperlipidemia, and coronary artery disease. Current trials have shown that weight loss, exercise, and restriction of sodium and alcohol have beneficial metabolic effects and enhance the effect of drug therapy.

6.   Diet and kidney disease has been discussed, focusing on the current controversy regarding protein restriction. Although a low protein diet may slow the progress of chronic renal disease, the nutritional adequacy of the diet must be considered first. Protein intake must be maintained to prevent low serum albumin levels, which are associated with a high mortality rate, and to balance the degree of proteinuria. A diet low in saturated fat and cholesterol will help to prevent atherosclerosis. The pilot studies have shown that lovastatin, a drug that inhibits cholesterol synthesis, significantly prevents progression of renal disease. Treatment with antihypertensive drugs is also effective in retarding the progression of renal disease but may not be as effective with a high-fat diet. Because diabetes is the leading cause of end-stage renal disease, adherence to a diabetic diet with strict control of blood glucose is very important in these patients. The progression of renal disease and development of other diabetic complications have been shown to be delayed by intensive insulin therapy and tight glucose control in the Diabetes Control and Complications Trial.

7.   The dietary guidelines for diabetes mellitus have been reviewed. The 1994 guidelines of the American Diabetes Association recommend a diet of 20% protein, 10% saturated fat, and 5% polyunsaturated fat with the remainder, 60% to 70% to be composed of carbohydrate plus monounsaturated fat. The amount of carbohydrate is listed without regard for its type and no specific role has been identified for fiber in the treatment of diabetes. Dr. Thomas M.S. Wolever, of the Department of Nutritional Sciences, University of Toronto, has stressed the importance of the nature of the carbohydrate, advocating foods with a low glycemic index and high fiber content. The beneficial effects of monounsaturated fatty acids have been discussed, with the point made

that a high-fat intake is not in accord with the recommendations for reducing the risk of obesity, cancer, and heart disease. Moreover, the beneficial effects of monounsaturated fatty acids on blood glucose can be produced without a high-fat intake by the use of soluble fiber and foods with a low glycemic index. The need for dietary advice based on food items rather than on the theoretical amounts of nutrients has been emphasized to improve compliance.

8.   The current concepts regarding the association between obesity and macronutrient balance show that nutrient balance occurs when the composition of the nutrients oxidized in the body corresponds to the nutrient composition of the food intake, and when the respiratory quotient (RQ) is equal to the food quotient (FQ). Weight gain and obesity result from excess intake, especially of fat, because dietary fat has a hyperphagic effect and is converted to body fat more readily than protein and carbohydrate. Excess protein and carbohydrate intake do not alter balances of body protein and carbohydrate; instead the excess is converted to fat. In contrast, body fat stores can expand enormously and do not appear to be tightly regulated despite the recent discovery of the fat-regulating hormone, leptin. In the developed countries, eating patterns present a metabolic stress due to overconsumption of fat, exacerbated by the high energy density of the foods. Alcohol, often consumed in addition to food, increases energy imbalance, promotes visceral obesity, and produces a synergistic effect with fat intake. The abnormal fat balance is probably the major contributor to the present epidemic of obesity.

9.   The immense economic and social burden of acute and long-term costs due to osteoporosis has been outlined. The key risk factors for osteoporosis are early menopause, family history, advanced age, and small body build or thinness. Calcium and vitamin D in childhood are important to maximize peak bone mass and retard bone loss in adult life. Weight-bearing exercise, maintenance of muscle mass, and good nutrition, with particular attention to lifelong calcium intake, will increase bone mass and decrease fracture rates. Animal protein was previously thought to increase urinary calcium loss, but now animal protein is considered important for maintaining nutritional adequacy and promoting trophic effects on bone, especially in the elderly. Calcium supplements decrease the rate of bone loss in postmenopausal women, and along with vitamin D significantly decrease the rate of fractures in elderly individuals. Calcium is best obtained from food sources and vitamin D by exposure to the sun, but supplements of both may be necessary, especially in view of the higher intakes recommended by the Osteoporosis Society.

10.   The deleterious effects of "empty" calories, vitamin interactions, and carcinogenesis due to alcohol intake have been highlighted. Because alcoholic beverages are often added to dietary intake, they will promote obesity, depending on lifestyle, diet, and drinking patterns. High alcohol intakes are classically associated with thiamin deficiency and deficiencies of folate, beta-carotene, retinoic acid, and pyridoxal phosphate; also, loss of antioxidant vitamins may be precipitated by high alcohol intake. Tissue damage caused by the oxidative stress of alcohol metabolism and the procarcinogenic action of ethanol can be moderated by the protective effects of antioxidants. The French paradox—the putative protective effects of moderate alcohol intake on ishemic heart disease—has also been discussed. This phenomenon is attributed to flavonoids in red wine that decrease lipid peroxidation. Although CHD is inversely related to intake of wine in European countries, correlation is also high with intake of alpha-tocopherol and positive for milk and lactose intake. Thus, several dietary constituents and confounding factors influence the risk of CHD, and the benefits of red wine are probably overrated.

11.   The consumption of an optimum diet by all the people would have a much greater chance of reducing avoidable illness. Dr. Ernst L. Wynder, president of the American Health Foundation, New York, expounded on the following three principles: (a) that most chronic diseases are due to metabolic overload, (b) that humans are meant to die not of disease, but of the natural interplay of genetic constitution and life cycle, and (c) that the known etiologies of these diseases must be used to develop preventive measures. A large portion of the decline in CVD and

cancer has been attributed to the strong social pressure against smoking. Experimental evidence clearly indicates the impact of type and amount of dietary fat in carcinogenesis. The importance of education, the media, and the food industry has been emphasized in optimizing nutrition for a given population. Hyperlipidemia and obesity begin during childhood, and smoking at a young age escalates the risk of heart disease, so preventive measures for children will have great impact. Nutritionists are urged to be more active and aggressive in order to provide proper nutrition education for children.

12.   The nutritional problems of elderly people have been discussed. As the proportion of senior citizens in developed countries will exceed all other age groups in the next 25 years, nutritional problems that arise with aging must be given increased attention. One primary problem is the malnutrition due to low overall dietary intake in senior citizens. The challenges of meeting their nutritional needs include identifying the population at risk and revising the recommended intakes to compensate for low intakes. The practical approach should encourage physical activity, seek to maintain appetite, assist in shopping and meal preparation, and utilize nutrient-dense foods.

13.   The isolation of carcinogenic heterocyclic amines that occur in cooked meats and fish has been emphasized. By analyzing urine samples, it has been shown that humans are continuously exposed to low levels of these amines, which cause mutations by forming DNA adducts. These have been detected in human colon, rectum, and kidney. This finding may account in part for the association between meat intake and colorectal cancer. The cooking time and temperature influence the formation of these carcinogens; antioxidants can suppress their formation. Exposure to heterocyclic amines can be reduced by limiting the intake of meats and fish cooked at high temperatures.

14.   The mortality rates for stomach cancer and stroke are highly correlated and both are positively associated with salt and negatively associated with consumption of fruits and vegetables. Some independent factors include nitrate intake, which is positively associated only with stomach cancer, whereas saturated fat intake is positively and polyunsaturated fat is negatively correlated with stroke mortality. The European Cancer Prevention (ECP)—Intersalt Study showed that nitrate intake is beneficial at salt intakes of less than 10 g per day but is harmful at higher levels. In low-salt diets, most of the nitrate is derived from vegetables, which also provide protective antioxidants. The incidence of stomach cancer is falling in different countries as refrigeration is becoming available, making the use of salt as a preservative unnecessary. The effect of chronic high-salt intake on blood pressure accounts for the relationship between salt intake and stroke mortality. The preventive strategies for both stomach cancer and stroke thus include low intake of salt and high intake of fruits and vegetables.

15.   The rates of both breast and colon cancer continue to be positively associated with fat and negatively associated with dietary fiber. Alcohol intake, inactivity, and increased body size are also risk factors for both types of cancer. Despite these common risk factors, the etiology of breast cancer is attributed to factors that alter estrogen levels, and the development of colorectal cancer is linked to fecal bile acids. However, a common mechanism may be involved in both types of cancer, viz., syndrome X, because cancer incidence is associated with diseases such as obesity and diabetes that feature insulin resistance. To minimize risk of breast and colon cancer, the slogan is " eat plants, not animals," to reduce fat intake, increase fruits and vegetables, minimize salt intake, and avoid carcinogens.

16.   The evidence demonstrating that tumor incidence is inhibited by caloric restriction has been reviewed. This effect may be due to prevention or relief from metabolic overload. Even the deleterious effect of dietary fat may be modified by restricting food intake in rats. Animal experiments have shown that a 20% restriction of energy intake results in decreased plasma insulin, increased insulin sensitivity, and higher antioxidant enzyme levels. In humans, there is a

positive relationship between obesity and cancer incidence; on the other hand, life-long vigorous activity is negatively related to cancer mortality. Energy restriction increases the activities of enzymes involved in antioxidant reactions, enhances DNA repair, and reduces expression of oncogenes. Thus, a modest reduction in energy intake may decrease cancer risk in humans.

In this symposium, the 1996 nutrition plan for Canada, Nutrition for Health: An Agenda for Action, was presented. Although the nutritional health of most Canadians is good, inequities exist and dietary patterns contribute to the high incidence of CVD, cancer, and obesity. Strategies identified are to reinforce healthy eating practices, to support nutritionally vulnerable populations, to enhance the availability of foods that support healthy eating, and to support nutrition research. This plan, it is hoped, will act as a catalyst for implementation of these strategies and will support the integration of nutrition considerations into health, agriculture, education, social, and economic programs (15).

V. VEGETARIANISM, AGING, AND LONGEVITY

According to a popular saying, "We are what we eat, nothing more, nothing less." Easton, as early as 1799, wrote a volume, 'Longevity,' in which biographical data are presented on individuals who lived to the age of 100 years or more. All these centenarians appeared to have one thing in common—they ate rather sparingly and were physically more active. Wynder et al. (16) have reviewed the role of diet in the maintenance of health throughout life and attempted to answer the question: What is the optimal diet that is conducive to the avoidance of illness and permits youthfulness throughout a long life? According to another popular saying in India, of what we eat, only half is required by the body, the remaining half is for the doctor (physician). Although deficiency diseases are virtually nonexistent in the developed world, nutrition-related diseases in the West are now largely a consequence of nutritional excesses. Most of the dietary problems of the developed world relate to a general problem of metabolic overload. Physiological systems of detoxification, packaging, and regulation cannot handle the onslaught of tobacco smoke to the respiratory organs, the deluge of a heavy alcohol intake on the liver and the excessive intake of macronutrients such as fat and cholesterol.

The mechanisms whereby nutritional overloads induce disease are being elucidated; however, the history of medicine has taught us that there is no need to understand fully the pathogenesis of a disease to prevent it. Therefore, the diets of the largely sedentary population must be modified to the extent that they become tuned to their metabolic capacities. The slogan that "medicine should help humans to die young as late in life as possible" can become a reality when the human race tunes its nutritional intake and other aspects of lifestyle to the basics of longevity. Perhaps humans need not die of disease but simply pass from life when the genetic time clock of biological existence has run its predetermined course. This goal appears to be medically feasible and physically imperative (16).

Vegetarian diets are rather heterogeneous, as are their effects on nutritional status, health, and longevity. Vegetarian diets avoid different animal foods and encompass various health-related attitudes and widespread philosophical and religious beliefs. According to Walter (17) vegetarianism is often considered to be a special lifestyle, because many vegetarian people do not smoke, drink little alcohol, and engage in more than average physical exercise. While evaluating results with vegetarians, these factors related to different lifestyle patterns must also be taken into account.

A vegetarian is often defined as a person who does not eat animal flesh (meat, poultry, fish) and a strict vegetarian, or vegan, specifically excludes all animal products, including milk and dairy products as well as eggs. This diet thus consists mainly of plant foods such as fruits, vegetables, legumes, grains, and nuts. A lacto-vegetarian eats dairy products, whereas a lacto-ovo-vegetarian consumes both dairy products and eggs. Considerable differences exist in the choice of plant foods, even within the classification of these diets. The "New Vegetarians" in parts of the Netherlands and the United States, for example, following the teachings of Ohsawa (18), prefer only natural, unprocessed foods, called macrobiotics, consisting of relatively large amounts of brown rice with smaller quantities of fruits. Vegan-fruitarians restrict their diet to raw fruits, nuts, and berries (17).

Good nutrition during growth is an essential basis for health in old age, and therefore nutritional risks should be avoided, especially during the early years of life. Even after the growing period, nutrition remains a crucial factor for maintenance of good health and prevention of disease in later years. Recent reviews of the literature (19–21) have shown more specific effects of vegetarian diets on human health, dealing with the risks on the one hand and with the beneficial effects on the other, both being important for longevity. Many recent studies have produced strong evidence for an inverse relationship between vegetable/fruit intake and various types of cancer, for a relationship between type of dietary fat and CHD (21), and for the effect of dietary fiber intake on mortality from CHD, cancer, and other disorders (22). These nutritional aspects are directly related to vegetarian diets.

A reasonably varied source of plant proteins can provide adequate amounts of the essential amino acids; e.g., maize, with a protein low in lysine, should be combined with beans, high in lysine. Soya protein, which has been found to be nutritionally as good as animal protein, can serve as a main source of protein intake. Vegetarians who eat eggs and dairy products often have adequate protein supplies, although vegans should be more careful to combine various plant proteins to avoid a deficiency of certain essential amino acids. The requirement of protein in the diet of adults has been debated (23). According to Young and Pellet (24), requirements for essential amino acids cannot be fulfilled by diets based only on cereals, unless at least 30% of total protein is obtained from animal sources or at least 40% of total protein is derived from animal sources plus a meat substitute such as soya protein.

Micronutrient deficiencies of vitamins B_{12} and D_3 as well as of iron and zinc are an important concern in vegetarian diets. Vitamin B_{12} is present in substantial quantities only in animal foods, and its deficiency is a matter of concern in diets that are partially or totally devoid of animal sources. Vegan diets are most likely to be deficient in vitamin B_{12} (25,26). Depletion of vitamin B_{12} stores in vegans is slow, depending on the initial body vitamin B_{12} pool. Thus, symptoms of vitamin B_{12} deficiency arise slowly but are nevertheless very dangerous. Children of vegan women with low vitamin B_{12} stores may be exposed to acute cobalamin deficiency (27,28).

The amount and type of vitamin B_{12} supplied by plants and microbial sources are not certain; e.g., fermented soya products such as *tempeh* contain many corrinoids (ring structure similar to vitamin B_{12} but have little activity in humans) (29). Rauma et al. (30) showed that vegans consuming *nori* or chlorella seaweed had double the vitamin B_{12} levels than those not eating the seaweed. However, these values were still significantly lower than normal. Walter (17) concluded that vitamin B_{12} from all these plant sources cannot possibly replace vitamin B_{12} from animal sources, and advised vegans and other strict vegetarians to consider supplementing their diets with vitamin B_{12} (use processed food fortified with B_{12}).

Because the standard microbiological assay for vitamin B_{12} in foodstuffs does not differentiate between inactive plant vitamin B_{12} derivatives and vitamin B_{12} from animal sources, experimental results on plant vitamin B_{12} content should be interpreted with caution.

Folic acid deficiency in vegetarians does not seem to be widespread. However, green leafy vegetables should not be boiled at high temperatures, to protect the folacin content. Lacto-ovo-vegetarians do not usually suffer from vitamin D_3 deficiency and lack of calcium, owing to their intake of milk and dairy products. However, strict vegans may be exposed to vitamin D_3 deficiency (21).

Vegetarians are often prone to iron-deficiency anemia because the bioavailability of iron in plant foods is low compared to that from meat. Vitamin C–containing foods can improve the absorption of nonheme iron among vegetarians having a limited intake of heme iron (31). Also, nonheme iron binds to phytates, tannins, and phosphates, commonly present in plant food diets. Phytates present in whole grain cereals, bran, and soya products strongly inhibit iron absorption (32). Similarly, oxalic acid, present in spinach, rhubarb, and other plants, decreases iron absorption by forming insoluble complexes with iron. Vegetarians therefore should consume plant foods that are rich in nonheme iron and low in substances that decrease absorption of iron. Children born to vegetarian mothers with lower iron stores, when breast-fed for a long period, may develop iron-deficiency anemia. Additional intake of iron before conception and during pregnancy is essential for vegetarians, because low iron status in the first trimester of pregnancy may increase the risk of premature birth (33,34).

Several studies have shown lower levels of plasma zinc in vegetarians and vegans compared with nonvegetarians eating red meat, eggs, and oysters and other seafoods that are rich sources of zinc (35–37).

It is known that n-3 fatty acids are vital for the development of the central nervous system and the retina. Infants born to vegan mothers and breast-fed may have a deficiency of n-3 fatty acids. Vegans and other vegetarians who do not eat seafoods may have very small intakes of eicosapentanoic and docosahexanoic acids, although the biological precursor of these two fatty acids, viz., alpha-linolenic acid, is present in some vegetable oils and the endogenous synthesis of the longer-chain derivatives may be sufficient (20). More research in this area is needed to draw exact conclusions (38,39).

Total vegetarians and vegans need to make sure that some good sources for riboflavin, vitamin D, vitamin B_{12}, calcium, iron, and zinc are consumed regularly. Riboflavin can be obtained by eating green leafy vegetables, whole grains, yeast, and legumes. Milk is a major source of riboflavin that is omitted from the vegan diet. Vitamin D can be obtained by regular exposure to sun or by eating foods supplemented with vitamin D. Vitamin B_{12} can be obtained by consuming fortified soyabean milk, soy proteins, or special yeast grown on media rich in vitamin B_{12}. By the time vitamin B_{12} deficiency is diagnosed, much nerve damage due to the deficiency may have taken place.

Vegans can obtain Ca by consuming fortified soy milk or fortified orange juice. Tofu, leafy greens, and nuts also contain calcium, but it is either not well absorbed or not very plentiful. Calcium supplements are another possibility. For iron, vegans can depend on whole grains, dried fruits, and legumes. The iron in these foods is not as well absorbed as that found in animal foods, but a good source of vitamin C consumed with these foods can greatly enhance iron absorption. Zinc is present in whole grains and legumes; however, the phytic acid present in whole grains limits its absorption. It is best if the grains are leavened, as in bread, to reduce the phytate influence. Of all these nutrients, it is most difficult to consume sufficient calcium. Veganism in childhood deserves special attention because the sheer bulk of a plant-based diet may make it difficult for a child to consume sufficient calories to meet the high energy needs. This is necessary so that dietary proteins can be used for the synthesis of body tissues, rather than energy needs.

Widdowson and McCance (40) showed that children will grow and develop normally on a diet consisting of plenty of bread and vegetables with minimum amounts of milk and meat. However, several reports have indicated that vegan children often fail to grow as well as omnivorous cohorts (41). Lower growth rates, especially in the first 5 years, have been reported for children reared on vegan (42) and on macrobiotic diets (43).

The intake of dietary fiber in vegetarians may have a greater negative effect on nutrient and energy balances in infants and children than in adults (41). Growing stage in vegetarians seems to be more critical because nutritional deficiencies that are rare in the general population have been reported in vegan and vegetarian children (44). Similarly, vegan mothers may run a risk of deficiency of vitamin B_{12}, vitamin D_3, iron, and n-3 fatty acids, needed for the development of babies (17).

According to Dwyer (19), mortality rates are similar or lower for vegetarians than for non-vegetarians and the risks of dietary-deficiency disease are higher for vegan, but not for all vegetarian diets. Both vegetarian dietary and lifestyle factors are involved, and evidence for decreased risks for certain chronic degenerative diseases varies. Data strongly support that vegetarians are at lower risk for obesity, constipation, and lung cancer. Also the risks for hypertension, CHD, type II diabetes, and gallstones are fairly lower. However, data are not sufficient to show that risks of breast cancer, diverticular disease of the colon, cancer, kidney stones, and osteoporosis are lower in vegetarians.

Taking mortality rates as in index for longevity, Kahn et al. (45), in a very large study with 27,530 vegetarian and nonvegetarian Seventh Day Adventists living in California, followed for 21 years, concluded that those with vegetarian food habits had lower age-specific mortality rates than those with omnivorous food habits. Also, the vegetarians had lower CHD mortality rates, and cancer rates were no higher than in the general population. In other studies, lower death rates for cancer and CHD were observed in some groups of Seventh Day Adventist (SDA) vegetarians (46,47). Walter (17) pointed out, however, that confounding factors, such as abstinence from smoking, alcohol, tea, and coffee may also have played a role. Fraser et al. (48) have shown that the lower rate of lung cancer in SDAs could be attributed to their abstinence from tobacco. Looking at a "healthy country lifestyle," which occasionally included meat products, Chang-Claude et al. (49) observed that mortality from all causes was reduced by 50% compared with the general population in the Federal Republic of Germany during an 11-year period. Cancer mortality was also reduced by 50% in men, but only by 25% in women. The deficit in cancer deaths was seen mainly for lung and gastrointestinal (G.I.) cancer in males, and for G.I. cancer in females. Deaths from diseases of the respiratory and digestive systems also decreased by around 50%, although deaths due to anemia increased slightly. Analyzing the strict and moderate vegetarians separately, it was found that ischemic heart disease was more than 50% less frequent among strict vegetarians for both sexes than for the control group, confirming earlier reports (50).

Walter (17) emphasized that vegetarians are seldom overweight, as also reported by several researchers (51,52). It is likely that vegetarian diets containing fiber and complex carbohydrates have a lower energy density and thus cause satiety at a lower calorie intake level. Less frequent overweight and obesity among vegetarians itself may be a reason for their greater longevity, as many studies have shown these two parameters to be important determinants for mortality (53,54).

Rosado (55) concluded that the plant-based diet consumed by a large proportion of the Mexican population is associated with a high incidence of micronutrient deficiencies. Although low ingestion of only some of these nutrients has been reported, the major mechanism that appears to be causing the deficiencies is low bioavailability of nutrients in the vegetarian diet, compounded by environmental factors such as parasitic infections. However, when a plant-based diet is consumed with an adequate mix of several foods, ingested in sufficient amounts—i.e., when a plant-based diet has variety and sufficiency—the result is a healthier complete diet with additional potential benefits to reduce the risk of chronic diseases (55).

According to Sanchez-Castillo (56), the limited evidence from studies in developing nations indicates that meat eating is especially beneficial if it is not associated with the other deleterious effects of the Western diet. Vegetarianism in developing nations probably evolved as an ecologic adaptation to limited food supplies and to the new availability of cereals. If a meat-rich diet that is low in fat and also rich in vegetables, roots, fruits, and nuts is the ideal diet, this may lead us to a scientific but uncomfortable view that few of the diets currently consumed in the world are ideal for both a healthy and a long life. Western diets often fail to meet new concepts of nutritional needs under ideal (i.e., uninfected) conditions. They also fail to cope with the everyday problems of parasitism and communicable infections. For practical reasons, the world population may have to continue to subsist on diets with an appreciable amount of energy derived from cereals, but meat as well as fruits and vegetables could prove, for reasons of both general health and longevity, to be desirable as prominent components of the diet (56).

Vegetarian diets seem to result in a lower risk for many diseases, such as obesity, cardiovascular disease, some types of cancer, constipation, hypertension, and type II diabetes. Considering lower mortality rates as a parameter, vegetarian diets seem to produce higher longevity, although vegan diets have an increased risk of iron, cobalamin, vitamin D_3, and calcium deficiency, and also of eventual deficits of zinc, n-3 fatty acids, and protein. Except for vitamin B_{12}, a vegan diet can fulfill nutritional requirements if one expertly selects fruits and vegetables containing the necessary nutrients (17).

According to current knowledge of human nutrition, high dietary contents of fruits, vegetables, and complex carbohydrates and low amounts of saturated fatty acids are correlated with a reduced risk of various diseases; even so, total abstinence from eating meat is not a major factor in the beneficial effects of vegetarian diets. However, in the sense of today's nutritional guidelines (57), a vegetarian-type diet with lots of vegetables, fruits, and complex carbohydrates can be considered "a prudent diet."

Although history has shown that vegetarians were right when they claimed more than 100 years ago that the vegetarian diet including fruits, vegetables, fiber, and complex carbohydrates is a healthy one, the inclusion of some low-fat meat and fish does not seem to be harmful. It could actually be beneficial in decreasing the risk of deficiencies encountered in some extreme cases of vegetarianism.

In view of the fact that about 40% of world grain production is diverted for meat production, and the increasing shortage of food in developing countries, it would be advisable, however, to lower the consumption of meat and increase consumption of cereal grains to improve the world's overall nutrition (17).

de Groot et al. (58) studied overall survival in men and women older than 70 years of age in relation to the Greek variant of the traditional Mediterranean diet. According to a dietary score based on eight characteristics, a significant 17% reduction in overall mortality was observed with each unit increase in diet score. The results of this investigation suggested that closer adherence to the traditional Greek diet favorably affects life expectancy among elderly people. The traditional Greek Mediterranean diet was defined in terms of food groups, with the addition of a moderate intake of alcohol and scored in terms of the following eight characteristics, using sex-specific median values as the cutoff point.

1. High monounsaturated: saturated fat ratio (1.6)
2. Moderate alcohol consumption (men: 10 g/day)
3. High consumption of legumes (men, 60 g/day; women 49 g/day)
4. High consumption of cereals (men, 291 g/day; women, 248 g/day)
5. High consumption of fruits (men, 249 g/day; women, 216 g/day)
6. High consumption of vegetables (men, 303 g/day; women, 248 g/day)
7. Low consumption of meat and meat products (men, 109 g/day; women, 91 g/day)
8. Low consumption of milk and dairy products (men, 200 g/day; women, 194 g/day)

A diet containing more of these characteristics was assumed to be more healthful, i.e., more closely related to the concepts of the Mediterranean diet. In the study sample, 57% of the subjects had at least four of the above-mentioned eight components.

An Italian study by Farchi et al. (59) also examined overall survival in relation to diet. Significant differences in mortality rates were found among elderly men characterized by different dietary scores. The lowest long-term (20-year) mortality rate coincided with diets meeting the recommendations, despite possible changes in dietary intake during the follow-up period.

Schroll et al. (60) have recently described the food patterns of elderly people across Europe, confirming the richness of the Southern diet in cereals, vegetables, fruit, lean meat, and olive oil. Future analyses will reveal whether scores developed in the studies by Trichopoulou et al. (61) and Farchi et al. (59) will be applicable to other European populations in order the examine differences in overall survival in relation to a variety of diets.

Immunological vigor is known to decline with age, contributing to increased morbidity and mortality in the elderly people. In addition, the elderly are at greater risk for low intake of several vitamins and minerals known to influence the immune response. Recent studies have indicated that supplementing the diets of the elderly with single nutrients or mixtures of vitamins and minerals at levels that exceed the recommended dietary allowances (RDAs) significantly improves certain indices of the immune response (62). In one such study, improved immune response was associated with decreased frequency of infectious diseases, indicating that nutrient-induced immunological improvement clinically enhances the health of elderly people (63). Numerous studies have demonstrated that significant improvements in the immune response of healthy elderly people can be achieved by nutrient supplementation, although the clinical significance of nutrient-induced immunological changes has been questioned by many researchers. However, Chandra (63) reported that immunological improvements following nutrient supplementation were associated with decreased frequency of infection-related illness (23 ± 5 vs. 48 ± 7 days). Also, the number of days antibiotics were used to treat infections was lower in the supplemented group (18 ± 4 vs. 32 ± 5 days). These findings clearly demonstrate that immunological improvements do seem to alter clinical outcomes, at least in elderly people (62).

Meager human studies have pursued the mechanism of nutrient-induced improvement in immune response. Meydani et al. (64) demonstrated that the vitamin E-induced enhancement of the immune response in the elderly was due at least in part to decreased production of suppressive factors, such as prostaglandin E_2, from macrophages. Similar mechanistic details for other nutrients remain to be elucidated.

It is not clear whether the supplements used (single or multi) act physiologically by correcting a marginal or severe nutrient deficiency (as defined by current standards) or act pharmacologically by decreasing production of suppressive factors, as reported by Meydani et al. (64), or increase production of certain stimulatory factors. Multivitamin/mineral supplementation trials, using moderate amounts (up to four times the RDAs) of several nutrients, have suggested a physiological role. However, in a study by Chandra (63), although specific nutrient deficiencies, as defined by current standards, were observed in only a small percentage of subjects (2–20%), improvements occurred in the majority of the subjects, even those who were not deficient. This indicates that the current nutrient standards might not adequately support optimal immune responsiveness and health in elderly people. Future research should be directed to these vital issues, to determine the mechanism(s) underlying the nutrient-induced improvement in immune response in the elderly (62).

Various foods, nutrients, and herbs have been examined for their ability to reverse or prevent the changes of immunosenescence (65). According to recent work in Chinese medicine, there is a group of polysaccharides that has the ability to improve the concanavalin A–induced proliferation of lymphocytes in aging mice, regulate interleukin-2 (IL-2) production, increase IL-2 receptor expression, and induce production of alpha, beta, and gamma interferons. According to Bradly and Xu (65), further studies on the effects of functional foods and herbs on the immune system may well prove to be beneficial.

VI. NEWER BIOTECHNOLOGICAL DEVELOPMENTS IN 1998

In recent years, biotechnology has contributed significantly to developments in food, nutrition, health, and medicines. For example, it is now possible to introduce human disease resistance in common foods such as bananas, corn, beans, tomatoes, potatoes, and sheep milk, eliminating the need for injections and oral drugs. Dr. Yasmin Thanawala of Buffalo University has successfully introduced the antigen of hepatitis-B virus into the potato, using biotechnological tools. The vaccine for dengue fever and nosal sprays to control common cold will soon be available in the commercial market.

Researchers in Petten (Netherlands) were successful in experimentally controlling the growth of cancer cells through neutron bambardment. Gene therapy is sucessfully being used to develop an AIDS vaccine and to administer insulin through the salivary glands. A gene responsible for balding in humans has been located. British researchers are trying to locate a gene responsible for aging, and a gene that regulates the immune system has been found by researchers in Israel; they have also successfully cloned this gene, using genetic engineering.

An enzyme known as telomerase controls the growth of cancerous cells. British scientists, Professor Newbold and associates from Brunell University, have identified a gene responsible for telomerase. Because most types of cancers involve telomerase activity, it is hoped that location of the gene responsible for telomerase will pave new ways of genetic treatment of cancers. Scientists from Texas University, Dallas Center, have also identified the DNA sequence of telomerase that is responsible for its aging. After each cell division, the length of the DNA chain decreases, and at one stage the cell division stops. It has been hypothesized that by altering the DNA sequence at the gene level, it may be possible to extend the youth period and to control aging. By using a "terminator" gene, it has now become possible to introduce disease resistance into agricultural crops such as wheat, rice, and cotton.

Bidlack (66) has presented "phytochemicals" as a new diet-health paradigm with the potential to evolve, one that would place more emphasis on the positive aspects of diet. The paradigm goes beyond the role of food constituents as nutrients required for sustaining life and growth to one of preventing or delaying the premature onset of chronic diseases later in life. Diets rich in fruits and vegetables appear to protect humans from disease; most likely, the phytochemicals, which developed as a part of the plant's own defense mechanism against environmental insult, fortuitously provide benefits to human beings.

The number of identified physiologically active such phytochemicals has increased dramatically in the past couple of decades. However, these compounds have not been systematically categorized or documented for their role in health promotion or disease prevention. Initially these agents were identified by epidemiological surveys that correlated a positive health benefit with specific food groups and then focused on specific dietary components. These phytochemicals have been further developed through chemical analyses, test tube reaction systems, cell and tissue culture, animal studies, and, in a few cases, human intervention data.

Certain phytochemicals that appear to have significant health potential are as follows (66):

1. Phytoestrogens that may decrease osteoporosis and estrogen-enhanced carcinogenesis, e.g., genestein and diadzein found in soy products. The phytoestrogens are thought to bind to the estrogenic receptor and thus either compete with or antagonize estradiol action; their health effect depends on the exposure level of the phytoestrogen, the binding constant relative to estradiol, and the selectivity of different tissue receptors.

2. Catechins present in tea may inhibit initiation and promotion of carcinogenic processes. It has been shown that these polyphenols express a broad spectrum of anticarcinogenic activity in multiple animal models, including the development of tumors at different sites, and affect a wide array of enzymes involved in cell proliferation. Data from animal experiments have

consistently indicated that the effective concentrations of these phenolics are equal to levels found in brewed green tea.

3. Tocotrionols exhibit characteristics different from those of alpha-tocopherol (vitamin E). Gamma-tocopherol is much more effective than alpha-tocotrionols in lowering cholesterol synthesis, whereas alpha-tocopherol is without effect. Gamma tocotrienol and alpha-tocopherol have been found to inhibit proliferation of cancer cells, and all tocopherols and tocotrienols effectively inhibit lipid peroxidation in food and biological systems.

4. Phenolic derivatives have been known to act as natural antimicrobial agents, e.g., antimicrobial compounds found in plants and species, such as benzoic acid, caffeic acid, catechin, catechol, rutin, vanillic acid, eugenol, and thymol. These chemicals occur naturally and have been used to protect foods from spoilage.

5. Organosulfur compounds found in garlic have antioxidant functions, decrease metabolic activation of carcinogens and adduct binding to DNA, and decrease platelet aggregation by diminishing the clotting mechanisms. The doses used in testing these agents are rather high

6. Prebiotics may enhance intestinal function, e.g., oligosaccharides, such as fructose oligosaccharides, produce specific physiological effects on immune function, tumorigenesis, and regulation of serum cholesterol. Some of the prebiotics have been incorporated into commercial products.

The foregoing examples represent the exciting potential of some phytochemicals as future physiologically active agents that may be incorporated into functional/health foods. Research is needed to clearly understand the actual health benefits of these agents, if any. Bidlack (66) has pointed out that a decision on efficacy must look at the lowest doses needed to produce their effects because higher doses increase the risk of toxicity. Also, it is important to determine whether the same dose of the agent in the food has the same health-promoting efficacy as the isolated compound. Safety must be assured, in all cases.

The phytochemicals must be evaluated on the basis of the best scientific evidence available as provided by cellular biology, animal studies, clinical trials, and epidemiological surveys. The interpretation must consider the quality, strength, and consistency of data, and the biological plausibility of the hypotheses.

While the confirmation of phytochemicals that may prevent human disease is eagerly awaited, the overpromotion of potential health benefits may create unrealistic expectations that may never be realized, resulting in decreased research efforts and support needed to identify these health-giving bioactive agents (66).

VII. CONCLUDING REMARKS

The history of human disease has to be based almost entirely on what is known about the changes in mortality and life expectancy. Illness and suffering do not lend themselves to hard statistics, but births and deaths can be counted (67). We have to look at mortality to learn how diseases have been conquered in the past. The major lethal diseases were conquered not so much by discovering how to treat them as by prevention, although discoveries such as antibiotics must be rightly admired. Humankind today considers it its right to live into old age, free from the misery of chronic illness and diseases.

REFERENCES

1. James, W.P.T., Historical perspective, *Human Nutrition and Dietetics* (J.S. Garrow and W.P.T. James, eds.), Churchill Livingstone, Edinburgh, London, 1993, p. 1.

2. Insull, W., T. Oiso, and K. Tsuchiya, The diet and nutritional status of Japanese, *Am. J. Clin. Nutr. 21*: 753 (1968).

3. FAO, Food balance sheets 1979–1981, Food and Agriculture Organization of the United Nations, Rome, 1984.

4. James, W.P.T., Policy and a prudent diet, *Human Nutrition and Dietetics* (J.S. Garrow and W.P.T. James, eds.), Churchill Livingstone, Edinburgh, London, 1993, p. 767.

5. Keys, A., *Seven Countries: A Multivariate Analysis of Death and Coronary Heart Disease*, Harvard University Press, Harvard, 1980.

6. Cannon, G., Food and health: the experts agree, Consumer's Association, London, 1992.

7. WHO, Diet, nutrition and the prevention of chronic diseases, WHO Technical Report No. 797, World Health Organization, Geneva, 1990.

8. James, W.P.T., and A. Ralph, What is a healthy diet? *Med. Intl. 82*: 3364 (1990).

9. WHO, Prevention of coronary heart disease, Tech. Rep. Series No. 678, World Health Organization, Geneva, 1982.

10. James, W.P.T., Healthy nutrition, WHO European Series No. 24, World Health Organization, Copenhagen, 1988.

11. WHO/FAO, Fats and oils in human nutrition: Report of a Joint Expert Consultation (WHO/FAO) 1994, *Nutr. Rev., 53*: 202 (1995).

12. FAO, Report of the Joint FAO/WHO Expert Consultation on Protein Quality Evaluation, 1989, Bethesda, Food and Agriculture Organization, Rome, 1990.

13. Young, U.R., D.M. Bier, and P.L. Peller, A theoretical basis for increasing current estimates of the amino acid requirements in adult man with experimental support, *Am. J. Clin. Nutr. 50*: 80 (1989).

14. Health of the Nation, A strategy for health in England, HMSO, London, 1992.

15. Behme, M.T., Diet, nutrition and health: an update, *INFORM 7*(11): 1233 (1996).

16. Wynder, E.L., J. Barone, and J.R. Hebert, The role of diet in the maintenance of health throughout life, *Diet, Nutrition and Health* (K.K. Carroll, ed.), McGill-Queen's Univ. Press, London, 1989, p. 141.

17. Walter, P., Effects of vegetarian diets on aging, and longevity, *Nutr. Rev. 55* (II Suppl.): 61 (1997).

18. Ohsawa, G. *Macrobiotics: An Invitation to Health and Happiness*, George Ohsawa Foundation, San Francisco, 1991.

19. Dwyer, J.T., Health aspects of vegetarian diets, *Am. J. Clin. Nutr. 48*: 712 (1988).

20. Dwyer, J.T. Nutritional consequences of vegetarianism, *Annu. Rev. Nutr. 11*: 61 (1991).

21. Willett, W.C., Diet and health: What should we eat? *Science 264*: 532 (1994).

22. Kromhout, D., E.B. Bosschieter, and C. De Lezenne Coulander, Dietary fibre and 10 year mortality from coronary heart disease, cancer and all causes, The Zutphen Study, *Lancet 2*: 518 (1982).

23. Margetts, B.M., and A.A. Jackson, Vegetarians and longevity, *Epidemiology 4*: 278 (1993).

24. Young, V.R., and P.L. Pellet, Current concepts concerning amino acids in adults and their implications for international planning, *Food Nutr. Bull. 12*: 289 (1990).

25. Campbell, M., W.S. Lofters, and W.N. Gibbs, Rastafarianism and the vegan syndrome, *Br. Med. J. 285*: 1617 (1982).

26. Dagnelie, P.C., W.A. Van Staveren, and F.J.V.R.A. Vergote, Increased risk of vitamin B_{12} and iron deficiency in infants on macrobiotic diets, *Am. J. Clin. Nutr. 50*: 818, (1989).

27. Sanders, T.A.B., Growth and development of British vegan children, *Am. J. Clin. Nutr. 48*: 822 (1988).

28. Lamberg-Allardt, C., M. Karkkainen, and R. Sepparen, Low serum 25-hydroxy vitamin D concentrations and secondary hyperparathyroidism in middle-aged white strict vegetarians, *Am. J. Clin. Nutr. 58*: 684 (1993).

29. Herbert, V., G. Drivas, and C. Manusselis, Are colon bacteria a major source of cobalamin analogues in human tissues? *Trans. Assoc. Am. Phys. 97*: 161 (1984).

30. Rauma, A.L., R. Torronen, and O. Hanninen, Vitamin B_{12} status of long-term adherents of a strict uncooked vegan diet ('living food diet') is compromised, *Am. Inst. Nutr. 25*: 11 (1995).

31. Hallberg, L., M. Brune, and L. Rossander-Huthen, Is there a physiological role of vitamin C in iron absorption? *Ann. N. Y. Acad. Sci. 498*: 324 (1987).

32. Hazell, T., Relating food composition data to iron availability from plant foods, *Am. J. Clin. Nutr. 42*: 509 (1988).

33. Kim, I., D.W. Hugerford, and R. Yip, Pregnancy nutrition surveillance system—United States, 1979–1990. *MMWR Center for Disease Control Surveillance Summaries (United States) 41*: 25 (1992).

34. Scholl, T.O., M.L. Hediger, R.L. Fischer, and J.W. Shearer, Anemia vs. iron deficiency: increased risk of preterm delivery in a prospective study, *Am. J. Clin. Nutr. 55*: 985 (1992).

35. Anderson, B.M., R.S. Gibson, and J.H. Sabry, The iron and zinc status of long term vegetarian women, *Am. J. Clin. Nutr. 34*: 1042 (1981).

36. King, J.C., T. Stein, and M. Doyle, Effect of vegetarianism on zinc status of pregnant women, *Am. J. Clin. Nutr. 34*: 1049 (1981).

37. Freeland-Graves, J., Mineral adequacy of vegetarian diets, *Am. J. Clin. Nutr. 48*: 849 (1988).

38. Sanders, T.A.B., and S. Reddy, Nutritional implications of a meatless diet, *Proc. Nutr. Soc. 53*: 297 (1994).

39. Reddy, S., T.A.B. Sanders, and O. Obeid, The influence of maternal vegetarian diet on essential fatty acid status of the newborn, *Eur. J. Clin. Nutr. 48*: 358 (1994).

40. Widdowson, E.M., and R.A. McCance, Studies on the nutritive value of bread and the effect of flour on the growth of undernourished children, MRC Special Report Series No. 287, London, 1954.

41. Acosta, P.B., Availability of essential amino acids and nitrogen in vegan diets, *Am. J. Clin. Nutr. 48*: 868 (1988).

42. Sanders, T.A.B., and J. Manning, The growth and development of vegan children, *J. Human Nutr. Dietet. 5*: 11 (1992).

43. Dagnelie, P.C., W.A. Van Staveren, J.D. Van Klaveren, and J. Burema, Do children on macrobiotic diets show catch-up growth. *Eur. J. Clin. Nutr. 42*: 1007 (1988).

44. Jacobs, C., and J.T. Dwyer, Vegetarian children: appropriate and inappropriate diets, *Am. J. Clin. Nutr., 43* (Suppl.): 811 (1988).

45. Kahn, R.H., R.L. Phillips, and D.A. Snowdon, Association between reported diet and all causes of mortality: Twenty-one year follow up on 27,530 adult Seventh Day Adventists, *Am. J. Epidemiol. 119*: 775 (1984).

46. Snowden, D.A., Animal product consumption and mortality because of all causes combined, coronary heart disease, stroke, diabetes and cancer in Seventh Day Adventists, *Am. J. Clin. Nutr. 48*: 739 (1988).

47. Fonnebo, V., Mortality in Norwegian Seventh Day Adventists, 1962–1986, *J. Clin. Epidemiol. 45*: 157 (1992).

48. Fraser, G.E., W.L. Beeson, and R.L. Phillips, Diet and lung cancer in California Seventh Day Adventists, *Am. J. Epidemiol. 133*: 683 (1991).

49. Change-Claude, J., R. Frentzel-Beyme, and U. Eilber, Mortality pattern of German vegetarians after 11 years of follow-up, *Epidemiology 3*: 395 (1992).

50. Burr, M.L., and P.M. Sweetmam, Vegetarianism, dietary fiber and mortality, *Am. J. Clin. Nutr. 36*: 873 (1982).

51. Burr, M.L., and B.K. Butland, Heart disease in British vegetarians, *Am. J. Clin. Nutr. 48*: 830 (1988).

52. Beilin, L.J., I.L. Rouse, B.K. Armstrong, Vegetarian diet and blood pressure levels: incidental or causal association, *Am. J. Clin. Nutr. 48*: 806 (1988).

53. Wilcosky, T., J. Hyde, and J.J.B. Anderson, Obesity and mortality in the Lipid Research Clinics Program follow-up study, *J. Clin. Epidemiol. 43*: 743 (1990).

54. Wienpahl, J., D.R. Ragland, and S. Sidney, Body mass index and 15-year mortality in a cohort of black men and women, *J. Clin. Epidemiol. 43*: 949 (1990).

55. Rosado, J.R., Invited comment, *Effects of vegetarian diets on aging and longevity* (P. Waltered), *Nutr. Rev. 55* (Suppl. 2): 61 (1997).

56. Sanchez-Castillo, C.P., Invited comment, *Effect of vegetarian diets on aging and longevity* (P. Waltered), *Nutr. Rev. 55* (Suppl. 2): 61 (1997).

57. Anonymous, Nutrition and your health, *Dietary Guidelines for Americans*, 3rd ed., USDA and USD-HHS, Washington, DC, 1990.

58. deGroot, C.P.G.M., W.A. Van Staveren, and J. Burema, Survival beyond age 70 in relation to diet, *Nutr. Rev. 54*: 211 (1996).

59. Farchi, G., F. Fidanza, S. Mariotti, and A. Menotti, Is diet an independent risk factor for mortality? 20

year mortality in the Italian rural cohorts of the Seven Countries Study, *Eur. J. Clin. Nutr. 48*: 19 (1994).

60. Schrool, K., A. Carbajal, B. Decarli, I. Martins, F. Grunenberger, Y.H. Blauw, and C.P.G.M. de Groot, Food patterns of elderly Europeans, *Eur. J. Clin. Nutr. 50* (Suppl. 2): 86 (1996).

61. Trichopoulou, A., A. Kouris-Blazos, M.L. Wahlqvist, C. Gnardellis, P. Lagiou, and E. Polychronopoulos, Diet and overall survival in elderly people, *Br. Med. J. 311*: 1457 (1995).

62. Meydani, S.N., Vitamin/mineral supplementation, the aging immune response and risk of infection, *Nutr. Rev. 51*: 106 (1993).

63. Chandra, R.K., Effect of vitamin and trace-element supplementation on immune response and infectious diseases in elderly subjects, *Lancet 340*: 1124 (1992).

64. Meydani, S.N., P.M. Barklund, and S. Liu, Vitamin E supplementation enhances cell-mediated immunity in healthy elderly subjects, *Am. J. Clin. Nutr. 52*: 557 (1990).

65. Bradley, J., and X. Xu, Diet, age and the immune system, *Nutr. Rev. 54* (Suppl. 2): 43 (1996).

66. Bidlack, W.R., Phytochemicals: A potential new health paradigm, *Food Technol. 52* (9):1 68 (1998).

67. Cairns, J., The history of mortality, *Diet, Nutrition and Health* (K.K. Carroll, ed.), McGill-Queen's Univ. Press, London, 1989, p. 309.

Index